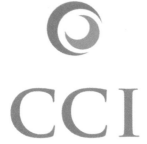

CCI
COMPETENCY & CREDENTIALING INSTITUTE

- **A Legacy of Leadership** Our continued mission of a personal commitment to extraordinary care reflects our values and expanded goals to promote safe patient care and quality outcomes for our institutional clients.

- **A Strong Identity** Our core services in credentialing, assessment and education will continue to combine the integrity of the credentialing system, the inspirations of healthcare professionals and the dedication to standards of excellence.

- **Our Personal Commitment** CCI is committed to healthcare competency, where value is placed on clinical competencies and the relationships created with patients and peers within the healthcare environment.

- **To Extraordinary Care** We support your personal commitment to your hospital, your patients and healthcare professionals through our credentialing and state of the art competency programs.

*"We are pleased to bring you **Competency for Safe Patient Care During Operative and Invasive Procedures**. Since its inception in 1979, CCI has been dedicated to promoting patient safety, and we continue to develop effective certification and competency products to promote quality outcomes. We hope you find this new resource beneficial to your perioperative education program and we look forward to continued service to you and your patients."*

The CCI Board of Directors

CCI proudly offers the following certification and competency products.
- CNOR and CRNFA Certifications
- Surgical Services Management Certificate
- Educator's Certificate Program (Fall 2009)
- Competency Education Modules
  - Age-Specific Care
  - Aseptic Technique
  - Care of the Bariatric Patient
  - Cultural Competency
  - Designing Competencies That Count
  - Electrosurgery
  - Moderate Sedation/Analgesia
  - Patient Positioning
  - Patient Safety
  - Sterilization
- Pharmacology Reference Guide

Another Important CCI Perioperative Textbook Coming in Fall of 2009
Assisting in Surgery: Patient Centered Care This book will be a valuable tool for all clinical professionals who are in the first assisting role and focuses on the needs of the surgical patient. Leading industry experts, Dr. Jane Rothrock and Trish Seifert, have made significant contributions to the content and editing of this book. We look forward to making this new resource available to you in the fall of 2009.

To learn about other CCI Certification and Competency Education Programs, visit our website at www.cc-institute.org.

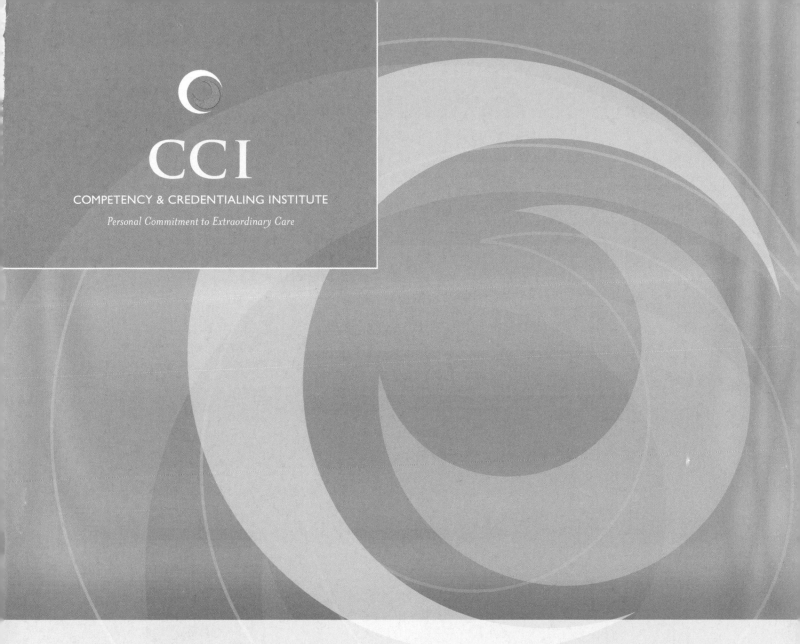

CCI

COMPETENCY & CREDENTIALING INSTITUTE

Personal Commitment to Extraordinary Care

Competency for Safe Patient Care
During Operative and Invasive Procedures

Mark L. Phippen, RN, MN, CNOR

Brenda C. Ulmer, RN, MN, CNOR

Maryann P. Wells, RN, PhD, FAAN

Library of Congress Cataloging-in-Publication Data

Competency for safe patient care during operative and invasive procedures/[edited by] Mark L. Phippen, Brenda C. Ulmer, Maryann P. Wells ; CCI/ Competency & Credentialing Institute.

   p. ; cm.

 Includes bibliographical references and index.

  ISBN 978-0-9787582-9-5 (casebound : alk. paper)

 1. Surgical nursing. I. Phippen, Mark L. II. Ulmer, Brenda C. III. Wells, Maryann M. Papanier. IV. Competency & Credentialing Institute.
[DNLM: 1. Perioperative Nursing—standards. 2. Clinical Competence. 3. Patient Care. WY 161 C7413 2009]
RD99.C715 2009
617'.0231—dc22

              2008055357

Published by
Competency & Credentialing Institute
2170 South Parker Road, Suite 295
Denver, CO 80231

ISBN-13: 978-0-9787582-9-5
ISBN-10: 0-9787582-9-3

Printed in the United States of America.

Contributors

CONTRIBUTORS

Molly McBrayer, MSN, RN-BC, CNOR
Clinical Nurse Specialist, Perioperative Services,
Bon Secour Saint Francis Hospital
Charleston, SC

Elizabeth Dvorsak, BSN, RN, CNOR
Clinical Educator, Medical University of South Carolina
Charleston, SC

Susan Ulmer DeWolf, RN, MSN, CNOR, CRNFA, NP-C
President/CEO Surgical First Assistants, Inc.
Marietta, GA

Patricia A. Mews, RN, MHA, CNOR
Manager Advanced Practices, Perioperative Services,
Scottsdale Healthcare System
Scottsdale, AZ

Michelle Byrne, RN, PhD, CNOR
Program Coordinator MS Nursing Education,
North Georgia College & State University
Dahlonega, GA

James (Jay) Bowers, RN, BSN, CNOR
Clinical Preceptor, Operating Room, West Virginia
University Hospital
Morgantown, WV

Mary Weis, RN, APRN-BC, CNOR, CRNFA
Clinical Nurse Specialist, Department of Surgery,
CentraCare Clinic
St. Cloud, MN

Rose Moss, RN, MN, CNOR
Perioperative Nurse Consultant
Del Norte, CO

Charles J. Moss, III, CRNA, MS
Director, Anesthesia Services, San Luis Valley Regional
Medical Center
Alamosa, CO

Deborah B. Hadley, RN, MSN, CNOR
Instructor, Department of Associate Degree Nursing,
Alcorn State University
Natchez, MS

Jeff Reichardt RN, MSN, FNP-BC
Family Nurse Practitioner, The Little Clinic
Brighton, MI

Cecil King, RN, MS, CNOR
Clinical Educator, Cape Cod Hospital
Hyannis, MA

Sophia Mikos-Schild, RN, EdD, CNOR
Educator, St. Mary & Elizabeth Medical Center
Chicago, IL

Kelly Kollar, RN, CNOR
Perioperative Staff Nurse, Level II, Children's Hospital
Boston, MA

BJ Hoogerwerf, RN, BSN, CNOR, CRNFA
RN First Assistant, Everett Clinic, Trask Surgery Center
Everett, WA

Joyce A. Cox, RN, MSN, CNOR, CRNFA, CNP
Adult Nurse Practitioner, Steven D. Cox, MD, Inc.
Lancaster, OH

Mary A. Rogers, RN, BSN, CNOR
Supervisor, Central Sterile, Fairfield Medical Center
Lancaster, OH

Joyce M. Stengel, RN, BSN, CNOR
Perioperative Staff Nurse, Hospital of the University
of Pennsylvania
Philadelphia, PA

Noel N. Williams, MD, FRCSI
Associate Professor of Surgery, Division of Gastrointestinal
Surgery, Hospital of University of Pennsylvania
Philadelphia, PA

Wendy Zander, RN, MSN/Ed, CNOR
Surgical & Anesthesia Services Performance Improvement
Manager, Palmetto Health Richland
Columbia, NC

Roberta C, Geiger, RN, BSN, CNOR
Clinical Educator, St. Joseph's Hospital
Atlanta, GA

Lillian H. Nicolette, RN, MSN, CNOR
Consultant, Faculty Perioperative Nursing,
Delaware County Community College
Newtown, PA

Susan K. Chandler, RN, BSN, CRNFA, CPSN
Nurse Clinician, Ambulatory Administration,
Virginia Commonwealth University Medical Center
Richmond, VA

Patricia C. Seifert, RN, MSN, CNOR, CRNFA, FAAN
Education Coordinator, CVOR, Inova Heart and Vascular
Institute
Falls Church, VA

Jill Collins, RN, BSN
Staff RN, CVOR, Inova Heart and Vascular Institute
Falls Church, VA

Mary O'Neale, RN, MN, CNOR
Director of Credentialing & Education,
Competency & Credentialing Institute
Denver, CO

Paula Bishop, RN, MSN, CNOR
Clinical Director, Perioperative Services
Canton, OH

Russell W. Todd, MGA, RCIS
Educational Coordinator
Inova Fairfax Hospital
Inova Heart and Vascular Institute
Falls Church, VA

Mark Phippen, RN, MN, CNOR
Global Senior Clinical Educator,
Covidien Energy-based Devices
Boulder, CO

Brenda Ulmer, RN, MN, CNOR
Global Manager, Professional Education
Covidien Energy-based Devices
Boulder, CO

Rose Moss, RN, MN, CNOR
Perioperative Nurse Consultant
Del Norte, CO

Donna Watson, RN, MSN, CNOR, ARNP-BC
Global Senior Clinical Educator,
Covidien Energy-based Devices
Boulder, CO

Mary Beth Kean, MSN, RN-BC, CRRN, CNS
Pain Management
Baylor University Medical Center
Houston, TX

Melissa James Browning, BA
Global Professional Education Manager for
Interventional Oncology
Boulder, CO

Reviewers

Rose Moss, RN, MN, CNOR
Perioperative Nurse Consultant
Del Norte, CO

Molly McBrayer, MSN, RN-BC, CNOR
Clinical Nurse Specialist, Perioperative Services,
Bon Secour Saint Francis Hospital
Charleston, SC

Lillian H. Nicolette, RN, MSN, CNOR
Consultant, Faculty Perioperative Nursing,
Delaware County Community College
Newtown, PA

Patricia C. Seifert, RN, MSN, CNOR, CRNFA, FAAN
Education Coordinator, CVOR, Inova Heart
and Vascular Institute
Falls Church, VA

Paula Bishop, RN, MSN, CNOR
Clinical Director, Perioperative Services
Canton, OH

Mary Beth Zaleski, RN, BSN, CNOR
Patient Care Specialist, Operating Room
Staff Development
Canton, OH

Stephen Wilkendorf, RT, RDMS
Senior Ultrasound Technologist
UC Davis Health System
Sacramento, CA

Elizabeth Dvorsak, BSN, RN, CNOR
Clinical Educator, Medical University
of South Carolina
Charleston, SC

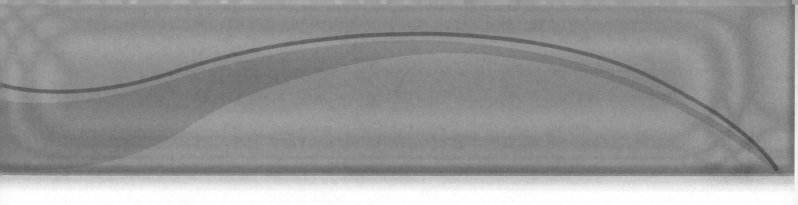

To Kat, Bishop, Zehr, and their grandmother, Cristina.
Your loving papa and husband.
Mark L. Phippen

To Samuel Mauldin, Erin Buckner, and Madison
Maudlin, with love.
Brenda Ulmer

To Alexandra, never stop searching for the rainbows
and moonbows in life. Enjoy the journey!
Maryann Papanier Wells

Table of Contents

Preface

Competency for Safe Patient Care During Operative and Invasive Procedures provides a model of practice for nurses caring for patients before, during, and after operative or invasive procedures. This book focuses on the basic competencies necessary for the provision of safe nursing practice and quality care for patients undergoing operative and invasive procedures. All nurses, whether they are practicing in the operative suite or other invasive procedure areas such as the cardiac catheterization laboratory, gastrointestinal laboratory, or interventional radiology, will find this text helpful in their goal to provide safe patient care.

Section 1, *Conceptual Fundamentals of Practice,* presents a conceptual model for nursing care of the patient undergoing an operative or invasive procedure. The model discussed in Chapter 1 presents a mental image of the realm of nursing as practiced by nurses caring for patients undergoing operative or invasive procedures. The second chapter focuses on competency assessment in the operative and invasive procedure setting and addresses competency assessment for members of the operative and/or invasive procedure nursing healthcare team. The chapter discusses practice frameworks for the delivery of nursing care in the operative and invasive procedure setting that can be used to develop competency assessment tools, presents a model for skill acquisition, discusses methodologies for assessing competency, and provides sample competency assessment tools.

Performance improvement in the operative and invasive procedure suite is the focus of Chapter 3. The chapter highlights the essential components of performance improvement.

Legal, regulatory, and ethical considerations are the focus of Chapter 4. The chapter covers topics such as the American legal system structure, criminal law, civil law, statutes and regulations, regulation of healthcare, key federal statutes, regulatory agencies, key not-for-profit bodies and regulations, federal agencies, non-governmental associations, and ethics.

Section 2, *Competencies for Safe Patient Care,* presents basic competencies necessary for providing safe patient care during an operative or invasive procedure. Each chapter in this section begins with a definition of the competency and identification of measurable criteria that indicate if the competency is being performed correctly. One or more nursing diagnoses are identified for each competency. The diagnoses describe the potential patient problems seen in the patients having operative or invasive procedures. These diagnoses will assist the practitioner in identifying patients at risk for experiencing an adverse outcome before, during, or after the operative or invasive procedure. Some competencies discussed in Section II are universal for all operative and invasive procedures, whether performed in the operative suite, interventional radiology, or the cardiac and gastrointestinal laboratories. These competencies include preparing the patient for the procedure; transferring the patient; assisting the anesthesia provider; positioning the patient; establishing and maintaining the sterile field; performing sponge, sharp, and instrument counts; providing instruments, equipment, and supplies; administering drugs and solutions; physiologically monitoring the patient; monitoring and controlling the environment; and handling cultures and specimens. A sample competency assessment checklist has been placed at the end of each chapter in this section. The reader is encouraged to implement and, if necessary, adapt these competencies to their particular practice area.

Chapters 16 and 17 of Section 2, which were written for nurses practicing in an advanced role, discuss handling of tissues with instruments and providing hemostasis. These chapters, although not a substitute for advanced practice clinical textbooks, nevertheless provide basic information concerning the skills needed to provide first and second assistant services. Nurses who have focused their practice on the scrub nurse and circulating nurse roles will also find these chapters helpful. Physician practice patterns are evolving because of changes in reimbursement. Consequently, more nurses will be called on to expand their practice in the future.

Chapter 18 of Section 2 describes how the advanced practice nurse can facilitate patient care after the procedure. This chapter includes information about critical variables that affect patient convalescence, the stages of wound healing, postprocedure wound and systemic complications, and assessment of the patient's physiological and psychological comfort level. The chapter includes information about how the nurse can help the patient and family make the transition between the acute healthcare setting and the community or convalescence in the home.

Section 3, *Operative and Invasive Procedures,* discusses common operative and invasive procedures performed in the operative suite, gastrointestinal and cardiac catheterization laboratories, and radiology department. Topics include general surgery, bariatric surgery, vascular surgery, thoracic surgery, cardiac surgery, transplantation surgery, plastic surgery, neurosurgery, urological surgery, orthopedic surgery, gynecological and obstetrical surgery, otorhinolaryngologic surgery, ophthalmic surgery, trauma care, cardiac catheterization and electrophysiology, gastrointestinal procedures, interventional radiology, and pain management.

Section 4 covers *Age Specific Care, Care of the Pediatric Patient and Care of the Geriatric Patient.* These chapters present concepts and discuss the challenges related to caring for these special populations.

The 21st century presents many new and exciting challenges for nurses responsible for the care of patients having operative and invasive procedures. We believe that you will find *Competency for Safe Patient Care During Operative and Invasive Procedures* to be an essential practice resource as you care for this very special patient population. In addition, this text can serve as a resource for nurses preparing for CNOR certification.

Mark L. Phippen
Brenda C. Ulmer
Maryann P. Wells

Section 1
Conceptual Fundamentals of Practice

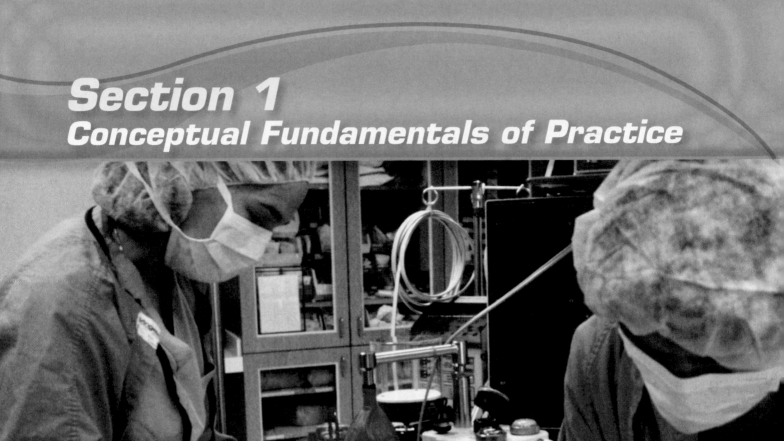

CHAPTER 1

Systems-in-Contingency

A Conceptual Model for Nursing Care of the Patient Undergoing an Operative and Invasive Procedure

Mark L. Phippen

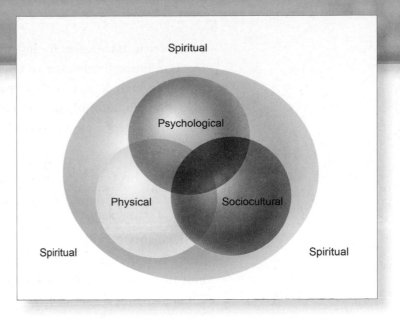

INTRODUCTION

The *Systems-in-Contingency Model* provides a framework for practice for the nurse providing care for patients undergoing operative or invasive procedures. The model describes the focus of nursing practice in the operative and invasive procedure setting and explains how the nurse relates with other members of the team when with the patient, who is the center and focus of all activities in the operative and invasive procedure setting.

CORE CONCEPTS

Person, environment, health, and *nursing* are the core concepts of the *Systems-in-Contingency Model*. These concepts theoretically describe the interaction of the patient with the environment, the goal of nursing care provided by the *registered nurse*[1], and the focus of all nursing interventions during the operative and invasive procedure period. The core concepts give direction to the nurse in collecting patient health data, analyzing health data, determining diagnoses, identifying expected outcomes, planning care that prescribes interventions to achieve expected outcomes, implementing interventions, and evaluating the patient's progress toward achievement of outcomes (AORN, 2008).

ASSUMPTIONS[2]

Supporting assumptions for the *Systems-in-Contingency Model* are based on the model's concepts of the person as a contingency system interacting with the environment and on the process of establishing and sustaining system equilibrium during the operative and invasive procedure period.

The term *nurse* refers to the nurse caring for a patient immediately before, during, and immediately after an operative and invasive procedure. Practice areas for the nurse include inpatient, outpatient, and office-based operating rooms, gastrointestinal laboratories, cardiac catheterization laboratories, interventional radiology departments, preprocedure preparation areas, and postprocedure care areas (discharge).

Assumption I

The person is a holistic system composed of physical, psychological, sociocultural, and spiritual components.

The theory of holism describes the universe in terms of interacting wholes that are more than the mere sum of elementary particles. The person, when viewed from a holistic perspective, is seen as an interacting system that is more than the total of the components of the system. Like other nursing models, the *Systems-in-Contingency Model* of care of the patient undergoing an operative or invasive procedure views the person as having a physical (biological) nature, a psychological nature, and a sociocultural nature. The model goes a step further, however, to describe the spiritual nature of the person (**Fig. 1.1**).

Specifically, the physical component describes the anatomical parts of the person and how they function physiologically. The psychological component focuses on the person's "perception, cognition, emotion, personality, behavior, and interpersonal relationships" (Wikipedia, 2008). The sociocultural component describes the behaviors common to all members of human society and those required for successful functioning in a particular segment of human society. Social behaviors refer to the interactions of a person with a group of people such as the family, a community, or a work group; and cultural behaviors refer to the customary beliefs, values, symbols, knowledge, attitudes, and habits of a specific social group. The spiritual component describes the incorporeal presence, the animating principle, or the actuating cause of a person's life. A person's view of the spiritual component is influenced by religious and philosophical beliefs.

Assumption 2

The physical, psychological, sociocultural, and spiritual components of the system exist in a state of contingency.

The physical, psychological, sociocultural, and spiritual components of a person are interrelated to, dependent on, and conditioned by one another. Furthermore, each component receives sustenance from the others, which leads to a state of interdependence (**Fig. 1.2**).

Assumption 3

The spiritual component of the person is the unifying force of the system.

The spiritual component holds the system together and continues to exist after biological death (**Fig. 1.3**). Some people believe the spiritual component exists in the form of a soul. Others believe that it exists through reincarnation or may continue to exist in one's family, religious institution, work, community, or school.

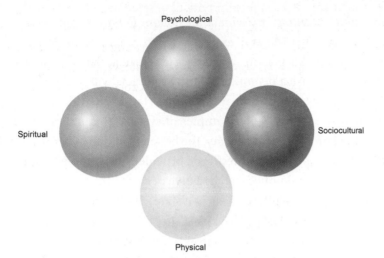

Figure 1.1

The person is a holistic system composed of physical, psychological, sociocultural, and spiritual components.

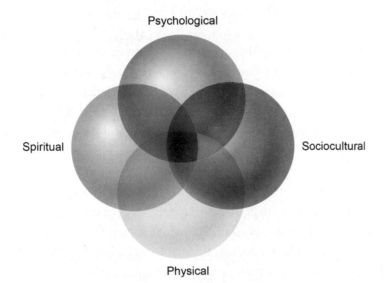

Figure 1.2

The physical, psychological, sociocultural, and spiritual components of the system exist in a state of contingency.

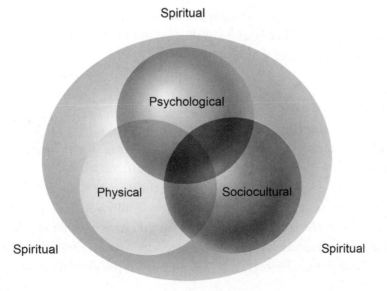

Figure 1.3

The spiritual component of the person is the unifying force of the system.

Assumption 4

The person exists in a state of contingency with other systems in the environment.

For each person, there are intrinsic and extrinsic environments. The intrinsic environment is located within the person, whereas the extrinsic environment is located outside the person. Because a person constantly interacts with the extrinsic environment, the person does not exist in a vacuum but in a state of contingency with other systems in the extrinsic environment. Examples of systems that interact with the person are a spouse, the family, the community, the hospital, and the operative or invasive procedure team (nurse, physician, anesthesia provider, and other personnel such as the surgical technologist and unlicensed assistive person). The person is also a component of other systems and therefore exists in a state of interdependence with the other components that compose the larger system. The relationships between the person and the systems of his or her extrinsic environment are dynamic.

Assumption 5

Health is dependent on the person's ability to cope with intrinsic and extrinsic environmental stressors.

Stressors have the potential for causing disequilibrium within the person and between the person and his or her environment. Intrinsic stressors originate within the person; extrinsic stressors originate outside the person. Examples of intrinsic stressors are incontinence, sensorimotor loss, and cognitive impairment. Prolonged pressure, friction, shearing force, and immobility caused by traction are examples of extrinsic stressors.

Health is a relative concept. A person is well if his or her physical, psychological, sociocultural, and spiritual components are united; if each of the components is successfully coping with intrinsic and extrinsic stressors; and if the person is in a state of equilibrium with the environment. A person becomes ill, however, when one or more of the physical, psychological, sociocultural, or spiritual components fail to cope adequately with intrinsic or extrinsic stressors, leading to a state of disequilibrium with the environment.

Illness is not limited to the physical and psychological components of the person. For example, a person who is physically and psychologically fit but experiencing a severe disturbance in role performance because of the loss of a job is not in a state of integrated wellness; this person is socioculturally ill.

Assumption 6

The person is in a constant state of movement along a life continuum.

The person is always moving along the life continuum toward biological death. Movement along the continuum is dynamic and is characterized by fluctuations between wellness and illness. Wellness or illness can occur at conception, at birth, during life, or at death. Some people believe that spiritual illness can occur in the afterlife. Spiritual illness may occur when a person biologically dies with bad memories, thoughts, or feelings toward family members, the community, or other significant people or systems that were part of the person's life experiences. Exit from the continuum can occur at any time. Furthermore, depending on the person's state of physical, psychological, sociocultural, and spiritual health, the person may exit in a state of wellness or illness. For example, a healthy young woman killed in an automobile accident by a drunk driver exits the continuum in a state of wellness. A person dying of cancer, however, exits the continuum in a state of illness.

Assumption 7

The physician performing the operative or invasive procedure and the anesthesia provider are therapeutic stressors.

Failure to cope adequately with intrinsic or extrinsic stressors can lead to conditions (stressors) that necessitate intervention with an operative or invasive procedure. In this case, the patient may seek a physician, who performs an operative or invasive procedure to eliminate, attenuate, or modify the stressor. In doing so, however, the physician becomes a stressor for the patient. For example, cigarette smoking (an extrinsic stressor), if not eliminated, can lead to the formation of a tumor in the respiratory tract. The tumor is an intrinsic stressor that, if not eliminated (removed), can lead to death. When the physician operates to remove the tumor, she or he becomes a stressor because she or he orders and performs tests and procedures that cause the patient pain and anxiety (**Fig. 1.4**).

Operative and invasive procedure intervention causes system disequilibrium (pain and alteration in body processes). The anesthesia provider initiates anesthesia to maintain system equilibrium. In doing so, however, the anesthesia provider, like the physician performing the procedure, becomes a stressor for the patient. For example, when the anesthesia provider administers a regional nerve block to anesthetize an extremity, he or she becomes a stress inducer because the administration of the nerve block causes the patient pain, discomfort, and anxiety.

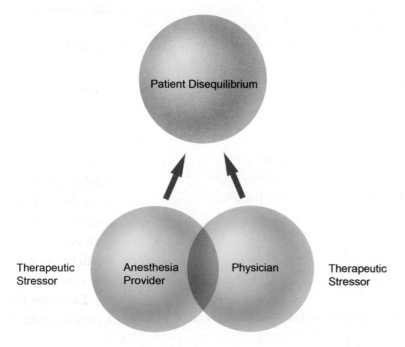

Figure 1.4

The physician performing the operative or invasive procedure and the anesthesia provider are therapeutic stressors.

VALUES OF THE *SYSTEMS-IN-CONTINGENCY MODEL*

Four basic values support the *Systems-in-Contingency Model's* goal.

1. Operative and invasive procedure nursing[3] is a socially significant specialty component of professional nursing practice that provides essential services needed by patients and families experiencing operative or invasive procedure intervention.
2. Establishing and sustaining system equilibrium during operative or invasive procedure interventions is essential for the patient's welfare.
3. Establishing and sustaining equilibrium during operative or invasive procedure intervention facilitates the rehabilitation process after the procedure.
4. Operative and invasive procedure nursing is unique because it focuses on the patient as a holistic system interacting with other systems in the operative and invasive procedure environment.

THE GOAL OF NURSING CARE DURING THE OPERATIVE AND INVASIVE PROCEDURE PERIOD

The goal of nursing care during the operative and invasive procedure is to establish and sustain system equilibrium. All nursing activities (assessment, diagnosis, outcome identification, planning, implementation, and evaluation) focus on establishing and sustaining the patient's equilibrium during the patient care events of the operative and invasive procedure period[4]. **Table 1.1** lists these patient care events.

THE RECIPIENT OF NURSING CARE

The *Systems-in-Contingency Model* describes the recipient of nursing care (the patient) as a holistic system composed of interrelated and interdependent physical, psychological, sociocultural, and spiritual components; the goal is to enhance, preserve, or achieve unity and equilibrium among the system components.

Table 1.1	Patient Care Events of the Operative and Invasive Procedure Period

Registered Nurses
- ☐ Prepare the Patient for the Procedure
- ☐ Transfer the Patient
- ☐ Assist the Anesthesia Provider
- ☐ Position the Patient
- ☐ Establish and Maintain the Sterile Field
- ☐ Perform Sponge, Sharp, and Instrument Counts
- ☐ Provide Instruments, Equipment, and Supplies
- ☐ Administer Drugs and Solutions
- ☐ Physiologically Monitor the Patient
- ☐ Monitor and Control the Environment
- ☐ Handle Cultures and Specimens
- ☐ Facilitate Care After the Procedure

Registered Nurses Practicing as First Assistants
- ☐ Handle Tissue with Instruments
- ☐ Provide Hemostasis

THE ROLE OF THE REGISTERED NURSE

The role of the registered nurse is to establish and sustain system equilibrium before, during, and after the procedure by assisting the patient in coping with the intrinsic and extrinsic stressors of the operative and invasive procedure environment and by facilitating the work of the physician and the anesthesia provider during the procedure. Specifically, the nurse assists the patient with coping by identifying the extrinsic and intrinsic stressors of the patient's operative and invasive procedure environment, formulating actual and potential nursing diagnoses, identifying expected outcomes, planning appropriate interventions, implementing the interventions, and evaluating the care given.

To illustrate, consider electrosurgery. Before the procedure, the nurse identifies electrosurgery as a potential extrinsic stressor because improper application of the patient return electrode may cause system disequilibrium (impaired skin integrity at the application site of the patient return electrode). Next, the patient is assessed for intrinsic stressors such as excessive hair, scar tissue, bony prominences, and metal implants that indicate his or her potential for experiencing injury related to electrosurgery, and then the nurse plans appropriate interventions. During the procedure, equilibrium is established by applying the patient return electrode to a site devoid of hair, scar tissue, bony prominences, and metal implants. The nurse sustains equilibrium by periodically checking the patient return electrode to ensure that it remains attached to the patient and by preventing tension on the electrode cord. After the procedure, the patient is assessed for signs of impaired skin integrity at the site of electrode application. If signs of impaired skin integrity are found, the nurse starts the process of reestablishing system equilibrium by referring the patient to the physician for appropriate treatment.

Another component of the nurse's role is facilitating the practice of the physician and the anesthesia provider during the procedure, which is essential for the patient's welfare. This role is derived from the assumption that the person exists in a state of contingency with other systems in the environment. During the procedure, the patient, as a holistic system, becomes dependent on the system identified as the operative or invasive procedure team: physician, anesthesia provider, circulating nurse, and scrub person. An operation that proceeds smoothly is performed by a team in a state of equilibrium with one another, and the patient. The key to this equilibrium is the nursing team. The scrub person facilitates the practice of the physician in the sterile field. The circulating nurse facilitates the practice of the physician and the anesthesia provider from outside the sterile field.

DEVIATIONS FROM THE DESIRED OUTCOMES

Deviations from the desired outcomes occur when the patient fails to cope with the intrinsic and extrinsic stressors during the operative and invasive procedure period, leading to system disequilibrium. For example, when an area of the body is exposed to prolonged pressure, such as when a person sits in one position for too long, the person adjusts by changing his or her position, which relieves the pressure. The patient under general or spinal anesthesia cannot change position; she or he loses the ability to cope and becomes vulnerable to system disequilibrium.

THE FOCUS OF INTERVENTIONS

The disequilibrium the patient may experience during the operative and invasive procedure period is the focus of interventions. Nursing diagnoses describe the types of potential or actual disequilibrium that can be prevented or treated by the nurse. **Table 1.2** lists the focus of interventions for patients undergoing operative and invasive procedures. Nursing diagnoses are categorized according to the patient care events.

THE INTERVENTIONS

Interventions prevent the potential problems or treat the actual problems. This is done by eliminating, attenuating, or modifying the intrinsic and extrinsic stressors confronting the patient (**Fig. 1.5**).

Elimination refers to the process of removing the stressor from the patient's environment. Removal of the stressor negates the potential or actual effect of the stressor on the patient. For example, foreign bodies are potential stressors. If items such as sponges, sharps, and instruments are retained, the patient experiences system disequilibrium after the procedure. Sponge, sharps, and instrument counts ensure that these potential stressors are eliminated from the immediate operative environment (wound) before closure.

Attenuation refers to the process of weakening or lessening the intensity of the stressor. By weakening or lessening the intensity of the stressor, the nurse decreases the potential or actual effect of the stressor on the patient. For example, the patient

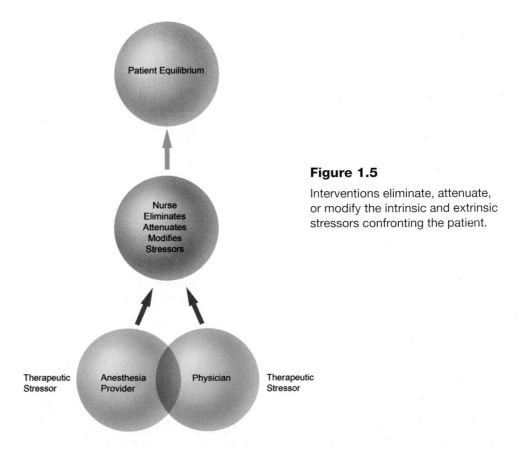

Figure 1.5

Interventions eliminate, attenuate, or modify the intrinsic and extrinsic stressors confronting the patient.

Table 1.2	The Focus of Interventions

Registered Nurses

Prepare the patient for the procedure

☐ Knowledge Deficit
☐ Fear related to the operative or invasive procedure experience
☐ Anxiety (Mild, Moderate, or Severe) related to the operative or invasive procedure experience
☐ Anticipatory Grieving related to the expected outcome of the operative or invasive procedure
☐ Ineffective Individual Coping related to the stress of the impending operative or invasive procedure

Transfer the patient

☐ Risk for Injury related to transfer to and from the operative and invasive procedure suite
☐ Risk for Hypothermia related to transfer to and from the operative and invasive procedure suite
☐ Risk for Ineffective Breathing pattern related to transfer to and from the operative and invasive procedure suite
☐ Risk for Discomfort or Pain related to transfer to and from the operative and invasive procedure suite

Assist the anesthesia provider

☐ Risk for Injury during the administration of general endotracheal anesthesia
☐ Risk for Injury secondary to malignant hyperthermia during the administration of general anesthesia
☐ Risk for Injury secondary to the administration of blood products during the operative or invasive procedure
☐ Risk of Hypothermia during the operative or invasive procedure
☐ Hyperthermia during the operative or invasive procedure

Position the patient

☐ Risk for Positioning Injury related to operative or invasive procedure positioning
☐ Risk for Impaired Skin Integrity related to operative or invasive procedure positioning
☐ Risk for Impaired Respiratory Function related to operative or invasive procedure positioning
☐ Risk for Ineffective Tissue Perfusion related to operative or invasive procedure positioning

Establish and maintain the sterile field

☐ Risk for Wound Infection
☐ Risk for Impaired Skin Integrity
☐ Risk for Hypothermia immediately before and during the procedure
☐ Risk for Ineffective Breathing Patterns
☐ Risk for Self-Esteem Disturbance

Perform sponge, sharp, and instrument counts

☐ Risk for Injury related to retained sponges, sharps, and instruments

Provide instruments, equipment, and supplies

☐ Risk for Infection
☐ Risk for Injury related to extended anesthesia time
☐ Risk for Hypothermia
☐ Risk for Injury related to the use of pneumatic tourniquet
☐ Risk for Injury related to electrosurgery

Administer drugs and solutions

☐ Risk for Infection related to the administration of drugs and solutions

☐ Risk for Injury related to hypersensitivity reaction because of improper identification of patient allergies

☐ Risk for Deficit Fluid Volume (blood loss) related to the use of heparin

☐ Risk for Deficit Fluid Volume related to the administration of hyperosmotic agents

☐ Risk for Injury related to an allergic reaction to local anesthetic

☐ Risk for Injury related to an allergic or adverse reaction because of patient sensitivity to otic medication

☐ Risk for Injury related to an allergic reaction to contrast media

☐ Risk for Injury related to toxicity from local anesthetic agents

☐ Risk for Decreased Cardiac Output related to toxicity from a local anesthetic

☐ Risk for Injury related to mydriatic agent administration causing an acute angle-closure glaucoma episode

☐ Risk for Impaired Skin Integrity related to the administration of skin medications

☐ Risk for Fluid Volume Excess related to the absorption of large amounts of endoscopic irrigating fluid into the systemic circulation

Physiologically monitor the patient

☐ Risk for Ineffective Airway Clearance and Ineffective Breathing Pattern during the operative or invasive procedure

☐ Risk for Impaired Tissue Integrity related to local infiltration of IV fluid

☐ Risk for Fluid Volume Excess related to IV therapy

☐ Risk for Decreased Cardiac Output related to air embolus from IV therapy

☐ Risk for Fluid Volume Deficit related to bleeding during the operative or invasive procedure

☐ Risk for Hypothermia operative or invasive

☐ Risk for Hyperthermia operative or invasive

☐ Risk for Ineffective Breathing Pattern related to moderate sedation/analgesia

☐ Risk for Impaired Tissue Integrity related to extravasation of IV medication

☐ Risk for Decreased Cardiac Output (Cardiodepression) related to the administration of local anesthetics

Monitor and control the environment

☐ Inadvertent hypothermia; risk for imbalanced body temperature; ineffective thermoregulation

☐ Risk for Injury related to the use of equipment during the operative or invasive procedure

☐ Risk for Injury related to chemical hazards

☐ Risk for Injury related to the use of electrical equipment

☐ Risk for Injury related to a fire during the operative or invasive procedure

☐ Risk for Injury/Impaired Skin Integrity related to the effects of radiation

☐ Risk for Injury/Impaired Skin Integrity related to the use of laser instruments and equipment

☐ Risk for Injury related to latex exposure; Allergic response to latex

☐ Risk for Anxiety or Fear due to sensory stimuli in the operative and invasive procedure room

☐ Risk for Infection

Handle cultures and specimens

☐ Risk for Injury related to improper handling of cultures and specimens obtained during the operative or invasive procedure

Facilitate care after the procedures

- ☐ Risk for Impaired Tissue Integrity related to abscess formation
- ☐ Risk for Impaired Tissue Integrity related to the formation of gas gangrene
- ☐ Potential for Impaired Skin Integrity: nonhealing wound
- ☐ Risk for Wound Infection
- ☐ Risk for Infection related to seroma formation in the postprocedure wound
- ☐ Risk for Potential Infection related to wound dehiscence or evisceration
- ☐ Risk for Postprocedure Hyperthermia (fever)
- ☐ Risk for Alteration in Postprocedure Cardiac Rate (tachycardia)
- ☐ Risk for Ineffective Airway Clearance during the postprocedure period
- ☐ Risk for Ineffective Breathing Patterns during the postprocedure period
- ☐ Risk for Acute Pulmonary Embolus
- ☐ Risk for Postprocedure Urinary Tract Infection
- ☐ Risk for Altered Postprocedure Bowel Function
- ☐ Risk for Alteration in Comfort (postprocedure pain)
- ☐ Risk for Alteration in Comfort related to nausea and vomiting
- ☐ Risk for Alteration in Comfort related to inadvertent hypothermia
- ☐ Risk for Injury related to devices used to assist patient recovery
- ☐ Deficient knowledge related to the rehabilitation process after the procedure
- ☐ Risk for ineffective therapeutic regimen management
- ☐ Risk for Noncompliance with prescribed therapeutic regimen after the procedure

Registered Nurses Practicing as First Assistants

Handle tissue with instruments

- ☐ Risk for Infection related to the handling of tissue with instruments during the operative or invasive procedure
- ☐ Risk for Injury related to handling of tissue with instruments during the procedure
- ☐ Risk for Impaired Tissue Integrity related to the handling of tissue with instruments during the procedure.

Provide hemostasis

- ☐ Risk for Deficient Fluid Volume related to related to alterations in clotting mechanisms
- ☐ Risk for Injury related to the use of mechanical methods to achieve hemostasis
- ☐ Risk for Injury related to the use of electrical devices to achieve hemostasis
- ☐ Risk for Injury related to the use of a laser to achieve hemostasis
- ☐ Risk for Injury related to the use of microfibrillar collagen hemostat, gelatin sponge, and oxidized cellulose
- ☐ Risk for Injury related to the use of collagen sponge
- ☐ Risk for Injury related to the use of oxidized cellulose for hemostasis
- ☐ Risk for Impaired Tissue Integrity related to the use of gelatin sponge
- ☐ Risk for Infection related to the use of electrical devices to achieve hemostasis
- ☐ Risk for Infection related to the use of microfibrillar collagen hemostat, gelatin sponge, and oxidized cellulose

Adapted from Carpentino-Moyet, L. J. (2008). *Handbook of nursing diagnosis* (12th Ed.). Philadelphia: Lippincott Williams & Wilkins, pp. 45–46, 364; *Perioperative nursing data set, the perioperative nursing vocabulary.* (Revised 2nd Ed.). Denver: AORN. Inc., p. 48.

has the potential for wound infection because of the presence of microorganisms in the immediate operative or invasive procedure environment, but complete elimination of microorganisms from this environment is impossible. The effect of microorganisms on the patient, however, can be minimized by decreasing their numbers. The nurse accomplishes the desired effect by preparing the patient's operative site with an antimicrobial solution and ensuring that the team members adhere to aseptic practices.

Modification refers to the process of altering how the stressor affects the patient during the operative and invasive procedure period. The stressor remains the same; the effect, however, is altered. For example, an elderly emaciated patient scheduled for a 6-hour operative procedure is confronted with the intrinsic stressors of inadequate adipose tissue, protruding bony prominences, and poor skin turgor. This patient is also confronted with the extrinsic stressors of a lengthy operative procedure, extended immobility while under anesthesia, and the surface of the operating bed. The nurse cannot eliminate these stressors. She or he can, however, modify the effect of the stressors by padding the operating bed and the bony prominences.

Because operative and invasive procedure nurses have traditionally focused on the prevention of potential health problems, such as potential infection and injury, the primary aim of interventions in the *Systems-in-Contingency Model* is the prevention of potential alterations in system equilibrium during the operative and invasive procedure period. This does not mean, however, that the nurse ignores actual health problems. On the contrary, treatment of actual health problems falls within the practice domain of the nurse caring for patients undergoing operative and invasive procedures. Examples of nurses treating actual health problems are interventions implemented for anxiety, anticipatory grieving, and body image disturbance; correction of knowledge deficit; and teaching of breathing and splinting techniques and dressing change technique (particularly for outpatients).

INTENDED OUTCOME

The intended outcome of the *Systems-in-Contingency Model* is system equilibrium during the operative and invasive procedure period. **Table 1.3** lists the intended outcomes for each patient care event.

CONCLUSION

The patient is a holistic system interacting with other systems in the operative and invasive procedure environment. The nurse is a strategic component of that environment. The *Systems-in-Contingency Model* for the care of the patient undergoing an operative or invasive procedure provides direction for the practice of nursing in the complex reality of this dynamic practice setting. This approach to the nursing paradigm provides a stimulus and direction for the development of operative and invasive procedure nursing curriculum, clinical practice, and research.

Table 1.3	Intended Outcomes of the *Systems-in-Contingency Model*
Patient Care Event	**Outcome**
Prepare the patient for the procedure	☐ The patient and family demonstrate knowledge of the expected responses to the operative or invasive procedure
	☐ The patient recognizes and manages fear during the operative or invasive period
	☐ The patient does not express feelings of apprehension and activation of the autonomic nervous system in response to the operative or invasive procedure experience
	☐ The patient recognizes the presence of anticipatory grief and engages in a functional grieving process
	☐ The patient is able to adequately manage internal and environmental stressors related to the impending operative or invasive procedure
Transfer the patient	☐ The patient is free from signs and symptoms of injury related to transfer/transport
	☐ The patient is free from evidence of a decrease in body temperature during transfer to and from the operative and invasive procedure suite
	☐ The patient is free from evidence of breathing difficulty
	☐ The patient is free from evidence of discomfort or pain during the transfer process
Assist the anesthesia provider	☐ The patient is free from evidence of injury secondary to the induction of general endotracheal anesthesia
	☐ The patient is free from evidence of injury secondary to malignant hyperthermia during the administration of general anesthesia
	☐ The patient is free from evidence of injury secondary to the administration of blood products during the operative or invasive procedure
	☐ The patient maintains normothermia during the operative or invasive procedure
Position the patient	☐ The patient is free from evidence of injury related to operative or invasive procedure positioning
	☐ The patient is free from evidence of impaired skin integrity related to operative or invasive procedure positioning
	☐ The patient is free from evidence of impaired respiratory function related to operative or invasive procedure positioning
	☐ The patient is free from evidence of ineffective tissue perfusion related to operative or invasive procedure positioning
Establish and maintain the sterile field	☐ The patient is free from evidence of wound infection
	☐ The patient is free from evidence of impaired skin integrity
	☐ The patient is free from evidence of hypothermia
	☐ The patient is free from evidence of ineffective breathing patterns
	☐ The patient is free from evidence of disturbed self-esteem
Perform sponge, sharp, and instrument counts	☐ The patient is free from signs and symptoms of injury caused by extraneous objects
Provide instruments, equipment, and supplies	☐ The patient is free from evidence of infection
	☐ The patient is free from evidence of injury resulting from an extended anesthesia time
	☐ The patient's body temperature is maintained within normal limits during the operative or invasive procedure
	☐ The patient is free from evidence of injury related to the use of a pneumatic tourniquet
	☐ The patient is free from evidence of injury related to the application of electrosurgery

Administer drugs and solutions	☐ The patient is free from evidence of infection related to the administration of drugs and solutions
	☐ The patient is free from evidence of hypersensitivity reaction because of improper identification of patient allergies
	☐ The patient is free from evidence of deficit fluid volume related to the use of heparin
	☐ The patient is free from evidence of deficit fluid volume related to the administration of hyperosmotic agents
	☐ The patient is free from evidence of injury related to allergic or adverse reaction to a local anesthetic
	☐ The patient is free from evidence of injury related to allergic or adverse reaction to otic medication
	☐ The patient is free from evidence of injury related to allergic or adverse reaction to contrast media
	☐ The patient is free from evidence of injury related to toxicity from a local anesthetic
	☐ The patient is free from evidence of decrease cardiac output related to toxicity from a local anesthetic
	☐ The patient is free from evidence of related to mydriatic agent administration causing an acute angle-closure glaucoma episode
	☐ The patient is free from evidence of impaired skin integrity related to the administration of skin medication
	☐ The patient is free from evidence of excess fluid volume related to the absorption of large amounts of irrigating fluid into the systemic circulation
Physiologically monitor the patient	☐ The patient is free from airway obstruction or ineffective breathing during the procedure
	☐ The patient's tissue integrity is maintained at the site of the IV infusion
	☐ The patient's fluid volume is maintained
	☐ The patient's cardiac output is maintained during the procedure
	☐ The patient's fluid volume is maintained during the procedure
	☐ The patient is at or returning to normothermia at the conclusion of the immediate operative and invasive procedure period
	☐ The patient is at or returning to normothermia at the conclusion of the immediate operative and invasive procedure period
	☐ The patient's breathing pattern is maintained during the procedure
	☐ The patient is free from tissue damage related to subcutaneous infiltration of medications and IV fluids
	☐ The patient's cardiac output is maintained during the procedure
Monitor and control the environment	☐ The patient is at or returning to normothermia at the conclusion of the immediate operative or invasive procedure period
	☐ The patient is free from signs and symptoms of injury caused by extraneous objects associated with equipment use
	☐ The patient is free from signs and symptoms of chemical injury
	☐ The patient is free from signs and symptoms of electrical injury
	☐ The patient is free from acquired physical injury due to fires during the operative or invasive procedure
	☐ The patient is free from signs and symptoms of radiation injury
	☐ The patient is free from signs and symptoms of laser injury
	☐ The patient is free from injury due to latex exposure
	☐ The patient is free from signs and symptoms of anxiety or fear
	☐ The patient is free from signs and symptoms of infection
Handle cultures and specimens	☐ The patient is free from evidence of injury related to the handling of specimens and cultures

Facilitate care after the procedures	☐ The patient experiences uncomplicated wound healing
	☐ The patient remains free from wound infection after the procedure
	☐ The patient is free from systemic postprocedure complications
	☐ The patient experiences physiological and psychological comfort after the operative or invasive procedure
	☐ The patient is free from injury related to the use of medical devices used to assist in recovery
	☐ The patient and family are compliant with the rehabilitation process and the therapeutic regimen after the procedure

Registered Nurses Practicing as First Assistants

Handle tissue with instruments	☐ The patient is free from evidence of postprocedure wound infection
	☐ The patient is free from evidence of injury related to handling tissue with instruments
	☐ The patient is free from evidence of impaired tissue integrity at the wound site
Provide hemostasis	☐ The patient is free from evidence of deficient fluid volume related to alterations in clotting mechanisms
	☐ The patient is free from evidence of injury related to mechanical hemostatic techniques used during the procedure
	☐ The patient is free from evidence of injury related to the use of electrical devices to achieve hemostasis used during the procedure
	☐ The patient is free from evidence of injury related to the use of laser equipment used to achieve hemostasis during the procedure
	☐ The patient is free from evidence of injury related to the use of microfibrillar collagen hemostat, gelatin sponge, and oxidized cellulose to achieve hemostasis during the procedure
	☐ The patient is free from evidence of impaired skin integrity related to the use of gelatin sponge to achieve hemostasis during the procedure
	☐ The patient is free from evidence of postprocedure infection related to thermal hemostatic techniques used during the procedure
	☐ The patient is free from evidence of postprocedure infection related to chemical hemostatic techniques used during the procedure

Adapted from Carpentino-Moyet, L. J (2008). *Handbook of nursing diagnosis* (12th Ed.). Philadelphia Lippincott Williams & Wilkins, pp. 45–46, 364. *Perioperative nursing data set, the perioperative nursing vocabulary* (Revised 2nd Ed.). Denver AORN Inc, p. 48.

ENDNOTES

1. The term *registered nurse* refers to the nurse caring for a patient immediately before, during, and immediately after an operative and invasive procedure. Practice areas for the nurse include inpatient, outpatient, and office-based operating rooms; gastrointestinal laboratories, cardiac catheterization laboratories, interventional radiology departments, preprocedure preparation areas, and postprocedure care areas (discharge).

2. An assumption is a statement that is taken for granted, as if it is true without proof (Free Dictionary, 2008).

3. Nursing practiced by perioperative, gastroenterology, cardiac catheterization laboratory, and interventional radiology nurses.

4. The patient care events serve as the focus for chapter content for chapters 5–18.

REFERENCES

1. AORN (2008). *Standards of Perioperative Clinical Practice, Standards, Recommended Practices, and Guidelines.* Denver, CO: AORN, pp. 19–22.
2. Wikipedia (2008). Psychology, http://en.wikipedia.org/wiki/Psychology. Accessed 13 June 2008.
3. The Free Dictionary (2008). Assumption, http://www.thefreedictionary.com/%20assumption. Accessed 13 June 2008.

CHAPTER 2

Competency Assessment

In the Operative and Invasive Procedure Setting

Michelle Byrne

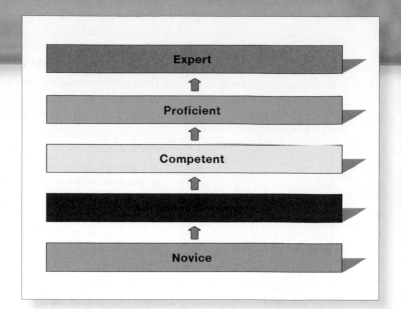

INTRODUCTION

As operative and invasive procedures and the associated technologies have evolved, becoming more sophisticated and complex, many procedures are being performed in settings such as offices, cardiac catheterization laboratories, interventional radiology suites, gastrointestinal laboratories, and free-standing clinics, as well as the traditional setting of the operating room.

Complexity and increased sophistication in the delivery of operative and invasive procedure services have led to advances in patient care and outcomes not imagined a decade ago. However, this complexity and sophistication have also stressed the delivery system, to include the human factor, to the point that agencies such as the Joint Commission and Centers for Medicare-Medicaid Services have focused attention on adverse outcomes and require facilities to provide definitive plans that address these unfortunate events. Competency assessment is one of the tools healthcare facilities can use to build a culture of quality patient care and potentially reduce the number of adverse outcomes.

Competency assessment within the operative and invasive procedure setting is a means of determining if nurses, surgical technologists, and other staff members, to include physicians and anesthesia providers, are proficient and have demonstrated the knowledge, cognitive skills, and psychomotor skills necessary to provide safe patient care relevant to their specific role function. This chapter will address competency assessment for members of the nursing team which includes registered nurses, licensed vocational nurses, surgical technologists, and others engaged in delivery, or supporting the delivery of nursing care, in the operative and invasive procedure

Chapter Contents

suite. The chapter will discuss practice frameworks for the delivery of nursing care in the operative and invasive procedure setting that can be used to develop competency assessment tools, a model for skill acquisition, methodologies for assessing competency, agencies that provide resources for assessing competency, and sample competency assessment tools.

NURSING ROLES IN THE OPERATIVE AND INVASIVE PROCEDURE SUITE

Nursing roles within the operative and invasive procedure setting are highly differentiated and include direct patient care as well as roles that indirectly address patient needs. The primary direct patient care roles for the registered nurse are scrubbing and circulating. When performing these roles the registered nurse provides care during patient care events that were previously described in Chapter 1. **Table 2.1** lists these patient care events which are common to most procedures performed in the operative and invasive procedure setting.

Another direct care role is first assistant. Registered nurses performing this role assist the surgeon during an operative procedure. Role functions include handling tissue with instruments and providing hemostasis during the procedure.

New knowledge impacts patient care. Informatics, sterile processing, genetics, and environmental issues have pushed the boundaries of nursing practice in the operative and invasive procedure suite. Nurses must continue to learn and integrate new knowledge into existing roles or tasks. Nurses in *Advanced Practice Registered Nursing* (APRN) roles in operative and invasive procedure settings continue to increase in numbers. Their roles are varied and continue to expand as more specialized knowledge is necessary due to the increasing complexity of patients and the technologies

APRN
Advanced Practice
Registered Nursing

Table 2.1	Patient Care Events of the Operative and Invasive Procedure Suite

Before the Procedure
1. Prepare the patient for the procedure

During the Procedure
2. Transfer the patient

3. Assist the anesthesia provider

4. Position the patient

5. Establish and maintain the sterile field

6. Perform sponge, sharp, and instrument counts

7. Provide instruments, equipment, and supplies for the procedure

8. Administer drugs and solutions

9. Physiologically monitor the patient

10. Monitor and control the environment

11. Handle cultures and specimens

After the Procedure
12. Facilitate care after the procedure

Table 2.2	Definitions of Roles in the Operative and Invasive Procedure Setting
Role	**Definition**
Circulating nurse	A registered nurse who coordinates and manages each surgical patient's operating room care by assessing, planning, intervening, evaluating and documenting patient care and patient outcomes. This nurse is the team leader in each operating room and the designated patient advocate.
Scrub person	A registered nurse, licensed practical nurse, or surgical technologist who performs hand asepsis and is considered a sterile member of the surgical team. This team member is responsible for maintaining the integrity of sterile instruments and supplies used at the surgical site and passing instruments to the surgeon and first assistant.
First assistant	Another MD or DO, a medical student, a registered nurse first assistant (RNFA), a nurse practitioner (NP), a physician's assistant (PA), or a surgical technologist (ST) who is designated to assist the surgeon at surgery. The first assistant's technical skills may include suturing, providing hemostasis, and retracting tissue depending on state's scope of practice laws, institutional policies, and education level of the individual. The first assistant is a sterile member of the surgical team.
Advanced practice nurses	Four primary roles include clinical nurse specialist (CNS), certified nurse midwife (CNM), certified registered nurse anesthetist (CRNA), and nurse practitioner (NP). These registered nurses have completed a master's or doctoral degree, have specialized in perioperative patient care, and may hold various roles in the perioperative arena.

used to care for them (King, 2007). **Table 2.2** lists of some of the current direct-care nurse roles found within the operative and invasive procedure setting.

Indirect patient care roles support the registered nurse in providing direct care. These roles include nurse educators, administrators, researchers, or industry consultants who can strongly impact patient care practices and decisions without having a direct hands-on relationship with the patient.

There are many professional and paraprofessional personnel with whom registered nurses must work and sometimes supervise. The operative and invasive procedure setting is interdisciplinary and multidisciplinary with physicians and anesthesia providers being integral team members who also provide patient care. Strategies must be developed to inspire teamwork and collaboration. These strategies include communication, patient advocacy, and leadership skills.

PRACTICE MODELS FOR THE DELIVERY OF NURSING CARE IN THE OPERATIVE AND INVASIVE PROCEDURE AREA

Practice models that provide frameworks for the delivery of patient care within the operative and invasive procedure area should serve as the foundation for the development of competency assessment strategies and tools. Two of these models are the *Systems-In-Contingency Model for the Patient Undergoing an Operative or Invasive Procedure* and the Association of periOperative Registered Nurses' (AORN) *Perioperative Patient-Focused Model.* Other resources for developing competency assessment tools are the *Perioperative Nursing Data Set* and the AORN *Competency Statements in Perioperative Nursing,* the *Perioperative Nursing Advanced Practice Nurse Competency Statements*, and *the Perioperative Care Coordinator Nurse Competency Statements.*

AORN
Association of periOperative Registered Nurses

The Systems-in-Contingency Model for the Patient Undergoing an Operative or Invasive Procedure

Chapter 1 provides an in-depth discussion of the *Systems-In-Contingency Model for the Patient Undergoing an Operative or Invasive Procedure.* This model is used in this text as the predominant framework for competency assessment within the operative and invasive procedure setting. As shown in **Table 2.1** there are twelve patient care events that the registered nurse performs or manages during the operative and invasive procedure period. Each event can be sub-divided into nursing care activities that range from the very simple to the complex. As an example, **Table 2.3** lists the activities for the patient care event titled *Provide Instruments, Equipment, and Supplies.* The list is not all-inclusive and may include other activities as identified by the facility.

Competency assessment tools developed using the *Systems-in-Contingency Model* focus on evaluating proficiency of the nurse and others, such as surgical technologists and attendants, doing these activities, or subsets of the activities, particularly if the activity is inherently risky to the patient, if not performed correctly, such as *Applying and Removing a Pneumatic Tourniquet.* See **Table 2.4** for an example of a competency assessment tool for Applying and Removing a Pneumatic Tourniquet.

Table 2.3	**Performance Criteria Provide Instruments, Equipment, and Supplies**

- ☐ Identifying the patient's risk for adverse outcomes related to the provision of instruments, equipment, and supplies
- ☐ Selecting appropriate instrumentation, equipment, and supplies for an operative or invasive procedure
- ☐ Delivering instruments and supplies to the sterile field
- ☐ Arranging instruments and supplies on the back table and Mayo tray
- ☐ Passing instruments and supplies to the physician or assistant
- ☐ Preparing and passing sutures to the physician or assistant
- ☐ Preparing and applying patient warming systems
- ☐ Applying and removing a pneumatic tourniquet
- ☐ Preparing air-powered instrumentation for use
- ☐ Implementing electrosurgical safety precautions
- ☐ Applying dressings
- ☐ Assisting with the application of casts and splints
- ☐ Preparing and operating endoscopic equipment

Table 2.4	COMPETENCY ASSESSMENT: Position the Patient

Name_____ Title_____

Unit_____ Date of Validation_____

Type of Validation: ☐ Initial (by educator)   ☐ Annual (by peer)

Method of Evaluation: Observation

COMPETENCY STATEMENT: The nurse demonstrates competency to position the patient for an operative or invasive procedure.

Score   **Performance Criteria**

Identifies physical alterations that require additional precautions for procedure-specific positioning

①②③④⑤ **1.** Identifies individuals at risk for positioning injury.

①②③④⑤ **2.** Reviews chart for information on patient's weight, preexisting medical conditions, and laboratory results.

①②③④⑤ **3.** Interviews patient for history of implanted devices.

①②③④⑤ **4.** Examines patient skin condition, Loss of Consciousness (LOC), perception of pain, presence of peripheral pulses, and mobility impairments.

①②③④⑤ **5.** Assesses external devices (eg, drains, catheters, orthopedic immobilizers).

①②③④⑤ **6.** Applies antiembolism stockings in a manner to minimize friction injuries.

①②③④⑤ **7.** Implements measures to prevent inadvertent hypothermia.

①②③④⑤ **8.** Maintains safe transport environment through use of elevated bed rails, safety straps applied, additional devices secured (eg, oxygen tanks, IV poles, Foley catheter, chest tube).

①②③④⑤ **9.** Supervises placement of equipment and/or surgical instruments on patient.

①②③④⑤ **10.** Monitors patient for external pressures applied by members of healthcare team.

Verifies presence of prosthetics or corrective devices

①②③④⑤ **11.** Identifies presence of or use of prosthetics or corrective devices and modifies nursing care as indicated for planned procedure.

①②③④⑤ **12.** Determines presence of metal and synthetic prostheses and implants, pacemakers, automated implanted cardioverter defibrillators (AICD), hearing augmentation devices, intraocular lenses, or plastic/fluid implants (eg, penile implants, testicular implants, breast implants) and notifies appropriate members of healthcare team.

①②③④⑤ **13.** Individualizes plan of care to accommodate prosthetic or corrective devices.

Positions the patient

①②③④⑤ **14.** Determines the need for, prepares, applies, and removes devices designed to enhance operative exposure, prevent neuromuscular injury, maintain skin and tissue integrity, and maintain body alignment and optimal physiological functioning.

①②③④⑤ **15.** Selects positioning devices based on patient's identified needs and the planned operative or invasive procedure.

①②③④⑤ **16.** Positions patient on stretcher with side rails up and wheels locked when:

☐ Awaiting admission to OR.

☐ Procedure is completed on the stretcher.

①②③④⑤ **17.** Determines that devices are readily available, clean, free of sharp edges, padded as appropriate, and in working order before placing patient on the OR bed.

① ② ③ ④ ⑤　**18.** Modifies OR bed as necessary before attaching positioning devices.

① ② ③ ④ ⑤　**19.** Reviews chart for information on patient's weight, preexisting medical conditions, previous surgeries, and laboratory results.

① ② ③ ④ ⑤　**20.** Assesses functional limitations while patient is awake and responsive.

① ② ③ ④ ⑤　**21.** Assesses patient for presence of skin conditions, LOC, perception of pain, presence of peripheral pulses, and mobility impairments while awake.

① ② ③ ④ ⑤　**22.** Adapts positioning plan to accommodate limitations.

① ② ③ ④ ⑤　**23.** Maintains body alignment.

① ② ③ ④ ⑤　**24.** Maintains proper alignment of legs (uncrossed).

① ② ③ ④ ⑤　**25.** Uses positioning devices to protect, support, and maintain patient position.

① ② ③ ④ ⑤　**26.** Attaches padded arm boards to bed at less than 90° angle.

① ② ③ ④ ⑤　**27.** Places patient's arms on boards with palms up and fingers extended or secures arms at patient's side in neutral position.

① ② ③ ④ ⑤　**28.** Places fingers in position clear of table breaks or other hazards.

① ② ③ ④ ⑤　**29.** Applies safety belt loosely so blood flow is not compromised.

① ② ③ ④ ⑤　**30.** Protects body parts from contact with metal portions of OR bed.

① ② ③ ④ ⑤　**31.** Protects patency of tubes, drains, and catheters.

① ② ③ ④ ⑤　**32.** Prevents limbs from dropping below bed level to prevent compression of peripheral nerves.

① ② ③ ④ ⑤　**33.** Rechecks body alignment, extremities, safety strap, and all padding if repositioning occurs.

① ② ③ ④ ⑤　**34.** Removes positioning devices cautiously after surgery while maintaining body alignment and homeostatic status.

Evaluates for signs and symptoms of injury as a result of positioning

① ② ③ ④ ⑤　**35.** Observes for signs and symptoms of injury to integumentary, neuromuscular, and cardiopulmonary systems as a result of the patient's position during the procedure.

① ② ③ ④ ⑤　**36.** Examines patient to assess peripheral pulses and/or neuromuscular impairments.

① ② ③ ④ ⑤　**37.** Examines sites related to positional devices for signs and symptoms of skin/tissue injury.

① ② ③ ④ ⑤　**38.** Examines pressure areas for signs of skin injury.

① ② ③ ④ ⑤　**39.** Assesses and monitors vital signs.

Scoring　① Did not demonstrate competency　② Minimal competency　③ Competency
④ Exceptional competency　⑤ Outstanding competency

Comments (mandatory for scores of 1, 2, 4, or 5)

_____
Validator's Signature

_____
Validator's Printed Name

_____
Employee's Signature

_____
Employee's Printed Name

The Perioperative Patient-Focused Model

The Perioperative Patient-Focused Model (**Fig 2.1**) was created to provide a framework for perioperative nursing practice (AORN, 2008). Similar to the *Systems-in-Contingency Model*, at the center of this model is the patient, thus emphasizing that the patient provides the focus for all activities. Four concentric circles move outward from the patient-centered model. These circles dissect three patient-centered domains addressing patient safety, physiologic responses to surgery, and behavioral responses of the patient and the family. The fourth quadrant addresses the healthcare system within which nursing care is provided. The healthcare system includes benchmarks, positive outcomes with reporting and structural elements all with the goal of providing patient-centered care (AORN, 2008).

The Perioperative Nursing Data Set (PNDS)

The Perioperative Patient Focused Model not only guides patient care but is the foundation for a clinical information infrastructure known as the Perioperative Nursing Data Set (PNDS; AORN, 2007). This data set has been used in perioperative nursing for over 10 years to support safe, outcome-oriented patient care. This PNDS provides perioperative nomenclature that can be used for communicating information that is reliable and valid. The language and taxonomy provide an objective and standardized method for communicating perioperative care across sites and disciplines. Software companies have adopted the PNDS as it provides a language of measurement indicators facilitating benchmarking data for system improvement.

PNDS
Perioperative
Nursing Data Set

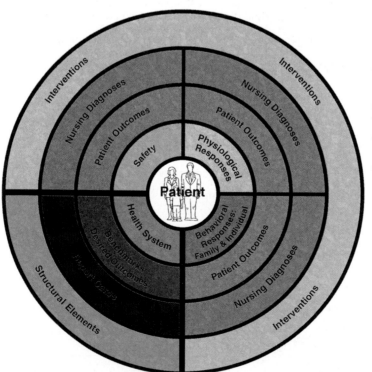

Figure 2.1

AORN Model for
Perioperative Nursing.

Source: Reprinted with permission from AORN's *Perioperative Nursing Data Set*, revised second edition, pages 16, 19. Copyright © 2007 AORN, Inc, 2170 South Parker Road, Suite 300, Denver, CO 80231.

Competency Statements in Perioperative Nursing

Another resource is the AORN *Competency Statements in Perioperative Nursing* which is directly linked to the PNDS. AORN has defined competency as "the knowledge, skills, and abilities necessary to fulfill the professional role functions of a registered nursing in the operating room" (AORN, 2007, p. 21). Competency statements are useful for employee orientation, continuing education, measurement and documentation for accrediting institutions. In addition to identifying competency statements for perioperative registered nurses, statements have also been articulated for Perioperative Advanced Practice Nurses and Perioperative Care Coordinators (AORN 2008).

Using the Perioperative Patient-Focused Model and the PNDS for Competency Assessment

The Perioperative *Patient-Focused Model* in conjunction with the *Perioperative Nursing Data Set* and *Competency Statements in Perioperative Nursing* provide a clear map for competency assessment, particularly in the domain of safety. As an example, the interpretive statements of Outcome 05, "*The patient is free from signs and symptoms of injury related to positioning*" provide critical information for staff and students learning how to position the patient, such as very specific indicators and examples of nursing interventions and activities. These interventions and activities provide criteria for assessing positioning competency, and can also be integrated into institutional policies, procedures, manuals, and educational offerings.

The PNDS is linked with the North American Nursing Diagnosis Association (NANDA) approved nursing diagnoses (Carpenito-Moyet, 2006). These diagnoses can be used as a framework for evaluating cognitive skills related to assessment and diagnosis of patients at risk for adverse outcomes during the operative and invasive procedure period, such as positioning-related injuries. The PNDS also provides consistent terminology that enhances benchmarking and multidisciplinary communication. PNDS taxonomy is the foundation for defining and communicating the activities that comprise nursing practice in the operative and invasive procedure setting. Table 2.4 shows an example of a competency assessment tool built on Domain 1, Outcome 05 Positioning Injury.

NANDA
North American
Nursing Diagnosis
Association

THE COMPETENCY CONTINUUM

As nurses gain experience, they advance in clinical competency. Consequently, clinical competency is not evaluated the same for all practitioners. Rather it is evaluated according to the practitioner's level of skill acquisition and role expectations.

A model frequently used to understand the process of experiential influences on nurse competency is the *Dreyfus & Dreyfus Model of Skill Acquisition*, which was applied to nursing by Benner (1984). This five-level model describes the process of skill development from no experience (*novice*) to very experienced (*expert*) (**Table 2.5**). The following describes characteristics of the five stages of the model as applied to student and practicing nurses. When designing competency assessment tools this model will provide guidance in crafting tools that are appropriate to the experience level of the practitioner.

Table 2.5	Dreyfus & Dreyfus Model of Skill Acquisition
Novice	The novice nurse has no prior experience upon which to base knowledgeable decision-making. Persons at this level seek concrete rules to follow and find it difficult when the rules do not apply exactly to the situation. When working with novices, it is important to be concrete and provide basic knowledge that can be applied to actions in practice.
Advanced Beginner	The advanced beginner nurse has some previous experiences upon which to base decisions. This nurse is able to see "gray" aspects in previously perceived black-and-white rules or procedures. Although this person acknowledges that situations may vary and actions cannot always be predicted, they usually have a difficult time anticipating subtleties in a situation and prioritizing nursing actions. Nurses at this level are very reactive rather than proactive.
Competent	The competent nurse has worked two to three years in the same practice area. Experience enables this nurse to discern commonalities and act toward meeting long-term outcomes or goals. Organization is a characteristic of this nurse and can be typically manifested in his or her deliberate plan for managing patient care priorities.
Proficient	Understanding the complete context rather than focusing on isolated tasks or pending actions is the hallmark of the proficient nurse. This nurse prioritizes easily and relies less on concrete rules and more on perceptions based on experience. Another characteristic is the ability to easily differentiate between the expected and the unexpected.
Expert	Intuitive knowing is a key characteristic of the expert nurse. Vast experience and cognition enables this nurse to provide high-quality nursing care by sensing subtle changes in the patient's conditions and acting swiftly in response to these changes.

Benner, P. (1984). *From Novice to Expert: Clinical Judgment-Making in Nursing.* Menlo Park, CA: Addison-Wesley.

Nurse Competency in the Operative and Invasive Procedure Setting

The *Dreyfus and Dreyfus Model of Skill Acquisition* demonstrates competency assessment tools need to be appropriate for the knowledge, cognitive skills, and psychomotor skill levels of the individual being assessed. Tools need to address minimum competency for the task and also include elements that evaluate staff members as they move along the competency continuum. As an example, *advanced beginner* to *expert* nurses might have in their job description the expectation of providing patient care as scrub and/or circulating nurses. In this case, a common element of practice such as *Perform Sponge, Sharp, and Instrument Counts* would be a focus for competency assessment. The *expert* nurse, however, may have an additional role expectation such as *Designs and Implements Continuing Nursing Education Programs,* which would be a focus of competency assessment for the expert nurse.

Within the operative and invasive procedure suite there are also overlapping functions that may be performed by staff with different levels of preparation based on education, certification, and licensure. As an example, both the registered nurse and the surgical technologist may transfer the patient, which presents a challenge in designing a competency tool that measures performance based on role function. Both the nurse and the surgical technologist need to demonstrate knowledge of the principles of transferring the patient as well as performing the psychomotor skills of implementing the transfer. Nurses would also need to demonstrate competency to identify the patient's risk for an adverse outcome related to the transfer episode and to demonstrate the ability to implement the nursing process related to this patient care event.

Designing the Tool

Competency Tools that Validate Expectations of Role Functions

Overall, a competency tool provides validation that a nurse or other healthcare worker is performing to minimum expectations for his/her designated role functions. Tool design is based on what needs to be assessed and who is going to do the assessment. Annual and peer evaluations, along with skills checklists are used to document nurse competency. One peer evaluation tool commonly used by managers is the 360-degree evaluation, which facilitates multiple perspectives contributing to one's competency. **Table 2.6** shows an example of a 360-degree feedback Survey. Clinical ladder programs, certificates, and professional education also promote professional development. As professionals, nurses have a moral mandate to demonstrate self-awareness of gaps in knowledge and then be proactive in pursuing lifelong learning opportunities and participating in the evaluation of competencies. Self-awareness and assessment of skills can be documented either via skills checklists or reflection forms. Many operative and invasive procedure suites use skills lists during orientation or at an annual evaluation. Reflective learning promotes learning from experience. Thinking about what worked well and what was problematic can enhance clinical decision-making during patient care as well as identify areas for additional knowledge that the nurse must obtain for competence. An example of a reflection form is provided in **Table 2.7**.

The portfolio is another means of validating competency, especially for nurses as they progress to the next level of the competency continuum. This tool is a "portable mechanism for evaluating competencies that may otherwise be difficult to assess, such as practice-based improvements, use of scientific evidence in practice, professional behavior and creative endeavors" (Byrne et al. 2007, pg 24–25). The portfolio can be a considered a scrapbook of professional accomplishments and may be kept in a paper or electronic format. As an example, the *Competency and Credentialing Institute* (CCI) recently initiated an evidence-based, peer-evaluated portfolio to assess the continued competency for perioperative nurses if they recertify or desire to reactivate their CNOR credential (CCI, 2008).

CCI
Competency and
Credentialing Institute

Tables 2.8 shows an example of a competency assessment tool for *Provide Instruments, Equipment, and Supplies.* This tool would be administered by the appropriate manager, educator, or peer. In this text, similar tools are listed for Chapters 5 through 18.

Competency Tools that Validate Performance of Critical Processes

Whereas competency validation previously discussed focused on evaluating the overall performance of the practitioner to determine if he or she is practicing

Table 2.6	**360-Degree Feedback Survey**

The purpose of this survey is to provide upward feedback from multiple sources. 360-degree feedback is a tool that can be used to provide feedback to managers from their superiors, peers, direct reports, and customers. Such feedback has been growing in popularity in a number of innovative and empowering organizations in recent years. Ultimately, improved managerial skills resulting from 360-degree feedback will further the goals of your organization.

As a part of this process, we would like you to fill out the attached survey that asks you to evaluate one of your peers in a number of areas. As a peer of this person, you have a unique perspective that could be very valuable as he/she tries to get a complete picture of how others evaluate his/her behavior. On the following pages you will find a series of statements relating to his/her behavior. For each statement, please provide a rating describing how often this person engages in each of the behaviors, or activities, listed. Use the nine-point scale shown to rate him or her. Indicate your answer by circling the number that describes how often he/she does the activity listed.

Note that the odd numbers (1, 3, 5, 7, and 9) have labels attached to them. These labels are just to give you some anchors or references when using the scale. You may use any number from 1 to 9 (including the even numbers) for your rating. The "not applicable" category should only be used if you do not think the behavior is applicable or you simply have not had an opportunity to observe it.

After you have responded to the statements, you may complete the two fill-in questions at the end of the form. When completing the fill-in section, please make specific, constructive comments about this employee's behavior that could be helpful to the person you are rating.

Be assured that your responses will remain anonymous. This survey must be completed and mailed by [date]. When mailing the survey, place it in an unmarked sealed envelop. Place this envelop in the addressed and stamped envelope provided. Thank you for your cooperation.

Please indicate how often this case manager engages in
each of the following activities or behaviors. This is a survey on: _____

(0) NA   (1) Never   (2)(3) Once in a While   (4)(5) Sometimes

(6)(7) Fairly Often   (8)(9) Always

PERSONAL EFFECTIVENESS

(0)(1)(2)(3)(4)(5)(6)(7)(8)(9)   Accepts feedback without becoming defensive (eg, making excuses, denial, getting angry).

(0)(1)(2)(3)(4)(5)(6)(7)(8)(9)   Makes tough decisions in a timely manner.

(0)(1)(2)(3)(4)(5)(6)(7)(8)(9)   Is available when needed.

(0)(1)(2)(3)(4)(5)(6)(7)(8)(9)   Provides valuable input into decisions.

INTERPERSONAL SKILLS

(0)(1)(2)(3)(4)(5)(6)(7)(8)(9)   Communicates information in a timely way.

(0)(1)(2)(3)(4)(5)(6)(7)(8)(9)   Keeps people informed about issues, changes, or problems that affect them.

(0)(1)(2)(3)(4)(5)(6)(7)(8)(9)   Is approachable.

(0)(1)(2)(3)(4)(5)(6)(7)(8)(9)   Makes it easy for people to tell him/her what they think.

INNOVATION, CHANGE AND RISK TAKING

⓪①②③④⑤⑥⑦⑧⑨   Creates an environment that supports change.

⓪①②③④⑤⑥⑦⑧⑨   Speaks positively about new initiatives.

⓪①②③④⑤⑥⑦⑧⑨   Helps others find new ways to get the job done.

CUSTOMER ORIENTATION

⓪①②③④⑤⑥⑦⑧⑨   Shows that internal and external customer satisfaction is a top priority.

⓪①②③④⑤⑥⑦⑧⑨   Treats all clients fairly, regardless of differences (eg, sex, ethnicity, beliefs, sexual orientation).

TEAMWORK

⓪①②③④⑤⑥⑦⑧⑨   Involves others in problem-solving and decision-making activities that have an impact on them.

⓪①②③④⑤⑥⑦⑧⑨   Promotes a spirit of of cooperation between members of the work group.

⓪①②③④⑤⑥⑦⑧⑨   Helps resolve conflicts when they occur in the work group.

⓪①②③④⑤⑥⑦⑧⑨   Works well with other supervisors and higher management.

LEADERSHIP

⓪①②③④⑤⑥⑦⑧⑨   Motivates and encourages others.

⓪①②③④⑤⑥⑦⑧⑨   Takes responsibility for the results of his/her actions.

⓪①②③④⑤⑥⑦⑧⑨   Displays a positive outlook and enthusiasm.

⓪①②③④⑤⑥⑦⑧⑨   Leads by positive example.

⓪①②③④⑤⑥⑦⑧⑨   Demonstrates behavior consistent with the organization's vision and values.

ADDITIONAL COMMENTS

In the spaces below you may make some additional comments to help the person you rated become a better leader. Any comments you write will be typed and given to this person along with all comments made by other peers rating the same person. Your name will NOT be attached to any of these comments. If you do wish to make comments, try to make them short and constructive so that this person will understand what you think his/her strengths are and in what areas he/she could improve.

A. List the three most effective strengths of the person you rated in this survey.

B. List the three areas in which the person you rated could use more development.

Table 2.7	**Reflection Form**

Reflection is the process of learning from experience. It allows you to use your experience to determine what you may do differently as a result of the learning. Reflection may raise new questions that will drive you to future learning. It aids in ongoing self-assessment and ensures that your ongoing learning is current and relevant to your practice.

This reflection form is designed to help you demonstrate how you incorporated these principles of reflection in the learning process. One completed reflection form must be included for each of the five (5) selected professional activities. Each reflection form must be accompanied by evidence supporting your role in the professional activity.

One form must be submitted for EACH activity. Make copies as needed or access the form electronically at www.cc-institute.org.

Professional Activity: _____

Date(s) of Activity: _____

Thoroughly describe the activity/project/event. What happened or occurred? Clearly describe your role.

What do you know now that you did not know before? (What have you learned? What do you do differently? Or how will you build on this experience?)

What are the implications for perioperative nursing practice?

Reprinted with permission. Competency & Credentialing Institute, Denver, CO.

competently at the expected level, tools that validate competency for performing critical processes focus on high-volume and high-risk processes; processes that if not done correctly, that is competently, may lead to an adverse patient outcome. As stated previously, this text uses the *System-in-Contingency Model* as a framework for competency assessment. Within the twelve patient care events are specific activities that are high-volume and high-risk, thus making them critical processes and the focus for evaluation. As an example, prepping the patient for an operative procedure is one of the activities of the patient care event *Establish and Maintain the Sterile Field*. Prepping the patient is a high-volume activity because it is a nearly universal occurrence for patients having an operative procedure. As for being a high-risk activity, if it is not done correctly, particularly for a patient diagnosed as high risk for wound infection, the patient could indeed experience a wound infection secondary to skin preparation. Additionally, if a flammable prepping solution is used, and preparation is not done according to the manufacture's Instructions for Use (IFU), the patient could be

IFU
Instructions for Use

Table 2.8	Competency Assessment: Provide Instruments, Equipment, and Supplies

Name_____   Title_____

Unit_____   Date of Validation_____

Type of Validation: ☐ Initial (by educator)   ☐ Annual (by peer)

Method of Evaluation: Observation

COMPETENCY STATEMENT: The nurse demonstrates competency to provide instruments, equipment, and supplies for an operative or invasive.

Score   **Performance Criteria**

① ② ③ ④ ⑤ **1.** Identifies the patient's risk for adverse outcomes related to the provision of instruments, equipment, and supplies.

① ② ③ ④ ⑤ **2.** Selects appropriate instrumentation, equipment, and supplies for an operative or invasive procedure.

① ② ③ ④ ⑤ **3.** Delivers instruments and supplies to the sterile field.

① ② ③ ④ ⑤ **4.** Arranges instruments and supplies on the back table and Mayo tray.

① ② ③ ④ ⑤ **5.** Passes instruments and supplies to the physician or assistant.

① ② ③ ④ ⑤ **6.** Prepares and passes sutures to the physician or assistant.

① ② ③ ④ ⑤ **7.** Prepares and applies patient warming systems.

① ② ③ ④ ⑤ **8.** Maintains safe transport environment through use of elevated bed rails, safety straps applied, additional devices secured (eg, oxygen tanks, IV poles, Foley catheter, chest tube).

① ② ③ ④ ⑤ **9.** Prepares air-powered instrumentation for use.

① ② ③ ④ ⑤ **10.** Implements electrosurgical safety precautions.

① ② ③ ④ ⑤ **11.** Applies dressings.

① ② ③ ④ ⑤ **12.** Prepares and operates endoscopic equipment.

Scoring   ① Did not demonstrate competency   ② Minimal competency   ③ Competency   ④ Exceptional competency   ⑤ Outstanding competency

Comments (mandatory for scores of 1, 2, 4, or 5)

_____   _____
Validator's Signature   Employee's Signature

_____   _____
Validator's Printed Name   Employee's Printed Name

the victim of a surgical fire. Clearly, those responsible for determining the elements of a competency assessment program would be prudent to target *prepping the patient* for evaluation. **Table 2.9** lists the patient care events of the operative and invasive procedure period and identifies potentially high-volume and/or high-risk activities that should be considered for targeted competency assessment.

Table 2.10 shows an example of a high-risk activity from the patient care event *Provide Instruments, Equipment, and Supplies.* Assuming that this example concerns a facility where infant and neonatal surgery is occasionally done, Performance Criteria 10, *Implement Electrosurgical Safety Precautions,* is selected as highrisk because of the infrequent use of return electrode contact quality monitoring (RECQM) infant and neonatal patient return electrodes. Manufacturer IFUs are very explicit about the application of RECQM infant and neonatal patient return electrodes, as well as generator power settings and activation times, indicating that the use of electro-surgery to achieve hemostasis is a potentially a high-risk activity. In this scenario it would be wise to have a focused competency evaluation concerning the patient return application, power settings, and activation times.

RECQM
Return Electrode
Contact Quality
Monitoring

Evidence-Based Practice as a Foundation for Nurse Competency

A current initiative in clinical practice and academic settings is evidence-based nursing practice. Simply, this means nurses make clinical decisions based on sound evidence for successful patient outcomes. Whether patient outcomes are defined as intact skin, successful wound healing, early ambulation, or adequate oral intake, the interventions done by the nurse should lead to positive patient outcomes. Nursing interventions can be guided by past experience, patient preference, and scholarly evidence resulting from clinical research.

Information Literacy

Information literacy is defined as the ability to access, evaluate and ethically use information. These three abilities should also be considered essential competencies for nurses practicing in the operative and invasive procedure setting.

Accessing Information

Computers have revolutionized accessing and communicating information. The historical act of physically going to a library, thumbing through a card catalog, and searching the Dewey decimal system for a specific book are long gone. With adequate computer and subscription databases and online journals, nurses can access journals and textbooks online. Specialty experts can be easily located on the Internet. Email and text messaging promotes prompt and ready communication with national and international experts. Websites are often used because they contain excellent resources for practicing nurses. **Table 2.11** lists organizations that can be used as resources for designing competency assessment tools and delineates some of the available resources.

Evaluating and Ethically Using Information

Many websites contain invaluable resources, yet the evaluation of information rests upon a nurse's discernment of knowledge claims (Hoss & Hanson, 2008).

Table 2.9	Examples of High-Risk Patient Care Activities of the Operative and Invasive Procedure Period	

Patient Care Event	High-Volume/High-Risk Activities
Prepare of the patient for the procedure	☐ Preparation of the cognitively impaired patient
Transfer the patient	☐ Patient and procedure site verification of cognitively impaired, sedated, or comatose patient ☐ Transfer of the bariatric patient ☐ Transfer of the patient in traction ☐ Transfer of the pediatric patient
Assist the anesthesia provider	☐ Awake induction ☐ Bariatric patient induction ☐ Trauma induction ☐ Use of uncuffed endotracheal tubes for airway procedures and procedures in the head and neck area
Position the patient	☐ Placing the elderly patient on a fracture table ☐ Placing the patient in the lateral decubitus position ☐ Placing the patient in the prone position ☐ Positioning the bariatric patient
Establish and maintain the sterile field	☐ Preparing the procedure site with alcohol-based prepping solution
Perform sponge, sharp, and instrument counts	☐ Open operative procedures
Provide instruments, equipment, and supplies for the procedure	☐ Applying the pneumatic tourniquet ☐ Applying warming devices ☐ Oral cavity electrosurgical safety precautions ☐ Pediatric electrosurgical safety precautions ☐ Suction coagulator safety precautions ☐ Use of ground referenced generators ☐ Use of isolated generators without return electrode contact quality monitoring
Administer drugs and solutions	☐ Identification of medications on sterile field
Physiologically monitor the patient	☐ Conscious sedation performed by registered nurse
Monitor and control the environment	☐ Evacuating endosurgical smoke ☐ Implementing fire safety precautions ☐ Flash sterilization ☐ Electrosurgery or laser use in oxygen enriched atmosphere
Handle cultures and specimens	☐ Procedures with multiple specimens
Facilitate care after the procedure	☐ Discharge instructions for cognitively impaired patients or family members

Table 2.10	COMPETENCY ASSESSMENT: Pediatric Electrosurgical Safety Precautions

Name_____ Title_____

Unit _____ Date of Validation_____

Type of Validation: ☐ Initial (by educator) ☐ Annual (by peer)

Method of Evaluation: Observation

COMPETENCY STATEMENT: The nurse demonstrates competency to implement pediatric electrosurgical safety precautions for an operative or invasive procedure.

Score | **Performance Criteria**

① ② ③ ④ ⑤ **1.** Describes the potential risk factors for adverse outcomes related to the application of electrosurgery.
Scar tissue, bony prominence and excessive hair at return electrode site; emaciation; use of a defective return electrode; impaired skin or tissue integrity or perfusion at site of return electrode; use of a ground-reference generator; use of an isolated generator without return electrode monitoring; use of inflammable agents to prepare the operative site.

① ② ③ ④ ⑤ **2.** Describes the ideal site for patient return electrode application.
Choose a well vascularized, convex area in close proximity to the surgical site; free of scar tissue, no bony prominences, and excessive adipose tissue; in an area where fluid will not pool.

① ② ③ ④ ⑤ **3.** Describes how to prepare the PRE site.
Clean and dry the application site as needed.

① ② ③ ④ ⑤ **4.** Describes how to check the return electrode expiration date and what to do it the PRE is expired.
Check the expiration date and discard the return electrode if expired.

① ② ③ ④ ⑤ **5.** Describes what to do after removing the liner from the PRE.
Lightly touch the surface of the return electrode to ensure the conductive adhesive is moist.

① ② ③ ④ ⑤ **6.** Describes when the return electrode would be used with or without the adhesive border around the exterior edge.
Would avoid using the adhesive border if the patient is impaired skin or has potential for an allergic reaction.

① ② ③ ④ ⑤ **7.** Describes what to do after applying the PRE.
Ensure the entire conductive surface of the return electrode is in contact with the patient. Apply finger pressure to massage the entire return-electrode surface (and adhesive border if used) to ensure secure contact with the patient's skin.

① ② ③ ④ ⑤ **8.** States the steps of connecting the PRE to the generator.
(1) Turn on the generator.
(2) Wait for the audible tone and the REM alarm indicator to display red and alarm to sound.
(3) Insert the return-electrode connector into the generator to correct the alarm condition.

① ② ③ ④ ⑤ **9.** Describes how to remove the PRE after the procedure.
Slowly remove the return electrode with one hand while supporting the skin with the other to avoid skin trauma.

① ② ③ ④ ⑤ **10.** States the outcome criteria for evaluating the PRE site following the procedure.
Redness indicating an allergic reaction to the patient return electrode conductive adhesive; evidence of postprocedure skin and tissue disruption/destruction at the patient return electrode site or at alternate pathway sites; and an ignition incident during the operative or invasive procedure.

Specific Considerations for the Infant Patient Return Electrode

① ② ③ ④ ⑤ **11.** States the weight parameters for using the infant PRE.
2.7 kg–13.6 kg (6 lbs–30 lbs)

① ② ③ ④ ⑤ **12.** Describes the preferred application site for infants.
The preferred sites are the back or torso.

① ② ③ ④ ⑤ **13.** States the parameters for power setting.
The power settings do not exceed 120 watts. Confirm proper electrosurgical generator settings with the surgeon prior to activation of the active electrode.

Specific Considerations for the Neonatal Patient Return Electrode

① ② ③ ④ ⑤ **14.** Specific Considerations for the Neonatal Patient Return Electrode.
States the weight parameters for using the neonatal PRE.
0.45 kg–2.72 kg (1 lb–6 lbs)

① ② ③ ④ ⑤ **15.** Describes the preferred application site for infants.
The preferred site is the back, inferior to the shoulder blades and superior to the sacrum.

① ② ③ ④ ⑤ **16.** States the parameters for generator selection.
Only use a generator that has been calibrated by biomedical engineer or technician and posted with the power settings as required by the manufacturer IFU.

① ② ③ ④ ⑤ **17.** States the parameters for power settings and application of current.
Not to exceed 300 milliamps nor be applied for longer than 30 seconds continually.

Scoring   ① Did not demonstrate competency   ② Minimal competency   ③ Competency
④ Exceptional competency   ⑤ Outstanding competency

Comments (mandatory for scores of 1, 2, 4, or 5)

_____   _____
Validator's Signature   Employee's Signature

_____   _____
Validator's Printed Name   Employee's Printed Name

Table 2.11	Resources for Design of Competency Assessment Tools for Registered Nurses Practicing in the Operative and Invasive Procedure Setting	
Organization	**Website**	**Resources**
American Academy of Ambulatory Care Nursing	www.aaacn.org	☐ Guide to Ambulatory Care Nursing Orientation and Competency Assessment
American College of Cardiovascular Nurses	www.accn.net	☐ ECG Competency Assessment Tool
American Radiological Nurses Association	www.arna.net	☐ Core Curriculum for Radiology Nursing
Association of periOperative Registered Nurses	www.aorn.org	☐ Perioperative Nursing Data Set (PNDA ☐ Competency Statements in Perioperative Nursing ☐ Outcome Standards for Perioperative Nursing
Competency and Credentialing Institute	www.cc-institute.org	COMPETENCY MODULES ☐ Age-Specific Care ☐ Aseptic Technique ☐ Care of the Bariatric Patient ☐ Cultural Competency ☐ Designing Competencies that Count ☐ Electrosurgery ☐ Moderate Sedation/Analgesia ☐ Patient Positioning ☐ Patient Safety
ECRI	www.ecri.org	PATIENT SAFETY, QUALITY, AND RISK MANAGEMENT DOCUMENTS ☐ Operating Room Risk Management System ☐ Bariatric Services: Safety, Quality, and Technology Guide ☐ Medication Safety Solutions
Society of Gastroenterology Nurses and Associates, Inc.	www.sgna.org	STANDARDS AND GUIDELINES ☐ Performance of Flexible Sigmoidoscopy by Registered Nurses for the Purpose of Colorectal Cancer Screening ☐ Guidelines for the Use of High Level Disinfectants and Sterilants for Reprocessing of Flexible Gastrointestinal Endoscopes ☐ Standards of Infection Control in Reprocessing of Flexible Gastrointestinal Endoscopes ☐ Guidelines for Preventing Allergic Reactions to Natural Rubber Latex in the Workplace ☐ Guidelines for Documentation in the Gastrointestinal Endoscopy Setting ☐ Standards of Clinical Nursing Practice and Role Delineation Statements

Nurses must be able to identify whether or not information is from a recognized authority. The suffix of a website provides preliminary information as to the reliability of the source. **Table 2.12** lists these website suffixes. **Table 2.13** lists questions that should be asked when authenticating information obtained from a website.

Table 2.12	Website Suffixes
.edu	Educational institution
.gov	Government website
.org	Nonprofit organization
.com	Commercial venture

Table 2.13	Questions to Ask When Authenticating Information from a Website
☐	What are the credentials and experience of the author?
☐	When was the site last updated?
☐	Are credible, known Internet links associated with the site?
☐	Who is advertising or sponsoring the website?
☐	Who profits?
☐	What types of science or scholarships support the website information?

MANUFACTURER INSTRUCTIONS FOR USE

The use of medical devices and patient care products, such as electrosurgery generators and alcohol-based prepping solutions, are the focus of some competency assessment tools that evaluate the performance of high-volume and or high-risk nursing care activities. For devices and products that could cause patient injury if not used correctly, the manufacturer Instructions for Use must be incorporated when designing competency assessment tools. These instructions can be found in user's guides and product inserts. Some manufacturers allow web access to this information. Additionally, some manufacturers provide documents that can be adapted as competency assessment tools.

CONCLUSION

Competency assessment is a means of validating the ability of nurses, surgical technologists, and others to safely perform nursing interventions and activities in the operative and invasive procedure suite. Assessment focuses on the individual's knowledge, cognitive, and psychomotor skills competency. For a detailed discussion concerning competency assessment refer the Competency and Credentialing Institute's Competency Module, *Designing Competencies that Count.*

REFERENCES

1. AHRQ (2007). Agency for Healthcare Research and Quality (AHRQ) FY08 Appropriations, http://www.aafp.org/online/en/home/policy/federal/background-on-federal-issues/ahrq.html. Accessed 6 June 2008.

2. AORN (2008). *Perioperative Standards and Recommended Practices.* Association of Operating Room Nurses. Denver.

3. AORN (2007). *Perioperative Nursing Data Set: The Perioperative Nursing Vocabulary.* Denver, CO: AORN.

4. Benner, P. (1984). *From Novice to Expert: Clinical Judgment-Making in Nursing.* Menlo Park, CA: Addison-Wesley.

5. Byrne, M., Delarose, T., King, C., Leske, J., Sapnas, K., & Schroeter, K. (2007). Continued Professional Competence and Portfolios. *Journal of Trauma Nursing* 14(1): 24–31.

6. Carpenito-Moyet, L. J. (2006). *Nursing Diagnosis: Application to clinical practice.* Philadelphia, PA: Lippincott, Williams & Wilkins.

7. Hoss, B. & Hanson, D. (2008). Evaluating the Evidence: Web Sites *AORN Journal* 28(1): 124–141.

8. King, C. (Ed). (2007, March). *Advanced Practice Nursing in Perioperative Nursing Clinics* Vol 2(1). WB Saunders.

9. NCLEX-RN The National Council Licensure Examination, http://www.a2zcolleges.com/exams/nclexrn.htm, Accessed 5 June 2008.

10. Sechrist, K., Valentine, W., & Berlin, L. (2006). Perceived Value of Certification among certified, noncertified and administrative perioperative nurses. *Journal of Professional Nursing,* 22(4): 242–247.

11. Vandewater, D. (2004). Best Practices in Competence Assessment of Health Professionals. College of Registered Nurses of Nova Scotia.

CHAPTER 3

Performance Improvement
In Operative and Invasive Procedure Suite

Wendy Zander

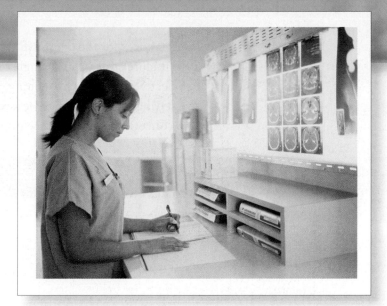

INTRODUCTION

The operative and invasive procedure area[1] must constantly change as technology improves or becomes obsolete, as employees come and go, as the departments are reorganized, and as healthcare consumers become more discerning. Change is fundamental to success. The performance improvement team is the change agent within the operative and invasive procedure area. Performance improvement begins as a study of a process or procedure, then moves on to the modification of the process in order to accomplish a more desirable result.

In any health care setting, departments must adapt to change while continuing an existing workload and providing an optimal level of care for patients. This is why it is critical to have a well-defined process in place to manage changes. Practices such as those contained in this chapter can provide guidance.

DEVELOPING A PERFORMANCE IMPROVEMENT PROGRAM

There are three ways to decide where to place your performance improvement efforts. They are best practices, occurrence trending, and clinical accidents. These strategies enable the performance improvement team to identify and address performance and process gaps in the delivery of patient care.

Best Practices

Best practices are those strategies and activities around patient care that have been proven through research and experience to be most effective in providing excellent results for patients. There are several organizations dedicated to providing information on evidence-based best practices. In this age of information and technology, learning the best practices for the operative and invasive procedure area are just a few keystrokes away. Before addressing a single organization, however, it is important to have some perspective of what is happening on a national or world-wide level in the perioperative setting. **Table 3.1** lists websites of organizations that provide valuable information concerning performance improvement.

Table 3.1	Websites with Performance Improvement Information	
Organization	**Website**	**Resources**
Association of periOperative Registered Nurses (AORN)	www.aorn.org	☐ Annual publication, Perioperative Standards and Recommended Practices ☐ Classic resource for perioperative practice ☐ Website has a large library, tool kits, research and articles with an easy-to-use search engine for key words
Institute for Healthcare Improvement	www.ihi.org	☐ Comprised of professionals who have an interest in improving healthcare ☐ Site is for all aspects of care ☐ A search for best practices related to the operative and invasive procedure area is required ☐ Links to other useful sites, a search engine for key words, improvement models and various tool kits
Quality Net	www.qualitynet.org	☐ Established by the Centers for Medicare and Medicaid Services (CMS) ☐ Provides news, resources and data reporting tools
US Department Health & Human Services	www.hospitalcompare.hhs.gov	☐ Site shows how area hospitals compare on compliance with various best practices ☐ Modern healthcare consumers are educated as to what hospitals should be doing for them ☐ Information is publicly reported and readily available
Joint Commission	www.jointcommission.org	☐ Accredits and certifies healthcare organizations in the United States ☐ Organization dedicated to health care quality ☐ Website provides standards and performance measures ☐ Site has valuable information about patient safety, including the national patient safety goals, sentinel event alerts, and more ☐ Comprehensive site with much to offer

Computer literacy and the ability to navigate the Internet are fundamental skills and necessary for those responsible for performance improvement activities in the operative and invasive procedure suite. The sites listed in **Table 3.1** are a small sample of the information available. There are many other sites and forums to gain insight and stay abreast of the current issues facing healthcare quality and best practices.

Occurrence Trending

Occurrence trending is another way of identifying potential performance and process gaps in the delivery of patient care. Staff-reported adverse events are categorized by type and then analyzed to determine which events are being reported most frequently. Occurrence trending is a good starting point, but do not use independently as it simply provides a means for gathering data to determine where processes commonly go amiss. For example, if a large number of occurrences identify incorrect operative counts as a potential problem, it might be tempting to note the same few people are involved in most of the reported occurrences; but it may be that the nurses in that area are simply more astute about filling out the occurrence reports than their counterparts in another area. Performance improvement initiatives should not focus on one person or a group of people using only reported occurrences.

Instead, when trending occurrences for incorrect surgical counts you might notice that most commonly it is a needle that is missing. Perhaps the process for keeping track of needles during the procedure deserves some attention.

When the response to occurrence reports is to focus on the people, the result is not better performance, but decreased reporting. Human error cannot be eliminated, and the removal or punishment of the individual does not change the environment that produced the error.

Occurrence reports are a valuable way to trend common causes in process errors. This knowledge of common causes is what will change the environment for better patient safety. As tempting as it may be to use reporting for punitive action against an individual, the result is skewed data from under-reporting and a loss of valuable information.

Clinical Accidents

Clinical accidents are events that result or might have resulted in harm to a patient (DHS, 2000). These events might be a patient fall, a patient return electrode site burn, a medication error or a wrong site surgery, to name a few.

Some clinical accidents are easy to distinguish as something preventable, like a retained sponge. Clearly that is something that should have been prevented. Other clinical accidents are more difficult to establish how the event could have been prevented. For example, if a patient had a reaction to a medication many factors might come in to play when trying to determine if the practitioners could have predicted the reaction.

There are three general categories that accidents can be considered: sentinel events, adverse events, and near misses (DHS, 2000). Sentinel events are accidents in which death or serious harm to a patient occurs (AORN, 2008). This type of event must be reported to Joint Commission through the hospital's risk manager. The performance improvement professional's responsibility is to get the hospital risk manager involved and assist with gathering information. Every sentinel event must have a case-by-case review and a root-cause analysis preformed (AORN, 2008).

Adverse events are accidents that result in harm of a less serious nature to a patient. A patient fall with a subsequent bruised knee is an example of such an event. Report these events to the hospital's risk manager, but not the Joint Commission. They should, however, be taken seriously because of the potential for litigation for the hospital. These types of events also provide an opportunity to examine how the patient safety system failed.

Near misses are incidents that had the potential to cause harm but did not, often because somebody intervened. For a performance improvement professional this is the most desirable of all clinical accidents. It is an opportunity to learn without harm actually coming to a patient. These are golden opportunities to prevent harm from ever taking place.

When an undesirable result occurs there is hardly ever one reason for it. Most accidents can be traced to the sequential failure of several safeguards. The Swiss cheese model (**Fig. 3.1**) of accidental causation has gained widespread acceptance and use in healthcare. Defenses or barriers against error are modeled as the slices of Swiss cheese. The holes in the slices are the weaknesses in each barrier. The system as a whole produces a failure when all of the holes in each of the slices line up allowing a hazard to pass through all of the layers of defense (Frosch, 2006).

For example, if two look-alike, sound-alike medications were not separated in the pharmacy, the first safety barrier has failed. If the pharmacist chooses the wrong medication, misreads it, and sends it on to the patient care area the second safety barrier has failed. If the nurse at the bedside misses the error the third barrier fails, and so forth. It is only when weaknesses in all of the safety barriers momentarily align that an accident occurs. The performance improvement team is tasked with eliminating as many weaknesses in those barriers as possible.

Human error is often cited as the leading cause of clinical accidents, but that is not a very useful answer in performance improvement. The most skilled, well-trained, and committed people sometimes make errors. Safeguards and processes in the workplace will influence how often errors occur and how severe the consequences

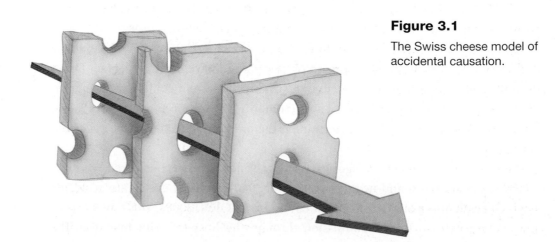

Figure 3.1

The Swiss cheese model of accidental causation.

are. This idea accepts that human error is inevitable and looks at the environment in which the errors occur to address the underlying problems.

Public reporting of these errors has greatly benefited healthcare quality. The weaknesses in barriers are not normally unique to the organization. If the error can occur in one institution it can occur in another. The Joint Commission is able to sound sentinel event alerts so that others can learn from the error without having to experience it in their own organization. This reporting also becomes the data from which the national patient safety goals are created and updated. Other organizations use publicly reported data to provide the best practices used throughout healthcare and in the operative and invasive procedure area.

WHERE TO BEGIN

There is no shortage of information when developing a performance improvement program. There are varied ways to approach performance improvement in the operative and invasive procedure setting. Knowing where to begin can be a challenge.

Use the organization's goals as the starting point. The organization's senior leadership and/or quality department should have stated annual goals to help direct the effort of the various hospital departments, including surgery. The performance improvement goals for the operative and invasive procedure area should support the goals of the organization.

If the organization has set a goal to improve patient satisfaction, the performance improvement team would also have a goal to improve patient satisfaction in operative and invasive procedure areas. The tool used by the organization to measure satisfaction should score different areas, and ambulatory surgery is often included.

The next step is to identify what patients scored as least satisfying and focus effort on those measures. Perhaps patients are most unhappy about wait times prior to their procedure. Maybe communication about delays was a problem. The goals for the operative and invasive procedure area would focus on these few things. The organization's goals will benefit from the effort. The goals are aligned.

Setting Goals

The best way to successfully accomplish something is to be clear about what result you want. The second habit of Steven Covey's *Seven Habits of Highly Effective People* (1989) is to "begin with the end in mind." The same can be said for a highly effective Performance Improvement program. The creation of a goal or an aim statement will provide structure to the change process. A stated goal is the "true north" as the improvement initiative unfolds. The more precisely the goal is stated, the more likely the initiative is to stay on course. For that reason the aim statement should meet the criteria for SMART goals (**Fig. 3.2**) (Nelson, Economy, & Blanchard, 2003).

Specific

Identify goals that are straightforward, focus effort, and clearly define what is to be accomplished. Make a goal specific, clear, and easy to understand. Instead of setting a goal to finish the day's caseload in a timelier manner, set a specific goal (eg, *As of*

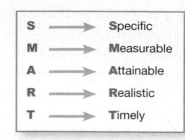

Figure 3.2

Smart Goals.

Adapted from Nelson, B., Economy, P., & Blanchard, K. (2003). *Managing for Dummies,* 2nd Ed. Wiley Publishing, Inc.

[identify the date], surgeons will make the incision for all first cases at the scheduled time 55 percent of the time).

The definitions included in the goal have to be specific too. To form this goal everyone involved must agree that the time on the surgical schedule is to be the incision time. Different practices may have far different definitions of what the scheduled time is. Having a specific definition may actually be half the battle. List the agreed upon definitions of the key components of the goal as part of the planning process.

Measurable

You can't manage what you don't measure is an old management adage that is just as accurate today. Create a way to measure success that can be answered with data. That means the change can be trended with numbers on a graph. If what you are measuring cannot be stated as a number then the goal is not measurable.

In the above example the first case of the day was to make incision by the scheduled time. How will this be measured? Look at the incision time and compare it to the time on the surgical schedule.

The measure is stated as a ratio or a percentage. The total number of first cases is the denominator and the number of times that incision is made by the scheduled time is the numerator. If there were sixty first cases in a given week and twenty-five of them made incision on time, it could be stated as shown in **Figure 3.3**.

Attainable

Identify attainable goals. If the goal is too far out of reach, it is hard to get a commitment from the staff and surgeons. Although the project may start with the best of intentions from all involved, if the people doing the work believe that it is too much for them the effort will not be as good.

Realistic

Realistic is not a synonym for easy; it just means that the goal is doable. The skills and resources needed to do the work have to be available. A realistic project may push the skills and knowledge of the people working on it but should not be impossible

Figure 3.3

Measurable Goal.

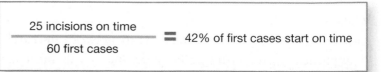

$$\frac{25 \text{ incisions on time}}{60 \text{ first cases}} = 42\% \text{ of first cases start on time}$$

for them. The idea is to set a goal that is possible to attain with some effort. Too difficult and the stage is set for failure, but too easy questions capability. Set the bar high enough for a satisfying achievement.

Timely

Without a time limit in the stated goal there is no urgency to start taking action. Putting an end point on the goal provides a clear target to work toward. Do not hesitate to make short commitments toward a larger target. Setting a very large goal for two years away can be overwhelming or too vague. Instead set smaller goals with short time tables.

The African proverb "*You can eat an elephant if you do it one bite at a time*" applies to performance improvement. Keep the long term goals in mind but set small attainable SMART goals that step the operative and invasive procedure area in the right direction.

MEASURING CHANGE

Measurement is fundamental to implementing change. What is going to be measured has all ready been defined within the well-written goal. Measurement will show movement toward desired change. Practitioners are usually most familiar with measurement for research. However, measurement for improvement looks much different.

The purpose of measuring for research is to discover new knowledge. The performance improvement team is measuring to bring that new knowledge into practice. The **Table 3.2** from the Institute for Health Care Improvement (2008) illustrates the differences well.

Effective Measures

The single most powerful measurement tool a team can use is to track a few key measures over time. Plotting measures on a graph to show how the change is progressing gives meaning to the project.

Provide all involved with a tangible record of how the initiative is progressing. This means posting or distributing a graph so all departments can follow trending and the progress being made with the initiative. This helps the project stay on track, reach the targeted date and provide the spirit of accomplishment that spurs on the continued effort that is needed to achieve goals.

Sampling is measuring a part of a large group. Sampling saves time and resources and gives a good representation of performance. For example, if you would like to know how compliant the operative and invasive procedure staff is with performing the pre-procedural time out, it would be labor intensive to monitor the beginning of every procedure. Instead, monitor the beginning of a few procedures to gather the data.

Sometimes it is possible to work data collection into the daily work routine. For such observational data collection as monitoring the time out, perhaps a staff

Table 3.2	Measurement for Research, Learning, and Process Improvement	
	Measurement for Research	**Measurement for Learning and Process Improvement**
Purpose	One large "blind" test	To bring new knowledge into daily practice
Tests	One large "blind" test	Many sequential, observable tests
Biases	Control for as many biases as possible	Stabilize the biases from test to test
Data	Gather as much data as possible, "just in case"	Gather "just enough" data to learn and complete another cycle
Duration	Can take long periods of time to obtain results	"Small tests of significant changes" accelerates the rate of improvement

IHI (2008). Institute for Healthcare Improvement. Retrieved January 11, 2008, from http://www.ihi.org/IHI/Topics/Improvement/ImprovementMethods/Measures.

member in orientation could be given a data collection tool with all of the components in the time out. This exercise has two benefits. The necessary data is collected and the orientee has the correct time out process reinforced. However, using staff engaged in patient care activities to collect data must be done sparingly and with the utmost consideration. In some instances, it can be beneficial but if overused can detract from patient care. That is never acceptable.

Collect *qualitative* data as well as *quantitative*. Qualitative data is valuable because it is often easier to access and is very informative. During performance improvement activities qualitative data is simply asking an opinion on how the change is working for an individual. The great thing about an interview approach to data collection is that in addition to a positive or negative response, information on how to improve the change process or make the desired result more feasible can be obtained. Listen carefully to the comments made by the ones working within the process that is changing and take action. Incorporate the staff's ideas into the change. They know how to make the project work for them. Not to capitalize on their insight is shortsighted. In addition, incorporating staff ideas into the change will give them ownership and increase the likelihood of success.

IMPROVEMENT METHODS

An improvement method is an approach to change that has been useful to others in developing changes that lead to improvement. The Associates in Process Improvement (2007) developed a model for improvement that has been successfully used in healthcare organizations around the world. The model is not meant to replace change models that the organization may all ready use but rather to accelerate the improvement process.

The first part of the model is to answer three questions about the improvement project.

1. What are we trying to accomplish?
2. How will we know that a change is an improvement?
3. What changes can we make that will lead to improvement?

The answer to the first question is the SMART goal. When using this model the goal is called an *Aim Statement*. This statement provides clear and precise direction.

Secondly, the performance improvement team uses quantitative data to trend the change as it moves toward the stated goal. This data tells if improvement is being made. Before any changes occur determine a baseline for the data. The baseline is important information to help create a goal that it is attainable and realistic.

Lastly, not all changes result in improvement or statistical movement toward the goal. To know what changes will produce the desired result best comes from the people working in the process that is to change. This is where the qualitative data is so important. It's not just important to "work hard" and "work smart," but also to work smart on the right things.

The right things come easily when the right people are part of the performance improvement team. Large projects require varied expertise. Depending on the project, the team may be made up of a different combination of people. Select team members who are familiar with all the different parts of the process, such as managers, administrators, physicians, pharmacists, and front-line workers. Always include someone who knows the hospital system, someone who has the technical experience in the process, and someone who is a day-to-day leader in the area to change, such as the manager or assistant nurse manager (IHI, 2008).

For smaller projects the expertise is still important so the performance improvement professional will rely heavily on interviewing and collection of qualitative data when a team is not possible.

TESTING CHANGE

The team is formed, the goal is written, how to measure change has been established and there is a baseline. The team has even decided what change may produce the desired result. Now what?

The next step is to test the change. The *Plan-Do-Study-Act* (PDSA) cycle (**Fig. 3.4**) is used to test change in the work setting (Deming, 2000). This test of change is what determines if the change is actually an improvement.

PDSA
Plan-Do-Study-Act

First the team plans the test or observation and then tries out the idea on a very small scale. The team then studies the results and refines the change based on what they learn. The PDSA cycle is a scientific method for learning. One cycle leads directly into the start of the next (IHI, 2008).

An Example

Imagine the following project goal "Patients who are on Beta Blockers at home will receive their medication the morning of surgery 95 percent of the time within six months."

Figure 3.4
PDSA Cycle.

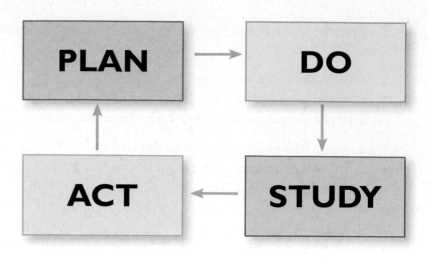

Deming, W. (2000). *The New Economics for Industry, Government, Education* (2nd Ed.). Cambridge, Massachusetts, MIT Press.

SCIP
Surgical Care
Improvement Project

This goal is a smaller part of a larger surgical services goal to decrease adverse cardiac events during surgery. The team decided on this because it is aligned with the organization's goal of a mortality rate reduction. This goal also was chosen because it is part of a care bundle recommended by a national quality initiative called the *Surgical Care Improvement Project* (SCIP). Continuation of a patient's beta blocker throughout the surgical experience is a best practice.

The team will know the change is an improvement if those patients taking beta blockers at home receive their medication the day of surgery. To measure the change the denominator is the number of patients who take beta blockers at home and the numerator is the number that received the medication the day of surgery. Currently the baseline data shows that 60 percent of the outpatients who take beta blockers at home are getting their medication the day of surgery.

Plan

The first step in the PDSA cycle challenges the performance improvement team to plan how they will present their idea for change into the work setting and how the data will be collected.

The team members have an idea that patients waiting for surgery in the preoperative area will identify themselves to the nurse if there is a sign listing the beta blockers along with a request that the patient let the nurse know if they are taking one of these medications. The change that will result in improvement, then, is to hang such signs in conspicuous places within the preoperative area such as patient cubicles or rooms.

The nurse caring for the patients in that cubicle or room will place a patient sticker on a sheet of paper for all patients who are processed through that cubicle or room during one day. Those patient's charts will be reviewed postoperatively to identify which patients were taking beta blockers at home. The number of all patients taking beta blockers that day is the denominator. The patients from that group who successfully identify themselves to the nurse will be the numerator.

Do

The second step in the PDSA cycle is the implementation of the plan. The sign is hung and the data collected for the patients that are processed through the one preoperative room for one day. The test of change is small. The nurse in the test room did nothing different than she normally would except she put the patient sticker on the collection tool for review by the performance improvement team. Five patients are processed through the test room with the beta blocker sign.

Study

The third step in the PDSA cycle is the time the team reviews results of the test. In our example the team reviewed the patient charts from the test room and found that only one of the five patients took beta blocker at home. However, this patient did not receive her beta blocker the day of surgery and did not identify herself to the nurse in response to the sign in the room. The team looked further to identify why the patient failed to notify the nurse. It turns out that the patient was there for cataract surgery and was unable to read a sign.

The team also spoke to the nurse in the room to gather qualitative data. The preoperative nurse liked the sign with the list of beta blockers on it. She said there were so many new medications out there that she had a hard time keeping up with them. She asked if the list of beta blockers could be hung at her workstation, too, so that when she reviewed the chart before speaking with the patient it would be easy for her to identify patients on beta blockers. She would then make sure the patient had taken it that morning. If they had not, she would get it for them.

Act

The fourth and final step in the PDSA cycle is the time for the team to refine the change based on what they have learned from the test. Even though the idea that the team originally had of hanging the beta blocker sign on the wall in the preoperative room did not work, they still learned much from the test. The preoperative nurse had good insight on how to modify the change. The team immediately began to plan the next test and the cycle started again with the sign moved to the workstation outside of the test room.

The PDSA cycles test a change quickly on a small scale to see how it works. The team refines the change as necessary before implementing it on a larger scale.

Spreading Change

Once the test of change has been refined and is successful it is time to spread the change from the pilot unit or population. The successful process is replicated on a broader scope.

In the example, there were several more cycles to refine the change. Eventually, the list of beta blockers were at the workstation outside of the test room and a reminder about the beta blocker was on the preoperative check sheet. A beta blocker reminder also went on the hand-off communication tool used between the preoperative and circulating nurses. Lastly, the workstations where nurses placed pre-admission phone calls to patients also had a list of beta blockers hung near each computer. When the nurse gathered information on the patient's home medications and the patient reported one of the beta blockers on the list the pre-admission nurse would ask the patient specifically to take that medication the day of surgery.

After the change process was refined the changes were spread to all of the preoperative area. The goal was that 95 percent of all patients who took beta blockers at home would receive beta blockers the day of surgery. The goal was surpassed within three months and has remained consistently above 95 percent since the implementation. Because receiving beta blockers is part of a national initiative the hospital's compliance is reported to CMS monthly.

As long as the compliance rate stays above 95 percent no further action will be taken. If the compliance rate falls below the 95 percent threshold, the performance improvement team will once again set a SMART goal, decide what type of change might bring about improvement and begin a new PDSA cycle.

CONCLUSION

Performance improvement in the operative and invasive procedure area is fluid and dynamic. It is a continuous process of assessment, planning, implementation, and evaluation. The performance improvement professional must stay abreast of what is happening in the perioperative profession and their own organization. Align operative and invasive procedure suite performance improvement goals with profession and the organizational goals.

Care in the operative and invasive procedure setting is in need of improvement. There are gaps between knowledge and practice. A performance improvement program in the operative and invasive procedure area attempts to narrow that gap; to bring the highest evidence-based care to patients, to reduce the waste of time and resources, and to help caregivers provide the excellent care they want for their patients.

The ability to change is essential for any operative and invasive procedure area that wants to improve. While all changes do not lead to improvement, all improvement requires change (IHI, 2008).

ENDNOTE

1. The term *operative and invasive procedure area* includes the perioperative, gastrointestinal laboratory, cardiac catheterization laboratory, and interventional radiology patient care areas.

REFERENCES

1. AORN (2008). *Perioperative Standards and Recommended Practices.* Association of Operating Room Nurses. Denver.

2. API (2007). Associates in Process Improvement. Retrieved February 12, 2008 from http://www.apiweb.org/API_home_page.htm.

3. Covey, S. (1989). *The Seven Habits of Highly Effective People.* Free Press.

4. Deming, W. (2000). *The New Economics for Industry, Government, Education* (2nd Ed.). Cambridge, Massachusetts: MIT Press.

5. DHS (2000). Improving Patient Safety in Victorian Hospitals, Department of Human Services, Victoria.

6. Frosch, R. (2006). "Notes toward a theory of the management of vulnerability", in Auerswald, P., Branscomb, L., La Porte, T., & Michel-Kerjan, E.: *Seeds of Disaster, Roots of Response: How Private Action Can Reduce Public Vulnerability.* Cambridge University Press.

7. IHI (2008). Institute for Healthcare Improvement. Retrieved January 11, 2008 from http://www.ihi.org/IHI/Topics/Improvement/ImprovementMethods/Measures/.

8. Nelson, B., Economy, P., & Blanchard, K. (2003). *Managing for Dummies,* 2nd Ed. Wiley Publishing, Inc.

CHAPTER 4

Legal, Regulatory, and Ethical Considerations

Ellen Murphy

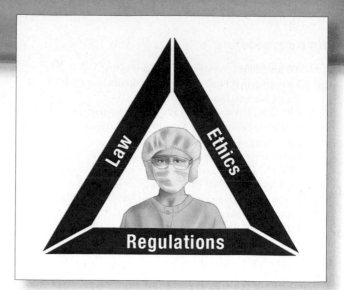

INTRODUCTION

Nurses providing care in the operative and invasive procedure setting[1] have long recognized the importance of the environment of care to the quality of the care the nurse delivers. The legal and ethical context of care is a part of the social environment within which care delivery occurs. While nurses cannot directly manage these systems in the same way they can manage other important elements in the environment of care (see Chapter 14), it is no less important that the nurse be cognizant of and incorporate these elements into care delivery in operative and invasive procedure settings.

The evolution of healthcare as a business, combined with the intimately personal type of service it is, has resulted in a near microcosm of American capitalist society at large—and operative and invasive care services, in turn, are a microcosm of the healthcare system. Almost every segment of the legal system has some application/relevance for the delivery and administration of these services. Ethics is also a part of the same society and ethical systems, too, interact and overlap with both the legal and healthcare systems.

Nurses and healthcare are part of this same society. In this representative democracy they have the power and, some would argue, the ethical duty, to influence laws and regulations to best benefit the provision of quality care to patients.

This chapter begins with a basic review of the American legal system structure, proceeds with application and examples of each structure to operative and invasive procedure services, and concludes with a review of ethical principles related to healthcare and how they are or are not reflected in the legal developments related to operative and

Chapter Contents

invasive procedure healthcare. It is intended as a survey chapter to alert the reader to many of the legal, regulatory, and ethical issues that influence perioperative practice and to provide web-based resources for detailed up-to-date information. No attempt is made or claimed to treat any one issue comprehensively because doing so would take volumes and outdate quickly.

Nurses should not expect themselves to be experts on every facet of the legal, regulatory, and ethical systems that influence their care. These areas are so many and so complex that most facilities designate compliance officers who keep current on legal and regulatory changes as part of their professional responsibilities. Most facilities also have access to ethics committees to review, discuss, and advise. Ethics committees, compliance officers, and risk managers can serve as the primary onsite resources for perioperative nurses needing more immediate and detailed information about how law and ethics frame the analysis of their specific situations.

THE AMERICAN LEGAL SYSTEM STRUCTURE
Sources of Law

The United States legal system is built around a tripartite form of government as set forth in the federal Constitution. The Constitution provides for three branches of government: the executive, legislative, and the judiciary. The Constitution also provides that individual states have the right to adopt their own constitutions within the limits of the federal constitutions. The states also have executive, legislative, and judicial branches although the states differ in how these are constituted and named. So, too, do cities, counties, and other local municipalities have some system of executive, legislative, and judicial branches within the confines of state laws.

The executive branches are headed by the president of the country and the governors of respective states and govern via executive actions and orders allowed by the respective constitutions. Fewer executive orders directly affect perioperative services as compared to the outcomes of the other branches, but some do, such as the mobilization of the armed forces or disaster declarations. The executive branches also appoint the directors and other top leaders or members of the administrative agencies that then provides indirect executive effects on healthcare.

The legislative branches (US Congress or state legislatures) govern through the passage of statutes. Statutes are written laws whose language is agreed upon by elected members of the Congress/legislature and signed by the executive or, if vetoed by the executive, overridden by the Congress or legislature. Because the federal Constitution leaves matters related to the public's health and safety to the states, more state statutes directly apply to operative and invasive procedure services than federal statutes. State statutes applying to healthcare are many and varied, most notably the Nurse Practice Act and its definition of what constitutes nursing practice in that state. However, many federal statutes do reach perioperative services through the administrative agencies they create (eg, Food and Drug Administration [FDA], Occupational Safety and Health Administration [OSHA]) and via the fact that the federal government pays for healthcare via Medicare and Medicaid, and thus can regulate the services it pays for.

The judicial branch adjudicates disputes between the other branches of government, between states, between individuals and the government, and between individuals pursuant to rules created by the government. The result of a compilation of judicial decisions are called constitutional law if it involves interpretation of the constitution, or more usually, common law or case law, when it refers to non-constitutional issues. The laws of negligence and malpractice are the most familiar examples of common law applicable to operative and invasive procedure services.

A hybrid of these branches has developed and is called administrative or regulatory law. Administrative or regulatory laws are promulgated by administrative agencies that are typically created by a statute from the legislature but led by appointees from the executive. These laws are subject to judicial review—but only to the extent that the regulation is reasonable related to the enabling legislation.

Increasingly, heretofore private, totally non-governmental organizations and coalitions have been integrated into the legal structure of the country, particularly through interface with administrative/regulatory law. The Joint Commission began as a voluntary organization for the accreditation of hospitals. Later the federal statutes that enacted the Medicare and Medicaid programs in 1965 extended what it called "deemed status" to the (then) JCAH (Joint Commission on Accreditation of Hospitals), which recognized Joint Commission accreditation as qualifying a hospital to receive federal payment. Even without formal "deemed status" recognition, private associations' and coalitions' recommendations for practice can and are used as evidence of the legal standard of care in common law negligence and malpractice cases. Thus, the Institute of Medicine (IOM), the Association of periOperative Registered Nurses (AORN's) recommended practices, the Surgical Care Improvement Project (SCIP) and the Joint Commission's National Safety Goals, among other like initiatives, are directly or indirectly being incorporated into legal expectations or regulations.

JCAH
Joint Commission on Accreditation of Hospitals

IOM
Institute of Medicine

AORN
Association of periOperative Registered Nurses

SCIP
Surgical Care Improvement Project

Categories of Law and Procedure

Law can be further categorized into the civil and criminal law, each of which has a different process of enforcement. The criminal law allows the government to apprehend, deter, punish, and rehabilitate individuals who commit acts that have been defined by state of federal statutes as crimes. Civil law involves disputes between individual parties and includes tort law, contract law, antitrust law, employment law, labor law—all of which have relevance to healthcare. Administrative law is sometimes also viewed as a separate category of law not only because of its hybrid origins but also because of its enforcement procedures that differ from the usual civil or criminal procedures.

The remainder of the legal section of this chapter is organized by these three categories of law: criminal, civil, and administrative.

CRIMINAL LAW

Governments or 'the state' can sue individuals for prohibited conduct under the criminal law. Crimes must be defined in statute, and traditionally required the element of intent and thus the perpetrator deserves punishment. Typically, actions such as murder and theft first come to mind as crimes. Statutes also recognize so called "white collar" crimes such as embezzlement and fraud. Criminal laws have also evolved to imply intent when behavior is so reckless that a crime could have been anticipated. Thus, driving while intoxicated can be a crime as is negligent manslaughter even though the perpetrator did not intend the deaths. Until about 10 years ago, criminal law's relevance to operative and invasive procedure services was limited to preservation of evidence and ensuring the chain of custody. More recently, a few state prosecutors have used the implied consent feature of the criminal law when a medical error caused severe injury or death resulted even though the professional did not intend to cause harm.

The Nurse as a Criminal Defendant

Until the late 1990s, nurses did not need to concern themselves with the criminal law except as an evidence collector and sometimes as a witness in the criminal trial of another (eg, forensic nursing). However, in 1998 three Colorado nurses were criminally charged in the death of a patient for infusing potassium chloride (KCL) instead of Lasix (furosemide; Smetzer, 1998). One of the three pled to a lesser charge and the two who went to trial were acquitted but the door was opened to the possibility of criminal charges for otherwise unintended medical error. In 2006, a Wisconsin labor and delivery nurse inadvertently hung buvipucaine instead of penicillin and hence administered the buvipucaine intravenously. This patient also died and the nurse was charged with a class H felony (*State* v *J.T, Criminal Complaint, Dane County* Circuit Ct No 2006CF2512, November 2, 2006; Denholm, 2007).

In 2007, 10 New York nurses were also criminally charged, this time not for a medication error, but for quitting their jobs in the same facility and thus "abandoning" their patients content (USA Today, 2008). Many scholars and groups have pointed out that criminalization of medical error is dangerous to the long-term public interest and it will interfere with the kinds of disclosure needed to promote patient safety and just culture initiatives (Just Culture, 2007). The AORN has adopted a position statement against attempts to criminalize nurses' actions not intended to cause harm for this same reason. Criminal prosecutions are not a sweeping trend, but as these examples indicate, are indeed possibilities. As these crimes are usually a matter of state law, the respective State Nurses' Association is the best resource for the nurse on issues related to criminalization or the need for a defense attorney.

Forensics in Nursing

The more common way nurses interact with the criminal law is their role in collection and preservation of evidence. Both victims and perpetrators of violent crime frequently become operative patients, sometimes without a stop in the emergency room where evidence is more usually collected, preserved, and cataloged. Evidence is crucial in a criminal case and operating rooms should have clear policies and procedures to guide nurses in evidence collection, preserving the chain of custody, and documenting descriptions of wounds. Trauma I facilities may have nurses who specialize in forensic evidence collection and preservation (eg, Sexual Assault Nurse Examiners) who can and should be used as resources. However, many facilities do not, and clear written procedures must be available. Websites such as www.iafn.org/ are also available.

Some parts of "routine" operative and invasive procedure nursing care (eg, clothing removal, specimen processing, and immediate pre and intraoperative documentation) will be done differently if the patient is a victim and/or a suspected perpetrator of a crime. For example, clothing must be removed very quickly but also very carefully to preserve any evidence such as hair fibers, blood, or chemicals that might be on the clothes. If clothes must be cut, care must be taken to avoid cutting through tears or holes in the fabric.

Each piece of clothing, including shoes, should be placed in separate paper (not plastic) bags and labeled with the item and the patient identified. These do not travel with the patient to the next care area. Rather, the chain of custody must be preserved. The chain of custody is a process to ensure that all evidence is what it is purported to be and has not been tampered with. Thus, until the evidence is turned over to the criminal investigation it must be documented, packed, preserved, and protected from any unidentified or unauthorized access. Should the patient die in the OR, similar care must be taken to preserve evidence. The body should not be cleaned in any way and all tubes, catheters, etc. should remain in the body, as they existed at time of death. Hands and feet may need to be encased in paper bags if not already done, before transport to the morgue.

These specifics are only a few examples of how usual practice is modified if criminal evidence is being collected and preserved. Again, every facility with emergency services should have a procedure reflecting the laws in that state and county regarding evidence collection and preservation.

CIVIL LAW

Civil law provides mechanisms to solve disputes between private parties. It includes contract, employment, and antitrust, but it is tort law that is most applicable to operative and invasive procedure practice.

Tort Law

Tort law deals with injury to persons (eg, battery, malpractice) or property (eg, trespass, automobile crash with property damage). Tort law includes both intentional (battery, trespass) and non-intentional acts (negligence and malpractice). The purpose of tort law is to compensate one party (the injured plaintiff) for injuries to persons or property caused by the unreasonable or imprudent actions of another (the defendant).

The section of tort law that first comes to mind to most nurses is negligence and malpractice[2], both unintentional torts under tort law. The legal duty of every nurse is 'simply' to do what a reasonable and prudent nurse of similar education and experience would have done under similar circumstances so as not to cause injury to a patient.

In order for patients to sue successfully for negligence or malpractice they must be able to produce evidence that proves:

1. What a reasonable and prudent nurse would have done;
2. That defendant failed to do what a reasonable and prudent nurse would do;
3. The failure of the nurse to act in a reasonable and prudent manner caused injury, usually a physical injury.

Nurse defendants cannot be found liable with the patient plaintiff proving all four elements. Conversely, nurses can use these same elements to analyze and prevent liability exposure.

Retrospective Analysis

If a situation arises that causes concern about possible liability for negligence or malpractice, nurses can analyze the likelihood of liability by asking:

1. Is there an injury? If yes,
2. Did the nurse's actions cause (or fail to prevent) the injury?
3. If yes, what did the nurse do or not do?
4. Were the nurse's actions consistent with what a reasonable and prudent nurse would have done as could be established by evidence (eg, expert witness, testimony, professional standards, statutory and regulatory requirements, current professional literature, and evidence-based practice)?

Typical suits against nurses practicing in the operative and invasive procedure setting involve retained foreign bodies, medication errors or the improper use of equipment with a typical result such as burns or pressure injuries (positioning aides and tourniquet).

Some suits for nurses' negligence are relatively straightforward; for example, the retained sponge case. It is easy to prove that a reasonable and prudent nurse counts sponges accurately and that failure to do so caused a retained sponge that in turn causes infection and a need for re-operation (injuries). Rarely are these cases litigated since liability is obvious. When they are litigated, the questions tend to center on whether the surgeon was reasonable and prudent in relying on the nurses' count or the amount demanded by the plaintiff is not reasonable for the injury incurred.

Other cases are less obvious, such as a positioning injury. If an injury results despite proper positioning and padding, it is difficult to demonstrate causation since length of procedure and/or patients pre-existing perfusion and tissue status may have caused the injury, not the actions of the nurse. Alternatively, it may not be clear whether the surgeon, anesthesia provider, or nurse had primary control over positioning. It is very hard, if not impossible, for the plaintiff to prevail in these cases if the nurse did what a reasonable and prudent nurse would have done because the plaintiff could not prove the nurse's failure to do so was the cause of the injury. As a practical matter, most injuries never become a court case, either because the patient chooses not to sue, because the facility chooses to settle the case, or because state laws requiring negotiation or affidavits preclude the patient from filing the case.

Prospective Analysis

Since the plaintiff (injured patient) must prove all four elements to sue successfully, these elements also present the nurse with preventive strategies. An injury is required for a patient to become a plaintiff, so the nurse's focus on patient safety and injury prevention also serves as a protection against negligence suits. Since the injury must be caused by the nurse's failure to do what a reasonable and prudent nurse would do, the nurse's compliance with regulatory and professional standards and recommended practices and evidence-based literature will make it unlikely the plaintiff (injured patient) can prove the nurse failed to do so. Moreover, of course, incorporating these standards into practice would have prevented injury in the first place. In short, the nurse's best protection against malpractice liability is the provision of safe nursing care that meets professional nursing standards.

Informed Consent

Informed consent emerged as a matter of state common law and, sometimes, state statutory law. Its underlying rationale is that adult competent patients have a right to self-determination. This principle was enunciated in 1914 in a case requiring the patient's consent to surgery and liability for battery (unconsented to touching) for failure to do so (*Schloendorff* v. *Society of N.Y. Hospital, 105 N.E. 92,* N.Y. 1914). After mid-century, a plethora of negligence cases emerged further requiring not only the patient's consent but also that the consent is informed.

A 1972 case, *Cobbs* v. *Grant* 104 Cal.Rptr. 505 (Cal. 1972), described the court's reasons for requiring an affirmative duty of the person performing the procedure to discuss and inform the patient of the risks, benefits, and alternatives. This court recognized that "except in rare cases, the knowledge of the patient and the physician are not in parity—the patient, being unlearned in the medical sciences, has an abject dependence upon and trust in his physician for the information upon which he relies in the decisional process" (Id. At 513). Thus, this California court imposed a requirement that not only must the patient consent before an operation but also the consent must be an informed one.

Cobbs began the sequence of cases shifting consent requirements from a case in the law of battery to informed consent cases in negligence law. Cases have differed on what and how much information a patient must receive (eg, what a reasonable patient would need [objective] what *this patient would need* [subjective], or what a reasonable surgeon would provide). Generally, case law is consistent that patients need to know: 1) risks, 2) benefits, and 3) alternatives to the proposed procedure.

It is also well established that the legal obligation to provide the information and obtain the consent lies with the person performing the procedure: namely, the surgeon, in the case of operative and invasive procedures. Since 1967, in a series of cases that began with *Fiorentino* v. *Wenger* 227 N.E.2d 296 (N.Y. 1967), courts have consistently refused to extend this physician obligation to nurses or facilities. Nurses, as well as facilities that allow operative and invasive procedures to be performed on their premises, however, may have a legal obligation to ensure that the patient's informed consent has been obtained (in contrast to obtaining the patient's consent).

Nurses can fulfill their legal obligation related to consent before the procedure by simply asking the patient whether he or she has had an opportunity to discuss the procedure with the physician and whether the patient has any questions or needs any further information before the procedure. If the patient has not discussed the procedure, the physician must be notified. If the patient has further questions, the nurse should inquire as to their nature. If the requested information relates to the medical nature of the procedure, such as its risks, benefits, and alternatives, those questions, too, should be referred to the physician. Nurses should use their judgment as to whether the needed information is something within the patient's knowledge base, so that the nurse is providing clarification or is actually providing new medical information. Different facilities have different methods of documenting the patient's consent. If the indicated method is to have the patient sign a consent form in the absence of the physician, the nurse can witness the signing of that form and attest to the fact that the patient said that he or she had discussed the procedure with the physician and had consented. The nurse is not legally obligated to probe the depth of the patient's understanding. Some facilities require that physicians themselves procure the patient's signature on the consent form.

CMS
Centers for Medicare and Medicaid Services

Some states have attempted statutory or regulatory clarification of the informed consent process. Most recently, informed consent has become a focus of the Centers for Medicare and Medicaid Services (CMS) survey processes with the result of having more prescriptive guidance on the informed consent process than had previously been the case (CMS, 2007a).

STATUTES AND REGULATIONS

As noted above, the United States Constitution provides that matters related to public health, and safety, are properly within the jurisdictions of the individual states. Different states have passed different state statutes and subsequent regulations relating to operative and invasive procedure nursing (eg, access to and confidentiality of medical records, informed consent, abuse and neglect, labor and employment laws). States may not have statutes on the same topic and the statutes and regulations they do have on the same topic (eg, regulation of nursing practice) will all differ, at least slightly. The statute that exists in all states most relevant to nursing is that regulating the practice of nursing.

The Nurse Practice Acts

Although called by different titles and situated in different parts of the state government structure, all states have a statute known in the nursing community as the Nurse Practice Act (NPA). Each state's NPA broadly defines the practice of nursing, establishes a regulatory agency usually called the state Board of Nursing and empowers it to regulate the practice of nursing in that state. The Board of Nursing then uses its rule-making authority to further define the scope of practice and standards of practice for nurses practicing in that state. For example, it would be a rare event for a state to include Registered Nurse First Assistant functions or conscious sedation administration or other questions of evolving practice in the Nurse Practice Act. The Board of Nursing would address these more specific issues within its rulings or regulations. Nurses must know both the NPA and the State board's rules and regulations that apply in the state where they practice. The National Council of State Boards of

NPA
Nurse Practice Act

Table 4.1	States That Subscribe to the Interstate Nursing Licensure Compact	
A mutual recognition model of nurse licensure allows a nurse to have one license (in his or her state of residency) and to practice in other states (both physical and electronic), subject to each state's practice law and regulation. Under mutual recognition, a nurse may practice across state lines unless otherwise restricted.		
Arizona	Maryland	South Carolina
Arkansas	Mississippi	South Dakota
Colorado	Nebraska	Tennessee
Delaware	New Hampshire	Texas
Idaho	New Mexico	Utah
Iowa	North Carolina	Virginia
Kentucky	North Dakota	Wisconsin
Maine		

Nursing's website can direct the reader to the website for individual states. (www.ncsbn.org).

Even states that subscribe to the interstate Nursing Licensure Compact will require that the nurse practice according to the laws of the state where the practice occurs, even if the nurse is licensed in another state participating in the compact (see **Table 4.1**).

The remainder of this chapter will deal with only federal statutes, agencies, and regulations. However, for every federal agency relating to healthcare, there is usually a corollary state agency that further applies to operative and invasive procedure practice in that state.

WHY REGULATE HEALTHCARE?

The 1970s has been described as the decade of regulation within the healthcare industry regulatory agencies, as well as regulations, proliferated. In recent years, regulation has increased even more because of concerns regarding the escalating costs of healthcare delivery, growing numbers of uninsured without access, and increased concerns about the safety of the healthcare delivered.

By the end of the 1980s, the United States spent in excess of $0.5 trillion on healthcare. By 2006, total health expenditures reached $2.1 trillion, which translated to $7,026 per person or 16 percent of the nation's Gross Domestic Product (GDP) (CMS 2006b).

Despite the large and ever-increasing healthcare expense, the number of people who are without health insurance continues to rise. The Census Bureau's data on the number of Americans without health insurance found: in 2006, the number of uninsured rose to 47 million, from 44.8 million in 2005.

GDP
Gross Domestic Product

There has been a constant tension, sometimes based on political philosophies, between the roles of the free market versus the need for further regulation in healthcare. While government and private sector interests may be willing to control a portion of their share of the healthcare market, neither sector is interested in paying the bill for the entire healthcare system. Yet without some sort of universal coverage, each will be constantly called upon to make up for the deficits of the other. As an evolving result, our present healthcare and financing systems are not systems at all but a combination of several methods of delivery and funding inclusive self, private insurance, federal and state payment, managed and capitated delivery.

KEY FEDERAL STATUTES

Health Insurance Portability and Accountability Act (HIPPA)

Congress enacted HIPAA in 1996 to address several concerns. It included protections of health insurance coverage for workers when they lose or change jobs (hence the title); required the establishment of national identifier numbers for providers and standards for electronic health transactions; and required the Department of Health and Human Services (DHHS) to establish rules for the protection of the privacy and security of healthcare data. It is this latter purpose of most concern to providers of operative and invasive procedure care. Although the Act was passed in 1996, implementation of the privacy rules datelines were set for the mid-2000s.

The rules that resulted are many and complex and have received much criticism despite their originally laudable purpose. Complete summary can be found at http://www.hhs.gov/ocr/privacysummary.pdf. The sections most familiar to practitioners in the operative and invasive procedure setting are those that (HIPAAdvisory, 2005):

- Conducting an impact assessment to determine gaps between existing information practices and policies and HIPAA requirements
- Reviewing functions and activities of the organization's business partners to determine where Business Associate Agreements are required
- Developing and implementing enterprise-wise privacy policies and procedures to implement the rule
- Assigning a Privacy officer who will administer the organizational privacy program and enforce compliance
- Training all members of the workforce on HIPAA and organizational privacy policies
- Updating systems to ensure they provide adequate protection of patient data

To further complicate matters, there may be other federal or state statutes that require or permit release of protected health information in order to protect the general public safety. Typically, these exceptions to HIPAA include child or elder abuse, gunshot wounds or other wounds reasonably believed to have occurred as a result of a crime. Many states have changed their statutes to be the same as HIPAA, but some have more restrictive statutes regarding patient privacy. In these cases, it is the most restrictive statute that prevails.

HIPPA
Health Insurance Portability and Accountability Act

DHHS
Department of Health and Human Services

As with any attempt to implement laudable general privacy rules, the devil is in the details. Nurses must be familiar with and implement whatever procedures the facility has implemented and work to change the procedures rather than attempt work-around if they are too unwieldy in operative and invasive procedure settings. For example, most facility policies require the nurse to log out every time the nurse leaves the computer. This is obviously necessary in settings where persons unconnected to the patient's treatment or even visitors can view the computer in the nurse's absence. It may not be necessary in the intraoperative setting if the facility's OR traffic control policy limits presence in the room to those persons involved with the patient's care, and thus allowed access under HIPAA.

Needlestick Safety and Prevention Act

Signed into law in 2000, the provisions of the Needlestick Safety and Prevention Act are relatively straightforward. The act revises 29 CFR [sections] 910.1030, which is part of the OSHA standards that apply to bloodborne pathogens. This section requires employers to use engineering controls to reduce employee exposure to bloodborne pathogens, and it mandates that these engineering controls be examined regularly to ensure their effectiveness. The act adds "safer medical devices" (eg, needleless systems, sharps with engineered sharps injury protectors) to this definition of engineering controls. By adding this language, required engineering controls will mean those that isolate or remove the bloodborne pathogen hazard from the workplace (eg, safer medical devices, sharps disposal containers, self-sheathing needles).

The Needlestick Safety and Prevention Act directs that the review and update of exposure control plans also reflect changes in technology that eliminate or reduce exposure to bloodborne pathogens. The Act further requires that the exposure control plans document annually consideration and implementation of appropriate commercially available and effective safer medical devices designed to eliminate or minimize exposure. The Act includes an additional record-keeping mandate that requires employers to keep a sharps injury log containing the type and brand of device involved, the department or work area where the exposure occurred, and an explanation of how the injury occurred. This log must be kept in a manner that protects the confidentiality of the injured employee.

Finally, the Needlestick Safety and Prevention Act adds an entirely new section to the OSHA bloodborne pathogen standards. This addition requires employers to solicit input from staff nurses and other non-managerial staff members responsible for direct patient care in the identification, evaluation, and selection of effective engineering and work practice controls (Murphy, 2001).

PATIENT SAFETY AND QUALITY IMPROVEMENT ACT OF 2005

Enacted as part of the response to the Institute of Medicine's 1999 report, To Err is Human, the Patient Safety and Quality Improvement Act, the goal of this federal statute is to improve patient safety by encouraging voluntary and confidential reporting of events that adversely affect patients. It creates *Patient Safety Organizations* (PSOs) to collect, aggregate, and analyze confidential information reported by healthcare providers. Currently, patient safety improvement efforts are hampered by the fear of discovery of peer deliberations, resulting in under-reporting of events and an inability to aggregate sufficient patient safety event data for analysis. By analyzing patient safety event information, PSOs will be able to identify patterns of failures and propose measures to eliminate patient safety risks and hazards (AHRQ, 2003). The law requires HHS to facilitate, through certified patient safety organizations, creation of a network of databases to collect, aggregate, and analyze voluntarily submitted reports of medical errors or near errors. The law also requires that analysis of regional and national statistics and trends be made public via annual reports from the patient safety organizations (Health Data Management, 2008).

PSO
Patient Safety
Organizations

Although passed in 2005, DHHS thru AHRQ had just begun implementation in 2008. Meanwhile, many states addressed patient safety concerns through patient safety acts of their own.

REGULATORY AGENCIES, KEY NOT-FOR-PROFIT BODIES, AND REGULATIONS

Regulations are the product of a state or federal statute that establishes the agency or assigns to a preexisting agency charges and rule-making authority. The result of agencies promulgating rules pursuant to this authority are called *legal regulations.*

Various areas of healthcare have long been subject to state and federal regulation. One of the first was the establishment of the Food and Drug Administration (FDA) of 1906. State licensure and other regulation of health professions emerged shortly afterward.

FDA
Food and Drug
Administration

Different states have passed statutes addressing a variety of components of operative and invasive procedure care over the succeeding decades, but for the most part, healthcare was a charitable enterprise left to its own surveillance and governance. Since 1965, however, there has been an escalation in federal and state regulatory involvement in healthcare and, more recently, there has been acceleration in the conflation of professional and legal standards as well as professional association, re-regulation and insurance-driven setting minimum standards.

FEDERAL AGENCIES

The Department of Health and Human Services (DHHS)

This is the umbrella department for many federal agencies related to healthcare and is represented at the President's Cabinet by the Secretary of the Department. Among the many divisions within this Department are (DHHS, 2008):

Administration on Aging (AOA)

Agency for Healthcare Research and Quality (AHRQ)

Agency for Toxic Substances and Disease Registry (ATSDR)

Centers for Disease Control and Prevention (CDC)

Centers for Medicare & Medicaid Services (CMS)

Food and Drug Administration (FDA)

Health Resources and Services Administration (HRSA)

Indian Health Service (IHS)

> National Institutes of Health (NIH)
>
> Substance Abuse and Mental Health Services Administration
>
> United States Public Health Services

Most of these centers or offices, in turn, are further divided into additional centers, offices and institutes. Agencies within this department with the closest connections to operative and invasive procedure practice are described below.

Centers for Disease Control and Prevention (CDC)

CDC
US Centers for
Disease Control and
Prevention

The US Centers for Disease Control and Prevention (CDC), which is located in Atlanta, Georgia, is an agency of the US Public Health Service. Its role is to protect the public health by way of national programs for the control and prevention of disease. The CDC was established in 1949 to provide health information and participate in research to locate the sources of epidemics. This agency also has been very involved with infectious diseases and works with associations such as the Association of Practitioners in Infection Control & Epidemiology (APIC) and the Association of periOperative Registered Nurses (AORN) through their Recommended Practices groups. This agency currently participates in worldwide activities. Within the CDC are 11 centers, institutes, and offices (CDC, 2008):

APIC
Association of
Practitioners in
Infection Control &
Epidemiology

> National Center for Chronic Disease Prevention and Health Promotion
>
> National Center for Environmental Health
>
> National Center for Health Statistics
>
> National Center for Infectious Diseases
>
> National Center for Injury Prevention and Control
>
> National Center for Prevention Services
>
> National Institute for Occupational Safety and Health (NIOSH)
>
> Epidemiology Program Office
>
> International Health Program Office
>
> Public Health Practice Program Office
>
> National Immunization Program

FOOD AND DRUG ADMINISTRATION (FDA)

The Food and Drug Administration (FDA) is an agency of the US Department of Health and Human Services. This agency oversees laws designed to guarantee pure food, safe cosmetics, and safe and effective biological products, pharmaceuticals, and therapeutic, radiological, and medical devices. The FDA also monitors clearances, marketing tactics, labeling and libeling claims, and safe packaging of products.

In 1971, the FDA assumed responsibility for enforcing the Radiation Control for Health and Safety Act of 1968. This called for the prevention of unnecessary exposure to radiation from electronic devices. In 1976, the Medical Device Amendments were made to the Food, Drug and Cosmetic Act, giving broader powers to the FDA, including the authority to regulate medical devices. The Safe Medical Devices Act

(SMDA) of 1990 provided the FDA with two additional activities, Post-market Surveillance for the monitoring of products after their clearance to market and Device Tracking for maintaining traceability of certain devices to the user level. While the primary responsibility for making these reports lie with the device manu-facturers, the nurse practicing in the operative and invasive procedure area should be alert to these requirements and follow facility policy to assure reportable events reach the FDA.

Other responsibilities of the FDA include the development of new methods of analyzing products and research on the effects of substances and devices on animals and for human use The FDA has been under a great deal of scrutiny by the healthcare community because of the long processing times for medical devices and pharma-ceutical agents (FDA, 2008).

NATIONAL INSTITUTE FOR OCCUPATIONAL SAFETY AND HEALTH

The National Institute for Occupational Safety and Health (NIOSH) is a federal agency established by the Occupational Safety and Health Act of 1970. NIOSH is the research arm of the CDC and is charged with conducting research and making recommendations for the prevention of work-related illness and injuries. Specifi-cally, it investigates potentially hazardous working conditions; evaluates hazards in the workplace; creates and disseminates methods for preventing disease, injury, and disability; and conducts research and provides scientifically valid recommendations for protecting workers. As an example, in September 1996, NIOSH released a hazard control bulletin that addresses the control of smoke generated from the use of laser and electro-surgery devices during operative and invasive procedures. Unlike OSHA, which is a part of the Department of Labor and which was established for creating and enforcing workplace safety and health regulations, NIOSH is in the Department of Health and Human Services and is a research agency (NIOSH, 2008).

NIOSH
National Institute for Occupational Safety and Health

OCCUPATIONAL SAFETY AND HEALTH ADMINISTRATION

The Occupational Safety and Health Act was passed in 1970. The purpose of the act was to ensure a safe and healthy workplace with jobs that would not subject the work environment and work force to hazards that could result in physical harm or even death.

Paving the way for this act were the politics of the 1960s, during which time there was renewed interest in the environment and concern about pollution and personal safety. Currently the Occupational Safety and Health Administration (OSHA) is considered to be an organization whose members wear a variety of hats. Employers have been unhappy with OSHA because of the seeming unconcern regarding the cost of meeting standards and the amount of paperwork required by the agency. Related to operative and invasive procedure services, OSHA develops and monitors issues such as standard precautions; the regulation of chemical germicides and dis-infectants used for cleaning, decontamination, and disinfection; and the use and monitoring of the carcinogenic and toxic effects of ethylene oxide, which is used

OSHA
Occupational Safety and Health Administration

for sterilization in healthcare facilities, and the use of personal protective equipment to guard against disease transmission in the operative and invasive procedure setting (OSHA, 2008).

CENTERS FOR MEDICARE & MEDICAID SERVICES (CMS)

CMS
Centers for Medicare & Medicaid Services

HCFA
Health Care Financing Administration

SCHIP
State Children's Health Insurance Program

CLIA
Clinical Laboratory Improvement Amendments

DRG
Diagnosis Related Groups

CMS is the Centers for Medicare & Medicaid Services. Formerly known as the Health Care Financing Administration (HCFA), it is the federal agency responsible for administering the Medicare, Medicaid, SCHIP (State Children's Health Insurance Program), HIPAA (Health Insurance Portability and Accountability Act), CLIA (Clinical Laboratory Improvement Amendments), and several other health-related programs.

As the administrative agency for a chief source of revenue (Medicare and Medicaid payments), the CMS has become a major player in regulation of the quality, cost, and access of the care it pays for. Its influence reaches to nearly all patients since most facilities need to comply for all patients in order to keep its Medicare payments. Additionally, many insurance companies adopt their own but similar requirements for payment under their private sector policies.

It was CMS' predecessor agency, HCFA, that first released Diagnosis Related Groups (DRGs) as the basis for inpatient prospective payment in the early 1980s in an attempt to control cost. This was a major shift from the previous fee-for-service reimbursement method that essentially paid for everything billed (albeit not at the billed amount).

Pursuant to deficit reduction mandates for Congress, by mid-2000, the CMS was actively structuring payments to incentivize desired behaviors related to both cost and quality. In accordance with its articulated vision, "the right care for every person every time," the CMS is moving to a Value Based Purchasing (VBP) system. Value-based purchasing, which links payment more directly to the quality of care provided, is a strategy to help transform the current payment system by rewarding providers for delivering high quality, efficient clinical care. Some examples of these initiatives included using Medicare payment as an incentive for hospitals to report on the care they provide all adults, regardless of payer (CMS, 2007b). In 2007, this incentive moved to a requirement that hospitals report their performance on 21 measures to obtain their full payment update. It is envisioned that this set of measures will expand over time. Failure to report will result in a reduction in payment for inpatient hospital services. In 2008, CMS expanded its incentives from requiring reporting to disincentivizing non-quality performance. In essence, the CMS identified eight preventable conditions that patients acquire in the hospital and refused to pay for the treatment of these conditions and disallowed the hospital to bill the patient for these costs. The initial eight identified conditions directly or could indirectly relate to operative and invasive procedure care. They were:

1. Foreign Object Retained After Surgery
2. Air Embolism
3. Blood Incompatibility
4. Stage III and IV Pressure Ulcers
5. Falls and Trauma

6. Fractures
7. Dislocations
8. Intracranial Injuries
9. Crushing Injuries
10. Burns
11. Catheter-Associated Urinary Tract Infection (UTI)
12. Vascular Catheter-Associate Infection
13. Surgical Site Infection-Mediastinitis after Coronary Artery Bypass Graft (CABG)

Nine additional conditions have been proposed for implementation in 2009, including deep vein thrombosis and surgical site infection for additional selected procedures.

Additional information regarding CMS and its programs is available at http://www.cms.hhs.gov/.

AGENCY FOR HEALTHCARE RESEARCH AND QUALITY (AHRQ)

Obviously, nurses should be familiar with federal agencies for familiarity with the legal regulations they promulgate. However, agencies also serve as valuable sources of information about quality practice in general that are not legally mandated.

Every nurse should bookmark the Agency for Healthcare Quality and Research (AHRQ) http://www.ahrq.gov. The AHRQ is the health services research arm of the US Department of Health and Human Services (HHS), complementing the biomedical research mission of its sister agency, the National Institutes of Health. It houses research centers that specialize in major areas of health care research related to:

AHRQ
Agency for Healthcare Research and Quality

- Quality improvement and patient safety.
- Outcomes and effectiveness of care.
- Clinical practice and technology assessment.
- Healthcare organization and delivery systems.
- Primary care (including preventive services).
- Healthcare costs and sources of payment.

It also works with the public and private sectors to build the knowledge base for evidence-based practice and to translate this knowledge into everyday practice and policymaking. The homepage is overwhelming as the agency disseminates its findings to the consumer and professional audience by populations as well as issues. Nurses will find the section titled Quality and Patient Safety most helpful. Unlike the regulations adopted by agencies with rulemaking authority, the position papers and information contained on the AHRQ website are not legal requirements per se. However, they can be used as evidence of the standard of care (what a reasonable and prudent nurse would have done) and can function to prevent patient injury in the first place thus 'protecting' the nurse from liability in negligence and malpractice cases.

A hybrid type of agency comprised of other agencies the Patient Safety Task Force. The Patient Safety Task Force serves as a special task force under the HHS Secretary's

Quality Improvement Initiative, the Patient Safety Task Force consists of representatives from the major regulatory agencies relevant to operative and invasive procedure practice:

- Agency for Healthcare Research and Quality (AHRQ).
- Centers for Disease Control and Prevention (CDC).
- Food and Drug Administration (FDA).
- Centers for Medicare & Medicaid Services (CMS).
- Other divisions of HHS, other interested Federal agencies, and other public- and private-sector organizations may also be involved (AHRQ, 2003).

NONGOVERNMENTAL ASSOCIATIONS

The Joint Commission

Formerly known as the Joint Commission for the Accreditation of Hospitals (JCAH), then the Joint Commission for the Accreditation of Healthcare Organizations (JCAHO), The Joint Commission establishes standards and surveys institutions for compliance with these standards. These surveys are required if an institution is seeking accreditation. Standards and surveys are currently in place for acute care hospitals, non-hospital-based psychiatric and substance abuse programs, long-term care facilities, home-care organizations, hospice programs, managed care providers, and ambulatory healthcare settings. The survey itself is designed to measure the degree to which an organization meets the established standards outlined in the accreditation manual. It is the responsibility of the organization being surveyed to provide documentation demonstrating compliance with the standards. If the institution is found to be in compliance, accreditation is provided even if the institution receives recommendations for improvement.

In 1973, the (then) JCAH included nursing and medical audits as a requirement for accreditation to verify that institutions were involved in continuous and ongoing evaluations of the quality of services provided. The nursing and medical professionals were then required to formulate criteria and implement means of evaluating care. This was to assure the public that they were receiving optimal quality services.

In the 2000s the Joint Commission established national patient safety goals and began surveying on their accomplishment. Goals have been added and in some cases include SCIP initiatives. **Table 4.2** lists the 2008 Patient Safety Goals related to the operative and invasive procedure setting.

Institute of Medicine (IOM)

The Institute of Medicine is a private, non-governmental organization and does not receive direct federal appropriations for its work. It is part of the National Academy of Sciences that was founded by the federal government in 1970 and is funded out of appropriations made available to federal agencies. Most of the studies carried out by the Academy complex are at the request of government agencies or as Prescription Drug, Improvement, and Modernization Act of 2003 (MMA) mandated that the Institute of Medicine (IOM) conduct a review of Medicare Quality Improvement Organization (QIO) Program (formerly referred to as the Medicare Utilization and

JCAH
Joint Commission for the Accreditation of Hospitals

JCAHO
Joint Commission for the Accreditation of Healthcare Organizations

Table 4.2	Joint Commission 2008 Patient Safety Goals
Goal 1	Improve the accuracy of patient identification.
1A	Use at least two patient identifiers when providing care, treatment or services. [Ambulatory, Assisted Living, Behavioral Healthcare, Critical Access Hospital, Disease-Specific Care, Home Care, Hospital, Lab, Long-Term Care, Office-Based Surgery]
1B	Prior to the start of any invasive procedure, conduct a final verification process, (such as a "time out,") to confirm the correct patient, procedure and site, using active—not passive—communication techniques. [Assisted Living, Home Care, Lab, Long-Term Care]
Goal 2	Improve the effectiveness of communication among caregivers.
2A	For verbal or telephone orders or for telephonic reporting of critical test results, verify the complete order or test result by having the person receiving the information record and "read-back" the complete order or test result. [Ambulatory, Assisted Living, Behavioral Healthcare, Critical Access Hospital, Disease-Specific Care, Home Care, Hospital, Lab, Long-Term Care, Office-Based Surgery]
2B	Standardize a list of abbreviations, acronyms, symbols, and dose designations that are not to be used throughout the organization. [Ambulatory, Assisted Living, Behavioral Healthcare, Critical Access Hospital, Disease-Specific Care, Home Care, Hospital, Lab, Long-Term Care, Office-Based Surgery]
2C	Measure and assess, and if appropriate, take action to improve the timeliness of reporting, and the timeliness of receipt by the responsible licensed caregiver, of critical test results and values. [Ambulatory, Behavioral Healthcare, Critical Access Hospital, Disease-Specific Care, Home Care, Hospital, Lab, Long-Term Care, Office-Based Surgery]
2E	Implement a standardized approach to "hand off" communications, including an opportunity to ask and respond to questions. [Ambulatory, Assisted Living, Behavioral Healthcare, Critical Access Hospital, Disease-Specific Care, Home Care, Hospital, Lab, Long-Term Care, Office-Based Surgery]
Goal 3	Improve the safety of using medications.
3C	Identify and, at a minimum, annually review a list of look-alike/sound-alike drugs used by the organization, and take action to prevent errors involving the interchange of these drugs. [Ambulatory, Behavioral Healthcare, Critical Access Hospital, Home Care, Hospital, Long-Term Care, Office-Based Surgery]
3D	Label all medications, medication containers (for example, syringes, medicine cups, basins), or other solutions on and off the sterile field. [Ambulatory, Critical Access Hospital, Hospital, Office-Based Surgery]
3E	Reduce the likelihood of patient harm associated with the use of anticoagulation therapy. [Ambulatory, Critical Access Hospital, Home Care, Hospital, Long-Term Care, Office-Based Surgery]
Goal 7	Reduce the risk of health care-associated infections.
7A	Comply with current World Health Organization (WHO) Hand Hygiene Guidelines or Centers for Disease Control and Prevention (CDC) hand hygiene guidelines. [Ambulatory, Assisted Living, Behavioral Healthcare, Critical Access Hospital, Disease-Specific Care, Home Care, Hospital, Lab, Long-Term Care, Office-Based Surgery]
7B	Manage as sentinel events all identified cases of unanticipated death or major permanent loss of function associated with a healthcare-associated infection. [Ambulatory, Assisted Living, Behavioral Healthcare, Critical Access Hospital, Disease-Specific Care, Home Care, Hospital, Lab, Long-Term Care, Office-Based Surgery]
Goal 8	Accurately and completely reconcile medications across the continuum of care.
8A	There is a process for comparing the patient's current medications with those ordered for the patient while under the care of the organization. [Ambulatory, Assisted Living, Behavioral Healthcare, Critical Access Hospital, Disease-Specific Care, Home Care, Hospital, Long-Term Care, Office-Based Surgery]

8B	A complete list of the patient's medications is communicated to the next provider of service when a patient is referred or transferred to another setting, service, practitioner or level of care within or outside the organization. The complete list of medications is also provided to the patient on discharge from the facility. [Ambulatory, Assisted Living, Behavioral Healthcare, Critical Access Hospital, Disease-Specific Care, Home Care, Hospital, Long-Term Care, Office-Based Surgery]
Goal 9	Reduce the risk of patient harm resulting from falls.
9B	Implement a fall reduction program including an evaluation of the effectiveness of the program. [Assisted Living, Critical Access Hospital, Disease-Specific Care, Home Care, Hospital, Long-Term Care]
Goal 10	Reduce the risk of influenza and pneumococcal disease in institutionalized older adults.
10A	Develop and implement a protocol for administration and documentation of the flu vaccine. [Assisted Living, Disease-Specific Care, Long-Term Care]
10B	Develop and implement a protocol for administration and documentation of the Pneumococcus vaccine. [Assisted Living, Disease-Specific Care, Long-Term Care]
10C	Develop and implement a protocol to identify new cases of influenza and to manage an outbreak. [Assisted Living, Disease-Specific Care, Long-Term Care]
Goal 11	Reduce the risk of surgical fires.
11A	Educate staff, including operating licensed independent practitioners and anesthesia providers, on how to control heat sources and manage fuels with enough time for patient preparation, and establish guidelines to minimize oxygen concentration under drapes. [Ambulatory, Office-Based Surgery]
Goal 12	Implementation of applicable National Patient Safety Goals and associated requirements by components and practitioner sites.
12A	Inform and encourage components and practitioner sites to implement the applicable National Patient Safety Goals and associated requirements. [Networks]
Goal 13	Encourage patients' active involvement in their own care as a patient safety strategy.
13A	Define and communicate the means for patients and their families to report concerns about safety and encourage them to do so. [Ambulatory, Assisted Living, Behavioral Healthcare, Critical Access Hospital, Disease-Specific Care, Home Care, Hospital, Lab, Long-Term Care, Office-Based Surgery]
Goal 14	Prevent healthcare-associated pressure ulcers (decubitus ulcers).
14A	Assess and periodically reassess each resident's risk for developing a pressure ulcer (decubitus ulcer) and take action to address any identified risks. [Long-Term Care]
Goal 15	The organization identifies safety risks inherent in its patient population.
15A	The organization identifies patients at risk for suicide. [Behavioral Healthcare, Hospital (applicable to psychiatric hospitals and patients being treated for emotional or behavioral disorders in general hospitals)]
15B	The organization identifies risks associated with long-term oxygen therapy such as home fires. [Home Care]
Goal 16	Improve recognition and response to changes in a patient's condition.
16A	The organization selects a suitable method that enables health care staff members to directly request additional assistance from a specially trained individual(s) when the patient's condition appears to be worsening. [Critical Access Hospital, Hospital]

Joint Commission 2008 Patient Safety Goals, www.jointcommission.org/PatientSafety/NationalPatientSafetyGoals/08_npsg_facts.htm.

Quality Control Peer Review Program) was created by statute in 1982 to improve quality and efficiency of services delivered to Medicare beneficiaries and how its impact could be enhanced. The IOM issued a report based on its study of quality and efficiency on March 9, 2006 (CMS, 2006a).

As previously noted, IOM's landmark report *To Err Is Human* (1999) served as the impetus for the renewed governmental and nongovernmental focus on patient safety seen in the 2000s.

Advanced Medical Technology Association (AdvaMed)

The Advanced Medical Technology Association (AdvaMed) is a trade association representing medical device manufacturers, makers of medical equipment, medical software and diagnostic equipment and supplies. Its mission is to advocate for a legal, regulatory, and economic climate that advances global healthcare by assuring patients can have access to the benefits of medical technology.

AdvaMed
The Advanced Medical Technology Association

In 2004, AdvaMed enacted a voluntary set of codes for ethical interactions with healthcare professionals. AdvaMed worked with the Department of Health and Human Services Inspector General to develop the codes that are designed to promote ethical and legal interactions in the medical devices industry. The code addresses the need to prevent the perception of undue influence or kickbacks in decisions to purchase items used in healthcare. The operative and invasive procedure setting uses a lot of expensive supplies and capital equipment and has been one area where marketing giveaways or enhancements to educational opportunities have been discontinued to avoid any such perceptions. The full text of the code and relevant AdvaMed press releases can be found at http://www.advamed.org/publicdocs/coe.html (AdvaMed, 2003).

Surgical Care Improvement Project (SCIP)

The Surgical Care Improvement Project (SCIP) is a national quality partnership of organizations focused on improving surgical care by significantly reducing surgical complications. It is a unique partnership that is proving to be a transformational undertaking in healthcare. The SCIP goal is to reduce the incidence of surgical complications nationally by 25 percent by the year 2010 (MedQIC, 2008). The SCIP Steering Committee comprises 10 national organizations. Note the combination of governmental agencies and non governmental professional associations:

- Agency for Healthcare Research and Quality
- American College of Surgeons
- American Hospital Association
- American Society of Anesthesiologists
- Association of periOperative Registered Nurses
- Centers for Disease Control and Prevention
- Centers for Medicare & Medicaid Services
- Institute for Healthcare Improvement
- Joint Commission on Accreditation of Healthcare Organizations
- Veterans Health Administration

SCIP has identified several key areas of practice requiring attention in order to reduce the incidence of surgical complications and has initially focused on controlling hypothermia, monitoring elevated blood glucose levels, using electric clippers to remove hair from the surgical site, and administering preoperative, procedure-specific antibiotics within an appropriate timeframe (Brendle, 2007).

The National Quality Forum (NQF)

The National Quality Forum (NQF) is a private, not-for-profit, open membership organization with broad participation from all parts of the healthcare system, including national, regional, state, and local groups representing consumers; public and private purchasers; physicians, hospitals, and other healthcare providers; accrediting bodies; supporting industries; and organizations involved in healthcare research or quality improvement. The NQF coordinates their efforts and achieve consensus on actions that can create meaningful, lasting change related to the quality of care delivered to America's patients (NQF, 2008).

Association of periOperative Registered Nurses (AORN)

The Association of periOperative Registered Nurses' (AORN) mission is to promote safety and optimal outcomes for patients undergoing operative and other invasive procedures by providing practice support and professional development opportunities to operative and invasive procedure nurses. AORN works with professional and regulatory organizations, industry leaders, and other healthcare partners who support this mission. It is the official voice of perioperative nursing at policy and regulatory tables, including the Joint Commission, CMS, CDC, the American College of Surgeons, and the American Medical Association, and represents nurses in SCIP and the NQF. Every reader, particularly nurses practicing in the operative and invasive procedure setting, committed to patient safety and quality care to patients in a supportive legal, regulatory, and ethical environment should be a member of this voluntary nonprofit organization.

National Fire Protection Agency (NFPA)

NFPA
National Fire
Protection Agency

The National Fire Protection Agency (NFPA) receives its membership from the scientific and education community. NFPA is an organization concerned with the causes, prevention, and control of destruction fires. This agency was first organized in 1896 and incorporated in 1930 as a private, voluntary, nonprofit organization. The NFPA is involved with the development of fire safety and technical standards, information exchange, technical advisory services, public education research, and service to public protection agencies through the provision of information and advice. For example, woven and nonwoven materials need to meet the standards for NFPA before they can be marketed to healthcare facilities.

SUMMARY—INTO THE FUTURE

This section briefly describes various criminal and civil laws, selected state and federal statutes, federal administrative agencies and nongovernmental associations, and combinations thereof that affect the delivery of operative and invasive procedure services in the United States. In addition, each state has its own statutes and regulations on which healthcare professionals and facilities are managed and measured for compliance.

External regulations result from a society that claims to want quality healthcare made available and accessible for everyone regardless of his or her financial status. Internal regulation (professional association recommendations and facility policies and procedures) comes, in part, as a response of healthcare providers to external regulations. Internal regulations also come from organizations that proactively establish standards and measure their performance against those standards. Individuals, departments, and facilities also create internal regulations by those who are concerned with providing optimal service to the best of their abilities. The 1990s and 2000s will be remembered as the decades of quality, cost, payment systems, and access concerns. All organizations are currently emphasizing quality in their mission, objectives, goals, and services and in their dealing with customers. Healthcare saw the rise of market forces after the failure of the Clinton healthcare plan in the mid-1990s. By the mid-2000s, dual concerns about patient safety and deficit reduction combined to increase regulation related to payment systems. The conflation of 'private' regulation by nongovernmental organizations and that of governmental agency regulation accelerated. How healthcare structure and regulation looks in the 2010s may well turn on the 2008 elections. Law both leads and reflects the needs and values of members of society. Whom members of society chose as their elected representatives to make laws will determine what those laws and regulations provide.

In pursuing optimal quality, nurses must continue to be mindful of the legal and regulatory requirements and their impact on practice. Federal and state and local laws and regulations guide facilities and professionals in the establishment of services, delivery of services, the monitoring of these services, and the evaluation of outcomes. They are also complex and ever changing, so efforts to stay current must be ongoing and comprehensive.

ETHICS

Law and ethics are two separate systems, but they do exist within the context of the same society. Because of this, what is legal may or may not be ethical (eg, sharing patients' medical information with clerks in billing processes without express patient consent) and what is ethical may or may not be legal (treating minors in non-emergencies without parental consent). That said, because the legal and moral/ethical systems exist within the same society and when that society is founded in democratic, representative governments (ie, elected law makers) law and morals/ethics will necessarily interact and, more often than not, overlap.

Moral Principles and Rules

According to Beauchamp and Childress (2009) the applicable principles in biomedical ethics are *respect for autonomy, nonmaleficence beneficence* and *justice*. From these principles flow the rules of Veracity; Confidentiality; Privacy; and Fidelity.

Autonomy

The autonomous individual is one that is free to make decisions affecting themselves that is free from control by others and free from limitations such as an inadequate understanding that prevents a meaningful choice. Respect for autonomy is reflected in the legal requirement for informed consent.

Nonmaleficence

Nonmaleficence is the obligation not to inflict harm. The equivalent phrase used in the healthcare professions is *Primum non nocere* or "first, do no harm." Most of what the nurse does during the operative or invasive procedure is founded in this principle. Nurses manage the environment to protect the patient from infection, or count sponges to avoid the harm of a retained foreign body, or properly ground the patient so there is no harm due to an electrocautery burn. The principle of nonmaleficence is legally enforceable via the law of negligence that allows harmed persons to sue the person inflicting the harm.

Beneficence

Beneficence is the affirmative corollary to nonmaleficence: Beyond avoiding the infliction of harm is the expectation that one should actually do good. This is the underlying reason most nurses chose nursing as a profession—in order to help others. Nurses practice beneficence when they hang blood or prepare medications or otherwise participate in affirmative roles in surgery; when they reassure the anxious patient; when they support the waiting family members.

Justice

Justice is simply fairness. Distributive justice refers to the fair and equitable allocation of benefits and burdens. Such simple definitions belie the complexity of what constitutes fair. Is it

- "To each an equal share?"
- "To each according to need?"
- "To each according to effort?"
- "To each according to contribution?"
- "To each according to merit?"
- "To each according to free market exchanges?"

Justice becomes most vexing when dealing with scarce resources. Nurses face choices of justice daily.

There are a limited number of 0800 start times: What is the fairest way to distribute them: According to need so the most seriously ill or children are scheduled first? According to merit so VIPs are scheduled first? According to free market exchange so the surgeon who does the most cases controls the most start times?

Organ transplant provides the most vivid example of distributional justice in surgical suites. Perhaps fortunately the nurse rarely is in a position to determine "who gets the heart." But if the recipient is someone the nurse thinks had less need and more merit—and the rest of the transplant team has decided differently, the nurse comes face to face with an ethical dilemma: the conflict of principles or rules.

There is no legal right to an 0800 start time; nor to an organ for transplant; nor in fact to healthcare at all (unless protected by the Emergency Medical Treatment and Labor Act). This is an area where law and ethics have yet to converge.

Veracity

Veracity refers to conveying accurate, objective information. It is related to the principle of autonomy—that persons deserve the respect of accurate and complete information—and the rule of fidelity or promise keeping, that what nurses say or write carries an implicit promise of being the truth. Documentation on the procedure record requires veracity to uphold the principles of beneficence and nonmaleficence of the nurse and other health team members who depend on the record to provide appropriate continued care. Veracity is also required for the information provided to third party payers; this obligation is legally enforced by laws relating to fraudulent business records. Other examples of veracity for operative or invasive procedure nurses are reports of lapses in sterile technique or the reports given to family members during the procedure; if the procedure is not going well, the nurse should not represent otherwise to the family.

Privacy

Privacy is a state of limited access to a person; it relates to a person's control or right to control access to him or herself. Ethicists recognize different forms of privacy that relate to limited access to a person. The forms most closely involved in operative and invasive procedure care are physical privacy and informational privacy or confidentiality. The intraoperative patient cannot control access to his or her body but does not surrender that ethical right by consenting to be sedated or anesthetized. The patient grants access to the parts of the body being operated on by consenting to the operation, but this access is limited to those the patient grants access to. The nurse plays a major role in protecting the patient's physical privacy by exposing only those areas of the body where access is required for a safe procedure and exposing them only during the time periods that access is necessary. Nurses also protect privacy by enforcing traffic control or visitor policies and assuring that only those persons the patient expects to be involved with the surgery actually do so. Some aspects of control of physical privacy must be foregone during a surgical, other invasive, or diagnostic procedure, but access to the information generated due to those procedures remains private as informational privacy, unless the patient grants informational access. The right of privacy precludes access of patient's healthcare data by unauthorized others. Persons who access patients' medical record information when they are not caring for them violate the patient's right to informational privacy. This underlies the practice of restricting access to the surgical schedule. Many of the regulations under HIPAA are designed to legally protect the patient's ethical right to informational privacy.

Confidentiality

Confidentiality is a subset of informational privacy. It prevents re-disclosure of information originally confided or learned within a confidential relationship. Nurses have a confidential relationship with patients and should not disclose those things that patients tell them unless necessary for the patient's care. For example, "My father died under anesthesia and I'm afraid I will too," should be disclosed to the surgeon and anesthesia provider; even then, the nurse should tell the patient this must be disclosed for her safety. Whereas, "My husband is not the father of this baby" should not, unless the patient consents to prevent his presence during a C-section. Workplace debriefing conversations that take place in social settings such as elevators, restaurants, other public places or even private gatherings of professionals can violate the patient's right to confidentiality. A nurse's own emotional need to tell a friend "I spent a lot of time with Ms. A before her procedure; she was so scared and so nice; I was devastated when her frozen came back positive" is nonetheless a violation of the nurse's confidential relationship with Ms. A.

Fidelity

Fidelity refers to faithfulness or loyalty to a significant relationship. The operative and invasive procedure setting is structured in such a way that nurses frequently find themselves with divided or conflicting loyalties. While the Nurse Code of Ethics directs that the "nurse's primary commitment is to the patient" (AORN, 2008, p. 638), the nurse also owes legal duties of loyalty to the employer. The AdvaMed code and its prohibition against accepting things of value from industry representatives as good-will gestures or inducements to sale speaks most directly to fidelity and avoiding conflicts of interest.

Like law and regulation, ethics and moral principles are many and complex and cannot be comprehensively treated within a few pages. Much of the above is adapted from Beauchamp, T. and Childress, J. (2009). *Principles of Biomedical Ethics*. Sixth Edition. Oxford University Press: New York. This highly respected, authoritative source for frameworks and analysis of moral/ethical issues in healthcare and is commended to the reader.

ANA CODE OF ETHICS AND PERIOPERATIVE EXPLICATIONS

The American Nurses Association has recognized that ethics is integral to the practice of nurses. The ANA has issued a Code of Ethics for nurses since 1950. In its most recent iteration, the Code incorporates nine provisions with interpretations, all of which reflect the principles and rules addressed above. Among the provisions and interpretations, the Code speaks to respect for human dignity (autonomy and privacy); conflicts of interests (fidelity); protection of health, safety, and rights of patients (nonmaleficence, privacy, confidentiality); responsibility for nursing practice (nonmaleficence, beneficence, veracity); improving the healthcare environment (beneficence).

Most helpful to the nurse are AORN's Explications of the Code for Perioperative Practice. The Explications parallel each provision and interpretation of the ANA

Code and provides explications and examples from the operative and invasive procedure setting for each. In doing so, the Explications not only reflect the ANA Code but also reflect the principles and rules of ethics, as found in the operative and invasive procedure setting. For example, an Explications' example of conflict of interest indicates the operative and invasive procedure nurse does not access of solicit items of value that could reasonable be inferred to influencing impartiality. Alternatively, provides auditory privacy and avoids needless exposure of the patient's body (AORN, 2008, pp. 633–660).

Nurses face ethical dilemmas or conflicts of ethical principles in their daily practice. Sometimes, they are not resolvable by referencing a book or a Code of Ethics. The Explications direct the nurse to 'formulate ethical decisions with assistance of available resources (eg, ethics committee, counselors, ethicists)' (AORN, 2008, p. 637). Most facilities have constituted ethics committees that are composed of persons with a variety of viewpoints (eg, pastoral, legal, consumer, other providers) to discuss difficult ethical conflicts and render their best thinking. Nurses can and should seek the advice of such groups when it seems the conflict cannot be resolved.

PATIENTS' BILL OF RIGHTS

The *Bill of Rights* as most Americans know it refers to the first 10 amendments to our Constitution, which had its origins in English law and declarations. As part of the Constitution, the *Bill of Rights* enjoys the highest legal protections in the land.

The *Patients' Bill of Rights* (p. 79) first became widely recognized in 1973 when the American Hospital Association (AHA) adopted and publicized a statement of principles related to patient care under that title. As a whole, it is not a statement of legal rights as the AHA has no legal enforcement authority. However, recalling the interaction of law and ethics, many individual 'rights' enumerated in the Patients' Bill of Rights have been incorporated into state statutes or reflect common law principles and thus are "legal" as well as ethical rights.

Since 1973, the AHA has updated its statement and several other professional associations or collations have made various similar statements of principles of care under the rubric of a *patients' bill of rights*. More recently, health plans third party payors have also adopted "patient/consumer bill of rights" statements after the President's Advisory Commission of Consumer Protections and Quality in the Health Care Industry in 1998 enumerated eight issues with consumer rights and responsibilities. Like the AHA's statement, some of these areas already have legal protection in state or federal statute while others remain statements of ethical principle.

The phrase *A Patients' Bill of Rights* has also been used as a title for House and Senate Congressional initiatives as yet not signed into law, but likely to be revisited as the country tries to address the cost/access/quality triad.

ETHICS SUMMARY

Ethics must be considered within any service profession, but most certainly one with as personal and intimate relationship with the patient as the nurse. Ethics carries its own obligations to the patient, some of which might also be legally enforced,

AHA
American Hospital Association

some not. A copy of the AORN Explications of the ANA Code is "a must" for every nurse providing operative and invasive procedure care. However, that alone cannot anticipate all the permutations that can arise within the context of practice. Keeping current with the literature and recommended practices is no less important in ethics than in any other area of practice.

ENDNOTES

1. The term *nurse* refers to registered nurses practicing in the perioperative, gastrointestinal, cardiac catheterization, and interventional radiology setting.

2. Malpractice is a subset of negligence: negligence by a professional in the performance of a professional act.

REFERENCES

1. AdvaMed (2003). Code of ethics on interactions with health care professionals. Retrieved June 25, 2008 from http://www.advamed.org/publicdocs/coe.html.

2. AHRQ (2003). Patient safety task force fact sheet. Retrieved June 25, 2008 from (http://www.ahrq.gov/qual/taskforce/psfactst.htm.

3. AORN (2008). AORN explications for perioperative nursing. *Perioperative Standards and Recommended Practices.* Denver, CO: AORN, Inc.: pp. 633–660.

4. Brendle, T.A. (2007). Surgical care improvement wproject and the perioperative nurse's role. *AORN Journal;* 86(1): pp. 94–95, 97–101.

5. CDC (2008). Coordinating center for health information and service (CCHIS). Retrieved June 25, 2008 from http://www.cdc.gov/about/organization/cchis.htm.

6. CMS (2007a). Revisions to the hospital interpretive guidelines for informed consent, http://www.cms.hhs.gov/SurveyCertificationGenInfo/downloads/SCLetter07-17.pdf (Accessed 25 June 2008).

7. CMS (2007b). US Department of Health and Human Services: Medicare hospital value-based purchasing plan development—Issues Paper. Retrieved June 25, 2008 from http://www.cms.hhs.gov/AcuteInpatientPPS/Downloads/Hospital_VBP_Plan_Issues_Paper.pdf.

8. CMS (2006a). Report to congress: Improving the Medicare quality improvement organization program—Response to the Institute of Medicine study. Retrieved June 25, 2008 from http://www.cms.hhs.gov/QualityImprovementOrgs/downloads/QIO_Improvement_RTC_fnl.pdf.

9. CMS (2006b). National health expenditure accounts—2006 highlights. Retrieved June 25, 2008 from http://www.cms.hhs.gov/NationalHealthExpendData/downloads/highlights.pdf.

10. Department of Health and Human Services (DHHS) (2008). HHS Family of Agencies. Retrieved June 25, 2008 from http://www.hhs.gov/

11. Denholm, C.R. (2007). Trust: The 5 Rights of the Second Victim. Solutions for leaders. *Journal of Patient Safety;* 3(2): pp. 107–119.

12. Food and Drug Administration (FDA) (2008). FDA overview. Retrieved June 25, 2008 from http://www.fda.gov/oc/opacom/fda101/sld001.html.

13. Health Data Management (2008). HHS issues Patient Safety Act Rule. Retrieved June 25, 2008 from http://www.healthdatamanagement.com/news/patient_safety25696-1.html.

14. HIPAAdvisory (2005). HIPAA primer. Retrieved June 25, 2008 from http://www.hipaadvisory.com/REGS/HIPAAprimer.htm.

15. Joint Commission. (2008). National Patient Safety Goals. Retrieved June 25, 2008 from www.jointcommission.org/PatientSafety/NationalPatientSafetyGoals/08_npsg_facts.htm.

16. MedQIC (2008). SCIP project information–other resource: about the project. Retrieved June 26, 2008 from http://www.medqic.org/dcs/ContentServer?cid=1136495755695&pagename=Medqic%2FOtherResource%2FOtherResourcesTemplate&c=OtherResource.

17. Murphy, E.K. (2001). Needlestick Safety and Prevention Act. *AORN Journal* 73(2): pp. 458, 461.

18. National Institute for Occupational Safety and Health (NIOSH). (2008). About NIOSH, Retrieved June 25, 2008 from http://www.cdc.gov/NIOSH.

19. National Quality Forum (NQF) (2008). About us. Retrieved June 25, 2008 from http://www.qualityforum.org/about/

20. Occupational and Safety Administration (OSHA) (2008). OSHA home page. Retrieved June 25, 2008 from http://www.osha.gov/

21. Smetzer, J. (1998) Lesson from Colorado: beyond blaming individuals. *Nursing Management,* 28(5): pp. 48–51.

22. The Just Culture Community (2007). Newsletter. Retrieved June 25, 2008 from http://www.justculture.org/downloads/newsletter_janfeb07.pdf.

23. USAToday (2008). Filipino nurses face criminal charges. Retrieved June 25, 2008 from http://www.usatoday.com/community/utils/idmap/28762781.story.

A Patient's Bill of Rights

INTRODUCTION

Effective healthcare requires collaboration between patients and physicians and other healthcare professionals. Open and honest communication, respect for personal and professional values, and sensitivity to differences are integral to optimal patient care. As the setting for the provision of health services, hospitals must provide a foundation for understanding and respecting the rights and responsibilities of patients, their families, physicians, and other caregivers. Hospitals must ensure a healthcare ethic that respects the role of patients in decision making about treatment choices and other aspects of their care. Hospitals must be sensitive to cultural, racial, linguistic, religious, age, gender, and other differences as well as the needs of persons with disabilities.

The American Hospital Association presents A Patient's Bill of Rights with the expectation that it will contribute to more effective patient care and be supported by the hospital on behalf of the institution, its medical staff, employees, and patients. The American Hospital Association encourages healthcare institutions to tailor this bill of rights to their patient community by translating and/or simplifying the language of this bill of rights as may be necessary to ensure that patients and their families understand their rights and responsibilities.

BILL OF RIGHTS

These rights can be exercised on the patient's behalf by a designated surrogate or proxy decision maker if the patient lacks decision-making capacity, is legally incompetent, or is a minor.

1. The patient has the right to considerate and respectful care.

2. The patient has the right to and is encouraged to obtain from physicians and other direct caregivers relevant, current, and understandable information concerning diagnosis, treatment, and prognosis.

    Except in emergencies when the patient lacks decision-making capacity and the need for treatment is urgent, the patient is entitled to the opportunity to discuss and request information related to the specific procedures and/or treatments, the risks involved, the possible length of recuperation, and the medically reasonable alternatives and their accompanying risks and benefits.

    Patients have the right to know the identity of physicians, nurses, and others involved in their care, as well as when those involved are students, residents, or other trainees. The patient also has the right to know the immediate and long-term financial implications of treatment choices, insofar as they are known.

A Patient's Bill of Rights was first adopted by the American Hospital Association in 1973.

This revision was approved by the AHA Board of Trustees on October 21, 1992.

American Hospital Association, October 21, 1992 http://www.patienttalk. info/AHA-Patient_Bill_of_ Rights.htm

3. The patient has the right to make decisions about the plan of care prior to and during the course of treatment and to refuse a recommended treatment or plan of care to the extent permitted by law and hospital policy and to be informed of the medical consequences of this action. In case of such refusal, the patient is entitled to other appropriate care and services that the hospital provides or transfer to another hospital. The hospital should notify patients of any policy that might affect patient choice within the institution.

4. The patient has the right to have an advance directive (such as a living will, healthcare proxy, or durable power of attorney for healthcare) concerning treatment or designating a surrogate decision maker with the expectation that the hospital will honor the intent of that directive to the extent permitted by law and hospital policy.

    Healthcare institutions must advise patients of their rights under state law and hospital policy to make informed medical choices, ask if the patient has an advance directive, and include that information in patient records. The patient has the right to timely information about hospital policy that may limit its ability to implement fully a legally valid advance directive.

5. The patient has the right to every consideration of privacy. Case discussion, consultation, examination, and treatment should be conducted so as to protect each patient's privacy.

6. The patient has the right to expect that all communications and records pertaining to his/her care will be treated as confidential by the hospital, except in cases such as suspected abuse and public health hazards when reporting is permitted or required by law. The patient has the right to expect that the hospital will emphasize the confidentiality of this information when it releases it to any other parties entitled to review information in these records.

7. The patient has the right to review the records pertaining to his/her medical care and to have the information explained or interpreted as necessary, except when restricted by law.

8. The patient has the right to expect that, within its capacity and policies, a hospital will make reasonable response to the request of a patient for appropriate and medically indicated care and services. The hospital must provide evaluation, service, and/or referral as indicated by the urgency of the case. When medically appropriate and legally permissible, or when a patient has so requested, a patient may be transferred to another facility. The institution to which the patient is to be transferred must first have accepted the patient for transfer. The patient must also have the benefit of complete information and explanation concerning the need for, risks, benefits, and alternatives to such a transfer.

9. The patient has the right to ask and be informed of the existence of business relationships among the hospital, educational institutions, other healthcare providers, or payers that may influence the patient's treatment and care.

10. The patient has the right to consent to or decline to participate in proposed research studies or human experimentation affecting care and treatment or requiring direct patient involvement, and to have those studies fully explained prior to consent. A patient who declines to participate in research or experimentation is entitled to the most effective care that the hospital can otherwise provide.

11. The patient has the right to expect reasonable continuity of care when appropriate and to be informed by physicians and other caregivers of available and realistic patient care options when hospital care is no longer appropriate.

12. The patient has the right to be informed of hospital policies and practices that relate to patient care, treatment, and responsibilities. The patient has the right to be informed of available resources for resolving disputes, grievances, and conflicts, such as ethics committees, patient representatives, or other mechanisms available in the institution. The patient has the right to be informed of the hospital's charges for services and available payment methods.

The collaborative nature of healthcare requires that patients, or their families/surrogates, participate in their care. The effectiveness of care and patient satisfaction with the course of treatment depend, in part, on the patient fulfilling certain responsibilities. Patients are responsible for providing information about past illnesses, hospitalizations, medications, and other matters related to health status. To participate effectively in decision making, patients must be encouraged to take responsibility for requesting additional information or clarification about their health status or treatment when they do not fully understand information and instructions. Patients are also responsible for ensuring that the healthcare institution has a copy of their written advance directive if they have one. Patients are responsible for informing their physicians and other caregivers if they anticipate problems in following prescribed treatment.

Patients should also be aware of the hospital's obligation to be reasonably efficient and equitable in providing care to other patients and the community. The hospital's rules and regulations are designed to help the hospital meet this obligation. Patients and their families are responsible for making reasonable accommodations to the needs of the hospital, other patients, medical staff, and hospital employees. Patients are responsible for providing necessary information for insurance claims and for working with the hospital to make payment arrangements, when necessary.

A person's health depends on much more than healthcare services. Patients are responsible for recognizing the impact of their lifestyle on their personal health.

CONCLUSION

Hospitals have many functions to perform, including the enhancement of health status, health promotion, and the prevention and treatment of injury and disease; the immediate and ongoing care and rehabilitation of patients; the education of health professionals, patients, and the community; and research. All these activities must be conducted with an overriding concern for the values and dignity of patients.

Section 2
Competencies for Safe Patient Care

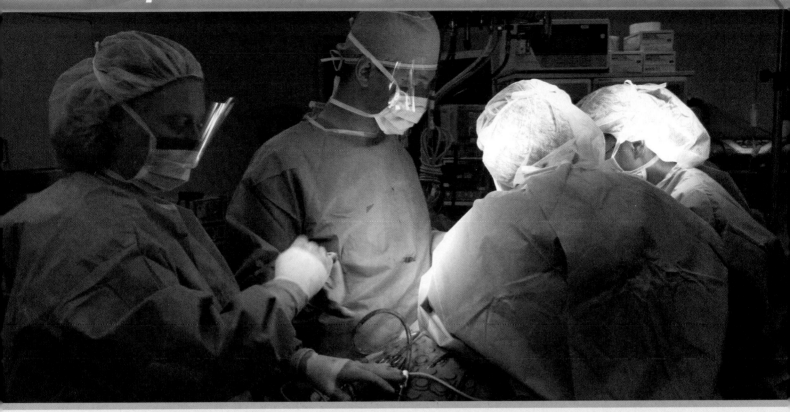

CHAPTER **5**

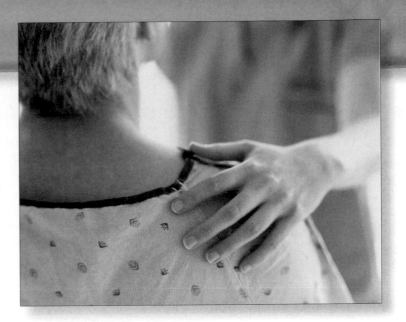

Preparation of the Patient for the Procedure:
Physical, Psychological, and Emotional Considerations

Charlotte Dorsey

INTRODUCTION

Over the past decades, preparation of the operative patient has drastically changed. At one time, the patient was admitted to the healthcare facility one to two days before the procedure during which time the preprocedure assessment and testing were completed. Today, the patient is admitted the day of the operative or invasive procedure, or the procedure is performed on an outpatient basis. Preprocedure preparation is critical to positive patient outcomes.

Preparing the patient for an operative or invasive procedure refers to the activities done by the registered nurse (RN) before the procedure to make the patient physically, psychologically, and emotionally ready for the procedure. The extent of involvement of the nurse in preparing the patient for the procedure depends on the practice expectations delineated in the position description. Responsibilities may include one or more of the following duties: admitting the patient, collecting laboratory specimens, obtaining the consent for treatment, and providing any ordered preprocedure treatment or care. Nurses providing these services may also provide patient care during and after the procedure.

MEASURABLE CRITERIA

The nurse demonstrates competency to prepare the patient for an operative or invasive procedure by:

- Facilitating patient admission to the healthcare facility;
- Identifying existing alterations in health status that contribute to the patient's risk for adverse outcomes before, during, and after the operative or invasive procedure;

Chapter Contents

RN
Registered
Nurse

- Identifying alterations in psychosocial and emotional health status; and
- Facilitating preprocedure care.

FACILITATING ADMISSION TO THE HEALTHCARE FACILITY

The physician, advanced practice nurse, office nurse, or physician's secretary may schedule the procedure with the hospital or healthcare facility. When scheduling the procedure, provide the clerk or secretary posting the case with the following information:

- patient's full name, age, date of birth, gender;
- physician's name;
- date and time of the procedure;
- planned procedure;
- preprocedure diagnosis;
- insurance information;
- preauthorization number from any insurance provider; and
- any special instrumentation, supplies, or equipment needed.

Operative and invasive procedure case posting varies by institution. In some institutions, the posting clerk obtains all the information noted above; in others, admitting personnel obtain information about insurance and preauthorization numbers. After posting the case, tell the patient when to report to the facility for pre-admission assessment and testing, as well as on the day of the operative or invasive procedure. Tell the patient to wear comfortable, loose-fitting clothing, leave valuables at home, and bring all home prescription medications to the healthcare facility when admitted. If an outpatient procedure is scheduled, the patient should ingest nothing by mouth after midnight or according to the protocol established by the anesthesia department. If the patient is a parent, instruct him or her to make plans for child care the day of the procedure. The patient should understand the requirement that after receiving sedation or anesthesia, he/she must be discharged in the company of a responsible, designated adult (The Joint Commission, 2007).

IDENTIFYING EXISTING ALTERATIONS IN HEALTH STATUS THAT CONTRIBUTE TO THE PATIENT'S RISK FOR ADVERSE OUTCOMES

Physical Assessment

The physical assessment evaluates the patient's health status through a health history and physical examination. The assessment is based on clinical and laboratory data, the medical history, and the patient's account of signs and symptoms (Taber's®, 2005). The physician,[1] anesthesia provider, and nurse use the assessment data. The physician uses the assessment data to diagnose acute or chronic medical conditions that may affect the performance of the procedure and to establish the patient's risk of postprocedure complications. The anesthesia provider uses the assessment data to formulate the anesthetic plan and determine the patient's anesthetic risk. Assessment data are used by the nurse to diagnose actual or potential alterations in health that may affect the patient during the operative and invasive procedure period. Careful evaluation and examination of major systems give the nurse an indication of the physical status of the patient. The nurse should be familiar with major symptom patterns and the probable changes in organ pathology causing the symptoms. **Table 5.1** outlines a sample preprocedure screening protocol.

Collecting Baseline Vital Data

Begin the assessment by introducing yourself to the patient and explaining the purpose of the assessment. Establish contact with the patient by touching or shaking the patient's hand during the introduction. This helps to establish rapport and puts the patient at ease. Continue contact by taking vital signs: pulse, temperature, blood pressure, and respirations. **Table 5.2** lists abnormal findings for vital signs, possible indications, and possible postprocedure complications. Communicate abnormal vital signs to the physician and the anesthesia provider. Postponement of the procedure may be necessary to treat the underlying problem associated with an abnormal vital sign.

Determine the patient's weight and height. If measurements are recorded in pounds and inches, also note the metric equivalents. Record the patient's chronological age. If the patient is younger than 2 years of age, record the age in months. An accurate weight is critical for calculating medication dosage, especially for pediatric patients. Both weight and height help determine the patient's risk for adverse outcomes during the operative and invasive procedure period.

Operative and Invasive Procedure History

Ask the patient about prior stays in healthcare facilities; obtain the date and reasons for the stays. Previous medical records, if available, should be obtained and included in the patient's chart. Determine whether the patient underwent operative and invasive procedures in the past. Obtain the dates of the past procedures and have the patient explain why the procedures were done. Ask the patient to describe the outcomes of past procedures, the types of anesthesia that were used, and whether there were any reactions to or complications from the anesthetics.

Laboratory and Diagnostic Studies

The extent and type of laboratory and diagnostic studies depend on a multitude of factors such as the patient's condition and medical diagnosis, the type of operative or invasive procedure planned, the physician's preference, and facility policy. Common laboratory and diagnostic studies include various blood studies, serological and microbiological studies, urinalysis, chest radiographs, electrocardiography, and other relevant studies.

Blood Studies

Common blood tests ordered for patients undergoing operative and invasive procedures are listed in **Table 5.3**. During any acute infection, the white blood cell count (WBC) is likely to be elevated. If the procedure is planned to treat an infectious condition (eg, acute appendicitis), an elevated WBC is not a contraindication to the procedure. On the other hand, high WBCs in patients undergoing elective

WBC
White Blood Cell count

Table 5.1	**Preprocedure Screening Protocol**

Recommended guidelines for asymptomatic patients. Additional test for symptomatic patients should be according to the physician.

Test	Type of Patient
History and Physical (*Valid for 30 days*)	☐ All Patients
HBG/HCT (*Valid 30 days if normal*)	☐ Male patients age 65 and older ☐ Female patients age 10 and older ☐ Pediatric patients less than 6 months ☐ Patients that fit the following criteria: recent autologous blood donation; surgical procedures which have the potential for significant blood loss; history of anemia; polycythemia; cancer; abnormal bleeding; renal disease; use of anticoagulants
ECG (*Valid for 1 year if normal; Valid for 1 month if abnormal, with cardiac clearance*)	☐ Age 50+ ☐ Any age with chest pain ☐ History of cardiac disease ☐ Treated for hypertension ☐ Morbid obesity ☐ History of congestive heart failure ☐ Diabetic patients
Chest X-Ray	☐ New onset of respiratory symptoms including dyspnea, orthopnea, wheezing, or hemoptysis ☐ Exacerbation of chronic pulmonary disease processes, including obstructive or reactive airway disease, or exacerbation of congestive heart failure within 2 months of surgical date (this would include increased use of medication) ☐ Pneumonia within 2 months of the planned surgical procedure ☐ Pulse oximetry of <92% on room air ☐ Patient that smokes ☐ Cardio-thoracic surgical patients should have chest x-ray per surgeons order
Basic Metabolic Panel (carbon dioxide, chloride, creatinine, glucose, potassium, sodium, urea nitrogen, calcium) (*Valid for 30 days*)	☐ Ages 65+ ☐ Diabetic patients ☐ Dialysis patient—post hemodialysis ☐ Patient on diuretics
Pregnancy Test	☐ Per physician order or guided by clinical history, last menstrual period or uncertain pregnancy history
Type and Screen	☐ Per physician order or clinical pathway
C-Spine Flexion/Extension X-rays	☐ Severe rheumatoid arthritis patient ☐ Being treated with more than NSAIDS ☐ Has had a joint replacement because of rheumatoid arthritis

Modified from Piedmont Hospital's Department of Anesthesia Protocols 2007, Piedmont, Georgia.

Table 5.2	Assessing Alterations in Vital Signs			
Vital Sign	**Normal Finding**	**Abnormal Finding**	**Possible Indication**	**Possible Postprocedure Complication**
Temperature	98.6°F (37°C)	Fever *temperature >101°F [38.3°C] in an adult*	☐ Dehydration (when accompanied by decreased skin turgor) ☐ Infection	☐ Fluid imbalance ☐ Shock ☐ Systemic infection ☐ Wound infection, dehiscence, or evisceration
Pulse	60–100 *beats per minute in a regular and strong pattern*	Tachycardia *>100 beats per minute*	☐ Anemia ☐ Dehydration ☐ Fever ☐ Hypoxia ☐ Pain ☐ Shock	☐ Anesthetic complications ☐ Cardiac arrhythmias ☐ Poor tissue perfusion ☐ Renal failure ☐ Shock ☐ Vascular collapse
		Bradycardia *<60 beats per minute*	☐ Drug effects (digitalis) ☐ Head injury ☐ Spinal injury	☐ Cardiac arrest ☐ Increased intracranial pressure ☐ Spinal shock
Respiration	12–20 *breaths per minute*	Tachypnea *>24 breaths per minute*	☐ Atelectasis ☐ Infection ☐ Pain or anxiety ☐ Pleurisy ☐ Pneumonia ☐ Renal failure	☐ Anesthetic complications ☐ Atelectasis ☐ Pneumonia ☐ Tissue hypoxia
		Bradypnea *<10 breaths per minute*	☐ Brain lesion ☐ Respiratory center depression	☐ Same as Tachypnea
Blood Pressure	Systolic *100–130 mm Hg*	Hypotension *<90 mm Hg systolic*	☐ Hemorrhage ☐ Myocardial infarction ☐ Shock ☐ Spinal injury	☐ Poor tissue perfusion ☐ Renal failure ☐ Shock ☐ Vasodilation
	Diastolic *60–80 mm Hg*	Hypertension *>140 mm Hg systolic and/or 90 mm Hg diastolic*	☐ Anxiety or pain ☐ Coronary artery disease ☐ Renal disease	☐ Hemorrhage ☐ Myocardial infarction ☐ Stroke

Adapted from Harkreader, Hogan, and Thobaben (2007). *Fundamentals of Nursing: Caring and Clinical Judgment;* and Ignatavicius and Workman (2006). *Medical-Surgical Nursing: Critical Thinking for Collaborative Care.*

procedures may be indicative of an unsuspected inflammatory process that could contraindicate the procedures. For example, an acute pneumonitis suspected on the basis of an elevated WBC and confirmed by chest radiograph necessitates cancellation of an elective procedure. Extremely high WBCs are rarely caused by infection

Table 5.3	**Common Preprocedure Blood Tests**		
		Abnormal Findings	
Test	**Normal Range**	**Increase**	**Decrease**
Hemoglobin	Females: 12–16g/dL Males: 14–18 g/dL		☐ Anemia ☐ Excessive blood loss
Hematocrit	Females: 37–47% Males: 42–52%	☐ Dehydration (hemoconcentration)	☐ Anemia ☐ Excessive blood loss
Potassium	3.5–5.0 mEq/L	☐ Dehydration ☐ Renal failure ☐ Acidosis ☐ Cellular/tissue damage ☐ Hemolysis of the specimen	☐ NPO status with inadequate potassium replacement ☐ Excessive use of non-potassium-sparing diuretics ☐ Vomiting ☐ Malnutrition ☐ Diarrhea ☐ Alkalosis
Sodium	135–145 mEq/L	☐ Cardiac or renal failure ☐ Hypertension ☐ Excessive amounts of IV normal saline ☐ Edema ☐ Dehydration	☐ Nasogastric drainage ☐ Vomiting ☐ Diarrhea ☐ Excessive use of laxatives or diuretics ☐ Excessive amounts of IV fluids containing water
Chloride	98–106 mEq/L	☐ Respiratory alkalosis ☐ Dehydration ☐ Renal failure ☐ Excessive amounts of NaCl IV fluids	☐ Excessive nasogastric drainage ☐ Vomiting ☐ Excessive use of diuretics ☐ Diarrhea
Carbon dioxide	23–30 mEq/L	☐ Chronic pulmonary disease ☐ Intestinal obstruction ☐ Vomiting or nasogastric suctioning ☐ Metabolic alkalosis	☐ Hyperventilation ☐ Diabetic ketoacidosis ☐ Diarrhea ☐ Lactic acidosis ☐ Renal failure ☐ Salicylate toxicity
Glucose (fasting)	70–105 mg/dL	☐ Hyperglycemia ☐ Excessive amounts of glucose in IV fluids ☐ Stress ☐ Steroid use ☐ Pancreatic or hepatic disease	☐ Hypoglycemia ☐ Excess insulin

White blood cell count	5000–10,000 cells/mm^3	☐ Infection ☐ Inflammation ☐ Autoimmune disorders ☐ Leukemia	☐ Prolonged infection ☐ Bone marrow suppression
Creatinine	0.6–1.2 mg/dL	☐ Renal damage ☐ Renal insufficiency ☐ Acute renal failure ☐ Chronic renal failure ☐ End-stage renal disease	☐ Atrophy of muscle tissue
Blood urea nitrogen (BUN)	10–20 mg/dL	☐ Dehydration ☐ Renal failure ☐ Excessive protein in diet ☐ Liver failure	☐ Overhydration ☐ Malnutrition
Prothrombin time (PT)	11–12.5 sec	☐ Coagulation defect	☐ Coagulation disorder, such as thrombophlebitis or pulmonary embolus
Partial thromboplastin time (PTT)	30–40 sec	☐ Coagulation defect ☐ Anticoagulant therapy (heparin) ☐ Liver disease	☐ Coagulation disorder, such as thrombophlebitis or pulmonary embolus ☐ Extensive cancer

Adapted from Harkreader, Hogan, and Thobaben (2007). *Fundamentals of Nursing: Caring and Clinical Judgment;* and Ignatavicius and Workman (2006). *Medical-Surgical Nursing: Critical Thinking for Collaborative Care.*

alone and may suggest a leukemia condition. Unusually low WBCs might suggest bone marrow depression, which also contraindicates an elective procedure.

Use the hematocrit or hemoglobin studies to assess the status of the patient's blood volume. An abnormal hematocrit reading, for example, may reveal an unsuspected anemia and force delay of the procedure. If an anemic state is suspected, as in gastrointestinal bleeding, the hematocrit level aids in determining the need for blood replacement before the procedure.

A fasting blood glucose study is usually ordered for patients suspected of having diabetes or with a family history of diabetes. A high fasting blood glucose level is suggestive of diabetes mellitus and necessitates further study.

Elevated blood urea nitrogen and creatinine levels may suggest poor renal function and be predictive of renal failure after the procedure.

Serological Studies

Serological blood determinations reflect heart and thyroid alterations, as well as the presence of syphilis and infectious mononucleosis.

Microbiological Studies

Sputum, urine, blood, spinal fluid, and stool cultures, as well as cultures in the throat, eye, ear, nasopharyngeal, vaginal, and urethral areas, are taken to identify pathogens and specific microorganisms.

Urinalysis

Urinalysis is an extremely important clearance test before any operative or invasive procedure. Much can be learned about the status of the kidneys, which infrequently remain asymptomatic in serious renal disease. When a urine specimen is collected, a clean and freshly voided urine specimen must be sent to the laboratory immediately. The diagnostic value of specimens decreases with the passage of time.

Use the urinalysis to determine several important things about the patient's health status. Red or white blood cells in the urine may suggest renal or bladder tumors, as well as chronic or acute infections of the urinary system. Casts, which develop from cast-off debris from various sites in the urinary tract, may, depending on their type and number, indicate severe chronic renal disease. An excessive spillage of protein into the urine is frequently associated with poor renal function secondary to chronic or acute renal disease. Spillage of glucose into the urine may be the first clue to the presence of a diabetic state. A low specific gravity (less than 1.01) may indicate poor renal function, in which the kidney is unable to concentrate its urine; a high specific gravity (greater than 1.025) may indicate a dehydrated state. This test often has to be repeated several times to validate the concentrating ability of the kidney. See **Table 5.4** for common preprocedure urine chemistry values.

Chest Radiography

Chest radiographs screen patients for diseases such as carcinoma, tuberculosis, and heart disease. The films provide information on the heart's position, the extent

Table 5.4	Common Preprocedure Urine Chemistry Values	
Characteristics/ Component	**Normal Finding**	**Significance of Abnormal Finding**
Color	☐ Pale yellow	☐ Dark amber indicates concentrated urine ☐ Pale yellow indicates dilute urine ☐ Dark red or brown indicated blood in the urine; brown also may indicate increased urinary bilirubin level ☐ Other color changes may result from diet or medications from many different angles
Odor	☐ Specific aromatic odor, similar to that of ammonia	☐ Foul smell indicates possible infection and/or dehydration
Turbidity	☐ Clear	☐ Cloudy urine indicates infection or sediment
Specific gravity	☐ Usually 1.015–1.025 ☐ Possible range: 1.01–1.03	☐ Changes reflect a disturbance in the concentrating and diluting function of the tubules; Specific gravity may become fixed in renal insufficiency
pH	☐ 6; possible range: 4.6–8	☐ Changes are caused by diet, medications, infection, acid-base imbalance, and altered renal function

Glucose	☐ None or <15 mg/dL	☐ Presence may indicate decreased tubular reabsorption capacity or hyperglycemia that exceeds this capacity
Ketones	☐ None	☐ Presence reflects incomplete metabolism of fatty acids, as in diabetes mellitus
Protein	☐ 2–8 mg/100 mL	☐ Increased levels may indicate stress infection, strenuous exercise, or glomerular disorders
Red blood cells	☐ 1 or 2 per high-power field	☐ Increased levels are normal with indwelling or intermittent catheterization or menses, but may reflect tumor, stones, or glomerular disorders
White blood cells	☐ 1 to 3 per high-power field	☐ Increased levels may indicate infectious or inflammatory processes
Bilirubin	☐ None	☐ Presence suggests hepatic or biliary disease or obstruction
Casts	☐ A few or none, composed of red or white blood cells, protein, or tubular cell casts	☐ Increased levels indicate presence of bacteria or protein, which is seen in severe renal disease
Crystals	☐ None	☐ Presence of normal and/or abnormal crystals may indicate that the specimen has been allowed to stand
Bacteria	☐ <1,000 colonies/mL	☐ Increased levels indicate need for urine culture to determine the presence of urinary tract infection
Creatinine (clearance)	☐ 0.8–2 g/24 hours ☐ Males: 1–2 g/24 hours ☐ Females: 0.6–1.8 g/24 hours	☐ Increased levels indicate glomerular dysfunction caused by renal disease, shock, or hypovolemia
Urea nitrogen	☐ 6–17 g/24 hours	☐ Increase levels commonly result from high-protein diet, dehydration, trauma, or sepsis
Sodium	☐ 40–180 mEq/24 hours	☐ Decreased levels are seen with hemorrhage, shock, and hyperaldosteronism ☐ Increase levels are common with diuretic therapy, excessive salt intake, and hypokalemia
Chloride	☐ 110–254 mEq/24 hours	☐ Decreased levels are seen with certain renal diseases
Calcium	☐ 50–300 mg/24 hours	☐ Increased levels are commonly seen with calcium renal stones and hypercalcemia ☐ Decreased levels indicate hypocalcemia

5

Adapted from Ignatavicius, D. and Workman, M. L. (2006). *Medical-Surgical Nursing: Critical Thinking for Collaborative Care.* 5th ed. Elsevier Saunders, St. Louis.

of calcium deposits (calcification), and the size of the chambers and great vessels. In addition, chest radiographs reflect alterations in the chest wall, the pleural spaces, the tracheobronchial tract, and the diaphragm. The films are used to determine the location of central venous pressure catheters, arterial catheters, pacemaker wires, and so on. Unsuspected acute and chronic pulmonary problems may manifest themselves only on chest radiographs. However, chest radiographs are not warranted for any asymptomatic patient who is less than 75 years of age and free of risk factors (Roizen, 2005).

Electrocardiography

ECGs
Electrocardiograms

Electrocardiograms (ECGs) reflect the heart's electrical activity. Alterations in the normal EGG pattern may indicate previous cardiac ischemia or infarction. A normal ECG does not eliminate the possibility of cardiac pathological changes because the heart's muscle strength is not measured in this study. For patients with known cardiac disease, a 12-lead ECG is often obtained to thoroughly evaluate electrical impulses in the heart. The 12-lead ECG also detects the presence of right ventricular infarction and the effects of chemical imbalances or drug therapy on cardiac function. **Figure 5.1** shows a normal ECG pattern and examples of ECG alterations that the nurse might observe during the operative or invasive procedure period. Every facility will have a policy on the medical necessity of performing a preprocedure ECG. In some cases, ECG exams are limited to patients undergoing cardiac procedures who have risk factors related to heart disease—with the result that anesthesiologists cannot obtain routine EKGs based solely on the patient's age (Bierstien, 2000). Further, the American Society of Anesthesiologists' (ASA) "Practice Advisory for Preanesthesia Evaluation" outlines the following (Bierstein, 2002):

ASA
American Society of
Anesthesiologists

> "The Task Force agrees with the consultants and ASA members that preoperative tests should not be ordered routinely. The Task Force agrees that preoperative tests may be ordered, required or performed on a selective basis for purposes of guiding or optimizing perioperative management. The indications for such testing should be documented and based on information obtained from medical records, patient interview, physical examination and type and invasiveness of the planned procedure."

Other Relevant Studies

IV
Intravenous

MRI
Magnetic Resonance
Imaging

These include radiological studies such as angiography and cholangiography; intravenous (IV) pyelography; myelography; computed tomography; magnetic resonance imaging (MRI); ultrasonography; biopsies and aspirations, such as liver biopsy and bone marrow aspiration; and endoscopic procedures, such as colonoscopy, esophagoscopy, and duodenoscopy.

The preprocedure tests performed depend on the patient, planned procedure, facility/anesthesia protocol, and physician preference. The nurse, physician, and anesthesia provider may collaborate to determine which laboratory and diagnostic studies are ordered. The preadmission testing nurse should review all test results and verify that they are within normal ranges. Abnormal findings are reported to the physician and the anesthesia provider.

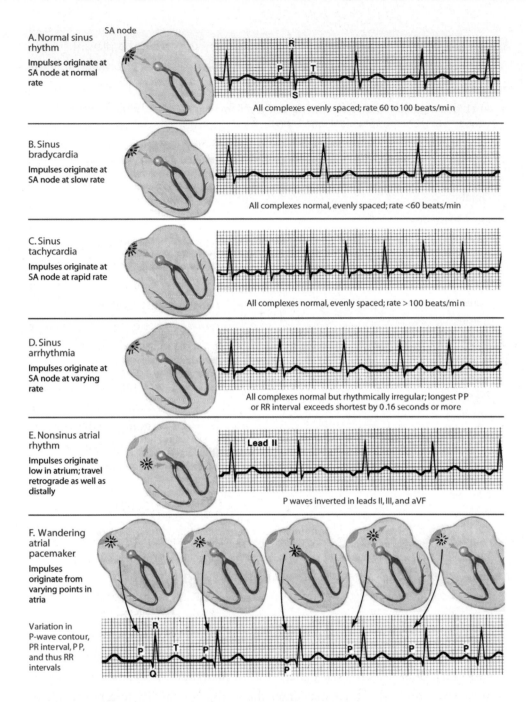

Figure 5.1

Normal ECG pattern and examples of ECG alterations.

A. Normal sinus rhythm

Impulses originate at SA node at normal rate

SA node

All complexes evenly spaced; rate 60 to 100 beats/min

B. Sinus bradycardia

Impulses originate at SA node at slow rate

All complexes normal, evenly spaced; rate <60 beats/min

C. Sinus tachycardia

Impulses originate at SA node at rapid rate

All complexes normal, evenly spaced; rate >100 beats/min

D. Sinus arrhythmia

Impulses originate at SA node at varying rate

All complexes normal but rhythmically irregular; longest PP or RR interval exceeds shortest by 0.16 seconds or more

E. Nonsinus atrial rhythm

Impulses originate low in atrium; travel retrograde as well as distally

Lead II

P waves inverted in leads II, III, and aVF

F. Wandering atrial pacemaker

Impulses originate from varying points in atria

Variation in P-wave contour, PR interval, PP, and thus RR intervals

Patient Allergies and Hypersensitivity Reactions

Ask the patient about allergies or hypersensitivity reactions to adhesives, radio-contrast media, opiates, antibiotics, local anesthetics, and other drugs. If the patient reports allergies or hypersensitivity reactions to food or chemical substances, determine which types of foods or substances and the type of reaction experienced. Note in the record and communicate to the anesthesia provider a history of anaphylaxis, asthma, or other respiratory difficulties related to the presence of allergens, toxins, or antigens. **Table 5.5** lists the most common agents that cause anaphylaxis.

Nutritional Status

Proper assessment of the nutritional status of the patient is an important aspect of care before the procedure. The patient may have an acute or chronic nutritional

Table 5.5	Common Agents That Cause Anaphylaxis

Drugs

☐ Antibiotics: penicillin, cephalosporins, tetracycline, sulfonamides, streptomycin, vancomycin, chloramphenicol, and others

☐ Adrenocorticotropic hormone, insulin, vasopressin, protamine

☐ Allergen extracts, muscle relaxants, hydrocortisone, vaccines

☐ Lidocaine, procaine, marcaine

☐ Opiates

Foreign Proteins

☐ Whole blood, cryoprecipitate, immune serum globulin

☐ Radiocontrast media

Food

☐ Bananas

☐ Berries

☐ Eggs

☐ Grains

☐ Legumes, nuts

☐ Preservatives

☐ Shellfish

Insects/Animals

☐ Bees

☐ Fire ants

☐ Hornets

☐ Wasps

Adapted from Ignatavicius, D. and Workman, M. L. (2006). *Medical-Surgical Nursing: Critical Thinking for Collaborative Care.* 5th ed. Elsevier Saunders, St. Louis

defect. The signs of depletion may be obvious or concealed. They may result from inadequate intake, absorption, or use of nutrients. Absence of teeth should alert the nurse to nutritional defects. Any patient with a malignancy, chronic infection, or chronic gastrointestinal disease may enter the healthcare facility in a poor state of nutrition. Under these conditions, the procedure is extremely hazardous because wounds do not heal properly, anesthesia is poorly tolerated by the liver, the kidneys fail to excrete toxins adequately, and blood-clotting mechanisms fail. Restoration of adequate nutritional status is frequently necessary to reduce the operative or invasive procedure risk. High-protein, high-carbohydrate diets are sometimes supplemented by enteral nutrition. If oral intake is impossible, as in patients with obstructing carcinoma of the esophagus, a feeding via jejunostomy may be necessary before a major procedure.

During the nutritional assessment, evaluate the patient's fluid and electrolyte status. Determine the presence of acute gastrointestinal disorders, such as vomiting and diarrhea, which may result in a serious imbalance of fluids and electrolytes.

A fluid and electrolyte imbalance must be corrected before the procedure. Accurate measurements of fluid intake and output must be assessed and recorded to help the physician decide on future allowances for fluids, as well as the patient's response to those already administered.

Determine whether the patient has had a high gas (methane)-producing diet before the procedure. The passage of flatus by the patient during a procedure could result in the accumulation of methane under drapes. In such cases, care must be exercised when electrosurgery is used. See Chapter 14 for a description of safety precautions that should be implemented when electrosurgery is used during an operative or invasive procedure.

INTEGUMENTARY SYSTEM

History

The integumentary system is the external covering of the body composed of the skin, hair, and nails. The skin is the largest organ of the body. Skin serves as a barrier to organisms, cushions and protects the deeper tissues, helps to regulate body temperature and maintains fluid and electrolyte balance (Ignatavicius & Workman, 2006).

Determine whether the patient's family has a chronic tendency toward skin disorders. Ask whether there have been recent complaints of skin problems. When assessing the patient for allergies or reactions to toxic substances, determine whether there have been skin reactions. Ask the patient about his or her occupation and whether he or she is exposed to irritants. Review the nutritional assessment data. If the patient has existing skin problems, determine when the problems began. If a skin problem exists, determine whether it is associated with itching, burning, stinging, numbness, pain, fever, nausea and vomiting, diarrhea, sore throat, cold, stiff neck, exposure to new foods, exposure to new soaps or cosmetics, exposure to new clothing or bed linens, or stressful situations. Describe what makes the skin problem worse and what makes it better (Ignatavicius & Workman, 2006).

Physical Examination

Perform the skin inspection in a well-lit room. During the skin examination, inspect each skin surface to include the scalp, the hair, the nails, and the mucous membranes. Observe the skin's color, temperature, and texture (see **Table 5.7**). Check the patient's skin for lesions. The initial skin reaction to a problem is called a *primary lesion,* and consists of an alteration in one of the structural components of the skin. A *secondary lesion* results with the normal progression of the disease that causes the primary lesion or the therapeutic intervention. For example, a primary lesion may consist of a contact dermatitis with vesicles. As the vesicles are disrupted because of scratching, the scrims exudate dries and a crust forms, resulting in the secondary lesion. Check the patient's nails (see **Table 5.6**).

Look for signs of edema (see **Table 5.7**). Edematous tissue appears shiny, taut, and paler than uninvolved skin. While looking for edema, check skin elasticity. Using moderate pressure, press the tip of the index finger against edematous tissue to determine the degree of indentation or pitting. Localized edema may be caused by inflammatory

Table 5.6	Assessing Nail Color	
Alteration	**Clinical Findings**	**Significance**
White	Horizontal white banding or areas of opacity Generalized pallor nail beds	☐ Chronic hepatic or renal disease ☐ Shock ☐ Anemia ☐ Early atherosclerotic changes (toenails) ☐ Myocardial infarction
Yellow-brown	Diffuse yellow to brown discoloration	☐ Jaundice ☐ Peripheral lymphedema ☐ Bacterial or fungal infections of the nail ☐ Psoriasis ☐ Diabetes ☐ Cardiac failure ☐ Staining from tobacco, nail polish, or dyes ☐ Long-term Tetracycline therapy
Red	Thin, dark-red vertical lines 1–3 mm long (splinter hemorrhages)	☐ Bacterial endocarditis ☐ Trichinosis ☐ Trauma to the nail bed ☐ Normal finding in some patients
Blue	Diffuse blue discoloration that blanches with pressure	☐ Respiratory failure ☐ Methemoglobinuria ☐ Venous stasis disease (toenails)

Adapted from Ignatavicius, D. and Workman, M. L. (2006). *Medical-Surgical Nursing: Critical Thinking for Collaborative Care.* 5th ed. Elsevier Saunders, St. Louis.

response and is usually confined to an area of injury. Dependent or pitting edema may be caused by fluid and electrolyte imbalance and by venous and cardiac insufficiency. Common sites of dependent or pitting edema are found on the dorsum of the foot and medial aspect of the ankle in ambulatory patients and on the buttocks, sacrum, and lower back of bedridden patients. An endocrine imbalance may cause nonpitting edema, which is generalized by more easily seen over the tibia. Pitting edema is evaluated by of scale of 1+ to 4+ to describe the severity of the edema. The nurse presses a finger into the area for 5 seconds. After releasing the pressure, note the depth of the indentation. The scale is 1+ is mild or 2mm indentation, 2+ is 4mm indentation, 3+ is 6mm indentation and 4+ is 8mm indentation. Assess the patient for cold or pale feet, absent or diminished peripheral pulses, cyanosis or flushing of the extremities, and leg cramps on walking (Harkreander, Hogan, & Thobaben, 2007).

Examine the patient's skin for moisture content (see **Table 5.7**). Autonomic nervous system stimulation may cause an increase in moisture. Look for increased

Table 5.7	Assessing the Integument System		
Alteration	**Cause**	**Location**	**Significance**
White color (pallor)	Decreased hemoglobin level Decreased blood flow to the skin (vasoconstriction)	Conjunctivae Mucous membranes Nail beds Palms and soles Lips	Anemia Shock or blood loss Chronic vascular compromise Sudden emotional upset Edema
Yellow-orange color	Increased total serum bilirubin level (jaundice)	Generalized Mucous membranes Sclera	Increased hemolysis of red blood cells Liver disorders
	Increased serum carotene level (carotenernia)	Perioral Palms and soles Absent in sclera and mucous membranes	Increased ingestion of carotene-containing foods Pregnancy Thyroid deficiency Diabetes
	Increased pigmentation	Generalized Absent in sclera and mucous membranes	Chronic renal failure (uremia)
Red color (erythema)	Increased blood flow to the skin (vasodilatation)	Generalized	Generalized inflammation
		Localized	Localized inflammation (sunburn, cellulites, trauma, and rashes)
		Face, cheeks, nose, upper chest	Fever; increased alcohol intake
		Area of exposure	Exposure to cold
Blue color	Increase in deoxygenated blood (cyanosis)	Nail beds Mucous membranes Generalized	Cardiopulmonary disease Methemoglobinemia
Reddish blue color	Increased overall amount of hemoglobin	Generalized	Polycythemia vera
	Decreased peripheral circulation	Distal extremities, nose	Inadequate tissue perfusion

5

Brown	Increased melanin production	Localized (to area of involvement)	Chronic inflammation
		Pressure points, areolae, palmar creases, and genitalia	Exposure to sunlight Addison's disease
		Face, areolae, vulva, and linea nigrae	Pregnancy; oral contraceptives
	Melanin and hemosiderin deposits bronze or grayish tan color)	Distal lower extremities	Chronic venous stasis
		Exposed areas or generalized	Hemochromatosis
Localized edema	Inflammatory response	Area of injury or involvement	Trauma
Dependent or pitting edema	Fluid and electrolyte imbalance Venous and cardiac insufficiency	Ambulatory—dorsum of foot and medial ankle Bedridden—buttocks, sacrum, and lower back	Congestive heart failure Renal disease Hepatic cirrhosis Venous thrombosis
Nonpitting edema	Endocrine imbalance	Generalized, but more easily seen over the tibia	Hypothyroidism (myxoedema)
Increased moisture	Autonomic nervous system stimulation	Face, axillae, skin folds, palms, and soles	Fever, anxiety, activity Hyperthyroidism
Decreased moisture	Dehydration Endocrine imbalance	Buccal mucous membranes with progressive involvement of other skin surfaces	Fluid loss Postmenopausal status Hypothyroidism Normal aging
Increased temperature	Increased blood flow to the skin	Generalized Localized	Fever, hypermetabolic states Inflammation
Decreased temperature	Decreased blood flow to the skin	Generalized	Impending shock, sepsis, anxiety Hypothyroidism
		Localized	Interference with vascular flow
Decrease turgor	Decreased elasticity of the dermis (tenting when pinched)	Abdomen, forehead, or radial aspect of the wrist	Severe dehydration Sudden, severe weight loss Normal aging

Roughness or thickness	Irritation, friction	Pressure points (soles, palms, and elbows)	Calluses Chronic eczema Atopic skin diseases
	Sun damage	Areas of sun exposure	Normal aging
	Excessive collagen production	Localized or generalized	Scleroderma Keloids
Softness or smoothness	Endocrine disturbances	Generalized	Hyperthyroidism

Adapted from Ignatavicius, D. and Workman, M. L. (2006). *Medical-Surgical Nursing: Critical Thinking for Collaborative Care.* 5th ed. Elsevier Saunders, St. Louis.

moisture on the face, in the axillae and skin folds, and on the palms and the soles of the feet. Fever, anxiety, activity, and hyperthyroidism are other conditions that may cause an increase in moisture. Fluid loss with subsequent dehydration, normal aging, and endocrine imbalance secondary to hypothyroidism may result in decreased skin moisture. Areas of decreased moisture include the buccal mucous membranes (Ignatavieius & Workman, 2006).

Nursing Diagnoses

Integumentary assessment provides data for identifying the patient's risk for impaired skin integrity, impaired skin integrity, and impaired tissue integrity.

CARDIOVASCULAR SYSTEM

History

The cardiovascular system is composed of the heart, blood vessels, and the cells and plasma that make up the blood. The blood vessels are a closed delivery system that functions to transport blood throughout the body, circulating substances such as oxygen, carbon dioxide, nutrients, hormones, and waste products.

Ask the patient whether she or he has experienced progressive weakness, shortness of breath, syncope, diaphoresis, nausea, or vomiting. If the patient has had these symptoms, ask under what circumstances they occurred. Determine whether the patient has a history of heart disease and, if so, ask what type of heart disease. Ask the patient whether family members have experienced heart disease, diabetes, stroke, or thromboembolism. Document the type of medications the patient is currently taking for existing cardiovascular disease, such as nitroglycerin, digitalis, diuretics, antihypertensives, and potassium supplements (Harkreander, Hogan, & Thobaben, 2007).

Assess the patient's social history. Look for occupation-related stress, type A behavior patterns, stress related to marital or family status, and recent stressful life events. Determine the patient's smoking and alcohol habits, as well as the amount of caffeine intake. Assess the patient's nutritional status to include typical eating patterns and salt intake. Ask about the patient's activity level. Note the type of exercise patterns, if any, and participation in cardiac rehabilitation activities.

Physical Examination

Physical examination of the cardiovascular system includes blood pressure, peripheral pulses, heart sounds, and circulatory perfusion; palpation and auscultation are used in the exam (Nursing Fundamentals, 2004):

- Blood Pressure—to obtain an accurate blood pressure reading, assure that the patient is relaxed, use a cuff that is not more than 20% wider than the diameter of the patient's limb, and that is long enough to encircle it completely. If the patient is very obese, it may be necessary to use a thigh cuff on his/her arm. If possible, take the blood pressure in two positions, supine or seated and standing.

- Peripheral Pulses—take the peripheral pulses with the patient in the supine position, using the index and middle fingers. **Figure 5.2** depicts the various peripheral pulse sites. Peripheral pulses are graded on a scale of 0–4 by the following system:

$$0 = \text{absent, without a pulse.}$$
$$+1 = \text{diminished, barely palpable.}$$
$$+2 = \text{average, slightly weak, but palpable.}$$
$$+3 = \text{full and brisk, easily palpable.}$$
$$+4 = \text{bounding pulse, sometimes visible.}$$

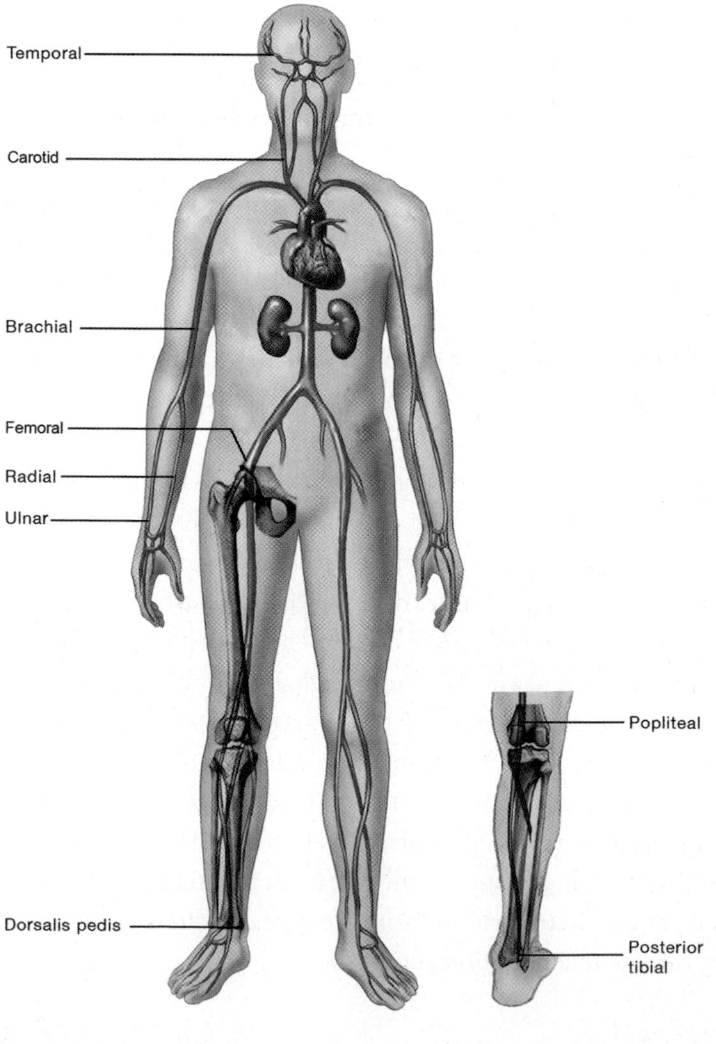

Figure 5.2

Various peripheral pulse sites.

- Heart Sounds—various heart sounds can be heard by auscultation. The first two heart sounds are produced by closure of the valves of the heart. The first heart sound (S1) occurs when the ventricles have been sufficiently filled and the right and left atrioventricular (A-V) valves close. S1 is heard as a single dull, low-pitched sound. After the ventricles empty their blood into the aorta and pulmonary arteries, the semilunar valves close, producing the second heart sound (S2). The second heart sound is shorter and has a higher pitch than S1. The two sounds occur within one second or less, depending on the heart rate. Normally, equal time elapses between heartbeats; any deviation from the normal pattern is arrhythmia. Murmurs, produced by turbulent blood flow, may occur at any cardiac auscultation site. The volume of blood flow, the force of the contraction, and the degree of valve compromise all contribute to murmur quality. **Table 5.8** describes various abnormal heart sounds.
- Circulatory Perfusion—this is the blood flow through the vessels of a specific organ or tissue. Close examination of the extremities will indicate the quality of the arterial and venous systems. Oxygen and food are supplied to the individual cells through capillary walls; to test capillary refill of the extremities, press on a toe or fingertip, then observe blanching and the time it takes the area to return to its original color. Document the time in seconds.

Review laboratory values (see **Table 5.9**) such as complete blood count, electrolytes, blood gases, cardiac enzymes, and coagulation studies. Obtain electrocardiographic readings and any other cardiac test such as angiography, scans, stress testing, pulmonary function tests, and other diagnostic tests.

Nursing Diagnoses

Cardiovascular assessment provides data for identifying the patient's risk for activity intolerance, activity intolerance, decreased cardiac output, and altered tissue perfusion.

RESPIRATORY SYSTEM

History

The respiratory system consists of the airways, the lungs, and the respiratory muscles that mediate the movement of air into and out of the body. The alveolar system of the lungs serves to passively exchange the oxygen and carbon dioxide in the lungs. Therefore, the respiratory system facilitates oxygenation of the blood and the removal of carbon dioxide and other gases and metabolic wastes from the blood (Piedmont Hospital, 2007). During the history, gather information about the patient's current and any previous respiratory problems, keeping in mind six important respiratory symptoms (Habel, 2006):

- cough;
- sputum production;
- dyspnea;
- hemoptysis;
- chest pain; and
- wheezing.

Table 5.8	Abnormal Heart Sounds
Diastolic Murmur	☐ Murmur that occurs in the filling phase of cardiac cycle
	☐ Caused by incompetent semilunar valves or stenotic AV valves
	☐ Almost always indicative of heart disease
	☐ Early diastolic murmurs usually result from insufficiency of a semilunar valve or dilation of the valvular ring.
	☐ Mid- and late-diastolic murmurs are usually caused by narrowed, stenosed mital and tricuspid valves that obstruct blood flow
	☐ A loud murmur accompanied by a thrill usually indicates a pathologic condition
Systolic Murmur	☐ Murmur that occurs during the ventricular ejection phase of the cardiac cycle
	☐ Vibration is heard during part or all of systole
	☐ Most systolic murmurs are caused by obstruction of the outflow of the semilunar valve (aortic, pulmonic) or by incompetent AV valves (mitral, tricuspid)
	☐ Other possible causes include structural deformities of the aorta or pulmonary arteries
Mid-Systolic Click	☐ Sound associated with mitral valve prolapse—the mitral valve leaflets not only close with contraction, but there is also a balloon backup into the left atrium; during ballooning, the sudden tensing of the valve leaflets and the chordae tendineae creates the click
	☐ It is best heard over the diaphragm, at the apex, but may also be heard at the left lower sternal border
	☐ The sound occurs in mid- to late-systole; it is a short, high-pitched sound with a click quality
	☐ The click is usually followed by a systolic murmur; the click and murmur move with postural changes
Pericardial Friction Rub	☐ Sound caused by a rubbing together of the inflamed visceral and parietal layers of the pericardium; this rubbing sound is usually present in both systole and diastole and is best heard over the apex
	☐ It can be heard during inspiration or expiration and does not change with the respiratory cycle
S3 (Ventricular Gallop)	☐ In some conditions, ventricular filling creates vibrations that can be heard over the chest (normally, diastole is silent)
	☐ These vibrations are the S3 heart sound, which occurs when the ventricles are resistant to filling during the early filling phase
	☐ This sound occurs immediately after the S2 when the AV valves open and the atrial blood pours into the ventricles
	☐ The S3 heart sound is a soft, low-pitched sound; it is best heard at the apex with the person in the left lateral position

Adapted from: O'Leary, P. (2008). Abnormal Heart Sounds. Retrieved June 4, 2008 from http://mtsu32.mtsu.edu:11259/abnormal_heart_sounds.htm.

The major symptoms that indicate alterations in the respiratory system include difficulty breathing, shortness of breath, cough, and pain. If the patient reports shortness of breath, ask when it occurs. If the patient has a cough, determine whether it is productive, hacking, habitual, or a nervous cough. The nurse should explore the patient's medical history for recent respiratory diseases such as pneumonia or an upper respiratory infection.

Table 5.9	Laboratory Studies for Cardiovascular Assessment	
Parameter	**Assessment**
Complete blood count	Check WBC count, hemoglobin level, and hematocrit to identify infectious or anemic trends.
Electrolytes	Check potassium to determine whether the patient is receiving diuretics or potassium supplements.
Blood gases	Check pH, oxygen pressure, and bicarbonate level for normal limits.
Cardiac enzymes	Check for trends in elevation of creatine kinase, lactate dehydrogenase, aspartate aminotransferase (formerly known as serum glutamic-oxaloacetic transaminase), and isoenzyme studies.
Coagulation studies	Check prothrombin time for oral anticoagulants, partial thromboplastin time for heparin therapy.
Urinalysis	Check specific gravity and look for the presence of protein.
Blood urea nitrogen	Check kidney function.
Serum drug levels	Check for presence of digitalis, lidocaine, procainamide, and quinidine.

Adapted from Ignatavicius, D. and Workman, M. L. (2006). *Medical-Surgical Nursing: Critical Thinking for Collaborative Care*. 5th ed. Elsevier Saunders, St. Louis.

Physical Examination

Once the history is completed, the respiratory physical exam is conducted by inspection, palpation, percussion, and auscultation (Habel, 2006). See **Table 5.10** for normal respiratory assessment findings. Check the patient's chest symmetry on inspiration, looking for abnormalities such as barrel, funnel or pigeon-shaped chest and spinal deformities. Evaluate the patient's skin color, warmth, turgor, and moisture. Cold, pale, clammy skin is a compensatory mechanism for oxygen deficit. Watch the patient's breathing pattern, checking for unusually quiet, labored, noisy, shallow breathing, shortness of breath, or dyspnea. The nurse needs to listen to the lungs for crackles, diminished sounds, rhonchi, and wheezes (Harkreander, Hogan, & Thobaben, 2007).

Normal breath sounds are classified as follows (Habel, 2006):

- Tracheal—these breath sounds are heard over the trachea; they are harsh and sound like air is being blown through a pipe.
- Bronchial—these sounds are present over the large airways in the anterior chest near the second and third intercostal spaces; they are more tubular and hollow-sounding than vesicular sounds, but not as harsh as tracheal breath sounds. Bronchial sounds are loud and high in pitch with a short pause between inspiration and expiration; expiratory sounds last longer than inspiratory sounds.
- Bronchovesicular—these sounds are heard in the posterior chest between the scapulae and in the center part of the anterior chest; they are softer than bronchial sounds, but have a tubular quality. Bronchovesicular sounds are about equal during inspiration and expiration; differences in pitch and intensity are often more easily detected during expiration.

Table 5.10	Normal Respiratory Assessment Findings
Inspection	☐ Relaxed posture ☐ Normal musculature ☐ Rate: regular; 10–18 breaths per minute ☐ Absence of cyanosis or pallor ☐ Anteroposterior diameter less than transverse diameter
Palpation	☐ Symmetric chest expansion ☐ Tactile fremitus present and equal bilaterally
Percussion	☐ Resonant
Auscultation	☐ Vesicular over peripheral fields ☐ Bronchovesicular over sternum (anterior) and between scapulae (posterior) ☐ Infant and child—bronchovesicular throughout ☐ No adventitious sounds

Adapted from: Habel, M. (2006). Respiratory assessment: Adult and child. Retrieved June 4, 2008 from http://www.rnceus. com/resp/respframe.html.

- Vesicular—these sounds are soft, blowing, or rustling sounds normally heard throughout most of the lung fields; they are normally heard throughout inspiration, continue without pause through expiration, and then fade away about one third of the way through expiration.

The patterns of normal breath sounds are created by the effect of body structures on air moving through airways; in addition to their location, breath sounds are also described by (Habel, 2006):

- duration (how long the sound lasts);
- intensity (how loud the sound is);
- pitch (how high or low the sound is); and
- timing (when the sound occurs in the respiratory cycle).

Abnormal breath sounds include (Habel, 2006):

- the absence of sound; and/or
- the presence of "normal" sounds in areas where they are normally not heard, (eg, bronchial breath sounds are abnormal in peripheral areas where only vesicular sounds should be heard).

Adventitious breath sounds refer to extra or additional sounds that are heard over normal breath sounds; they are most commonly described as follows (Habel, 2006):

- Crackles (rales)—crackles are caused by fluid in the small airways or atelectasis. They are referred to as discontinuous sounds (ie, they are intermittent, nonmusical, and brief). Crackles may be heard on inspiration or expiration.

The popping sounds produced are created when air is forced through respiratory passages that are narrowed by fluid, mucus, or pus. Crackles are often associated with inflammation or infection of the small bronchi, bronchioles, and alveoli. Crackles that don't clear after a cough may indicate pulmonary edema or fluid in the alveoli due to heart failure or adult respiratory distress syndrome (ARDS). Crackles are often described as:

- Fine—these are soft, high-pitched, and very brief. This sound can be simulated by rolling a strand of hair between your fingers near your ear, or by moistening your thumb and index finger and separating them near your ear.
- Coarse—these crackles are somewhat louder, lower in pitch, and last longer than fine crackles. Some describe them as sounding like opening a Velcro fastener.

ARDS
Adult Respiratory
Distress Syndrome

- Wheezes—these are sounds that are heard continuously during inspiration or expiration, or during both inspiration and expiration. They are caused by air moving through airways narrowed by constriction or swelling of airway or partial airway obstruction.
- Wheezes that are relatively high-pitched and have a shrill or squeaking quality may be referred to as sibilant rhonchi. These sounds are often heard continuously through both inspiration and expiration and have a musical quality; they occur when airways are narrowed, such as during an acute asthmatic attack.
- Wheezes that are lowerpitched sounds with a snoring or moaning quality may be referred to as sonorous rhonchi. Secretions in large airways, such as with bronchitis, may produce these sounds; they may clear somewhat with coughing.
- Pleural friction rubs—these are low-pitched, grating, or creaking sounds that occur when inflamed pleural surfaces rub together during respiration. More often heard on inspiration than expiration, the pleural friction rub is easy to confuse with a pericardial friction rub. In order to determine whether the sound is a pleural friction rub or a pericardial friction rub, ask the patient to briefly hold his/her breath; if the rubbing sound continues, its a pericardial friction rub because the inflamed pericardial layers continue rubbing together with each heart beat—a pleural rub stops when breathing stops.
- Stridor—this term refers to a high-pitched harsh sound heard during inspiration. Stridor is due to obstruction of the upper airway and is a sign of respiratory distress that requires immediate attention.

Detection of adventitious sounds is an integral component of the respiratory examination, as it often leads to the diagnosis of cardiac and pulmonary conditions; if adventitious sounds are heard, it is important to assess (Habel, 2006):

- their loudness;
- the timing in the respiratory cycle;
- location on the chest wall;
- persistence of the pattern from breath to breath; and
- whether or not the sounds clear after a cough or a few deep breaths.

Review laboratory results, especially complete blood count since it will provide information about the oxygen-carrying capacity of the blood. The arterial blood gas results also need to be checked, since they indicate respiratory function. The arterial blood gas provides the following values (Orlando Regional Healthcare, Education, & Development, 2004):

- **pH**
  Measurement of acidity or alkalinity, based on the hydrogen (H+) ions present.
  Normal range: 7.35 to 7.45
- **PaO_2**
  The partial pressure of oxygen that is dissolved in arterial blood.
  Normal range: 80 to 100 mm Hg.
- **SaO_2**
  The arterial oxygen saturation.
  Normal range: 95% to 100%
- $PaCO_2$
  The amount of carbon dioxide dissolved in arterial blood.
  Normal range is 35 to 45 mm Hg.
- HCO_3
  The calculated value of the amount of bicarbonate in the bloodstream.
  Normal range is 22 to 26 mEq/liter
- Base Excess (BE)
  The BE indicates the amount of excess or insufficient level of bicarbonate in the system. A negative base excess indicates a base deficit in the blood.
  Normal range: −2 to +2 mEq/liter.

BE
Base Excess

Table 5.11 outlines the steps in interpreting arterial blood gas results.

Nursing Diagnoses

Respiratory assessment provides data for identifying ineffective airway clearance, ineffective breathing pattern, and impaired gas exchange.

GASTROINTESTINAL SYSTEM

History

GI
Gastrointestinal

The gastrointestinal (GI) system is the system that is used to eat and digest food and rid the body of waste after digestion. The GI system is made up of the mouth, pharynx, esophagus, stomach, small intestines, large intestines, rectum, and anus. Other organs that assist with the digestion of food include the liver and gallbladder, pancreas, salivary glands, lips, teeth, and tongue. The major symptoms indicating alterations in the gastrointestinal system include belching, heartburn, bowel habit changes, weight loss, past history of ulcers, gastrointestinal bleeding, and jaundice. Postprocedure gastrointestinal complications include bleeding ulcers, liver failure, and intestinal obstruction.

Assess the patient for gastrointestinal pain (see **Table 5.12**). Look for the presence of nausea, vomiting, and diarrhea. Determine when episodes of gastrointestinal

Table 5.11	Arterial Blood Gas Interpretation

Arterial blood gas analysis is used to evaluate both acid-base balance and oxygenation, each of which represents separate conditions. Acid-base assessment requires a focus on three of the reported components: pH, $PaCO_2$ and HCO_3. There are three steps involved in the interpretation process.

Step I
- ☐ Assess the pH to assess if the blood is within normal range, alkalotic or acidotic
- ☐ Results above 7.45—the blood is alkalotic
- ☐ Results below 7.35—the blood is acidotic

Step 2
- ☐ If blood is alkalotic or acidotic, determine if the cause is primarily a respiratory or metabolic problem by assessing the $PaCO_2$ level
- ☐ Compare the pH and the $PaCO_2$ values: if pH and $PaCO_2$ are moving in *opposite directions,* the problem is primarily respiratory in nature

Step 3
- ☐ Assess HCO_3 value
- ☐ Compare the pH and HCO_3 values; if pH and HCO_3 are moving in the *same direction,* the problem is primarily metabolic in nature

Analysis Chart

	pH	$PaCO_2$	HCO_3
Respiratory Acidosis	↓	↑	normal
Respiratory Alkalosis	↑	↓	normal
Metabolic Acidosis	↓	normal	↓
Metabolic Alkalosis	↑	normal	↑

Adapted from: Orlando Regional Healthcare, Education, & Development (2004). Interpretation of arterial blood gas. Retrieved June 4, 2008 from www.nursing4all.com/forum/attachment.php?attachmentid=1792&d=1196178040.

distress occur, such as before or after meals. Search for precipitating factors such as emotional stress, medications, specific foods, treatments, and exercise. If the patient reports vomiting or diarrhea, describe the frequency, amount, color, odor, and consistency. Determine whether the patient is constipated. Ask about the time of the last bowel movement. Determine whether laxatives or enemas are used. Assess the patient for episodes of belching, gas, and flatulence. Determine their frequency. Ask the patient whether he or she has had episodes of gastrointestinal bleeding and, if so, to describe the type of bleeding. For example, did the vomitus contain any bright red blood: Was it blood tinged, brown, or have a coffee ground appearance; Was it positive for occult blood? Was the stool blood tinged, dark, or tarry; contain bright red blood; and test positive for occult blood? Inquire about recent weight gain or loss. Determine whether the patient has a history of gastrointestinal problems and, if so, inquire about the type of therapy used and whether it was effective. Ask whether the patient has experienced gastrointestinal problems related to allergies. List all medications that the patient uses for gastrointestinal problems, such as over the-counter antacids, proton pump inhibitors, laxatives, and sodium bicarbonate. Determine the patient's normal bowel and bladder habits and if there has been a recent change in either.

Table 5.12	Primary Causes of Abdominal Pain	
Common, recurrent	☐	Irritable bowel syndrome
	☐	Lactose intolerance and celiac disease
	☐	Constipation
	☐	Myofascial pain syndrome
Referred	☐	Cardiac pain
	☐	Lower lobe pneumonias, pulmonary emboli, pleurisy
	☐	Spinal and hip pain
Metabolic	☐	Diabetic ketoacidosis
	☐	Lead toxicity
	☐	Hypercalcemia
Infection	☐	Urinary tract sepsis
	☐	Intestinal sepsis
Neurogenic	☐	Herpes zoster postherpetic neuralgia
	☐	Tabes dorsalis
	☐	Spinal degeneration or injury
Other Causes	☐	Peptic ulceration
	☐	Psychogenic
	☐	Side effects of common drugs

Adapted from: Stephenson, M. (2008). Non-surgical causes of abdominal pain. Retrieved June 4, 2008 from http://student.bmj.com/issues/08/06/education/246.php.

Physical Examination

Before the examination, instruct the patient to empty his/her bladder. Position the patient in the supine position. Expose the abdomen, being sure to cover the breasts with the gown and the pubic area with the bed sheet. Observe the patient's skin color, looking for jaundice. Inspect the skin for rashes, pigmentations, or operative scars. Assess the patient for asymmetry, masses, hernias, visible peristalsis, or pulsations. Look at the contour of the patient's abdomen and describe in terms of obesity, flatness, and distention. Auscultate the abdomen using the diaphragm of the stethoscope. Normal bowel sounds should be heard in all four quadrants every 5 to 20 seconds. Hypoactive bowel sounds are less than one per minute and could indicate paralytic ileus, peritonitis, obstruction, hemorrhage, post-abdominal surgery, or no food in the bowel.

Hyperactive bowel sounds are continuous sounds and may occur with vomiting or diarrhea, above bowel obstruction, or after eating. The abdomen can be lightly palpated for areas of tenderness, masses, and involuntary guarding.

Review laboratory results, especially the complete blood count, electrolyte values, and blood urea nitrogen level. Other diagnostic tests the patient might have include barium enema and barium swallow examinations, sigmoidoscopy, endoscopy, nuclear scans, and ultrasonography.

Nursing Diagnoses

Gastrointestinal assessment provides data for identifying constipation, diarrhea, bowel incontinence, regurgitation, and/or gastric reflux.

MUSCULOSKELETAL SYSTEM

History

The musculoskeletal system is made up of bones that are attached to other bones with joints, and the skeletal muscle system in which muscles are attached to the skeleton by tendons.

Obtain information about the patient's previous illnesses and accidents related to the musculoskeletal system. Ask about traumatic incidents such as sprains and fractures. Explore the patient's family history because osteoporosis often occurs in several generations and bone cancer also tends to be genetically linked. Evaluate the patients nutritional and exercise habits. Inactive patients, who do not get regular exposure to sunlight and have an inadequate intake of calcium or protein are predisposed to bone and muscle tone loss. Patients with an inadequate intake of vitamin C have inadequate bone and tissue healing.

Note the patient's weight. Obese patients with musculoskeletal problems are at risk for respiratory and circulatory complications. Obesity also places excessive strain and stress on joints and bones, which may lead to fractures and cartilage degeneration.

Physical Examination

Observe the patient's posture, gait, and general mobility for gross deformities or impairment (see **Table 5.13**). First, evaluate the patient's posture by examining body build and alignment when standing and walking. Assess the curvature of the spine and the length, shape, and symmetry of extremities. Second, evaluate the patient's gait including patient's balance. The nurse should determine the patient's need for ambulatory assistive devices. Lastly, evaluate the patient's mobility including ability

Table 5.13	Assessing Posture, Gait, Mobility
Posture	☐ Evaluate the patient's body build and alignment when standing and walking
	☐ Look for curvature of the spine: lordosis, scoliosis, kyphosis
	☐ Inspect the extremities for length, shape, and symmetry
Gait	☐ Evaluate the patient's balance and steadiness
	☐ Determine the patient's ease and length of stride
	☐ Look for limp or other asymmetrical leg movements or deformities
	☐ Determine the patient's need for ambulatory assistive devices
Mobility	☐ Assess the patient's ability to perform activities of daily living
	☐ Determine the extent of range of motion by having the patient demonstrate active movement of major joints

Adapted from: Ignatavicius, D. and Workman, M. L. (2006). *Medical-Surgical Nursing: Critical Thinking for Collaborative Care.* 5th ed. Elsevier Saunders, St. Louis.

Table 5.14	Assessing the Skeletal System
Head and Neck	☐ Inspect and palpate the skull for shape, symmetry, tenderness, and masses.
	☐ Evaluate the temperomandibular joints by palpating while the patient opens his or her mouth. Common abnormal findings are tenderness or pain, crepitus, and a spongy swelling caused by excessive synovium and fluid, which can be palpated.
	☐ Observe and palpate each vertebra in the neck.
Vertebral Spine	☐ Observe and palpate the thoracic, lumbar, and sacral spine. Look for malalignment, tenderness, and inability to flex, extend, and rotate.
	☐ Check for discomfort in the lower back by placing both hands over the lumbosacral area and applying pressure with the thumbs to elicit tenderness.
Upper Extremities	☐ Assess both extremities concurrently.
	☐ Starting with the shoulders and moving to the elbows and then the wrists, check for size, swelling, deformity, malalignment, tenderness or pain, and mobility.
	☐ Assess hand function by palpating the metacarpophalangeal, proximal interphalangeal, and distal interphalangeal joints. Compare the same digits on the right and left hands.
	☐ Determine range of motion for each joint.
Lower Extremities	☐ Evaluate the hip joints by determining the degree of mobility.
	☐ Assess the knee joints with the patient in a sitting position with then knees flexed. Look for fluid accumulation, or effusion, and limitations in movement with accompanying pain.
	☐ Inspect the ankles and feet. Observe, palpate, and test each joint for range of motion.

Adapted from: Ignatavicius, D. and Workman, M. L. (2006). *Medical-Surgical Nursing: Critical Thinking for Collaborative Care.* 5th ed. Elsevier Saunders, St. Louis.

to perform activities of daily living. The nurse should determine the extent of range of motion by having the patient demonstrate active movement of all major joints. The nurse should also assess the patient's grip strength. Assess head and neck, vertebral spine, and the upper and lower extremities (see **Table 5.14**).

Review laboratory studies, especially serum calcium, phosphorus, and phosphate levels, and erythrocyte sedimentation rate (see **Table 5.15**). The nurse will review any other diagnostic studies, such as radiography, myelography, computed tomography, biopsy, bone scan, magnetic resonance imaging, ultrasonography (see **Table 5.16**).

Nursing Diagnoses

Musculoskeletal assessment provides data for identifying the patient's risk for injury related to musculoskeletal impairment, impaired physical mobility, and self-care deficit. Before the procedure the nurse must also individualize positioning needs based on the presence of musculoskeletal problems or limitations.

URINARY SYSTEM
History

The urinary system includes the two kidneys, two ureters, the bladder, and the urethra and is responsible for the production, storage, and alimentation of urine.

Table 5.15	Laboratory Studies for Musculoskeletal Assessment	
Test	**Normal Ranges (Adults)**	**Interpreting Abnormal Ranges**
Serum calcium level	9.0–10.5 mg/dL, decreased in older adults	Hypercalcemia ☐ Metastatic cancers of the bone ☐ Paget's disease ☐ Bone fractures in healing stage Hypocalcemia ☐ Osteoporosis ☐ Osteomalacia
Serum phosphorus	3.0–4.5 mg/dL, decreased in older adults	Hyperphosphatemia ☐ Bone fractures in healing stage ☐ Bone tumors ☐ Acromegaly Hypophosphatemia ☐ Osteomalacia
Alkaline phosphatase (ALP)	30–120 units/L, slightly higher in older adults	Elevations may indicate: ☐ Metastatic cancers of the bone ☐ Paget's disease ☐ Osteomalacia
Erythrocyte sedimentation rate (Sed Rate)	Normal values vary depending on the laboratory procedure used ☐ 20–40 mm/hr—mild inflammation ☐ 40–70 mm/hr—moderate inflammation ☐ 70–150 mm/hr—severe inflammation	Elevations may indicate: ☐ Infection ☐ Inflammation ☐ Carcinoma ☐ Cell or tissue destruction

Adapted from Ignatavicius, D. and Workman, M. L. (2006). *Medical-Surgical Nursing: Critical Thinking for Collaborative Care.* 5th ed. Elsevier Saunders, St. Louis.

Note the patient's age and sex. Some urinary tract disorders are related to the age or sex of the patient. For example, sudden hypertension in a patient older than 50 years of age may indicate the presence of renovascular disease. Another example is polycystic disease, which typically occurs in patients in their 40s or 50s. Men older than 50 years of age may experience dysfunctional urinary patterns as a result of prostatic disease. Women, because of the short urethra, may experience cystitis.

Assess the patient's personal and family history. Ask the patient about a history of urinary tract infections or urological procedures. Note any history of arthritis, hypertension, and diabetes mellitus. Arthritis medication may result in injury to renal tissue. Hypertension, especially if untreated or uncontrolled, may result in nephrosclerosis, leading to renal failure. Diabetes mellitus may lead to renal failure. Determine whether the patient's family has a history of renal disease.

Table 5.16	Diagnostic Studies of the Musculoskeletal System	
Examination or Test	**Purpose**	**Method**
Standard radiography	☐ Visualize the skeleton and supporting structures ☐ Observe bone denslty, alignment, swelling, and intactness ☐ Determine condition of joints, including size of the joint space, the smoothness of articular cartilage, and synovial swelling ☐ Determine soft tissue involvement	☐ Standard x-ray imaging
Tomography and xeroradiography	☐ Tomography—helpful in musculoskeletal assessment because it produces planes, or slices, for focus and blurs the images of other structures ☐ Xeroradiography highlights the contrast between structures, allowing margins and edges to be clearly seen	☐ X-ray imaging with higher doses of radiation
Myelography	☐ Visualize the vertebral column, intervertebral disks, spinal nerve roots, and blood vessels	☐ Injection of a contrast medium into the subarachnoid space of the spine
Diskography	☐ Visualize an intervertebral disk	☐ Injection of a contrast medium directly into the target disk
Arthrography	☐ Visualize a joint	☐ X-ray imaging of a joint after injection of a contrast medium (air or solution) to enhance visualization
Computerized tomography	☐ Detect musculoskeletal problems (used with or without contrast medium)	☐ Scanner produces a narrow x-ray beam for imaging body sections from many different angles. ☐ A computer produces a three-dimensional picture of the structure being studies ☐ Small tumors may not be detected without the use of oral or intravenous contrast medium.
Bone biopsy	☐ Confirm the presence of infection or neoplasm	☐ Collection of a bone specimen for microscopic examination via needle or open extraction
Muscle biopsy	☐ Diagnose muscle atrophy (as in muscular dystrophy) and inflammation (as in polymyositis)	☐ Collection of a muscle specimen for microscopic examination via needle or open extraction

Electromyography	☐ Determine the electrical potential generated in an individual muscle	☐ The patient performs activities to measure muscle potential during minimal and maximal contractions
	☐ Usually accompanied by nerve conduction studies	☐ Nerve and muscle activity is recorded on an oscilloscope
	☐ Helpful in the diagnosis of neuromuscular, lower motor neuron, and peripheral nerve disorders	☐ When done in conjunction with nerve conduction studies, flat electrodes are placed along the nerve to be evaluated, and small doses of electrical current are passed via the electrodes to the nerve and muscle innervated. It the muscle contracts, nerve conduction is confirmed
Bone scan	☐ Radionuclide test used to detect tumors, arthritis, osteomyelitis, osteoporosis, vertebral compression fractures, and unexplained bone pain	☐ The radioactive isotope technetium (^{99m}Tc) is injected intravenously for visualization of the entire skeleton
Gallium scan	☐ This test is similar to the bone scan but is more specific and sensitive in detecting bone problems	☐ Radioactive medium used is gallium citrate (^{67}Ga), which is administered *3 days before* the test, owing to the slow absorption rate of the material
Indium imaging	☐ Use primarily to detect bone infection	☐ The patient's leukocytes are separated from a blood sample, tagged with indium (^{111}In), and injected intravenously. In acute bone infections (osteomyelitis), the tagged leukocytes accumulate and can be seen on scanning
Magnetic resonance imaging	☐ Identify problems with muscle, tendons, and ligaments	☐ The image is produced through the interaction of magnetic fields, radiowaves, and atomic nuclei showing hydrogen density. The lack of hydrogen ions in cortical bone makes it easily distinguishable from soft tissues
Ultrasonography	☐ Detect soft tissue disorders such as masses and fluid accumulation	☐ Use of sound waves to produce an image of the tissue being studied

Adapted from Ignatavicius, D. and Workman, M. L. (2006). *Medical-Surgical Nursing: Critical Thinking for Collaborative Care.* 5th ed. Elsevier Saunders, St. Louis.

Review nutritional assessment data. Symptoms such as changes in appetite and taste acuity or an inability to discriminate tastes are associated with the accumulation of nitrogenous waste products from renal failure. High protein intake can result in transient renal problems. Some patients are prone to renal calculi formation secondary to excessive calcium intake.

Review the patient's medication history. Determine whether the patient has taken medications for chronic health problems such as diabetes mellitus, hypertension, cardiac disorders, hormone deficiencies, and arthritis. Medications used to treat these disorders may lead to renal dysfunction. Antibiotics such as gentamicin are also associated with sudden renal dysfunction. Determine whether the patient takes over-the-counter medications; some (eg, analgesics), especially when combined with other agents, can affect renal function.

Assess the patient's urinary patterns. Ask whether the patient has experienced changes in the color of the urine, the pattern of urination, and the ability to start or control urination. Determine whether the patient has experienced alterations in the appearance of the urine. Ask whether the patient has experienced oliguria, anuria, polyuria, hesitancy, dysuria, or urgency (see **Table 5.17**). Document if the patient has experienced alterations in the appearance of the urine or experienced oliguria, anuria, polyuria, hesitancy, dysuria, urgency, or urinary incontinence (Ignatavicius & Workman, 2006).

Physical Examination

Assess the general condition of the patient. Examine at the skin to determine if there is any type of discoloration, such as yellow tinges, rashes, or ecchymoses. Check the pedal, pretibial, presacral, and periorbital tissues, which are common sites for edema in renal disorders. Assess the patient's level of consciousness. Deficits in concentration, impaired thought processes or memory, dysarthria (the inability to speak clearly and distinctly), and an altered level of alertness may indicate the presence of renal disease. Document any deficits in concentration, impaired thought process or memory since these cognitive changes could result from accumulation of waste products from renal disease (Ignatavicius & Workman, 2006). Check the patient's gait and hand coordination, which may also be affected by the presence of renal disease.

Assess the kidneys, ureters, and bladder in conjunction with the abdominal assessment (see **Table 5.18**). Inspect the urethra by checking the meatus for discharge,

Table 5.17	Terms for Urinary Dysfunction	
Oliguria	☐	Decrease in urine output, specifically an output of 100–400 mL/24 hours
Anuria	☐	Absence of urine output, specifically less than 100 mL/24 hours
Polyuria	☐	Increase in urine output, usually greater than 1,500 mL/24 hours
Dysuria	☐	Any discomfort associated with urination
Hesitancy	☐	Difficulties in initiating the flow of urine
Urgency	☐	Sensations experienced when there is a sudden need to urinate; may be associated with urinary incontinence
Renal Colic	☐	Severe or spasmodic pain associated with renal or ureteral irritation that radiates into the perineal area, groin, scrotum, or labia

Adapted from: Ignatavicius, D. and Workman, M. L. (2006). *Medical-Surgical Nursing: Critical Thinking for Collaborative Care.* 5th ed. Elsevier Saunders, St. Louis.

Table 5.18	Assessing the Kidneys, Ureters, and Bladder
Auscultation	☐ Listen to the aorta and renal arteries for the presence of a *bruit* (an audible sound produced when the volume of blood or the diameter of the blood vessel is changed).
	☐ If a bruit is detected, listen for a *thrill* (a palpable sensation of blood that is similar to a rippling pulse).
Palpation	☐ Lightly palpate all quadrants of the abdomen. Note areas of tenderness or discomfort. If severe bladder distention is present, the outline of the bladder may be identified as high as the umbilicus.
	☐ The ureters are not palpable; however, a spasm of the ureteral musculature results in flank or low abdominal pain that is severe, excruciating, and similar to colic.
	☐ Do not palpate the kidneys unless appropriately trained. The ability to palpate the kidneys requires special training and practice under the guidance of a qualified practitioner and is usually reserved for advance practice nurses.
Percussion	☐ Gently palpate the outline of the distended bladder; then place the fingertips of one hand on the lower abdomen. Use the fingertips of the other hand to thump over the top of the fingers of the hand resting on the abdomen. A distended bladder sounds dull when percussed. Move the hand resting on the bladder toward the umbilicus until the dull sounds are no longer heard.
	☐ Usually, the patient complains of discomfort or a constant, dull ache with inflammation or infection of the kidney, the renal capsule, or the adjacent fascia. If the patient has not identified flank pain, percuss the nontender costovertebral angle, which is the lower portion of the rib cage and the vertebral column. Have the patient assume the sitting, lateral, or supine position for this percussion. Clench the examining hand into a fist. With the heel of the hand and the little finger, quickly and firmly thump the costovertebral area. The elicitation of costovertebral tenderness is highly suggestive of kidney infection or inflammation.

Adapted from: Ignatavicius, D. and Workman, M. L. (2006). *Medical-Surgical Nursing: Critical Thinking for Collaborative Care.* 5th ed. Elsevier Saunders, St. Louis.

such as blood, mucus, or purulent drainage. Check the surrounding tissues for the presence of lesions, rashes, or other abnormalities of the penis or scrotum or of the labia or vagina. Suspect urethral irritation if the patient reports discomfort when initiating urination.

Nursing Diagnoses

Urinary system assessment provides data for identifying the patient's risk for fluid volume deficit, fluid volume excess, altered patterns of urinary elimination, and incontinence (functional, stress, and total).

IDENTIFYING ALTERATIONS IN PSYCHOSOCIAL AND EMOTIONAL HEALTH STATUS

Psychosocial and emotional health status has an impact on the patient throughout the operative and invasive procedure period. For example, a patient with a diagnosed knowledge deficit may not have sufficient knowledge to implement preprocedure instructions, adhere to therapeutic regimens before and after the procedure, and implement self-care activities before or after the procedure. Likewise, a patient experiencing anticipatory anxiety may not be able to implement preprocedure instructions. Assess the patient's and the family's psychosocial and emotional health status by determining the patient's and/or family's knowledge about the operative or invasive procedure experience and their ability to handle fear, deal with anticipatory anxiety, recognize and resolve body image disturbance, grieve success fully, and cope effectively with the stress associated with an operative or invasive procedure.

The following nursing diagnoses are examples of alterations in psychosocial and emotional health status that may increase the patient's risk for adverse outcomes during the operative and invasive procedure period. Refer to **Table 5.19** for more information about these diagnoses.

Deficient Knowledge

Deficient knowledge is defined as state in which a person or the family experiences a deficiency in cognitive knowledge or psychomotor skills concerning the disease, preprocedure testing, and/or treatment plan (Carpenito-Moyet, 2008). Knowledge deficit can lead to adverse outcomes (eg, aspiration, pneumonia, infection), particularly in the outpatient setting. This occurs when the patient does not correctly perform the desired or prescribed activities prior to the procedure (eg, nothing by mouth [NPO] after midnight, or bowel preparation). Knowledge deficit can be due to a lack of exposure and understanding of medical test and language, lack of recall of the activities to be performed, or a misinterpretation of written or verbal instructions. Because of knowledge deficit, it is important to include the patient's family or significant others in preprocedural teaching.

Due to the changes in healthcare delivery today, with more patients being treated on an outpatient basis, or having the procedure the same day as admission, nurses have a limited interaction with the patients before the procedure. Many characteristics influence a patient's ability to learn, such as age, race, gender, diagnosis, religious beliefs, and culture. Other important assessment factors include literacy, education, developmental level, readiness to learn, and learning style.

NAAL
National Assessment of Adult Literacy

Literacy is defined as using printed and written information to function, to achieve one's goals, and to develop one's knowledge and/or potential (National Center for Education Statistics, 2006). The National Assessment of Adult Literacy (NAAL) divides literacy into four levels—Below Basic, Basic, Intermediate, and Proficient; furthermore, the 2003 NAAL found that a total of 22% of adults were classified as being below basic (National Center for Education Statistics, 2006). For this reason, patient education material should be published at a forth grade readability. The other challenge nurses face today is the growing number of patients for whom English is not their primary language. Therefore, it is important to have an interpreter present during the interview and have all forms and education material translated into the various languages.

Also associated with literacy is the developmental level; this means is that the teaching should be appropriate for the patient's specific developmental levels. Teaching and learning for a child, an adolescent, adult, or an older adult are different for each. Therefore, it is important to develop education materials and teaching plans that are appropriate for the patient population.

Table 5.19	Preparing the Patient for an Operative or Invasive Procedure Does Not Compromise or Cause Injury to the Patient

Outcome 1   The patient and family demonstrate knowledge of the expected responses to the operative or invasive procedure.

Diagnosis	Risk Factors	Outcome Indicators
Deficient Knowledge	☐ Limited understanding of the injury or disease process and of the operative or invasive procedure ☐ Poor performance of a required skill related to the operative or invasive procedure period ☐ Inaccurate or inappropriate responses to questions about the operative or invasive procedure period ☐ Inability to perform skills or follow through after instruction ☐ Low readiness to learn about the operative or invasive procedure ☐ Lack of interest or motivation to learn about the operative or invasive procedure ☐ Uncompensated memory loss ☐ Sensory deficit (visual or auditory) making it difficult to read or hear instructions and see skill demonstrations ☐ Inability to use materials or information resources because of cultural or language differences	☐ Do the patient and family describe the sequence of the planned procedure and prescribed postoperative regimen; repeat instructions correctly; ask questions based on the information provided; and participate in the plan of care? ☐ Do the patient and family verbalize realistic expectations regarding recovery from the procedure? ☐ Do the patient and family accurately identify signs and symptoms to report to the physician/healthcare provider? ☐ Was the patient calm, cooperative, exhibited relaxed facial muscles, verbalized the ability to cope? ☐ Does the patient correctly demonstrate deep breathing, coughing, leg exercises, if applicable, and verbalized wound care requirements?

Outcome 2   The patient recognizes and manages fear during the operative or invasive period.

Diagnosis	Risk Factors	Outcome Indicators
Fear related to the operative or invasive procedure experience	☐ Feelings of dread, nervousness, or concern about the operative or invasive procedure ☐ Verbal statements about expecting danger to self ☐ Increased questioning or information seeking ☐ Voice tremors, pitch changes ☐ Increase in quantity of verbalization ☐ Increased rate of verbalization ☐ Hand tremor ☐ Increased muscle tension ☐ Narrowing focus of attention, progressing to fixed ☐ Diaphoresis ☐ Increased heart rate ☐ Increased respiratory rate ☐ Knowledge deficit about the impending event or health status ☐ Perceived inability to control the process or outcome of the operative or invasive procedure	☐ Does the patient verbally recognize the presence of fear? ☐ Is the patient able to talk rationally about his or her feelings of fear? ☐ Are physical signs (such as hand tremor, muscle tension, diaphoresis, increased heart and respiratory rates) present, indicating that the patient is not managing his or her feelings of fear?

5

Outcome 3   **The patient does not express feelings of apprehension and activation of the autonomic nervous system in response to the operative or invasive procedure experience.**

Diagnosis

Anxiety (Mild, Moderate, Severe, or Panic) related to the operative or invasive procedure experience

Risk Factors

☐ Verbalization of apprehension, uncertainty, fear, distress, or worry; painful and persistent feelings of increased helplessness, inadequacy, regret

☐ Expressions of concern (change in life events)

☐ Fear of unspecified consequences

☐ Overexcited, rattled, jittery, scared state

☐ Restlessness, focus on self, insomnia, increased perspiration

☐ Increased wariness, glancing about, poor eye contact, facial tension, quivering voice

☐ Increased tension, foot shuffling, hand or arm movements, trembling, hand tremor, shakiness

☐ Increased heart and respiratory rates

☐ Perceived threat of death related to the operative or invasive procedure experience

☐ Unconscious conflict (essential values, life goals) triggered by an operative or invasive procedure

☐ The operative or invasive procedure perceived by the patient as a threat to self-concept, health status, socioeconomic status, role functioning, interaction patterns, or environment

Outcome Indicators

☐ Does the patient verbally recognize feelings of anxiety?

☐ Is the patient able to talk rationally about his or her feelings of anxiety?

☐ Are physical signs (such as hand tremor, facial muscle tension, diaphoresis, increased heart and respiratory rates) present, indicating that the patient is not managing his or her feelings of anxiety?

Outcome 4   **The patient recognizes the presence of anticipatory grief and engages in a functional grieving process.**

Diagnosis

Anticipatory Grieving related to the expected outcome of the operative or invasive procedure

Risk Factors

☐ Verbal expression of distress at potential (anticipated) loss

☐ Anger

☐ Sadness, sorrow, crying

☐ Crying at frequent intervals, choked feeling

☐ Change in eating habits

☐ Difficulty with sleeping

☐ Change in activity level

☐ Change in libido

☐ Ideation of anticipated loss

☐ Developmental regression

Outcome Indicators

☐ Does the patient verbally recognize that he or she is experiencing anticipatory grief?

☐ Is the patient able to identify the source of anticipatory grief?

☐ Is the patient able to talk rationally about his or her feelings of anticipatory grief?

☐ Alterations in concentration
   or pursuit of task

☐ Expected loss or change related
   to anticipated operative result

☐ Operative procedure for removal
   of a body part significant to
   sexual identity

☐ Operative procedure resulting
   in a change in the appearance
   of body parts visible to others
   (face, neck, hands)

☐ Amputation

☐ Unavailable support systems

Outcome 5   The patient is able to adequately manage internal and environmental stressors related to the impending operative or invasive procedure.

Diagnosis	Risk Factors	Outcome Indicators
Ineffective Individual Coping related to the stress of the impending operative or invasive procedure	☐ Verbalization of inability to cope ☐ Inability to ask for help or to effectively solve problems ☐ Anxiety, fear, anger, irritability, tension ☐ Presence of life stress (such as a major operative experience or disease process) ☐ Inability to meet role expectations (such as a permanent or temporary loss of employment as a consequence of the procedure) ☐ Inability to meet basic needs ☐ Changes in social participation ☐ Destructive behavior toward self and others ☐ Inappropriate or ineffective use of defense mechanisms ☐ Change in usual communication patterns ☐ Excess food intake, alcohol consumption, smoking ☐ Digestive, bowel, appetite disturbance; chronic fatigue or sleep pattern disturbance ☐ Situational crises such as an operative or invasive procedure ☐ Personal vulnerability ☐ Knowledge deficit concerning an operative or invasive procedure ☐ Problem-solving skills deficit, particularly in relation to dealing with the outcome of an operative or invasive procedure	☐ Does the patient verbalize that he or she is coping? ☐ Is the patient able to ask for help with coping? ☐ Does the patient demonstrate effective problem solving? ☐ Is the patient able to meet basic needs? ☐ Does the patient demonstrate functional societal participation? ☐ Is there an absence of destructive behavior toward self and others? ☐ Are defense mechanisms appropriate and effective? ☐ Are communication patterns functional and effective?

Adapted from Carpentino-Moyet, L. J. (2008) *Handbook of Nursing Diagnosis* (12th ed.) Philadelphia: Lippincott Williams & Wilkins; Petersen C. (2007). *Perioperative Nursing Data Set, the Perioperative Nursing Vocabulary.* (Revised 2nd ed.). Denver: AORN. Inc.

The patient must be ready to learn. The nurse needs to assess the patient's readiness to learn before teaching. There are three factors that influence a patient's readiness to learn:

1. physical comfort—if a patient is not physically comfortable because of pain, nausea, fatigue or weakness, it is hard for the patient to listen;
2. psychological comfort—if the patient is psychologically uncomfortable because of fear, anxiety, or worry, he/she will only hear part of what is taught; and
3. motivation—the patient must be motivated in order to learn.

Learning styles involve the type of learning environment that is most conducive to learning. The three most common learning styles are auditory, visual, or hands-on. Some patients prefer to hear the instructions; others prefer to read a pamphlet or handout, or view a videotape. Certain teaching needs to be hands-on instruction and practice so that the skill can be done repeatedly until the patient is comfortable performing the task correctly.

Fear Related to the Operative or Invasive Procedure Experience

Unlike the patient with anticipatory anxiety, the patient experiencing fear knows the reason for the fear: he or she is afraid of the impending procedure. Fear is a common reaction to operative and invasive procedures, even though patients are becoming more knowledgeable about their healthcare alternatives. The patient may be able to discuss the rationale for the procedure and accept the event as inevitable, and yet the knowledge that his or her body will be surgically or diagnostically violated instills a feeling of dread. Elimination of fear is an unrealistic expectation because it is a human response to threat and impending danger. The nurse, however, can help the patient recognize and manage fear. This process can begin in the physician's office when the patient consents to the procedure. At this time, the patient's knowledge level about the procedure should be determined and appropriate teaching about the operative or invasive procedure begun. Nurses providing outpatient and inpatient care should also look for the defining characteristics of fear. Interventions aimed at calming the patient should be implemented during the preprocedure period (see Anxiety below).

Anxiety (Mild, Moderate, Severe, Panic) Related to the Operative or Invasive Procedure Experience

An operative or invasive procedure often causes the patient to experience a mild, moderate, severe, or panic anxiety reaction; knowledge or anticipation of possible complications, anesthesia, diagnosis, postprocedure pain or incapacitation—no matter how brief—and therapeutic treatment regimens such as chemotherapy and radiation may trigger an anxiety reaction.

A person undergoing sterilization provides an example of unconscious conflict associated with his/her basic values. Religious norms or values may prohibit sterilization, whereas the economic reality of controlling the size of the family may necessitate the procedure. An example of unconscious conflict associated with life goals can be seen in a patient facing a permanent operative outcome that limits mobility. If a patient has a life goal that focuses on a career entailing the use of the legs, such as a career in professional sports, the fact that the person will have to rely on career skills that do not entail the use of the legs may precipitate unconscious conflict. Because most patients experience some form of anxiety when confronted with an operative or invasive procedure, the nurse can help the patient identify the source of anxiety and suggest strategies for managing it. The nurse in practice with a physician should start the intervention process early in the patient's operative or invasive procedure experience. An assessment that focuses on the identification of the anxiety as soon as the patient consents to the procedure provides an opportunity to work with the patient and family in developing a plan of care that addresses anxiety management. Interventions should focus on providing information about the impending procedure, clarifying misinformation that the patient may have, teaching relaxation techniques, helping the patient explore the source of anxiety, and communicating the patient's psychosocial status to the outpatient and/or inpatient nursing staff.

Registered nurses with practices limited to the outpatient or the inpatient setting should also identify defining characteristics that indicate when a patient is experiencing anxiety. For these nurses, anxiety may be easier to identify because the patient is more likely to exhibit signs of anxiety when the procedure is imminent. Developing a plan of care with interventions to manage the anxiety, however, may be more difficult because of the immediacy of the situation. Interventions should focus on providing support, particularly during the immediate preprocedure period. Gentle physical contact, a quiet and unhurried environment, soothing words, a warm blanket, a pillow, and headphones for listening to music help the patient deal with anxiety.

Anticipatory Grieving Related to the Expected Outcome of the Operative or Invasive Procedure

In their zeal to care and cure, healthcare providers some times forget that an operative or invasive procedure is a disruptive event in the life of a patient that may lead to an anticipatory grief response. Patients consenting to the procedure for removal of a body part often grieve before the procedure because of the anticipated loss. For example, it is not uncommon for a patient to grieve before hysterectomy for the expected loss of her uterus, even if she is past childbearing years. For some, the loss of the uterus signifies the loss of femininity.

Grieving is part of the human experience. When a person is confronted with a precipitating event, functional grieving is necessary for good physical, psychological, sociocultural, and spiritual health. Dysfunctional grieving, in contrast, has a negative impact on the holistic well-being of the individual. Such grief can lead to physical, psychological, and sociocultural imbalances and damage the human spirit.

The nurse who has extensive interaction with the patient before the procedure has the opportunity to identify the presence of anticipatory grieving. Helping the patient move along the grief continuum to the point of acceptance places the patient in a position in which he or she is better able to deal with the physiological and psychosocial stressors of the procedure. If the patient exhibits signs of anticipatory grieving, the nurse should help him or her get in touch with the grief and understand that the experience is not uncommon. The nurse should discuss the stages of grieving with the patient and encourage him or her to set goals in response to the expected loss.

Registered nurses in the inpatient and outpatient settings should look for the defining characteristics of anticipatory grieving. If these are present, nurses should document and communicate the findings to the appropriate members of the health-care team such as pastoral care personnel, social workers, and psychologists. If the patient exhibits behaviors such as crying or expresses anger, sorrow, or sadness, the nurse should respond appropriately by listening and showing sympathy. If not contraindicated because of the patient's cultural practices or preference, establish body contact with the patient by touching the hand, the shoulder, or the side of the face. Prepare the patient for the sensations that she or he will experience during and after the procedure. Explain that feelings of loss and grieving are normal.

Ineffective Individual Coping Related to the Stress of the Impending Procedure

While effective individual coping is not a guarantee for successful rehabilitation and recuperation, it is nonetheless an important contributing factor. Ineffective coping on the part of the patient affects the control of anxiety and fear. The inability to cope may also interfere with the patient's compliance with the postprocedure treatment regimen.

For many people, an operative or invasive procedure is a significant crisis. Suddenly, they are personally vulnerable in that they must submit, even though willingly, to therapeutic interventions or diagnostic procedures. They lose control over their senses and sometimes their normal body functions. Interventions that focus on eliminating knowledge deficit and strengthening problem-solving skills as they relate to the procedure enable the patient to cope better with the procedure. Intervene by identifying the patient's past experiences and coping strategies as they relate to the procedure or illness, and then encourage the patient to implement those strategies. Facilitate open communication. Encourage the patient to participate in the decision-making process concerning the procedure. Promote acknowledgment of the possible outcomes of the procedure. Encourage the patient to share the fears and anxieties related to both the act and the outcome of the procedure. Facilitate the implementation of relaxation and meditation techniques.

FACILITATING PREPROCEDURE CARE

Before operative and invasive procedures, patients require special preparation. This is done so that patients will experience the procedures with the least amount of risk, discomfort, and fear and will recover from them with a minimum of pain and other complications. A patient should also have an understanding of how he or she can assist in speeding recovery and convalescence. Before the patient's admission to the healthcare facility, or soon after, the physician writes orders specifying the type of preparation necessary for the patient. These orders may vary and are designed to meet the specific needs of each patient relating to the planned procedure. The orders may address all or some of the following aspects of care.

Patient Education

Patient education begins in the physician's office when the procedure is scheduled. When the patient arrives for testing in the pre-admission testing area, the nurse continues with the patient education regarding the care the patient will receive during the before, during, and after the operative or invasive procedure. Patient education prior to the day of procedure relieves anxiety, speeds recovery, reduces cost of hospitalization, prevents complaints about care, and increases patient compliance. If available, include the patient's family and/or support person in the preprocedure education. By educating the family members with the patient, the family members have a better understanding of the operative or invasive procedure and the postprocedure care. It helps alleviate the family member's anxiety and fear.

Preprocedure Skin Antisepsis

Preprocedure skin antisepsis is the first step in reducing the risk of postprocedure operative site infection (AORN, 2008). The patient may be instructed to take two preprocedure showers with chlorhexidine gluconate (CHG), when appropriate (AORN, 2008). The patient should be instructed not to shave or use a depilatory on the operative site prior to the procedure; removing hair at the operative site abrades the surface of the skin and also enhances microbial growth (AORN, 2008). Chapter 9 discusses preparing the patient's skin for the operative or invasive procedure.

CHG
Chlorhexidine
Gluconate

Preprocedure Hair Preparation

The patient should be instructed to wash his or her hair the night before the procedure and not to put oil or hair spray on the hair prior to the procedure, particularly if the patient is going to have a procedure in the head or neck area. Oil and hair spray are fuel sources and increase the patient's risk for injury secondary to a fire, especially in an oxygen-enriched atmosphere. If the patient has long hair, braiding will help in keeping the hair contained within the head covering.

Diet

By withholding food and fluids before an operative or invasive procedure, the patient reduces the risk of aspiration if protective reflexes are compromised during the procedure, particularly during the induction of and emergence from anesthesia. Also, if the procedure involves the upper gastrointestinal tract, the absence of food and liquids facilitates performance of the procedure. All patients are instructed to be NPO for a specified period of time prior to the procedure; these times may vary according to the anesthesia protocol of the healthcare facility. **Table 5.20** outlines the ASA Fasting Recommendations.

Gastrointestinal Tract Preparation

Bowel preparation is usually required only for patients having major abdominal, pelvic, perineal, or perianal procedures. The type and amount of bowel preparation depends on the physician's preference and the type of procedure scheduled. The common bowel preparations include oral laxatives and enemas. Depending on the results the physician needs, the patient may have only one bowel preparation or multiple types and multiple doses. Occasionally, oral antibiotics are given prior to operative procedures to help sterilize the bowel.

In certain types of abdominal operations, particularly those on the intestinal tract, it is necessary to have a nasogastric tube inserted through the nose to the esophagus and into the stomach. The tube is fastened in place and aids in removing fluid and gas, which can cause distention and postprocedure discomfort. If a patient has gastrointestinal obstruction, a nasogastric tube is passed before the procedure, and the stomach is aspirated or placed on continuous suction to reduce the possibility of regurgitation and aspiration during the induction of anesthesia. If an emergency procedure is to be performed on a patient who has eaten within 12 hours of the procedure, insertion

Table 5.20	Summary of Preprocedure Fasting Guidelines*

*These recommendations apply to healthy patients who are undergoing elective procedures; following these guidelines does not guarantee complete gastric emptying. These guidelines are not intended for women in labor.

Ingested Material	Minimum Fasting Period (Hours)
Clear Liquids	2—applies to all ages
— examples include water, fruit juices without pulp, carbonated beverages, clear tea, black coffee	
Breast Milk	4
Infant Formula	6
Non-Human Milks	6
— since non-human milk is similar to solids in *gastric* emptying time, the amount ingested must be considered when determining an appropriate fasting period.	
Light Meal	6
— A light meal typically consists of toast and clear liquids; meals that include fried or fatty foods or meat may prolong gastric emptying time. Both the amount and type of foods ingested must be considered when determining an appropriate fasting period.	

Adapted from: ASA (1999). Practice guidelines for preoperative fasting and the use of pharmacologic agents to reduce the risk of pulmonary aspiration: application to healthy patients undergoing elective procedures. *Anesthesiology;* 90: pp. 896–905.

of a nasogastric tube is advisable. When there is no indication for a nasogastric tube before the procedure and one is needed during the procedure, the anesthesia provider can pass the tube into the stomach after the patient is anesthetized.

Preprocedure Medications

The patients should be told which medications to take prior to the procedure, which medications need to be stopped, and when to stop taking them. It is common to have the patient stop taking aspirin-containing products, anticoagulants, and herbal medications several days prior to the procedure. Outpatients as well as patients being admitted the morning of the procedure should be instructed which medications to take the morning of procedure with a sip of water. The physician may order a barbiturate or sleeping pill for the night before the procedure to alleviate anxiety and to ensure a restful night's sleep. Immediately prior to the procedure, the anesthesia provider will usually administer IV midazolam (Versed) to reduce anxiety and if needed, an analgesic, typically fentanyl (Sublimaze).

Blood Transfusion

If the physician anticipates using blood or blood products during or after the operative or invasive procedure, the patient must have a type and screen or a type and crossmatch. This can be done during the preprocedure appointment in the admission testing area. Instruct the patient to wear the blood arm band until after the procedure and discharge home. If the patient removes the blood arm band prior to the procedure, another type and screen or type and crossmatch must be done. During the preprocedure visit to the physician, the patient can be given the option to donate his or her own blood. Usually the amount donated is two units. The patient can donate two weeks apart. But, the physician needs to make arrangements for the autologous blood transfusion donations. See Chapter 7 for more information concerning blood transfusion.

Urinary Bladder Preparation

If urinary retention is anticipated or if there is a need for hourly monitoring of urine output before, during, or after the procedure, a Foley catheter can be inserted for constant bladder drainage. If bladder distention interferes with exposure in the pelvis, a catheter, should be placed before the procedure. Catheterization can be done in the patient's room before the patient leaves the holding area, although it may preferably be done after the patient has been anesthetized.

Intravenous Therapy

For procedures associated with marked blood loss, a 14- or 16-gauge intravenous catheter is used for the rapid administration of blood, fluid, or medication. Intravenous therapy may be needed before the procedure for providing hydration as well as for maintaining adequate fluid and electrolyte balances. Intravenous access is advisable for conscious patients receiving local anesthetics, analgesics, and sedatives, as well as for patients receiving general or regional anesthetics.

Discharge Planning

Discharge planning begins during the preprocedure visit in the physician's office and in the preadmission testing area. With the tremendous increase of outpatient operative and invasive procedures, same day admission procedures, and shorter hospital stays, the preadmission testing area and the preprocedure nurses have an increased responsibility for discharge planning. The nurse can identify patients at risk for self-care deficit and noncompliance with treatment regimens. Discharge instructions includes that outpatients must have a responsible adult to drive them home and to stay with them for at least the first 24 hours. Other topics for the discharge instructions include diet, pain control, wound and dressing care, activity limitations, when to return to the physician, what to do or who to call for questions or an emergency.

Preprocedure Telephone Assessment

It is not always possible for the patient to have a preadmission testing appointment. For this reason, many facilities utilize preprocedure telephone assessments for suitable patients. Suitable patients are those who are healthy and need minimal testing that can be done the morning of surgery (such as, just a hemoglobin and hematocrit). The nurse conducting the telephone assessment will ask the same questions as she/he would ask if the assessment was being conducted face-to-face. If during any of the interview, the nurse identifies something that would indicate the need for additional preprocedure testing, the patient is instructed to visit the preadmission testing area prior to surgery. One of the major benefits for patients is that they do not need to visit the hospital prior to the day of procedure. For many patients this eliminates the need to take more time off work and struggle with car parking and child care. Assessments are completed by phone at a convenient time for the patient. For the preadmission testing area, this has resulted in a smoother patient flow since fewer many patients are being seen and there is a decreased waiting time. The preadmission testing area is able to assess a greater number of patients with more complex medical needs. The patients receiving the preprocedure telephone assessment receive the same verbal patient education as the face-to-face patients. If the patient request written materials, they can be mailed to the patient's home.

CONCLUSION

The nurse plays a crucial role in the physical, psychological, and emotional preparation of the patient for an operative or invasive procedure. Central to this role is facilitating the patient's admission to the healthcare facility, performing a preprocedure assessment, and facilitating preprocedure care. Through effective preprocedure preparation, the nurse can promote both a positive operative experience, as well as optimal patient outcomes.

COMPETENCY ASSESSMENT
Preparation of the Patient for the Procedure:
Physical, Psychological, and Emotional Considerations

Name: _____ Title: _____ Unit: _____ Date of Validation: _____

Type of Validation: ☐ Initial ☐ Annual ☐ Bi-annual

COMPETENCY STATEMENT: The nurse demonstrates competency to prepare the patient for an operative or invasive procedure

Performance Criteria	Met	Not Met
1. Facilitates patient admission to the healthcare facility	☐	☐
2. Identifies existing alterations in health status that contribute to the patient's risk for adverse outcomes	☐	☐
3. Identifies alterations in psychosocial and emotional health status	☐	☐
4. Facilitates preprocedure care	☐	☐

_____   _____

Validator's Signature   Employee's Signature

_____

Validator's Printed Name

ENDNOTE

1. The term physician refers to the Doctor of Medicine, Doctor of Podiatry, and Doctor of Osteopathy who may perform an operative or invasive procedure in the operating room suite, gastroenterology laboratory, interventional radiology suite, and cardiac catheterization laboratory.

REFERENCES

1. AORN (2008). Recommended practices for preoperative skin antisepsis. *Perioperative Standards and Recommended Practices.* Denver, CO: AORN, Inc; pp. 537–555.
2. ASA (1999). Practice guidelines for preoperative fasting and the use of pharmacologic agents to reduce the risk of pulmonary aspiration: application to healthy patients undergoing elective procedures. *Anesthesiology;* 90: pp. 896–905.
3. Bierstein, K. (2000). Miscellany: Pain, critical care and preop services. Retrieved June 16, 2008 from http://www.asahq.org/Newsletters/2000/03_00/practmang0300.html.
4. Bierstein, K. (2002). Preoperative visits—Should I bill for them? Retrieved June 16, 2008 from http://www.asahq.org/Newsletters/2002/2_02/pm202.htm.
5. Carpentino-Moyet, L. J. (2008) *Handbook of nursing diagnosis* (12th ed.) Philadelphia: Lippincott Williams & Wilkins.
6. Habel, M. (2006). Respiratory assessment: Adult and child. Retrieved June 4, 2008 from http://www.rnceus.com/resp/respframe.html.
7. Harkreader, H., Hogan, M., & Thobaben, M. (2007). *Fundamentals of Nursing: Caring and Clinical Judgment,* 3rd ed. St. Louis, MO: Saunders.
8. Ignatavicius, D. & Workman, M. (2006). *Medical-Surgical Nursing: Critical Thinking for Collaborative Care.* 5th ed. St. Louis, MO: Elsevier Sanders.
9. National Center for Education Statistics. (2006). Fast facts. Retrieved June 4, 2008 from http://nces.ed.gov/fastfacts/display.asp?id=69.
10. Nursing Fundamentals (2004). Components of a physical assessment. Retrieved June 4, 2008 from http://64.78.42.182/sweethaven/MedTech/FraPkr02.asp?iCode=040607.
11. O'Leary, P. (2008). Abnormal Heart Sounds. Retrieved June 4, 2008 from http://mtsu32.mtsu.edu:11259/abnormal_heart_sounds.htm.
12. Orlando Regional Healthcare, Education, & Development (2004). Interpretation of arterial blood gas. Retrieved June 4, 2008 from www.nursing4all.com/forum/attachment.php?attachmentid=1792&d=1196178040.
13. Petersen, C. (2007). Perioperative nursing data set, the perioperative nursing vocabulary, revised 2nd ed. Denver, CO: AORN. Inc.
14. Piedmont Hospital (2007). Surgical Services Policy and Procedure Manual, Respiratory System. Retrieved February 22, 2008 from http://en.wikipedia.org/wiki/Respiratory_system.
15. Roizen, M. F. (2005). Preoperative evaluation. In *Miller's Anesthesia,* 6th ed. R. Miller, Ed. Philadelphia, PA: Elsevier, pp. 927–997.
16. *Taber's® Cyclopedic Medical Dictionary,* 20th ed. (2005). D. Venes, ed. Philadelphia, PA: F.A. Davis Company.
17. The Joint Commission (2007). Standards sampler for ambulatory surgery centers. Retrieved June 16, 2008 from http://www.jointcommission.org/NR/rdonlyres/A88E7A36-0C20-4C37-B67D-CD8638538E09/0/ASC_stdsampler_07.pdf.

CHAPTER 6

Transfer the Patient

Roberta (Bobbie) Geiger

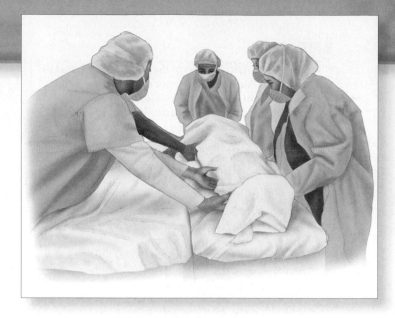

Chapter Contents

INTRODUCTION

Transfer the patient describes the activities of the nurse and other members of the operative and invasive procedure nursing team in moving the patient to and from the operative suite without compromising or causing injury to the patient.

Before transferring the patient, the nurse[1] assesses the patient's risk for adverse outcomes related to the transfer process, identifies nursing diagnoses that describe the patient's degree of risk, identifies expected outcomes that delineate criteria for determining whether the patient experienced an adverse outcome, and plans for patient care, which includes the identification of needed transfer equipment and the assignment of trained personnel to perform transfer activities. The nurse evaluates the patient after the procedure according to the criteria delineated in the expected outcomes.

Transferring the patient is the responsibility of the nurse. Other personnel, such as the surgical technologist, orderly, or nursing assistant, participate, especially during transfer between the nursing unit and the operative and invasive procedure suite. The nurse, however, has ultimate responsibility for the welfare of the patient during the preprocedure transfer process and when the patient is moved to the bed[2] from the gurney. This responsibility continues into the postprocedure transfer process when the patient is returned to the nursing unit or transferred to the postanesthesia care unit (PACU). When the nurse transfers the patient with the anesthesia provider, both share in the responsibility for patient welfare.

MEASURABLE CRITERIA

The nurse demonstrates competency to transfer the patient by:

- Identifying the patient's risk for adverse outcomes related to transfer activities.
- Performing or directing the transfer of the patient from the nursing unit to the operative and invasive procedure suite holding area.
- Implementing handoff communication protocols at time of transfer.
- Admitting the patient to the operative and invasive procedure suite.
- Performing or directing the transfer of the patient from the operative and invasive procedure suite holding area to the procedure room.
- Implementing the *Universal Protocols for Preventing Wrong Site, Wrong Procedure, and Wrong Person Surgery.*
- Assisting with the transfer of the patient from the operative and invasive procedure suite to the PACU.
- Performing or directing the transfer of the patient from the operative and invasive procedure suite to the nursing unit.
- Performing or directing the transfer of the patient with special needs.
- Documenting and communicating risk factors, nursing diagnoses, expected outcomes, the plan of care, interventions, and evaluation.

PACU
Postanesthesia
Care Unit

CONSIDERATIONS

Transferring the patient to and from the operative and invasive procedure suite is often viewed as a simple and tedious task that anyone can perform. Taking the transfer process lightly can lead to an adverse outcome for the patient.

Nurse Coordinating Transfer Activities

For the reason that each patient is unique and has different needs, the nurse coordinating the patient's transfer must ensure that only qualified personnel who have demonstrated competency to implement appropriate safety measures, such as the nurse, surgical technologist, or unlicensed assistive person, perform transfer activities. Additionally, when planning for a transfer, the nurse ensures that an adequate number of personnel are available to implement the transfer activity.

The nurse coordinating transfer activities determines the skill set required for a patient transfer. For some transfers the presence of a nurse, in some cases, an anesthesia provider, will be required. For routine transfers, such as low-risk patients having an elective procedure, the assignment for the transfer is given to a qualified unlicensed assistive person.

Personnel Assigned to Implement Transfer Activities

Personnel performing a transfer activity should know and apply the principles of body mechanics, which will help in reducing the risk for injury to the patient and staff. Prior to the transfer, the assigned personnel verify that all transfer equipment is functioning according to manufacturers' specifications. In the event restraints and other safety devices are required, they are used in accordance with regulatory standards, facility policy and procedure, and manufacturers' written instructions.

IDENTIFYING THE PATIENT'S RISK FOR ADVERSE OUTCOMES RELATED TO TRANSFER ACTIVITIES

Transfer activities have potential for compromising or causing injury to the patient. **Table 6.1** identifies outcome statements, diagnoses, risk factors, and outcome indicators related to this patient care event.

TRANSFERRING THE PATIENT TO THE OPERATIVE AND INVASIVE PROCEDURE SUITE HOLDING AREA

This section describes the patient care activities used to transfer the patient to the operative and invasive procedure suite. The nurse, surgical technologist, or other qualified assistive person may implement these patient care activities. The supplies and equipment needed are a gurney (a wheeled stretcher) with functional side rails and safety strap, an intravenous (IV) pole, a coversheet and blanket, and a patient pickup slip.

IV
Intravenous

Preparing for the Transfer

After receiving the patient transfer assignment, confer with the nurse coordinating the transfer or review the nursing care plan to check for orders concerning transportation equipment requirements and planned patient care activities during the transfer.[3] Obtain the transfer (pickup) slip, which identifies the patient by name, hospital number, and location. Note the time of departure from the operative and invasive procedure suite according to facility policy. After obtaining the needed transportation equipment and checking for proper functioning, go to the designated nursing unit.

Arriving on the Nursing Unit

After arriving on the nursing unit, report to the patient's nurse; ask if the patient is ready to depart for the operative and invasive procedure suite, and request that unit personnel assist with moving the patient to the gurney, if needed.

Reviewing the Patient's Chart

If the nurse is transferring the patient, before entering the patient's room or cubicle, the nurse will review the patient's chart, paying particular attention to the preprocedure checklist. If unlicensed assistive personnel are transferring the patient, this chart review will take place upon arrival in the operative and invasive procedure suite holding area. Check the procedure consent form for patient and witness signatures according to healthcare facility policy. Review the preprocedure checklist to ensure that the patient's jewelry has been removed, that the patient has voided and had nothing by mouth for the required length of time, and that all prostheses (eg, dentures, hearing aids) have been removed. Some healthcare facilities allow the patient to wear prostheses to the procedure suite. In such cases, the holding area and/or the circulating nurse will need to secure the prostheses during the procedure. Check the chart for x-ray films, electrocardiogram, laboratory reports, and other routine preprocedure reports specific to the facility.

Table 6.1	**Transfer Activities Implemented During the Operative and Invasive Procedure Period Do Not Compromise or Cause Injury to the Patient**

Outcome 1 The patient is free from signs and symptoms of injury related to transfer/transport.

Diagnosis	**Risk Factors**	**Outcome Indicators**
Risk for Injury related to transfer to and from the operative and invasive procedure suite	☐ Neuromuscular impairment ☐ Musculoskeletal impairment ☐ Vascular impairment ☐ Cognitive impairment ☐ Sensory/perceptual impairment (vision, hearing) ☐ Speech impairment ☐ Safety violations by the transporter ☐ Equipment malfunction ☐ Extraneous objects (hanging intravenous [IV] bags, patient drainage devices)	☐ Does the patient or family verbally identify an injury related to the transfer process? ☐ Does the patient show signs of injury such as broken or bruised skin?

Outcome 2 The patient is free from evidence of a decrease in body temperature during transfer to and from the operative and invasive procedure suite.

Diagnosis	**Risk Factors**	**Outcome Indicators**
Risk for Hypothermia related to transfer to and from the operative and invasive procedure suite	☐ Extremes in age (neonate, elderly) ☐ Extremes in weight ☐ Fluid deficit (dehydration) ☐ Altered metabolic rate ☐ Impaired temperature regulation secondary to illness or injury ☐ Vasoconstriction or vasodilation secondary to medication ☐ Cold environment ☐ Inadequate covering	☐ Does the patient indicate through verbal statements or nonverbal clues that he or she is experiencing discomfort due to cold? ☐ Does the patient show signs of temperature decrease (shivering or chattering teeth)?

Outcome 3 The patient is free from evidence of breathing difficulty.

Diagnosis	**Risk Factors**	**Outcome Indicators**
Risk for Ineffective Breathing Pattern related to transfer to and from the operative and invasive procedure suite	☐ Obesity ☐ Neuromuscular impairment ☐ Musculoskeletal impairment ☐ Perceptual or cognitive impairment ☐ Anxiety ☐ Preprocedure sedation ☐ Pain ☐ Improper position of the patient during transfer ☐ Pregnancy (third trimester)	☐ Does the patient state that he or she is having difficulty breathing? ☐ Does the patient show signs of difficulty breathing such as orthopnea, dyspnea, and shortness of breath, use of accessory muscles, altered chest excursion, tachypnea, cough, and nasal flaring?

6

Outcome 4	The patient is free from evidence of discomfort or pain during the transfer process.	

Diagnosis	**Risk Factors**	**Outcome Indicators**
Risk for Discomfort or Pain related to transfer to and from the operative and invasive procedure suite	☐ Existing injury ☐ Chronic physical disease such as osteoarthritis ☐ Neuromuscular impairment ☐ Musculoskeletal impairment ☐ Cognitive or perceptual impairment ☐ Anxiety ☐ Operative wound ☐ Presence of traction devices ☐ Equipment malfunction (imbalanced gurney wheels, which cause an uneven ride) ☐ Careless maneuvering of the gurney or the patient's bed by the transporter	☐ Does the patient verbally indicate the presence of discomfort or pain? ☐ Does the patient demonstrate nonverbal expressions such as facial masks of pain, guarded movement, crying, or moaning indicating discomfort or pain?

Adapted from Carpentino-Moyet, L. J. (2008). *Handbook of Nursing Diagnosis* (12th ed.) Philadelphia: Lippincott Williams & Wilkins, pp. 45–46, 364; *Perioperative Nursing Data Set, the Perioperative Nursing Vocabulary.* (Revised 2nd ed.). Denver: AORN. Inc., p. 48.

Arriving at the Patient's Room

Unit nursing personnel should accompany the transporter to the patient's room or cubicle to perform the preliminary identification to the patient and assist with the transfer process. After arriving at the patient's room, allow the unit nurse to tell the patient it is time to depart for the operative and invasive procedure suite.

Identifying the Patient

Identify the patient before transport to the operative and invasive procedure suite and holding area. This is done to ensure that the correct patient is transported at the appropriate time with all necessary paperwork completed and in the chart.

Alert and Oriented Patient

After entering the patient's room or cubicle, identify yourself and then ask the patient to say his or her name and what procedure she or he is having done. Ask open-ended questions, such as what is your full name please? And what procedure are you having done today? Patients are frequently anxious when being prepared for the procedure and this anxiety can impair their thought processes. The open-ended question requires the patient to think about the answer and allows the transporter to determine whether the patient is alert and oriented.

As the patient states her or his name, read the name on the transfer slip obtained from the operative and invasive procedure suite. Make a second identity check comparing the name and number on the patient's identification bracelet. Also, check the patient's name on the transfer slip with the name on the patient's chart.

The consent form is checked again to ensure that the procedure identified on the consent form is the same as that identified by the patient. Discrepancies should be corrected before the patient is transferred from her or his bed to the gurney. If discrepancies are found, call the operative procedure suite for guidance.

Child

When identifying a child, follow the steps for identifying an alert and oriented adult. The difference is to whom the questions are directed, which is based on the development of the child. Establish initial contact simultaneously with the child and parents or legal guardian. The parents or legal guardian signed the consent authorizing the procedure; therefore, they *must* participate in identifying the patient. Ask the parents or legal guardian the child's name and the procedure being done. If the child is old enough to respond, also ask the child the questions. This allows the child to participate in the care process.

If a parent or legal guardian is unavailable, rely on the unit nursing staff to identify the patient. This does not negate the need to check the transfer slip against the patient's hospital bracelet and chart.

Comatose or Disoriented Patient

With modification, use the same steps followed for identifying an alert adult when identifying the comatose or disoriented patient. If a family member or a significant other is present, ask him or her to identify the patient. In the absence of family members or significant other, ask the unit nursing staff or other personnel to identify the patient. Again, it is important to compare the transfer slip with the patient's identification bracelet and chart.

Transferring the Patient to the Gurney

After explaining to the patient what is going to happen, cover the patient up to the neck with a sheet or blanket. Next, position the gurney adjacent to the bed and lock the wheels of the bed and the gurney. Stand next to the gurney. Unit nursing personnel stand opposite, next to the bed. After raising the bed to the level of the gurney, tell the patient to move from the bed to the gurney, buttocks first, then the shoulders second, and feet last. During the transfer, the unit nursing personnel stabilize the bed by leaning against it. At the same time, raise the side rails. The possibility of side rails' becoming dislodged or falling is an ever-present danger; therefore instruct the patient to keep fingers, hands, arms, and legs, including the knees, away from the side rails.

IMPLEMENTING HANDOFF COMMUNICATION PROTOCOLS AT TIME OF TRANSFER

Handoff communication should take place at this time between the nurse in the patient care unit and the nurse picking up the patient. If other personnel, other than an anesthesia provider or nurse, are transporting the patient, handoff communication should take place via written checklist/document and signed by the patient care unit nurse. This ensures continuity of care and proper patient identification. **Table 6.2** describes handoff protocols applicable to transferring the patient.

Table 6.2	Handoff Communication Protocols

Any time the patient is transferred from one unit to another, a handoff communication protocol should be used. Patient safety and quality care can be improved with appropriate communication at each patient transfer.

Handoff communication should:

- ☐ Be interactive, structured and standardized for the facility and include an opportunity to ask and respond to questions
- ☐ Include information such as patient/problem, assessment/actions, continuing treatments and changes, and evaluations
- ☐ Occur verbally
- ☐ Have a written component such as a checklist or template
- ☐ Have a process for verification of the received information, including repeat-back or read-back and verify, as appropriate
- ☐ Be done with limited interruptions to minimize the possibility of information failing to be conveyed or forgotten
- ☐ Provide an opportunity for personnel receiving the patient to review relevant patient data, including historical and current care data, treatment, medication administration, operation reports, laboratory and imaging reports
- ☐ Document in writing the person signing off, the personnel accepting the patient, and the means/mode of transportation at the time of transfer

TRANSPORTING THE PATIENT TO THE OPERATIVE AND INVASIVE PROCEDURE SUITE

If present, family members or significant others should accompany the patient to the operative and invasive procedure suite. This may help minimize the patient's anxiety about the impending procedure.

Always push the gurney through the corridors feet first. This allows the patient to see where he or she is going. Also, some patients may experience motion sickness if moved backward. When turning corners, watch for unexpected obstacles or people. If using an elevator, pull the gurney in headfirst to avoid having the patient's head too close to the opening and closing elevator doors. After arriving at the designated floor, pull the gurney out of the elevator. When pulling the gurney out of the elevator, hold the elevator doors back to prevent inadvertent closure on the gurney.

On arrival in the operative and invasive procedure suite holding area, allow visitors, if not permitted in the holding area, to interact with the patient before he or she enters the suite. Tell or, if possible, show the significant others where to wait while the patient is having the procedure. Let them know that the physician will be told that they are in the waiting room so that he or she may speak to them after the procedure.

When in the holding area, lock the wheels of the gurney and tell the holding area nurse and suite patient care coordinator that the patient has arrived. Before leaving the holding area, document the method of transfer, who transported the patient, safety measures used, and the time when the patient arrived in the operative and invasive procedure suite. In some suites, the time when the patient arrived in the operative and invasive procedure suite is noted on the master schedule and/or the patient's chart.

ADMITTING THE PATIENT TO THE OPERATIVE AND INVASIVE PROCEDURE SUITE HOLDING AREA

The nurse implements the patient care activities used to admit the patient to the procedure suite. The supplies required are procedure documents, laboratory test results and the patient's data information card or labels. Admitting equipment includes blood pressure cuff and sphygmomanometer; temperature probes and recording devices; suction devices; emesis basins, urinals, and bedpans; warm blankets, preparation equipment such as depilatory and hair clippers; and IV needles, tubing, and bags. Many holding areas have electrocardiographic monitors and pulse oximeters. For pediatric patients, one or two rocking chairs, story books, and safe toys are appropriate. Adult and adolescent patients appreciate headphones and cassette players.

Reviewing the Patient's Chart

After the patient has arrived in the invasive procedure suite holding area, the holding area nurse assumes responsibility for care. The holding area nurse should ask open-ended questions, as well, to the patient. Greet the patient and review the chart for completeness and the patient data card for accuracy. Review the preprocedure checklist to determine whether the patient has voided, removed jewelry and prostheses, and received prescribed preprocedure medications. Check the chart for prescribed test reports, the history, and physical examination. Question the patient about allergies, and check the chart for information regarding allergies. Validate nothing-by-mouth status by asking the patient the last time he or she had something to eat or drink. Investigate items on the checklist not initialed as complete, and take appropriate corrective action before transferring the patient to the invasive procedure room.

Carefully review the consent forms for accuracy and completeness according to facility policy. Make every effort to ensure that the patient gave legal and informed consent. Ensure that all appropriate consents are signed, completed, and accurate. Consents should include: operative and/or invasive procedure consent, anesthesia consent, blood products consent, general consent, and hospital consent for treatment. If facility protocols have not been followed (barring emergency situations), obtain a valid consent before beginning the procedure. Patients with a cognitive impairment or altered sensorium secondary to preprocedure medication should not sign a consent form. When the patient is no longer affected by the medication, the physician counsels the patient; again, a new consent form is signed and witnessed according to facility policy.

Check the preprocedure orders for blood and blood products. If blood has been ordered, check with the patient care coordinator to ensure that the blood is available. If the blood is not available, call the laboratory to ensure the order has been received and to check blood availability. This information should be communicated in the handoff communication upon transfer of the patient to the invasive procedure suite.

Performing a Holding Area Assessment

If a nurse has had the opportunity to perform an assessment before the patient arrives in the operative and invasive procedure suite, review the assessment data. Add new assessment data to the record as necessary.

If an assessment has not been done, perform an assessment. Chapter 5 provides information on performing an assessment. After completing the assessment, give the assessment data to the nurse assigned to give patient care during the procedure.

Preparing the Paperwork for the Procedure

Prepare documentation paperwork before transferring the patient to the procedure room. Using the data card or labels, prepare the following records: anesthetic record, procedure report, nursing record (if separate from procedure report), charge slips, labels, and slips from the pathology, laboratory, operative progress note, intraoperative physician orders, and radiology departments. Organize the records and place them in the chart. Patient care records vary in number and content according to facility policy. Many facilities use electronic records to document patient care. In such cases, follow facility electronic record protocols.

TRANSFERRING THE PATIENT FROM THE OPERATIVE AND INVASIVE PROCEDURE SUITE HOLDING AREA TO THE PROCEDURE ROOM

The nurse implements the patient care activities used to transfer the patient from the holding area to the procedure room. The anesthesia provider may also accompany the nurse. Surgical technologists and other assistive personnel assist the nurse as necessary. The supplies and equipment needed are the bed, a draw (lift) sheet, armboards, safety strap for the legs and arms, IV poles, warm sheets, and headrest.

Preparing for the Transfer

After invasive procedure team members are ready to receive the patient, go to the holding area and check with the holding area nurse about the status of the patient. The holding area nurse reports pertinent findings from the patient assessment. Greet the patient and let him or her know that it is time to go to the procedure room. After verifying the patient's identity, allergies, and nothing-by-mouth status and the planned procedure, check the chart for the consent form and the presence of laboratory and radiology department reports. At this time an additional handoff communication should take place.

Transporting the Patient to the Procedure Room

Unlock the wheels of the gurney and push it feet first. On entering the procedure room, announce to team members that the patient is entering the room. Staff in the room must keep noise to a minimum. Introduce the patient to the staff in the room. After lowering the side rail next to the bed, position the gurney next to the bed and lock the wheels. Before moving the patient, check the wheels of the bed and lock them. Lower the side rail.

Mobile Patient

Stand next to the gurney. Ask the anesthesia provider or assistive person to stand on the opposite side of the bed to protect the patient from falling off the bed during transfer. Remove any blankets that were wrapped around the patient during the transfer to the operative and invasive procedure suite. Leave the cover sheet over the patient. Move the IV bags to the IV pole near the head of bed. If the patient has drainage devices, hold them during the transfer process or place them on the patient. Ask the patient to move to the bed, moving buttocks first, shoulders second, and feet last. Protect the patient's privacy by keeping the cover sheet in place during the transfer.

Immobile Patient

Depending on the patient's size, at least four people should move the immobile patient. The nurse and assistants should place themselves at the sides of the patient, two at the head and two toward the foot of the gurney, with legs apart, one ahead of the other, and as close to the bed and gurney as possible. The anesthesia provider remains at the head of the bed and directs the transfer. Place the patient's arms across the chest. After rolling the patient to the side toward the lifters stationed by the gurney, place a lifting sheet or transfer device under the patient (**Fig. 6.1**). The patient is supported and on the count of three moved from the gurney to the bed (**Fig. 6.2**). During the transfer, the anesthesia provider supports the head and the lifters at the foot of the bed support the feet (**Fig. 6.3**). After the patient is moved to the bed, gently roll him or her to the side and remove the transfer sheet or transfer device (**Fig. 6.4**).

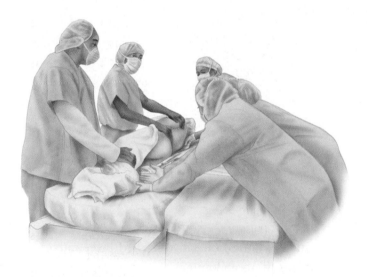

Figure 6.1

The nurse and assistants position themselves for the transfer and prepare the patient for the transfer.

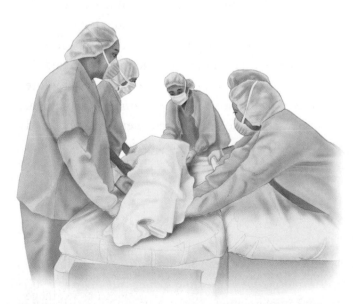

Figure 6.2

The nurse and assistants are ready to transfer the patient from the gurney to the bed.

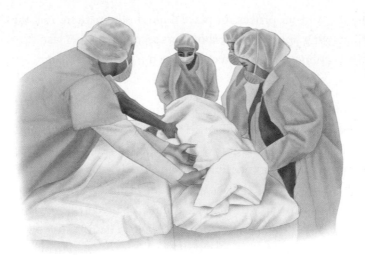

Figure 6.3
The head and feet are supported during the transfer.

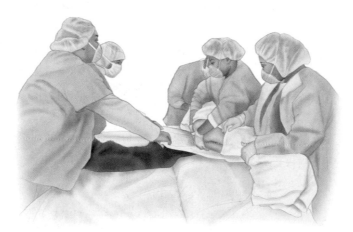

Figure 6.4
The transfer sheet is removed.

Securing the Patient on the Procedure Bed

After the patient is on the bed, center the patient's hips and check the body alignment of the patient's shoulders, abdomen, and feet along the length of the bed. Place and secure a safety strap across the patient's thighs, if an abdominal procedure, approximately 2 inches (5 cm) above the knees. Check the strap for excessive tautness or looseness by placing one hand between the thighs and the strap. The strap should not be so tight as to prevent the hand from being placed between the thighs and the strap. Securing the strap is crucial, especially as the patient enters the excitement phase of anesthesia and emerges from the anesthesia at the end of the procedure. Patients employed in physically demanding occupations or aggressive hobbies sometimes respond more combatively during the excitement phase than do other patients. Improperly securing the safety strap on these patients could result in patient injury. Place the patient's hands and arms on the armboards and secure with arm straps as per facility policy.

IMPLEMENTING UNIVERSAL PROTOCOLS FOR PREVENTING WRONG SITE, WRONG PROCEDURE, AND WRONG PERSON SURGERY

After the patient has been placed on the procedure bed and prior to the initiation of the procedure, the *Universal Protocols for Preventing Wrong Site, Wrong Procedure, and Wrong Person Surgery* are implemented. This is a prime responsibility of all team members and must be diligently performed for every operative and invasive procedure. **Table 6.3** highlights the Joint Commission on Accreditation of Healthcare Organizations protocols and describes the purpose and the process for *preoperative verification, marking the operative site* and *time out* immediately before starting the procedure. *Preoperative verification* begins when the transfer process starts and continues as the patient moves through the perioperative continuum leading up to the procedure. Marking the operative site should take place prior to the patient entering into the procedure room.

Once all members are present in the operating room, a universal *time out* must take place just before starting the procedure. Members present must include: the surgeon, anesthesia personnel, registered nurse circulator, and scrub person. The *time out* information is an active communication between all team members. This communication should include: name of patient's allergies, medical record number, procedure and site, including laterality, level, and structure, if applicable, correct patient position, availability of implants, special equipment, ex-rays as applicable, hung for review by the physician. **Table 6.4** describes how to implement the protocols.

Table 6.3	Universal Protocol For Preventing Wrong Site, Wrong Procedure, Wrong Person Surgery™

Preoperative Verification Process

Purpose: To ensure that all of the relevant documents and studies are available prior to the start of the procedure and that they have been reviewed and are consistent with each other and with the patient's expectations and with the team's understanding of the intended patient, procedure, site, and, as applicable, any implants. Missing information or discrepancies must be addressed before starting the procedure.

Process: An ongoing process of information gathering and verification, beginning with the determination to do the procedure, continuing through all settings and interventions involved in the preoperative preparation of the patient, up to and including the *time out* just before the start of the procedure.

Marking the Operative Site

Purpose: To identify unambiguously the intended site of incision or insertion.

Process: For procedures involving right/left distinction, multiple structures (such as fingers and toes), or multiple levels (as in spinal procedures), the intended site must be marked such that the mark will be visible after the patient has been prepped and draped.

Time Out Immediately Before Starting the Procedure

Purpose: To conduct a final verification of the correct patient, procedure, site and, as applicable, implants.

Process: Active communication among all members of the surgical/procedure team, consistently initiated by a designated member of the team, conducted in a *fail-safe* mode (ie, the procedure is not started until any questions or concerns are resolved).

Adapted from "Universal Protocol For Preventing Wrong Site, Wrong Procedure, Wrong Person Surgery," Joint Commission on Accreditation of Healthcare Organizations, http://www.jointcommission.org/NR/rdonlyres/ E3C600EB-043B-4E86-B04E-CA4A89AD5433/0/universal_protocol.pdf (accessed on 11 April 2008).

Table 6.4	Implementation Expectations for the Universal Protocol for Preventing Wrong Site, Wrong Procedure, and Wrong Person Surgery™

Preoperative Verification Process

Verification of the correct person, procedure, and site should occur (as applicable):

- ☐ At the time of surgery/procedure is scheduled.
- ☐ At the time of admission or entry into the facility.
- ☐ Anytime the responsibility for care of the patient is transferred to another caregiver.
- ☐ With the patient involved, awake, and aware, if possible.
- ☐ Before the patient leaves the preoperative area or enters the procedure/surgical room.

A preoperative verification checklist may be helpful to ensure availability and review of the following, prior to the start of the procedure:

- ☐ Relevant documentation (eg, H&P, invasive procedure consent, general consent, blood product consent, laboratory values, anesthesia consent).
- ☐ Relevant images properly labeled and displayed.
- ☐ Any required implants and special equipment.

Marking the Operative Site

Marking the operative site can take place in the preoperative holding area or the admission area.

- ☐ Make the mark at or near the incision site. Do NOT mark any non-operative site(s) unless necessary for some other aspect of care.
- ☐ The mark should be unambiguous (eg, use initials or "YES" or a line representing the proposed incision; consider that "X" may be ambiguous).
- ☐ The mark should be positioned to be visible after the patient is prepped and draped.
- ☐ The mark should be made using a marker that is sufficiently permanent to remain visible after completion of the skin prep. Adhesive site markers should not be used as the sole means of marking the site.
- ☐ The method of marking and type of mark should be consistent throughout the organization.
- ☐ At a minimum, mark all cases involving laterality, multiple structures (fingers, toes, lesions), or multiple levels (spine). Note: In addition to pre-operative skin marking of the general spinal region, special intraoperative radiographic techniques are used for marking the exact vertebral level).
- ☐ The person performing the procedure should do the site marking.
- ☐ Marking should take place with the patient involved, awake and aware, if possible.
- ☐ Final verification of the site mark should take place during the "time out."
- ☐ A defined procedure should be in place for patients who refuse site marking.

Exemptions

- ☐ Single organ cases (eg, Cesarean section, cardiac surgery).
- ☐ Interventional cases for which the catheter/instrument insertion site is not predetermined (eg, cardiac catheterization).
- ☐ Teeth—BUT, indicate operative tooth name(s) on documentation OR mark the operative tooth (teeth) on the dental radiographs or dental diagram.
- ☐ Premature infants, for whom the mark may cause a permanent tattoo.

Time Out **Before Starting the Procedure**

Conduct *time out* just before starting the procedure. It should involve the entire operative team (including the surgeon, anesthesia provider, circulator, surgical technician), using active communication, be briefly documented, such as in a checklist and/or visible item, such as a board, (organization should determine the type and amount of documentation) and should include:

- ☐ Correct patient identity.
- ☐ Correct side and site.
- ☐ Agreement on the procedure to be done.
- ☐ Correct patient position.
- ☐ Availability of correct implants and any special equipment or special requirements.
- ☐ Allergies.
- ☐ Medications on sterile and antibiotic given and time given.

The organization should have processes and systems in place for reconciling differences in staff responses during the *time out.*

Procedures for non-OR Settings (Including Bedside Procedures)

- ☐ Site marking should be done for any procedure that involves laterality, multiple structures or levels (even if the procedure takes place outside of an OR).
- ☐ Verification, site marking, and *time out* procedures should be as consistent as possible throughout the organization, including the OR and other locations where invasive procedures are done.
- ☐ Cases in which the individual doing the procedure is in continuous attendance with the patient from the time of decision to do the procedure and consent from the patient through to the conduct of the procedure may be *exempted* from the site marking requirement. The requirement for a *time out* final verification still applies.

Adapted from "Implementation Expectations for the Universal Protocol for Preventing Wrong Site, Wrong Procedure, and Wrong Person Surgery," Joint Commission on Accreditation of Healthcare Organizations, http://www.jointcommission.org/NR/rdonlyres/DEC4A816-ED52-4C04-AF8C-FEBA74A732EA/0/up_guidelines.pdf (accessed on 11 April 2008).

TRANSFERRING THE PATIENT FROM THE PROCEDURE ROOM TO THE POSTANESTHESIA CARE UNIT

This section describes the patient care activities used to transfer the patient from the procedure room to the PACU. Transfer from the procedure room to the PACU is potentially the most dangerous time for the patient during the transfer progress. The patient may not be fully recovered from the effects of the anesthetic agents and thus is dependent on the procedure team members for basic support such as airway management. Therefore, the nurse must implement the patient care activities with the anesthesia provider. Surgical technologists and other assistive personnel assist the nurse as necessary. The supplies and equipment needed are recovery bed with an IV pole and functional side rails; an oxygen tank with delivery valve and tubing and at least 500–1000 pounds per square inch in the tank; an oral airway; a warm sheet and blanket, and a patient body roller.

Preparing to Transfer the Patient from the Bed

Four people are needed as described for transferring the immobile patient to the bed. Place the patient's arms across the chest. The side lifter on the side opposite the recovery bed holds the patient's arms across the chest. Remove the armboards from the bed and move the recovery bed adjacent to the bed. Lock the wheels of the recovery bed. For the unresponsive patient or one unable to control his or her arms, the lifter on the opposite side of the bed from the recovery bed ensures that the patient's arms remain across the chest. Move the IV bags to the IV pole on the recovery bed. Do not lower the IV bags below the level of the patient's heart. Next, move drainage tubes to the recovery bed. Keep the bags below tube exit sites. Remove safety strap. **Figure 6.5** shows patient care team members ready to move the patient to the recovery gurney. The anesthesia provider directs the transfer.

Transferring the Patient to the Recovery Bed
Mobile Patient

The anesthesia provider tells the alert patient who is physically capable of moving to move to the recovery bed, buttocks first, shoulders second, and feet last. While the patient is moving, lean against the recovery bed and assist the patient. Keep the patient covered during the move. Center and align the patient after he or she moves to the recovery bed. Raise the side rails. If indicated, the anesthesia provider places an oxygen mask or nasal cannula on the patient and opens the oxygen tank valve.

Immobile Patient: Bed Tilt Technique

For this transfer technique, assistive personnel stand next to the bed and the nurse stands next to the recovery bed. Raise the bed above the level of the recovery bed. The side lifter standing next to the bed reaches across the patient and grasps the draw sheet. He or she brings the sheet over the patient and uses it to hold the patient in position while the bed is tilted.

Move the recovery bed slightly away from the bed to allow the anesthesia provider to operate the lever and thus tile the bed. The anesthesia provider tilts the bed toward the recovery bed. After the anesthesia provider tilts the bed as much as possible, move the recovery bed back against the bed.

As the side lifter holding the patient releases the end of the draw sheet, which was used to hold the patient in place, grasp the free end of the draw sheet during this maneuver, place one foot in front of the other, bend slightly at the waist, and keep the upper torso straight. On the anesthesia provider's count, pull the draw sheet and patient toward the recovery bed. While pulling the patient, shift your body weight from the front foot to the back foot and simultaneously raise the upper torso, which is kept straight.

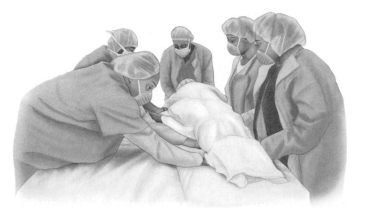

Figure 6.5

The patient is safely positioned and covered for transfer from the operating suite.

The side lifter on the opposite side places one foot in front of the other and shifts weight in the back foot. He or she pulls the draw sheet taut under the patient and positions his or her hands against the patient, one at the shoulders and the other at the hips. On the anesthesia provider's count, the lifter shifts weight to the front foot, bends slightly at the waist while keeping the upper torso straight, and moves the patient down the incline created by the tilted bed to the recovery bed. During this maneuver, the anesthesia provider moves the patient's head and the lifter at the foot of the bed moves the patient's legs and feet.

Roller/Slide Technique

Assistive personnel stand next to the procedure bed as described for transferring the immobile patient to the bed. The circulating nurse stands next to the recovery bed. Remove the safety strap. The side lifter next to the procedure bed reaches across the patient and grasps the draw sheet. With permission from the anesthesia provider, the side lifter pulls the sheet up. The patient will roll toward the lifter. After the side lifter rolls the patient on his or her side, position the body roller under the draw sheet as far as possible, between the patient's shoulders and thigh. The roller should not extend above the head or foot of the recovery bed. Next, lower the patient onto the roller/slide.

Standing with one leg slightly ahead of the other, the circulating nurse reaches across the recovery bed and grasps the draw sheet. The upper torso must remain straight and not bent along the spine during this maneuver. On the anesthesia provider's count, the nurse steps backward and slightly raises his or her torso while pulling the draw sheet. The lifter on the other side of the bed also moves the patient on the anesthesia provider's count. This lifter takes one step forward while bending slightly at the waist keeping the torso straight. The lifter then moves the patient at the shoulder and hip over the roll in the recovery bed. The anesthesia provider moves the patient's head, and the lifter at the foot of the bed moves the patient's feet.

After moving the patient, have the lifter move to the recovery bed. On the anesthesia provider's count, as the lifter removes the roller, roll the patient toward you with the draw sheet. After removing the roller, push the draw sheet under the patient as far as possible. Next, roll the patient onto her or his back and gently remove the draw sheet. At this time, remove residue preparation solution, blood, and other secretions with a warm wet towel or sponge. Also, assess the patient's skin integrity. Dry and cover the patient with a warm blanket. Raise the recovery bed side rails and transfer the patient to the PACU.

Transferring the Patient to the PACU

After collecting the chart, nursing notes, and x-ray films, accompany the patient to the PACU. The anesthesia provider pushes the recovery bed feet first. During the transfer, pull the recovery bed and help the anesthesia provider to maneuver the bed. In the PACU, give a report to the postanesthesia nurse. At a minimum, the report should include the patient's condition, nursing care provided during the procedure, and the location of dressing and drainage devices.

TRANSFERRING THE PATIENT FROM THE OPERATIVE AND INVASIVE PROCEDURE SUITE TO THE NURSING UNIT

Occasionally, a patient will be returned to the nursing care directly from the operative and invasive procedure room, bypassing the postanesthesia care unit. In such cases, the nurse is responsible for coordinating this transfer and depending on the patient's condition, may participate in the transfer activities. The supplies and equipment needed are a gurney with functional side rails and safety straps, an IV pole, an emesis basin, a warm covering for the patient, and oxygen if warranted by the patient's condition.

Preparing for the Transfer

After transferring and securing the patient to the gurney, gather the chart, nursing notes, and x-ray films. Unlock the gurney wheels. If transport to the nursing unit is delayed, take the patient to the holding area to await transfer back to the nursing unit.

Giving a Patient Status Report to the Nursing Unit Nurse

Contact the unit nurse by telephone. Tell the unit nurse about the patient's condition, including an overview of vital signs during the procedure, the medications given during the procedure and the dosage, drainage devices, and physician's orders that must be implemented immediately after the patient returns to the nursing unit.

Transferring the Patient to the Nursing Unit

Before departure, assess the patient to determine whether a nurse should accompany the patient to the unit. Transfer the patient as described for transporting the patient to the operative and invasive procedure suite holding area. After arrival on the nursing unit, the transporter ensures that nursing personnel know that the patient has returned to the unit.

TRANSFERRING THE PATIENT WITH SPECIAL NEEDS

Depending on the patient's risk for adverse outcomes during the transfer process, the nurse, surgical technologist, or other qualified assistive person may implement these patient care activities. The nurse assesses the patient's risk for adverse outcomes before the transfer process and then decides who should implement the activities. Supplies and equipment needed are a gurney with functional side rails and safety strap, an IV pole, a cover sheet and a head cover for the patient, a warm infant gurney for neonates, a crib for young children, oxygen tanks with delivery devices, and a portable monitor and defibrillator unit.

Intensive Care Patient

A nurse from the operative and invasive procedure suite or intensive care nurse should accompany all patients from the intensive care unit. If the patient requires respiratory assistance, an anesthesia provider or a respiratory therapist should also accompany the critically ill patient to the operative and invasive procedure suite.

Before transporting the patient from the intensive care unit, contact the intensive care unit nurse to determine transfer needs. After collecting the appropriate equipment and ensuring its proper functioning, go to the intensive care unit with an assistive person and an anesthesia provider or respiratory therapist, if warranted.

Before departing from the intensive care unit, coordinate with the operative and invasive procedure suite patient care coordinator to ensure that the patient will immediately be taken into the designated procedure room on arrival. Do not begin the transfer until the room is ready.

Patient with Major Orthopedic Injuries

Before transporting the patient with an orthopedic injury, assess the patient to determine the extent of injury, the traction or immobilization devices in use, and the appropriate vehicle for transfer. In general, patients with extensive injuries and multiple skeletal support devices are transported to the operative and invasive procedure suite in their orthopedic bed. This minimizes disruption in the skeletal traction that is being used.

Orthopedic beds with traction devices are not designed for transporting patients to the operative and invasive procedure suite and therefore are not easy to handle. Additional personnel are needed to move the bed through hospital corridors and onto elevators. When transferring the patient with traction devices, ensure that the transfer is accomplished without compromise of the patient's traction-induced skeletal alignment.

Infants

Like intensive care patients, infants should be taken directly to the procedure room, unless the holding area is equipped and staffed to provide care. This requires prior coordination with the operative and invasive procedure suite patient care coordinator. Perform a preprocedure assessment to determine the extent of care required. A warmed infant transport vehicle provides a protective environment for the neonate during the transfer. Depending on the condition of the patient, the nurse, the pediatrician, or the anesthesia provider accompanies the patient to the operative and invasive procedure suite. Equipment needed for the neonate may include an oxygen tank with appropriate delivery equipment, a portable monitor and defibrillator, and an IV infusion device. Parents or a guardian should accompany the infant to the operative and invasive procedure suite if they desire. Do not transfer the infant until the procedure room is warmed and prepared for the procedure.

Toddlers

Toddlers and other children who are uncooperative, such as those refusing to remain lying and secured with a safety strap, should be transported in a crib with a bubble top and side rails up. The parents or guardian should accompany the child to the operative and invasive procedure suite, and, if possible, carry the child while the transporter pushes the crib. On arrival in the operative and invasive procedure suite holding area, the parents or guardian may stay with the patient until it is time to bring him or her into the procedure room and stay with the child during the induction of anesthesia.

DOCUMENTATION AND COMMUNICATION PROCEDURES

Documentation begins with the preprocedure assessment. The nurse records assessment data, identifies nursing diagnoses and expected outcomes that pertain to transferring the patient, the plan for care, and the results of the evaluation. Transporters are informed by the nurse about the patient's needs during transfer. The transporter documents transfer activities according to the hospital policy and procedure. At a minimum, documentation by the transporter must include the method of transfer, the time of arrival in and departure from the operative and invasive procedure suite, and the identification of who transported the patient.

COMPETENCY ASSESSMENT
Transfer the Patient

Name: _____ Title: _____ Unit: _____ Date of Validation: _____

Type of Validation: ☐ Initial ☐ Annual ☐ Bi-annual

COMPETENCY STATEMENT: The nurse demonstrates competency to transfer the patient during the operative and invasive procedure period.

	Performance Criteria	Met	Not Met
1.	Identifies the patient's risk for adverse outcomes related to transfer activities	☐	☐
2.	Performs or directs the transfer of the patient from the nursing unit to the operative and invasive procedure suite holding area	☐	☐
3.	Implements handoff communication protocols at time of the transfer	☐	☐
4.	Admits the patient to the operative and invasive procedure suite	☐	☐
5.	Performs or directs the transfer of the patient from the operative and invasive procedure suite holding area to the procedure room	☐	☐
6.	Implements Universal Protocols for Preventing Wrong Site, Wrong Procedure, and Wrong Person Surgery	☐	☐
7.	Assists with the transfer of the patient from the operative and invasive procedure suite to the PACU	☐	☐
8.	Performs or directs the transfer of the patient from the operative and invasive procedure suite to the nursing unit	☐	☐
9.	Performs or directs the transfer of the patient with special needs	☐	☐
10.	Documents and communicates risk factors, nursing diagnoses, expected outcomes, the plan of care, interventions, and evaluation	☐	☐

_____ _____
Validator's Signature   Employee's Signature

_____
Validator's Printed Name

ENDNOTES

1. The term "the nurse" refers to a registered nurse.
2. The term "bed" refers to the operating room bed (table) and to the invasive procedure bed (table).

3. If transfer activities are performed by nursing unit personnel, the unit nurse is responsible for the transfer and related communication.

REFERENCES

1. "Implementation Expectations for the Universal Protocol for Preventing Wrong Site, Wrong Procedure, and Wrong Person Surgery," Joint Commission on Accreditation of Healthcare Organizations, http://www.jointcommission.org/NR/rdonlyres/DEC4A816-ED52-4C04-AF8C-FEBA74A732EA/0/up_guidelines.pdf (accessed on 11 April 2008).
2. "Universal Protocol for Preventing Wrong Site, Wrong Procedure, Wrong Person Surgery," Joint Commission on Accreditation of Healthcare Organizations, http://www.jointcommission.org/NR/rdonlyres/E3C600EB-043B-4E86-B04E-CA4A89AD5433/0/universal_protocol.pdf, (accessed on 11 April 2008).

3. AORN Standards, *Perioperative Standards and Recommended Practices* (2008), Patient Outcome Standards, Denver, CO: AORN.
4. Carpentino-Moyet, L.J. (2008) *Handbook of Nursing Diagnosis* (12th ed.) Philadelphia, PA: Lippincott Williams & Wilkins.
5. Johnson, M., Bulechek, G., McCloskey-Dochterman, J., Maas, M., Moorhead, S. *NANDA, NOC, and NIC linkages: Nursing diagnoses, outcomes, & interventions.* (2005). St. Louis, MO: Mosby.
6. *Perioperative nursing data set, the perioperative nursing vocabulary* (2007) (Revised 2nd ed.). Denver: AORN.

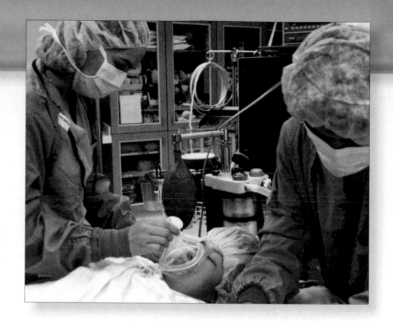

CHAPTER 7

Assist the Anesthesia Provider

Charles J. Moss

Rose Moss

INTRODUCTION

Assist the anesthesia provider refers to the activities performed by the registered nurse to support the anesthesia provider during the administration of anesthesia. During an operative or invasive procedure, the patient is usually anesthetized or sedated, and therefore is incapable of making decisions on his/her own behalf. Through effective collaboration with and assisting the anesthesia provider, the nurse serves as the patient's advocate at a time when he/she is most vulnerable; this aspect of operative and invasive procedure nursing care is critical to the promotion of positive patient outcomes.

HISTORICAL PERSPECTIVE

The starting point from which anesthesiology emerged as a medical specialty was the public demonstration of ether anesthesia by William T.G. Morton in 1846 (Larson, 2005). Prior to this event, operative procedures were associated with unimaginable pain and the high probability of death. Historical accounts, including those by Ashhurst (1896), document that over hundreds of years, the search for pain-relieving techniques was undertaken by cultures worldwide. Various pain-relieving modalities ranged from botanical preparations of belladonna, marijuana, and jimsonweed; hypnosis; to actually striking the person to induce unconsciousness. By the 1800s, opium and alcohol were only partially effective and often accompanied by serious side effects such as vomiting and death. Since the 1800s, there have been both enormous progress and change in the specialty of anesthesiology, including increased understanding of cardiopulmonary physiology, intravascular pressures, autonomic nervous system

Chapter Contents

and neurohumoral transmission; the development of pain theories, and the introduction of the various types of anesthesia. In fact, the majority of operative procedures in today's operating rooms (OR) could not have been performed before the progress in anesthetic practice that took place between the years of 1925 and 1960 (Larson, 2005).

OR
Operating Room

OVERVIEW

The administration of anesthesia is an integral part of operative and invasive procedure patient care, not only in hospital-based operative suites, but also in ambulatory surgery centers, physicians' offices, and other outpatient facilities. Therefore, assisting the anesthesia provider is an important role of the nurse providing care to the patient undergoing operative and invasive procedures requiring anesthesia. The anesthesia provider may be an anesthesiologist, a certified registered nurse anesthetist (CRNA), anesthesia assistant (AA), a physician in an anesthesiology residency program, or a registered nurse in a nurse anesthesia program. Anesthesia technicians or other unlicensed assistive personnel may also provide assistance to the anesthesia provider. The skills required by the nurse to assist the anesthesia provider range from patient assessment, knowledge of disease processes and medical treatment modalities, the objectives of the operative intervention to critical thinking skills in order to effectively anticipate patient care needs.

CRNA
Certified Registered Nurse Anesthetist

AA
Anesthesia Assistant

The nurse should also be familiar with the definition of the scope of anesthesia practice; the various types of anesthesia, including the equipment and supplies needed for each type; and also the level of assistance required to meet the anesthetic needs of the patient. In order to better understand the scope of the specialty of anesthesiology, it is helpful to review the definition promulgated by the American Board of Anesthesiology (2004):

> Anesthesiology and perioperative management are defined as the continuity of patient care involving preoperative [preprocedure] evaluation, intraoperative and postoperative [postprocedure] care and the management of systems and personnel that support these activities.

MEASURABLE CRITERIA

The nurse demonstrates competency to assist the anesthesia provider during the operative or invasive procedure by:

- Identifying the patient's risk for potential adverse outcomes related to the administration of anesthesia;
- Describing the various types of anesthesia;
- Assisting the anesthesia provider with induction of anesthesia;
- Assisting the anesthesia provider with proper positioning for regional anesthesia;
- Describing the potential physiologic changes that may occur during monitored anesthesia care;
- Assisting the anesthesia provider with administering blood component therapy;

- Assisting the anesthesia provider during emergency procedures;
- Assisting the anesthesia provider with the management of a malignant hyperthermia crisis;
- Implementing measures to maintain the patient's body temperature;
- Assisting with parental presence during induction of anesthesia for pediatric patients according to facility policy;
- Controlling and monitoring the environment to minimize noise and conversations in the operative or invasive procedure room, especially during induction of and emergence from general anesthesia; and
- Assisting the anesthesia provider in preventing anesthesia awareness.

IDENTIFYING THE PATIENT'S RISK FOR POTENTIAL ADVERSE OUTCOMES RELATED TO THE ADMINISTRATION OF ANESTHESIA

The preprocedure assessment is the initial step toward identifying the patient's risk for potential adverse outcomes related to the administration of anesthesia (**Table 7.1**). This assessment ensures that the patient is ready for an operative or invasive procedure from both the nursing and anesthesia perspectives. A complete assessment is necessary and helpful in determining the patient's medical

Table 7.1 Outcomes Related to Assisting the Anesthesia Provider

Outcome 1 The patient is free from evidence of injury secondary to the induction of general endotracheal anesthesia.

Diagnosis	Risk Factors	Outcome Indicators
Risk for Injury during the administration of general endotracheal anesthesia.	☐ Emergency procedure, (eg, trauma, ectopic pregnancy, ruptured abdominal aortic aneurysm) ☐ Maxiofacial trauma ☐ Cervical spine trauma ☐ Full stomach at time of induction ☐ Ineffective airway clearance ☐ History of cardiac disease ☐ ASA classification of P3–P5	☐ Did the patient experience interruptions in breathing patterns during intubation? ☐ Did the patient aspirate gastric contents during intubation? ☐ Did the patient experience injury or exacerbation of existing injury secondary to intubation?

Outcome 2 The patient is free from evidence of injury secondary to malignant hyperthermia during the administration of general anesthesia.

Diagnosis	Risk Factors	Outcome Indicator
Risk for Injury secondary to malignant hyperthermia during the administration of general anesthesia.	☐ One parent with autosomal dominant trait ☐ Family history of malignant hyperthermia	☐ Did the patient experience a malignant hyperthermia reaction during the procedure?

- ☐ Exposure of susceptible individual to a triggering agent such as inhalation anesthetics and succinylcholine
- ☐ Muscular dystrophy
- ☐ Central core disease
- ☐ First time administration of general anesthesia
- ☐ Neuromuscular disorders, such as
  - ☐ Duchenne muscular dystrophy
  - ☐ King-Denborough syndrome
  - ☐ Becker muscular dystrophy
  - ☐ Other myopathies
  - ☐ Periodic paralysis
  - ☐ Myotonia congenita
  - ☐ Schwartz-Jampel syndrome
  - ☐ Fukuyama-type congenital muscular dystrophy
  - ☐ Mitochondrial myopathy
  - ☐ Sarcoplasmic reticulum adenosine triphosphate deficiency.

Outcome 3 The patient is free from evidence of injury secondary to the administration of blood products during the operative or invasive procedure.

Diagnosis	**Risk Factors**	**Outcome Indicator**
Risk for injury secondary to the administration of blood products during the operative of invasive procedure.	☐ Recipient of allogenic blood ☐ Emergency procedure ☐ Operative hemorrhage	☐ Did the patient have a transfusion reaction during the procedure?

Outcome 4 The patient maintains northermia during the operative or invasive procedure.

Diagnosis	**Risk Factors**	**Outcome Indicators**
Risk of Hypothermia during the operative of invasive procedure.	☐ Trauma or large open wound ☐ Exposure of internal organs and body cavities ☐ Extremes in age ☐ Malnutrition ☐ Sedation ☐ Decreased metabolism ☐ Use of cool fluids for irrigation and infusion ☐ Inadequate warmth during the operative procedure	☐ Does the patient have a decrease in body temperature below range? ☐ Does the patient's skin feel cool? ☐ Does the patient show evidence of mental confusion? ☐ Does the patient have a decrease in pulse and respiration rates?

Risk for Hyperthermia during the operative of invasive procedure.	☐ Dehydration	☐ Did the patient experience body temperature increase above the normal range?
	☐ Illness resulting in fever	
	☐ Use of warm fluids for irrigation and infusion	☐ Was the patient's skin Hushed?
	☐ Use of medication causing vasoconstriction or adverse reaction	☐ Did the patient have an increase in respiratory rate (particularly the non-ventilated patient)?
	☐ Endocrine disorders such as thyroid disease	☐ Was there evidence of tachycardia?
	☐ Intracranial infection or injury to the hypothalamus	☐ Did the patient have a seizure or convulsion?

Adapted from Carpentino-Moyet, L. J. (2008) *Handbook of Nursing Diagnosis* (12th ed.) Philadelphia: Lippincott. Williams & Wilkins; Petersen C. (2007). *Perioperative Nursing Data Set, the Perioperative Nursing Vocabulary.* (Revised 2nd ed.). Denver: AORN. Inc.; AORN (2008) Malignant Hyperthermia Guideline, *Perioperative Standards and Recommended Practices.* Denver: AORN, Inc.

and operative and invasive procedure history, as well as his/her present physical, mental, and emotional status. The assessment is not only a requirement outlined by the Joint Commission, but it also documents, from a legal point of view, the patient as he/she presented before the procedure.

Effective preprocedure assessment improves outcomes by ensuring that patients are adequately prepared for anesthesia, the operative or invasive procedure, as well as the postprocedure period; it can also improve overall efficiency by decreasing patient waiting times and enabling early discharge. Preprocedure assessment for patients having elective operative or invasive procedures has become recognized as a valuable method of ensuring a safe and well-planned hospital experience (Beck, 2007).

Vital health information can be obtained by reviewing the information in the medical record before meeting with the patient. A preprocedure assessment is performed by a member of the anesthesia care team prior to the patient's arrival in the operative and/ or invasive procedure holding area; this assessment is then documented in the patient's record. The anesthetic plan is based on the assessment data, as well as the planned procedure, patient and/or family concerns, and the results of the laboratory tests, radiographs, electrocardiogram, and any other tests performed before the procedure. The assessment is usually completed on an outpatient basis for those patients who arrive the day of the procedure; the anesthesia assessment of inpatients usually takes place the night before the procedure. During the assessment, the anesthesia care team discusses and educates the patient and patient's family on the anesthetic options, expectations, risks and benefits, and also answers questions pertaining to the anesthetic plan.

As part of this initial assessment, the patient's American Society of Anesthesiology (ASA) classification (**Table 7.2**) (ASA, 2008), used to determine risk factors based on the patient's current physical/health status, should be used as a guide to aid both the anesthesia provider and nurse in anticipating potential adverse events that may occur as a result of anesthetic intervention and/or the procedure.

ASA
American Society of Anesthesiology

Table 7.2	ASA Physical Status Classification System	
P1	A normal healthy patient	
P2	A patient with mild systemic disease	
P3	A patient with severe systemic disease	
P4	A patient with severe systemic disease that is a constant threat to life	
P5	A moribund patient who is not expected to survive without the operation	
P6	A declared brain-dead patient whose organs are being removed for donor purposes	

Source: American Society of Anesthesiologists. ASA physical status classification system. Retrieved January 5, 2008 from http://www.asahq.org/clinical/physicalstatus.htm.

Other key components of patient preparation are the operative site verification process and "time out," which are outlined in the Joint Commission's Universal Protocol for Preventing Wrong Site, Wrong Procedure, Wrong Person Surgery™. The Universal Protocol requires active communication and involvement of the entire operative team. The "time out" can be recorded by checklist or other methods specified by organizational policy and must, at the least, include (Joint Commission, 2008):

- Correct patient identity;
- Correct side and site;
- Agreement on the procedure to be done;
- Correct patient position; and
- Availability of correct implants and any special equipment or special requirements.

The use of a preprocedure or anesthesia induction room is increasing in popularity. Mean turnover times, as well as the time spent in the OR, have been shown to be reduced by the concurrent induction of anesthesia (Sokolovic et al, 2002). While previous studies of anesthesia induction outside the OR focused either on anesthesia-controlled time or turnover time, a recent study investigated the impact of an induction room model on the entire operative process, including its phases and delays between the phases, and the number of cases performed during the seven-hour working day (Torkki et al, 2005). The authors conducted a prospective analysis of OR times for five weeks with the traditional induction-in-the-OR model followed by four weeks with the new model—a team of two nurses and one anesthesiologist was added to one OR to perform parallel anesthesia induction in a separate induction room. The durations of phases of operative process, number of completed cases between 7:45 AM and 3:00 PM, and daily raw utilization of the OR were assessed; the data were compared to those measured before the intervention. The results indicated that operative time remained unchanged while the mean nonoperative time was reduced by 45.6%. The time savings contributed to the concurrent anesthesia induction and the decrease in delays between the phases. The new model allowed one additional case to be performed during the seven-hour working day.

TYPES OF ANESTHESIA

In order to effectively assist the anesthesia provider, the nurse must be aware of the nursing implications of the various types of anesthetic interventions. Throughout the patient's operative or invasive procedure experience, the nurse should remain alert to the potential adverse reactions to anesthesia and be prepared to assist the anesthesia provider in all phases of general, regional, or monitored anesthesia care.

General Anesthesia

General anesthetics depress the central nervous system (CNS), alleviate pain, and cause loss of consciousness. General anesthesia involves the management of a complex array of anesthetic agents that act in an intricate web of neural connections or neural nexus. Inhaled and intravenous anesthetics must intervene at some level of the neural nexus in order to produce amnesia, immobility, hypnosis, and suppression of noxious reflexes; this intervention occurs at the spinal and supraspinal level and involve spinal pathways and centers of arousal and memory formation centrally. Currently research does not support the concept of a single mechanism of action for general anesthetics, but instead suggest that anesthetics act by altering neuronal ion channels and neural communication; in general, anesthetics act by either enhancing inhibitory transmission or blocking excitatory conduction in neural impulses (Villars, Kanusky, & Dougherty, 2004).

Intravenous (IV) induction agents may be opioid or non-opioid; these agents include propofol (Diprivan®); etomidate (Amidate®); barbiturates such as thiopental sodium (Pentothal®) and methohexital (Brevital®); benzodiazepines such as diazepam (Valium®), lorazepam (Ativan®), and midazolam (Versed®) are used both for preanesthesia sedation and induction of anesthesia; and ketamine (Ketalar®). Inhalation anesthetic agents used today include isoflurane (Forane®), desflurane (Suprane®), sevoflurane (Ultane®), and nitrous oxide.

Muscle relaxants are also an important component of general anesthesia. These agents cause skeletal muscle contractions to cease. Muscles relaxants work by blocking the effect of acetylcholine at the neuromuscular junction; they are used to enable endotracheal intubation and facilitate both mechanical ventilation and the operative procedure through muscle relaxation. The muscle relaxants commonly used today are pancuronium (Pavulon®), rocuronium (Zemuron®), vecuronium (Norcuron®), and succinylcholine chloride (Anectine®).

The nurse should also be familiar with the laryngeal mask airway (LMA) in order to assist the anesthesia provider during induction of general anesthesia (**Fig. 7.1**). The LMA is a supraglottic airway device that is designed to provide and maintain a seal around the laryngeal inlet for spontaneous ventilation and allow controlled ventilation at modest levels of positive pressure and are available in a variety of sizes (Gal, 2005). Before insertion, the cuff of the mask is deflated and lubricated. After the patient is anesthetized, his/her neck is extended and then the mouth is opened widely. The apex of the mask, with its open end pointing downwards toward the tongue, is pushed backwards towards the uvula. The LMA device follows the natural bend of the oropharynx, coming to rest over the pyriform fossa. Once in place, the cuff around the mask is inflated with air in order to create a tight seal; the entry of air into the lungs is confirmed by ausculatation, or by the presence of end tidal carbon

CNS
Central Nervous System

LMA
Laryngeal Mask Airway

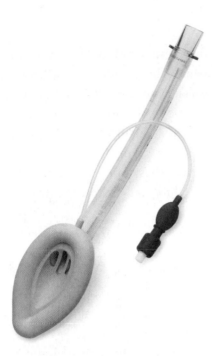

Figure 7.1

Laryngeal mask.

Source: Courtesy of LMA North America, Inc.

dioxide. When the anesthesia provider is using an LMA, the nurse can best assist him/her by remaining at the head of the bed and assisting with inflation of the cuff or as needed.

During induction and maintenance of general anesthesia, the nurse should be aware of the potential patient responses and be prepared to assist appropriately. For example, during induction, the patient's hearing becomes intensified. The nurse should reduce extraneous noise by closing the procedure room doors and reduce talking and unnecessary movement in the room (see below for additional information on conversations and noise in the procedure room). In addition, he/she should remain at the head of the bed to provide emotional support to the patient and assist the anesthesia provider as needed with endotracheal intubation, including obtaining and preparing a different size endotracheal tube (ETT) upon request, removing the stylet, and providing cricoid pressure as directed.

ETT
Endotracheal
Tube

Regional/Blocks

Local anesthetics are pharmacologic agents that suppress pain by blocking impulse conduction along axons; conduction is blocked only in the neurons located close to the administration site. By blocking axonal sodium channels, local anesthetics stop sodium entry, thereby preventing conduction. In comparison to general anesthetics, the primary advantage of local anesthetics is that pain can be suppressed without causing the generalized depression of the entire nervous system. Therefore, local anesthetics allow selected operative or invasive procedures to be performed with less risk than that which is associated with general anesthesia. Agents used for regional anesthesia include bupivacaine (Marcaine®, Sensorcaine®), chloroprocaine (Nesacaine®), lidocaine (Xylocaine®), mepivacaine (Carbocaine®), and ropivacaine (Naropin®).

During the administration of regional anesthesia, the nurse should assist the anesthesia provider with proper positioning of the patient, adjust lighting as needed for optimal visualization, and assist with preparing the anesthetic agents upon request.

MAC
Monitored
Anesthesia Care

Monitored Anesthesia Care

Monitored anesthesia care (MAC) is defined as the combination of local anesthesia with intravenous (IV) sedative and analgesic agents. This term is used when an anesthesia provider monitors a patient receiving local anesthesia or administers supplemental agents to the patient undergoing a diagnostic or therapeutic procedure. The primary objective of MAC is to ensure patient comfort, safety, and satisfaction during the procedure. The standard of care for the patient receiving MAC is the same as that for a patient undergoing regional or general anesthesia, that is, a complete preprocedure assessment, monitoring during the procedure, and postprocedure care (White & Freire, 2005).

Anesthetic agents, as well as various sedative-hypnotic drugs, are administered during MAC with the goal of providing analgesia, sedation, and anxiolysis, as well as ensuring a quick recovery without adverse effects. The sedative-hypnotic agents used include barbiturates, benzodiazepines, ketamine, and propofol; these may be administered by a variety of delivery systems, such as intermittent bolus, variable-rate infusion, or target-controlled infusion (White & Freire, 2005).

During MAC, the nurse should be aware of any sudden or unanticipated physiologic changes in the patient, such as bradycardia, hypotension, or hypoventilation, and assist the anesthesia provider as directed.

POSTPROCEDURE CARE

Recovery from anesthesia and an operative or invasive procedure intervention is usually a smooth, uneventful process. Staff in the postanesthesia care unit (PACU) must simultaneously care for the patient as he/she is emerging from general anesthesia or recovering from regional anesthesia and must be experienced and flexible to ensure proper recovery and eventual discharge (Feeley & Marcario, 2005). Today, the use of shorter-acting agents and the prompt initiation of effective pain relief measures, in combination with the recognized standards for PACU admission and discharge, have changed the approach to anesthetic recovery (Apfelbaum, 2002).

PACU
Postanesthesia
Care Unit

Once the care of the patient has been transferred from the anesthesia provider to the PACU registered nurse and all questions have been answered, the nurse assesses and monitors the patient until the following critical elements are met (ASPAN, 2008):

1. patent airway without assistance,
2. initial assessment completed, and
3. hemodynamic stability.

The PACU registered nurse consults with the anesthesia provider as the patient's condition warrants, based on continual assessment of the patient and his/her responses to nursing interventions.

BLOOD COMPONENT THERAPY

A survey conducted by the ASA's Committee on Blood and Blood Products demonstrated that much of all blood given to patients is done so during the operative and invasive period (Nuttall, Stehling, & Beighley, 2003). Therefore, the anesthesia provider and nurse must remain aware of the implications and potential complications associated with blood transfusions. Blood transfusions are given to increase oxygen-carrying capacity and intravascular volume. The American College of Surgeons (ACS) has classified blood loss into four groups based on the amount of blood loss and the patient's physiologic response (**Table 7.3**) (Miller, 2005).

ACS
American College of Surgeons

Compatibility testing (including the ABO-Rh type, crossmatch, and antibody screen) is designed to establish any harmful antigen-antibody interactions in vitro, in order to prevent harmful in vivo antigen-antibody interactions (Miller, 2005). Although the safety of the nation's blood supply is promoted by rigid standards and the American Red Cross guidelines for collection, storage, and transfusion, allogenic blood product administration still carries with it small, but acknowledged risks from infection and immunologic changes. To make a sound decision about transfusing and to quantify the numbers and types of units, knowledge of the estimated blood loss is critical. Communication between the anesthesia provider and nurse about estimated blood loss on sponges, on drapes, and in suction canisters should be ongoing, as should estimates when circumstances such as the use of irrigation solutions prevents a more accurate accounting.

The use of autologous blood, donated by the patient several weeks before an elective operative procedure, is assumed to be much safer than allogenic blood, primarily

Table 7.3	Classes of the American College of Surgeons (ACS) for Acute Hemorrhage			
Parameter	**Class I**	**Class II**	**Class III**	**Class IV**
Blood loss (mL)	≤750 mL	750–1,500 mL	1,500–2,000 mL	≥2,000 mL
Blood loss (as percent total blood volume)	≤15%	15–30%	30–40%	≥40%
Pulse	>100	>100	>120	≥140
Blood pressure (BP)	Normal	Normal	Decreased	Decreased
Pulse pressure	Normal or increased	Decreased	Decreased	Decreased
Capillary refill	Normal	Delayed	Delayed	Delayed
Respirations	14–20	20–30	30–40	>35
Urine output	≥30 mL/h	20–30 mL/h	5–10 mL/h	Minimal
Mental status	Slightly anxious	Mildly anxious	Anxious and confused	Confused and lethargic
Intravenous replacement solutions	Crystalloid	Crystalloid	Crystalloid & blood (in ratio of 3:1)	Crystalloid & blood (in ratio of 3:1)

Adapted from: Miller R. D. (2005). Transfusion therapy. In *Miller's Anesthesia*, 6th ed. RD Miller, ed. Philadelphia, PA: Elsevier; 1799–1930.

because of the decreased risk of infection (Miller, 2005). Complications are still associated with autologous blood transfusions and include (Domen, 1998):

- Anemia
- Preprocedure myocardial ischemia due to anemia
- Administration of the wrong units
- The need for more frequent blood transfusions
- Febrile and allergic reactions

In order to assist with the safe administration of either allogenic or autologous blood, strict adherence to blood bank rules for checking units with a second person continue to be important. Likewise, the administration of cell-saver blood should be accompanied by policies on verifying the origin of the unit. Both a blood warmer and filter are commonly used, and assistance with their setup may be requested by the anesthesia provider. A filter is used to remove microaggregates of fibrin and platelets that form during storage; facility policy will outline the pore size of the filter to be used.

Transfusion reactions are rare, but potentially serious. The classic signs and symptoms of a transfusion reaction—fever, chills, chest and flank pain, and nausea—are masked by anesthesia; under general anesthesia, the only signs that may be present are hemoglobinuria, bleeding diathesis, or hypotension (Miller, 2005).

In the event of a suspected reaction, the anesthesia provider will stop the transfusion immediately and send a sample of the patient's blood to determine the presence of hemoglobinemia and urine for analysis of hemoglobinuria. Cardiovascular support may require rapid volume expansion and administration of vasoactive agents, while ongoing operative blood loss may worsen the situation. Assistance with resuscitation efforts and information on measured blood loss and laboratory results will improve the anesthesia provider's ability to manage this serious event. The nurse can assist the anesthesia provider in taking appropriate action when a reaction is suspected or confirmed; a protocol for the management of a hemolytic transfusion reaction is outlined in **Table 7.4** (Miller, 2005).

EMERGENCY PROCEDURES

Management of the patient undergoing an emergency operative or invasive procedure varies depending on the nature of the emergency and the hemodynamic stability of the patient. In every emergency the nurse must be prepared to act quickly because changes in the patient may occur acutely. Emergency procedures are performed for a number of clinical conditions, such as traumatic injuries, ruptured aneurysm, and ectopic pregnancy. In an emergency, there is little time to prepare, and it is essential that all members of the operative team work together in an expedient manner to provide safe and effective care for the patient. In-depth assessments are often not possible, and underlying medical diseases such as diabetes or hypertension may be uncontrolled and/or exacerbated as a result of the emergent situation and with the impending procedure.

Induction of general anesthesia on these patients must be quick and yet accomplished safely. If the patient arrives in the procedure room awake, his/her anxiety level

Table 7.4	Protocol for Management of a Hemolytic Transfusion Reaction

1. STOP THE TRANSFUSION

2. Maintain urine output at a minimum of 75–100 mL/hour by:
   - generously administering IV fluids and possibly Mannitol (12.5–50 g, administered over 5–15 minutes)
   - if IV fluids and mannitol are ineffective, administer furosemide (Lasix®) IV (20–40 mg)

3. Alkalinize the urine:
   - administer sodium bicarbonate (40–70 mEq per 70 kg of body weight)
   - repeat urine pH determinations to determine the need for additional bicarbonate

4. Assay urine and plasma hemoglobin concentrations.

5. Determine platelet count, partial thromboplastin time, and serum fibrinogen level.

6. Return unused blood to blood bank for repeat crossmatch.

7. Send the patient's blood and urine samples to the blood bank for examination.

8. Prevent hypotension to ensure adequate renal blood flow.

Adapted from: Miller R. D. (2005). Transfusion therapy. In *Miller's Anesthesia*, 6th ed. RD Miller, ed. Philadelphia, PA: Elsevier; 1799–1930.

may be greatly increased, due to the unanticipated operative or invasive procedure. The patient requires emotional support to calm the fear and anxiety related to the impending procedure and its possible outcomes. Frequently, the patient may arrive from the emergency department in an unstable condition, possibly with a full stomach; occasionally the patient may already be intubated. Effective assistance to the anesthesia provider by the nurse is of utmost importance in emergencies; expeditious interventions by the entire operative team may indeed save the life of the patient.

Vomiting of stomach contents and subsequent aspiration is a real danger in these patients because the anesthesia evaluation of the patient may be brief with little information available about the NPO status of the patient. If aspiration does occur, the patient may experience acute respiratory compromise, which may ultimately lead to cardiac arrest. The nurse must stay focused with the anesthesia provider during induction and intubation. Cricoid pressure is applied as soon as the patient loses consciousness, and constant pressure must be maintained until the airway is safely secured. If there is traumatic injury to the neck, intubation may be quite difficult and therefore require the strategies and equipment for difficult airway management. Ideally, at the beginning of an emergency procedure there should be two circulating nurses, or a circulating nurse and a qualified assistive person, to accomplish all that is needed to provide safe patient care.

The induction method of choice for these patients is a rapid sequence induction (RSI), which is the use of pharmacologic agents to aid in establishing a definitive airway; it is intended for those patients who are considered at risk of aspiration of stomach contents, the so-called "full stomach" patients, as an effort to decrease the potential occurrence of pulmonary aspiration (Pousman, 2008). RSI involves:

RSI
Rapid Sequence Induction

- Induction—the use of pharmacologic agents, whether it be intravenous solutions or inhaled gases, that act on the brain to *quickly* move from consciousness to unconsciousness; to create a plane or level of anesthesia.
- Preoxygenation—the application of oxygen to the patient prior to attempting intubation.
- Premedication—the administration of medications prior to the induction of anesthesia; usually chosen with a particular purpose in mind.
- Cricoid Pressure—the use of gentle, continuous downward pressure on the cricoid cartilage of the larynx; intended to aid in protection from aspiration by compressing the larynx against the posteriorly located esophagus.
- Neuromuscular Relaxing Agents—drugs that produce a chemical paralysis of skeletal muscle. It must always be remembered that these agents only paralyze skeletal muscle; they offer *no* benefit of sedation or analgesia. Also called paralytic agents, neuromuscular blockers, and skeletal muscle relaxants.

The difference in the performance of RSI from induction in a non-emergent situation is the exclusion of assisted ventilation once the patient is induced. The induction agent is immediately followed by administering the paralytic agent, thus the name "rapid sequence induction." Preoxygenation is done before administering any agents and cricoid pressure is applied until airway establishment has been confirmed. A sample RSI sequence is as follows (Pousman, 2008):

ECG
Electrocardiogram

- All equipment is available and functional—this includes laryngoscopes, ETTs, suction, No. 11 blade, pulse oximeter/end tidal CO_2 monitor, electrocardiogram (ECG), and BP monitors.
- IV access is established.
- Preoxygenation with non-rebreather mask or AMBU bag—valve-assisted ventilations with the application of cricoid pressure.
- Premedications, if any, are administered.
- The induction agent is administered.
- The paralytic agent is given immediately following induction.
- Laryngoscopy and intubation is performed.
- ETT placement is confirmed (listening for bilateral equal breath sounds, absence of breath sounds over the stomach, esophageal detector, presence of end tidal CO_2, observing symmetrical chest expansion).
- Cricoid pressure is then released.
- ETT is secured.
- Patient is ventilated with additional paralysis and sedation as needed.

Airway management is the critical first step in preparing a patient for an emergency procedure; unless the airway is safely secured, other efforts toward saving the patient's life may be futile. Patients are compromised in a number of ways when they present for an operative and/or invasive procedure under emergency circumstances. As stated earlier, the patient may not have had an in-depth assessment and therefore laboratory tests and sometimes radiographs may be necessary. Laboratory test results are needed immediately and may be performed on portable machinery outside the operative or invasive procedure suite. The same laboratory standards and procedures apply, but results are obtained in a *stat* mode. Often blood component therapy must be initiated quickly; in extreme emergencies, non-cross-matched type-specific blood may be given. Cell-saver units and other blood pump team efforts may need to be initiated quickly. Maintenance of body temperature may also be a major concern, especially for trauma patients. Appropriate warming methods (ie, increasing the ambient temperature of the procedure room, forced-air warming blankets, warmed IV fluids and irrigation solutions, warmed and humidified anesthetic gases) must be implemented as appropriate to achieve and maintain normothermia.

MALIGNANT HYPERTHERMIA

Malignant hyperthermia (MH) is a serious, and potentially fatal, complication of general anesthesia that often occurs without warning and requires immediate attention by all members of the operative team. In its classic form, MH occurs during anesthesia with a volatile inhalation agent such as halothane and the depolarizing muscle relaxant succinylcholine, and produces rapid increases in temperature (rising by as much as 1°C every 5 minutes) and severe acidosis. MH is a dominantly inherited trait, but remains latent until one of the triggering agents or conditions activates the self-disseminating crisis. Malignant hyperthermia is a myopathy, characterized by an acute loss of control of intracellular calcium ions (Gronert, 2005). The triggering agent causes an increase in intracellular calcium ion concentration; this elevated calcium level causes a sequence of reactions, producing the signs and symptoms related to hypermetabolism, including, but not limited to, tachycardia, dysrhythmias, tachypnea, hypercarbia, respiratory acidosis, metabolic acidosis, muscle rigidity, elevated body temperature, cyanosis, skin mottling, hyperkalemia, diaphoresis, rapid temperature elevation, hemodynamic instability, and coagulopathy (AORN, 2008a).

MH
Malignant
Hyperthermia

In order to effectively assist the anesthesia provider, it is prudent for the nurse to be knowledgeable about MH and also to be prepared for an MH crisis, even though its occurrence is rare. All operative patients should be screened for a family history of MH. The nurse assesses, documents, and reports any MH risk factors identified in the preprocedure evaluation to the anesthesia provider and other members of the operative team. The nurse should also develop a plan of care with appropriate interventions to attain the expected outcomes; the interventions should be implemented as needed. For example, in the event of an MH crisis, the nurse should assist the anesthesia provider in turning off all anesthetic agents and replacing the anesthesia machine. A protocol for the management of an MH crisis, as well as an MH crisis cart, stocked with all the necessary supplies, drugs and solutions should be readily available in all clinical practice settings where anesthesia is administered.

The AORN Malignant Hyperthermia Guideline provides a resource for nurses and outlines the key nursing responsibilities during an MH crisis. The following are some of the nursing interventions may be indicated (AORN, 2008a):

- Recognize and report deviations in diagnostic studies;
- Use supplies and equipment within safe parameters;
- Identify physiological status; report variances from normal (electrocardiogram, vital signs, lab values);

- Assess skin condition;
- Implement protective measures to prevent skin/tissue injury due to thermal sources;
- Administer prescribed medications and solutions:
  - Dantrolene sodium (Dantrium®)
    - At the present time, dantrolene sodium (Dantrium®) is the only known drug that treats MH. It impairs calcium-dependent muscle contraction and controls the hypermetabolism manifestations associated with MH.
    - Dantrolene sodium (Dantrium®) should be mixed with sterile water for injection (without a bacteriostatic agent; 60 mL per 20 mg ampule) and shaken vigorously
    - Rapidly administer IV dantrolene sodium (Dantrium®) 2–3 mg/kg initial bolus
  - Sodium bicarbonate
    - Used to correct metabolic acidosis (as indicated by blood gas analysis)
    - Initial dose of 1–2 mEq/kg—repeat as indicated
  - Glucose and insulin
    - Used to treat hyperkalemia—give either:
      - 10 units regular insulin in 50 mL 50% glucose titrated to potassium level; or
      - 0.15 u/kg regular insulin in 1 cc/kg 50% glucose
  - Calcium chloride
    - 2–5 mg/kg to treat hyperkalemia
  - Anti-arrhythmic agents
    - Used if dysrhythmias persist following treatment of acidosis and hyperkalemia
  - AVOID solutions containing potassium
- Implement thermoregulation measures;
- Consult with appropriate members of the healthcare team to implement new treatments or change existing treatments;
- Monitor physiological parameters (vital signs, ie, blood pressure, pulse rate, body temperature; oximetry; capnometry; core temperature, ie, esophageal, tympanic, axillary, rectal, bladder; urine color and output; diaphoresis; mottling of the skin);
- Administer intravenous therapy—DO NOT use lactated Ringer's solution, as it may contribute to the patient's acidosis; and
- Provide postprocedure instructions to patient/significant other/support person.

Another resource for consultation in patient management of an MH crisis is the MH Hotline (1.800.MH-HYPER—1.800.644.9737). The nurse should report patients who have had acute MH episodes to the North American MH Registry of Malignant Hyperthermia Association of the United States (MHAUS) by means of a confidential report (1-412-692-5464). The nurse can also refer patients and families to MHAUS for additional information and/or to be included in the registry database (see www.mhreg.org).

MHAUS
Malignant
Hyperthermia
Association of the
United States

TEMPERATURE MANAGEMENT

Temperature management of the patient during the operative or invasive procedure period is another area of increased awareness for all members of the operative team. The Perioperative Nursing Data Set (PNDS) describes a desired outcome related to the maintenance of normothermia, Outcome 012, as "the patient is at or returning to normothermia at the conclusion of the immediate postprocedure period." (Beyea, 2002). This outcome is defined as: "the patient's core body temperature is within expected or therapeutic range" (Beyea, 2002).

While there are no standardized definitions of normothermia and hypothermia in the literature, the most widely accepted definitions are (ASPAN, 2002):

- Normothermia: core body temperature range of 36°C to 38°C (96.8°F to 100.4°F)
- Hypothermia: core body temperature less than 36°C (96.8°F)

Hypothermia can be further defined in three levels (Rolfe, 2008):

- Mild: 34°C–36°C (93.2°F–96.8°F)
- Moderate: 30°C–34°C (86° F–93.2°F)
- Severe: <30°C (<86°F)

It is important to remember that hypothermia may be present, despite the patient's temperature, if the patient expresses feeling cold or presents with common signs and symptoms of hypothermia, such as shivering, peripheral vasoconstriction, and piloerection (Frank, Raja et al, 1999).

To understand how hypothermia develops in the patient, knowledge of the four mechanisms of heat loss and their implications within the operative and invasive procedure environment is vital. Heat can be transferred from a patient to the environment in four ways: radiation, convection, conduction, and evaporation (Moss, 2000; Sessler, 2005):

- Radiation—this is the greatest source of the body's heat loss, in the form of radiant energy from a warmer surface (i.e., the body) to a cooler one (i.e., the environment) although the two are not in direct contact (**Fig. 7.2**). Radiation accounts for about 65% of heat loss.
- Convection—this is the loss of heat through circulating air currents; it is dependent on a temperature gradient between the body and the ambient air (**Fig. 7.3**). In the OR, it is often called the "wind chill factor" and is due to the required ventilation and air exchanges. Convention accounts for approximately 25% of the body's heat loss.
- Conduction—conduction is the loss of heat from a warmer surface through direct contact with a cooler one (**Fig. 7.4**). In the operating room, the patient loses heat to the cooler bed, sheets, and drapes. Conduction accounts for only about 5% of the body's heat loss.
- Evaporation—with evaporation, heat is transferred or lost as surface fluid converts to gas (**Fig. 7.5**). Most evaporative heat loss during a procedure is due to exposed viscera, perspiration, respiration, and evaporation of skin prep solutions. Evaporative heat loss accounts for approximately 5% of the body's heat loss.

In addition to recognizing the mechanisms of heat loss, the effects of anesthesia in the redistribution of body heat and subsequent development of hypothermia

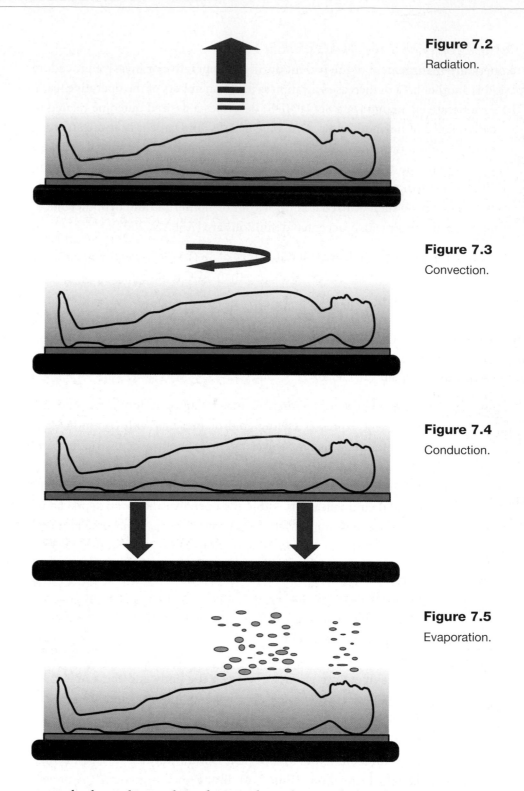

Figure 7.2
Radiation.

Figure 7.3
Convection.

Figure 7.4
Conduction.

Figure 7.5
Evaporation.

must also be understood. Inadvertent hypothermia during the operative or invasive procedure period results from anesthetic-impaired thermoregulation and exposure to the cold environment of the procedure room (Sessler & Kurz, 2006). Anesthetics inhibit thermoregulation in a dose-dependent manner and inhibit vasoconstriction and shivering approximately three times as much as they restrict sweating (Sessler, 1997). During general anesthesia, there is a characteristic pattern to the development of hypothermia:

- first, there is an initial rapid reduction in the core temperature;
- secondly, there is a slow decrease in the core temperature;

- finally, the core temperature stabilizes and remains practically unchanged (Sessler, 2000).

The redistribution effect, which is defined as the transfer of heat from the warmer core to the colder periphery and vice versa, is responsible for the development of hypothermia after induction of anesthesia (**Fig. 7.6**). Research has demonstrated that the greatest core temperature drop occurs during the first hour of operative, as a direct result of anesthesia (Sessler, Schroeder et al, 1995). Prior to the induction of anesthesia, the patient often becomes cold in the preprocedure area. As a result, peripheral vessels vasoconstrict, in an effort to keep warm blood at the core to protect the vital organs. The induction of anesthesia subsequently triggers vasodilatation of the smooth muscle in the veins and arteries; this vasoconstriction then allows the warm blood to flow out of the core to the cold periphery (ie, the arms and legs) and also sends cold blood from the periphery back to the core. As a result, the core temperature decreases quickly; during the first hour of general anesthesia, the core temperature decreases 1°C–1.5°C as the result of the redistribution of body heat from the core to the periphery. After the first hour of general anesthesia, the core temperature usually decreases at a slower rate; this occurs because the body's heat loss exceeds metabolic heat production. Approximately 90% of all heat loss occurs through the surface of the skin, typically due to radiation and convection more so than conduction or evaporation. After three to five hours of anesthesia, the core temperature reaches a thermal plateau that reflects a steady state in which heat loss equals heat production; this steady state is most likely to occur in patients who are well-insulated or who have been effectively warmed. It is important to note that patients undergoing regional anesthesia are also at risk for developing hypothermia, since regional anesthesia impairs both central and peripheral thermoregulation; a patient who becomes sufficiently hypothermic during spinal or epidural anesthesia will shiver (Sessler, 1997). The danger for these patients is that they may often feel warmer and more comfortable, while they are most likely becoming hypothermic.

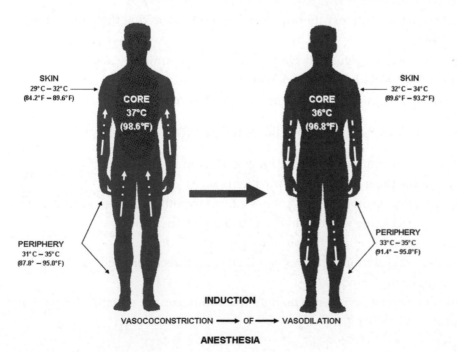

Figure 7.6

Redistribution of Body Heat.

The nurse can assist the anesthesia provider in the prevention of inadvertent hypothermia during the operative or invasive procedure period by assessing the patient's risk of unplanned perioperative hypothermia and developing a plan of care to minimize the risk in those patients (AORN, 2008b). Assessment factors before the procedure include (ASPAN, 2002):

- Identifying patient's risk factors for unplanned hypothermia.
- Measuring patient temperature on admission.
- Determining the patient's thermal comfort level (ask the patients if they are cold).
- Assessing for other signs and symptoms of hypothermia (shivering, piloerection, and/or cold extremities).

Prewarming, the application of heat prior to the procedure in order to increase the total body temperature, is one method to assist with temperature management in the patient. Active prewarming for as little as 30 minutes likely prevents substantial redistribution (Sessler, Schroeder et al, 1995). Other interventions before the procedure include (ASPAN, 2002):

- Instituting preventive warming measures for patients who are normothermic. A variety of measures may be used, unless contraindicated. Passive insulation may include warmed cotton blankets, socks, head covering, limited skin exposure, circulating water mattresses and increase in ambient temperature (minimum 20°C–24°C or 68°F–75°F).
- Instituting active warming measures for patients who are hypothermic. Active warming is the application of a forced-air convection warming system. Apply appropriate passive insulation and increase the ambient room temperature (minimum 20°C–24°C or 68°F–75°F); consider warmed intravenous fluids.

Assessment parameters during the procedure include (ASPAN, 2002):

- Identifying patient's risk factors for unplanned hypothermia;
- Determining the patient's thermal comfort level, (ie, asking the patient if he/she is cold);
- Assessing for other signs and symptoms of hypothermia, (eg, shivering, piloerection, and/or cold extremities); and
- Monitoring the patient's temperature during the procedure.

Nursing interventions during the procedure include (AORN, 2008b):

- Consider prewarming the patient for a minimum of 15 minutes immediately prior to induction of anesthesia for patients at risk;
- Using effective methods to prevent unplanned hypothermia such as forced-air warming, circulating water blankets, and energy transfer pads;
- Consider warming intravenous and irrigation solutions;
- Using skin preparation solutions at a temperature recommended by the solution manufacturer; and
- Using all warming devices in a manner that minimizes the potential for patient injuries.

Patient assessment after the procedure should include (ASPAN, 2002):

- Identifying patient's risk factors for unplanned hypothermia.
- Assessing temperature on admission to the Phase I PACU.
- If hypothermic, monitoring serial temperatures at a minimum of every 30 minutes until normothermia is achieved.
- If normothermic, assessing temperature again prior to discharge and as ordered by physician.
- Determining patient's thermal comfort level (ask the patients if they are cold).
- Assessing for signs and symptoms of hypothermia (shivering, piloerection, and/or cold extremities).

Nursing interventions after the procedure include (ASPAN, 2002):

- If normothermic: institute preventative warming measures:
  - Apply appropriate passive insulation: warm blankets, socks, head covering, limited skin exposure, and circulating water mattress.
  - Increase ambient room temperature (minimum 20°C–24°C or 68°F–75°F).
  - Assess patient's thermal comfort level every 30 minutes.
  - Observe for signs and symptoms of hypothermia (shivering, piloerection, and/or cold extremities).
  - Reassess temperature if patient's thermal comfort level decreases and/or signs of hypothermia are present.
  - Measure patient's temperature prior to discharge.

- If hypothermic, initiate active warming measures:
  - Apply forced-air warming system.
  - Apply passive insulation: warm blankets, socks, head covering, limited skin exposure, and circulating water mattress.
  - Increase ambient room temperature (minimum 20°C–24°C or 68°F–75°F).
  - Warm IV fluids.
  - Humidify and warm gases (oxygen).
  - Assess temperature and patient's thermal comfort level every 30 minutes until normothermia is reached.

PARENTAL PRESENCE DURING INDUCTION OF PEDIATRIC PATIENTS

Another area of increasing attention is parental presence during induction of pediatric patients, as family-centered care is becoming an integral part of both nurse anesthesia and perioperative nursing practice (Romino, Keatley et al, 2005). Numerous studies have been conducted, demonstrating the benefits, as well as the controversy, of parental presence during induction.

One study demonstrated that parental presence during induction of anesthesia enhanced the effect of oral midazolam on emergence behavior of children undergoing general anesthesia (Arai, Ito et al, 2007). In another study conducted to identify child and parental characteristics that are associated with low anxiety and good compliance during induction of anesthesia when parents are present, the authors concluded that children who benefit from parental presence are older, had lower levels of activity in

PPIA
Parental Presence
During Induction
of Anesthesia

their temperament, and had parents who were calmer and who valued preparation and coping skills for medical situations (Kain, Mayes et al, 2006). Another study (Astuto, Rosano et al, 2006) noted that while the issue of parental presence during induction of anesthesia has been a controversial topic for many years, the potential benefits from parental presence during induction include reducing or avoiding the fear and anxiety that might occur in both the child and its parents, thereby reducing the need for preprocedure sedatives and improving the child's compliance. The presence of other figures, such as clowns in the procedure room, together with one of the child's parents, is an effective intervention for managing child and parental anxiety during the operative and invasive procedure period. One study (Kain, Caldwell-Andrews et al, 2006) demonstrated that anxious children who received parental presence during induction of anesthesia (PPIA) from a calm parent were significantly less anxious during induction as compared with anxious children who did not receive PPIA. On the contrary, calm children who received PPIA from an overly anxious parent were considerably more anxious as compared with calm children who were not accompanied by a parent; there was no effect of PPIA on children's anxiety during induction of anesthesia when calm parents accompanied calm children into the OR or when overly anxious parents accompanied anxious children. These authors concluded that the presence of a calm parent does benefit an anxious child during induction of anesthesia and the presence of an overly anxious parent has no benefit. A measure was developed to determine whether maternal motivation to be present during induction (Motivation for Parental Presence during Induction of Anesthesia [MPPIA]) is related to children's anxiety during the induction process (Caldwell-Andrews, Kain et al, 2005). These authors found that mothers with high MMPIA-Desire and low MPPIA-Hesitancy had children with significantly higher anxiety during induction of anesthesia, as compared with mothers with low MPPIA-Desire and MPPIA-Hesitancy. The authors also found that highly motivated mothers reported significantly higher levels of anxiety. Therefore, they concluded that clinicians should be aware that many mothers who have a high desire to be present in the OR are very anxious and that their children are likely to display high anxiety levels during induction of anesthesia.

MPPIA
Motivation for
Parental Presence
during Induction of
Anesthesia

Each facility will have its policy on parental presence during induction of anesthesia. If parental presence during induction is allowed, the nurse can best facilitate this process by assessing the parents' level of anxiety, as well as their desire to be present, and instruct the parent on the guidelines as well as what to expect. In collaboration with the anesthesia provider, the nurse must provide support for both the parent and child in this scenario in order to provide the safest possible anesthetic and operative or invasive procedure experience.

CONVERSATIONS/NOISE IN THE PROCEDURE ROOM

As noted above, extraneous noise and conversations in the procedure room should be kept to a minimum, especially during induction of anesthesia. The operative and invasive procedure environment presents unique challenges for all members of the operative team as they work amidst the noises typical in this setting, such as background music, as well as noise from drills, anesthesia machines, and other pieces of commonly used equipment. Such excessive noise levels can affect patient safety, for example, a clinician may not be able to hear the correct name of a requested medication, or the noise may distract or interrupt the clinician and therefore indirectly lead to an error. Noise can also adversely affect staff members by increasing stress levels and decreasing job satisfaction (Beyea, 2007). In addition to the safety issues related to excess conversations and noise in the procedure room noted above, talking and the number of people present should be kept to a minimum during procedures, as an increase in the number of people can increase the number of airborne microorganisms (AORN, 2008c).

Effective management of noise in the operative and invasive procedure environment requires a collaborative effort by all members of the operative team. The nurse can best assist the anesthesia provider and other team members by (Beyea, 2007):

- Gaining agreement that excessive noise creates a risk for both staff members and patients;
- Identifying the various sources of noise in order to determine whether and how these sources can be reduced;
- Accepting the personal responsibility to manage how much noise he/she produces, including conducting casual conversations outside of patient care areas;
- Being aware of personal vocal levels;
- Investigating noxious sounds to determine how they can be decreased in number or frequency.

AWARENESS UNDER ANESTHESIA

Awareness under anesthesia, or patient awareness under general anesthesia, is a rare condition that occurs when a patient having an operative or invasive procedure can recall his/her surroundings or an event—sometimes even pressure or pain—related to the procedure while he/she is under general anesthesia (AANA, 2008).

Due to the routine use of muscle relaxants during general anesthesia, the patient is often unable to communicate with the operative team if awareness occurs (Joint Commission, 2004). The frequency of awareness under anesthesia has been documented in various studies to range from 0.1% to 0.2% of all patients undergoing general anesthesia (Sebel, Bowdle, et al, 2004; Lennmarken & Sandin, 2004; Ostgerman, Hopper et al, 2001). The administration of general anesthesia to 21 million patients in the United States each year translates to the occurrence of 20,000 to 40,000 cases of anesthesia awareness. Patients experiencing awareness report auditory recollections (48%), sensations of not being able to breathe (48%), and pain (28%) (Sebel, Bowdle et al, 2004). Over half of these patients are also reported to experience mental distress after the procedure, including an undetermined number with post-traumatic stress syndrome (Lennmarken & Sandin, 2004; Ostgerman, Hopper et al, 2001).

The incidence of awareness is reported to be greater in patients in whom the dose of general anesthetic must be smaller and carefully titrated to decrease significant side effects, for example, in a patient who is hemodynamically unstable. Procedures that are typically identified in this category include some cardiac, obstetric, and major trauma cases (Ghoenim, 2000). Factors that contribute to the risk of awareness under anesthesia include the increasing use of intravenous delivery of anesthesia, as opposed to inhalation, and the premature lightening of anesthesia at the end of the procedures to facilitate OR turnover (Joint Commission, 2004). The significance of the problem of awareness under anesthesia, including both the under-recognition and under-treatment, led the Joint Commission to issue a Sentinel Event Alert in 2004 on preventing and managing its impact.

Awareness is often difficult to recognize while it is occurring. The indicators of physiologic and motor responses, for example, an elevation in blood pressure, increased heart rate, movement, or hemodynamic changes, are often masked by the use of paralytic agents and the other agents needed for appropriate patient management, such as beta-blockers or calcium channel blockers. New methods to detect awareness under anesthesia, ones that are less affected by the agents used in general anesthesia, are being developed to overcome the limitations that exist with the current detection methods. Consciousness monitors—also known as level-of-consciousness monitors, sedation-level monitors, and anesthesia-depth monitors—measure brain activity via electroencephalography (EEG) devices, rather than measuring physiological responses to anesthesia. These EEG-based technologies include the Bispectral Index (BIS)®, spectral edge frequency (SEF) and median frequency (MF) monitors (Joint Commission, 2004). These devices may have a role in preventing and detecting anesthesia awareness in patients with the highest risk, thereby ameliorating the impact of anesthesia awareness.

It is important to note that consciousness monitoring is still an emerging technology; a body of evidence has not yet been developed to definitely define the role of these devices in detecting and preventing anesthesia awareness (Joint Commission, 2004). In its review of the BISx (Bispectral [BIS] Index monitor), the United States Food and Drug Administration (FDA) determined that (FDA, 2008):

> "The BIS may be used as an aid in monitoring the effects of certain anesthetic agents. Use of BIS monitoring to help guide anesthetic administration may be associated with the reduction of the incidence of awareness with recall in adults during general anesthesia and sedation."

The nurse can effectively assist the anesthesia provider in the prevention and management of awareness under anesthesia by:

- Conducting a thorough preprocedure assessment to identify patients at increased risk for awareness. Prior to the procedure, the patient should have the opportunity to meet with the anesthesia provider to discuss the possibility of awareness, the approach to anesthesia that will be used, monitoring during the procedure, and any other concerns. It is also important for ask the patient about current medications (including herbal supplements), alcohol and drug consumption, physical conditions, and other factors that could affect the body's reaction to anesthesia (AANA, 2008).

- Assisting with care and monitoring during the procedure. Both the ASA and the American Association of Nurse Anesthetists (AANA) provide guidelines for administering and monitoring anesthesia; specifically, these recommendations include (Ghoneim, 2000):
  - Be alert to patients on beta-blockers, calcium channel blockers, and other drugs that can conceal physiologic responses to inadequate anesthesia;
  - Conduct periodic maintenance of the anesthesia machine and its vaporizers; thoroughly check the machine and its ventilator before administering anesthesia;
  - Consider premedication with amnesic drugs (ie, benzodiazepines or scopolamine) especially when light anesthesia is likely;
  - Administer more than just a "sleep dose" of induction agents if they will be followed immediately by tracheal intubation; and

EEG
Electro-encephalography

BIS
Bispectral Index

SEF
Spectral Edge Frequency

MF
Median Frequency

BISx
Bispectral [BIS] Index monitor

FDA
Food and Drug Administration

AANA
American Association of Nurse Anesthetists

- Avoid muscle paralysis unless absolutely necessary and, even in this situation, avoid total paralysis by using only the amount clinically required.
- Conducting a postprocedure assessment for anesthesia awareness. The primary screening tool should be a structured interview after the procedure, asking the patient:
  - What is the last thing you remember before going to sleep?
  - What is the first thing you remember after waking up?
  - Do you remember anything between going to sleep and waking up?
  - Did you dream during your procedure?
  - What was the worst thing about your procedure?

For patients who report awareness (Ghoneim, 2000), an apology should be given to the patient; the patient should also be assured of the credibility of his/her account; and an explanation of what happened and its reasons, (eg, the necessity to administer light anesthesia in the presence of significant cardiovascular instability) should also be given. Additionally, the patient should be offered psychological or psychiatric support, including referral to a mental health professional. The surgeon should also be notified, along with the nurses and other key personnel about the incident and the subsequent interview with the patient. Operative and invasive procedure team members should also be educated about anesthesia awareness and its management.

The Joint Commission recommendations to assist in the prevention and management of awareness under anesthesia for healthcare organizations which perform procedures under general anesthesia are (Joint Commission, 2004):

1. Develop and implement an anesthesia awareness policy that addresses the following areas:
   - Education of the clinical staff about anesthesia awareness and management of patients who have experienced awareness.
   - Identification of patients at proportionately higher risk for an awareness experience; discussion with these patients, prior to the procedure, of the potential for anesthesia awareness.
   - The effective use of available anesthesia monitoring techniques, including the timely maintenance of anesthesia equipment.
   - Appropriate postprocedure follow-up of all patients who have undergone general anesthesia, including pediatric patients.
   - The identification, management and referral (if appropriate) of patients who have experienced awareness.
2. Ensure access to the necessary counseling or other support for patients who are experiencing post-traumatic stress syndrome or other type of mental distress.

CONCLUSION

The operative and invasive procedure environment presents special challenges for the patient; anesthesia represents one of the more significant of these challenges. As the patient's advocate, the nurse must effectively assist the anesthesia provider in safely caring for the patient requiring anesthesia for an operative and/or invasive procedure. The nurse is in the unique role of assisting the anesthesia provider and coordinating the activities of other personnel in appropriately preparing the patient for anesthesia and operative or invasive procedure intervention and also evaluating the patient's responses to that intervention. Through these collaborative efforts, the anesthesia care team can promote both an optimal operative or invasive procedure experience as well as positive patient outcomes.

COMPETENCY ASSESSMENT
Assist the Anesthesia Provider

Name: _____ Title: _____ Unit: _____ Date of Validation: _____

Type of Validation: ☐ Initial   ☐ Annual   ☐ Bi-annual

COMPETENCY STATEMENT: The nurse demonstrates competency to assist the anesthesia provider during the operative or invasive procedure.

	Performance Criteria	Met	Not Met
1.	Identifies the patient's risk for adverse outcomes related to the administration of anesthesia.	☐	☐
2.	Describes the various types of anesthesia.	☐	☐
3.	Assists the anesthesia provider with induction of general anesthesia.	☐	☐
4.	Assists the anesthesia provider with proper positioning for regional anesthesia.	☐	☐
5.	Describes the potential physiologic changes that may occur during monitored anesthesia care.	☐	☐
6.	Implements blood component therapy.	☐	☐
7.	Describes appropriate interventions for emergency procedures.	☐	☐
8.	Assists the anesthesia provider with proper positioning for regional anesthesia.	☐	☐
9.	Describes appropriate interventions in the management of a malignant hyperthermia crisis.	☐	☐
10.	Assists with parental presence during induction of anesthesia for pediatric patients according to facility policy.	☐	☐
11.	Minimizes noise in the operative and invasive procedure suite, especially during induction of and emergence from general anesthesia.	☐	☐
12.	Assists the anesthesia provider in preventing anesthesia awareness.	☐	☐

_____   _____
Validator's Signature   Employee's Signature

_____
Validator's Printed Name

REFERENCES

1. American Association of Nurse Anesthetists (AANA). (2008). Anesthesia awareness fact sheet. Retrieved January 6, 2008 from http://www.anesthesiapatientsafety.com/patients/ss/aware_factsheet.asp.

2. American Board of Anesthesiology (2004). Booklet of information. (Raleigh: American Board of Anesthesiology).

3. American Society of Anesthesiologists (ASA). (2008). Physical status classification system. Retrieved January 5, 2008 from http://www.asahq.org/clinical/physicalstatus.htm.

4. American Society of PeriAnesthesia Nurses (2002). Clinical guideline for the prevention of Unplanned perioperative hypothermia. Retrieved January 6, 2008 from http://www.aspan.org/PDFfiles/HYPOTHERMIA_GUIDELINE10-02.pdf.

5. American Society of PeriAnesthesia Nurses (ASPAN). (2008). Resource 3: Patient classification/recommended staffing guidelines. Retrieved January 16, 2008 from http://www.aspan.org/PDFfiles/Resource%203%202006-08%20Standards.pdf.

6. Apfelbaum, J.L., Walawander, C.A., Grasela, T.H., et al. (2002). Eliminating intensive postoperative care in same-day surgery patients using short-acting anesthetics. *Anesthesiology*; 97(1): pp. 66–74.

7. Arai, Y.C., Ito, H., et al. (2007). Parental presence during induction enhances the effect of oral midazolam on emergence behavior of children undergoing general anesthesia. *Acta Anaesthesiologica Scandinavica*; 51(7): pp. 858–861.

8. Ashhurst, J. (1896). Surgery before the days of anesthesia. *Boston Medical and Surgical Journal*; 135(16): pp. 378–380.

9. Association of periOperative Registered Nurses (AORN). (2008a). AORN malignant hyperthermia guideline. In *Perioperative Standards and Recommended Practices*. (Denver: AORN, Inc.): pp. 103–139.

10. Association of periOperative Registered Nurses (AORN). (2008b). Recommended practices for the prevention of unplanned perioperative hypothermia. In *Perioperative Standards and Recommended Practices*. (Denver: AORN, Inc): pp. 407–420.

11. Association of periOperative Registered Nurses (AORN). (2008c). Recommended practices for traffic patterns in the perioperative practice setting. In *Perioperative Standards and Recommended Practices*. (Denver: AORN, Inc.): pp. 613–617.

12. Astuto, M., Rosano, G., et al. (2006). Preoperative parental information and parents' presence at induction of anaesthesia. *Minerva Anaestesiologica*; 72(6): pp. 461–465.

13. Beck, A. (2007). Nurse-led pre-operative assessment for elective surgical patients. *Nursing Standard*; 21(51): pp. 35–38.

14. Beyea, S. (2007). Noise: A distraction, interruption, and safety hazard. *AORN Journal*; 86(2): pp. 281–285.

15. Beyea, S, ed. (2002). *Perioperative Nursing Data Set: The Perioperative Nursing Vocabulary*, 2nd ed. (Denver: AORN, Inc,): p. 121.

16. Caldwell-Andrews, A.A., Kain, Z.N., et al. (2005). Motivation and maternal presence during induction of anesthesia. *Anesthesiology*; 103(3): pp. 478–483.

17. Domen, R.E. (1998). Adverse reactions associated with autologous blood transfusions. *Transfusion*; 38(3): pp. 296–300.

18. Food and Drug Administration (FDA). (2008). 510k Summary. Retrieved January 6, 2008 from http://www.fda.gov/cdrh/pdf4/k040183.pdf.

19. Feeley, T.W. & Macario, A. (2005). The postanesthesia care unit. In *Miller's Anesthesia*, 6th ed. RD Miller, ed. (Philadelphia: Elsevier); pp. 2703–2727.

20. Frank, S.M., Raja, S.N., et al. (1999). Relative contribution of core and cutaneous temperature to thermal comfort and autonomic responses in humans. *Journal of Applied Physiology*; 86(5): pp. 588–1593.

21. Gal, T.J. (2005). Airway management. In *Miller's Anesthesia*, 6th ed. RD Miller, ed. (Philadelphia: Elsevier); pp. 1617–1652.

22. Ghoneim, M.M. (2000). Awareness during anesthesia. *Anesthesiology*; 92(2): pp. 597–602.

23. Gronert, G.A., Pessah, I.N., Muldoon, S.M., Tautz, T.J. (2005). Malignant hyperthermia. In *Miller's Anesthesia*, 6th ed. RD Miller, ed. (Philadelphia: Elsevier): pp. 1169–1190.

24. Joint Commission (2004). Sentinel Event Alert. Issue 32, October 6, 2004. Preventing, and managing the impact of, anesthesia awareness. Retrieved January 6, 2008 from http://www.jointcommission.org/SentinelEvents/SentinelEventAlert/sea_32.htm.

25. Joint Commission (2008). Universal Protocol for Preventing Wrong Site, Wrong Procedure, Wrong Person Surgery.™ Retrieved January 5, 2008 from http://www.jointcommission.org/NR/rdonlyres/E3C600EB-043B-4E86-B04E-CA4A89AD5433/0/universal_protocol.pdf.

26. Kain, Z.N., Caldwell-Andrews, A.A., et al. (2006). Predicting which child-parent pair will benefit from parental presence during induction of anesthesia: a decision-making approach. *Anesthesia & Analgesia*; 102(1): pp. 81–84.

27. Kain, Z.N., Mayes, L.C., et al. (2006). Predicting which children benefit most from parental presence during induction of anesthesia. *Paediatric Anaesthesia*; 16(6): pp. 627–634.

28. Larson, M.D. (2005). History of anesthetic practice. In *Miller's Anesthesia*. 6th ed. Miller RD, ed. (Philadelphia: Elsevier); pp. 3–52.

29. Lennmarken, C. & Sandin, R. (2004). Neuromonitoring for awareness during surgery. *Lancet*; 363(9423): pp. 1747–1748.

30. Miller, R.D. (2005). Transfusion therapy. In *Miller's Anesthesia*, 6th ed. RD Miller, ed. (Philadelphia: Elsevier): pp. 1799–1930.

31. Moss, R. (2000). *Inadvertent Perioperative Hypothermia*. (Denver: AORN, Inc); pp. 7–8.

32. Nuttall, G.A., Stehling, L.C., Beighley, C.M., et al. (2003). Current transfusion practices of members of the American Society of Anesthesiologists. *Anesthesiology*; 99(6); pp. 1433–1443.

33. Osterman, J.E., Hopper, J., et al. (2001). Awareness under anesthesia and the development of posttraumatic stress disorder. *General Hospital Psychiatry*; 23(4): pp. 198–204.

34. Pousman, R.M. (2008). Rapid sequence induction for prehospital providers. Retrieved January 6, 2008 from http://www.uam.es/departamentos/medicina/anesnet/journals/ijeicm/vol4n1/rapid.htm#V.%20Rapid%20Sequence%20Induction.

35. Rolfe, S. (2008). Hypothermia and the trauma patient. Retrieved January 6, 2008 from http://www.umc-cares.org/Health_Info/article.asp?Category=General&ArticleID=388.

36. Romino, S.L., Keatley, V.M., et al. (2005). Parental presence during anesthesia induction in children. *AORN Journal*; 81(4): pp. 780–792.

37. Sebel, P.S., Bowdle, T.A., et al. (2004). The incidence of awareness during anesthesia: A multicenter United States study. *Anesthesia & Analgesia*; 99(3): pp. 833–839.

38. Sessler, D., Schroeder, B., et al. (1995). Optimal duration and temperature of prewarming. *Anesthesiology*; 82(3): pp. 674–681

39. Sessler, D.I. (1997). Mild perioperative hypothermia. *New England Journal of Medicine*; 336(24): pp. 1730–1737.

40. Sessler, D.I. (2000). Perioperative heat balance. *Anesthesiology*; 92(2): pp. 578–596.

41. Sessler, D.I. & Kurz, A. (2006), Mild perioperative hypothermia. *Anesthesiology News Special Edition*; pp. 25–31.

42. Sessler, D.I. (2005). Temperature monitoring. In *Miller's Anesthesia*, 6th ed. RD Miller, ed. (Philadelphia: Elsevier): pp. 1571–1597.

43. Sokolovic, E., Biro, P., Wyss, P., Werthemann, C., Haller, U., Spahn, D., Szucs, T. (2002). Impact of the reduction of anaesthesia turnover time on operating room efficiency. *European Journal of Anaesthesia*; 19(8): pp. 560–563.

44. Torkki, P.M., Marjamaa, R.A., Torkki, M.I., Kallio, P.E., Kirvela, O.A. (2005). Use of anesthesia induction rooms can increase the number of urgent orthopedic cases completed within 7 hours. *Anesthesiology*; 103(2): pp. 401–405.

45. Villars, P.S., Kanusky, J.T., Dougherty, T.B. (2004). Stunning the neural nexus: mechanisms of general anesthesia. *AANA Journal*;72(3): pp. 197–205. Retrieved January 16, 2008 from http://www.general-anaesthesia.com/mechanisms.html.

46. White, P.F. & Freire, A.R. (2005). Ambulatory (outpatient) anesthesia. In *Miller's Anesthesia*, 6th ed. RD Miller, ed. (Philadelphia: Elsevier): pp. 2589–2635.

CHAPTER 8

Position the Patient

Paula Bishop

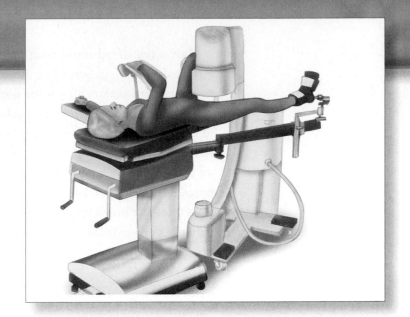

INTRODUCTION

Position the Patient provides information to the registered nurse about positioning patients for operative and invasive procedures. The nurse must perform many activities when positioning the patient on the operating room or the invasive procedure bed. Proper positioning is extremely important because it allows for accurate operative site preparation, appropriate draping, and adequate exposure of the operative site. The nurse must have knowledge of anatomy and physiology as well as the operative or invasive procedure involved to facilitate proper patient positioning. Proper positioning must be accomplished while maintaining the patient's musculoskeletal and neurological safety, skin and tissue integrity, body alignment, and optimal physiological functioning of the respiratory and circulatory system during the operative or invasive procedure.

Before the procedure, the nurse makes a complete assessment of the patient. This assessment must include skin integrity, range of motion, including restrictions or previous injury, age, medical conditions, and the presence of implants or prostheses. This assessment supports the actions in the nursing plan of care that promote optimal outcomes. The care plan includes specific actions to take during positioning, including the appropriate positioning devices to use, special precautions to take when moving the patient, avoiding nerve injury, and the number of assistants needed. The goal is to avoid adverse outcomes while providing optimal positioning for the procedure. The nurse evaluates the patient at the end of the procedure based on the expected outcome criteria.

Chapter Contents

Only a registered nurse with proven competency should position the patient for a procedure. Delegation of positioning activities to surgical technologists or assistive personnel occurs only if the nurse determines that the patient's risk for adverse outcomes related to positioning is low. When delegating any part of the positioning to another party, the nurse must reassess the patient before the procedure begins. Reassessment of the patient during the procedure occurs when patient or environmental variables change. These changes may include change in position, extended procedure time, pooling of body fluids, or team members leaning against a body structure. The nurse must remain vigilant in observing changes and reassessing the patient as needed. The nurse maintains accountability for the patient throughout the procedure.

MEASURABLE CRITERIA

The nurse demonstrates competency for positioning a patient by

- Identifying the patient's risk for adverse outcomes related to positioning
- Selecting the appropriate supplies and equipment based on the patient's identified needs
- Preparing the bed
- Centering the patient on the bed
- Placing the arms on arm boards
- Using positioning devices according to the established practice recommendations and the manufacturer's recommendations
- Padding bony prominences
- Moving the anesthetized patient
- Communicating and documenting risk factors, nursing diagnoses, expected outcomes, the plan of care, interventions, and evaluation
- Placing the patient in various positions for operative and invasive procedures
  - Supine
  - Trendelenburg
  - Reverse Trendelenburg
  - Lithotomy (high and low)
  - Prone
  - Jackknife
  - Lateral
  - Fowler (sitting)
  - Semi-Fowler (beach chair)
  - Fracture table
  - Spine table

IDENTIFYING THE PATIENT'S RISK FOR ADVERSE OUTCOMES RELATED TO POSITIONING

Positioning for the procedure has the potential for compromising or causing injury to the patient. **Table 8.1** identifies outcome statements, diagnoses, risk factors, and outcome indicators related to this patient care event.

Table 8.1	Positioning the Patient Does Not Compromise or Cause Injury to the Patient

Outcome 1 The patient is free from evidence of injury related to operative or invasive procedure positioning.

Diagnosis

Risk for Positioning Injury related to the operative or invasive procedure

Risk Factors

- ☐ Anemia
- ☐ Ascites
- ☐ Cancer
- ☐ Cardiovascular disease
- ☐ Chronic disease
- ☐ Compromised immune system
- ☐ Dehydration
- ☐ Diabetes mellitus
- ☐ Disorientation
- ☐ Edema
- ☐ Elderly
- ☐ Existing or previous trauma or accidental injury
- ☐ External skeletal traction or immobilization device
- ☐ History of thrombosis
- ☐ Hypothermia
- ☐ Impaired judgment
- ☐ Inadequate or shortage of equipment
- ☐ Incoordination
- ☐ Infant
- ☐ Infection
- ☐ Internal skeletal prosthetic device
- ☐ Lack of safety precautions attributed to inadequate, untrained, or inattentive staff
- ☐ Limited range of motion
- ☐ Loss of protective response secondary to anesthesia
- ☐ Muscle weakness
- ☐ Obesity
- ☐ Osteoporosis, rheumatoid arthritis
- ☐ Paralysis
- ☐ Peripheral vascular disease
- ☐ Pregnancy
- ☐ Procedure of 2 hours or longer
- ☐ Radiation therapy
- ☐ Renal, hepatic function
- ☐ Sensory and/or perceptual deterioration due to disease, medication, or anesthesia
- ☐ Thin body frame
- ☐ Tobacco use

Outcome Indicators

- ☐ Is the patient able to resume preprocedure patterns of ambulation?
- ☐ Does the patient report tingling, numbness, cramping, pain, or ache in the joints?
- ☐ Does the patient report weakness and stiffness in the upper or lower extremity?
- ☐ Can the patient abduct, adduct, flex, and extend the upper and lower extremities without experiencing pain or discomfort?

8

Outcome 2 The patient is free from evidence of impaired skin integrity related to operative or invasive procedure positioning.

Diagnosis	Risk Factors	Outcome Indicator
Risk for Impaired Skin Integrity related to operative or invasive procedure positioning	☐ Altered pigmentation ☐ Altered tissue perfusion, arteriosclerosis ☐ Anemia ☐ Change in skin turgor ☐ Edema ☐ Inattentive staff leaning on the patient ☐ Lack of position change especially when the procedure lasts more than 2 hours ☐ Nutritional deficit such as protein or ascorbic acid deficiency ☐ Obesity or emaciation ☐ Physical immobilization secondary to anesthesia ☐ Pooling of patient body fluids ☐ Pooling of skin preparation or irrigation solutions ☐ Pressure on the peripheral nervous or vascular systems ☐ Prolonged pressure on the bony prominences ☐ Shearing force during procedure	☐ Does the patient show signs of disruption or breakdown of skin layers, especially over bony prominences?

Outcome 3 The patient is free from evidence of impaired respiratory function related to operative or invasive procedure positioning.

Diagnosis	Risk Factors	Outcome Indicators
Risk for Impaired Respiratory Function related to operative or invasive procedure positioning	☐ Decreased respiratory function related to mechanical restriction of the rib cage and abdomen in various positions ☐ Elderly ☐ General or spinal anesthesia ☐ Inattentive staff leaning on the patient ☐ Neuromuscular or musculoskeletal impairment ☐ Obesity ☐ Perceptual or cognitive impairment (conscious patient) ☐ Pregnancy (third trimester)	☐ Does the conscious patient report shortness of breath or difficulty breathing? ☐ Does the conscious patient demonstrate labored breathing, such as dyspnea? ☐ Does the conscious patient report feeling anxious or apprehensive? ☐ Does the patient demonstrate changes in respiratory rate and/or depth? ☐ Are arterial blood gas values within normal range (pH 7.35–7.45, PCO_2 35–45 mm Hg, PO_2 75–100 mm Hg, HCO_3 24–28 mEq/L)? ☐ Is the patient's O_2 saturation within normal limits (95% or greater)? ☐ Is the patient cyanotic?

> **Outcome 4** **The patient is free from evidence of ineffective tissue perfusion related to operative or invasive procedure positioning.**
>
> | Diagnosis | Risk Factors | Outcome Indicators |
> |---|---|---|
> | Risk for Ineffective Tissue Perfusion related to operative or invasive procedure positioning | ☐ Decrease in blood pressure related to anesthetic agent use

☐ Interruption of arterial or venous blood flow secondary to compression of the extremities against positioning devices or bed accessories, or staff leaning on the patient

☐ Reduced perfusion to bony prominences and limbs related to changes in vessel compliance | ☐ Do the patient's extremities feel cool?

☐ Is there decreased capillary refill?

☐ Does the patient have diminished arterial pulsations?

☐ Are there blood pressure changes in the extremities?

☐ Is edema present?

☐ Are the patient's extremities discolored? |

Adapted from Carpentino-Moyet, L. J. (2008). *Handbook of Nursing Diagnosis* (12th ed.) Philadelphia: Lippincott Williams & Wilkins; Petersen C. (2007). *Perioperative Nursing Data Set, the Perioperative Nursing Vocabulary.* (Revised 2nd ed.). Denver: AORN, Inc.

Body Structures at Risk

Positioning places many of the patient's body structures at risk for injury. During the assessment, the nurse identifies at-risk body structures through evaluation of the following systems: respiratory, circulatory, neurological, musculoskeletal, and integumentary. Thorough assessment will determine if the patient has an existing impairment. Awareness of vulnerable body structures will help the nurse plan for the positioning episode. As an example, the hip joint is an at-risk structure for the patient being placed in the lithotomy position. The nurse would determine the extent of range of motion in the hip and the presence of existing disease processes such as rheumatoid arthritis, of edema, and of prosthetic devices. Other factors that the nurse would consider in the assessment include age, height, weight, skin condition, and nutritional status. Procedure type and length must also be factored into planning appropriate positioning interventions for an operative or invasive procedure (AORN, 2008). Specific body structures at risk are shown in **Table 8.2.**

Pressure

Some of the areas at risk during patient positioning are created by changes in the skin and underlying tissue, the musculoskeletal system, the nervous system, the cardiovascular system, and the respiratory system. Other areas of vulnerability include the eyes, breasts, perineum, and fingers (Rothrock, 2007).

The skin and underlying tissue may be injured during positioning as a result of external pressure and time. When sitting or lying, the body weight is borne by the tissue overlying the bony prominences. Pressure over the bony prominence and the support structure is called external pressure. This pressure can also occur from a retractor or positioning device exerting force against the patient's tissue. When external pressure exceeds capillary pressure, capillary flow is obstructed.

Table 8.2 Body Structures at Risk in Various Patient Positions

	Supine	Trendelenburg	Reverse Trendelenburg	High & Low Lithotomy	Lateral Decubitus	Prone Jackknife	Sitting
Integumentary System and Other Structures							
Scalp	✓	✓	✓	✓	✓		✓
Eyelids					✓	✓	
Cornea						✓	
Ear					✓	✓	
Skin layers, especially over bony prominences	✓	✓	✓	✓	✓	✓	✓
Skin layers, especially over pendulous abdomen						✓	
Breasts and genitalia						✓	
Nervous System							
Cervical spinal cord						✓	✓
Optic nerve						✓	
Facial nerve						✓	
Brachial plexus	✓	✓	✓	✓	✓		✓
Suprascapular nerve					✓		
Radial, ulnar, and medial nerves	✓	✓	✓	✓	✓	✓	✓

Nervous System

Structure	Supine	Trendelenburg	Reverse Trendelenburg	High & Low Lithotomy	Lateral Decubitus	Prone Jackknife	Sitting
Lateral femoral cutaneous nerve	✓				✓		
Common peroneal nerve	✓	✓	✓	✓	✓		
Tibial nerve		✓	✓	✓			
Sciatic nerve				✓	✓		
Femoral nerve				✓			
Obturator nerve				✓			
Saphenous nerve				✓			

Skeletal System and Bony Prominences

Structure	Supine	Trendelenburg	Reverse Trendelenburg	High & Low Lithotomy	Lateral Decubitus	Prone Jackknife	Sitting
Occiput	✓	✓	✓	✓			
Temporal area					✓	✓	
Zygomatic arch					✓	✓	
Acromion process					✓	✓	
Clavicle						✓	
Scapula	✓	✓	✓	✓			✓
Spinous process	✓	✓	✓	✓			
Sacrum	✓	✓	✓	✓			
Anterior superior iliac spine (ASIS)						✓	✓
Lateral chest wall						✓	✓

8

	Supine	Trendelenburg	Reverse Trendelenburg	High & Low Lithotomy	Lateral Decubitus	Prone Jackknife	Sitting
Skeletal System and Bony Prominences							
Greater tubercle of humerus					✓		
Olecranon process	✓	✓	✓	✓	✓	✓	✓
Styloid process of ulna and radius	✓	✓	✓	✓	✓		
Iliac crest							
Ischial tuberosities					✓		✓
Greater trochanter of femur					✓		
Patella					✓		
Tibial tuberosity						✓	
Lateral femoral epicondyle					✓	✓	
Medial femoral epicondyle				✓	✓	✓	
Tibial condyles				✓	✓		
Lateral malleolus					✓		
Medial malleolus					✓		
Calcaneous	✓	✓	✓			✓	✓
Dorsum of foot							
Muscles							
Calf and strap muscles				✓			
Neck					✓	✓	✓
Respiratory system							
Diaphragm	✓	✓		✓		✓	✓
Chest wall					✓		

Circulatory system

	Supine	Trendelenburg	Reverse Trendelenburg	High & Low Lithotomy	Lateral Decubitus	Prone Jackknife	Sitting
Cerebrovascular		✓					
Carotid artery		✓					
Jugular vein		✓					
Superficial temporal artery		✓				✓	✓
Occipital artery		✓					✓
Heart	✓	✓	✓	✓	✓	✓	
Abdominal aorta				✓		✓	
Inferior vena cava	✓						
Axillary artery					✓		
Brachial artery	✓	✓	✓	✓	✓	✓	✓
Popliteal artery	✓	✓	✓	✓			✓
Femoral artery				✓			
Saphenous vein				✓			

Sources: AORN, 2008; Rothrock, 2007; Krettek & Aschemann, 2006; Phillips, 2007; Nagelhout & Zaglaniczny, 2005.

8

This obstructed flow results in diminished circulation to the area. Capillary blood flow disruption for more than two hours results in cellular destruction and irreversible tissue damage (Mills, 2006). High pressure over a shorter duration is as significant in development of tissue injury as long periods with less extrinsic pressure.

Based on research, the most significant factors in predicting the risk of pressure ulcer development during operative procedures are increasing age, a medical diagnosis of diabetes or vascular disease, and vascular procedures. These findings support the belief that patients who have poor peripheral circulation, based on their decreased tissue tolerance, would be more at risk of developing pressure ulcers. Other risk factors for tissue injury include poor nutrition and smaller body size as well as obesity (Shultz, 2005).

Nerve Injury

Stretching and compressing nerves can result in serious neuropathies occurring in the upper and lower extremities, head and neck, and pelvis and spine. Peripheral nerve injury can cause sensory or motor injury or both. There are some patients who have an increased risk for nerve injury based on metabolic conditions including diabetes mellitus, cancer, alcoholism, smoking, vitamin deficiencies, previous nerve injuries, limitations in range of motion, obesity, and malnutrition (Nagelhout & Zaglaniczny, 2005; Rothrock, 2007, p. 136).

Stretch

Stretching a peripheral nerve causes ischemia or nerve disruption, resulting in nerve injury. Peripheral nerves have a high degree of flexibility and laxity, but prolonged stretching beyond the normal range can result in intraneural pressure increase great enough to cause ischemia and tissue death (Nagelhout & Zaglaniczny, 2005).

Compression

Injury induced by pressure is dependent on both on the amount and duration of pressure. Typically, duration of pressure is of more significance than the quantity of pressure, but extremely high pressure can cause injury (Nagelhout & Zaglaniczny, 2005).

Ulnar Nerve

The ulnar nerve is at high risk for injury due to the anatomic position of the nerve in the medial epicondyle. The nerve lacks adequate cover from connective tissue or muscles, thus exposing it to higher risk from pressure. Extreme flexion or pronation increases pressure risk (Krettek & Aschemann, 2006). Padding should be placed around the elbow to prevent direct pressure on the olecranon process.

Brachial Plexus

The brachial plexus exits the intervertebral foramina of the cervical spine and runs through the anterior and middle scalene muscles. The plexus divides into trunks that run through the narrow space between the clavicle and the first rib to the axilla

(Krettek & Aschemann, 2006). The plexus travels in close proximity to bony structures and immobile soft tissue structures and is fixed in two locations. The anatomical structure of the brachial plexus increases the risk for injury related to stretch and direct nerve compression (Rothrock, 2007).

Causes of injury to the brachial plexus include hyperabduction of the arm and the use of shoulder braces. The position of the cervical spine and the head are factors that greatly influence the development of injury. Guidelines for positioning the upper extremity include:

- Limit abduction to a maximum of 90 degrees
- Avoid simultaneous abduction, supination, and extension
- Maintain the head and cervical spine in neutral position
- Avoid dorsal extension and lateral flexion of the head to the side opposite of the arm being positioned
- Avoid extension and abduction of the arms above the head (Rothrock, 2007)

Use caution when positioning the arms in the prone position, preferably tucking the arms at the side.

Shoulder braces are used to support the patient positioned in head-down tilt or Trendelenburg. The shoulder braces can compress the brachial plexus against the bony structures within the shoulder complex. While there are newer techniques to minimize the use of shoulder braces, such as non-slip mattresses and modifying operative techniques, the need to use shoulder braces still exists. When braces are used, the following guidelines are recommended:

- Use only when absolutely necessary
- Pad shoulder braces well and position over the acromion and not the clavicle or the root of the neck
- Use a non-slip mattress for the head-down tilt position
- Avoid the use of wrist straps
- Avoid abduction of arms greater than 90 degrees
- Tuck arms at the sides whenever possible
- Adjust the shoulder braces before tilting the table
- Recheck the position of the braces and torso after tilting the table (Nagelhout & Zaglaniczny, 2005)

Lower Extremity

Injury to the nerves of the lower extremities can occur because of compression or stretching most commonly experienced when placed in the lithotomy position. The nerves at risk include the peroneal, posterior tibial, femoral obturator, and sciatic nerves. Pressure exerted on the lateral aspect of the knee from a stirrup bar or other foot holder against the peroneal nerve can result in foot drop. Care should be taken when placing popliteal knee supports, as pressure on the posterior tibial nerve in this area can result in numbness of the foot. Pressure placed against the medial tibial condyle produces compression of the femoral obturator nerve and can result in paralysis and numbness of the calf muscle. This can occur when the medial side of the knee is pressed against a metal knee-supporting device. Excess flexion of the hips with high extension, such as in high lithotomy position, can create both compression and stretching injury to the sciatic nerve (Spry, 2005).

Physical Limitations

Physical limitations for patient positioning are a risk factor for injury and should be considered when preparing the patient for surgery. Such limitations include:

- Decreased range of motion
- Previous operative procedures
- Preexisting medical conditions (arthritis or diabetes)
- Presence of joint prosthesis
- Patient's height and weight (O'Connel, 2006)

An awake and alert patient can restrict range of motion to prevent injury. The anesthetized patient does not have this safety mechanism, therefore the nurse and the operative or invasive procedure team must be alert to situations in which injury could occur. Moving the patient from the stretcher to the bed should be performed while maintaining the patient in proper body alignment. Avoid jerking motions and support the extremities as much as possible during the transfer and positioning process.

Respirations

The respiratory system can be compromised during positioning due to an upward shift in the viscera placing pressure against the diaphragm, typically in the lithotomy and Trendelenburg positions. The lateral position results in decreased lung capacity due to the weight of the body putting pressure on the lower chest. This creates mechanical interference with the chest wall, diaphragm, and abdominal wall. The prone position creates a decreased cardiac index and stroke volume with increased systemic and pulmonary vascular resistance (Nagelhout & Zaglaniczny, 2005). The operative or invasive procedure team must be aware of the effect of the patient's position and compensate appropriately.

Throughout the positioning process, attention must be paid to the areas at risk for injury. The appropriate measures to reduce risk for injury are detailed as each position is discussed later in this chapter.

NURSING ACTIVITIES COMMON TO ALL POSITIONS
Selecting Supplies and Equipment

Supplies and equipment needed for positioning the patient depend on patient variables such as height, weight, physiological condition, and the required position for the procedure. The nurse plans for the positioning equipment prior to the procedure. This is accomplished by looking at the planned procedure, the physician's preferences, and the patient condition. Further evaluation of the specific case such as the length of procedure, the operative approach, and the use of radiological equipment provides more information for appropriate planning (AORN, 2008). Universal Protocol dictates that the operative or invasive procedure team verifies the correct patient position and equipment during the "time out" (Joint Commission, 2008).

Basic positioning supplies and equipment include arm boards, arm restraints, pillow or headrest, padding for bony prominences, safety strap, and overlays for bed mattresses. Padding may include gel pads, foam, and blankets. The nurse should be aware that foam pads might not provide effective padding when used in areas of heavy weight, as this compresses the foam quickly and negates the pressure reducing effect. Convoluted foam mattress overlays (egg crate mattress) may be more effective in reducing pressure, but not for obese patients. Pillows, blankets, and molded foam devices are less effective during long procedures and provide only minimal pressure reduction. Towel rolls and sheets do not decrease pressure and linen may actually cause tissue damage (AORN, 2008). Both foam or gel mattresses and viscoelastic overlays prevent skin changes more effectively than standard mattresses (Schultz, 2005).

Some supplies are procedure specific and include items such as protective leg coverings (foam boots, stockings, and towels), stirrups, and stirrup holders for lithotomy positioning. Other specialized supplies such as a padded footboard, pelvic wedge, table extension, beanbag, padded knee rests, supporting frames, backrest or face rest, and toboggans are identified on an as needed basis in the nursing care plan.

Preparing the Bed

Before transferring the patient, check the bed for proper functioning. Ensure that the bed can he elevated and lowered, flexed up and down, placed in the Trendelenburg and reverse Trendelenburg positions, horizontally rotated to the left and the right, and modified for the lithotomy and sitting positions.

On electrically operated beds, look for frayed cords. Make sure that the control box is clearly marked and operational.

Inspect the bed for cleanliness. Check the underside of the foot of the bed, the base of the bed, and the bed railings. During bed cleaning these areas may be overlooked and harbor dried blood, body fluids, or prepping solutions and tissue debris. Look for cracks or tears in bed pad covers. Crack or tears may present an infection control hazard.

Look for hazards on the bed such as sharp edges and loose screws, nuts, and bolts. Confirm that devices used to secure bed pads to the bed are intact. Loose securing devices may result in pad movement while the patient is being transferred to the bed or while being positioned. Bed pads should be of equal height. Modify the bed for the procedure and lock it in place. Transfer the patient to the bed, as described in Chapter 5, *Transfer the Patient.*

Centering the Patient on the Bed

Align the patient's head, spine, and legs. The patient's legs should not be crossed. Apply the safety strap at least 2 inches (5 cm) above the knees. Insert a hand between the strap and the thighs to check for excessive pressure.

Placing the Patient's Arms on the Arm Boards or Tucking at Side

Position arm boards at less than a 90-degree angle to the patient's body (Phillips, 2007). Caution must be exercised for patients with restricted range of motion. Ensure that the arm boards and bed pad are of the same height to prevent the arms from falling below the body or being elevated. This helps to prevent the potential for stretch and possibly compression injuries. Secure each arm onto a padded arm board with a safety strap.

When placing the arms at the sides, turn the palms toward the patient's sides with the fingers extended. Pad the hands and arms and tuck them in with the draw sheet or a padded arm-securing device, often referred to as a toboggan or sled. The arms should be tucked in a manner that prevents them from sliding off the side of the bed or contacting any parts of the bed edge or attachments (Rothrock, 2007). Using a draw sheet for tucking the arms is an effective technique for securing the arms. The draw sheet is brought up and over the arm, taking care to avoid wrinkles or bunching, and then tucked under the patient's body (**Fig. 8.1**).

Using Positioning Devices

Before positioning the patient on the bed, ensure that positioning devices are readily available, clean, free of sharp edges, padded as appropriate, and in working order. Make necessary modifications to the bed before attaching positioning devices. When attaching the devices to the bed or applying them to the patient, follow manufacturer's written instructions, the nurse's plan of care, and applicable institutional practice guidelines. Maintain the patient's body alignment and physiological status when removing positioning devices from the patient and the bed.

Padding Bony Prominences

Pad bony prominences to help prevent excessive pressure that could result in tissue and nerve injury. Pad areas that will contact positioning devices as well, to avoid unnecessary pressure. Select padding that is thick enough to provide sufficient cushioning. Padding made from hypoallergenic material will reduce the patient's risk for skin sensitivity or development of an allergic reaction. When applying the padding, ensure that it is wrinkle-free and dry. Reusable padding that has been decontaminated with a germicidal solution should be rinsed with water before use. Dried germicidal solution may leave a film that may irritate the patient's skin. After

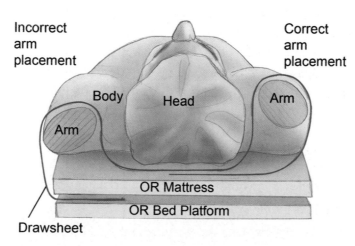

Incorrect arm placement

Correct arm placement

Figure 8.1

Correct method for tucking arms at the side.

Body Head Arm

Arm

Arm

OR Mattress

OR Bed Platform

Drawsheet

padding is applied, the nurse assesses the patient to determine if the padding is providing the intended integumentary protection and pressure relief.

Moving the Anesthetized Patient

The patient may require repositioning on the bed after the induction of anesthesia. Safe patient positioning requires coordination of the entire operative or invasive procedure team. The team must use clear communication to assure that each member knows his or her responsibility during the positioning process. Check with the anesthesia provider before positioning or repositioning the anesthetized patient. Move the patient only with adequate assistance. Before the move, remove or loosen the leg safety strap. Leaving the strap attached during a move may result in skin trauma from pinching or shearing force. When moving the patient, do so slowly and as a coordinated team, maintaining proper body alignment and supporting the patient's extremities and joints to minimize potential injury. Prevent excessive abduction of the patient's arms during the move. If necessary, cross the patient's arms across his or her chest during the move. After the move is complete, reapply or tighten the safety strap as applicable. Check that it is secure and not constrictive. Reassess the patient for body alignment and tissue integrity before draping (AORN, 2008).

Communication and Documentation

Communication with the patient and members of the operative or invasive procedure team is essential. The nurse should inform the patient of the positioning procedure during the patient teaching session. Specific patient requirements should be communicated with other members of the team.

Documentation of positioning is a professional responsibility. At a minimum, the documentation should include a preprocedure assessment that notes the patient's overall skin condition upon arrival to the operative or invasive procedure suite, identified risk factors, nursing diagnoses with expected outcomes, patient position/reposition, positioning devices, personnel positioning the patient, incidents of reassessment, and postprocedure assessment for signs and symptoms of injury due to positioning (AORN, 2008).

PATIENT CARE ACTIVITIES FOR SPECIFIC POSITIONS

Staffing Requirements

Patient positioning is a team effort and should be coordinated through effective communication of each team member's responsibilities. The number of people required to assist in positioning is dependent upon the type of position, the parts of the body that must be moved and supported, and the need to move in tandem (such as in raising legs for the lithotomy position). The nurse should take an active role as a participant in the safe positioning of the patient (AORN, 2008). The nurse maintains the patient's dignity by providing privacy during the transfer and positioning. This may include such actions as keeping doors closed, keeping the patient exposed only to the extent necessary for the procedure, restricting access to the procedure room to authorized personnel, and providing care without prejudicial behavior (AORN, 2008). The anesthesia provider should always have responsibility for the patient's airway and coordinating the movement of an anesthetized patient. The nurse verifies that appropriate actions are taken to promote skin integrity and body alignment while using the correct positioning devices to promote operative exposure. Final inspection and approval of the patient's position is the responsibility of the physician or the licensed independent practitioner involved in the operative or invasive procedure.

SUPINE POSITION

The supine position, also known as the dorsal recumbent position, is the most frequently used position for patients undergoing an operative or invasive procedure. The patient is placed flat on the back. The neck and spine are in a horizontal line with hips parallel to each other. The legs are extended and the arms rest either on arm boards or at the sides (**Fig. 8.2**). The supine position is routinely used for any procedure that requires an anterior approach such as abdominal, thoracic, vascular, head and neck, and orthopedic procedures (Spry, 2005).

Supplies and Equipment

- Arm boards
- Arm restraints
- Pillow or headrest
- Padding for bony prominences
- Safety strap
- Supplementary supplies
  - Padded footboard
  - Pelvic wedge
  - Table extension
  - Toboggans or sleds
  - Antiembolism stockings and/or sequential compression stockings (as identified in the nursing care plan)

Positioning Procedure

The patient is transferred onto the bed. If the patient is conscious, he or she can actively assist with the transfer. If the patient is heavily sedated or already anesthetized, the operative or invasive procedure team must coordinate efforts to assure a safe and efficient transfer. The neck and spine form a horizontal line with the hips parallel and legs extended. Verify that the legs are uncrossed and slightly apart. Tall patients may require a table extension. Care must be taken to avoid allowing the heels to hang beyond the end of the bed, which could injure the Achilles tendon.

A small donut or headrest supports the head to avoid stretching the neck muscles. It may also help prevent loss of hair secondary to prolonged pressure on the occiput.

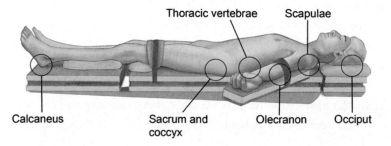

Figure 8.2

Supine position with arms extended.

Thoracic vertebrae   Scapulae

Calcaneus   Sacrum and coccyx   Olecranon   Occiput

Arms are placed on padded arm boards or tucked at the side. Be sure that the fingers of tucked arms are free from the bed breaks and attachments. Follow the guidelines described earlier for placement of the arms.

For long procedures, place a small pillow behind the back in the lumbar curvature to help prevent back strain that can occur when the muscles become relaxed during anesthesia. A pillow may also be placed under the knees to lessen strain on the back. The pillow should be placed above the popliteal space to avoid pressure on the popliteal artery, common peroneal nerve, and the tibial nerve, which run superficially through the popliteal space. A padded footboard may be required to avoid plantar flexion and resulting foot drop and should be used for any debilitated patient. The footboard must extend beyond the toes to prevent crushing injuries. Procedures expected to take longer than 2 hours increase the risk for skin injury, particularly from pressure duration. It is important to pad the bony prominences and other areas at risk for pressure (Spry, 2005).

Apply the table strap loosely over the upper thighs, at least 2 inches (5 cm) above the knee to prevent hyperextension of the knees. Make sure the strap is secure, but not constricting and that a sheet or blanket is placed between the patient's skin and the safety strap.

Increased pressure on the vena cava occurs from compression by abdominal viscera in obese patients, abdominal masses, or a fetus in a pregnant woman resulting in decreased blood return to the heart and lowered blood pressure. To relieve some of this pressure, a wedge is placed under the right flank area causing the patient to tilt slightly to the left (Rothrock, 2007).

Potential Adverse Effects of the Supine Position

Every patient position has the potential for adverse effects. Each position discussed in this chapter will have a table listing these adverse effects. **Table 8.3** lists the potential adverse effects of the supine position.

TRENDELENBURG POSITION

The Trendelenburg position is a modification of the supine (dorsal recumbent) position. Also referred to as the head-down tilt position, the patient is placed in the supine position and the bed is modified to varying degrees of the head-down tilt. The lower section of the bed may be altered to lower the knees (**Fig. 8.3**). This position causes the abdominal organs to move out of the pelvis, improving the view of the pelvic organs. However, because of the risk for physiological stresses or abnormalities, this position should be used with caution (Nagelhout & Zaglaniczny, 2005).

Supplies and Equipment

- Arm boards
- Arm restraints
- Pillow or headrest
- Padding for boney prominences
- Safety strap
- Supplementary supplies and equipment
  - Padded foot board
  - Pelvic wedge

Table 8.3	Potential Adverse Effects of the Supine Position	
Cause		**Effect**
Prolonged (greater than 2 hours) pressure on tissue	→	Skin breakdown at heels, elbows, and sacrum
Crossed ankles throughout the procedure	→	Peroneal nerve damage
Positioning pressure on the popliteal space from positioning aids such as pillows and straps that are not appropriately placed	→	Common peroneal nerve injury
Arms abducted greater than 90 degrees	→	Brachial plexus injury—sensory and motor loss ranging from a portion of to the entire arm
Prolonged arm pronation or flexion of the elbow greater than 90 degrees	→	Ulnar nerve compression injury
Organs resting against the upper abdominal wall	→	Decreased diaphragmatic excursion
Position-induced	→	Hypotension
Reduction of venous pressure, poor venous return	→	Venous pooling in legs
Induction of anesthesia	→	Decreased mean arterial pressure, heart rate, and peripheral resistance
Vena cava and aortic compression/obstruction	→	Pregnant patients—risk of hypotension and diminished placental and uterine perfusion

Sources: AORN, 2008; Rothrock, 2007; Krettek & Aschemann, 2006; Phillips, 2007; Nagelhout & Zaglaniczny, 2005.

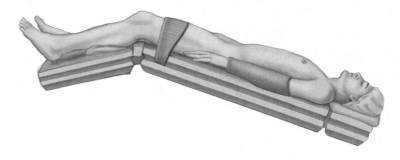

Figure 8.3

Trendelenburg position with knees flexed.

- Table extension
- Toboggans or sleds
- Antiembolism stockings and/or sequential compression stockings (as identified in the nursing care plan)
- Shoulder braces (not recommended)

Positioning Procedure

Position the patient as described for the supine position. If lowering the knee section of the bed to minimize pressure on the calves and knee joints, position the knees over the break in the bed so that safe anatomical positioning is maintained (Rothrock, 2007). Tilt the bed, feet up and head down, to the desired angle. When tilting the bed, be sure equipment is clear of the bed to avoid catching or tipping the equipment. The Mayo stand should be raised to prevent pressure to the feet. Shoulder braces may be used, with caution, to secure the patient. The braces should be applied carefully in the appropriate position, as described earlier, to minimize the risk of brachial plexus injury.

Potential Adverse Effects of the Trendelenburg Position

Table 8.4 lists the potential adverse effects of the Trendelenburg Position

REVERSE TRENDELENBURG POSITION

The reverse Trendelenburg position is a modification of the supine position. The patient is placed in the supine position, and the bed is adjusted to a head-up tilt (**Fig. 8.4**). This position is used for procedures of the head and neck.

Supplies and Equipment

- Arm boards
- Arm restraints
- Padded foot board
- Pillow or headrest
- Padding for bony prominences
- Safety strap
- Supplementary supplies and equipment

Table 8.4	Potential Adverse Effects of the Trendelenburg Position	
Cause		**Effect**
Prolonged (greater than 2 hours) pressure on tissue	→	Skin breakdown at vulnerable weight-bearing bony prominences
Increased venous pressure	→	Retinal detachment or cerebral edema
Improper positioning of shoulder braces	→	Brachial plexus injury
Displaced abdominal contents exerting pressure against the diaphragm; Increased in obese individuals	→	Increased work of spontaneous ventilation
Unrecognized blood loss due to gravitational flow of blood away from the operative field, reduced cardiac output	→	Hypotension
Congestion of cerebral arteries	→	Venous thrombosis
Positioning and restraining devices or flexed knees diminish blood flow	→	Occlusion of superficial veins and thrombophlebitis
Dependent position of head and thorax	→	Increased intracranial pressure
Dependent position of head, abnormal cranial circulation	→	Increased intraocular pressure

Sources: AORN, 2008; Rothrock, 2007; Krettek & Aschemann, 2006; Phillips, 2007; Nagelhout & Zaglaniczny, 2005.

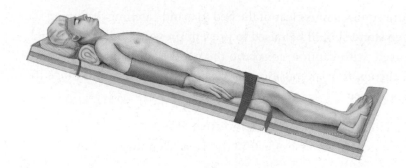

Figure 8.4
Reverse Trendelenburg position.

Table 8.5	Potential Adverse Effects of the Reverse Trendelenburg Position	
Cause		**Effect**
Prolonged (greater than 2 hours) pressure on tissue	→	Skin breakdown at vulnerable weight-bearing bony prominences
Shearing forces from patient sliding toward the foot of bed	→	Impaired skin integrity
Arms placed at side with misalignment or compression of arms against bed	→	Radial, median, or ulnar nerve damage
Decreased circulating blood volume during procedure	→	Hypotension
Venous pooling in the legs	→	Cardiovascular overload at the completion of the case and return to supine position

Sources: AORN, 2008; Rothrock, 2007; Krettek & Aschemann, 2006; Phillips, 2007; Nagelhout & Zaglaniczny, 2005.

- Pelvic wedge
- Table extension
- Toboggans or sleds
- Antiembolism stockings and/or sequential compression stockings (as identified in the nursing care plan)

Positioning Procedure

Position the patient as described for the supine position. Attach a padded footboard to the foot of the bed to keep the patient from sliding toward the foot of the bed. This intervention will help prevent shearing force as the bed is tilted. Tilt the bed, feet down and head up, to the desired angle.

Potential Adverse Effects of the Reverse Trendelenburg Position

Table 8.5 lists the potential adverse effects of the Reverse Trendelenburg position.

LITHOTOMY POSITION

The lithotomy position is primarily used for gynecological and urological procedures, but may be used for any procedure requiring a perineal approach. There are variations of the position, including standard, high, and low lithotomy positions.

The patient begins in the supine position. The legs are raised and abducted to expose the perineal region and secured in leg holders. The foot of the bed is lowered to allow access by the physician.

The thighs are flexed approximately 90 degrees for standard lithotomy. This is the position used for most gynecologic procedures. In high lithotomy position, used for extreme perineal exposure, the thighs are flexed beyond 90 degrees in relation to the trunk and the legs are extended high toward the ceiling with a slight flex in the knee. Low lithotomy position is used for most urological procedures and for procedures that require access to the abdomen and perineum simultaneously. The thighs are flexed approximately 30–45 degrees in this position. When the physician prefers to have the legs completely out of the way of the operative field, the exaggerated lithotomy position may be used. In this position, the thighs are flexed toward the abdomen, the calves are vertical, and the pelvis is propped on a pillow or pad to flex it vertically at the spine (Rothrock, 2007). **Figure 8.5** illustrates the various lithotomy positions

Supplies and Equipment

- Arm boards
- Arm restraints
- Pillow or headrest
- Padding for bony prominences
- Safety strap
- Protective leg coverings (foam boots, towels)
- Leg positioning devices (stirrups or boots—matched pair)
- Supplementary supplies and equipment
- Antiembolism stockings and/or sequential compression stockings (as identified in the nursing care plan)

Discussion of Lithotomy Positioning Devices

There are a variety of devices used to position the legs in the lithotomy position. These devices support either the heel, the foot and heel, or the heel and calf. Complications can result from the use of any lithotomy positioning device, with each

8

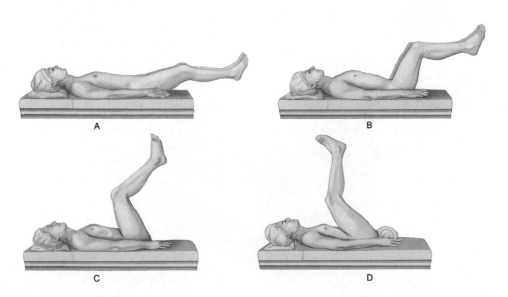

Figure 8.5

Various lithotomy positions. A) Standard, B) Low, C) High, and D) Exaggerated.

A

B

C

D

one possessing its own unique risks. In lithotomy position, regardless of the positioning device used, nerve injury can occur. Excessive abduction of the thigh results in femoral nerve entrapment and hyperflexion of the thigh can cause damage to the sciatic and obturator nerves due to stretch injury (Rothrock, 2007).

The heel-supporting device is commonly referred to as the candy cane stirrup, consisting of a strap that wraps around the ankle and the plantar surface of the foot. The stirrup is secured to a pole that is attached to the side of the bed. When using the candy cane stirrups, uncontrolled abduction of the leg can occur, allowing the knee or calf to rest on the pole. This can result in pressure over the common peroneal nerve that curves over the fibula (Rothrock, 2007).

Providing support at the knee area reduces the uncontrolled abduction, but care must be used to avoid pressure on the peroneal, tibial, and saphenous nerves in the popliteal space or the medial or lateral aspects of the knee.

The calf-supporting device supports the entire weight of the leg on the calf and places it at great risk for developing compartment syndrome. Compartment syndrome is a complication that can be attributed to prolonged direct pressure on the muscles of the calf. The prolonged pressure increases the pressure within the muscle compartment. This is a critical complication and frequently requires operative intervention (Nagelhout & Zaglaniczny, 2005). While the calf-supporting device may provide more stability than the ankle strap stirrup, it is still not optimal.

The heel and calf devices provide support at the heel and calf of the leg, dispersing pressure over a greater area. This decreases the risk for developing compartment syndrome (Rothrock, 2008). There are a variety of heel and calf supporting devices available on the market today (**Fig. 8.6**). One particular device has the appearance of a boot and provides padding and support to the entire foot and calf. The newer boot devices move easily without removing them from the side rail socket and can be placed in any configuration desired to obtain the appropriate level of lithotomy. This ease of manipulation helps reduce the risk of injury to the patient and staff.

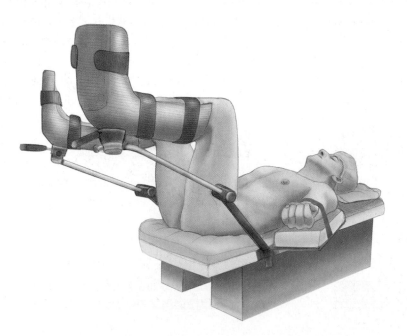

Figure 8.6

Lithotomy position using the boot type positioning device.

Regardless of the device selected to maintain the lithotomy position, care must be exercised to avoid injury. Placing padding over all areas in contact with any part of the positioning device is very important. Following the proper procedure for placing the patient in lithotomy position will also help minimize the risks for injury.

Positioning Procedure
Adjust the Bed and Transfer the Patient

Before transferring the patient, adjust the bed. Begin by releasing the head section of the mattress pad. Pull the headpiece and mattress pad out. Attach the headpiece and mattress to the foot of the bed. Refit the bed sheet to the bed. Transfer and prepare the patient for anesthesia administration in the supine position. Apply protective padding to the patient's feet and lower legs. Other protective padding is used as described for interventions common for all positions.

Attach the Stirrup/Boot

The common verbiage used to describe any positioning device for placing the patient in the lithotomy position is *stirrup*. The term *stirrup* typically connotes the ankle strap device. The use of this term can be confusing, as this may not be the appropriate device to use. This chapter uses the terms *stirrup* and *boot* to describe positioning devices as appropriate to the discussion.

Attach the positioning device holders, also called side rail sockets, to the bed above the knee break hinge. These holders are designed to fit on the bed and allow insertion of the device at the desired location on the bed. Insert the positioning device into the holders and tighten. Adjust the stirrups or boots to the appropriate height for the level of lithotomy desired; ensure that they are level and secure and are a matched pair.

Place the Patient in Lithotomy Position

After the patient is anesthetized, remove the safety strap from the legs. Grasp the sole of one foot in one hand, supporting the leg at the knee with the other hand. Instruct the assistant to perform the same maneuver for the other leg. Together with the assistant, *slowly* flex the legs toward the abdomen, then slightly externally rotate the hips and secure the feet in the stirrup strap or boot (Rothrock, 2007). Do not allow the knees to drop outward, externally rotating, to minimize the potential for joint dislocations or nerve or muscle injury. When using ankle strap stirrups, ensure that the legs and thighs do not touch the stirrup poles and that the feet and ankles are well padded at the strap points. When boots are used, be sure they are at the same angle and level before placing the legs. The knees should always remain flexed in the lithotomy position and never be allowed to straighten to minimize pressure on the knee joints (Rothrock, 2007). Cover the patient's genitalia and perineum with a towel or sheet.

Complete the Bed Modification

Remove the headrest and the leg section of the bed. Place the headrest and the leg section on a clean surface outside the sterile field. Touch the patient's hands to ensure that the patient's fingers are not in the hinges of the bed. Lower the leg section of the bed.

Reposition if Necessary

Remove the arm board straps and fold the patient's arms across the abdomen. Coordinate with the anesthesia provider before any patient movement. Stand between the patient's legs. Place the hands and arms under the patient's buttocks. Gently lift using proper body mechanics and move the patient to the edge of the bed break. Take care to lift instead of dragging the patient to minimize the risk of shearing forces on the skin of the patient's back and buttocks. Be sure that the anesthesia provider protects the arms during movement. An alternative method includes the use of an assistant to lift the patient. Both team members may stand on opposite sides of the bed and move the patient using the draw sheet underneath the patient to lift and move the patient. Move the arm boards and re-secure the patient's arms. Reassess leg and stirrup position. Palpate the patient's inner thighs to check for tension or stretching of ligaments and tendons. Check again for any pressure points before draping the patient.

Reposition After the Procedure

Check that the patient's hands and fingers are not extending beyond the bedbreak. Elevate the leg section to the horizontal position. Replace the mattress pad on the leg section. Reattach the head section and mattress pad to the foot of the bed. Have the assistant stand on the opposite side of the bed and prepare to reposition the patient. When given clearance by the anesthesia provider, both team members simultaneously grasp the patient's legs and remove the stirrup straps or remove the leg from the boot. With one hand under the patient's heel and the other under the knee, *slowly* bring the knees back to alignment with the body; extend the legs and then lower them together. Lowering the legs too rapidly can cause the patient's blood pressure to drop significantly, so ensure that the anesthesia provider is ready for the legs to be repositioned. Reapply the safety strap securely across the thighs. Cover the patient with a warm sheet or blanket. Remove the positioning equipment from the bed.

Potential Adverse Effects of the Lithotomy Position

Table 8.6 lists potential adverse effects of the lithotomy position.

LATERAL DECUBITUS POSITION

The lateral decubitus position, also known as lateral recumbent or Sims position, is used for access to the upper chest, the kidney, the upper section of the ureter, and the hip. The patient lies on one side to expose the area required for the procedure (**Fig. 8.7**). The reference to left or right lateral indicates which side on which the patient is lying. In right lateral, the patient is lying on the right side to expose structures on the left side. In left lateral, the patient is lying left side down.

Supplies and Equipment

- Headrest
- Pillows for between the legs and supporting structures
- Bath blankets
- Padding for bony prominences
- Arm boards: regular and over-arm
- Safety strap (several)

- Beanbag positioning device
- Kidney rest braces
- Axillary roll
- Adhesive tape

Table 8.6	Potential Adverse Effects of the Lithotomy Position	
Cause		**Effect**
Prolonged pressure (greater than 2 hours) on tissue	→	Skin breakdown at vulnerable weight-bearing bony prominences
Elevation of legs and decreased venous return	→	Venous pooling in the lumbar region
Thigh flexion	→	Vein compression in the groin
Positioning equipment	→	Vein compression in the legs
Thighs pressing against the abdomen, especially in obese patients	→	Increased intra-abdominal pressure—subsequent reduction in diaphragmatic movement
Blood draining from the torso into the legs upon lowering legs from lithotomy position	→	Severe hypotension
Pressure from thighs on the abdomen and pressure from viscera on the diaphragm restrict thoracic expansion, causing reduced respiratory efficiency	→	Reduced vital capacity and tidal volume
Acute flexion of the thighs	→	Injury to obturator and femoral nerves
Misplaced or unpadded stirrups/boots	→	Injury to saphenous and common peroneal nerves
Hyperextension of arms when moving patient toward break in bed during positioning	→	Brachial plexus injury
Excessive abduction of legs during positioning, especially in elderly or those with prosthetic devices	→	Hip injury
Prolonged use of exaggerated lithotomy position	→	Muscle injury
Improperly positioned buttocks over the break of the bed	→	Lower back strain
Prolonged contact and pressure from leg supports	→	Compartment syndrome in the calf

Sources: AORN, 2008; Rothrock, 2007; Krettek & Aschemann, 2006; Phillips, 2007; Monti-Sieber & Dorman, 2005; Spry, 2005.

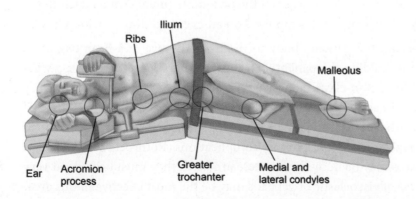

Ilium
Ribs
Malleolus
Ear   Acromion process   Greater trochanter   Medial and lateral condyles

Figure 8.7

Lateral decubitus position.

Positioning Procedure
Transfer the Patient to the Bed

Transfer and prepare the patient for anesthesia administration in the supine position.

Prepare the Assistants

Ensure that the assistants understand their individual roles. The anesthesia provider has control of the patient's head and airway. The nurse and one assistant stand on one side of the bed. Two other assistants stand on the opposite side of the bed. One assistant stands at the foot of the bed to control the feet and legs. The patient is turned so that the operative side is up.

Turn and Position the Patient

The anesthesia provider controls the head and neck and initiates the movement. After the patient's arms are placed at his or her sides, the circulating nurse and an assistant reach under the patient's shoulders and hips, lift slightly, and draw the patient's far shoulder and hip toward the middle of the bed. They concurrently rotate the patient to the lateral position. Two assistants help rotate the patient. The assistant at the foot of the bed controls the patient's legs. Support the patient until after the anesthetist has reestablished ventilation. Place a rolled towel or other type of padding (axillary roll) under the patient below the axilla, not in the axilla (Nagelhout & Zaglaniczny, 2005). Secure the patient with tape, beanbags, rolls, or other type of support. Flex the downside leg at the hip and knee to add stability. Ensure the dependent leg is well padded, especially at the knee and ankle. Place pillows or padding between the patient's legs.

The lateral decubitus position may be modified to provide better exposure for a particular procedure. Modifications include more lateral tilt creating the semi prone position or flexion at the kidney break to create the flexed kidney position. The principles for turning and positioning the patient remain the same.

After positioning the patient, verify the following:

- the patient's head, neck, and spine are in proper alignment
- the axillary roll is in the proper position below the axilla
- the genitals and dependent breast are free from pressure
- the legs and knees are padded
- no part of the patient's anatomy is resting on an unpadded surface
- the extremities are secured away from the bed joints (breaks) and attachments
- the nondependent arm is well supported on an over bed sling or with pillows

Stabilize and secure the patient's body to the bed. The use of a bean bag positioner is effective in holding the patient stable and disperses pressure over a wide area (Rothrock, 2007). Non-elastic adhesive tape and Velcro type safety straps may be used for stability in addition to the bean bag or alone. For positioning in a flexed or kidney position, the kidney rest is elevated. Make sure the iliac crest is positioned over the kidney break to prevent respiratory complications (Rothrock, 2007). The use of kidney rest braces may be necessary. If these are used, they must be padded very thoroughly. The use of viscoelastic or gel pads may be the most effective in this area.

Potential Adverse Effects of the Lateral Decubitus Position

Table 8.7 lists the potential adverse effects of the Lateral Decubitus Position

PRONE POSITION

For the prone position (also known as the ventral recumbent or ventral decubitus position), the patient is placed face down, resting on his or her abdomen and chest (**Fig. 8.8**). This position and modifications of this position, such as the Kraske (Jackknife) position, are used for procedures of the spine, back, rectal area, and posterior aspects of the lower extremities. Typically, the patient is placed under general anesthesia on the transport stretcher before being transferred to the bed. However, the patient may be anesthetized on the bed and then rotated into the prone position.

Supplies and Equipment

- Pillows
- Head rest
- Chest rolls or supporting frame
- Padding for bony prominences
- Padding or pillows for feet

Table 8.7 Potential Adverse Effects of the Lateral Decubitus Position	
Cause	**Effect**
Pressure and stretching forces	→ Injury to dependent brachial plexus
Pressure points and insufficient padding	→ Injury to median, radial, ulnar, and peroneal nerves
Prolonged pressure, decreased circulation to tissue in dependent position	→ Pressure sore development on tissues overlying the dependent greater trochanter of the femur
Possible shift in heart position	→ Potential interference with cardiac action
Kidney rests compressing the flank	→ Vena cava occlusion
Lateral flexion of the head and stretching of cervical nerve structures	→ Injury to cervical sympathetic nerves—ptosis of eyelid, flushing of the face
Excessive pressure on dependent eye—improperly placed positioning device	→ Retinal artery thrombosis

Sources: AORN, 2008; Rothrock, 2007; Krettek & Aschemann, 2006; Phillips, 2007; Nagelhout & Zaglaniczny, 2005.

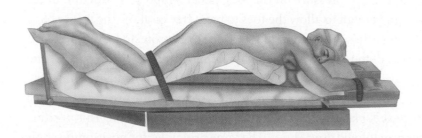

Figure 8.8

Prone position.

- Arm boards
- Arm board restraints
- Safety strap
- Face rest (horseshoe, Mayfield, other)
- Padded knee rest (donut or other gel type pad)
- Supplementary supplies and equipment
- Antiembolism stockings and/or sequential compression stockings (as identified in the nursing care plan)

Positioning Procedure
Transfer the Patient to the Bed

Transfer and prepare the patient for anesthesia administration in the supine position.

Turn the Patient on the Bed

Prepare the assistants by communicating their individual roles and confirming that they understand them. The circulating nurse and one assistant stand on one side of the bed, and the other two assistants stand on the opposite side of the bed. One assistant stands at the foot of the bed to control the legs and feet. The anesthesia provider controls the head and neck and initiates the movement. After the patient's arms are placed at his or her sides, the circulating nurse and assistant reach under the patient's shoulders and hips, lift slightly, and draw the patient's far shoulder and hip toward the middle of the bed. The nurse and assistant concurrently rotate the patient to the lateral position. The assistants across from the circulating nurse help rotate the patient. The assistant at the foot of the bed maintains control of the legs, keeping them in alignment with the hips and spine. Continue rotating the patient while centering the trunk on the positioning device (eg, Wilson frame, chest rolls). Support the patient until after the anesthesia provider has reestablished ventilation. Place supplemental positioning devices under the patient's extremities (Phillips, 2007). Care should be taken to avoid pulling any tubes such as catheters, IV access, or breathing circuit hoses so that patency is maintained.

Place the Patient in Position

After turning the patient, make certain that the chest rolls extend from the acromioclavicular joint to the iliac crest and that they do not impinge on the chest expansion and decrease abdominal pressure (AORN, 2008). Position the breasts so that they are displaced medially on the chest rolls. Check that the head, neck, spine, and legs are in proper alignment. Ensure that the legs are uncrossed and slightly apart. Check and free genitals from pressure and torsion. Pad iliac crests to decrease abdominal pressure on the vena cava, which is especially important with obese patients (Rothrock, 2007). To prevent pressure on the toes, either support the dorsum of the foot with a pillow high enough to allow the toes to hang free or allow the feet to hang over the end of the bed. Be sure the dorsum of the foot is protected from pressure. Make sure that no part of the patient's anatomy is resting on an unpadded surface and that the extremities are secured away from the bed joints (breaks) and attachments.

The Jackknife or Kraske position is a modification of the prone position in which the table is reverse flexed, placing the patient in an inverted V position. This position is typically used for proctologic procedures. The same principles for positioning apply to this position. Because the patient is flexed in this position, the risk for respiratory and circulatory compromise is increased. The potential adverse effects of Jackknife position are listed in **Table 8.8**.

Position the Arms

If arm boards are used, the arms are positioned above the patient's head with the elbows flexed, as seen in **Figure 8.8**, and secured to the arm boards (Phillips, 2007). If the arms are placed at the patient's side, the palms should be turned toward the body. The full length of the arms needs to be secured by a draw sheet or padded toboggan. Pressure points at the elbow and wrist should be carefully padded.

Reassess the Patient

Reassess the patient before draping. Make a final inspection of the areas at risk for increased pressure, verifying that all padding is still in place. Confirm the placement of the chest rolls or support and that the breasts and genitalia are not impinged.

Table 8.8	Potential Adverse Effects of the Prone and Jackknife Position	
Cause		**Effect**
Increased intra-abdominal pressure from pressure of lying on abdomen results in venous engorgement and venous congestion of the epidural veins	→	Potential rapid, massive blood loss in spinal procedures if vessel is cut
Improperly placed support devices, improper placement of arms	→	Injury to brachial plexus
Compression against the pelvic support device	→	Injury to the lateral femoral cutaneous nerves
Improperly placed support devices	→	Injury to facial motor nerves
Improper arm placement, ineffective padding	→	Injury to ulnar nerves
Feet resting on edge of bed	→	Injury to nerves and tendons of the dorsum of the foot
Improper placement on spinal frame or chest rolls, impingement of tissue	→	Injury to genitalia and breasts
Interference in diaphragm movement from weight of patient's body	→	Decreased tidal volume
Manipulation of patient's arm while performing the turning maneuver during positioning	→	Potential for shoulder dislocation
Compression for prolonged periods	→	Injury to tissue in areas of dependent bony prominences such as cheeks, shoulders, elbows, iliac crests, knees, and ankles
Head at or below heart level	→	Conjunctival edema
Related to opening eyes during position maneuvering	→	Corneal abrasion
Improper positioning/padding of the head	→	Injury to lingual and buccal nerves

Sources: AORN, 2008; Rothrock, 2007; Krettek & Aschemann, 2006; Phillips, 2007; Nagelhout & Zaglaniczny, 2005.

Check the body for proper alignment and make sure the safety strap is in place. Reassess the arms for proper placement and security and verify that the dorsum of the foot is supported to prevent pressure on the toes. If any aspect of the patient's position appears unsatisfactory, the nurse has an obligation to the patient to question this with the physician and anesthesia provider and to follow through until the situation has been addressed to everyone's satisfaction.

Spinal Frame or Spinal Surgery Table

There are devices that are designed to place the patient in a kneeling position to improve exposure to the spine while taking pressure off the abdomen, decreasing the risks associated with increased intra-abdominal pressure. The Andrews frame is a well-known spinal positioning device. It consists of a body lift, where the patient's head and chest rest; a tibial support with leg restraints to allow the patient's weight to be evenly distributed over the pretibial area; iliac crest supports and bolsters to level the lumbar spine; and a support strap that goes across the patient's thighs and the support frame to provide security (Phillips, 2007; O'Connell, 2006). The arms are placed on arm boards and flexed at the elbows so that they are positioned next to the head. The face rests in a cut-out foam pad or face rest designed to avoid pressure on the face, eyes, and ears.

The spinal table is designed to allow surgery with imaging access and is often used for lumbar and cervical surgery, providing cervical traction. The patient is positioned using a variety of supporting pads and attachments (Rothrock, 2007). The spinal table can be rotated with precise control, allowing the patient to be turned from supine to prone and back by rotating the table.

The same safety precautions exist when using the spinal frame or spinal surgery table. Extra care should be taken when positioning the legs on the tibial support in the kneeling position to avoid excess pressure on the knees and pretibial areas. The patient must be secured with care before rotating position when using the spinal table. While the spinal frame and table do help reduce the intra-abdominal pressure and the associated complications from this, there are still associated risks when positioning the patient. These are listed in **Table 8.8.**

Potential Adverse Effects of the Prone and Jackknife Positions

Table 8.8 lists the potential adverse effects of the prone and jackknife positions.

SITTING POSITION

The sitting position is used for cranial surgery requiring a posterior or occipital approach and for some ear and nose procedures. In this position, the patient's back is raised approximately 90 degrees, the knees are slightly flexed, and the legs lowered (Rothrock, 2007, p. 153). **Figure 8.9** depicts the patient in sitting position.

Supplies and Equipment

- Head holder (skull clamp, Mayfield, Gardner)
- Padding for bony prominences
- Padded footboard
- Safety strap
- Supplementary supplies and equipment

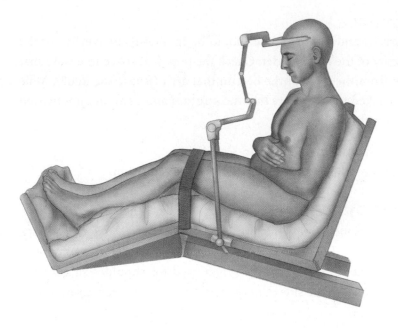

Figure 8.9
Sitting position with cervical head holder.

- Antiembolism stockings and/or sequential compression stockings (as identified in the nursing care plan)
- Table extension

Positioning Procedure
Transfer the Patient to the Bed
Transfer and prepare the patient for anesthesia administration in the supine position.

Prepare the Patient
Before placing the patient in the sitting position, apply compression stockings. The physician may request sequential compression stockings be applied as well to prevent postural hypotension and pooling of blood in the lower extremities (Spry, 2005). Generously pad the patient under the buttocks, as the ischial tuberosities support the majority of the patient's weight in this position. Place padding under each heel. A padded footboard should be attached to the end of the bed to provide support and help prevent foot drop. If cranial surgery is planned, after the patient is anesthetized, the cervical head holder is applied to the patient.

Modify the Bed to the Sitting Position
Raise the upper portion of the bed to elevate the torso into the sitting position, then lower the foot of the bed slowly, flexing the knees and the pelvis. The feet are supported by the padded footrest. The head end of the bed is then tilted to attain the desired position for the physician. Place the patient's arms, flexed at the elbow on a pillow in the patient's lap. The torso and arms should be secured with a body strap. Adhesive tape may be used. Pad each elbow with foam padding. If available, place the patient's arms in arm holders at the side of the bed. For cranial surgery, the head of the bed is removed and a special craniotomy headrest is attached to the bed to place the head in the appropriate position for the surgery (Rothrock, 2007). For ear or nose procedures, a bolster or other padded positioning device may be used.

Reassessing the Patient

The cervical, thoracic, and lumbar spine should be in alignment. Verify correct placement and security of the head holder. Check the popliteal space to ensure that there is no pressure from the edge of the bed on that area (Rothrock, 2007). Male patients should be checked to make sure that the scrotum and penis are not twisted or compressed between the legs.

Potential Adverse Effects of the Sitting Position

Table 8.9 lists the potential adverse effects of the sitting position.

SEMI-SITTING/FOWLER/BEACH CHAIR POSITION

The semi-sitting position is most frequently used for shoulder, nasal, abdominoplasty, and some cranial surgery. It differs from the sitting position in that the amount of elevation of the torso is about half as much. When used for shoulder surgery, the patient may be moved closer to the side of the bed on the operative side to allow better access for the physician.

Supplies and Equipment

The supplies and equipment for the semi-sitting position are the same as for the sitting position except for the additional item for shoulder surgery.

- Traction device for suspending the operative extremity for prepping and surgery

Positioning Procedure

Preparation of the bed and the patient is the same as for the sitting position. The torso is elevated approximately 45 degrees and the knees are flexed with the leg section lowered slightly. The bed is tilted so that the head is not so erect, reducing sliding and shearing forces on the patient. A footrest is used and the arms are secured on the patient's lap on a pillow.

Table 8.9	Potential Adverse Effects of the Sitting and Semi-Sitting Position	
Cause		**Effect**
Pooling of blood in lower torso and legs	→	Orthostatic hypotension and diminished perfusion to the brain
Venous pooling in legs, decreased venous return	→	Risk of venous thrombosis
Gravity causes negative venous gradient between operative site and right atrium—creates potential for air embolus if a venous sinus is opened	→	Venous air embolism
Increased weight bearing on this area due to sitting position	→	Pressure sore development on ischial tuberosities
Improper positioning of legs with prolonged extension of the knees	→	Stretch injury to sciatic nerve
Positioning of head after intubation when placed into head holder and excessive flexion occurs	→	Displacement of endotracheal tube

Sources: AORN, 2008; Rothrock, 2007; Krettek & Aschemann, 2006; Phillips, 2007; Nagelhout & Zaglaniczny, 2005.

For shoulder surgery, the team must carefully move the patient to the edge of the bed before elevating the back and lowering the legs. The anesthesia provider controls the move while maintaining the airway. Two assistants on each side lift the patient using a draw sheet and place the body on the edge of the bed on the operative side. Care must be taken to prevent dropping or injury to the operative extremity when moving. The non-operative arm will rest next to the patient and should be padded and tucked with the palm facing in to prevent injury. The operative arm will be secured in a device that allows operative access. This is often some form of traction device or sling.

As with the supine position, verify appropriate spinal alignment, padding, and freedom from pressure or impingement of any tissue, including the male genitalia.

Potential Adverse Effects of the Semi-Sitting Position

Table 8.9 lists the potential adverse effects of the semi sitting position. In the lower sitting position, the risk of venous pooling of blood and the risk of hypotension may be less.

SPECIAL CONSIDERATIONS

Fracture Table

The orthopedic fracture table is used to provide access for hip surgery such as fracture repair, femoral nailing, or total hip replacement. The table is configured in such a way as to provide exposure of the affected hip with full access for radiographic equipment (C-arm) while maintaining traction on the affected extremity (**Fig. 8.10**).

Typically, the patient is anesthetized on the transport cart and then transferred to the fracture table. The same safety principles apply to this process as they do for transferring any anesthetized patient. Care should be taken to have enough personnel present and appropriate transfer devices, such as a roller or smooth board to avoid risk of dropping the patient. The team must coordinate activities and communicate the roles clearly before beginning the patient transfer.

The patient is placed supine on the fracture table. The perineum rests against a vertical perineal post. This post must be very well padded to avoid any nerve injury to that area. This perineal post maintains the patient's torso and pelvis in position against the traction of the operative leg.

The operative leg is placed in traction using a boot type device that secures the foot and ankle. This is connected to a gear device that allows the physician to apply as much traction and rotation as necessary to reduce a fracture or provide exposure. The boot must provide padding to all areas of the foot, particularly the medial and lateral malleoli and the dorsum of the foot.

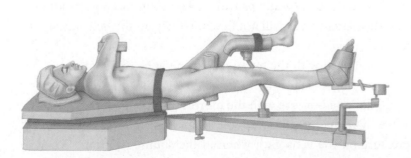

Figure 8.10

Fracture table position.

The unaffected leg is flexed at the hip and knee and is placed in a holder such as a well or sling. The holder must also be well padded to avoid injury to the extremity. The leg should be secured in the holder with a safety strap (Rothrock, 2007).

The arm on the operative side is secured either against the patient's torso or over the body in a padded sling or on an arm holder. The purpose is to avoid obstruction of the operative site. Pressure must be avoided over the ulnar nerve regardless of the method used. When securing the arm to the torso, avoid extreme flexion of the elbow to prevent ulnar nerve injury and keep circumduction of the shoulder unforced, to avoid a stretch injury to the suprascapular nerve. When securing the arm to the torso, place padding between the arm and the body. Use caution when securing the arm in an arm holder above the patient to also avoid stretching the suprascapular nerve (Rothrock, 2007). The arm on the non-operative side can be secured on a padded arm board at the side, following the practices previously discussed.

Upon final positioning, be sure that all areas are padded, pulses are present in all extremities, and positioning devices are secure.

The Morbidly Obese Patient

The morbidly obese patient, one with a BMI over 40 or weight of 100 pounds (45.36 kg) over the recommended weight, presents some special considerations when being positioned for a procedure. Some of these have been previously discussed. The physiological issues associated with morbid obesity include respiratory and circulatory.

Respiratory issues:

- Short, thick neck causes airway compromise
- Risk of difficult intubation
- Increased risk for hypoxia
- Increased risk of aspiration
- Increased risk for intra-abdominal pressure on the diaphragm

Circulatory issues:

- Increased cardiac output
- Increased pulmonary artery pressure
- Risk for inferior vena cava compression (AORN, 2008)

The AORN Recommended Practices for Positioning the Patient in the Perioperative Practice Setting (2008) provide several guidelines for protecting the morbidly obese patient. These practices include using a procedure bed that will support patients weighing 800–1000 pounds and that has hydraulics that can lift a patient in that weight range. Mattresses on the bed should provide enough support and padding to avoid compression. If the patient's legs will not fit completely on the bed, stirrups or side extensions should be used.

Supplies and equipment used with the obese patient must be extra large or extra long, provide greater padding capability, and be able to withstand greater weight. Use only items that are designed for use with the morbidly obese patient.

As described earlier, a wedge or pillow should be placed under the right flank area to decrease pressure on the vena cava when in the supine position. When in the prone position, verify that the upper chest and pelvis are supported to free the abdominal viscera so that pressure is reduced on the diaphragm and the vena cava. The lateral position may be preferable over the prone position when possible because the weight of the panniculus can be displaced off the abdomen. Caution must be exercised to prevent the risk of falling in this position. Lithotomy position should be avoided if possible because the pressure of the thighs on the abdomen creates increased intra-abdominal pressure. If it is used, be sure the leg holders can support the extra weight. Trendelenburg position should be avoided since increased pressure on the diaphragm produces respiratory compromise and increased blood flow from the lower extremities into the pulmonary and central circulation causes vascular congestion (AORN, 2008).

While this discussion focuses on the morbidly obese patient, care should be taken with any overweight patient to assure proper equipment is used and to prevent complications.

Robotic Surgery

In robotic surgery, the physician sits at an operative console consisting of hand-held controls and three-dimensional imaging, while robotic arms at the operative site hold instruments and respond to the physician's commands from the console.

The use of robots in surgery presents a unique situation in patient positioning. The robot must be located either on the sides or at the foot of the bed. The base of the patient side cart containing the robotic arms has a large footprint and once it is placed, the bed cannot be moved (Intuitive Surgical, 2007). Access to the patient becomes restricted once the side cart is in place, so final assessment of the patient's position should take place prior to this. A study performed to review an institution's experience with robot-assisted laparoscopy determined that one disadvantage is the bulkiness of the robot arms. These arms can interfere with the assistant's movements (Miller, Schlinkert, & Schlinkert, 2004).

The conventional positions are still used for robotic operative procedures and the same precautions to prevent injury must be taken. Additionally, the perioperative nurse should be especially vigilant in observing the procedure to assure that the robotic arms do not disrupt the patient's position in any way. Careful preparation is essential when positioning the patient for any procedure, especially robotic surgery.

CONCLUSION

Positioning a patient for operative and invasive procedures requires assessment skills, knowledge of anatomy and physiology, an understanding of the planned procedure, and familiarity with the positioning devices and various positions used in surgery. The nurse uses the information obtained during the assessment to plan the care during the positioning event. Injury to the patient's integumentary, circulatory, respiratory, musculoskeletal, and neurological structures can be prevented by identifying patients at risk for injury before initiating positioning activities.

Careful planning and cooperation with clear communication of assigned roles and responsibilities supports safety for the patient and the team positioning the patient. Teamwork is essential to help avoid adverse outcomes related to positioning.

COMPETENCY ASSESSMENT
Position the Patient

Name: _____ Title: _____ Unit: _____ Date of Validation: _____

Type of Validation: ☐ Initial ☐ Annual ☐ Bi-annual

COMPETENCY STATEMENT: The nurse demonstrates competency to position the patient for an operative or invasive procedure.

Performance Criteria	Met	Not Met
1. Identifies the patient's risk for adverse outcomes related to positioning	☐	☐
2. Selects the appropriate supplies and equipment based on the patient's identified needs	☐	☐
3. Prepares the procedure bed	☐	☐
4. Centers the patient on the bed	☐	☐
5. Places the patient's arms on arm boards	☐	☐
6. Uses positioning devices according to the established practice recommendations and the manufacturer's recommendations	☐	☐
7. Pads bony prominences	☐	☐
8. Move the anesthetized patient	☐	☐
9. Communicates and documents risk factors, nursing diagnoses, expected outcomes, the plan of care, interventions, and evaluation	☐	☐
10. Places the patient in the supine position	☐	☐
11. Places the patient in the Trendelenburg position	☐	☐
12. Places the patient in the reverse Trendelenburg position	☐	☐
13. Places the patient in the low lithotomy position	☐	☐
14. Places the patient in the high lithotomy position	☐	☐
15. Places the patient in the prone position	☐	☐
16. Places the patient in the jackknife position	☐	☐
17. Places the patient in the Fowler position	☐	☐
18. Places the patient in the semi-Fowler position	☐	☐
19. Positions the patient on the fracture table	☐	☐
20. Positions the patient on the spine table	☐	☐

_____
Validator's Signature

_____
Employee's Signature

_____
Validator's Printed Name

REFERENCES

1. AORN (2008). Recommended practices for positioning the patient in the perioperative practice setting. In *Perioperative standards and recommended practices, 2008 edition*. Denver: AORN, Inc. pp. 497–520.

2. Beyea, S. C. (2002). *Perioperative Nursing Data Set: The perioperative nursing vocabulary, 2nd ed.* Denver: Association of Perioperative Registered Nurses.

3. Intuitive Surgical (2007). DaVinci sacropopexy procedure card. Intuitive Surgical, Sunnyvale, CA.

4. Krettek, C., & Aschemann, D. (2006). *Positioning techniques in surgical applications*. Heidelberg, Germany: Springer Medizin Verlag.

5. Miller, D. W., Schlinkert, R. T., & Schlinkert, D. K. (2004, Sep). Robot-assisted laparoscopic cholecystectomy: Initial mayo clinic Scottsdale experience. *Mayo Clinic Proceedings*, 79(9), pp. 1132–1136.

6. Mills, E.J. (ed.) (2006). *Handbook of medical-surgical nursing, 4th ed.* Philadelphia: Lippincott, Williams, & Wilkins. pp. 739–742.

7. Monti-Siebert, E.J., Dorman, L., & Hill, D. (2005). Positioning for anesthesia and surgery. In J.J. Nagelhout and K.L. Zaglaniczny, *Nurse anesthesia, 3rd ed.* St. Louis: Elsevier Saunders. pp. 390–408.

8. O'Connel, M. P. (2006). Positioning impact on the surgical patient. *Nursing clinics of North America*, 41, pp. 173–192.

9. Phillips, N. (2007). *Berry & Kohn's operating room techniques, 11th ed.* St. Louis: Mosby. pp. 492–530.

10. Rockrock, J. (2007). Positioning the patient for surgery. In *Alexander's care of the patient in surgery, 13th ed.* St. Louis: Mosby, pp. 130–158.

11. Schultz, A. (2005). Predicting and preventing pressure ulcers in surgical patients. *AORN Journal*, 81(5), pp. 986–1006.

12. Spry, C. (2005). *Essentials of perioperative nursing (3rd ed.)*. Sudbury: Jones and Bartlett Publishers.

13. The Joint Commission. (2008). Universal protocol for preventing wrong site, wrong procedure, wrong person surgery. Available at http://www.jointcommission.org/NR/rdonlyres/E3C600EB-043B-4E86-B04E-CA4A89AD5433/0/universal_protocol.pdf Accessed February 25, 2008.

CHAPTER 9

Establish and Maintain the Sterile Field

Pat Mews

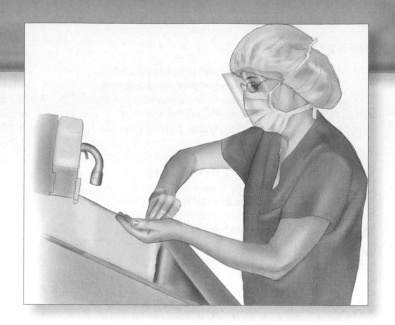

INTRODUCTION

As patient advocates, nurses are responsible for providing a safe environment for patients undergoing operative and invasive procedure intervention. Establishing and maintaining a sterile field can directly influence patient outcomes. Patient care activities that adhere to aseptic practices by all individuals involved in the procedure aid in fulfilling the professional responsibility to protect patients from injury. Implementation of aseptic practices before, during, and after the procedure minimizes wound contamination and reduces the patient's risk for an operative site infection (AORN, 2008a). One of the fundamental components of providing a safe environment is the practice of *strict aseptic technique*. Rigorous adherence to the principles of asepsis is the foundation for preventing an operative site infection.

MEASURABLE CRITERIA

The nurse demonstrates competency to establish and maintain a sterile field by

- Identifying patients at risk for adverse outcomes related to establishing and maintaining a sterile field
- Donning and wearing appropriate operative attire
- Preparing supplies, instruments, and equipment for the sterile field
- Scrubbing the hands and forearms
- Donning sterile gown and gloves
- Preparing the patient's skin for the procedure
- Draping the patient and equipment

Chapter Contents

CONSIDERATIONS FOR PREPARING A STERILE FIELD AND LOWERING THE RISK OF OPERATIVE SITE INFECTIONS

Surgical Site Infections

Establishing and maintaining a sterile environment during the procedure minimizes the patient's risk for an operative (surgical) site infection. Based on the National Nosocomial Infection Surveillance (NNIS) system, surgical site infections (SSI) are the third most common cause of healthcare-acquired (ie, nosocomial) infections, accounting for 38% of all such infections in the United States (Mangram, 1999) The CDC's NNIS system has developed standardized surveillance criteria for defining SSIs (**Table 9.1**). By these criteria, SSI are classified as being either incisional or organ/space. Incisional SSIs are further divided into those involving only skin and subcutaneous tissue (superficial incisional SSI) and those involving deeper soft

NNIS
National Nosocomial Infection Surveillance

SSI
Surgical Site Infections

Table 9.1	Criteria for Defining a Surgical Site Infection (SSI)

Superficial Incisional SSI

Infection occurs within 30 days after the operation *and* infection involves only skin or subcutaneous tissue of the incision *and* at least *one* of the following:

1. Purulent drainage, with or without laboratory confirmation, from the superficial incision.
2. Organisms isolated from an aseptically obtained culture of fluid or tissue from the superficial incision.
3. At least one of the following signs or symptoms of infection: pain or tenderness, localized swelling, redness, or heat *and* superficial incision is deliberately opened by surgeon, *unless* incision is culture-negative.
4. Diagnosis of superficial incisional SSI by the surgeon or attending physician.

Do *not* report the following conditions as SSI:

1. Stitch abscess (minimal inflammation and discharge confined to the points of suture penetration).
2. Infection of an episiotomy or newborn circumcision site.
3. Infected burn wound.
4. Incisional SSI that extends into the fascial and muscle layers (see deep incisional SSI).

Note: Specific criteria are used for identifying infected episiotomy and circumcision sites and burn wounds.

Deep Incisional SSI

Infection occurs within 30 days after the operation if no implant[†] is left in place or within 1 year if implant is in place and the infection appears to be related to the operation *and* infection involves deep soft tissues (eg, fascial and muscle layers) of the incision *and* at least *one* of the following:

1. Purulent drainage from the deep incision but not from the organ/space component of the surgical site.
2. A deep incision spontaneously dehisces or is deliberately opened by a surgeon when the patient has at least one of the following signs or symptoms: fever (>100.4°F [38°C]), localized pain, or tenderness, unless site is culture-negative.
3. An abscess or other evidence of infection involving the deep incision is found on direct examination, during reoperation, or by histopathologic or radiologic examination.
4. Diagnosis of a deep incisional SSI by a surgeon or attending physician.

Notes:

1. Report infection that involves both superficial and deep incision sites as deep incisional SSI.
2. Report an organ/space SSI that drains through the incision as a deep incisional SSI.

> **Organ/Space SSI**
>
> Infection occurs within 30 days after the operation if no implant[†] is left in place or within 1 year if implant is in place and the infection appears to be related to the operation *and* infection involves any part of the anatomy (eg, organs or spaces), other than the incision, which was opened or manipulated during an operation *and* at least *one* of the following:
>
> 1. Purulent drainage from a drain that is placed through a stab wound[‡] into the organ/space.
> 2. Organisms isolated from an aseptically obtained culture of fluid or tissue in the organ/space.
> 3. An abscess or other evidence of infection involving the organ/space that is found on direct examination, during reoperation, or by histopathologic or radiologic examination.
> 4. Diagnosis of an organ/space SSI by a surgeon or attending physician.

Horan TC et al.† National Nosocomial Infection Surveillance definition: a nonhuman-derived implantable foreign body (eg, prosthetic heart valve, nonhuman vascular graft, mechanical heart, or hip prosthesis) that is permanently placed in a patient during surgery. ‡ If the area around a stab wound becomes infected, it is not an SSI. It is considered a skin or soft tissue infection, depending on its depth.

CDC
Centers for Disease Control and Prevention

HICPAC
Hospital Infection Control Practices Advisory Committee

tissues of the incision (deep incisional SSI). Organ/space SSIs involve any part of the anatomy (eg, organ or space) other than incised body wall layers opened or manipulated during an operation (Mangram, 1999). Preventing SSI is critical to patients and everyone within the healthcare system.

The Centers for Disease Control and Prevention (CDC) and the Hospital Infection Control Practices Advisory Committee (HICPAC) developed practice guidelines with the main objective to reduce the incidence of SSI and improve patient outcomes. The CDC guidelines consist of an overview of the issues related to the incidence of surgical site infections and provide recommendations aimed at preventing these infections (**Table 9.2**). Each recommendation is categorized based on existing scientific data, theoretical rationale, and applicability; and include suggestions for antimicrobial prophylaxis. In addition, the recommendations support the Surgical Care Improvement Project initiatives to reduce SSIs.

Table 9.2	Recommendations for Prevention of Surgical Site Infections (SSI)
Rankings	
CDC/HICPAC system for categorizing recommendations is as follows:	
Category IA	Strongly recommended for implementation and strongly supported by well-designed experimental, clinical, or epidemiologic studies.
Category IB	Strongly recommended for implementation and supported by certain experimental, clinical, or epidemiologic studies and a strong theoretical rationale.
Category IC	Required for implementation, as mandated by federal or state regulation or standard.
Category II	Suggested for implementation and supported by suggestive clinical or epidemiologic studies or a theoretical rationale.
No Recommendation (NR)	Unresolved issue. Practices for which insufficient evidence or no consensus regarding efficacy exist.

Preparation of the Patient	Category
Whenever possible, identify and treat all infections remote to the surgical site before elective operation and postpone elective operations on patients with remote site infections until the infection has resolved.	IA
Do not remove hair preoperatively unless the hair at or around the incision site will interfere with the operation.	IA
If hair is removed, remove immediately before the operation, preferably with electric clippers.	IA
Adequately control serum blood glucose levels in all diabetic patients and particularly avoid hyperglycemia perioperatively.	IB
Encourage tobacco cessation. At minimum, instruct patients to abstain for at least 30 days before elective operation from smoking cigarettes, cigars, pipes, or any other form of tobacco consumption (eg, chewing/dipping).	IB
Do not withhold necessary blood products from surgical patients as a means to prevent SSI.	IB
Require patients to shower or bathe with an antiseptic agent on at least the night before the operative day.	IB
Thoroughly wash and clean at and around the incision site to remove gross contamination before performing antiseptic skin preparation.	IB
Use an appropriate antiseptic agent for skin preparation.	IB
Apply preoperative antiseptic skin preparation in concentric circles moving toward the periphery. The prepared area must be large enough to extend the incision or create new incisions or drain sites, if necessary.	II
Keep preoperative hospital stay as short as possible while allowing for adequate preoperative preparation of the patient.	II
No recommendation to taper or discontinue systemic steroid use (when medically permissible) before elective operation.	NR
No recommendation to enhance nutritional support for surgical patients solely as a means to prevent SSI.	NR
No recommendation to preoperatively apply mupirocin to nares to prevent SSI.	NR
No recommendation to provide measures that enhance wound space oxygenation to prevent SSI.	NR

Hand/Forearm Antisepsis for Surgical Team Members	Category
Keep nails short and do not wear artificial nails.	IB
Perform a preoperative surgical scrub for at least 2 to 5 minutes using an appropriate antiseptic (Table 6). Scrub the hands and forearms up to the elbows.	IB
After performing the surgical scrub, keep hands up and away from the body (elbows in flexed position) so that water runs from the tips of the fingers toward the elbows. Dry hands with a sterile towel and don a sterile gown and gloves.	IB
Clean underneath each fingernail prior to performing the first surgical scrub of the day.	II
Do not wear hand or arm jewelry.	II
No recommendation on wearing nail polish.	NR

Management of Infected or Colonized Surgical Personnel	Category
Educate and encourage surgical personnel who have signs and symptoms of a transmissible infectious illness to report conditions promptly to their supervisory and occupational health service personnel.	IB
Develop well-defined policies concerning patient care responsibilities when personnel have potentially transmissible infectious conditions. These policies should govern (a) personnel responsibility in using the health service and reporting illness, (b) work restrictions, and (c) clearance to resume work after an illness that required work restriction. The policies also should identify persons who have the authority to remove personnel from duty.	IB

9

	Category
Obtain appropriate cultures from, and exclude from duty, surgical personnel who have draining skin lesions until infection has been ruled out or personnel have received adequate therapy and infection has resolved.	IB
Do not routinely exclude surgical personnel who are colonized with organisms such as *S. aureus* (nose, hands, or other body site) or group A *Streptococcus,* unless such personnel have been linked epidemiologically to dissemination of the organism in the healthcare setting.	IB
Antimicrobial Prophylaxis	**Category**
Administer a prophylactic antimicrobial agent only when indicated, and select it based on its efficacy against the most common pathogens causing SSI for a specific operation.	IA
Administer by the intravenous route the initial dose of prophylactic antimicrobial agent, timed such that a bactericidal concentration of the drug is established in serum and tissues when the incision is made. Maintain therapeutic levels of the agent in serum and tissues throughout the operation and until, at most, a few hours after the incision is closed in the operating room.	IA
Before elective colorectal operations in addition to administering a prophylactic antimicrobial agent, mechanically prepare the colon by use of enemas and cathartic agents. Administer nonabsorbable oral antimicrobial agents in divided doses on the day before the operation.	IA
For high-risk cesarean section, administer the prophylactic antimicrobial agent immediately after the umbilical cord is clamped.	IA
Do not routinely use vancomycin for antimicrobial prophylaxis.	IB

CDC/HICPAC Centers for Disease Control and Prevention & Health Infection Control Practices Advisory Committee (2001).

SCIP
Surgical Care
Improvement Project

Surgical Care Improvement Project (SCIP) Initiatives

SCIP is a national quality partnership of organizations committed to improving the safety of surgical care through the reduction of surgical complications, thus improving the health outcomes of surgical patients. The ultimate goal of the partnership is to save lives by reducing the incidence of surgical complications by 25% by the year 2010. **Table 9.3** highlights the seven initiatives that concentrate on the reduction of SSIs. The goal of SCIP is to prevent SSI by implementing four components of care. These components of care are supported by clinical trials and experimental evidence and, if implemented consistently, significantly reduce the incidence of preventable surgical site infections (**Table 9.4**).

Table 9.3	Surgical Care Improvement Project (SCIP)*
Infection	
SCIP INF 1	Prophylactic antibiotic received within one hour prior to surgical incision
SCIP INF 2	Prophylactic antibiotic selection for surgical patients
SCIP INF 3	Prophylactic antibiotics discontinued within 24 hours after surgery end time (48 hours for cardiac patients)
SCIP INF 4	Cardiac surgery patients with controlled 6 a.m. postoperative serum glucose
SCIP INF 5	Postoperative wound infection diagnosed during index hospitalization (OUTCOME)
SCIP INF 6	Surgery patients with appropriate hair removal
SCIP INF 7	Colorectal surgery patients with immediate postoperative normothermia

Cardiac

SCIP CARD 2 Surgery patients on a beta-blocker prior to arrival that received a beta-blocker during the perioperative period

SCIP CARD 3 Intra- or postoperative acute myocardial infarction (AMI) diagnosed during index hospitalization and within 30 days of surgery (OUTCOME)

VTE

SCIP VTE 1 Surgery patients with recommended venous thromboembolism prophylaxis ordered

SCIP VTE 2 Surgery patients who received appropriate venous thromboembolism prophylaxis within 24 hours prior to surgery to 24 hours after surgery

SCIP VTE 3 Intra- or postoperative pulmonary embolism (PE) diagnosed during index hospitalization and within 30 days of surgery (OUTCOME)

SCIP VTE 4 Intra- or postoperative deep vein thrombosis (DVT) diagnosed during index hospitalization and within 30 days of surgery (OUTCOME)

* SCIP is a national quality partnership of organizations committed to improving the safety of surgical care through the reduction of postoperative complications. The ultimate goal of the partnerships is to save lives by reducing the incidence of surgical complications by 25% by the year 2010. SCIP Project information: http://www.medqic.org/dcs/ContentServer?cid=112290493 0422&pagename=Medqic% 2FContent%2FParentShellTemplate&parentName=Topic&c=MQParents (Accessed March 15, 2008).

Table 9.4	**Four Components of Care to Reduce Incidence of SSI**	
Appropriate use of antibiotics	☐	Selection of the appropriate drug
	☐	Timing of the administration of the antibiotic, within one hour prior to the time of the incision
	☐	Discontinuation of the antibiotic within 24 hour
Appropriate hair removal	☐	Using clippers
	☐	Eliminating shaving with razors for hair removal
Maintenance of postoperative glucose control	☐	Major cardiac surgery patients
Maintenance of postoperative normothermia	☐	Colorectal surgery patients

100k lives, The prevention of SSI a component of Surgical Care Improvement Project (SCIP) http://www.medqic.org/dcs/ContentServer?cid=1136495723627&pagename=Medqic%2FOtherResource%2FOtherResourcesTemplate&c=OtherResource (Accessed May, 2008).

Importance of Aseptic Technique

In order to establish and maintain a sterile field operative and invasive procedure team members must focus on inhibiting the microbial contamination of the surgical site. Preventing surgical site infection requires the flawless application of aseptic technique by all members of the patient care team[1]. Practicing aseptic technique (methods by which contamination with microorganisms are prevented) helps reduce the risk of postprocedure infections in patients by decreasing the likelihood that microorganisms will enter the body during the procedure. Aseptic technique also helps reduce the team member's risk of exposure by acting as a barrier against potentially infectious tissue, blood, or other body fluids during the procedure.

Because many hospital-acquired infections can be traced to the operative or invasive procedure suite, patient care team members practice strict aseptic techniques at all times. *Sterile* is defined as being maximally free of all living microorganisms. Perfect asepsis, the absence of disease-causing microorganisms, is the ideal toward which team members should strive.

Skin is the patient's first line of defense against infection. Disruption of the skin surface from an operative incision or trauma compromises that line of defense by creating an entry for microorganisms. Sources of infection can be either endogenous or exogenous. Endogenous infection comes from the large number of microorganisms produced within or caused by factors within or on the patient's body. After the skin is incised, certain factors or conditions, including age, nutritional status, impaired defense mechanisms, preexisting disease, and length and type of procedure, can influence a patient's risk of infection.

To control endogenous infection a number of steps may be taken. To achieve maximum antiseptic effectiveness, patients, unless contraindicated, should shower twice with 4% chlorhexidine gluconate (CHG) before arriving at the facility. Prior to entering the operative or invasive procedure suite, the patient changes into a clean gown and covers the hair with a bouffant cap. Gastrointestinal cleansing and preparations with laxatives and enemas are often given before intestinal procedures.

Exogenous infection is acquired from organisms originating outside or caused by factors outside the patient's body. Supplies, instruments, equipment, and personnel are sources that contribute to SSIs. People are a major source of contamination and thus are responsible for maintaining good personal hygiene. Restricting personnel to the minimum contact necessary for the procedure and limiting talking minimize the spread of microorganisms. In addition, to protect the patient from microorganisms, all personnel must wear proper operative attire, which includes a head cover or hood, scrub top and pants, warm-up jacket if not scrubbed, and masks, to minimize the chance of spreading microorganisms.

Although the operative or invasive procedure suite is considered a clean environment, it does contain microorganisms in the air and on any permanent structures in the room, such as floors, walls, cabinets, and overhead lights. All are potential sources of infection. Chapter 14 describes the procedures for a safe environment of care.

The nurse plays a key role in the ongoing maintenance of aseptic technique during the procedure. The nurse may function as the circulating or scrub nurse during the procedure. The scrub nurse maintains the integrity, safety, and efficiency of the sterile field throughout the procedure. While performing this nursing activity the nurse wears a mask with a protective shield, sterile gown, and gloves. Role functions include assisting the surgeon and assistants by providing the sterile instruments and supplies required for the procedure. The circulating nurse acts as the patient's

CHG
Chlorhexidine Gluconate

advocate, coordinates and documents all activities during the procedure, manages the patient's nursing care, and assists in controlling the physical and emotional atmosphere of the room. Because the circulating nurse is able to view the sterile field from a distance, she or he is better able to observe the entire field and must remain alert to catch any breaks in aseptic technique that other personnel may not have seen.

Surgical Conscience

Whether scrubbing or circulating, the nurse and other team members must immediately respond to any break in aseptic technique during the procedure. Surgical conscience involves a concept of self-inspection coupled with moral obligation. Involving both scientific and intellectual honesty, it is self-regulation in practice according to a deep personal commitment to the highest values. Do not make compromises when it comes to sterility. As advocates for the patient, the circulating nurse and every other member of the patient care team must maintain both an individual and a collective surgical conscience.

The collective surgical conscience does not excuse error but admits readily to and rectifies any breaks in aseptic technique in order to serve the patient better (Phillips, 2004). Team members attend to the activities of everyone else in the operative or invasive procedure suite. They consistently observe the events that may compromise the sterile field, and when comprised they initiate corrective action.

"*Perioperative Standards and Recommended Practices (2008) Maintaining a Sterile Field*" delineates basic principles and guidelines for maintaining a sterile field (**Table 9.5**).

Table 9.5	Principles and Guidelines for Establishing and Maintaining a Sterile Field
Principles	**Guidelines**
Scrubbed persons function within a sterile field.	☐ Don appropriate operative attire.
	☐ Perform surgical hand antisepsis per AORN's RPs and manufacturer's instructions.
	☐ Don sterile gown and gloves from a sterile area away from the main instrument table to prevent contamination of the sterile field.
	☐ Use sterile gowns and gloves within the sterile field.
	☐ Inspect gloves for integrity after donning.
	☐ Consider gowns sterile in front from the chest to the level of the sterile field.
	☐ Consider gown sleeves sterile from 2 inches (5 cm) above the elbow to the cuff circumferentially.
	☐ After donning the original gloves, consider the gown cuffs contaminated.
	☐ Sleeve cuffs should be considered contaminated when the scrubbed person's hands pass beyond the cuff.
	☐ Sterile gloves that become contaminated should be changed as soon as possible using the assisted gloving method.
Use sterile items within a sterile field.	☐ Inspect all items immediately before presentation to the sterile field. All items should be inspected before presentation to the sterile field for proper packing, processing, seal, package container integrity, and inclusion of a sterilization indicator, and expiration date, if indicated.

Open, dispense, and transfer all items onto a sterile filed by methods that maintain sterility and integrity.	☐ Unscrubbed persons open wrapped supplies by opening the wrapper flap farthest away from the body first and the wrapper flap nearest to the body last.
	☐ Secure wrapper edges when delivering items to the sterile field.
	☐ Deliver sterile items to the scrub person, or place them securely on the sterile field.
	☐ Deliver sharps, heavy objects, directly to the scrub person, or open on a separate surface.
	☐ Open rigid container systems on a separate surface and inspect locks for security and check filter.
	☐ When delivering solutions to the sterile field, have the scrub person hold the solution receptacle, or place it near the table edge.
	☐ Pour solutions slowly to avoid splashing.
	☐ The edge of a solution container is contaminated; therefore, discard solutions remaining in the container.
Constantly monitor and maintain the sterile field.	☐ Cover nonsterile equipment with sterile barriers before placing them in or over the sterile field.
	☐ Dispense medications to the sterile field utilizing transfer devices (eg, sterile vial spike, filter straws).
	☐ Follow AORN's RPs for safe medication practice.
	☐ Prepare the sterile field as close as possible to the time of use.
	☐ Prevent the spread of moisture droplets by limiting conversation in the presence of a sterile field.
	☐ Use nonperforating devices to secure tubing and equipment to the sterile field.
Move within or around the sterile field in a manner that maintains sterility of the field.	**Scrubbed Person**
	☐ Remain close to the sterile field.
	☐ Move from sterile areas to sterile areas.
	☐ When changing positions with another scrubbed person, turn back to back or front to front while maintaining a safe distance.
	☐ Keep arms and hands within the sterile field at all times.
	☐ Avoid changing levels, and sit only when the entire procedure Sis done at the sitting level.
	Unscrubbed Person
	☐ Face sterile fields on approach.
	☐ Do not walk between two sterile fields.
	☐ Keep a safe distance from the sterile field.
	☐ Do not reach over a sterile field when delivering supplies.

Adopted from AORN (2008). Maintaining a Sterile Field, *Perioperative standards and recommended practices.* Denver, CO: AORN.

IDENTIFYING PATIENTS AT RISK FOR ADVERSE OUTCOMES RELATED TO ESTABLISHING AND MAINTAINING A STERILE FIELD

The nurse establishes and maintains the sterile field without compromising or causing injury to the patient. If done incorrectly, this patient care event has potential for causing adverse patient outcomes, particularly for high-risk patients. **Table 9.6** lists potential nursing diagnoses and associated patient risk factors and identifies indicators that validate achievement of the desired outcomes.

Table 9.6	Establishing and Maintaining a Sterile Field During the Operative or Invasive Procedure Does Not Compromise or Cause Injury to the Patient

Outcome 1   The patient is free from evidence of wound infection.

Diagnosis	Risk Factors	Outcome Indicators
Risk for Wound Infection	☐ Impaired skin and tissue integrity ☐ Altered tissue perfusion ☐ Decreased hemoglobin concentration ☐ Leukopenia ☐ Suppressed inflammatory response ☐ Immunosuppression ☐ Inadequate acquired immunity ☐ Existing infection ☐ Increased environmental exposure as a result of the length of operative or invasive procedure ☐ Break in aseptic technique; improper wearing of operative attire, resulting in shedding of or spraying of microorganisms from the operative or invasive procedure team into the sterile field	☐ Does the patient show evidence of wound infection 72 hours after the procedure? ☐ Does the patient have cellulitis at the wound site? ☐ Does the wound have signs that indicate abscess formation? ☐ Does the patient have lymphangitis? ☐ Are there signs of gas gangrene formation? ☐ Does the patient have signs that indicate the presence of a Meleney's ulcer? ☐ Did the patient have a wound dehiscence episode after the procedure?

Outcome 2   The patient is free from evidence of impaired skin integrity.

Diagnosis	Risk Factors	Outcome Indicators
Risk for Impaired Skin Integrity	☐ Impaired tissue perfusion at the operative or invasive site ☐ Allergy or sensitivity to the prepping solution ☐ Allergy or sensitivity to an adhesive agent in the draping materials ☐ Obesity ☐ Gross underweight ☐ Poor skin turgor ☐ Pooling of prepping solutions ☐ Improper application of towel clips	☐ Was the patient's skin punctured by towel clips? ☐ Did adhesive drapes cause an allergic reaction or injure the patient's skin? ☐ Did the patient experience skin breakdown because of pooled prepping solution?

Outcome 3   The patient is free from evidence of hypothermia.

Diagnosis	Risk Factors	Outcome Indicators
Risk for Hypothermia immediately before and during the procedure	☐ Existing hypothermia ☐ Impaired skin integrity ☐ Low body weight (malnutrition) ☐ Age: very young or very old ☐ Inability to shiver ☐ Decreased metabolic rate ☐ Low temperature in the procedure room ☐ Limited application of covers	☐ Was the patient's temperature within normal limits during draping and during the procedure? ☐ Did the patient shiver while being draped and during the procedure? ☐ Did the patient's skin feel cold? ☐ Did the patient's behaviors indicate mental confusion? ☐ Did the patient experience decreases in the pulse and respirations?

☐ Cold solutions such as intravenous fluids, skin preparation solutions, and wound irrigation solutions

☐ Medication causing vasoconstriction

Outcome 4   The patient is free from evidence of ineffective breathing patterns.

Diagnosis	Risk Factors	Outcome Indicators
Risk for Ineffective Breathing Patterns	☐ Type of anesthesia (local, regional, spinal, or general) ☐ Neuromuscular impairment ☐ Musculoskeletal impairment ☐ Anxiety related to procedure ☐ Pain during the procedure secondary to the incision or positioning ☐ Perceptual or cognitive impairment ☐ Claustrophobia ☐ Drapes covering a nonventilated patient's face ☐ Nonfunctioning oxygen delivery devices (masks, nasal prongs)	☐ Does the patient have shortness of breath or dyspnea? ☐ Does the patient use accessory muscles to breathe? ☐ Is there evidence of altered chest excursion? ☐ Is tachypnea present? ☐ Does the patient have nasal flaring? ☐ Does the patient have pursed-lip breathing or a prolonged expiration phase? ☐ Does the patient say he or she is experiencing difficult breathing?

Outcome 5   The patient is free from evidence of disturbed self-esteem.

Diagnosis	Risk Factors	Outcome Indicators
Risk for Self-Esteem Disturbance	☐ Cultural or religious beliefs (ie, prohibitions against nudity in presence of opposite sex ☐ Location of the operative site, such as genitalia or breasts for female patients ☐ Consciousness during the procedure ☐ Derogatory comments or joking by the staff concerning the patient's appearance, weight, or physical condition ☐ Mixed gender of the staff ☐ Unnecessary traffic flow in the operative and invasive procedure suite.	☐ Does the patient make statements that indicate that he or she is experiencing anxiety or shame during the preparation or draping? ☐ Is the patient restless? ☐ Is the patient perspiring? ☐ Does the patient have a tense look, clenched hands, or shakiness in the extremities?

Adapted from Carpentino-Moyet, L. J. (2008) *Handbook of Nursing Diagnosis* (12th ed.) Philadelphia: Lippincott Williams & Wilkins; Petersen C. (2007). *Perioperative Nursing Data Set, the Perioperative Nursing Vocabulary.* (Revised 2nd ed.). Denver: AORN, Inc.

DONNING AND WEARING APPROPRIATE OPERATIVE ATTIRE

Considerations

All personnel entering the semi-restricted and restricted patient areas of the operative suite must wear proper operative attire. While in semi-restricted areas, personnel should wear operative attire and head gear that covers all head and facial hair. In the restricted areas, in addition to operative attire, personnel should wear masks if open sterile instruments, supplies, equipment, or scrubbed personnel are present (AORN, 2008c).

Skin, hair, and mucous membranes constantly shed microorganisms, thus increasing the patient's risk for wound infection. By wearing barriers such as head covers, masks, operative attire, and gowns, team members decrease microorganism shedding and spraying into the air and thus reduce the patient's risk for wound contamination. When not scrubbed, wear a fastened long-sleeved jacket. Complete closure of the jacket avoids accidental contamination of the sterile field. Long-sleeved attire is advocated to prevent bacterial shedding from bare forearms and is included in the Occupational Safety and Health Administration (OSHA) regulation for the use of personal protective equipment (PPE) (OSHA, 2008). Other garments should be contained completely within or covered by the operative attire. Do not wear clothing that cannot be covered by the operative attire.

The nurse ensures that personnel comply with operative attire policies and procedures. Likewise, operative or invasive procedure patients should also wear attire that reduces particulate shedding during procedures. Appropriate patient attire includes a clean gown, clean linen coverings, and clean hair covering. The patient, however, does not wear a mask in the presence of opened sterile instruments, supplies, equipment, and scrubbed personnel. The mask can limit access to the patient's face and airway. Furthermore, for some patients the presence of a mask may increase anxiety or contribute to feelings of fear. Minimize the possibility of contamination by keeping the patient's head away from the sterile field until the patient is draped and/or intubated.

Good hygiene, including daily bathing and frequent hair washing, by patient care team members helps control microorganism shedding into the patient's immediate operative or invasive procedure environment. Team members with an infectious disease, such as an upper respiratory tract illness, or with skin lesions, boils, and infected lesions should not participate in direct patient care activities or work in the restricted area of the operative or invasive procedure suite.

"Perioperative Standards and Recommended Practice (2008) Surgical Attire" describes the type of attire that should be worn within the semi-restricted and restricted areas of the operative or invasive procedure environment. **Table 9.7** highlights these guidelines.

OSHA
Occupational Safety and Health Administration

PPE
Personal Protective Equipment

Table 9.7	Principles and Guidelines for Wearing Operative Attire
Principles	**Guidelines**
Wear facility approved operative attire when entering the semi-restricted and restricted areas of the operative and invasive procedure suite.	☐ Wear approved, clean, and freshly laundered operative attire.
	☐ Don operative attire in a designated dressing area of the facility upon entry to the facility.
	☐ Change daily or whenever operative attire becomes visibly soiled, contaminated, or wet.
	☐ Worn operative attire is not to be hung or placed in a locker for wearing at another time.
	☐ Remove visibly soiled, contaminated, or wet operative attire as soon as possible and replace with fresh, clean ones.

☐ Operative attire contaminated with visible blood or body fluid must remain at the facility and be laundered by hospital or commercial laundry.

☐ Home laundering of operative attire is not recommended.

☐ Wear operative attire consisting of a two-piece pantsuit. Secure the top of pantsuit at the waist by tucking into the pants or securing it to fit closely to the body.

☐ When not scrubbed, wear a long-sleeved button or snap-closed jacket.

Cover head and facial hair, including sideburns and neckline, when in the semi-restricted and restricted areas of the operative and invasive procedure suite.

☐ Before donning operative attire, cover all hair with a facility-approved bouffant hat or hood that covers the side hair above the ears and hair at the nape of the neck.

☐ Discard used hair covers in an appropriate container.

Wear a mask in the restricted area of the operative and invasive procedure suite when open sterile items, equipment, or scrubbed personnel are present.

☐ When wearing a mask, cover both the mouth and nose and secure it in a manner that prevents venting.

☐ Remove mask carefully by handling only the ties and discard immediately.

☐ Do not let a mask hang from the neck.

☐ Do not tuck a mask into a pocket for future use.

☐ Use of double masks does not increase filtration: therefore, it is unacceptable.

Wear protective eyewear, masks or face shields when splashing or spraying is likely.

☐ Apply protective eyewear (eg, goggles, glasses with solid side shields, chin-length face shields whenever eye, nose, or mouth contamination reasonably can be anticipated as a result of splashes, spray or splatter of blood droplets or other infectious materials.

Confine or remove all jewelry and watches when entering the semi-restricted and restricted areas of the operative and invasive procedure suite.

☐ Remove rings and bracelets.

☐ Confine or remove watches.

☐ Confine or remove earrings.

Keep fingernails short, clean, and healthy.

☐ Keep fingernails short and in good condition.

☐ If nail polish is worn, ensure that it is fresh and intact.

☐ Do not wear artificial nails.

Wear protective barriers to reduce the risk of exposure to potentially infective materials.

☐ Wear sterile gloves when performing sterile procedures.

☐ Wear nonsterile gloves when performing procedures that may result in exposure of blood, body fluids, and/or sources of contamination.

☐ Change gloves between each patient contact.

☐ Wear protective eyewear, masks, or face shields during any activity that has potential for splashing or spraying.

☐ Wear additional protective attire such as liquid-resistance aprons, gowns, and shoe covers when anticipating exposure to blood, body fluids, and/or sources of contamination.

☐ Wear shoes that provide protection from sharps and fluids.

☐ Change shoe covers whenever they become torn, wet, or soiled and remove before leaving the operative area.

Adapted from AORN (2008). Surgical Attire, *Perioperative standards and recommended practices*, Denver, CO: AORN.

Laundering of Operative Attire

Always wear operative attire within the semi-restricted and restricted areas of the operative suite. Policies for laundering, wearing, covering, and changing operative attire vary greatly. Some policies restrict the laundering of operative attire to the facility, while other facilities have policies that allow laundering by employees. Well-controlled studies, however, that evaluate operative attire laundering as a Surgical Site Infection (SSI) factor do not exist (Killen, 2006); therefore, avoid home laundering operative attire that was worn while providing patient care during an operative or invasive procedure (AORN, 2008c). Without clear evidence about the safety for patients, health care workers, and their family members, it is prudent to restrict laundering of operative attire to a facility that can guarantee the implementation of consistent and appropriate laundering parameters. If a facility requires home laundering of operative attire, follow the guidelines listed in **Table 9.8**.

SSI
Surgical Site Infection

Operative attire contaminated with visible blood or body fluids must remain at the facility. The hospital or a hospital-contracted commercial laundry must launder this attire. Controlled laundering of attire contaminated by blood or body fluids reduces the risk of transferring pathogenic microorganisms from the facility to the home or the public (AAMI, 2003a; OSHA, 2008; CDC, 2003).

Supplies and Equipment

When dressing for the restricted or semi-restricted areas, wear a scrub top and pants that are easy to don and remove. Wear a closed long-sleeved warmup jacket if unscrubbed, to minimize shedding from bare forearms. A disposable bouffant hat or hood; shoe covers (optional); protective eyewear; and disposable mask complete the attire (**Fig. 9.1**). Wear attire made of fabrics that meet or exceed the requirements

Table 9.8	Criteria for Home Laundering Soiled Operative Attire

- ☐ Use an automatic washer and hot air dryer
- ☐ Use water temperature of 110° F to 125° F (43.33° C to 51.67° C) to facilitate microbial kill
- ☐ Use chlorine bleach (ie, sodium hypochlorite)
- ☐ Use detergent according to manufacturer's instructions
- ☐ Launder operative attire in a separate load with no other items
- ☐ Launder operative attire as the last load after all other items have been laundered
- ☐ Wash hands immediately after placing laundry in the washing machine
- ☐ Keep laundry items completely submerged during the entire wash and rinse cycle to facilitate removal of soil and microorganisms
- ☐ Avoid placing hands or forearms in the laundry or rinse water to keep items submerged
- ☐ Thoroughly clean the door and lid of the washing machine before removing the laundered attire to prevent reintroduction of contaminants on clean attire when removing it from the washing machine and before placing it in the dryer
- ☐ Use the highest drying setting possible that is safe for the material of attire construction
- ☐ Promptly remove attire when dry to avoid desiccation of materials

Adapted from AORN (2008). Surgical Attire, *Perioperative standards and recommended practices*, Denver, CO: AORN.

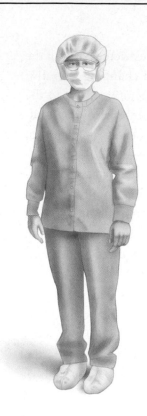

Figure 9.1
Operative attire.

NFPA
National Fire Protection
Agency

of the National Fire Protection Agency (NFPA) regulations. Disposable hats and hoods should be comfortable, lint free, and made of a soft fabric. Reduce risk from exposure to blood, body fluids, and other potentially infectious materials by wearing protective eyewear during operative and invasive procedures. Select a mask based on the documented quality of microorganism filtration and comfort. An acceptable mask has at least a 95% efficiency rating. Mask designs include the pleated mask with pliable nosepiece, the cone-shaped mask with an elastic band, the anti-fog mask for wear with glasses, the laser mask that helps protect against electrosurgery and laser plume contaminants, and the fluid shield mask with a splashguard visor to protect the wearer against body fluid splashes and aerosolization. Double masking creates an impediment to breathing and does not increase filtration; therefore making this practice unacceptable (Friberg, 2001). After the procedure, place reusable operative attire in a post-use container. Laundering operative attire after each use in a laundry facility approved and monitored by the practice setting will prevent potential spread of pathogens to the home environment.

Procedure

Obtain a clean scrub top, clean pants, and a disposable hat or hood. Select a top and pants for proper fit and comfort. Avoid tight-fitting operative attire; such garments rub against the body surfaces and may increase the dispersal of body scurf. Remove street clothes and remove or confine jewelry. Street clothes and jewelry may harbor microorganisms, thus increasing the patient's risk for a hospital-acquired infection.

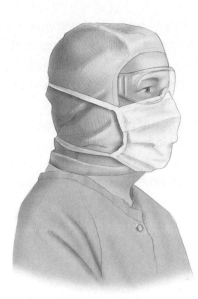

Figure 9.2

Hood for covering facial hair or long sideburns.

Prevent the possible dispersal of microorganisms and scalp hair onto the operative attire by covering hair with a bouffant hat or hood before donning the shirt. Adjust the hat or hood to cover all scalp hair. Personnel with beards or long sideburns should obtain a beard cover to contain all facial hair (**Fig. 9.2**). After donning the pants, tuck the top into the pants to prevent the possible dispersal of body scurf from beneath the shirt. Also, tuck pants' ties to prevent inadvertent contamination of the sterile field by loose, swinging ties. Pants should not touch the floor during dressing. To prevent cross-infection, change operative attire when it becomes soiled or wet.

Change to comfortable, supportive, protective footwear to protect the feet against falling items such as sharps and heavy instruments. Footwear should also allow quick and safe movement in an emergency. When contamination of footwear with blood and body fluids is a risk, wear disposable shoe covers to protect footwear from gross contamination. Avoid tracking blood and debris throughout the operative or invasive procedure suite by removing shoe covers that become moist or contaminated with body fluids or tissue before leaving the room.

Apply a mask on entering the restricted area where opened sterile instruments, supplies, and equipment are present and in the presence of scrubbed personnel, including personnel in the process of scrubbing. Form the pliable nosepiece of the mask over the bridge of the nose; tie the mask at the back of the head and behind the neck, allowing the mask to fit securely and preventing venting at the sides. A properly applied mask minimizes the transmission of nasopharyngeal and respiratory bacteria from the patient care team to the patient. Discard the mask after the procedure and if it becomes soiled or wet. When removing the mask, do so by handling only the mask strings. Avoid touching the filter portion of the mask, and dispose of it in an appropriate receptacle. Masks are either on or off; do not wear a mask around the neck, on top of the head, or in a pocket.

Before scrubbing, apply protective eyewear or a mask with a protective splashguard visor to protect against uncontrolled body fluid splashes (OSHA, 2008). During laser procedures, wear laser masks[2] and protective eyewear specified for the type of laser in operation. Clean eyewear with an antimicrobial agent between procedures.

If personnel don laboratory coats or cover gowns when leaving the operative or invasive procedure suite, they should wear freshly laundered coats or gowns that have long sleeves, can be completely closed, and hang below the knees. Research supporting the wearing of cover attire is limited; therefore, the decision to wear cover attire or uncovered scrub attire depends on the culture in each operative or invasive procedure suite, and determined by institution policies and procedures, the manager's priorities, and applicable state regulations. Wearing scrub attire is an element of environmental control that promotes high-level cleanliness and hygiene within the semi-restricted and restricted areas of the operative or invasive procedure suite.

PREPARING SUPPLIES, INSTRUMENTS, AND EQUIPMENT FOR THE STERILE FIELD

Considerations

Maintaining a sterile field demands comprehensive attention to detail before and during the procedure. When preparing for the procedure, verify the sterility of the equipment, instruments, and supplies intended for use in the sterile field. Create the sterile field, including skin preparation and draping of the patient, to prevent contamination. Once created, maintain the sterile field throughout the procedure. Before handling sterile supplies or having contact with the wound, the operating team dons gowns and gloves. Finally, keep the procedure room clean using three main methods: (1) concurrent cleaning (prompt cleanup of items contaminated with blood, tissue, or body fluids); (2) end-of-case cleaning (immediately following the procedure); and (3) terminal cleaning (end of day when scheduled procedures are completed and should occur each 24-hour period during regular workweek) (Mangram, 1999).

Supplies, Instruments, and Equipment

All supplies, instruments and equipment used during an operative or invasive procedure.

Procedure

Principles of Aseptic Techniques

EO
Ethylene Oxide

Wrap and sterilize needed items prior to the procedure. Sterilizing agents used to kill microorganisms include steam under pressure, low-temperature hydrogen peroxide gas plasma, peracetic acid, ozone, ethylene oxide (EO), dry heat, and radiation. Use only items packaged, labeled with the sterilization date, and stored in a manner to ensure sterility. The shelf life of sterile packages is event-, not time-related. Shelf life depends in part on the type of packaging used, frequency of handling of the item, and events such as moisture exposure that may compromise the sterility of the package contents. Prior to opening a sterile package, verify package integrity by looking for holes, tears, punctures, or moisture. For items sterilized in a container system, inspect for intact filters and sealed valves or gaskets. Verify compliance with the manufacturers' Instructions for Use (IFU). Check for expiration dates and for any sterilizing chemical process indicators. Allow racks of sterile items freshly removed from the sterilizer to cool thoroughly to prevent steam condensation and contamination. Consider any package with a dry stain contaminated and take appropriate action.

IFU
Instructions for Use

Flash Sterilization

Keep flash sterilization of unwrapped instruments and porous items to a minimum. Use this type of sterilization only when time does not permit sterilization by the preferred wrapping method. Avoid flash sterilization for reasons either of time, convenience, or as an alternative to purchasing additional instrument sets time (Mangram, 1999). Flash sterilization may be associated with increased risk of infection to patients because of the pressure on personnel to eliminate one or more of the steps in the cleaning and sterilization process. Speed reduces the margin of safety, in terms of both operator error and the reliability of the sterilizer. If flashing of instruments is necessary, strictly follow the guidelines delineated in the AORN *Recommended Practices for Sterilization in Perioperative Practice Setting* (AORN, 2008b).

Do not flash sterilize implantable devices except in cases of emergency when no other option is available. When flash sterilization of an implant is unavoidable, run the load with a rapid-action biological indicator (BI) with a Class 5 chemical integrating indicator (or enzyme only indicator) (AAMI, 2006). Using a closed container system for flash sterilization and transport of items eliminates the need for the scrubbed person to leave the sterile field to retrieve instruments from a sterilizer. Refer to Chapter 14, Sterilization and AORN Recommended Practices for Sterilization in the Perioperative Practice Setting guidelines (AORN, 2008b).

BI
Biological Indicator

When working with sterile and nonsterile items and areas in the operative or invasive procedure room the patient care team maintains a safety margin. Nonsterile team members should not lean or reach over the sterile field and should never walk between two sterile fields. Prepare sterile fields as close as possible to the time of the procedure. Once established, continually monitor the sterile field for possible contamination. Continual sterility of an open sterile field is event related; contamination does not depend on a specified time, such as two hours. However, long exposure of a sterile item to the environment increases the chance for contamination. Consequently, consider an unattended sterile field contaminated; sterility cannot be verified if the field is not under constant supervision. Do not cover the sterile field; it is difficult to remove the drape without bringing the portion of the drape that hung below the horizontal surface of the table over the sterile field. Additionally, the nurse cannot verify the sterility of an unobserved covered sterile field.

Present sterile items to the scrubbed person. If this is not possible, place the item securely on the sterile field (AORN, 2008a). For linen or nonwoven wrappers the area considered sterile is the inside area, immediately surrounding the sterile item (**Fig. 9.3**). Open a sterile package from the far side first and the near side last

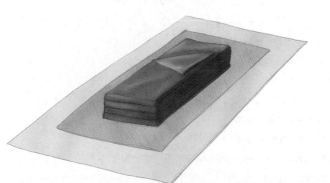

Figure 9.3

For linen or nonwoven wrappers the area considered sterile is the inside area.

(**Fig. 9.4**). Secure any loose flaps; this prevents spring back and possible contamination of the sterile contents. Pull back the outside wrapper of small peel pouches and then flip the contents onto the sterile field (**Fig. 9.5**). When presenting larger peel pouches, the scrubbed person pulls the contents straight up and out of the wrapper (**Fig. 9.6**). If the contents touch the edge of the package or the package tears during opening, consider the contents contaminated and discard.

Open larger packs on a separate table by opening first the back, then the front flaps, and then the side flaps. Take care to walk around the pack, rather than reach over the sterile field (**Fig. 9.7**). When a sterile wrapper also serves as a table cover,

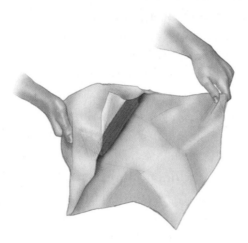

Figure 9.4

Open a sterile package from the far side first.

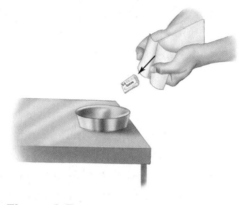

Figure 9.5

Pull back the outside wrapper of small peel pouches and then flip the contents onto the sterile field.

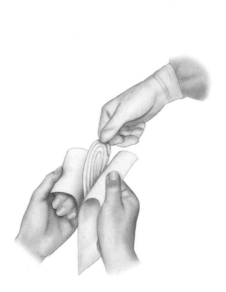

Figure 9.6

Pull the contents straight up and out of the wrapper.

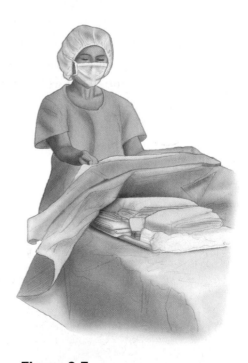

Figure 9.7

For larger packs open the sides last.

consider only the interior and surface levels as sterile. Carefully pour solutions; this will reduce the amount of splashing. When pouring, the solution should not run down the sides of the container. The scrub person should hold the container or place it close to the edge of the sterile table. After removing the cap from the container pour the entire contents and discard any remaining solution.

Discard[3] any item dropped below the waist; the item is contaminated. Avoid changing table heights, as in sitting, unless performing the entire procedure while seated. Consider the edges and sides of table drapes as nonsterile; they are out of sight and cannot be monitored. Scrubbed persons should not allow their hands to fall below their waist or the sterile field. Consider any item that falls over the edge of the table as contaminated. Secure items that remain on the drapes during the procedure to prevent the item from sliding below the level of the sterile field, such as cords[4] and tubing. Discard any item if sterility is in doubt. Even though a sterile package may appear undamaged, for the safety of the patient, consider the item contaminated.

SCRUBBING THE HANDS AND FOREARMS

The foremost potential source of Surgical Site Infections (SSI) is the microbial contamination of health care workers' hands. A critical step in preventing infections is good hand hygiene by all members of the patient care team. Good hand hygiene is the single most effective and important step to prevent the transmission of microorganisms and healthcare-associated infections (Pittet, 2001).

SSI
Surgical Site
Infection

Hand Hygiene

The term *general hand hygiene* refers to decontamination of the hands by one of two methods: hand washing with either an antimicrobial or plain soap and water; or use of an antiseptic hand rub (CDC, 2002). The *CDC/HICPAC Recommendations for Hand Hygiene in Health Care Settings* listed in **Table 9.9** highlights these recommendations.

All operative personnel should practice general hand hygiene. Members of the operative team who have direct patient contact should wash their hands between patients, and after handling equipment, assisting anesthesia providers, or whenever they are soiled. For hands not contaminated with blood or body fluids, use an alcohol-based hand rub. Alcohol-based rubs have added emollients and skin softeners and users that routinely disinfect their hands with these rubs have fewer complaints of dry and cracking skin. The CDC hand hygiene guideline clearly states that alcohol-based hand rubs are preferred over washing with antimicrobial soap and water for routine hand hygiene when clinician's hands are not visibly soiled or contaminated with blood or body fluid (proteinaceous material) (CDC, 2002). Studies indicate that accessibility of hand-hygiene facilities affect the frequency of handwashing or alcohol-based hand rubs by personnel (Bischoff, 2000). Therefore, alcohol-based hand rub dispensers should be readily available in the operative and invasive areas.

Gloves do not serve as a substitute for effective hand hygiene. Always wear gloves when possible contact with blood or other potentially infectious materials, mucous membranes, and non-intact skin could occur. Remove gloves after caring for a patient. Do not wash gloves between patients; rather remove the gloves, perform

Table 9.9	Recommendations For Hand Hygiene In Health Care Settings

The Center for Disease Control/Healthcare Infection Control Practices Advisory Committee (CDC/HICPAC) guidelines, each recommendation is categorized on the basis of existing scientific data, theoretical rationale, applicability, and economic impact.

CDC/HICPAC SYSTEM FOR CATEGORIZING RECOMMENDATIONS IS AS FOLLOWS:

Category IA	Strongly recommended for implementation and strongly supported by well-designed experimental, clinical, or epidemiologic studies.
Category IB	Strongly recommended for implementation and supported by certain experimental, clinical, or epidemiologic studies and a strong theoretical rationale.
Category IC	Required for implementation, as mandated by federal or state regulation or standard.
Category II	Suggested for implementation and supported by suggestive clinical or epidemiologic studies or a theoretical rationale.
No Recommendation (NR)	Unresolved issue. Practices for which insufficient evidence or no consensus regarding efficacy exist.

Indications for Handwashing and Hand Antisepsis	Category
When hands are visibly dirty or contaminated with proteinaceous material or are visibly soiled with blood or other body fluids, wash hands with either a non-antimicrobial soap and water or an antimicrobial soap and water.	IA
If hands are not visibly soiled, use an alcohol-based hand rub for routinely decontaminating hands in all other clinical situations described in items 1C–J. Alternatively, wash hands with an antimicrobial soap and water in all clinical situations described in items 1C–J.	IA IB
Decontaminate hands before having direct contact with patients.	IB
Decontaminate hands before donning sterile gloves when inserting a central intravascular catheter.	IB
Decontaminate hands before inserting indwelling urinary catheters, peripheral vascular catheters, or other invasive devices that do not require a surgical procedure.	IB
Decontaminate hands after contact with a patient's intact skin (eg, when taking a pulse or blood pressure, and lifting a patient).	IB
Decontaminate hands after contact with body fluids or excretions, mucous membranes, nonintact skin, and wound dressings if hands are not visibly soiled.	IA
Decontaminate hands if moving from a contaminated-body site to a clean-body site during patient care.	II
Decontaminate hands after contact with inanimate objects (including medical equipment) in the immediate vicinity of the patient.	II
Decontaminate hands after removing gloves.	IB
Before eating and after using a restroom, wash hands with a non-antimicrobial soap and water or with an antimicrobial soap and water.	IB
Antimicrobial-impregnated wipes (ie, towelettes) may be considered as an alternative to washing hands with non-antimicrobial soap and water. Because they are not as effective as alcohol-based hand rubs or washing hands with an antimicrobial soap and water for reducing bacterial counts on the hands of HCWs, they are not a substitute for using an alcohol-based hand rub or antimicrobial soap.	IB
Wash hands with non-antimicrobial soap and water or with antimicrobial soap and water if exposure to Bacillus anthracis is suspected or proven. The physical action of washing and rinsing hands under such circumstances is recommended because alcohols, chlorhexidine, iodophors, and other antiseptic agents have poor activity against spores.	II
No recommendation can be made regarding the routine use of nonalcohol-based hand rubs for hand hygiene in healthcare settings. Unresolved Issue.	NR

CDC/HICPAC (2001). Centers for Disease Control and Prevention & Health Infection Control Practices Advisory Committee.

hand hygiene, and don a fresh pair. Change gloves during patient care if moving from a contaminated body site to a clean body site. After removing gloves wash/ clean hands before undertaking any further activities.

A majority of microorganisms harbor in the subungual area of the hands. Keep fingernails short, not extending beyond the fingertips clean and healthy (Moolenar et al, 2000), Remove debris from under fingernails using a disposable nail cleaner under running water. Do not wear artificial or sculptured nails in the operative or invasive procedure suite; nails may harbor microorganisms. Studies demonstrate that fungal growth occurs frequently under artificial nails because of trapped moisture between the natural and artificial nail (Mangram, 1999; Moolenaar et al, 2000). Research data show no increase in microbial growth when nail polish is fresh. Chipped nail polish or polish worn longer than four days, however, has a tendency to harbor bacteria, and may present a surgical site infection risk to the patient (Baumgardner et al, 1993).

Remove jewelry, such as rings, bracelets, and watches before performing hand hygiene. Removal of all jewelry from the hands and forearms permits full skin contact with an antimicrobial agent. Contain pierced earrings within the head cover. Do not wear hanging earrings, they are inappropriate and may break and fall into a wound or contaminate the sterile field.

Skin breakdown becomes a significant deterrent for hand hygiene compliance. Check the hands, cuticles, and forearms for impaired skin integrity. Open lesions and breaks in skin integrity increase the risk of patient and surgical team member infection. Because of the potential danger of wound contamination, do not serve as a member of the sterile team when cuts or abrasions on the hands or forearms are present.

Preprocedure Surgical Hand Antisepsis/Hand Scrub

The term *surgical hand antisepsis* refers to the surgical alcohol-based hand rub or the traditional water-based scrub performed before donning sterile attire and gloves (AORN, 2008d). Both of these methods remove debris and transient microorganisms from the nails, hands, and forearms; reduce the resident microbial count to a minimum; and inhibit rapid rebound growth of microorganisms (AORN, 2008d).

Transient and resident microorganisms inhabit the skin. Washing the hands and forearms thoroughly with soap and water easily removes the loosely attached transient microorganisms on the skin surface. Resident microorganisms, however, survive and multiply in superficial skin layers and hair follicles and can cause surgical site infection when allowed to enter deep tissues during the procedure. To reduce the potential risk of surgical site infections, surgical team members complete a regimen of hand scrubbing to remove gross contaminants, dirt, skin oil, and microbes from the skin; to eliminate transient bacteria on the skin while reducing the resident colony count; and to leave an antimicrobial residue on the skin to inhibit the regrowth of microorganisms.

Surgical hand antisepsis practice should follow a written standardized hand scrubbing procedure approved by the healthcare facility. The procedure should also follow the manufacturers' written IFU. Both the alcohol-based surgical hand rub products should meet FDA requirements as outlined in the Tentative Final Monograph (TFM) for Health-Care Antiseptic Drug Products (US Government, 1994) and the traditional water-based surgical hand scrub using FDA-compliant traditional antimicrobial scrub agents.

TFM
Tentative Final
Monograph

Surgical Hand Rub (Preprocedure Hand/Forearm Antisepsis)

Perform the hand rub immediately before donning sterile gowns and gloves. Brushless/waterless alcohol rubs and cleansers do not use mechanical action or friction, or a water rinse to remove microorganisms; the main action is chemical. Before the hand rub, however, remove gross soil by washing the hands and forearms with soap and running water. For the subungual areas, use a disposable nail cleaner under running water. Following this wash, dry the hands and forearms. Products that have superior antimicrobial action and promote skin hygiene can reduce the amount of time needed to scrub, reducing skin trauma, and resulting in less water consumption. A 60% to 95% alcohol preparation provides the most rapid and effective reduction of microorganisms on the skin but has no persistent activity or cumulative effect. The addition of other agents, such as 0.5% to 1% chlorhexidine gluconate, creates a surgical hand antiseptic product with persistent and cumulative properties that prevents microbial regrowth. Alcohol-based hand rubs have been shown to have greater antimicrobial efficacy against both transient and resident hand flora, compared with plain or antimicrobial soaps (Kampf & Kramer, 2004; Rotter, 2001). The CDC, as well as European guidelines, recommends these products for hand hygiene and surgical hand disinfection (Boyce & Pittet, 2002; Labadie et al, 2002).

Traditional Surgical Scrub (Preprocedure Hand/Forearm Antisepsis)

Members of the surgical team who have direct contact with the sterile operating field wash their hands and forearms by performing a traditional procedure known as scrubbing (or the surgical scrub) immediately before donning sterile gowns and gloves. When performing the traditional scrubbing of hands and forearms always use mechanical action and an antimicrobial agent, which inhibits microbial growth and/or kills resident microorganisms during procedures. Use either the anatomical timed[5] scrub or the counted brush[6] stroke method to scrub the hands and forearms. When performed correctly, both methods ensure sufficient exposure of all skin surfaces to friction and an antimicrobial agent. The anatomical timed scrub specifies a prescribed amount of time for each anatomical area. The counted brush stroke denotes a set number of brush strokes to each surface of the fingers, hands, and forearms.

Considerations

The AORN *"Recommended Practices for Surgical Hand Antisepsis/Hand Scrub"* (**Table 9.10**) highlights guidelines for surgical hand antisepsis. Additionally, policies and procedures for surgical hand antisepsis should be developed, reviewed periodically, and readily available in the practice setting.

Supplies and Equipment

FDA
Food and Drug Administration

Limit choice of surgical hand antiseptic/scrub agents to an FDA-compliant, surgical hand antiseptic agent (ie, surgical hand scrub/rub) approved by the facility's infection control.

The surgical hand antiseptic agent should

- significantly reduce microorganisms on intact skin;
- contain a nonirritating, antimicrobial preparation;

Table 9.10	Guidelines for Preoperative Surgical Antisepsis Hand/Forearm Scrub

Alcohol-Based Surgical Hand Rub	**Traditional Water-Based Surgical Hand Scrub**
A standardized protocol for alcohol-based surgical hand rubs should follow manufacturers' written instructions and include, but may not be limited to, the following.	A standardized protocol for traditional, standardized, surgical hand antisepsis scrub should follow manufacturers' written instructions and include, but may not be limited to, the following.
☐ Wash hands and forearms with soap and running water immediately before beginning the surgical hand antisepsis procedure.	☐ Wash hands and forearms with soap and running water immediately before beginning the surgical scrub.
☐ Clean the subungual areas of both hands under running water using a nail cleaner.	☐ Clean the subungual areas of both hands under running water using a disposable nail cleaner.
☐ Rinse hands and forearms under running water.	☐ Rinse hands and forearms under running water.
☐ Dry hands and forearms thoroughly with a paper towel.	☐ Dispense the approved antimicrobial scrub agent according to the manufacturer's written directions.
☐ Dispense the manufacturer-recommended amount of the surgical hand rub product.	☐ Apply the antimicrobial agent to wet hands and forearms. Some manufacturers may recommend using a soft, nonabrasive sponge.
☐ Apply the product to the hands and forearms, following the manufacturer's written directions. Some manufacturers may require the use of water as part of the process.	☐ Visualize each finger, hand, and arm as having four sides. Wash all four sides effectively. Repeat this process for opposite fingers, hand, and arm.
☐ Rub thoroughly until dry.	☐ Repeat this process if directed to do so by the manufacturer's written directions for use.
☐ Repeat the product application process if indicated in the manufacturer's written directions.	☐ Avoid splashing operative attire. For water conservation, turn water off when it is not directly in use, if possible.
☐ In the OR, don a sterile surgical gown and gloves.	☐ Hold hands higher than elbows and away from operative attire.
	☐ Discard sponges, if used, in appropriate containers.
	☐ In the OR, dry hands and arms with a sterile towel before donning a sterile surgical gown and gloves.

Adapted from AORN (2008). Surgical Hand Antisepsis, *Perioperative standards and recommended practices*. Denver, CO: AORN.

- be broad spectrum and fast acting; and
- have a persistent effect (US Government, 1994).

When evaluating product efficacy, determine if the effects of the product are immediate and persistent. US guidelines recommend that agents used for surgical hand scrubs should substantially reduce microorganisms on intact skin, contain a non-irritating preparation, have broad-spectrum activity, and be fast-acting and persistent (HICPAC, 1995). The hand scrub products that are US Food and Drug Administration (FDA) compliant have a documented ability to kill organisms immediately upon application, provide antimicrobial persistence to reduce regrowth of microorganisms, and have a cumulative effect over time (US Government, 1994).

Procedure

Surgical Hand Rub and Traditional Hand Scrub

Scrub the hands and forearms in an area adjacent to the scrub sink with automatic controls. Set the water at a comfortable temperature and moderate flow to prevent spraying of operative attire. High-filtration masks, scrub brushes, disposable nail cleaners, antimicrobial agents, and alcohol-based hand rubs should be within easy reach of the sink. Inspect the operative attire by adjusting the hat or hood to cover and contain all hair. The mask should completely cover both the nose and mouth and fit securely to prevent venting at the sides. Apply protective eyewear or a mask with a protective splashguard visor to protect against uncontrolled body fluid splashes (OSHA, 2008). Tuck all loose operative attire and strings into the scrub pants. Replace or adjust shoe covers (worn in anticipation of high fluids or gross contamination on the floor) to completely protect shoes. Examine the hands and forearms for good skin integrity; remove all jewelry. Nails should be short, non-artificial, and free from chipped and cracked polish and cuticles should be in good condition.

Hand Rub

Turn on the water, and adjust the temperature and spray so that operative attire does not become wet. Immediately prior to the alcohol-based hand rub, wash hands and forearms with soap and running water. Clean the subungual area of both hands under running water using a disposable nail cleaner. Dry hands and forearms completely with a paper towel. Apply alcohol-based hand rub following the manufacturer's recommendations. Dispense one pump (ie, 2 mL) of alcohol product in the palm of one hand. Dip the fingernails of the opposite hand into the solution and work it under the nails (**Fig. 9.8**). Spread the remaining solution over the hand and up the forearm. Dispense another pump of the product into the palm of the other hand and

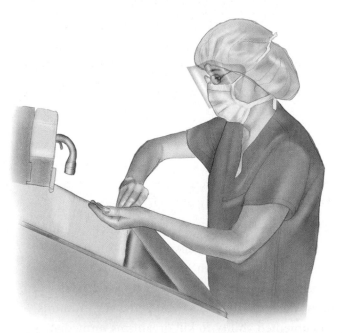

Figure 9.8

Dispense one pump of alcohol product in the palm of one hand.

repeat the same process for the other hand. Dispense a final pump of solution into the palm of either hand and reapply to both hands up to the wrist. Allow to air dry completely before donning gown and gloves.

Traditional Hand Scrub

Turn on the water and adjust the temperature. Regulate the spray so that operative attire does not become wet. Wash and rinse the hands for the initial wash with water and a small amount of soap or antimicrobial agent to remove transient flora and gross contaminants (**Fig. 9.9**). Clean the nails and cuticles under running water with the disposable nail cleaner, paying special attention to the subungual areas of both hands (**Fig. 9.10**). Select either the anatomical timed scrub or the counted brush stroke method. Each takes about 2 minutes to complete. Beginning at the fingertips and, using the sponge side of a disposable scrub brush, scrub with vertical strokes. Proceed to the palm and the back of the hand. Scrub all four sides of each digit, including the web space. Proceed to the wrist; with a circular motion, continue scrubbing up the forearm to 2 inches (5 cm) above the elbow. Scrub each anatomical area, exposing all surfaces to friction and an antimicrobial agent; repeat for the other hand, and discard the scrub brush in an appropriate receptacle. Rinse the hands and forearms thoroughly under running water, keeping the hands elevated to allow the water to drain off the flexed elbows (**Fig. 9.11**). Do not touch the faucet, clothing, or other objects. Avoid splashing water onto operative attire. If the hands or forearms are touched, repeat the scrubbing procedure to correct the contamination. Proceed to the operative or invasive procedure room, with the hands held upward to allow water to drip off the elbows (**Fig. 9.12**).

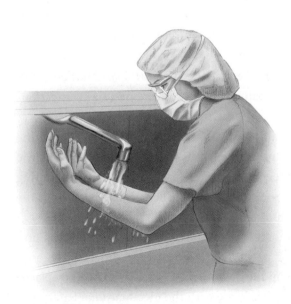

Figure 9.9

Wash and rinse the hands for the initial wash with water and a small amount of soap or antimicrobial agent.

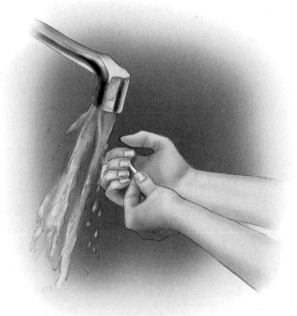

Figure 9.10

Clean the nails and cuticles under running water.

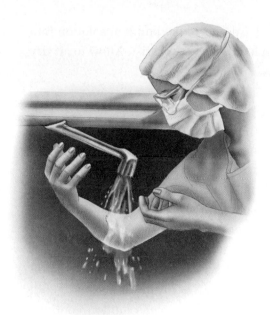

Figure 9.11

Hold hand upward to allow water to drip off the elbows.

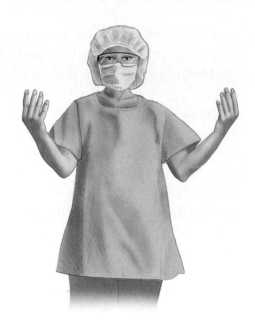

Figure 9.12

Move to the gowning and gloving area with hands held upward.

DONNING STERILE GOWN AND GLOVES

Gowning and gloving are essential components of establishing and maintaining a sterile field. Surgical team members within the sterile field should wear sterile gowns and gloves according to AORN's "*Recommended Practices for Surgical Attire*" (AORN, 2008c) and *Recommended Practices for Standard and transmission-based precautions*" (AORN, 2008e). Team members wear gowns and gloves, referred to as Personal Protective Equipment (PPE), to prevent transfer of microorganisms from the skin and clothing to the sterile field, operative site, and the patient during the operative or invasive procedure. Gowns and gloves also reduce the surgical team member's risk of occupational exposure to bloodborne pathogens and other potentially infectious materials (APIC, 2002).

Don the sterile gown after the alcohol-hand rub has evaporated, or if using the traditional hand scrub method, after drying the hands and forearms with a sterile towel. Once the gown is on, immediately don the sterile gloves. When performing unassisted gowning and gloving don from a separate sterile surface away from the main instrument table to prevent contamination of the sterile field.

Wear surgical gowns made of disposable single-use or reusable materials and of the wrap-around style, *sterile back* gown. The type of gown material chosen depends on the proposed procedure and the degree of blood and body fluid splashing expected during the procedure in accordance with the Occupational Safety and Health Administration (OSHA) guidelines for use of personal protective equipment (Federal Register, 1991; Belkin, 2002). At a minimum, the gown should serve as a barrier to fluids, thus preventing the passage of microorganisms from nonsterile to sterile areas.

PPE
Personal
Protective
Equipment

OSHA
Occupational
Safety and Health
Administration

Table 9.11	Levels for Classifying Protective Apparel
Level 1	Lumps and bumps
Level 2	Simple orthopedic procedures with a tourniquet, or hernias, breast biopsies, etc
Level 3	Procedures with more substantial fluid or blood loss such as mastectomy
Level 4	Trauma, open heart, AAA (Abdominal Aortic Aneurysm), total joint

Koch (2004). Interview—Koch, "New standard aids in selecting barriers." *OR Manager* Vol. 20, No 5 (May 2004), 1–4.

Use the Association of Medical Instrumentation (AAMI; AAMI, 2003b) standard that classifies surgical gowns when evaluating the barrier protective qualities of gowns and selecting the level of protection needed for anticipated blood and body fluids exposure. **Table 9.11** lists four levels for classifying protective apparel based on industry-accepted test methods and provide consistent definitions for measuring barrier performance of gowns. In addition to the barrier protection, surgical gowns should maintain structural integrity, be durable, and resistant to tears, punctures and abrasions. They should be as lint-free as possible, free of toxic ingredients and allergens and resist combustion. Limited memory is a desired characteristic, as is flexibility, which allows the gown to conform loosely to the wearer's body. The gown should also have the ability to maintain an isothermic environment for the surgical team member. Gown size should allow for complete closure in the back and sleeve length adequate to prevent cuff exposure outside the glove.

AAMI
Association of Medical Instrumentation

Use the closed-gloved technique when donning sterile gown and gloves. This technique prevents exposure of bare skin during gowning and donning of sterile gloves, thereby lessening the chance of contamination. Use disposable gloves. Do not rewash or reuse gloves. Wear two pairs of gloves during operative or invasive procedures. Double gloving significantly reduces the number of perforations through the innermost glove, when compared to the outer glove or single gloves. Wearing standard-thickness colored gloves under standard-thickness white gloves helps the wearer's rapid recognition of perforations to the outer glove (Tanner & Parkinson, 2004). Orthopedic gloves have thicker latex, thus providing the same protection as does two pair of standard latex gloves (Turnquist et al, 1996). The CDC and the American Academy of Orthopedic Surgeons (AAOS) support double gloving during operative or invasive procedures (AAOS, 2008; CDC 1999). Only use the open-glove technique when donning gloves for procedures not requiring sterile gowns.

AAOS
American Academy of Orthopedic Surgeons

Supplies and Equipment

Use the following supplies and equipment when gowning and gloving; sterile absorbent towels, sterile gown with appropriate barrier protection, sterile disposable gloves, and a separate sterile area for the gowning and gloving procedure.

Procedure

Unassisted Gowning

The prevention of contamination while donning a sterile gown and gloves requires skill and attention to detail. After completing the alcohol-hand rub, and hands and forearms are completely dry, proceed to the operative or invasive procedure room to don the sterile gown and gloves. After completing the traditional hand scrub, proceed to the operative or invasive procedure room, grasp the sterile folded towel near the corner with one hand, and pull straight up (**Fig. 9.13**). Pay careful attention not to drip water onto the sterile field. Step back from the sterile field, extend the forearms, and lean slightly forward at the waist to prevent the towel from touching operative attire. Unfold the towel; begin drying one hand with half the towel, and move to the wrist and forearm, using a rotating motion, being careful not to retrace any surface. Grasp the untouched end of the towel with the dry hand; repeat the process on the other hand and forearm. Discard the towel in an appropriate receptacle. If the sterile towel touches the operative attire, discard the contaminated towel and begin with another sterile towel.

Grasp the inside of the folded gown at the neckline and step back from the sterile field, allowing the gown to unfold completely, with the inside toward you. Holding the arms at shoulder level, slide both forearms simultaneously into the armholes (**Fig. 9.14**). The circulating nurse assists by reaching inside and pulling the gown up over the shoulders for proper sleeve adjustment. Leave the cuffs extended over the hands for the closed-glove technique (**Fig. 9.15**). Pull the cuffs up to expose the hands for the assisted gloving technique.

The circulating nurse ties the inside ties at the waist (**Fig. 9.16**) and secures the gown at the neckline (**Fig. 9.17**). After the scrub person dons gloves, the circulating

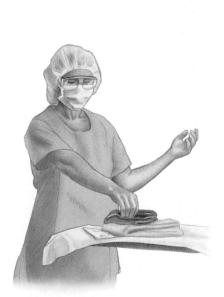

Figure 9.13

Grasp the sterile folded towel near the corner with one hand.

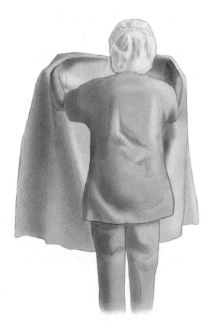

Figure 9.14

Slide both forearms simultaneously into the armholes.

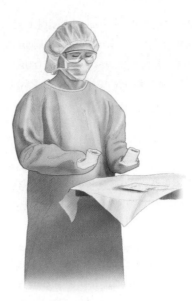

Figure 9.15

Leave the cuffs extended over the hands for the closed-glove technique.

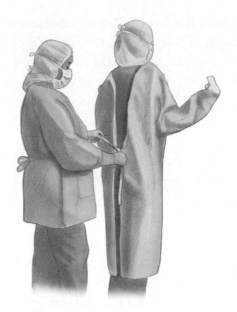

Figure 9.16

Circulating nurse ties the inside ties at the.

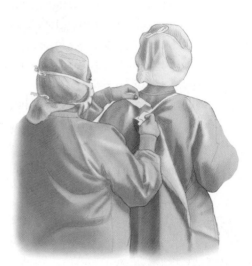

Figure 9.17

Circulating nurse secures the gown at the neckline.

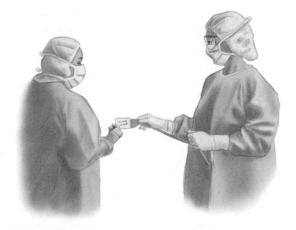

Figure 9.18

The scrub persons hands the circulating nurse the prepackaged card of the gown tie.

nurse secures the final tie on a wraparound gown. When closing the sterile back, do so in three ways:

1. Grasp the belt tie (reusable gown) and hand it to another sterile team member.
2. For a disposable gown, hand the prepackaged card securing the belt tie to the circulating nurse (**Fig. 9.18**).
3. If scrubbed, secure the belt tie with an instrument and hand it off to the circulating nurse.

While the circulating nurse holds the prepackaged card or sterile instrument, pivot to the left, thereby completing the back closure of the gown. Pull the belt tie free and tie it while the circulating nurse retains the cardboard or instrument.

Flex the forearms at the elbows and hold in front with both hands in sight at all times (**Fig. 9.19**). Do not drop gloved hands below table or waist level. Consider gowns sterile in the front from shoulder to table level. Sleeves are sterile from 2 inches (5 cm) above the elbow to the wrist, excluding the stockinet cuff (**Fig. 9.20**). The scrubbed person cannot view the back of a wrap-around, sterile back gown; therefore, consider the back as unsterile.

Closed-Glove Technique

While donning a sterile gown, slide the fingers into the sleeves, paying close attention not push fingers beyond the proximal edges of the stockinet cuffs. After the hands touch the stockinet cuff, consider the cuffs as contaminated; gloves must cover them. With the fingers still inside the sleeves, open the inner glove wrapper on a sterile field. Position the gloves palm side up, with the glove labeled L on the left and the glove labeled R on the right (**Fig. 9.21**). If right-handed, don the left glove first. Turn your left hand palm side up, and flip the left glove onto your left palm. Place the folded glove cuff even with the gown cuff seam; the thumb of the glove is on the thumb side of your hand and the fingers of the glove are on the ulnar side of your wrist, with the glove fingertips pointing toward your elbow (**Fig. 9.22**). Grasp the lower edge of the glove cuff with your left thumb and index finger. Secure the upper edge of the glove cuff with your right thumb and index finger, and stretch the entire glove cuff over the stockinet opening, being careful not to touch the edge of the stockinet cuff (**Fig. 9.23**). Work your fingers into the glove, and then grasp the left glove and gown at the seam with your right hand and pull up over your wrist (**Fig. 9.24**).

Turn your right hand palm side up, and flip the right glove onto your right palm. Place the folded glove cuff even with the gown cuff seam; the thumb of the glove is

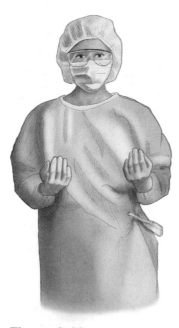

Figure 9.19

Flex the forearms at the elbows and hold in front with both hands in sight.

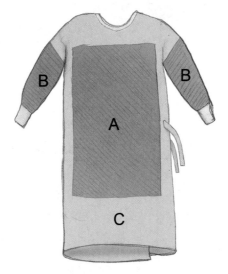

Figure 9.20

"A" and "B" signify the parts of the gown that are sterile.

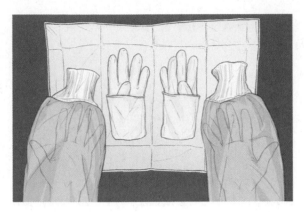

Figure 9.21

Position the gloves palm side up, with the glove labeled L on the left and the glove labeled R on the right.

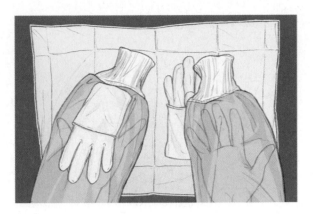

Figure 9.22

Place the folded glove cuff even with the gown cuff seam.

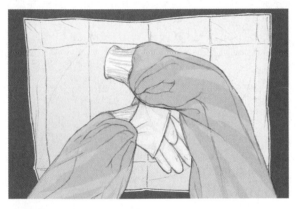

Figure 9.23

Secure the upper edge of the glove cuff with your right thumb and index finger.

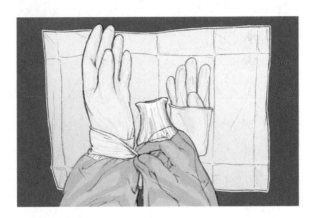

Figure 9.24

Work your fingers into the glove.

on the thumb side of your hand and the fingers of the glove are on the ulnar side of your wrist, with the glove fingertips pointing toward your elbow (**Fig. 9.25**). Grasp the lower edge of the glove cuff with your right thumb and index finger. Secure the upper edge of the glove cuff with your left thumb and index finger, and stretch the entire glove cuff over the stockinet opening, being careful not to touch the edge of the stockinet cuff (**Fig. 9.26**). Work your fingers into the glove (**Fig. 9.27**), and then grasp the right glove and gown at the seam with your left hand and pull up over your wrist (**Fig. 9.28**). Adjust both gloves for comfort and fit.

Wipe gloves with a sponge moistened with sterile water to remove any powder from gloves. Hold gloved hands at or above waist level and kept in sight at all times. Keep gloved hands away from the face and from under the axillary areas. Keep elbows close and perpendicular to the body sides.

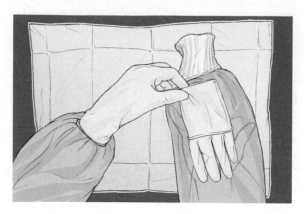

Figure 9.25
Place the folded glove cuff even with the gown cuff seam.

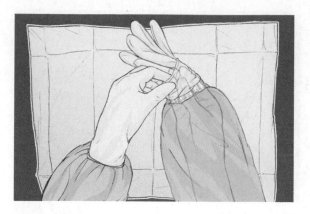

Figure 9.26
Place the folded glove cuff even with the gown cuff seam.

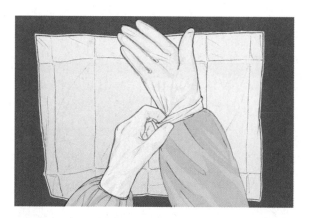

Figure 9.27
Work fingers into the glove.

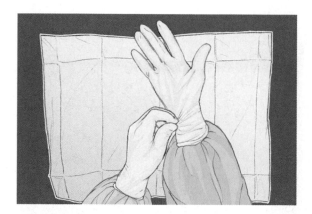

Figure 9.28
Pull the glove onto the wrist.

Open-Glove Technique

Open the inner glove wrapper carefully to expose the gloves, making sure that the wrapper does not flip back and contaminate the gloves (**Fig. 9.29**). If right-handed, grasp the right glove cuff on the fold with your left thumb and index finger, touching only the *interior* of the glove (**Fig. 9.30**). Insert your right hand into the glove and gently pull it on by the cuff. Leave the cuff turned down until after the left hand is gloved (**Fig. 9.31**).

To glove left hand, slide the fingers of your gloved right hand under the fold of the left glove cuff, touching only the *exterior* of the glove, and insert your left hand into the glove (**Fig. 9.32**). Gently pull it on, avoiding inward rolling of the glove cuff (**Fig. 9.33**). Slide the fingers of your left gloved hand under the fold of the right cuff and pull it up avoiding inward rolling of the glove cuff.

Assisted Gowning

After the surgical team member finishes the traditional hand scrub, place an open sterile towel over his or her outstretched hand (**Fig. 9.34**). Pick up the gown

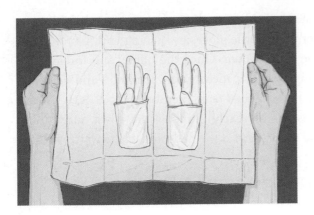

Figure 9.29

Open the inner glove.

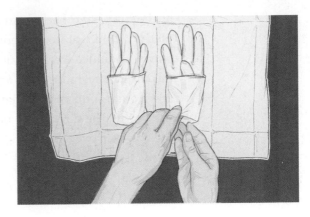

Figure 9.30

If right handed, grasp the right glove cuff on the fold with your left thumb and index finger.

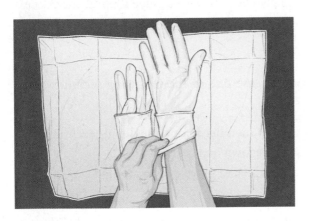

Figure 9.31

Insert your right hand into the glove and gently pull it on by the cuff.

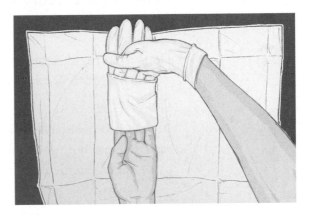

Figure 9.32

To glove left hand, slide the fingers of your gloved right hand under the fold of the left glove cuff.

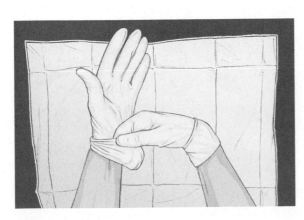

Figure 9.33

Gently pull the glove on.

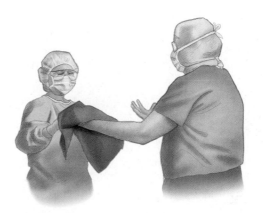

Figure 9.34

Place an open sterile towel over his or her outstretched hand.

at the neck, step back from the sterile field, and allow the gown to unfold completely. Form a protective cuff over your sterile gloves by placing your hands at the gown's shoulder level exterior side of the gown. Once the hands and forearms of the surgical team member are completely dry, identify the armholes and place the gown on the outstretched hands of the scrubbed team member (**Fig. 9.35**). Release the gown. The circulating nurse assists by reaching inside the gown and pulling the gown up over the shoulder and securing it at the neck and at the waist with the inside tie.

Assisted Gloving

Grasp the right glove under the inverted cuff[7]. Stretch the cuff while protecting your sterile thumbs and fingers by placing them under the cuff on the exterior side of the glove. Hold the stretched glove open, palm side toward the surgical team member. Assist the team member's hand into the glove by gently pulling the glove upward as the surgical team member pushes his or her hand into the glove (**Fig. 9.36**). Cover the gown stockinet cuff completely with the sterile glove. Repeat the process for the other hand.

Regowning and Regloving

When a glove becomes contaminated, use one of the following techniques for regloving:

- Ask for assistance from a sterile team member in open regloving technique
- Remove both gown and gloves and regown and reglove
- Apply a sterile glove over the contaminated glove until a sterile team member can assist with open gloving

To remove a contaminated glove, extend the glove out of the sterile field. The circulating nurse wearing protective gloves pulls off the contaminated glove leaving

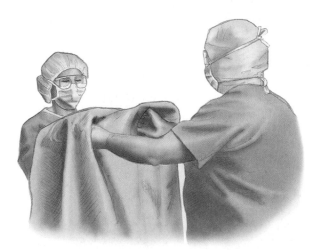

Figure 9.35

Place the gown on the outstretched hands of the scrubbed team member.

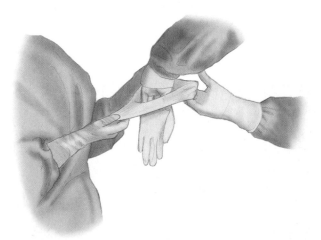

Figure 9.36

Assist the team member's hand into the.

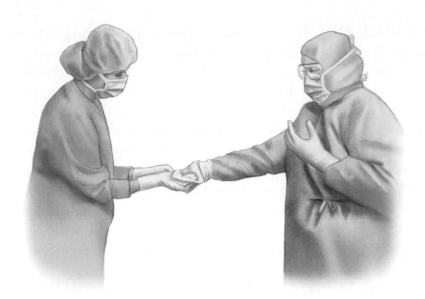

Figure 9.37

The circulating nurse wears protective gloves to pull off a contaminated glove.

the stockinet cuff in place (**Fig. 9.37**). Do not use the closed-glove technique for regloving; the stockinet cuff is contaminated. Ask a sterile team member to assist you in open gloving; if this is not feasible at the time; apply a sterile glove over the contaminated glove.

When a gown becomes contaminated, don protective gloves, untie the scrub person's gown, face the scrubbed team member, and then grasp the gown at the shoulders. While inverting the gown, pull it off. Next, remove the scrub person's contaminated gloves by touching the interior of the gloves without touching the scrubbed hands, and remove the gloves. During removal, turn the gloves inside out. The scrubbed team member is ready to regown and reglove. After the patient has arrived in the operative or invasive procedure room, consider the gown and gloves worn as contaminated. Do not wear these gloves outside the operative or invasive procedure suite.

PREPARING THE PATIENT'S SKIN FOR THE PROCEDURE

Correctly preparing the patient's skin can help reduce the risk of a surgical site infection. Skin preparation may include a shower or bath, hair removal, the removal of foreign substances (adhesives, tar, grease), and the cleansing of the incision site and surrounding area with an antimicrobial agent.

A preprocedure antiseptic shower or bath decreases skin microbial colony counts. Clinical trials support the use of preprocedure antiseptic showers to reduce the number of microorganisms on the skin, including *Staphylococcus aureus* (Garibaldi, 1998). In 1999, the CDC recommended requiring patients to "shower or bathe with an antiseptic agent at least the night before the operative day" (Category IB) (Kaiser et al, 1988). Unless contraindicated, patients should perform two showers with four percent chlorhexidine gluconate (CHG) to achieve maximum antiseptic effectiveness (Garibaldi, 1988; Hayek et al, 1987). Use only CHG approved or cleared for use as a general cleansing agent by the US Food and Drug Administration (FDA) for preprocedure (Federal Register, 1994).

CHG
Chlorhexidine Gluconate

FDA
Food and Drug Administration

Focus on maintaining the patient's skin integrity during the skin preparation. Skin is the major source of contaminants for many operations, and it is a source of pathogens for all procedures. Skin acts as a mechanical barrier to microorganisms and is composed of the epidermis, dermis, and subcutaneous tissues (**Fig. 9.38**). The most superficial layer, the epidermis, is thin, devoid of blood vessels, and divided into two layers; an outer horny layer of dead keratinized cells and an inner cellular layer in which both melanin and keratin are formed. Transient microorganisms, which are easy to remove with soap and water, reside on the epidermis. The epidermis depends on the underlying dermis for its nutrition. Well supplied with blood, the dermis contains connective tissue, the sebaceous glands, and some of the hair follicles. Resident microorganisms survive and multiply in the dermis, can be repeatedly cultured, and cause wound infection when allowed to enter deep tissues during the procedure. The dermis merges below with the subcutaneous tissues, which contain fat, the sweat glands, and the remainder of the hair follicles. Skin has many functions: it protects the deeper tissues from drying and injury, regulates body temperature, maintains fluid balance, and houses the sensory nervous system (Bevis, 2008).

To maintain skin integrity when preparing the patient's operative site, the nurse should consider the patient's overall physical condition, allergies, skin sensitivities and the anatomy involved during the proposed procedure. Determine whether the patient showered or bathed with an antimicrobial agent before admission to the facility and the degree of bioburden within the operative site. Check the patient's skin condition in and around the operative site. Determine whether the patient will be awake or anesthetized during the skin preparation. When performed correctly, the skin preparation removes gross contaminants, dirt, skin oil, and microbes from the skin and eliminates transient bacteria while reducing the resident colony count in the shortest period, with the least amount of tissue irritation. The prep should leave an antimicrobial residue on the skin to inhibit rebound growth of microorganisms during the procedure. Ensure that the types of supplies and antimicrobial agents

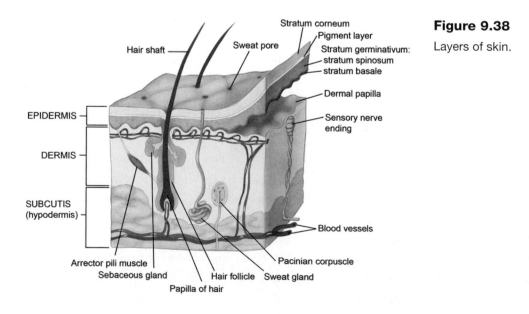

Figure 9.38

Layers of skin.

required for the preparation are available. Assess the need for extra personnel to help stabilize fractures, support an extremity, or assist with multiple traumas, extensive skin prep, or multiple preps.

Hair Removal

The Surgical Care Improvement Project (SCIP) recommendations for preventing Surgical Site Infections (SSIs) include appropriate hair removal (**Table 9.3**). Staphylococcus aureus is one of the most common microorganisms found on the skin; hence, it also is one of the most common pathogens associated with SSIs (Mangram, 1999). Shaving the skin in the operative area with a razor can result in small cuts and hair follicle disruption. This creates a perfect environment for microbial growth. Do not remove hair unless it is so thick that it will interfere with the incision. No hair removal is the preferred technique. If removing hair, however, do not use a razor; shaving increases the risk of surgical site infections (Segal, 2006) A large study demonstrated the following infection rates in wounds classified in the clean wound category: shaving hair with razor, 2.5%; clipping with scissors, 1.7%; removal of hair with an electric clipper, 1.4%; and no hair removal, 0.9% (Kjonniksen et al, 2002).

If hair removal is necessary, do it either by clipping or with a depilatory rather than shaving. Clipping hair with electric clippers or scissors and using depilatories lower the risk of surgical site infections. This is the least irritating way to remove hair from an operative site. Use a disposable clipper head. If using a reusable clipper head, disinfect between uses. Remove the hair immediately before the operative procedure and away from the area where the procedure will be performed. Loose hair and skin debris have the potential to contaminate the surgical site and sterile field.

Most pediatric and female facial procedures do not require shaving because of the relative lack of body hair. Remove hair around the eye with caution and avoid shaving the eyebrows because they often do not grow back completely.

Considerations

AORN's (2008) *Perioperative Standards and Recommended Practices for Preoperative Patient Skin Antisepsis* provides guidelines for preparing the patient's skin for operative or invasive procedures. **Table 9.12** highlights these recommended practices.

Supplies and Equipment

Nonsterile supplies include nonsterile gloves, terminally sterilized reusable clippers or a battery operated clipper with a disposable clipper head, small scissors, tape, and hand towels, and agents used for disinfection of the skin. A depilatory cream can also be used. The prep should also be performed in adequate lighting.

Sterile supplies include sterile gloves and antiseptic agents. Iodophors (eg, povidine-iodine), alcohol-containing products, and chlorhexidine gluconate are the most commonly used agents. If using flammable solutions, use agents packaged for controlled delivery, such as unit–dose applicators or swabs. See **Table 9.13** for information concerning the mechanism and spectrum of activity of antiseptic agents.

SCIP
Surgical Care Improvement Project

SSIs
Surgical Site Infections

Table 9.12	Guidelines for Preparing the Patient's Skin for an Operative or Invasive Procedure

- ☐ Perform two consecutive showers with 4% chlorhexidine gluconate (CHG) for open Class I operative procedures
- ☐ Avoid CHG contact with the eyes, inside ears, meninges, and mucous membranes
- ☐ Assess patient allergies and operative site before the skin preparation
- ☐ Use clippers (clipper head that can be disinfected between uses or a disposable clipper head) to remove hair from the operative site
- ☐ Remove jewelry (eg, body piercing ornaments) at the operative site before prep begins
- ☐ Remove soil, debris, exudates and transient microorganisms prior to the sterile prep
- ☐ Clean the umbilicus (abdominal surgery) before the antiseptic skin preparation
- ☐ Prepare the operative site and surrounding skin area (when indicated) with an antimicrobial agent (in preprocedure holding area immediately prior to the operative procedure)
- ☐ Clean traumatic orthopedic injuries with a pulse lavage, high-pressure parallel water-jet suction irrigation
- ☐ Remove alcohol-based hair products (hair spray) when preparing patient for head and neck surgery
- ☐ Use FDA and infection control approved preoperative skin antiseptic agents for all skin preparation
- ☐ Don sterile gloves prior to skin preparation
- ☐ Apply antiseptic agent over the operative site surrounding area in a manner to minimize contamination, preserve skin integrity, and prevent tissue damage
- ☐ Apply skin antiseptic agent progressing from the incision site to the periphery
- ☐ Prepare the skin area to extend large enough to accommodate potential extension of the incision, additional incisions and drain sites
- ☐ Protect all items from dripping and pooling of prep agents beneath and around the patient
- ☐ Remove all items where prep solution has dripped or pooled
- ☐ Refer to manufacturer's instructions to ensure uniform distribution of the antiseptic agent
- ☐ Allow prep agent (alcohol-based) to dry and fumes to dissipate before draping
- ☐ Document patient skin preparation according to AORN's Recommended Practices for Documentation of Perioperative Nursing Care

Adapted from AORN (2008). Skin Antisepsis, *Perioperative standards and recommended practices,* Denver, CO: AORN.

Procedure

Nonsterile Patient Skin Preparation

Use clippers to remove hair from the operative site. Shaving the site with a razor creates skin abrasions and injury associated with increased SSI. Do not remove hair the evening before the procedure by any method because colonization of the numerous skin nicks and abrasions will increases the chances of a SSI. Verify physician's order for area of hair removal. Double check clipper equipment and time length of the battery and proper clipper heads. Identify the patient with two identifiers; verify patient procedure with patient verbal confirmation and the patient's chart. Check the patient care area for adequate lighting and patient privacy. Explain the procedure to the patient. Inquire about allergies, scars, moles, or other skin abnormalities

Table 9.13	**Mechanism and Spectrum of Activity of Antiseptic Agents for Preoperative Skin Preparation and Surgical Scrubs**									
							USE ON			
Antiseptic Agent	Mechanism of Action	Gram + Bacteria	Gram − Bacteria	Viruses	Rapidity of Action	Persistent/ Residual Activity	Eye or Ear	Mucous Membrane	Contraindi-cations	Cautions
Alcohol	Denatures proteins.[1]	Excellent[1]	Excellent[1]	Good	Excellent[1]	None	No—Can cause corneal or nerve damage.[1]	No	Known allergies to isopropyl alcohol	Flammable. Does not penetrate organic material. Optimum concentration is 60% to 90%.[1]
Chlorhexidine gluconate	Disrupts cell membrane	Excellent[1]	Good[1]	Good	Moderate[1]	Excellent[1]	No—Can cause corneal damage deafness if in contact with inner ear	Use with caution[2]	Known hypersensitivity to drug or any ingredient.[2] Lumbar puncture and use on meninges.[2]	Prolonged skin contact may cause irritation in sensitive individuals. Rare severe hypersensitivity reactions have been reported.[2] Use with caution on mucous membranes.

9

Antiseptic Agent	Mechanism of Action	Gram + Bacteria	Gram – Bacteria	Viruses	Rapidity of Action	Persistent/Residual Activity	USE ON		Contraindications	Cautions
							Eye or Ear	Mucous Membrane		
Povidine-iodine	Oxidation/substitution with free iodine	Excellent[1]	Good[1]	Good	Moderate[1]	Minimal	Yes—Moderate ocular irritant	Yes	Sensitivity to povidone-iodine. (Shellfish allergies are not a contraindication).[6]	Prolonged skin contact may cause irritation. May cause iodism in susceptible individuals; avoid use in neonates.[3,4] inactivated by blood.[7,8]
Chlorhexidine gluconate with alcohol	Disrupts cell membrane and denatures proteins.[1,2]	Excellent[1]	Excellent[1]	Good	Excellent[1]	Excellent[1]	No—Can cause corneal damage & deafness if in contact with inner ear.	No	Known hypersensitivity to drug or any ingredient. Lumbar puncture and use on meninges.	Flammable
Iodophor with alcohol	Oxidation/substitution by free iodine denatures proteins.[1,3]	Excellent[1]	Excellent[1]	Good	Excellent[1]	Moderate[1]	No—Can cause corneal damage or nerve damage.	No	Sensitivity to povidone-iodine. (Shellfish allergies are not a contraindication.)	Flammable

Antiseptic Agent	Mechanism of Action	Gram + Bacteria	Gram − Bacteria	Viruses	Rapidity of Action	Persistent/ Residual Activity	USE ON		Contraindications	Cautions
							Eye or Ear	Mucous Membrane		
Parachloroxylenol (PCMX)	Disrupts cell membrane.	Good[1]	Fair	Fair	Moderate[1]	Moderate[1]	Yes[5]	Yes[5]	Known hypersensitivity to PCMX or any ingredient[5]	Minimally effective in the presence of organic matter. The FDA has classified PCMX as a Category III (data are insufficient to classify it as safe and effective). The FDA continues to evaluate PCMX.[5]

[1] Mangram A. J., Horan T. C., Pearson M. L., Silver L. C., Jarvis W. R., Guideline for prevention of surgical site infection, 1999. *Infect Control Hosp Epidemiology. 1999;* 20:250–278.

[2] Denton G. W., Chlorhexidine. In: *Disinfection, Sterilization and Preservation.* 5th ed. Block SS, ed. Philadelphia, PA: Lippincott Williams & Wilkins; 2001: 321–36.

[3] Bryant W. P., Zimmerman D. Iodine-induced hyperthyroidism in a newborn. *Pediatrics.* 1995; 95:434–436.

[4] Smerdely P., Lim A., Boyages S. C., et al. Topical iodine-containing antiseptics and neonatal hypothyroidism in very-low-birthweight infants. *Lancet.* 1989; 2:661–664.

[5] EnviroSystems, Incorporated. Technical Overview, Biocides. *http://www.envirosi.com/TechInfo/technical overview.html.* Accessed November 6, 2007.

[6] American Academy of Allergy Asthma and Immunology. Academy Position Statement: *The Risk of Severe Allergic Reactions from the Use of Potassium Iodide for Radiation Emergencies.* *http://www.aaaai.org /media/resources/academy_statements/position_statements/potassium_iodide.asp.* Accessed August 28, 2007.

[7] Zamora J. L., Price M. F., Chuang P., Gentry L. O., Inhibition of povidone iodine's bactericidal activity by common organic substances: an experimental study. *Surgery.* 1985; 98:25–9.

[8] Gottardi W. Iodine and iodine compounds. In: *Disinfection Sterilization and Preservation.* 5th ed. Block SS, ed. Philadelphia, PA: Lippincott Williams & Wilkins; 2001:159–83.

9

that may interfere with the hair removal. Expose the operative area, and assess the patient's skin condition. Don nonsterile gloves, and place a towel beneath the area to be clipped. When removing hair with clippers or scissors, clip only the hair that may interfere with the procedure. If necessary, trim long hair surrounding the incisional area so it does not interfere with the procedure or the application of the dressing after the procedure.

After clipping the area, pat area with tape to remove stray hairs and make the patient comfortable. When removing hair with a depilatory cream, perform a skin sensitivity test before applying the cream. Apply the cream according to the manufacturer's instructions (IFU). After the specified time, remove the cream and hair. Clean, rinse, and dry the skin. Document the patient's skin condition before and immediately after the hair removal, noting any redness, nicks, or skin abrasions. Some procedures require a pre-surgical skin prep of the incisional and surrounding area with an antimicrobial solution in the preprocedure area before entering the operating room.

Sterile Patient Skin Scrub

Even though sterilization of the skin is impossible, use aseptic technique when preparing the patient's skin for an operative or invasive procedure. Thoroughness is essential to reduce potential pathogens that colonize the patient's skin and will help prevent the introduction of environmental pathogens to the operative area. Prepare sterile supplies for skin preparation on a separate, small movable table. Select broad-spectrum antimicrobial agents capable of reducing and inhibiting both transient and resident microorganisms. Use fast-acting, long-acting, and easily applied agents. In addition, use agents that are nonirritating and nonsensitizing, and remain effective in the presence of soaps, detergents, organic matter, or alcohol. Apply only agents approved by the US Food and Drug Administration (FDA). When using an antimicrobial agent, always read the manufacturer's instructions, some agents can be neurotoxic and some may be toxic or harmful at various body sites. Eye injury from chlorhexidine gluconate has been reported, and chlorhexidine gluconate can cause ototoxicity if instilled directly into the middle ear.

FDA
Food and Drug
Administration

If the patient is awake, explain the procedure and provide privacy and comfort. Make every effort to allay fears. Answer questions in a reassuring manner. If the patient has been anesthetized, check with the anesthesia provider before starting the preparation. After the patient has been positioned, move the small table with the sterile skin prepping supplies close to the patient. Expose the area to be prepared. Assess the skin condition and the effectiveness of hair removal. Don sterile gloves, and arrange supplies for the procedure. Place absorbent towels on each side of patient to absorb excess prepping solution and to prevent pooling under the patient, electrodes, and the electrosurgical patient return electrode. To prevent pooling under tourniquets, seal off with an impervious U-drape or towel. Pooling of solutions may result in skin burn or irritation from chemical action. Also, place impervious pads under extremities to prevent solutions from saturating the patient's linen.

Begin cleansing at the incision site in a circular motion, moving out toward the periphery. Work from the cleanest to the least clean area. Upon reaching the preparation site edges, discard the used sponge. Repeat the process with a new sterile sponge. Never bring a soiled sponge back toward the incisional site. Prepare at least 6–8 inches (15–20 cm) beyond the incisional site in all directions unless otherwise stated for a specific procedure (see the next section for specific anatomical areas). The cleansing of the operative site should last long enough to cleanse the skin thoroughly. Use cotton-tipped applicators to clean the umbilicus and hard-to-reach areas.

Cleansing should proceed from clean to dirty, scrubbing an area of high bioburden last and discarding the sponge. Areas of high bioburden are the umbilicus, the axillary area, the vagina, the anus, open skin lesions, soiled traumatic wounds, and stomas. If the incisional site includes a stoma as an integral part of the procedure, cover the stoma with a sterile gauze, cleanse the area surrounding the stoma, and cleanse the stoma last. If the stoma is in the operative area, yet not included in the incision, isolate the stoma with a clear plastic adherent drape and then begin the skin preparation. Most open traumatic wounds, burns, or denuded areas need copious amounts of sterile solutions to flush contaminants out of the wound. Prepping after removal of a cast or a large dressing may require soaking with sterile solutions to remove adherent dressings. Exercise care in this situation because of the possibility of sensitive and denuded skin. Prepping for procedures involving skin or bone grafts requires separate setups. If the area is small, one preparation setup may be used. When using one preparation setup, cleanse the donor site first. When preparing an area with a possible malignancy (eg, a breast mass), omit scrubbing, in order to avoid the possible spread of carcinoma, and only apply an antimicrobial paint or gel to the operative area.

After scrubbing, wipe off the lather with a dry sponge or blot dry with an absorbent towel. When removing the towel, grasp the edges farthest away and lift it up away from the skin. Pay careful attention not to contaminate the prepared area with the edges of the towel. Using a sponge stick and an outward circular motion, apply the antimicrobial solution starting at the incisional area and move to the periphery. If necessary, use a second and third sponge stick to cover the operative area completely.

If using flammable solutions (alcohol, acetone, alcohol-based prepping solutions, fat solvents), allow adequate time for the solution to dry and the vapors to disperse before draping and/or activating electrosurgical or laser equipment. Evaporation times vary according to the type and amount of solution, used, room temperature, and humidity level. If an adherent drape is immediately applied after prepping with a flammable solution, the risk of trapping solution is significant. In such cases, an extreme fire hazard exists. Do not allow solutions to pool; pooled solutions evaporate, and drapes trap the vapors, thus creating a fire hazard in the presence of an ignition source.

After the prep is completed remove the impervious pad from under the extremities, the absorbent towels from each side of the patient, and any linen soiled with prepping solution. Avoid bringing towels over the prepared area. Remove the gloves, and discard all preparation materials in a proper receptacle. Document the patient's skin condition and the effectiveness of hair removal before the skin preparation began; state the antimicrobial agent used, the area prepped, and the person performing the prep.

On completion of the procedure, assess the patient's skin in and around the operative site, and document on the record any redness, abrasions, or burns. Communicate the findings to the physician and the postanesthesia care nurse. A skin preparation procedure manual should specify the type of agent, the anatomical areas, and the process for each type of operative or invasive procedure.

The following are skin preparations procedures used for different anatomical areas of the body. These are recommendations for many of the most common procedures.

ONE-STEP SCRUB PROCEDURE

In a one-step method, the detergent type agent is eliminated. The prep solution is contained in a sterile single-use kit that includes a pre-filled tube-like applicator with the solution and cotton-tipped applicators.

Perform hand hygiene immediately before initiating the surgical prep. Use sterile gloves and supplies for patient skin preparation. Place sterile absorbent towels for specific anatomical areas as described in the two-step prep method to absorb any pooling or excess solution.

Hold the applicator unit in an upright position with the sponge face parallel to the floor; press the cap end of the applicator. Solution will begin to flow into the sponge. Once the applicator sponge has been primed with solution, it is ready for use. Apply preparation to clean, dry, residue-free, intact skin and carefully follow manufacturers' specific written instructions. Start at the incision and apply a thin even coat in the same stroke direction as for the two-step prep to the operative site. Do not blot or wipe away. Allow the solution to dry 2–3 minutes on the skin before draping or using ignition sources. Many of the one-step prep applications contain alcohol; therefore, follow strict fire precautions.

TWO-STEP SCRUB PROCEDURE FOR SPECIFIC ANATOMICAL AREAS

Eye

Confine the patient's hair within a disposable bouffant hat or towel. Secure the patient's head in a head support to prevent rolling or moving. Squeeze sponges almost dry when cleansing, to prevent pooling of the solution in the eye. Using a nonirritating aqueous antimicrobial solution and sponges, cleanse the periorbital area, the eyelid, the lashes, and at least a 1-inch (2.5 cm) diameter area beyond the periphery of the eye (**Fig. 9.39**). Begin at the center of the eyelid and continue to the periphery, using cotton-tipped applicators for difficult-to-reach areas. Irrigate the periorbital area with a small bulb syringe and sterile water. Contain irrigating solution in a basin or with a towel at the side of the patient's head. Blot the area dry with a sterile sponge.

Lower Face and Nose

Confine the patient's hair within a disposable bouffant hat or towel. Secure the patient's head in a head support to prevent rolling or moving. Protect the patient's eyes with sponges or eye pads. Squeeze the sponges almost dry when cleansing, to prevent pooling of the solution in the patient's eyes or ears. Begin cleansing at the bridge of the nose in a circular motion, moving out toward the hairline and down to the mandible (**Fig. 9.40**). Use cotton-tipped applicators to cleanse the nostrils and hard-to-reach areas. Squeeze excess antimicrobial solution from the sponge stick and paint from the nose to the periphery.

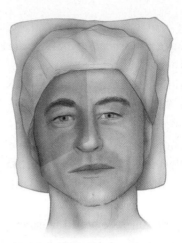

Figure 9.39

Eye prep.

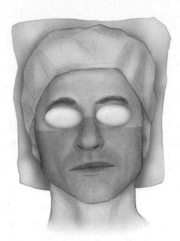

Figure 9.40

Lower face and nose prep.

Ear

Confine the patient's hair within a disposable bouffant hat or towel. Turn the patient's head to the side, with the ear to be operated on up, and secure in a head support to prevent rolling or moving. Secure the hair and define the operative area with tape or adhesive plastic towels. Squeeze the sponges almost dry when cleansing, to prevent pooling of the solution in the ear. Using a nonirritating antimicrobial solution, prepare from the center of the ear. Extend the prep onto the face and neck area (**Fig. 9.41**). Use cotton-tipped applicators to cleanse the external ear canal. A small piece of cotton may be placed in the external ear to absorb solution and prevent pooling of prepping solution. Squeeze excessive antimicrobial solution from the sponge stick and paint from the center of the ear. Extend the prep on to the face and neck area.

Neck and Combined Head and Neck

Expose the operative area to the nipple line. Place an impervious pad at the table line beneath the patient's head. Begin cleansing in a circular motion from the incisional site to the periphery. Prepare the neck anteriorly and laterally from the mandible to midsternum, including the tops of the shoulders (**Fig. 9.42**). For a combined head and neck procedure, also cleanse the lower portion of the face and the areas of the head around the ears. Continue the scrubbing long enough to cleanse the area thoroughly. Blot the area dry with absorbent sterile towels. Paint with an antimicrobial solution.

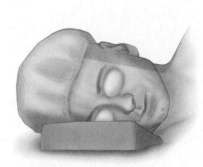

Figure 9.41

Ear prep.

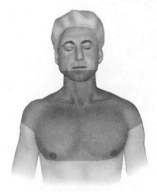

Figure 9.42

Head and neck prep.

Chest or Breast

Support the fingers in a hand-holder device, or have an assistant elevate the patient's hand and arm. Expose the operative area to the waistline. Place an absorbent towel over the nonoperative side and an impervious preparation pad on the table under the axilla and shoulder of the operative side. Begin cleansing in a circular motion from the incisional site to the periphery. Prepare from the top of the shoulder to below the diaphragm and from the edge of the nonoperative breast to the table line, including the upper arm to elbow circumferentially and the axilla (**Fig. 9.43**). Cleanse the axillary area last or use a separate sponge and discard it because of the high bioburden in that area. Prepare both sides of the chest for a bilateral procedure. Paint with an antimicrobial solution. For a breast biopsy, prepare the breast from the incisional area, to include an approximately 3-inch (7.5 cm) diameter area beyond the breast. When preparing a breast with a possible malignancy, omit scrubbing, to avoid possible spread of carcinoma; gently apply an antimicrobial paint or gel to the operative area only.

Abdomen, Supine Position

Expose the operative area from the nipple line to the pubis. Place absorbent towels alongside the patient at the table line to absorb any solution and prevent pooling. Begin cleansing in a circular motion from the incisional site to the periphery. Prepare from the breast line to the groin area and from table line to table line (**Fig. 9.44**). Continue scrubbing long enough to cleanse the area thoroughly. Blot the area dry with absorbent sterile towels. Paint with an antimicrobial solution.

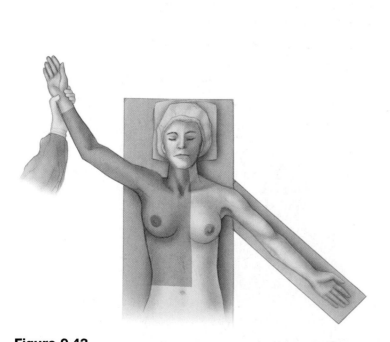

Figure 9.43

Chest or breast prep.

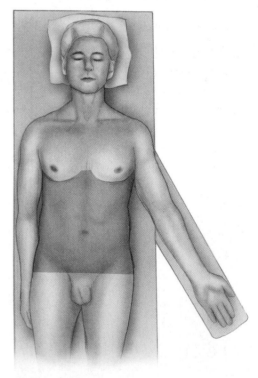

Figure 9.44

Abdomen prep.

Back, Prone Position

Expose the operative area from the shoulders to the top of the buttocks. Place absorbent towels alongside the patient at the table line to absorb any solution and prevent pooling. Place a plastic adhesive towel over the buttocks area. Begin cleansing in a circular motion from the incisional site to the periphery. Prepare from the shoulders to the top of the buttocks and from table line to table line (**Fig. 9.45**). Continue scrubbing long enough to cleanse the area thoroughly. Blot the area dry with absorbent sterile towels. Paint with an antimicrobial solution.

Chest and Kidney, Lateral Position

Expose the operative area to the ileum. Place absorbent towels anteriorly and posteriorly under the chest at the table level. Begin cleansing in a circular motion from the incisional site to the periphery. Prepare the area from the shoulders to the ileum and the anterior and posterior chest wall for thoracic procedures (**Fig. 9.46**). Prepare the patient from mid-chest to the hip, anteriorly and posteriorly for kidney procedures. Blot the area dry with absorbent sterile towels. Paint with an antimicrobial solution.

Perineum or Vagina

Expose the perineal area, and place an impervious pad under the buttocks and form a funnel into a kick bucket to collect fluids. Prepare from the pubis to the anus, including the vulva, labia, perineum, inner aspects of the thighs, and the vagina

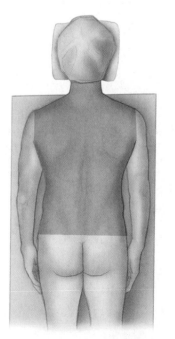

Figure 9.45

Back prep.

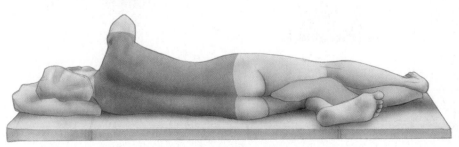

Figure 9.46

Kidney procedure prep.

(Fig. 9.47). Cleanse from the pubis area downward over the vulva and the perineum and past the anus; always discard the sponge after touching the anus because of the high bioburden in that area. Scrub the inner aspects of the thighs beginning at the labia majora and moving outward. Insert a narrow sponge stick saturated with an antimicrobial agent gently into the vagina and, using a rotating motion, cleanse the many folds of the vaginal mucosa. Repeat the procedure, discarding the sponge stick after each use. Insert a dry narrow sponge gently into the vagina to absorb any pooling of antimicrobial agent. Pay special attention to the gluteal cleft because prepping solution may have pooled.

Figures 9.48 A and B shows the prep area for a patient undergoing a procedure involving the abdomen and perineal area such as a laparoscopy assisted vaginal hysterectomy.

Catheterization in Conjunction with Perineal-Vaginal Preparation

Remove the gloves; they are considered contaminated from the prep. Don sterile gloves and insert a sterile catheter.

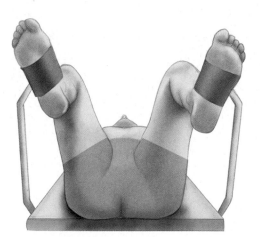

Figure 9.47

Perineum prep.

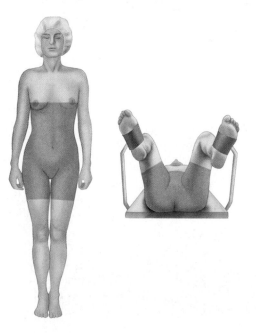

Figure 9.48

Abdomen-perineum/
vaginal prep.

Hand or Forearm

Apply a tourniquet to the upper arm, when ordered (see Chapter 11). Place the patient's arm on a hand table, which is protected with an impervious pad. Elevate the forearm on an extremity support. Begin cleansing at the fingertips and continue to the elbow circumferentially, paying close attention to areas under the nails and the cuticles (**Fig. 9.49**). If the nail beds are dirty, soak a sudsy solution under the nails and clean with a nail cleaner and brush. Blot the area dry with absorbent sterile towels. Paint with an antimicrobial solution from the fingertips to the elbow.

Elbow and Upper Arm

Apply a tourniquet to the upper arm, when ordered (see Chapter 11). Support the fingers in a hand-holder device, or have an assistant elevate the patient's hand and arm. Apply an impervious adhesive U-drape, sealing off the tourniquet to prevent the prepping solution from running or pooling under tourniquet. Begin cleansing in a circular motion from the incisional site to the periphery. Prepare from the wrist to the axilla or to the tourniquet, if applied, circumferentially (**Fig. 9.50**). Continue the scrubbing long enough to cleanse the area thoroughly. Blot the area dry with absorbent sterile towels. Paint with an antimicrobial solution from the incisional site to the periphery.

Shoulder

Support the fingers in a hand-holder device, or have an assistant elevate the patient's shoulder from the table. Place an impervious pad under the shoulder and axilla. Begin cleansing in a circular motion from the incisional site to the periphery. Prepare from mid neck to the elbow circumferentially, including the shoulder, the

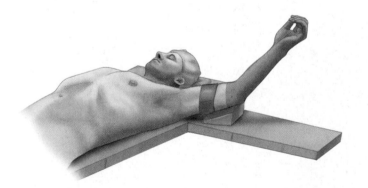

Figure 9.49
Hand or forearm prep.

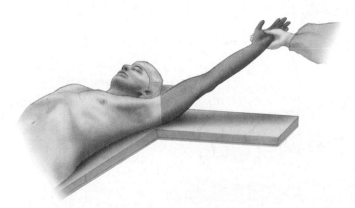

Figure 9.50
Elbow and upper arm prep.

scapula, the chest to the nipple, and the axilla (**Fig. 9.51**). Cleanse the axillary area last, or use a separate sponge and then discard, because of the high bioburden in that area. Continue scrubbing long enough to cleanse the area thoroughly. Blot the area dry with absorbent sterile towels. Paint with an antimicrobial solution from the incisional site to the periphery.

Hip, Semi-Lateral Position

Support the foot in an extremity-holder device, or have an assistant elevate the patient's entire leg from the groin to the ankle. Apply an impervious adhesive U-drape, isolating the perineal-rectal area. Begin cleansing in a circular motion from the incisional site to the periphery. Prepare from the waist to mid buttocks and to the lower outer aspect of the abdomen, and include the leg circumferentially from the hip to the ankle (**Fig. 9.52**). Blot the area dry with absorbent sterile towels. Paint with an antimicrobial solution from the incisional site to the periphery.

Hip, Fracture Table

Position the patient on a fracture table with the affected leg in traction. Apply an impervious adhesive U-drape, isolating the perineal-rectal area. Place an impervious pad between the affected hip and the top of the fracture table. Begin cleansing in a circular motion from the incisional site to the periphery. Prepare from the waist to the abdominal midline and to the table level, and include the leg circumferentially from the hip to the knee (**Fig. 9.53**). Continue scrubbing long enough to cleanse the area thoroughly. Blot the area dry with absorbent sterile towels. Paint with an antimicrobial solution from the incisional site to the periphery.

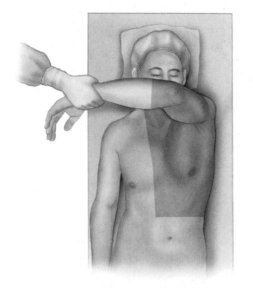

Figure 9.51

Shoulder prep.

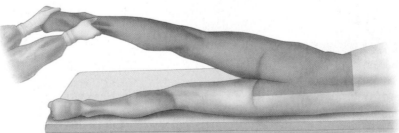

Figure 9.52

Hip in the semi-lateral position prep.

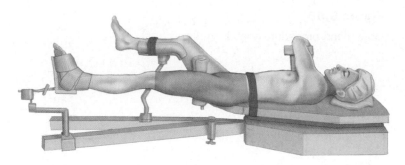

Figure 9.53

Hip prep with the patient on the fracture table.

Knee

Support the foot in an extremity-holder device, or have an assistant elevate the entire leg from the table. Apply a tourniquet to the upper thigh, when ordered (see Chapter 11). Apply an impervious U-drape, sealing off the tourniquet to prevent the solution from running or pooling under the tourniquet. Prepare circumferentially from the ankle to the tourniquet **(Fig. 9.54)**. Begin cleansing at the knee in a circular motion, moving up toward the tourniquet, and discard sponges. Begin cleansing again at the knee in a circular motion to the ankle and discard sponges. Continue scrubbing long enough to cleanse the area thoroughly. Blot the area dry with absorbent sterile towels. Paint with an antimicrobial agent from the knee to the tourniquet, and discard the paint stick. With another paint stick, paint from the knee to the ankle.

Foot or Ankle

Apply a tourniquet to the upper thigh, when ordered (see Chapter 11). Elevate the lower leg on an extremity support. Place an impervious pad under the foot. Begin cleansing at the toes and move up toward the lower leg. Prepare from the tip of the toes to the midcalf circumferentially, paying close attention to the area under and around the nails **(Fig. 9.55)**. Blot the area dry with absorbent sterile towels. Paint with an antimicrobial solution, starting at the toes and moving up toward the calf.

Figure 9.54

Knee prep.

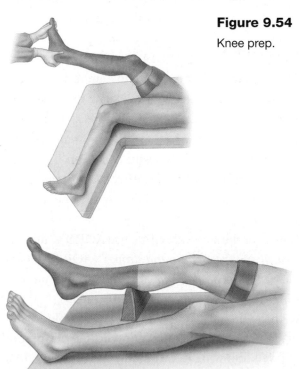

Figure 9.55

Foot or ankle prep.

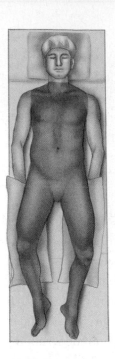

Figure 9.56
Open-heart procedure prep.

Open Heart

Expose the operative area from the neck to the toes. Elevate the legs on an ankle support. Place an impervious pad under the legs and towels alongside the patient at the table line to absorb excessive solution. Prepare from the chin to the toes, including both legs circumferentially (**Fig. 9.56**). Begin cleansing in a circular motion at the sternum and move toward the periphery of the torso. Prepare the leg circumferentially, beginning at the incision area and continuing to the periphery of the legs. Prepare the genital area separately, and isolate the area with an impervious towel. Continue scrubbing long enough to cleanse the area thoroughly. Blot the area dry with absorbent sterile towels. Paint with an antimicrobial solution from the incisional site to the periphery. Separate preps may be done for the chest area and the leg areas.

DRAPING THE PATIENT AND EQUIPMENT

Sterile drapes cover the patient and equipment in order to define and establish the sterile field during the operative or invasive procedure. Drapes isolate the incisional site and prevent microbial migration from nonsterile to sterile areas. In theory, this sterile zone is free of microorganisms at the start of and throughout the procedure. The area draped includes the patient from the anesthesia screen including arm boards to the foot of the bed, team members in sterile attire, Mayo stand, back table, ring stand, and any other furniture or equipment used during the operative or invasive procedure.

When selecting the gowns and drapes for the surgical setting use AORN's "*Recommended practices for selection and use of surgical gowns and drapes*"(AORN, 2008f) and the AAMI guideline "*Liquid barrier performance and classification of protective apparel and drapes intended for use in health care facilities.*" (AAMI, 2003b)

To prevent moist bacterial strike-through and to contain and control blood and body fluids, use impervious barrier drapes. Packaging that contains barrier drapes should be identified with the barrier levels following AAMI guidelines (**Table 9.11**).

Most operative suites use a disposable or reusable draping system or a combination of both for procedures. When selecting the sterile drapes for the proposed procedure, whether reusable or disposable, use fluid-proof fabrics with impervious barriers that avoid strike-through when soaking with blood and body fluids is a risk, or fluid-resistant fabrics when splashing or spraying of blood and body fluids is a risk, thereby eliminating microorganism penetration. Lint-free fabrics minimize airborne contamination and the dissemination of particles into the wound. Select fabrics strong enough to resist abrasions, tears, or punctures; yet porous enough to prevent heat buildup. Such fabrics maintain an isothermic environment that is appropriate for the patient's body temperature. Drape fabrics should also be memory free, have anti-slick surfaces, not allow light absorption or reflection, be nonabrasive, be free from toxic agents, inhibit the transfer of additives, and be permeable to sterilizing agents. All materials, both reusable woven linens and nonwoven disposables, create a fire hazard, especially in the presence of an oxygen-enriched environment. In the presence of ignition sources such as electrosurgical active electrodes, stray radio-frequency current, laser beams, and endoscopic light sources, woven and nonwoven fabrics are equally susceptible to ignition. Note and heed manufacturers' labels and instructions. Request that suppliers document the degree of safety of their drapes because all materials are capable of igniting and burning. Members of the patient care team must comprehend the true flammability properties of drape fabrics so that they can take the necessary precautions.

Strike-through occurs when fluids penetrate sterile drapes from a sterile to a non-sterile area or vice versa, thus breaking the sterile barrier and allowing microbial transfer to and from the patient. The types of draping material and degree of barrier selection for each specific procedure depends on the anatomical area involved, the position required, the amount of moisture inherent during the proposed procedure and the protection required for anticipated blood and body fluids' exposure to the surgical team members.

When assessing the patient and the proposed procedure before draping, consider the *patient critical zones.* These zones are the areas that immediately surround the operative site; sites with potential for increased amounts of blood and irrigation, and sites where soaking with blood and body fluids are potential risks (**Fig. 9.57**). To prevent strike-through and inhibit microbial transfer to maintain a sterile field for the duration of the procedure, use fluid-proof fabrics with impervious barriers.

The use of instruments or medical devices may cause tears, punctures, or abrasions of the drapes, thus allowing strike-through and causing a break in the sterile field; this allows microbial transfer to and from the patient. Draped areas at risk for compromise include the back table, Mayo stand, hand table; areas under or around extremities, areas of friction from retractors, areas involved in trauma procedures; and any other area where there is a potential risk of strike-through. These draping areas require special attention: fluid-proof fabrics with impervious barriers and added strength or plastic pouches that are necessary for containing and controlling blood and body fluids.

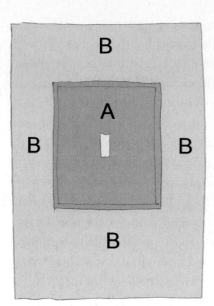

Figure 9.57

"A" highlights the critical zone for a laparotomy drape.

The *patient peripheral area* is the draping area that covers the entire patient and surrounds the critical zone. The area includes armboards, the anesthesia screen, and area over the foot of the bed, and an adequate length beyond the bed level. In these areas, splashing and spraying of body fluids are a risk, but the chance of fluid strike-through is lower than in the other two areas because of the small amount of moisture anticipated. A fluid-resistant fabric provides an effective sterile barrier in these areas.

Equipment draping areas include equipment and medical devices used in and around the sterile field. Mayo stands and back tables where sterile instruments and supplies are placed require a fluid-proof fabric with impervious barriers to prevent strike-through and to prevent microbial transfer and contamination. Drape equipment in the periphery of the sterile field, where splashing and spraying of body fluids is a risk, with a fluid-resistant fabric to provide an effective sterile barrier. Plastic, transparent, impervious drapes provide ideal sterile barriers for cameras, microscopes, laser forearms, power equipment, and imaging equipment.

When draping the patient fire safety is of utmost concern. Drapes are made of synthetic or natural fibers. They may burn or melt depending on the fiber content. Do not touch drapes with activated or recently de-activated[8] ignition sources (eg, laser, electrosurgical unit, light sources, high-powered drills) (ECRI, 2006). Ensure that oxygen, chemicals, or fumes, (prepping solutions containing alcohol) do not accumulate beneath the drapes. Provide moistened towels and sponges that are in close proximity to ignition sources and a container of fluid on the back table.

Considerations

See **Table 9.14** for the basic principles for draping.

Supplies and Equipment
Reusable Drapes

Reusable drapes are made of woven materials of various thread counts and are designed for multiple uses. Tightly woven, polyester-cotton blends, treated with chemicals, were developed to improve barrier properties. This treatment renders

Table 9.14	Basic Principles of Draping

- [ ] Aseptically prepare the procedure site before applying sterile surgical drapes.
- [ ] Allow 2–3 minutes for the alcohol-based prep to completely dry and fumes to evaporate before applying sterile drapes.
- [ ] Use impervious fluid-proof drapes to provide an effective sterile barrier when soaking, splashing, or spraying of blood and body fluids are a potential risk.
- [ ] Handle sterile drapes as little as possible; avoid shaking, fanning, or haphazard unfolding.
- [ ] Carry folded drapes to the operative site. Consider the drapes nonsterile if allowed to fall below the waist or table level.
- [ ] Drape the area around the incision first (critical zone) and then the periphery.
- [ ] When placing drapes, never reach across the nonsterile area to drape the other side; go around. All draping is done from the appropriate side.
- [ ] Form a cuff with the sterile drape to protect the sterile gloved hands when draping the periphery or equipment.
- [ ] Hold the drapes high enough to avoid touching the nonsterile areas of the bed.
- [ ] Do not move or reposition a drape once it is placed. The circulating nurse removes incorrectly placed or contaminated drapes, being careful not to contaminate the operative site or other drapes.
- [ ] Do not reposition or remove a towel clip that has been placed through a drape; its tips are contaminated. If the towel clip must be removed hand it off the sterile field and cover the area with a sterile drape.
- [ ] If the sterility of a drape is questionable, discard the drape.
- [ ] Once draping is complete and before the procedure begins a "TIME OUT" is conducted to assure—correct patient identification, correct site (and side if applicable) match the consent, and fire safety precautions taken.

them non-wicking and liquid resistant. Fabrics of polyester microfibers are durable, cool, breathable, and have a water-repellent finish. In most cases, the barrier effectiveness achieved through waterproofing of reusable drapes deteriorates with multiple processing. The repeated processes of laundering and sterilization gradually disrupt the integrity of the fabrics. As they experience wear, and then swell and shrink repeatedly in the laundering process, the threads begin to loosen, permanently altering their ability to protect the patient and the patient care team. Tests have shown that treated materials lose their barrier quality after being laundered and sterilized 75 times. GoreTex, a barrier fabric laminate bonded between two layers of lightweight polyester, is liquid proof, durable, breathable, and prevents strike-through.

When selecting a reusable woven system for operative or invasive procedures, pay attention to the barrier quality of the fabric. Determine which fabric provides the best possible protection for the patient and the patient care team. Fabrics should consistently provide protection, be cost effective, and not cause harm to the environment.

When considering a reusable draping system, ask the following questions.

- What are the initial purchase, inventory, and subsequent replacement costs?
- Do the barrier materials being considered meet the criteria listed in the AORN *Recommended Practices for Selection and Use of Gowns and Drapes*?

- How many supplies will be needed to construct linen packs (tape, sterilizing indicators, wrappers, etc.)?
- Is there an isolated area available for de-linting, inspection of gowns and drapes over a light table, folding and assembling packs?
- Will a grid system be needed to monitor the number of times that drapes are used and processed?
- Is there an adequate laundry facility available?
- What will be the cost per pound to launder the drapes?
- What are the sterilization, labor, equipment, and utilities costs?
- Is there an area available for storing the sterile packs and gowns?

When making a decision as to what type of fabric to purchase, ask the following questions:

- During the laundering process, do detergents cause a loss of barrier properties, and are a specific wash cycle and specific temperature required?
- How is the loss of effective barrier and repellency measured?
- Is the sterilization process for barrier drapes the same as for drapes without barriers?
- What are the manufacturer's test methods and published clinical data for evaluating barrier effectiveness?
- What effect does the processing have on the environment?[9]

Disposable Drapes

Disposable drapes made of nonwoven materials are designed for one-time use and may not be resterilized unless the manufacturer provides written instructions for reprocessing. Disposable nonwoven drapes are composed of both natural and synthetic fibers of various types. The most widely used are a spun-laced, wet-laid wood pulp, and polyester fiber blend and a spun-bonded melt-blown polyethylene. Both of these fabrics have polyethylene film laminated beneath the nonwoven fabric in the critical areas of the drapes, thereby providing an effective fluid-proof sterile barrier. Areas that are not laminated with polyethylene provide an effective fluid-resistant sterile barrier.

Some nonwoven drapes are made with special reinforcement around the fenestrations to reduce instrument slippage. They also offer antimicrobial, absorbent reinforcements and attached plastic pouches in the critical zones to contain and control body fluids. When these types of drapes are used, the handling of fluid-saturated linen is eliminated, thereby reducing the staff's exposure to fluid-borne contaminants. Nonwoven or disposable drapes streamline the task of draping the patient. Many are designed for specific procedures and feature elastic fenestrations, built-in incise, and adhesives (Manz, 2006). Disposable drapes reduce setup time and provide barriers with less material. Conduct a cost analysis before selecting a disposable nonwoven draping system using the following criteria.

- Ask each manufacturer to submit published clinical data to provide comparisons of impermeability on the various qualities and brands of their fabrics.

- Use the AORN *Recommended Practices for Selection and Use of Gowns and Drapes* as a reference and guideline for evaluating disposable nonwoven sterile draping systems.
- Investigate such factors as packaging, maintenance of sterility, cost effectiveness, storage space, delivery capabilities, and the cost of disposal.
- Take into consideration the fact that some companies recycle disposable drapes and gowns.

There are multiple designs of drapes for all types of procedures. **Table 9.15** the types of drapes used for operative or invasive procedures.

Drapes cannot withstand thermal laser beam impact. Use wet towels as a safety precaution around the area where the laser will be used to decrease the potential for fire (NFPA, 1999). Apply fluid-proof drapes under the wet towels to prevent strikethrough and microbial migration. The patient care team must determine how critical a given zone is and then use the proper type of fabrics and drapes to achieve the desired barrier protection.

Procedure
Draping the Patient and Equipment

Inspect the area in the operative or invasive procedure room where the sterile field will be set up. Assemble furniture and equipment to be draped within the sterile field. Check the surfaces of tables and equipment for cleanliness and dryness. Gather all necessary draping supplies for the proposed procedure. Many suites have a case cart system, in which all supplies and drapes for the procedure are assembled in advance and placed on a cart. Verify the correct surgical packs and drapes for the proposed procedure and anatomical area involved. Inspect the outer package for holes or damage that may compromise the integrity of the package, therefore rendering it nonsterile. Consider packages with defects as nonsterile and discard. Effective sterile barriers for back tables and Mayo stands are fluid-proof barrier drapes with impervious backings because these areas are considered critical zones.

Draping of the Back Table by a Nonsterile Team Member

Remove the drape pack from the outer package and place it on the center of the back table. Tear the seal and open toward the back of the table first, and then open toward the front of the table. Open the flap farthest away from you first and the nearest flap last. Walk to either end of the table, grasp the cuff below table level, and unfold the back table cover toward yourself. Move to the other side of the table and repeat the same movements. The area touched falls below the nonsterile table level, leaving the surface of the table sterile while the pack contents are exposed.

Draping of the Back Table by a Sterile Team Member

Open the table drape toward you to cover the nonsterile front edge of the table first, to minimize the possibility of contaminating the front of the gown. Protect gloved hands in the folded cuffs, and place a drape over the back of the table and then laterally to each side.

Table 9.15	Types of Surgical Drapes

Type	Purpose
Aperture Drape	Small clear plastic film drape with adhesive around the fenestration, which helps secure the drape to the skin around the incision.
Barrier Drapes	Drape made of impervious material, predominantly made of plastic. Essential in providing fluid-proof barriers when soaking with blood and body fluids is a risk.
Separate Sheets ☐ Medium Sheets ☐ ¾ Sheets ☐ Half Sheets	Separate sheets, usually fan folded and used in free draping (squaring off the incision site with all separate sheets). Used for draping large areas (eg, equipment, armboards, foot of the bed, back table).
Equipment Drapes	Plastic transparent drapes that covers cameras, microscopes, C-arm, x-ray equipment, and other equipment used within the sterile field.
Fenestrated Drapes	Drape with a specific opening for designated procedures (eg, laparotomy, thyroid, hand, and extremity. Area surrounding the fenestration should have an impervious barrier of 8–10 inches (20–25 cm) to prevent soaking of blood and body fluids.
Fluid Collection Pouches	Plastic transparent pouches utilized to contain and control blood and body fluids. May be applied on top of disposable or reusable drapes or may be incorporated into disposable drapes. Also used for high-volume irrigation and arthroscopy procedures.
Isolation Drape	Plastic transparent hanging drape used to isolate the C-arm, x-ray equipment, and or other nonsterile equipment from the sterile operative field.
Incise Drape	A self-adhering plastic film applied directly to the prepared dry skin. It provides a sterile surface up to the wound edge. The incision is made directly through the plastic film. It also helps stabilize other drapes, eliminates the need for towel clips, and isolates potential sources of infection such as stomas, colostomies and fistulas. It may be applied as a separate sheet or incorporated into a disposable fenestrated sheet.
Incise Antimicrobial Drape	A self-adhering plastic film drape that incorporates an antimicrobial agent in the adhesive and provides continuous antimicrobial activity that cannot be washed away.
Leggings	Drape utilized to cover the feet and legs in the lithotomy position.
U-Drape	Plastic drape with adhesive strips used predominantly on extremities to seal off the perineal area, the tourniquet, and the axillary area to provide a totally impervious sterile barrier.
Stockinette	Seamless tubing of stretchable impervious or woven material used to isolate an extremity draped within the sterile field.
Towel Drape	Small drape with a band of adhesive along one end of a towel, made of either disposable nonwoven or clear plastic.
Nonsterile plastic drapes	Used to wall off dirty area (stoma, colostomy, perineal area) before the prep begins.

Draping of the Mayo Stand by a Sterile Team Member

Place both hands under the cuff, palms down. A Mayo stand cover is a long tube (pillowcase-like) drape. Slide the cover over the Mayo stand, allowing it to unfold as it is being applied and taking precautions not to let it fall below waist level (**Fig. 9.58**). Stabilize the Mayo stand by placing one foot on its base while sliding the cover on. A nonsterile team member adjusts the lower open end of the Mayo stand cover by pulling the cuff down the stand.

Arrange all drapes on the sterile field in sequence of their use, and handle them as little as possible. Drapes must be correctly folded and have directional markings for ease in positioning and opening. The surgeon may elect to drape the patient, assisted by other sterile team members, or the surgeon may indicate the proposed field of delineation and charge the sterile team members with the responsibility for draping the patient. It is the responsibility of the patient care team members to have all the appropriate drapes ready for the proposed procedure. The circulating nurse should observe and direct the sterile patient care team members as necessary and watch carefully for breaks in aseptic technique during the process of draping the patient.

DRAPING FOR SPECIFIC PROCEDURES AND ANATOMICAL AREAS

Abdomen or Flat Surface

Prepare drape towel by folding one third of the towel lengthwise with the folded edge toward you and hand it to the surgeon or first assistant (**Fig. 9.59**), or place the towel, folded edge toward the patient, to outline the operative site. Secure towels with clips or an incise drape that provides a sterile surface up to the wound edge. When applying the incise adhesive drape the surgeon unfolds and hands it to the first assistant. While holding it taut, another assistant removes the release liner backing. Both surgeon and first assistant apply it to the patient's skin while using a folded towel, applies slight pressure to smooth it out and eliminate bubbles and/or wrinkles (**Fig. 9.60**).

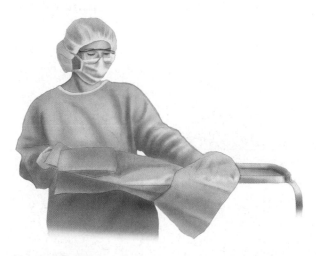

Figure 9.58

Draping the Mayo stand.

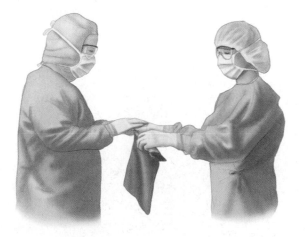

Figure 9.59

Handing the drape towel to the surgeon.

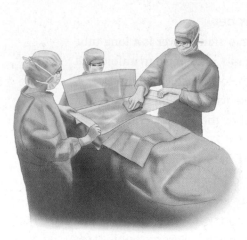

Figure 9.60

Smoothing the bubbles/wrinkles from the incise drape.

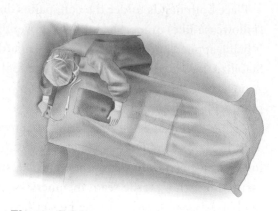

Figure 9.61

Placing the drape fenestration over the operative site.

If using a fenestrated laparotomy sheet remove the release liners from the adhesive strips around the fenestration; place the folded laparotomy sheet with the fenestration directly over the operative site (**Fig. 9.61**). Unfold the drape to each side, keeping it at table level until it is unfolded toward the patient's head, including arm boards, and toward the patient's feet, including an adequate length over the end of the bed (**Fig. 9.62**).

Eye, Ear, Nose, and Face

Place the gloved hands, palms down, under the cuff of the head or bar drape. Place the head or bar drape under the patient's head while a nonsterile team member lifts up the patient's head (**Fig. 9.63**). Remove the release liner tabs from adhesive strips and draw the drape up separately on each side of the patient's face (turban style) and secure with adhesive. Place a split sheet on the patient's chest with the tails toward the head, and unfold to the sides and then to the feet. Remove release liners from adhesive strips and simultaneously position the tails while securing them around the operative site (**Fig. 9.64**). Apply a small aperture drape

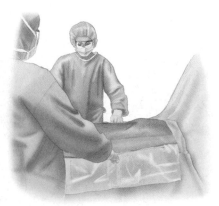

Figure 9.62

Unfolding the drape to each side of the patient.

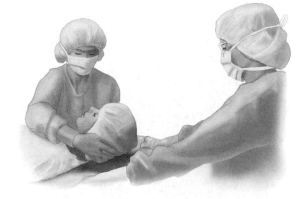

Figure 9.63

Placing the head or bar drape under the patient's head.

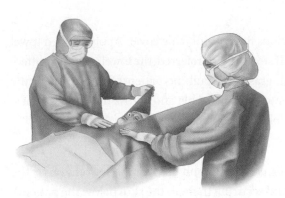

Figure 9.64

Securing the split sheet around the patient's head.

by removing the release liner from the adhesive and then securing the edges to the skin around the operative site. When applying drapes around the head and face of an awake patient, provide adequate breathing space and avoid making the patient feel claustrophobic. On minor EENT procedures, a half body drape may be used to isolate the operative field.

Lithotomy

Separate Leggings and Sheet. Place the gloved hands, palms up, under the cuff of the under buttocks drape and position it under the patient's buttocks. Protect the gloved hands in the legging cuff and allow adequate fold in the cuff as not to contaminate the legging opening while applying it over the leg and stirrup. The telescope fold allows for ease of application. Repeat this process for the other leg. Place the sheet on the abdomen (firmly pressing the adhesive strip to the skin to stabilize the drape), unfold laterally over the perineal area, and then unfold to the head.

One-Piece Drape with Attached Leggings. Remove the release liner from the adhesive strip. Place the fenestration over the perineal area. Unfold the drape toward the patient's head while firmly pressing the adhesive strip to patient's abdomen to stabilize the drape. Grasp the legging marked "toe" with the right hand and pull it up over the patient's right leg and stirrup. Touching only the underside of the drape, the nonsterile team member assists in placing the drape over the patient's leg and stirrup. Repeat with the left hand for the left leg. Some drapes are designed with plastic pouches to help contain and control blood and body fluids (**Fig. 9.65**).

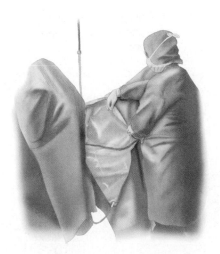

Figure 9.65

Arranging the plastic pouch used to contain and control blood and body fluids.

Hand

Drape the hand table with an impervious fluid-proof table cover. Apply a rolled towel around the arm and secure it with a clip. If stockinet is preferred, the towel may be omitted. Position the hand drape over the hand; grasp and pull the patient's hand through the elastic fenestration. Unfold the drape onto the hand table and across the patient's chest unfold toward the patient's feet, and unfold to the patient's head (**Fig. 9.66**).

Shoulder

With the patient's arm and shoulder elevated, apply a U-drape by removing the release liners from the adhesive strips and securing them to the skin below the patient's arm, sealing off the axillary area. Apply impervious stockinet if the arm is draped within the sterile field. Twist it to achieve a better fit and to expel the air as it is rolled up the arm. Apply a sterile incise drape around the support apparatus if the arm is in traction. Position the body split sheet below the arm at the axilla; unfold the sheet side to side, then toward the patient's feet. Fold back the tails and remove the release liner from the adhesive strips (**Fig. 9.67**). Seal the adhesive tails around the patient's shoulder and toward the patient's head. Position the shoulder drape with the pouch above the shoulder (**Fig. 9.68**). The arrow points toward the patient's feet. Unfold the drape from side to side and up to create the anesthesia screen. Unfold the tails toward the anesthesia screen to expose the incise release liner, remove the release liner, bring both tails down around the shoulder simultaneously, and seal the adhesive to the bottom split sheet.

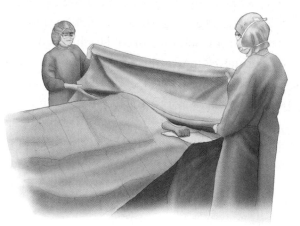

Figure 9.66

Draping the hand.

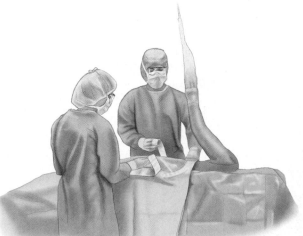

Figure 9.67

Removing the release liners from the adhesive strips of the U-drape.

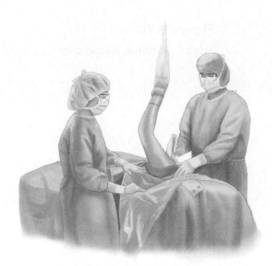

Figure 9.68

Positioning the pouch above the shoulder.

Hip, Semi-Lateral Position

With the patient's leg elevated, apply a U-drape by removing the release liner from the adhesive strips and securing them to the patient's skin, sealing off the perineal area and crossing the tails up over the iliac crest to complete the fenestration. (**Fig. 9.69**) Apply an impervious stockinet, twisting it to achieve a better fit and to expel the air as it is rolled up the leg, apply an elastic bandage up to the operative site to secure the stockinet. While the leg is extended, position the nonwoven split sheet under the patient's leg with the tails toward the operative site. Unfold the drape to each side and then to the feet. Fold back the tails, remove the release liners from the adhesive strips, and simultaneously position the tails, attaching them around the operative site. Position the top sheet with the arrow toward the incision, unfold to the side, remove the release liners from the adhesive strip, and seal to the split sheet, completing the fenestration around the operative site. Unfold upward to create the anesthesia screen. When using an elastic fenestrated hip sheet, apply an impervious U-drape and stockinet first. Slip the fenestration over the patient's foot and unfold to each side and then toward the foot and up to create the anesthesia screen. When using an incise drape, apply it over the operative site, securing the stockinet and all drapes in place (**Fig. 9.70**).

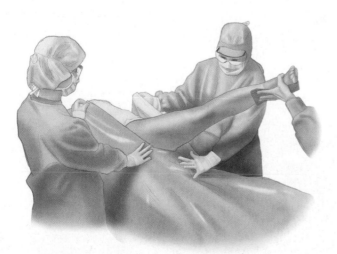

Figure 9.69

Sealing off the perineal area while draping the hip.

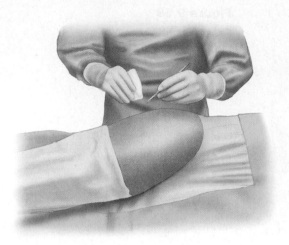

Figure 9.70

The incise drape placed over the hip.

Hip, Fracture Table

Square off the operative site with adhesive drape towels. Apply an isolation-hanging drape by removing the release liner from the incision area of the drape and firmly pressing the adhesive onto the operative site to stabilize the drape. Unfold laterally to each side. Unfold to top toward the support bar. While touching only the underside of the drape, the nonsterile team member assists in adhering the wall drape (shower curtain) to the support bar (**Fig. 9.71**). Unfold the drape toward the floor.

Arthroscopy

With the patient's leg elevated, apply a U-drape by removing the release liner from the adhesive strips and securing them to the leg above the knee, sealing off the tourniquet and the leg-holder device. Apply an impervious stockinet, twisting it to achieve a better fit and to expel the air as it is rolled up the leg. Position the arthroscopy drape with the fluid control pouch at the knee. Grasp the foot and pull the patient's leg through the double elastic fenestrations with the pouch. Unfold the drape to each side, then to the head and to the feet. To form a pouch, place one

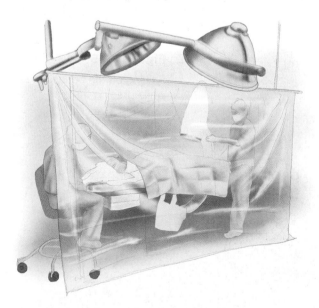

Figure 9.71

Isolation-hanging drape in place.

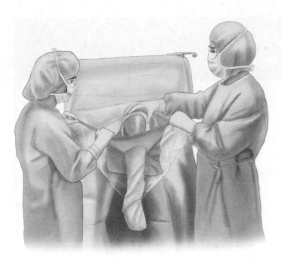

Figure 9.72

Draping for an arthroscopy of the knee.

elastic fenestration above the knee and the other below the knee (**Fig. 9.72**). If an elastic fenestrated arthroscopy drape is used without a pouch, apply an impervious U-drape and stockinet first. Slip the fenestration over the patient's foot and unfold to each side and then to the head and to the feet.

Ankle or Foot

With the patient's foot elevated, place an impervious fluid-proof barrier drape under the operative extremity. Apply a rolled towel around the patient's thigh and secure it with a clip. If stockinet is preferred, the towel may be omitted. Position the elastic fenestrated extremity sheet over the foot. Grasp and pull the patient's foot through the elastic fenestration. Unfold the drape to each side, then to the head and to the foot.

Open Heart

With the patient's legs elevated, place an impervious fluid-proof barrier drape under the legs. Place a stockinet on each foot, or cover the feet with a small drape. Lower the patient's legs onto the sterile barrier. Seal off the perineal area with an impervious towel or drape. Apply adhesive drape towels along the sides of the patient's chest and legs. Apply a large incise sheet to cover the chest and the abdomen. Apply another large incise sheet over both legs and the groin area. Position a cardiovascular split drape on the patient's chest; remove the release liners from adhesive and secure to the patient's chest.

CONCLUSION

Establishing and maintaining a sterile field is a core competency for the operative or invasive procedure nurse. The nurse and other members of the patient care team implement actions aimed at preventing the transmission of microorganisms that are present in the environment of the patient. Diligent application of the principles of asepsis and the nursing actions listed as measurable criteria for this competency reduce the patient's risk of acquiring a SSI (surgical site infection). It is everyone's job to help in reducing the incidence of SSIs. It is therefore essential that surgical infection reduction efforts be practiced by everyone in the operative or invasive suite.

COMPETENCY ASSESSMENT
Establish and Maintain a Sterile Field

Name: _____   Title: _____   Unit: _____   Date of Validation: _____

Type of Validation: ☐ Initial   ☐ Annual   ☐ Bi-annual

COMPETENCY STATEMENT: The nurse demonstrates competency to establish and maintain a sterile field for an operative or invasive procedure.

Performance Criteria	Met	Not Met
1. Identifies patients at risk for adverse outcomes related to establishing and maintaining a sterile field	☐	☐
2. Dons and wears appropriate operative attire	☐	☐
3. Prepares supplies, instruments and equipment for the sterile field	☐	☐
4. Scrubs the hands and forearms	☐	☐
5. Dons a sterile gown and gloves	☐	☐
6. Prepares the patient's skin for the procedure	☐	☐
7. Drapes the patient and equipment	☐	☐

_____

Validator's Signature

Employee's Signature

_____

Validator's Printed Name

ENDNOTES

1. Operative and invasive procedure team members include the physician, circulating nurse, scrub person, anesthesia provider, and others engaged in care in the operative and invasive procedure care areas.
2. Laser masks are also appropriate for wear during procedures that generate excessive electrosurgery plume.
3. Do not reprocess single-use items unless approved by the manufacturer. Facilities choosing to reprocess single-use items should follow the *AORN Guidance Statement: Reuse of Single-Use Devices.*
4. Do not secure electrosurgery or other electrical device cords with metal instruments such as a towel clip or hemostat. See Chapter 11 for further information.
5. Studies suggest that scrubbing for at least 2 minutes is as effective as the traditional 10-minute scrub in reducing hand bacterial colony counts (Boyce & Pittet, 2002).

6. Evidence continues to build that a lengthy scrubbing (10 minutes) procedure is unnecessary (Labadie et al, 2002). Similarly, use of a brush or sponge is counterproductive and causes skin damage and increased shedding (Hobson, 1998). There is increasing evidence that alcohol-based surgical hand preparations are efficacious as or better than conventional scrubs, and their use may actually increase compliance with proper antisepsis technique (Parienti et al, 2002).
7. The right hand is usually gloved first in assisted gloving.
8. Recently de-activated ignition sources such as an electrosurgical active electrode or the metal tip of a fiber optic light cord pose an ignition hazard because of residual heat.
9. Laundering and sterilizing of reusable drapes consumes water and chemicals, creates detergent waste, uses a great deal of energy, and contributes to air pollution.

REFERENCES

1. 100k lives, The prevention of SSI a component of Surgical Care Improvement Project (SCIP) http://www.medqic.org/dcs/ContentServer?cid=1136495723627&pagename=Medqic%2FOtherResource%2FOtherResourcesTemplate&c=OtherResource (Accessed May, 2008).

2. AAMI (2003a). "Safe handling and biological decontamination of reusable medical devices in health care facilities and in nonclinical settings," ANSI/AAMI ST35:2003 (Arlington, Va: Association for the Advancement of Medical Instrumentation, 2003) 11–12, 51–57.

3. AAMI (2003b). Association for the Advancement of Medical Instrumentation, Liquid Barrier Performance and Classification of Protective Apparel and Drapes Intended for Use in Health Care Facilities, ANSI/ AAMI PB70 (Arlington, VA: Association for the Advancement of Medical Instrumentation, 2003).

4. AAMI (2006). Association for the Advancement of Medical Instrumentation. ANSI/AAMI ST79: 2006—Comprehensive Guide to Steam Sterilization and Sterility Assurance in Health Care Facilities. Arlington, VA: Association for the Advancement of Medical Instrumentation, 4, 24–25, 36–37, 39, 54, 60, 62–74, 77–80, 83, 87, 90, 110.

5. AAOS (2008). "Advisory statement: Preventing the transmission of bloodborne pathogens," American Academy of Orthopedic Surgeons, http://www.aaos.org/wordhtml/papers/advistmt/1019.htm (accessed 17 May 2008).

6. AORN (2008a). "Recommended Practices for Maintaining a Sterile Field" in *Perioperative Standards and Recommended Practices* (Denver: AORN) 565–573.

7. AORN (2008b). "Recommended Practices for Sterilization in Perioperative Practice Setting" *Standards and Recommended Practices* (Denver: AORN) 575–598.

8. AORN (2008c). Recommended Practices for Surgical Attire" in *Perioperative Standards and Recommended Practices* (Denver: AORN) 285–291.

9. AORN (2008d). "Recommended Practices for Surgical Hand Antisepsis/Hand Scrubs" in *Perioperative Standards and Recommended Practices* (Denver: AORN) 397–405.

10. AORN (2008e). "Perioperative Standards and Recommended Practices for Prevention of Transmissible Infections in the Perioperative Practice Setting," in *Perioperative Standards and Recommended Practices* (Denver: AORN) 619–629.

11. AORN (2008f). "Recommended practices for selection and use of surgical gowns and drapes," in *Perioperative Standards, Recommended Practices* (Denver: AORN) 391–395.

12. APIC (2002). Association for Professionals in Infection Control and Epidemiology, APIC Text of Infection Control and Epidemiology (Washington, DC: Association for Professionals in Infection Control and Epidemiology, 2002) 27–1 to 27–4.

13. Baumgardner, C.A., et al, "Effects of nail polish on microbial growth of fingernails," *AORN Journal* 58 (July 1993) 84–88.

14. Belkin, N.L. (2002). "A historical review of barrier materials," *AORN Journal* 76 (October 2002) 648–653.

15. Bischoff, W.E., Reynolds, T.M., Sessler, C.N., Edmond, M.B., Wenzel, R.P. (2000). Handwashing compliance by healthcare workers. The impact of introducing and accessible, alcohol-based hand antiseptic. *Arch Intern Med;* 160: 1017–1021.

16. Boyce, J.M., Pittet, D. (2002). Guideline for hand hygiene in health-care settings: recommendations of the Healthcare Infection Control Practices Advisory Committee and the HICPAC/SHEA/APIC/IDSA HAND Hygiene Task Force. *Infection Control and Hospital Epidemiology;* 23(12 suppl): S3–S40.

17. CDC (1999). Centers for Disease Control and Prevention, "Guideline for prevention of surgical site infection, 1999," Infection Control and Hospital Epidemiology 20 (April 1999) 247–277. www.cdc.gov/ncidod/dhqp.pdf/guidelines/SSI.pdf. Accessed May 3, 2008.

18. CDC (2002). Centers for Disease Control and Prevention, "Guidelines for Hand Hygiene in Health-Care Settings, Recommendations and Reports," Morbidity and Mortality Weekly Report 51 (RR-16) (Oct 25, 2002).

19. CDC (2003). Centers for Disease Control and Prevention (CDC), "Guidelines for environmental infection control in health-care facilities: Recommendations of CDC and the Healthcare Infection Control Practices Advisory Committee (HICPAC)," Morbidity and Mortality Weekly Report 52 (June 6, 2003) 27–29.

20. ECRI, "Surgical fire safety", *Health Devices* 35 no 2 (February 2006) 45–66.

21. Federal Register (1991). "Occupational exposure to bloodborne pathogens; Final rule," Federal Register 56 (Dec 6, 1991) 640004–64182.

22. Friberg, B. et al, "Surgical area contamination—Comparable bacterial counts using disposable head and mask and helmet aspirator system, but dramatic increase upon omission of head-gear: An experimental study in horizontal laminar air-flow," *Journal of Hospital Infection* 47 (February 2001) 110–115.

23. Garibaldi, R.A. (1988). Prevention of intraoperative wound contamination with chlorhexidine shower and scrub. J Hosp Infect; 11 (Suppl B): 5–9.

24. HICPAC. Hospital Infection Control Practices Advisory Committee (1995). Recommendations for preventing the spread of vancomycin resistance. Infect Control Hosp Epidemiol; 16: 105–113.

25. Hobson, D.W., et al, "Development and evaluation of a new alcohol-based surgical hand scrub formulation with persistent antimicrobial characteristics and brushless application," American Journal of Infection Control 26(October 1998) 507–512.

26. Kaiser, A.B., Kernodle, D.S., Barg, N.L., Petracek, M.R. (1988). Influence of preoperative showers on staphylococcal skin colonization: a comparative trial of antiseptic skin cleansers. *Ann Thorac Surg.*; 45: 35–39.

27. Kampf, G., Kramer, A., (2004). Epidemiological background of hand hygiene and evaluation of the most important agents for scrubs and rubs. *Clin Microbiol Rev.* 17: 863–893.

28. Killen, A.R., (2006). Presentation "Evidence Based Protocols —Does Home-Laundering vs Hospital-laundering of individual scrubs influence infection rate?" *Managing Today's OR Suite.*

29. Kjonniksen, J., Anderson, B.M., Sondenna, V.G., Segadal, L. (2002). Preoperative hair removal—a systematic literature review. *AORN Journal* (May 2002; 928–940.

30. Koch (2004). Interview—Koch "New standard aids in selecting barriers" *OR Manager* Vol. 20 No 5 (May 2004) 1–4.

31. Labadie, J.C., Kampf, G., Lejeune, B., et al. (2002). Recommendations for surgical hand disinfection: requirements, implementation and need for research: a proposal by representatives of the SFHH, DGHM AND DGKH for a European discussion. *J Hosp Infect;* 51: 312–315.

32. Mangram, A.J., et al, "Guideline for prevention of surgical site infection, 1999, "Hospital Infection Control Practices Advisory Committee 20 (April 1999) 247–279.

33. Manz, E.A., Edgar, B.L., "Examining Draping Practices for Cost-Effectiveness," *Surgical Services Management,* (August 1998) 41–47.

34. Moolenaar, R.L., et al. "A Prolonged Outbreak of Pseudomonas aeruginosa in a neonatal intensive care unit: Did staff fingernails play a role in disease transmission?" *Infection Control and Hospital Epidemiology* 21 (February 2000) 80–85.

35. NFPA 115: Recommended Practice on Laser Fire Protection (Quincy, Mass: National Fire Protection Association, 1999).

36. OSHA (2008). "Regulations (Standards 29 CFR) Bloodborne pathogens—1910–1030," US Department of Labor, Occupational Safety and Health Administration (OSHA), http://www.oshaslc.gov/pls/oshaweb/owadisp.showdocument?p_table=STANDARDS&p_id=10051 (accessed 15 February 2008) 15–16.

37. Parienti, J.J., Thibon, P., Heller, R., et al. Hand-rubbing with an aqueous alcoholic solution vs. traditional surgical hand scrubbing and 30-day surgical site infection rates, *JAMA* 2002; 288:722–727.

38. Phillips (2004). Berry & Kohn's Operating Room Technique Edition 11, St. Louis, MO 2004, Mosby, Inc. 48–49.

39. Pittet, D., "Improving adherence to hand hygiene practice: A multidisciplinary approach," *Emerging Infectious Disease* 7 March/April 2001) 234–240.

40. Revis, D.R., Skin, Anatomy, eMedicine Specialties, Plastic Surgery, Department of Surgery, Division of Plastic and Reconstructive Surgery, University of Florida College of Medicine (accessed 14 March 2008)1–11.

41. Rotter, M.L., Arguments for alcoholic hand disinfection. *J Hosp Infect* 2001; 48(suppl A): S4–S8.

42. Segal, C.G., Infection Control: Start with skin. *Nursing Management.* April 2006; 46–51.

43. Tanner, J., Parkinson, H., "Double gloving to reduce surgical cross-infection," (Cochrane Review) *The Cochrane Library,* Issue 3 (Oxford: John Wilson & Sons, 2003).

44. Turnquist, M., et al. "Perforation rate using a single pair of orthopedic gloves vs. a double pair of gloves in obstetric cases," *Journal of Maternal-Fetal Medicine* 5 no 6 (November-December 1996) 362–365.

45. FDA (1994). US Department of Health and Human Services, Food and Drug Administration. Tentative final monograph for health care antiseptic drug products proposed rule. CFR.21.333, CFR.21.369. *Federal Register.* June 17, 1994: 31402–31452.

46. US Government (1994). "Topical antimicrobial drug products for over-the-counter human use; tentative final monograph for health-care antiseptic drug products," in Code of Federal Regulations (CRF) 21: Food and Drugs, Parts 333 and 369 (Washington, DC: US Government Printing Office, 1994) 31402–31452.

CHAPTER 10

Perform Sponge, Sharp, and Instrument Counts

Mary O'Neale

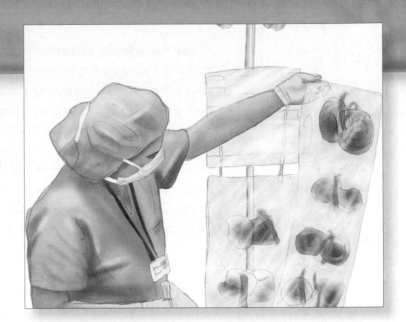

INTRODUCTION

Sponge, sharp, and instrument counts are performed by the registered nurse to reduce the potential for injury to the patient as a result of a retained foreign body. This crucial activity is an integral component of safe patient care during the operative and invasive procedure.

Because nurses have a critical responsibility to provide safe patient care, they should determine the patient's risk for poor outcomes related to the retention of foreign bodies before every procedure.

MEASURABLE CRITERIA

The nurse demonstrates competency to ensure that the patient is free from injury related to retained sponges, instruments, and sharps by:

- Identifying the patient's risk for adverse outcomes related to the retention of extraneous objects;
- Initiating count procedures that reduce the patient's risk for retained extraneous objects;
- Initiating incorrect count procedures; and
- Documenting count procedures according to facility policy.

ROLE OF THE NURSE

Members of the surgical team are responsible for taking the measures necessary to provide safe patient care. The circulating nurse makes certain that the facility's counting policies and procedures are followed and that the required counts are performed. The scrub person collaborates with the circulating nurse to account for all sponges, sharps, and instruments.

Chapter Contents

The Association of periOperative Registered Nurses (AORN) in its "Recommended Practices for Sponge, Sharp, and Instrument Counts" states "legislation does not prescribe how counts should be performed, who should perform them, or even that they need to be performed; the law requires only that foreign bodies not be negligently left in patients" (AORN, 2008, p. 293). Further, complete and accurate counts help promote optimal perioperative patient outcomes and also demonstrate the commitment to patient safety (AORN, 2008, p. 293). All members of the surgical team should be committed to establishing policies and procedures related to surgical counts. In the event of a lost counted item, the circulating nurse implements facility policy and procedures for reconciliation of count discrepancies.

AORN RECOMMENDED PRACTICES

The AORN "Recommended Practices for Sponge, Sharp, and Instrument Counts" (AORN, 2008) are intended as guidelines for the development of policies and procedures and are adaptable to various practice settings. These recommended practices help promote an optimal level of practice. Each practice setting should use the recommended practices to develop count policies and procedures tailored for its particular practice environment. For example, Recommended Practice III states that "instruments should be counted on all procedures in which the likelihood exists that an instrument could be retained" (AORN, 2008, p. 296). This recommended practice enables the facility to define what types of procedures require instrument counts. Instrument counts may be deferred for pediatric patients when there is no perceived risk of retained instruments (AORN 2008, p. 297).

FACILITY POLICIES AND PROCEDURES

Facilities must define policies and procedures for counts. The registered nurse must know and carry out the facility's policies and procedures. Failure to do so places the patient at risk for injury and the surgical team at risk for legal action. The facility's policies and procedures should describe:

- Items to be counted;
- The sequence for performing counts (ie, start at the incision, surrounding sterile area, Mayo stand, back table, discarded items);
- Procedures for which subsequent counts can be omitted after a baseline count is performed;
- Miscellaneous items that should be counted; and
- Nursing actions and procedures for count discrepancy reconciliation.

LEGAL ISSUES

Protecting patients from injury is one of the nurse's most critical roles. If a sponge, sharp, or instrument is left in a patient and the patient sues, and if the suit goes to trial, the jury will determine if the nurse did what any reasonable and prudent nurse would have done to account for the item before closure of the wound. Jury members will be instructed to base their decision on the evidence presented at the trial, such as expert witness testimony, AORN's recommended practices, and the

Figure 10.1

Nurse counting sponges.

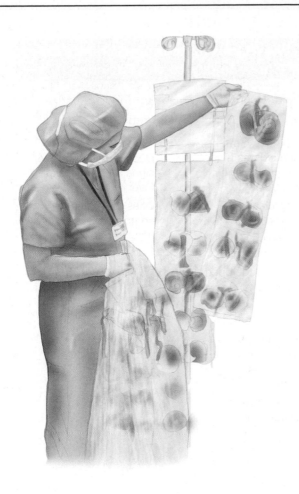

facility's policy. Retention of sponges, sharps, and instruments may result in a verdict of negligence against the nurse (Murphy, 1991). The following cases of retained foreign bodies were reported between the years of 2002 and 2003 (Murphy, 2004):

- A Babcock clamp was left in a patient after a gastric bypass;
- A sponge was left in a patient after a Cesarean section (**Fig. 10.1**);
- An instrument was left in a patient during a cholecystectomy; and
- An epicardial retractor was left in a patient's heart after a triple bypass surgery.

IDENTIFYING THE PATIENT'S RISK FOR ADVERSE OUTCOMES RELATED TO THE RETENTION OF EXTRANEOUS OBJECTS

Table 10.1 identifies the desired outcome for the patient care event of performing sponge, sharp, and instrument counts. Listed in the table are criteria for this outcome with the applicable nursing diagnosis, risk factors, and outcome indicators specific to the nursing diagnosis. Scrub and circulating nurses will find the information delineated in this table useful as they assess the patient for risk factors, plan care, and apply interventions to ensure that items are accounted for prior to wound closure.

10

Table 10.1	Performing Sponge, Sharp, and Instrument Counts Does Not Compromise or Cause Injury to the Patient
Outcome	The patient is free from evidence of signs and symptoms of injury caused by extraneous objects.

Diagnosis	Risk Factors	Outcome Indicators
Risk for Injury related to retained sponges, sharps, and instruments	☐ Emergency procedures that preclude counting sponges, sharps, and instruments ☐ Abdominal, retroperitoneal, and thoracic procedures ☐ Procedures in which a cavity within a cavity is entered ☐ Procedures with a large open wound or extensive operative area ☐ Patient obesity ☐ Hemorrhaging during the procedure necessitating the immediate use of a large number of sponges ☐ Procedure that involve the packing of cavities with sponges ☐ Change of nursing staff during the procedure ☐ Lenient institutional count policies and procedures	☐ Does the patient have signs and symptoms of fever? ☐ Does the patient complain of pain unrelated to incisional pain? ☐ Are there signs of intestinal obstruction? ☐ Are there signs of abscess formation? ☐ Do patient radiographs indicate the presence of a retained foreign body?

Adapted from Carpentino-Moyet, L. J. (2008). *Handbook of Nursing Diagnosis* (12th ed.). Philadelphia: Lippincott Williams & Wilkins; Petersen C. (2007). *Perioperative Nursing Data Set, the Perioperative Nursing Vocabulary.* (Revised 2nd ed.). Denver: AORN, Inc.

INITIATING COUNT PROCEDURES THAT REDUCE THE PATIENT'S RISK FOR RETAINED EXTRANEOUS OBJECTS

Counting Sponges

Sponges should be counted on all procedures in which the possibility exists that a sponge could be retained; sponges should be counted (AORN, 2008, p. 293):

- Before the beginning of the procedure to establish a baseline;
- Before closure of a cavity within a cavity;
- Before wound closure begins;
- At skin closure or the end of the procedure;
- At the time of permanent relief of either the scrub person or the circulating nurse; and
- When adding sponges to the sterile field.

The count should be performed by two individuals, and one of whom should be the registered nurse circulator. Count the sponges out loud, viewing each sponge as it is separated. Use only x-ray detectable sponges during the procedure. Count sponges in units of 5 or 10, depending on how they are packaged. Remove packages of sponges from the sterile field that contain more or less than the packaged number. Do not remove counted sponges from the operating room (OR) until the end of the procedure. Contaminated sponges must be handled and disposed of according to the Bloodborne Pathogens Standard of the Occupational Safety and Health Administration (OSHA) and in accordance with the facility's policies and procedures. Contaminated sponges should be placed in a leak-proof, tear-resistant container. Personnel handling contaminated sponges should use appropriate personal protective equipment (PPE).

OR
Operating Room

OSHA
Occupational Safety and Health Administration

PPE
Personal Protective Equipment

Counting Sharps

Sharps and other miscellaneous items should be counted on all procedures (AORN, 2008, p. 295). Sharps and miscellaneous items such as vessel clip bars, vessel loops, umbilical or hernia tapes, vascular inserts, cautery scratch pads, and trocar sealing caps should be counted (AORN, 2008):

- Before the beginning of the procedure to establish a baseline;
- Before closure of a cavity within a cavity;
- Before wound closure begins;
- At skin closure or the end of the procedure;
- At the time of permanent relief of the scrub person and/or circulating nurse; and
- When adding sharps to the sterile field.

The count should be performed by two individuals, one of whom should be the registered nurse circulator. Suture needles should be counted out loud with the scrub person and documented according to the number on the outer package. When the scrub person opens the package, the number of needles is verified. Do not remove counted sharps from the OR during the procedure. Use of a disposable puncture-resistant container on the sterile field ensures containment and decreases the risk of injury. When possible, sharps should be handed to and from the surgeon using a "neutral zone" or "hands-free" technique. These techniques help prevent injury to all members of the surgical team scrubbed at the sterile field. If sharps, suture needles, or other miscellaneous items break, all broken pieces must be accounted for to prevent unintentional retention of a foreign body in the patient (AORN, 2008, p. 296).

Counting Instruments

Instruments should be counted for all procedures in which the likelihood exists that an instrument could be retained; instruments should be counted (AORN, 2008, p. 296):

- Before the beginning of the procedure to establish a baseline;
- Before wound closure;
- When feasible, at the time of permanent relief of the scrub person and/or circulating nurse; and
- When adding instruments to the sterile field.

The count should be performed by two individuals, one of whom should be the registered nurse circulator. Instruments should be counted when they are assembled for sterilization and documented on an instrument count sheet. The initial instrument count is performed in the OR to establish a baseline for subsequent counts. If there are parts to an instrument such as pieces of a retractor (blades, wing nuts, etc.) they should be accounted for and documented on the count sheet. If an instrument is broken, the pieces of the instrument should be accounted for to avoid unintentional retention of a foreign body. Hospitals performing surgery on pediatric cases should determine when instruments counts should be performed (AORN, 2008, p. 297).

INITIATING INCORRECT COUNT PROCEDURES

In the event of an incorrect count, the surgical team does everything possible to locate the missing item. The following steps include, but are not limited to:

- Inform the surgeon and the surgical team of the discrepancy;
- Repeat the count;
- Search for the missing item by inspecting the operative site, surrounding sterile field including the Mayo stand, back table, floor, trash, and linen containers;
- If indicated in the facility's policies and procedures, request an x-ray before the patient is taken from the room (**Fig. 10.2**); and
- Document incorrect counts and actions taken according to the facility's policies and procedures.

DOCUMENTATION AND COMMUNICATION PROCEDURES

The registered nurse circulator and the scrub person should communicate regularly during the procedure about the status of sponges, sharps, and instruments. The surgeon must be notified of the results of the counts and acknowledge the results of the counts to the registered nurse circulator. Documentation of the results of the counts should be recorded in the patient's record according to the facility's policies and procedures using uniform perioperative nursing vocabulary. According to AORN's "Recommended Practices for Sponge, Sharp, and Instrument Counts," documentation should include, but not be limited to (AORN, 2008, p. 299):

- Types of counts (ie, sponge, sharps, instruments, miscellaneous items) and number of counts taken;
- The names and titles of the surgical team members performing the counts;

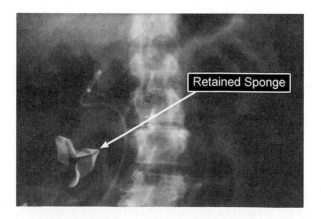

Figure 10.2

X-ray showing a retained radiopaque sponge.

Retained Sponge

- The results of the counts;
- Notification of the surgeon;
- Any instruments or sponges intentionally remaining with the patient;
- Actions taken in the event of discrepancies;
- Outcomes of actions taken;
- The rationale for not performing or finishing counts as outlined in policy.

The registered nurse circulator, as the responsible person, and the scrub person should sign the patient record as prescribed by the facility's policy.

CONCLUSION

Legislation does not require sponge, sharp, and instrument counts be performed, nor does legislation identify those who should do the counts. The law does require, however, that members of the surgical team do not negligently leave foreign bodies in patients. Follow the steps listed in this chapter and review the current AORN "Recommended Practices for Sponge, Sharp, and Instrument Counts." In doing so, you will greatly reduce the patient's risk for retained foreign bodies after an operative or invasive procedure. The surgical team members should view counts from the interdisciplinary perspective and collaborate in writing and follow sensible and safe count policies and procedures (AORN, 2008, p. 299).

COMPETENCY ASSESSMENT
Perform Sponge, Sharp, and Instrument Counts

Name: _____ Title: _____ Unit: _____ Date of Validation: _____

Type of Validation: ☐ Initial ☐ Annual ☐ Bi-annual

COMPETENCY STATEMENT: The nurse demonstrates competency to perform sponge, sharps, and instrument counts during the operative or invasive procedure.

Performance Criteria	Met	Not Met
1. Identifies the patient's risk for adverse outcomes related to the retention of extraneous objects	☐	☐
2. Initiates count procedures that reduce the patient's risk for retained extraneous objects	☐	☐
3. Initiates incorrect count procedures	☐	☐
4. Documents count procedures according to facility policy	☐	☐

_____   _____
Validator's Signature   Employee's Signature

_____
Validator's Printed Name

10

REFERENCES

1. Association of periOperative Registered Nurses. Recommended practices for sponge, sharp, and instrument counts. *Perioperative Standards and Recommended Practices.* Denver: AORN, Inc, 2008: pp. 293–302.

2. Murphy, E.K. (1991). OR nursing law: Counts, documentation revisited. *AORN Journal;* 54(4): p. 878.

3. Murphy, E.K. (2004). OR nursing law: Protecting patients from potential injuries. *AORN Journal,* 79(5): pp. 1014–1015.

4. PNDS. Extraneous objects. *Perioperative Nursing Data Set: The Perioperative Nursing Vocabulary.* Denver; AORN, Inc, 2007: pp. 31–37.

5. The conceptual framework of the PNDS. In *Perioperative Nursing Data Set; the Perioperative Nursing Vocabulary:* (Denver: AORN, Inc, 2007), 19, 25.

CHAPTER 11

Provide Instruments, Equipment, and Supplies

Darin M. Prescott

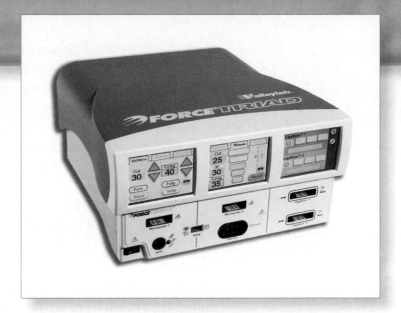

INTRODUCTION

Emerging technologies continue to raise the bar of operative and invasive procedure care and challenges the nursing care team to be knowledgeable of instruments, equipment and supplies. This chapter describes the competencies necessary for the nurse to safely and efficiently provide these items before, during, and after operative and invasive procedures.

After identifying the patient's risk for adverse outcomes related to the provision of instruments, equipment, and supplies, the nurse may delegate appropriate tasks to qualified surgical technologists or assistive personnel. The nurse is responsible for knowing that surgical technologists and assistive personnel are competent to perform the task that is being delegated and the nurse must provide appropriate supervision.

MEASURABLE CRITERIA

The nurse demonstrates competency to safely and efficiently provide instruments, equipment, and supplies by:

- Identifying the patient's risk for adverse outcomes related to the provision of instruments, equipment and supplies;
- Selecting appropriate instrumentation, equipment, and supplies for an operative or invasive procedure;
- Delivering instruments and supplies to the sterile field;
- Arranging instruments and supplies on the back table and Mayo tray;
- Passing instruments and supplies to the physician or assistant;
- Preparing and passing sutures to the physician or assistant;
- Preparing and applying patient warming systems;

Chapter Contents

- Applying and removing a pneumatic tourniquet;
- Preparing electrical instrumentation and equipment for use;
- Preparing air-powered instrumentation for use;
- Implementing electrosurgical safety precautions;
- Applying dressings;
- Assisting with the application of casts and splints; and
- Preparing and operating endoscopic equipment.

IDENTIFYING THE PATIENT'S RISK FOR ADVERSE OUTCOMES RELATED TO THE PROVISION OF INSTRUMENTS, EQUIPMENT AND SUPPLIES

Providing instruments, equipment, and supplies has the potential for compromising or causing injury to the patient. If done incorrectly the patient could experience infection, extended anesthesia time, alterations in body temperature, thermal injury secondary to use of a warming device, injury related to tourniquet use, injury related to the application of electrosurgery, and injury related to the inappropriate use of endoscopic video equipment. **Table 11.1** identifies outcome statement, diagnosis, risk factors, and outcome indicators related to this patient care event.

Table 11.1	Providing Instruments, Equipment, and Supplies Does Not Compromise or Cause Injury to the Patient

Outcome 1   The patient is free from evidence of infection.

Diagnosis	Risk Factors	Outcome Indicators
Risk for Infection.	☐ Remote site of infection	☐ Does the patient have a wound infection?
	☐ Abdominal of thoracic operative procedure	☐ Does the patient have a urinary tract infection?
	☐ Procedure lasting longer than 2 hours	☐ Does the patient have an upper respiratory infection?
	☐ Transected organ systems such as the gastrointestinal or urological system	
	☐ Instrumentation/presence of devices (ventilator, suction, catheters, nebulizers, tracheostomy, invasive monitoring)	
	☐ Implants	
	☐ Anesthesia	
	☐ Age (less than 1 year or more than 65 years)	
	☐ Underlying disease conditions (chronic obstructive pulmonary disease, diabetes, cardiovascular blood dyscrasia)	
	☐ Substance abuse	
	☐ Medications (steroids, chemotherapy, antibiotics) than modify the immune system	
	☐ Nutritional status (intake less than minimum daily requirements or more than minimum daily requirements)	
	☐ Smoker	
	☐ Compromise of the immune system	
	☐ High white blood cell count, low platelet count, and anemia	

- [ ] Impaired skin and tissue integrity
- [ ] Failure of sterilization or disinfection process
- [ ] Nonadherence to aseptic technique
- [ ] Failure of environmental sanitation processes

Outcome 2   The patient is free from evidence of injury resulting from an extended anesthesia time.

Diagnosis	**Risk Factors**	**Outcome Indicators**
Risk for Injury related to extended anesthesia time	<ul><li>[ ] Inaccurate and outdated physician preference cards</li><li>[ ] Inadequate inventory of necessary supplies and implants</li><li>[ ] Equipment not procured or checked for function before induction of anesthesia</li><li>[ ] Instruments not preprocessed and sterilized in a timely manner</li><li>[ ] Inaccurate checking of case carts or inventories</li></ul>	<ul><li>[ ] Was anesthesia time extended because instruments, equipment, or supplies were not available?</li><li>[ ] Was anesthesia time extended because instruments, equipment, or supplies were not functioning properly?</li></ul>

Outcome 3   The patient's body temperature is maintained within normal limits during the operative or invasive procedure.

Diagnosis	**Risk Factors**	**Outcome Indicators**
Risk for Hypothermia	<ul><li>[ ] Cold operating room</li><li>[ ] General and regional anesthesia</li><li>[ ] Undergoing an operative or invasive procedure</li><li>[ ] Cool skin preparations</li><li>[ ] Use of unwarmed infusion or irrigating solutions</li><li>[ ] Operative exposure of the abdominal or thoracic cavities</li><li>[ ] Preexisting medical conditions (eg, hypothyroid or hyperthyroid problems)</li><li>[ ] Extremes in age, particularly infants, small children, and geriatric patients</li><li>[ ] Decreased body fat for insulation</li><li>[ ] Malnourishment</li><li>[ ] Debilitation or chronic illness</li><li>[ ] Anticipated long operative or invasive procedure time</li><li>[ ] Intracranial procedure</li><li>[ ] Multiple trauma injuries</li><li>[ ] Hypovolemia</li><li>[ ] Rapid insufflation of cold CO_2 gas to create pneumoperitoneum</li></ul>	<ul><li>[ ] Does the patient have a core body temperature of less than 96.8°F (36°C)?</li><li>[ ] Does the conscious patient complain of feeling uncomfortably cold?</li><li>[ ] Is the patient shivering during the procedure?</li><li>[ ] Does the patient's skin feel cool, have pallor, or have piloerection?</li><li>[ ] Does the patient have decreased pulse and respiration rates?</li></ul>

Outcome 4   The patient is free from evidence of injury related to the use of a pneumatic tourniquet.

Diagnosis	**Risk Factors**	**Outcome Indicators**
Risk for Injury related to the use of a pneumatic tourniquet.	<ul><li>[ ] Improper cuff size</li><li>[ ] Inadequate or wrinkled padding</li><li>[ ] Improper cuff positioning</li><li>[ ] Cuff rotation after positioning</li></ul>	<ul><li>[ ] Does the patient have bruising, blistering, pinching, or necrosis of skin?</li><li>[ ] Are there skin abrasions or welling?</li></ul>

11

☐ Pooling of prep solutions under the cuff	☐ Does the patient have signs indicating a chemical skin burn?
☐ Excessive cuff pressure	
☐ Excessive cuff inflation time	☐ Does the patient have signs indicating paralysis or other signs of nerve damage?

Outcome 5   The patient is free from evidence of injury related to the application of electrosurgery.

Diagnosis	Risk Factors	Outcomes Indicators
Risk for Injury related to electrosurgery	☐ Excessive hair at the patient return electrode site ☐ Scar tissue at the patient return electrode site ☐ Internal or external prosthetic device at the patient return electrode site ☐ Impaired skin or tissue integrity at the patient return electrode site ☐ Presence of a pacemaker or an automatic implantable cardioverter-defibrillator (ACID) ☐ Obesity ☐ Emaciation ☐ Use of a ground reference generator ☐ Use of an isolated generator *not* equipped with a contact quality monitoring system ☐ Procedure done in the presences of an oxygen-enriched environment ☐ Use of a flammable prepping agent ☐ Coiling, clamping, or twisting of active and patient return electrode cords ☐ Failure to use a non-conductive safety holster ☐ Contact of a electrode shaft (suction coagulator, electrode extensive) with adjacent tissue during activation	☐ Is there evidence of impaired skin integrity at the patient return electrode site? Is the skin discolored? Does the skin appear to have an allergic reaction to the patient return electrode conductive adhesive? ☐ Does the patient show evidence of postprocedure skin and tissue disruption/destruction at the patient return electrode site or at alternate pathway sites? ☐ Was there an ignition incident during the operative or invasive procedure? ☐ Does the patient fail to make reasonable progress after a laparoscopic procedure? Are there signs of fever? ☐ Does the patient complain of abdominal pain?

Adapted from Carpentino-Moyet, L. J. (2008). *Handbook of Nursing Diagnosis* (12th ed.) Philadelphia: Lippincott Williams & Wilkins; Ulmer, B. C. (2008). *Electrosurgery Self-Study Guide.* Boulder, CO: Covidien.

SELECTING INSTRUMENTATION, EQUIPMENT, AND SUPPLIES FOR AN OPERATIVE OR INVASIVE PROCEDURE

Selecting instruments, equipment, and supplies for an operative or invasive procedure requires knowledge of the procedure, physician preferences, facility protocols, and patient needs. Organization is paramount to the effective execution of the provision for instrumentation, equipment, and supplies. Without organization, delays may cause complications and untoward outcomes for the patient. Also, delays may result in extended anesthesia time, which has the potential of adversely affecting the cardiac, respiratory, neurological, and integumentary systems. Providing instrumentation, equipment, and supplies that are prepared for use and functioning appropriately will decrease the risk Sof extended anesthesia time.

Operative and invasive procedure team members, including sterile processing personnel, assemble instrument sets, or trays. Most operative and invasive procedure departments possess a standard tray of basic instrumentation used on many cases (eg, minor or major set). Additional specialty sets are also assembled specific to physician preference and case needs (eg, basic orthopedic or laparoscopy tray).

All sterile items should be packaged according to AORN *Recommended Practices for Selection and Use of Packaging Systems for Sterilization* and applicable manufacturer packaging Instructions for Use (IFUs) specific to the method of sterilization.

When gathering instruments and supplies for a procedure check the packaging for signs of moisture, compromise of package integrity, such as pinhole and tears, and for the presence of sterilization indicators. Do not use items if a defect in packaging is found. Sterility indicators verify that the parameters of sterilization were met. If sterilization cannot be verified discard the item or return it for re-sterilization. Adhere to outdates listed on the item packaging. For most items shelf life of sterile packaged items is event related (AORN, 2008). Some items, however, particularly commercially prepared items, are made from materials that may degrade over time; thus they are stamped with an expiration date. If the item is outdated, do not use it.

Return items not immediately used during setup of a sterile field to the appropriate location. Because patient charges may be generated by items used, the nurse has an ethical responsibility for making the appropriate adjustments to the patient charge record.

IFUs
Instructions for Use

DELIVERING INSTRUMENTS AND SUPPLIES TO THE STERILE FIELD

General Guidelines

Persons establishing or working in the presence of a sterile field should wear caps, gloves, and masks. In addition, persons functioning in the scrub role working in a sterile field should also wear a sterile gowns and gloves (AORN, 2008). Prior to opening a sterile item, check items for signs of moisture, appropriate packaging and processing, seal integrity, compromise of packaging material, expiration dates (if applicable), and the presence of indicators that sterilization parameters have or have not been met. Any defects found render the package contaminated and indicate that it should not be used as part of the sterile setup. Establish sterile fields with sterile drapes that are impervious to fluids and resistant to tears or holes.

Once the sterile field is established, do not bring items below the level of the field up to the level of the sterile field. Additionally, unsterile personnel should not reach over sterile fields. Any items that are dropped on the floor should be considered contaminated and not used.

Wrapped Items

Break the indicator tape on wrapped items. Position the package to open the flap furthest away from your body. Proceed opening the second and third flaps to the right and left. Open the last flap toward you without passing over the sterile exposed item. The edge of the wrapper is considered contaminated, thus secure wrapper edges to prevent contamination from edges touching the sterile item. Place the item on the sterile field or hand to the scrubbed person. Follow facility policy with regard to whether the inner wrapper of double-wrapped items is opened when being delivered to the sterile field. Open large, bulky, or heavy items on a separate surface, such as a table or Mayo stand, or hand the item directly to the scrubbed person (AORN, 2008).

Peel Packaged Items

Open peel packaged items by peeling the edges apart. Present the item to the scrubbed person. The item is then removed by the scrubbed person lifting it upward from the package, or it is flipped onto the sterile field. The contents must not touch the inner sealed surfaces of the package during opening or removal. In the event this happens, consider the contents contaminated.

Rigid Container Systems

Rigid container systems offer an opportunity to reduce the amount of waste generated from disposable wrapped items. Use rigid container systems according to manufacturer's IFUs. Manufacturer chemical indicators located on the outside of the rigid container must be turned to the appropriate color. If the indicator has not turned, consider the contents contaminated and return for reprocessing. Place the rigid container on a flat surface such as a table or Mayo stand. Be mindful of the tray weight with regard to the surface in which it is placed. Place the container in a position where the inner contents can be removed by the scrubbed person without compromising sterility. Remove the lid by lifting it straight up and away from the container. The scrubbed person removes the contents without touching the outer sides of the container. The filter placement and effectiveness should be evaluated during assembly and when opening the sterilized container. Consider damaged, dislodged, or damp filters contaminated and return the container and its contents for reprocessing.

Solutions

Place solution receptacles near the edge of the sterile field or have the scrubbed person hold the receptacle. Pour solutions slowly to avoid splashing. Do not fill receptacles to the top; this will reduce the potential for splashing and the spilling of solution over the side of the receptacle. The edge of the fluid container is considered contaminated after the cap has been removed and should not touch the receptacle. Containers should not be held directly over the receptacle during pouring. The scrub person labels the receptacle according to facility policy. Any remaining fluid in the container should be considered contaminated and discarded.

ARRANGING INSTRUMENTS AND SUPPLIES ON THE INSTRUMENT TABLE AND MAYO TRAY

General Guidelines

Check chemical indicators or integrators on all items prior to transfer to the back table. If the indicator or integrator has not changed or is missing, consider all contents of the tray or package unsterile. In this event, it is necessary to re-gown and re-glove.

The following guidelines provide an example of organizing a back table and a Mayo tray. Depending on the number of instruments and equipment required, the scrub person may need more instruments and equipment than can be contained on back table and Mayo tray. In such cases additional back tables and Mayo trays may be required. To facilitate the continuity of care during staff changes, all specialties should have standard back table and Mayo tray setups. Facility policies and procedures should include orientation to this standard (**Fig. 11.1** and **11.2**). Setups may be specialty specific and altered according to the procedure.

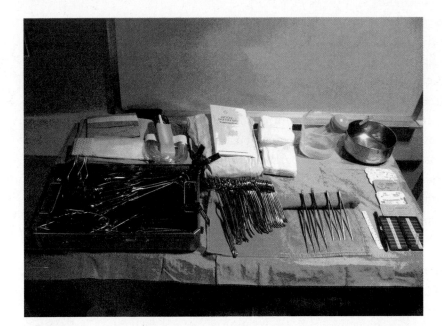

Figure 11.1
Back table setup.

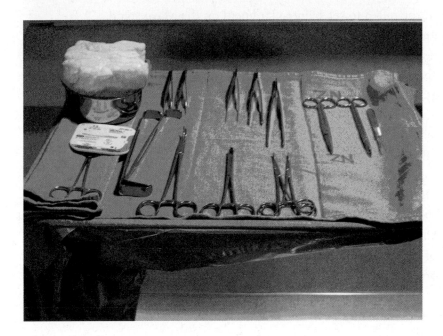

Figure 11.2
Mayo tray setup.

Back Table

One or more back tables may be set up, depending on the number of instruments required for the procedure. If scrubbed, mentally divide the back table into four quadrants and stand next to the left and right lower quadrants. Place instruments and supplies by frequency and order of use, and in close proximity for easy retrieval. Items that are used infrequently, such as drapes and gowns, are placed in the left upper quadrant of the table. Stack drapes, gowns and gloves in the order of use. Frequently used items are placed in the right rear and front quadrants. Set a large basin of saline or sterile water in the upper right quadrant of the back table. Put counted sponges near this basin.

11

Using **Figure 11.1** as an example, remove stringed instruments from the instrument pan and place on a rolled towel in the front quadrants of the back table. Close towel clips and box locks to prevent accidental puncture of gloves and injury. Arrange retractors in order of use and size in the lower left quadrant of the back table. Organize tissue and dressing forceps according to type and size to the right of the hinged instruments. Arrange sutures according to use and type on the right lower quadrant of the table. Place an emesis basin in the lower right quadrant. Use the emesis basin for specimens, separating sharp instrumentation or collecting small trash items and tissue. Place the irrigation pitcher at the back of the instruments. Attach the suction tip to the tubing and the appropriate electrode tip to the electrosurgical pencil.

Mayo Tray

Selection of the appropriate size Mayo stand depends on the type of case, amount and weight of instrumentation to be needed at the field. Cover the Mayo stand with a sterile drape.

Initial sponge, sharps and instrument counts are performed while instrument sets are together on the rolled towel, before placement on the Mayo stand.

Arrange suture ties on the covered Mayo stand using a drape or towel to separate the suture types. This may be accomplished by either draping a towel over the ties and tucking it under the Mayo tray or placing a fan-folded suture towel to the back of the Mayo tray (**Fig. 11.2**) for the absorbable ties. Place them in order by gauge and type.

Arrange clamps and hemostats according to order of use on a rolled towel or on the edge of the tray.

Load the scalpel blades on the knife handles by holding the scalpel handle in your non-dominant hand. With your dominant hand, grasp the blade on the dull edge with a needle holder at its widest point, avoiding the cutting edge. Point the blade and handle down and away from you and slide the blade into the handle groove until it is secured. Place loaded scalpels in the lower right quadrant or other established neutral zone of the Mayo tray with the blade facing away from you.

Place scissors between the scalpels and the tissue forceps. Arrange forceps by size and order of use. Use a small basin or folded towel to hold moistened, counted laparotomy sponges.

PASSING INSTRUMENTS AND SUPPLIES TO THE PHYSICIAN

Use the hands-free technique to pass scalpels, needles or other sharp instruments to reduce the risk for injury. When using this technique, set sharp items or needle holders down in a designated neutral zone on the sterile field (AORN, 2008). Pass tissue forceps and ringed or box-locked instruments in the position of function. Assemble retractors prior to handing to the physician or assistant. When passing a retractor, pass it handle first.

Place sponges close to the operative site. Moisten and wring out sponges as requested by the physician. Moisten sponges for the abdominal or thoracic cavity with warm sterile saline. During the procedure, keep these sponges moist. Dried sponges create a fire hazard in the presence of an ignition source such as electrosurgery. Pass Kittner dissector sponges held in a Kelly clamp or Rochester-Pean forceps and stick sponges on a sponge forceps. Pass instruments by gently snapping them into the hand of the physician or assistant. As soon as the physician or assistant has a firm grip, release the instrument.

PREPARING AND PASSING SUTURES TO THE PHYSICIAN

Nonabsorbable Suture

Nonabsorbable sutures are strands of material that effectively resist enzymatic deterioration in living tissue. Tear the suture pack at the notch and remove the suture strands from the package as a unit. Unfold the strands of suture to its full length. Avoid pulling silk suture between gloved fingers. This technique prevents the buildup of static electricity in the suture. Place the strands under the towel on the Mayo tray according to type and size.

Absorbable Suture

Absorbable sutures are digested by body tissues during the healing process. Surgical gut is packaged in an alcohol solution. Carefully tear the foil package to prevent fluid from dripping onto the sterile field. Place the center of the suture over two fingers of your nondominant hand and unwind it to half length. Gently pull to straighten the suture. Fold and cut the suture into equal segments if necessary. Place the strands under the towel on the Mayo tray according to type and size.

Free Tie

Hold both ends of the suture securely with one end in each hand. Press the tie firmly into the palm of the physician or assistant. Release the suture as physician or assistant closed his or her hand.

Tie to Pass Ligature

Place the tip of the suture strand into the tip of a tonsil, Schnidt, or right-angled-clamp and lock the clamp. Hold the box lock of the clamp between the thumb and the index finger. Snap the rings of the clamp into the hand of the physician or assistant so that the tip of the clamp points toward the center of his or her body.

PREPARING AND APPLYING PATIENT WARMING SYSTEMS

General Guidelines

Patient hypothermia is defined as a core temperature of 36°C (96.8°F) or less (Cooper, 2006). The first line of defense is maintaining an environmental temperature between 20°C (68°F) and 22.2°C (72°F). Forced-air warming for 15 minutes before the procedure can also prevent hypothermia by maintaining the core body temperature as much as two hours post-anesthesia.

Follow the manufacturer's IFUs when selecting, applying, and using warming devices. Select the appropriate type of device based on patient size and body area to be covered. Prior to applying the warming device assess the patient's skin integrity and temperature. While the warming device is in use periodically assess the patient due to the risk of thermal burns.

Preparing the Convective Air Warming System

Convective air warming systems transfer heat to the patient by blowing warm air through micro-perforation on the underside of a lightweight blanket that covers the patient. The warming blanket warms the air surrounding the patient without making the room uncomfortable for the operative team. Convective warming devices should be used with caution on patients with compromised vascular perfusion.

Thermal injuries are possible with the use of convective air warming systems and adverse outcomes have been reported when blankets were used without being attached to the hose. This practice is called *free-hosing* and, when done, allows warm air to blow directly onto the patient. Reports of injuries include 2nd- and 3rd-degree burns to the lower extremities and muscle necrosis secondary to a lower leg burn to the lower leg, which eventually lead to an above-the-knee amputation (Marders, 2008).

Preparing the Hyperthermia or Hypothermia Unit for Use

Hypothermia or hyperthermia units and blankets are used to maintain, increase, or decrease the patient's temperature. Before using these units, ensure that the fluid reservoir is filled according to the manufacturer's IFUs. Check controls for proper functioning prior to use.

Inspect the blanket surfaces and tubing for holes and kinks before placing the blanket on the bed. Attach the blanket tubing to the hypothermia or hyperthermia unit. Set the controls to the desired heating or cooling temperature and activate the unit. As the unit pumps fluid through the tubing and blanket, check for leaks. Prevent folds and creases in the blanket, which hinder the proper filling of fluid through the blanket and may cause hot or cold spots on the blanket's surface. Thermal burns or pressure necrosis may occur with a hyperthermia or hypothermia blanket; therefore, unless the blanket is designed for direct skin contact, cover the blanket with an absorbable pad or sheet. During use, periodically check that the unit is functioning properly. Feel for excessive heat or cold radiating from the tubing and the blanket. Continue to monitor the temperature controls.

APPLYING AND REMOVING A PNEUMATIC TOURNIQUET

General Guidelines

Pneumatic tourniquets are used to assist in providing a bloodless field on procedures involving the extremities. Pneumatic tourniquet equipment includes a pressure source, pressure gauge, regulator, tubing, connectors and an inflatable cuff. Follow the manufacturer's IFUs for inspecting, testing, applying, and operating the pneumatic tourniquet. Before use, inspect and test the tourniquet. When checking the tourniquet system, verify cleanliness, and look for defects, such as cracks or holes in the tubing. This should be done before and after each use. Also, ensure that the inner tube of the cuff is completely encased in the tourniquet sleeve (AORN, 2008).

Selecting the Tourniquet Cuff

Assess the patient for extremity size and then select a cuff that overlaps the ends by at least three, but no more than six, inches (7.6- to 15-cm). A wide bladder occludes blood flow at a lower pressure. Additional overlap may cause increased pressure and potential rolling or wrinkling of the soft tissue (AORN, 2008).

Applying the Tourniquet Cuff

Apply wrinkle-free, non-shedding, soft padding or a limb-protection sleeve prior to placing the tourniquet. Padding should protect the skin under the cuff from mechanical injury. Select a location that has adequate muscle mass, which will help protect nerves and blood vessels. **Table 11.2** describes correct placement of the tourniquet for the upper and lower extremities. Exercise caution when placing the cuff below the elbow or knee. The thin layer of soft tissue between underlying bones and the cuff may not be sufficient to protect the nerves and blood vessels. Avoid an incomplete or overly aggressive seal of the cuff. Improper cuff seals may cause bruising, blistering, pinching, or necrosis of the skin. Secure the tourniquet by tying the cuff strings in a bow. Avoid tying in a knot to expedite removal. Plan cuff placement to facilitate the connections being placed in the optimal location based on position and tourniquet location. Avoid rotating the cuff after the tourniquet is applied. Cuff rotation potentially causes shearing forces which may result in skin injury (AORN, 2008).

Preparing and Draping the Extremity After Tourniquet Application

Apply an impervious barrier around the extremity prior to skin preparation. Pooling of antimicrobial solutions with the subsequent pressure of the inflated cuff may result in chemical burns. If preparation solutions seep under the cuff, remove the cuff and wet padding, use a moist cloth to remove the prepping solution from the extremity, dry the extremity, and reapply the padding and cuff. During draping, ensure that the scrubbed team members do not puncture the cuff. Do not use piercing towel clips. Holes may not immediately affect cuff inflation; however, cuff effectiveness could be diminished and hemostasis potentially compromised.

Table 11.2	Applying the Tourniquet
Upper arm and thigh	Place on the limb at the point of maximum circumference proximal to the incision.
Forearm	Place mid-forearm.
Calf	Place with proximal edge on the largest area of calf circumference.
Ankle	Place over the lower third of the low leg, with the distal edge proximal to the malleoli.

Adapted from: AORN (2008). Recommended Practices for the Use of the Pneumatic Tourniquet in the Perioperative Practice Setting. *Perioperative Standards and Recommended Practices*. Denver, CO: AORN, p. 486.

Preparing the Limb for Tourniquet Inflation

The physician or assistant may tightly wrap the extremity with a 4- to 6-inch (10- to 15-cm) Esmarch or elastic bandage before inflating the tourniquet cuff. This action compresses the veins and drains the blood from the limb. Starting with the most distal part of the limb, the physician or assistant elevates and tightly wraps the limb toward the cuff. The limb is unwrapped by reversing the procedure and rewinding the bandage, which is saved for later use.

Inflating the Tourniquet

LOP
Limb Occlusion
Pressure

Base the tourniquet pressure setting on *limb occlusion pressure* (LOP), which is the "unique cuff pressure required to occlude arterial flow in the limb" (AORN, 2008, p. 493). Occlusion can be achieved using lower pressure when using the LOP method. The application of lower pressures results in less pain after the procedure. **Table 11.3** describes how to manually use LOP method for inflating the tourniquet. Tourniquet systems are available that automatically determine LOP and allow for fluctuations in blood pressure during the procedure. **Figure 11.3** shows a manual LOP measurement with a Doppler stethoscope and lower leg cuff.

Inflate the tourniquet rapidly. This will occlude "the arteries and veins almost simultaneously, preventing filling of superficial veins before occlusion of arterial blood flow" (AORN, 2008, p. 488).

Monitoring the Tourniquet during the Procedure

Ensure that the operating screen and gauges are visible to the staff caring for the patient. Monitor the cuff at regular intervals for pressure fluctuations. Excessive or insufficient tourniquet pressure may cause nerve damage. Hemorrhagic infiltration of extremity nerves secondary to passive venous congestion of the limb is another complication of insufficient tourniquet pressure. Tourniquet inflation time should be kept to a minimum to prevent paralysis. Less than one hour is the recommended maximum inflation time for an upper extremity and less than two hours for a lower extremity. A period of five minutes for every thirty minutes of tourniquet application is the recommended time for reperfusion (AORN, 2008).

Documentation of Nursing Interventions Related to Tourniquet Use

Table 11.4 provides guidelines for documenting pneumatic tourniquet use.

PREPARING POWERED INSTRUMENTS FOR USE
General Guidelines

The use of powered instrumentation within the operative and invasive procedure setting has eliminated the need for many hand-operated instruments; in turn reducing the time required for the procedure. Hazards of using powered instrumentation include possible injury to the patient or to the operative team, possible contamination of the sterile field, and possible exposure of the operative team to aerosolized blood and body fluids. Inspect, test, and use powered instruments according to manufacturer's IFUs (AORN, 2008).

Worn or damaged air hoses pose a hazard to personnel and can cause delays in the procedure. Meticulously inspect hoses before using air-powered instruments.

Table 11.3	Determining Limb Occlusion Pressure (LOP)

General Guidelines

1. Make LOP measurement after the blood pressure has been stabilized to the level expected during the procedure

   ☐ Measure before or after induction of anesthesia

   ☐ Document the blood pressure at the time of LOP measurement

2. Confirm the LOP and pressure setting with the physician

Procedure

1. Apply the tourniquet cuff over the limb protection material

2. Use a Doppler stethoscope to locate the arterial pulse distal to the cuff

   ☐ Radial artery for the arm

   ☐ Posterior tibial artery or dorsalis pedis artery for the leg

3. Increase cuff pressure slowly until the arterial pulse stops and remains stopped for several heartbeats

4. Note the cuff pressure, which is the LOP

5. Deflate the cuff and assess the limb for the return of the distal pulse

6. Adjust the cuff pressure setting by adding a safety margin to the LOP before inflating the cuff

   ☐ Add 40 mm Hg for LOP less than 130 mm Hg

   ☐ Add 60 mm Hg for LOP between 131–190 mm Hg

   ☐ Add 80 mm Hg for LOP greater than 190 mm Hg

   ☐ For pediatric patients add 50 mm Hg

Adapted from: AORN (2008). Recommended Practices for the Use of the Pneumatic Tourniquet in the Perioperative Practice Setting. *Perioperative Standards and Recommended Practices.* Denver, CO: AORN, p. 487.

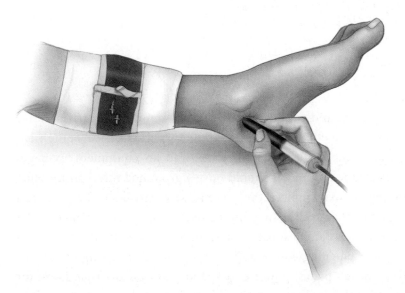

Figure 11.3

A manual LOP measurement with a Doppler stethoscope and lower leg cuff.

11

Table 11.4	Guidelines for Documenting Pneumatic Tourniquet Use

- ☐ Pneumatic tourniquet system identification serial number;
- ☐ Calibrations;
- ☐ Cuff pressure;
- ☐ Skin protection (stockinet, gel lining, cast padding);
- ☐ Location of tourniquet;
- ☐ Skin and tissue integrity under the cuff before and after use of the pneumatic tourniquet;
- ☐ Person placing tourniquet cuff; and
- ☐ Assessment and evaluation of the entire extremity.

Adapted from: AORN (2008). Recommended Practices for the Use of the Pneumatic Tourniquet in the Perioperative Practice Setting. *Perioperative Standards and Recommended Practices.* Denver, CO: AORN, p. 484.

Secure air hoses on the sterile field to avoid contamination. Do not use perforating towel clips, as a puncture to the hose could be dangerous to the patient and operative and invasive procedure team. Securely connect attachments to the handpiece before activating the device. This will prevent the attachment from being thrown from the handpiece, resulting in possible injury to the patient or personnel. Place triggers in the safety position when not in use.

Use medical-grade compressed air or compressed dry nitrogen (99.97% pure) for air-powered instruments. Check the manufacturer's IFUs for the recommended psi for operating the instrument. Check tank pressure prior to use. At least 1000 psi should register on the pressure gauge. Set psi while the instrument is running or as described by the manufacturer's IFUs. Do not exceed the recommended psi setting because excessive gas pressure can damage the air-powered instruments and place a great amount of stress on the hose (AORN, 2008). Also, when the instrument is sluggish or erratic, do not automatically exceed the recommended psi setting. In such cases, check the instrument for proper functioning.

PREPARING ELECTRICAL INSTRUMENTATION AND EQUIPMENT FOR USE

General Precautions

Electrical instrumentation and equipment are used commonly during operative and invasive procedures. Biomedical personnel should inspect electrical equipment before initial use within the institution and enter into an equipment management program. All electrical equipment should have a grounded three-prong plug. Non-grounded equipment may subject the patient to microshock. Prepare and operate electrical equipment according to manufacturer's IFUs (AORN, 2008). Affix attachments to the instrument and test before use. Place equipment on/off switches in the off position when plugging equipment in to an outlet or changing attachments. Check outlets, switch plates, power cords, and plugs for damage. Look for fraying on the cord and at the cord and plug interface. Damaged cords may result in injury to patients and the operative and invasive procedure team. Place power cords in a position that minimizes risk of tripping hazard or inadvertent unplugging.

Electrical Powered Instruments

Similar cautions apply as described with air-powered instrumentation; the difference being that electrical current is the power source of this instrumentation. Avoid placing controls near water. If water comes in contact with electrical powered instruments, biomedical personnel should inspect the equipment for damage prior to its continued use. Electrical contacts should be inspected; clean, dry, and free of corrosion.

Battery Powered Instruments

Cordless powered instruments are easier to handle than corded instruments and decrease the chance of contamination of the sterile field. Sterile batteries are used for these types of instruments. Ensure that an adequate number of fully charged sterile batteries are available to run the equipment and to provide backup. Follow the manufacturer's IFUs for care, charging and sterilization of the batteries. After repeated use, batteries gradually lose the ability to hold a charge and must be replaced. Follow facility policies when recycling or disposing of batteries.

IMPLEMENTING ELECTROSURGICAL SAFETY PRECAUTIONS

Electrosurgery is common to most operative and invasive procedures whenever there is a need to cut or coagulate tissue. Operative and invasive procedure team members should possess comprehensive knowledge in the safe use of electrosurgery technology. The electrosurgical unit (ESU) comes in basic models (**Fig. 11.4**) to integrated technology models (**Fig. 11.5**). Potential patient injuries can include:

ESU
Electrosurgical Unit

- patient return electrode burns
- alternate electrical pathway site injuries
- unintended burns at the active electrode site
- tissue injuries caused by insulation failure, capacitive coupling, or direct coupling during laparoscopic procedures
- tissue injuries caused by stray radiofrequency current
- injury caused by an ignition incident

See Chapter 17 for additional information about electrosurgery technologies and the use of electrosurgery during an operative or invasive procedure.

Bipolar Electrosurgery

Bipolar electrosurgery units use alternating electrical current. The active electrode and return electrode functions are performed at the site of surgery. Only the tissue grasped is included in the electrical circuit. Bipolar instruments are available in many different configurations (**Fig. 11.6**). Because the electrical current only travels through the tissue grasped between the tines of the bipolar forceps, voltages are lower. There is no need to use a patient return electrode when using bipolar.

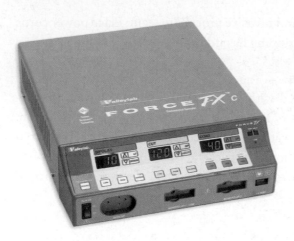

Figure 11.4

Force FX™ C Electrosurgical Generator with Instant Response™.

Source: Copyright © Covidien. All rights reserved. Reprinted with the permission of the Energy-based Devices and Surgical Devices divisions of Covidien.

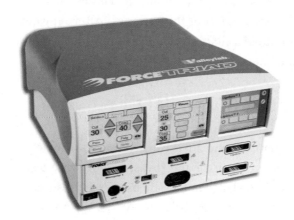

Figure 11.5

Force Triad™ Energy Platform with TissueFect Sensing Technology.

Source: Copyright © Covidien. All rights reserved. Reprinted with the permission of the Energy-based Devices and Surgical Devices divisions of Covidien.

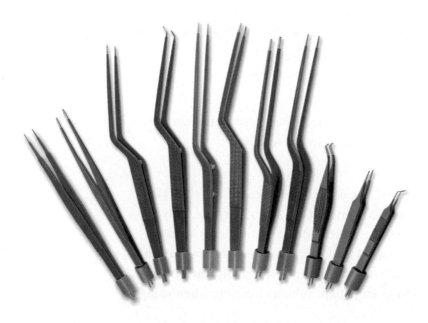

Figure 11.6

Bipolar electrosurgery forceps.

Source: Copyright © Covidien. All rights reserved. Reprinted with the permission of the Energy-based Devices and Surgical Devices divisions of Covidien.

Monopolar Electrosurgery

The most frequently used type of electrosurgery is monopolar because it has a greater range of tissue effects and it is more powerful. When using monopolar electrosurgery the generator produces the current, which travels through an active electrode into patient tissue. The current is collected by a patient return electrode which carries it safely back to the generator. That is the intended pathway for the electrical current flow. The type of monopolar generator used, along with appropriate physician and nursing interventions, can help assure that this is the path the current takes.

Electrosurgical Accessories

The generator only makes up 25% of the electrosurgical system. The remaining 75% of the system includes the pencil, the patient return electrode, and the user. Nurses and physicians should be knowledgeable about electrosurgical accessories and their safe and effective use (Ulmer, 2007).

Active Electrodes

The active electrode delivers concentrated electrical current to patient tissues. Many types of active electrodes are available for use with both bipolar and monopolar electrosurgery, including needles, blades, balls, and loops (**Fig. 11.7**). Electrosurgery pencils (**Fig. 11.8**) or forceps may be controlled by hand switches or by foot pedals. Active electrodes are available for laparoscopic use, and some active electrodes combine suction and coagulation in the same handpiece (**Fig. 11.9**).

A potential hazard associated with the active electrode tip is buildup of eschar on the tip. Eschar buildup increases the resistance to electrical flow through the tip,

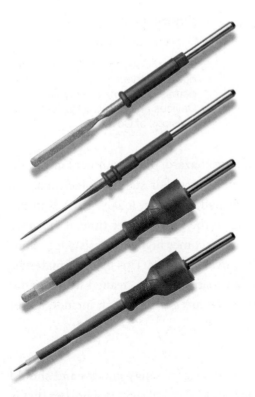

Figure 11.7

Valleylab EDGE electrodes (blade, needle, insulated blade, and insulated needle).

Source: Copyright © Covidien. All rights reserved. Reprinted with the permission of the Energy-Based Devices and Surgical Devices divisions of Covidien.

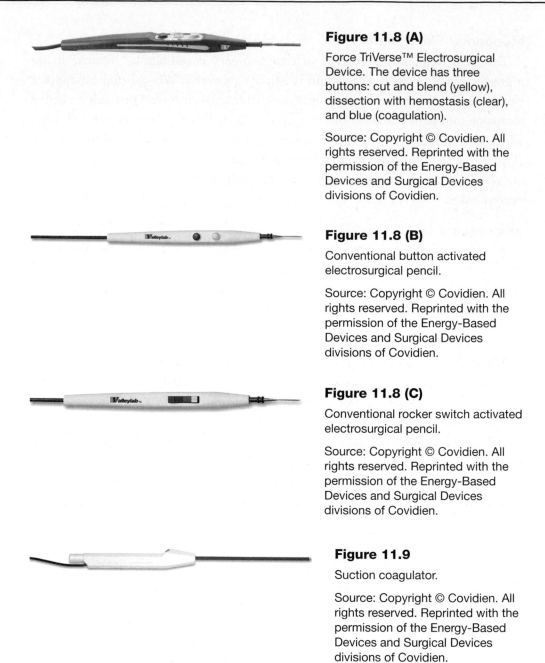

Figure 11.8 (A)

Force TriVerse™ Electrosurgical Device. The device has three buttons: cut and blend (yellow), dissection with hemostasis (clear), and blue (coagulation).

Source: Copyright © Covidien. All rights reserved. Reprinted with the permission of the Energy-Based Devices and Surgical Devices divisions of Covidien.

Figure 11.8 (B)

Conventional button activated electrosurgical pencil.

Source: Copyright © Covidien. All rights reserved. Reprinted with the permission of the Energy-Based Devices and Surgical Devices divisions of Covidien.

Figure 11.8 (C)

Conventional rocker switch activated electrosurgical pencil.

Source: Copyright © Covidien. All rights reserved. Reprinted with the permission of the Energy-Based Devices and Surgical Devices divisions of Covidien.

Figure 11.9

Suction coagulator.

Source: Copyright © Covidien. All rights reserved. Reprinted with the permission of the Energy-Based Devices and Surgical Devices divisions of Covidien.

which causes heat buildup and, potentially, a fire hazard. The scrub person should watch for eschar buildup and remove it as necessary. For stainless steel tips, use scratch pads to remove the eschar. The coarse pad, however, makes grooves in the active electrode tip and causes eschar buildup in the groves. Over time, it becomes impossible to remove all the eschar and the tip becomes higher in resistance. Non-stick active electrode tips can facilitate the removal of eschar. Tips made of materials such as Teflon® (PTFE) or elastomeric silicone coating can be cleaned with a damp sponge. Use coated tips according to the manufacture's IFUs, which include use of appropriate power settings (Ulmer, 2007).

PTFE
Teflon®

Holsters

Holsters are one of the most important electrosurgery safety devices and should be routinely used. When the active electrode is not in use, place it in a holster that is recommended by the manufacturer as being safe. It should be visible to the operative team and in easy reach of the physician and scrubbed personnel. Never use plastic pouches, folded towels, or other makeshift devices, as they are a threat to patient safety (Ulmer, 2007).

Patient Return Electrodes

Dry adhesive patient return electrodes are a layer of foam, the conductive thin metal plate covered by a layer of adhesive, which looks similar to tape. Dry electrodes are less adherent than gelled patient return electrodes and do not fill in voids on the skin surface, which could result in limitations on the number of potential application sites. Dry adhesive return electrodes use acrylic-based adhesives made from pure polymers that stick to skin. They may require additional preparation, such as hair removal and cleaning for removal of oils and lotions prior to placing on the skin. Electrical characteristics of polymers used in dry adhesive are generally measured in terms of insulation rather than conduction capabilities.

The thermal performance of some dry adhesive return electrodes is affected by the electrode's ability to uniformly distribute current and maintain contact with the skin. Dry adhesive return electrodes may require specific positioning on the patient to prevent the buildup of electrical current (Hotline News, 2003).

Some dry adhesive patient return electrode packaging specifies that the nurse must not touch the adhesive area. Touching the electrode can lead to spots on the adhesive that are higher in resistance due to salt and oils from the fingers. Dry adhesive electrode is more susceptible to fluid invasion, which could pose a problem if prep solutions, body fluids, or irrigation fluids invade the patient the return electrode site.

The benefits of a dry adhesive electrode include thinness and pliability, longer shelf life, ability to store the electrode vertically, and is potentially less expensive than water-based gel and low-impedance hydrogel electrodes.

Another type of patient return electrode is made with *water-based gel*. A water-based gel return electrode has a thick coating that adheres to the skin, it is potentially less expensive than low impedance hydrogel electrodes, and its pliability allows adherence to patient contours. Unlike the dry adhesive patient return electrode, the water-based gel fills in voids in the patient's skin and overcomes the natural resistance of the epidermis. It also helps to cool the skin, as heat can build up underneath the pad during electrosurgery activation. These are important safety considerations.

Water-based gel patient return electrodes must be stored flat. If not stored flat, the gel has a tendency to migrate from the pull of gravity. When this happens there may be exposed areas on the return electrode surface creating areas where a burn could occur. Short shelf life is a concern with water-based patient return electrodes. Instructions for the water-based pads specify a number of preparation requirements, such as hair clipping or cleansing the return electrode site. Like the dry adhesive return electrode, water-based pads may require specific ways of positioning on the patient. Care must be exercised when working with water-based gel patient return electrodes. The nurse should never touch the gel. The gel may also leave a residue on the patient after the return electrode is removed. Like dry adhesive, water-based gel uses acrylic-based adhesives made from pure polymers (Hotline News, 2003).

Hydrophilic conductive adhesive patient return electrodes, like the water-based gel electrodes, provide a thick coating that adheres to the skin. The hydrophilic conductive adhesive is a blend material formulated with deionized water and polyvinylpyrrolidone (PVP). It is a water-insoluble, hydrophilic (water loving) material, with pressure-sensitive adhesive that enhances conductivity between patient skin and the electrode. The high concentration of deionized water in the hydrophilic conductive adhesive increases electrode conductivity, lowers skin resistance, and decreases thermal concentration to minimize the risk of a return electrode site burn. This return electrode has a shorter shelf life than dry return electrodes. Unlike the water-based gel, the polymer-based conductive adhesive gel does not migrate under gravity, so it can be stored flat or vertically. The PVP component provides unique elongation properties that allow the hydrogel to stretch, accommodating the skin's surface irregularities. This conformability permits the gel to surround any hair and adhere only to the skin underneath, minimizing contact voids and improving the total area of electrical conductivity. When the return electrode is removed, the gel gently stretches as it releases its hold on the skin, reducing skin trauma. No sticky residue is left behind. The gel can be touched by the nurse prior to application to ensure that the adhesive is moist. It can be placed at any angle on the patient, giving the greatest flexibility in patient return electrode site selection (Hotline News, 2003).

Another type of return electrode available for clinical use is the large, *reusable capacitive return electrode*. The electrode is placed on the OR bed and covered with a layer of linen. The patient lies on top of this electrode and forms a capacitive bond. This pad bypasses the electrosurgical generator contact quality system (Hotline News, 2008).

The operative and invasive procedure staff should follow the manufacturers' IFUs when using a capacitive-coupled patient return electrode with a compatible electrosurgical generator. Do not use the pad on patients under 25 pounds. Ensure that there is adequate pad contact with the patient's body. Do not place extra linen between the pad and the patient. Confirm that small metal material, such as snaps on gowns, is not in contact with the patient's skin. If this occurs current can concentrate at the site of metal contact (AORN, 2008).

Return Electrode Contact Quality Monitoring

One of the most important safety innovations in electrosurgery was the development of return electrode contact quality monitoring (RECQM) in 1981. With this system, the patient return electrode and the electrosurgery generator work together and continuously monitor the quality of the contact between the pad and the patient interface. The generator sends an interrogation current through the pad. If a situation develops under the patient return electrode that could cause a patient injury, the RECQM system inactivates the generator. The pad has a split, which can

PVP
Polyvinylpyrrolidone

RECQM
Return Electrode
Contact Quality
Monitoring

be horizontal or vertical, depending on the manufacturer of the pad. There is also a pin on the end of the pad cord that activates the RECQM system when the cord is plugged into the generator. RECQM is the safest system for the patient during electrosurgery use (Rothrock, 2007).

Applying the Patient Return Electrode

Place the patient return electrode after positioning the patient. Attach the electrode to a clean, dry skin surface, over a well-vascularized, large muscle mass, and in a convex area close to the procedure site. **Figure 11.10** shows suggested placement areas for a hydrophilic conductive adhesive electrode. The shorter the distance between the procedure site and the patient return electrode site, the lower the power setting that is needed. Avoid bony prominences, scar tissue, hairy surfaces, pressure points, and adipose tissue; all of these areas are high in impedance. Do not place it over metal prostheses. Scar tissue surrounding the implant increases resistance to the flow of electrical current. Placing the electrode over a high-impedance area may necessitate higher power settings.

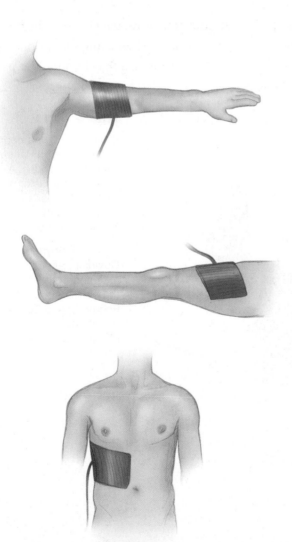

Figure 11.10

Potential sites for patient return electrode placement.

IED
Implantable Electronic Device

Never apply the patient return electrode should where fluids can pool during the procedure. Besides causing a chemical burn hazard, fluid may cause the electrode to detach during the procedure.

Use of electrosurgery with caution in the presence of an implantable electronic device (IED). These devices include pacemakers, defibrillators and ventricular assist devices. "Electronic interference is the most common safety issue noted when caring for patients with existing cardiac IEDs" (AORN, 2008, p. 186). Pacemakers should be programmed to an asynchronous mode to avoid malfunction. In the presence of an implanted electrical device, assure that placement of the patient return electrode does not draw current through the path of the device. Device manufacturers should be consulted prior to the use of electrosurgery to determine whether or not the pacemaker is susceptible to electrical interference. Bipolar is always a safer alternative when patients have IEDs.

Figure 11.11 shows various sizes of patient return electrodes. Select an electrode appropriate to the size of the patient. If the electrosurgery generator is equipped with a RECQM system, always use a RECQM pad. Do not bypass this safety system. See Chapter 37, Care of the Pediatric Patient, for information concerning infant and neonatal patient return electrodes.

Read and follow manufacturer's IFUs for the patient return electrode being used. These instructions are legal and binding instructions when using the product. Failure to follow the manufacturer's IFUs could constitute negligence should a patient injury incident occur (Ulmer, 2007).

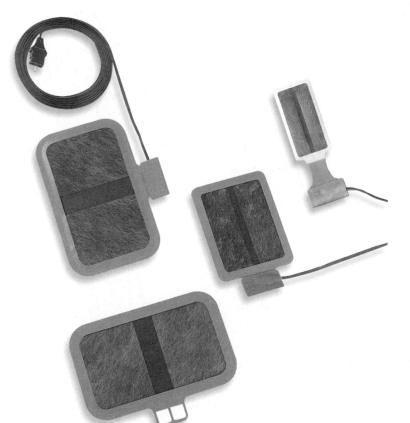

Figure 11.11

Adult, infant, and neonatal PolyHesive™ II Patient Return Electrodes. A reusable cord is applied to the adult patient return electrode shown without an attached cord.

Source: Copyright © Covidien. All rights reserved. Reprinted with the permission of the Energy-based Devices and Surgical Devices divisions of Covidien.

Nursing Care of the Patient During Electrosurgery

Nursing care of the patient during electrosurgery can be enhanced by following routine and systematic procedures. **Tables 11.5, 11.6,** and **11.7** discuss nursing considerations before, during, and after the procedure. **Table 11.8** provides guidelines for the routine care and maintenance of electrosurgical generators.

Smoke Evacuation

In 1994 AORN (the Association of periOperative Registered Nurses) first published a recommended practice stating that patients and operative and invasive procedure personnel should be protected from inhaling the smoke generated during the use of electrosurgery. The recommendation to evacuate and appropriately filter surgical smoke has remained a standard supported by AORN since that time. In 2008 AORN adopted an Official Position Statement on Surgical Smoke recommending that all surgical smoke is evacuated filtered (AORN, 2008). The recommended practice and the position statement are applicable whenever smoke plume is produced, whether it is from laser or electrosurgery or any other surgical devices that aerosolizes human tissue. Toxic fumes and carcinogens have been isolated from surgical smoke (Ulmer, 2008a). Formaldehyde and benzene are two of the long list of substances that are contained in smoke. Acrylonitrile and hydrogen cyanide are toxic, colorless gases present in smoke that are easily absorbed through the skin and lungs. Acrylonitrile

AORN
Association
of periOperative
Registered Nurses

Table 11.5	Electrosurgery Nursing Considerations: Before the Procedure

- ☐ Know which ESU the surgeon prefers and how to use it safely. Consult the instruction manual for specific instructions or questions.
- ☐ All equipment and accessories should be available. Use only accessories designed and approved for use with the unit.
- ☐ Test all alarm systems.
- ☐ Never cut a disposable patient return electrode.
- ☐ Avoid the use of flammable anesthetics during electrosurgery use.
- ☐ Place EKG electrodes away for the surgery site.
- ☐ Do not use needles as monitoring electrodes during electrosurgery procedures; unintended electrosurgical burns may occur.
- ☐ Check the cord and plug on the ESU. DO NOT use extension cords.
- ☐ Do not use power or accessory cords that are broken, cracked, frayed, or taped.
- ☐ Check biomedical sticker to ensure the generator has undergone a current inspection.
- ☐ Cover the foot pedal with a plastic bag.
- ☐ Document generator serial number on the operative and invasive procedure record.
- ☐ Record exact anatomical pad position and skin condition of the pad site. Consult the manufacturer's recommendations for proper placement.

Ulmer, B. C. (2007). *Electrosurgery Self Study Guide.* Boulder: Valleylab/Covidien; Covidien (2007). *Force Triad*™ *Users Guide.* Boulder: Valleylab/Covidien.

Table 11.6	Electrosurgery Nursing Considerations: During the Procedure

- ☐ If using an alcohol-based skin prepping agent, allow the solution to dry prior to draping.
- ☐ Do not allow the patient to lay in pooled prep solutions.
- ☐ Use the lowest possible power settings to achieve the desired tissue effect. The need for abnormally high settings may indicate a problem within the system.
- ☐ Confirm power settings with the surgeon.
- ☐ Position cords to avoid a tripping hazard.
- ☐ Avoid putting tension on the patient return electrode cord when it is connected to the generator.
- ☐ Do not roll equipment over electrical cords.
- ☐ Place the generator close enough to the sterile field so that power settings and display screen information can be viewed by the operative and invasive procedure team.
- ☐ If the patient has an implanted medical device such as a pacemaker or automatic cardioverter defibrillator, avoid laying the cord of the active electrode on the device, device leads, and heart.
- ☐ Use monopolar electrosurgery with extreme caution on delicate structures and appendages. The use of electrosurgery in small operative fields, or on small appendages could result in thermal injury. Bipolar is a safer alternative.
- ☐ Avoid touching the electrosurgery activate electrode to metal clamps or forceps. Doing so may cause a burn in an unintended area such as the patient's lip during a tonsillectomy.
- ☐ If the patient is moved or repositioned, check that the patient return electrode is still in good contact with the patient. Do not reposition patient return electrodes. If the patient return electrode is removed for any reason, apply a new pad.
- ☐ Never lay an active electrode on a patient. If not in use remove it from the sterile field.
- ☐ Use an insulated holster recommended by the manufacturer. Place the holster in a location that is visible and easily accessible to surgical team members.
- ☐ Do not coil active electrode cords as this can increase and concentrate leakage current and may present a potential danger to the patient.
- ☐ Do not "buzz" hemostats in a way that creates metal-to-metal arching, such as open circuit activation. If "buzzing" a hemostat is necessary, touch the hemostat with the active electrode and then activate the active electrode.
- ☐ Use endoscopes with insulated eyepieces.
- ☐ Keep active electrodes clean. Eschar buildup will increase resistance, reduce performance, and require higher power settings.
- ☐ Do not submerse active accessories in liquid to avoid inadvertent activation of active electrodes that are not sealed against fluid invasion.
- ☐ Note the type of active electrode used on the operative and invasive procedure record.
- ☐ If an ESU alarm occurs, check the system to assure proper function of the entire electrosurgery circuit.
- ☐ Do not use electrosurgery generator surfaces for storage space for fluids. Spills could invade the generator and cause malfunctions.

Ulmer, B. C. (2007). *Electrosurgery Self Study Guide.* Boulder: Valleylab/Covidien; Covidien (2007). *Force Triad*™ *Users Guide.* Boulder: Valleylab/Covidien.

exerts its toxicity by liberating the cyanide, while the cyanide combines with other substances to impair tissue oxygenation (Barrett, 2004). Air in hospitals and operating rooms has been described as a "chemical soup" which can cause symptoms such as shortness of breath, eye and respiratory irritation, rhinitis, contact dermatitis,

Table 11.7	Electrosurgery Nursing Considerations: After the Procedure

- ☐ Turn all controls to one or zero—whichever is the lowest setting
- ☐ Turn off the electrosurgical unit
- ☐ Disconnect all cords by grasping the plug, not the cord
- ☐ Inspect patient return electrode site to be sure it is clear and unremarkable
- ☐ Inspect the patient return electrode after removal from the patient. If an undetected problem has occurred, such as a burn, evidence of the injury may appear on the pad surface
- ☐ Discard all disposable items according to hospital policy
- ☐ Remove and discard the plastic bag covering the foot pedal
- ☐ Clean the ESU, foot pedal, and power cord with an appropriate cleaner
- ☐ Coil power cords for storage in a way that will prevent damage
- ☐ Clean all reusable accessories according to hospital policy

Ulmer, B. C. (2007). *Electrosurgery Self Study Guide.* Boulder: Valleylab/Covidien; Covidien (2007). *Force Triad*™ *Users Guide.* Boulder: Valleylab/Covidien; AORN (2008), Recommended Practices for Electrosurgery. *Perioperative standards and recommended practices,* Denver, CO: AORN, pp. 315–329.

Table 11.8	Routine Care and Maintenance of ESU Equipment

- ☐ Routinely inspect all reusable cables and active electrodes and repair/replace as necessary
- ☐ A qualified Biomedical Engineer should inspect electrosurgery units at specified intervals to assure proper function; maintenance of electrosurgical equipment can prolong its life and reduce costly repairs, thereby making the units safer for patients and staff
- ☐ If an ESU is dropped or damaged, do not use it until it can be inspected by a Biomedical Engineer
- ☐ Replace adapters that do not provide tight connections
- ☐ Use adaptors recommended by the manufacturer with the electrosurgical unit
- ☐ Inspect permanent cords and cables for cracks or breaks in the insulation
- ☐ Proper use and maintenance of electrosurgical equipment can prolong its life and reduce costly repairs, thereby making the units safer for patients and staff

Ulmer, B. C. (2007). *Electrosurgery Self Study Guide.* Boulder: Valleylab/Covidien; Covidien (2007). *Force Triad*™ *Users' Guide.* Boulder: Valleylab/Covidien; AORN (2008). Recommended Practices for Electrosurgery. *Perioperative standards and recommended practices,* Denver, CO: AORN, pp. 315–329.

headaches, join pain, memory problems, and difficulty concentrating, to name a few (Wilburn, 2006). **Table 11.9** lists the chemicals found in surgical smoke. There has been no quantitative way to measure the long-term effects on healthcare workers, but as with cigarette smoking, the effects of inhaling surgical smoke is cumulative and most dangerous to susceptible people. In September 1996 the National Institute for

Table 11.9	Chemical Contents of Surgical Smoke		
Acetonitrile	3-Butenenitrile	Furfural	Methyl pyrazine
Acetylene	Carbon Monoxide	Hexadecanoic acid	Phenol
Acrolein	Creosol	Hydrogen cyanide	Propene
Acrylonitrile	1-Decene	Indole	2-Propylene nitrile
Alkyl benzene	2,3-Dihydro indene	Isobutene	Pyridine
Benzaldehyde	Ethane	Methane	Pyrrole
Benzene	Ethene	3-Methyl butenal	Styrene
Benzonitrile	Ethylene	6-Methyl indole	Toluene
Butadiene	Ethyl benzene	4-Methyl phenol	1-Undecene
Butene	Formaldehyde	2-Methyl propanol	Xylene

Ulmer, B. C. (2008). *Surgical Smoke Self Study Guide.* Boulder: Valleylab/Covidien.

NIOSH
National Institute for Occupational Safety and Health

CDC
Centers for Disease Control

Occupational Safety and Health (NIOSH) issued a hazard alert through the Centers for Disease Control's (CDC) healthcare facility network. The alert recommended that laser and electrosurgical smoke be evacuated and filtered to protect all healthcare workers (CDC/NIOSH, 2006).

Patients are also at risk from surgical smoke during laparoscopic procedures. When smoke is absorbed through the peritoneal membrane during laparoscopic surgery, elevated levels of methemoglobin and carboxyhemoglobin are produced in the patient's bloodstream. This can pose a potential risk to patients during surgery (Ulmer, 2008b).

Scrubbed team members are also at increased risk from inhaling surgical smoke during laparoscopic procedures due to a surge of concentrated smoke being released from the cannula system. It is recommended that a smoke evacuation laparoscopic handpiece be used to maintain visualization throughout the procedure through metered smoke evacuation. Any air that is released from the cannula should be collected by a smoke evacuator (HealthStream, 2004).

The toxic chemicals contained in surgical smoke is reason enough to institute a policy that all smoke be evacuated and filtered Before the procedure the nurse should determine the volume of smoke that will be produced and select the appropriate smoke evacuation system. The vacuum source should be portable, easy to set up and use. A filtration system with a triple filter offers the greatest protection. The systems consists of a prefilter to filter out large particles; an ULPA (Ultra Low Penetrating Air) filter to capture microscopic particles; and a charcoal filter to adsorb, or bind to toxic gases produced during the procedure (Ulmer, 2008b). The vacuum source should be able to adequately pull sufficient air through the system to efficiently capture the smoke. A system powerful enough to handle the amount of smoke produced during all surgical procedures is the most effective evacuator and offers the operative and invasive procedure staff the flexibility to select the appropriate capture device. A smoke evacuator with variable power settings will be of most use in a wide variety of surgical procedures.

ULPA
Ultra Low Penetrating Air

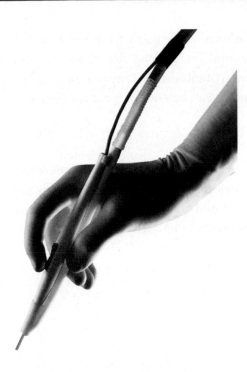

Figure 11.12

AccuVac™ Smoke Evacuation Attachment for use with an electrosurgery pencil.

Source: Copyright © Covidien. All rights reserved. Reprinted with the permission of the Energy-based Devices and Surgical Devices divisions of Covidien.

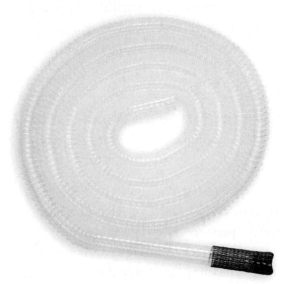

Figure 11.13

7/8" smoke evacuation tubing with sponge guard.

Source: Copyright © Covidien. All rights reserved. Reprinted with the permission of the Energy-based Devices and Surgical Devices divisions of Covidien.

There are also different capture devices that can be attached to the smoke evacuator. The most convenient is the smoke carriage that attaches to the electrosurgical pencil (**Fig. 11.12**). This has the advantage of being in direct proximity to where the smoke originates, which is the recommended location to most efficiently capture smoke. During procedures that produce larger volumes of smoke, larger tubing may be needed (**Fig. 11.13**). The system configuration that is the most efficient and effective is the one that should be selected for every surgical procedure where smoke is produced (Ulmer, 2008a).

APPLYING DRESSINGS

Preparation of the Incision Site

Before removing the drapes, the scrub person cleans the incision site with a wet sterile sponge or towel to remove dried prep solution, blood, other body fluids, and tissue. Avoid potential for wound contamination by using fresh sterile water. The scrub person carefully dries the skin around the incision site. Application of tape over dried prep solution may lead to skin irritation and a chemical burn. Also, application of tape over blood, fluids, or tissue creates an environment conducive to microorganism growth.

Applying the Dressing

The scrub person applies the dressing according to the physician's preference. Do not use radiopaque sponges as surgical dressings. The scrub person holds the dressing in place with the nondominant hand and removes the drapes with the dominant hand. The circulating nurse secures the dressing with tape. Do not stretch skin while tape is applied, to prevent skin trauma and blisters. If the tape is applied by a physician or scrub person, they should don clean gloves to prevent cross-contamination.

ASSISTING WITH THE APPLICATION OF CASTS AND SPLINTS

Postprocedure immobilization may require the use of a cast or splint. This is accomplished with plaster or synthetic materials (eg, fiberglass). A cast or splint is applied to immobilize a bone proximally and distally to the area of injury and repair. A variety of types of casts exist.

Preparing the Area

Prior to the application of casting material, prepare the area by placing an impervious covering on the floor. This will enhance cleanup of dried casting materials and avoid damage to the floor.

Using Casting Materials

Fill a basin with warm water no warmer than 75° F (24° C) (Halanski, et al, 2007). Padding is indicated to reduce the risk of pressure sores development in tissues located over bony prominences under the cast. For a close-fitting cast, apply stockinet as the first layer of padding. This first layer of padding may also reduce the incidence of itching (Smith et al, 2005). Apply the padding smoothly over the stockinet in one to three layers with turns overlapping about one half the width of the bandage.

Plaster of Paris

Plaster of Paris is made from hydrous calcium sulfate. Hardening times vary according to the chemicals added to the plaster. As the plaster sets, long cylindrical crystals form and interlock to form the hard cast. Do not move or manipulate the cast before it is dry; the crystals may break and not interlock, causing the cast to weaken.

Synthetic Casting Material

Fiberglass knit casting and splinting products are impregnated with a water-activated polyurethane resin. These fiberglass products come in a variety of colors and prints. Manufacturer IFUs should be followed with the specific product. Upon preparation, the casting material is applied wrapping the limb spirally, overlapping each piece by one half the width of the tape. The cast is molded and typically dries quickly.

Preparing the Bandage Roll

The plaster or fiberglass roll is selected based on the provider's preferences. Hold the roll in a vertical position, allowing air to escape through the core of the roll as it is dipped in water. Squeeze the roll gently to remove excess water. The application may be accelerated by removing excess water from the roll, rubbing and working with the material as it is applied or by immersing the roll in warmer water.

Preparing the Splint

Splints may be applied to areas that require additional strength or support. Select the appropriate splint material and size based on the provider's preference. Dip the splints in the water and rapidly withdraw them. Draw each side of the splint through the index and middle fingers and pass to the applier.

Molding the Cast

The physician rubs and molds the cast over the contour of the body part. Water may be applied to a plaster cast to smooth or remove plaster crumbs. Molding continues until the casting material begins to set. Use the palms of both hands to handle a wet cast. Avoid creating indents in the cast which in turn could create pressure points in the dried cast. The cast is trimmed and edges covered by padding and stockinet, which is incorporated into the ends of the cast.

After cast application, elevate the extremity on a pillow and protect the cast from rough surfaces. Exposing the cast to air while it dries will help dissipate the heat that is generated as the casting material sets.

Removing the Cast

An electric cast cutter with an attached vacuum is used to remove a cast. Use of the cast saw is recommended outside the restricted areas of the operative and invasive procedure suite to confine dust generated from plaster or fiberglass. Use care cutting over bony prominences. Assure the patient that he or she will not be cut during cast removal.

PREPARING AND OPERATING ENDOSCOPIC EQUIPMENT

General Guidelines

Minimally invasive surgery has continued to evolve around the world, improving efficiency; enhancing quality of care; and decreasing postprocedure pain, facility stay, and recovery time. The basic video system includes a scope, light cable, light source, video camera, camera cord, camera-scope coupler, camera control unit, and video monitor. Additional equipment may be necessary for recording and transmitting electronic media. The nurse is responsible for ensuring that equipment functions correctly. This requires a thorough understanding of the equipment, its operation, and troubleshooting. Staff and physicians should be oriented to all video equipment. Virtual reality training centers offer specific training and may be available from endoscopic equipment manufacturers. Some training centers provide education and training for the entire operative team. Some facilities also employ specific technical personnel to operate video equipment. Standardization of video equipment facilitates provision of efficient and reliable operation among staff members. Only knowledgeable and conscientious personnel should operate video equipment due to the high cost involved with repairs or replacement.

Endoscopic Lenses

Endoscopes come in either a rigid or flexible form, depending on the procedure for which they are indicated. The endoscope may have an eyepiece for direct visualization or one that connects to a camera. Some endoscopes connect directly to the camera and video projection system bypassing the eyepiece. A light cable attachment may be indicated via a connection located on the endoscope. Some units have the light cable and camera built into a single unit to facilitate cleaning, protection, and efficiency. Endoscopic equipment and instrumentation should be handled carefully during use. Follow the manufacturer's IFUs when processing at the end of a procedure, and ensure that the endoscope is packaged in appropriate protective material. Do not place other instruments on top of the endoscope during packaging, and avoid placing instrument sets on top of packaged endoscopes. Check endoscopes with an eyepiece before sterilization and just before use. To do this, grasp the endoscope by the eyepiece. Carefully hold the endoscope with two hands and look through the eyepiece at the room light for clarity. If the lens does not appear clear, follow manufacturer recommendations for repair. The lens should also be warmed prior to insertion into a body cavity to prevent fogging. This may be done by using hot sterile water on the field, or using a commercial scope warmer or antifogging solution. Follow the manufacturer's IFUs for the use of antifogging solutions.

Video Cameras

The video camera is the interface of the video system. The camera cable transfers the signal to a camera control unit which then transmits the image to a video monitor, recorder, or hard-copy picture. Digital processing allows for the image to be enhanced and manipulated to specific parameters. It also allows for multiple images to be projected and altered at one time. Light intensity is also adjustable on most camera units from the point of use and/or on the camera control unit. Automatic adjustment is a feature available on most camera systems on the market. Other controls include white balancing, recording, or taking pictures.

Once the camera is attached and ready for use, perform a white-balance to adjust the color produced by the camera to the colors of the light source. The scrub person holds the lens up to a white object, such as a white sponge, and completes the protocol according to the manufacturer's IFUs.

During packaging, loosely coil the cable; avoid pinching or stretching the cable. Inspect all cables by running a gloved hand along the surfaces to detect any breach in the cable integrity. Cameras may come sterile or have a sterile drape applied for use on the sterile field. Best practice is to use sterile endoscopes and endoscopic instruments (AORN, 2008). If sterilization is not possible, prepare the endoscope and instruments using high-level disinfection. However, endoscopic instrumentation that can withstand steam or other sterilization methods is becoming more available. Follow the manufacturer's IFUs for sterilization or high-level disinfection.

Video Monitors

High-definition video monitors have become the standard with video endoscopy. Video monitors used in endoscopy typically receive input only through direct cables compared with standard television sets. Monitors should match closely to the quality of picture with the camera being used. Many procedures require two or more video monitors. Endoscopic suites may also offer additional panels for viewing the procedure by team members. Common sizes of monitors are 19 and 20 inches (48 and 51 cm) and are measured diagonally from screen corner to screen corner. Placement may depend on the physician and procedure being performed. Standard placement includes the foot or head of the patient bed.

Video Lighting

Lighting affects the picture within the cavity. Endoscopic light sources produce a high-intensity light delivered through a fiberoptic light cord. Fiberoptic light cables are made of fine strands of glass; handle these cables according to the manufacturer's IFUs. Check light cable effectiveness by holding the light cable up to room light. Breaks in the fibers can be seen as dark spots. Consider replacing based upon manufacturer recommendations. Ensure that appropriate connectors are available for the light cord prior to use. The light source uses a xenon high-intensity lamp that provides a pure white light. Most light sources have intensity adjustment capability. An illuminated light cord or endoscope creates temperatures high enough to ignite the drapes, particularly in an oxygen-enriched atmosphere; therefore, do not lay the light cord or endoscope on the draped patient or allow contact with flammable materials. Activate the light source only when the endoscope is going to be used.

Recording Documentation

Recording devices may include video printers, disc burners (eg, DVD or CD ROM), video cassette (eg, VHS) or electronic media storage. Digital recording may also be linked to the patient electronic medical record in facilities utilizing that technology. Electronic transmission of images or video may also be sent to physician offices or other authorized entities for consultation purposes. Facility policy should determine the appropriate recording, storage, and ownership of any recorded documentation.

Video printers provide a still photograph. The printer stores the image and then prints it onto paper. Printer picture units offer programming such as number of pictures per sheet of paper as well as patient information that is input by the physician or staff. Prints can be used for teaching purposes and/or remain part of the medical record.

The disc burner records the video feed onto a disc that can be replayed for teaching purposes or become part of the medical record. The VCR also records the video feed on a video cassette (eg, VHS tape). The VCR does not offer the capability for editing that the disc recording does. The electronic medical record also may offer storage for video feed or pictures to be stored.

Video conferencing is also an option for two-way interaction using live audio and video signals. This may be of particular value with regard to diagnosis or expert opinion. Video conferencing technology must be present on both ends of transmission to accommodate effective communication.

Video Storage Systems

Video equipment should be secured to a video cart or equipment boom. A video cart is a stable, mobile device that allows for secure transport of the video equipment to various locations. An equipment boom is a device attached to the room ceiling which is designed to hold the necessary equipment of the room. The equipment boom is stationary to the specific operative suite in which it is installed. Therefore, careful consideration as to placement of equipment booms and the amount of equipment occupying shelf space must be considered when considering installation of an equipment boom in the operative suite. Consideration must also be made for level of security required and space for either a video cart or equipment boom.

Laparoscopic Insufflator

CO_2
Carbon Dioxide

Pneumoperitoneum is created to assist in the visualization of the abdominal and pelvic cavities during laparoscopic procedures. A Veres needle is inserted into the abdomen at a 45° angle. The physician protects abdominal structures from punctures while establishing the pneumoperitoneum by grasping the abdomen and holding it away from the abdominal organs during the insertion of the Veres needle. Placement is typically verified by aspiration negative aspiration and saline instillation without resistance. The space created allows for the carbon dioxide (CO_2) gas to inflate the abdominal and peritoneal cavities; thus creating visualization for the procedure. CO_2 is used for insufflation as it does not support combustion, is cost effective, and can be absorbed in large quantities without adverse effects; although rare instances of gas emboli with CO_2 have been reported (Kirby, 1998). It is important to review facility policies and procedures with regard to the use of insufflation gas storage and use.

Before the procedure, check tank gas levels to assure adequate supply for the procedure. Tanks should be stored and used in an upright position and secured at all times in a holding apparatus. The insufflator should display current settings including rate or flow of CO_2, volume delivered and intraabdominal pressure.

The CO_2 begins to flow through the Veres needle at a low setting. Once flow begins, monitor intraabdominal pressure and maintain it between 14 and 16 mm Hg. Delivery ranges of 15 to 20 L/min will offer adequate expansion. The faster that CO_2 can be replaced, the less time spent waiting for the abdominal cavity to re-expand. Once adequate pneumoperitoneum is reached, the endoscopic trocars are introduced. Adjustment to the insufflator may be necessary upon incision and insertion of the trocars.

Trocar openings should be covered when introducing and withdrawing instrumentation. This will prevent inadvertent spraying of aerosolized blood and body fluids. Appropriate smoke evacuation for procedures using electrosurgery or laser should also be provided to promote a clear field to work in, prevent staff from breathing in plume, including aerosolized blood and body fluids; and decrease the risk of false oxygen saturation levels by increased carboxyhemoglobin and methemoglobin blood levels.

CONCLUSION

The chapter has provided an overview of instrumentation, equipment and supplies that the nurse may provide during operative or invasive procedures. Some of the tasks discussed may be delegated to appropriately trained team members; the nurse, however, maintains the accountability for these delegated functions.

The nurse has the responsibility for identifying patients at risk for adverse outcomes related to providing instrumentation, equipment, and supplies. If this responsibility is fulfilled, the nurse will have taken the steps necessary to reduce the patient's risk for experiencing alterations in temperature; thermal injury; hospital-acquired infection; extended anesthesia time due to delays; and tissue trauma related to the provision of instrumentation.

COMPETENCY ASSESSMENT
Provide Instruments, Equipment, and Supplies

Name: _____ Title: _____ Unit: _____ Date of Validation: _____

Type of Validation: ☐ Initial   ☐ Annual   ☐ Bi-annual

COMPETENCY STATEMENT: The nurse demonstrates competency to provide instruments, equipment, and supplies during the operative or invasive procedure.

Performance Criteria	Met	Not Met
1. Identifies the patient's risk for adverse outcomes related to the provision of instruments, equipment, and supplies	☐	☐
2. Selects appropriate instrumentation, equipment, and supplies for an operative or invasive procedure	☐	☐
3. Delivers instruments and supplies to the sterile field	☐	☐
4. Arranges instruments and supplies on the back table and Mayo tray	☐	☐
5. Passes instruments and supplies to the physician or assistant	☐	☐
6. Prepares and passes sutures to the physician or assistant	☐	☐
7. Prepares and applies patient warming systems	☐	☐
8. Applies and remove a pneumatic tourniquet	☐	☐
9. Prepares air-powered instrumentation for use	☐	☐
10. Prepares electrical instrumentation and equipment for use	☐	☐
11. Implements electrosurgical safety precautions	☐	☐
12. Applies dressings	☐	☐
13. Assists with the application of casts and splints	☐	☐
14. Prepares and operates endoscopic equipment	☐	☐

_____   _____

Validator's Signature   Employee's Signature

_____

Validator's Printed Name

11

REFERENCES

1. Altizer, L. (2004, March/April). Casting for immobilization. *Orthopaedic Nursing* (23) 2, p. 136–141.

2. Alp, E., Biji, D., Bleichrodt, R.P., Hansson, B., & Voss, A. (2006). Surgical smoke and infection control. *Journal of Hospital Infection* 62, p. 1–5. Elsevier: The Hospital Infection Society.

3. AORN (2008). *Perioperative standards and recommended practices.* Association of periOperative Registered Nurses: Denver.

4. AORN (2008). Recommended Practices for Electrosurgery. *Perioperative standards and recommended practices,* Denver, CO: AORN, pp. 315–329.

5. AORN (2008). Recommended Practices for the Use of the Pneumatic Tourniquet in the Perioperative Practice Setting. *Perioperative Standards and Recommended Practices.* Denver, CO: AORN, pp. 483–495.

6. Barrett W.L. & Garber S.M. (2004). Surgical smoke—a review of the literature. *Surgical Endoscopy* 17(6): p. 979–987.

7. Bragg, K., VanBalen, N., & Cook, N. (2005, December). Future trends in minimally invasive surgery. *AORN Journal* 82 (6), p. 1006–1018.

8. CDC/NIOSH (2006). Control of smoke from laser/electric surgical procedures. HC11 DHHS (NIOSH) Publication No. 96–128. Available at: http://www.cdc.gov/niosh/hc11.html. Accessed September 11, 2006.

9. Capacitive-coupled patient return electrodes (December, 2007). *Hotline News,* Vol. 12, No 2.

10. Cooper, S. (2006, May). The effect of preoperative warming on patients' postoperative temperatures. *AORN Journal* 83 (5) p. 1074–1085.

11. Cunnington, J. (2006). Facilitating benefit, minimizing risk: responsibilities of the surgical practitioner during electrosurgery. *Journal of Perioperative Practice* 16 (4) p. 195–202.

12. Electrosurgery safety update: Patient return electrode warming (March, 2003). *Hotline News,* Vol. 8, No. 1.

13. Goldberg, J. (2006, October). Brief laboratory report: surgical drape flammability. *AANA Journal* 74 (5) pp. 352–354.

14. Halanski, M.A., Halanski, A.D., Ashish, O., Vanderby, R., Munoz, A., & Noonan, K.J. (2007). Thermal injury with contemporary cast-application techniques and methods to circumvent morbidity. *Journal of Bone and Joint Surgery, Inc.* (89) p. 2369–2377.

15. HealthStream (2004). *No Smoking in the OR Study Guide.* Denver, CO. March 2004: p. 14–15.

16. Hill, J. (2006, March/April). *Understanding the safety features of electrosurgical units. Biomedical Instrumentation & Technology.* Alliance Communications.

17. Jones, C.M., Pierre, K.B., Nicoud, I.B., Stain, S.C. & Melvin III, W.V. (2006). Electrosurgery. Current Surgery. Association of Program Directors in Surgery: Elsevier.

18. Khraim, F.M. (2007, June). The wider scope of video-assisted thoracoscopic surgery. *AORN Journal* 85 (6) p. 1199–1208.

19. Kirby, R.R. (1998). Unusual causes of air embolism. *Reviews for nurse anesthetists* 21 (12) p. 106–111.

20. Marders, J. (2008) FDA encourages the reporting of medical device adverse events: free-hosing hazards. Article available at http://www.apsf.org/resource_center/newsletter/2002/fall/09reportevents.htm, Accessed 10 May 2008.

21. Massarweh, N.N., Cosgriff, N., & Slakey, D.P. (2006). Electrosurgery: history, principles and current and future uses. *J Am Coll Surg;* 202(3); p. 520–530.

22. O'Connor, C. & Murphy, S. (2007, August). Pneumatic tourniquet use in the perioperative environment. *Journal of Perioperative Practice.* 17 (5) p. 391–397.

23. Olivecrona, C., Tidemark, J., Hamberg, P., Ponzer, & Cederfjall, C. (2006). Skin protection underneath the pneumatic tourniquet during total knee arthroplasty. *Acta Orthopaedica* 77 (3) p. 519–523.

24. Olympus Winter & Ibe GmbH (2005). *System-related instruction manual system guide endoscopy.* Olympus Surgical & Industrial America, Inc. New York: Orangeburg.

25. Rothrock, J.C. (2007). *Alexander's Care of the Patient in Surgery,* 13th Ed. St. Louis: Mosby; p. 222.

26. Smith, G.D., Hart, R.G., & Tsu-Min, T. (2005). Fiberglass cast application. *American Journal of Emergency Medicine.* (23) p. 347–350.

27. Stanton, C. (2007, June). Assessing the impact of surgical smoke in the OR. *AORN Connections.* Denver, CO.

28. 3M Health Care (2007). Package insert Scotchcast casting products. St. Paul, MN: 3M Health Care.

29. Ulmer, B.C. (2007). *Electrosurgery Self Study Guide.* Boulder: Valleylab/Covidien.

30. Ulmer, B.C. (2008a). The hazards of surgical smoke. *AORN J.* 84(4); p. 721–738.

31. Ulmer, B.C. (2008b). *Surgical Smoke Self Study Guide:* Boulder: Valleylab/Covidien.

32. Wang, K. & Advincula, A.P. (2007). Current thoughts in electrosurgery. *International Journal of Gynecology and Obstetrics,* 97 p. 245–250.

33. Wilburn S. (2006). Is the air in your hospital making your sick? Nursing World, July 1999. Available at www.nursingworld.org/ajn/1999/july/heal079b.htm. Accessed September 11, 2006.

CHAPTER 12

Administer Drugs and Solutions

Deborah B. Hadley

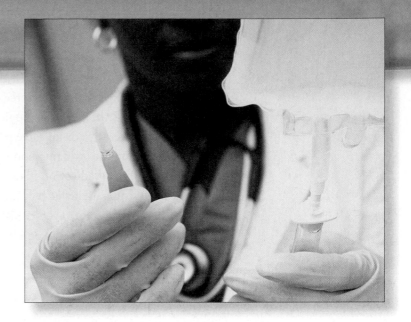

INTRODUCTION

The nurse must ensure that drugs or solutions are administered to the patient according to hospital policy, manufacturers' recommendations, applicable federal and state regulations and laws, and recommended nursing practices. Before administering drugs and solutions, the nurse identifies the patient's risk for adverse outcomes related to the administration of drugs and solutions, the nursing diagnoses that describe the degree of risk, and expected patient outcomes. After the identification of risks, diagnoses, and outcomes, the nurse plans interventions for care. After administering drugs and solutions the nurse evaluates the effectiveness of interventions according to criteria delineated in the expected outcomes.

Proper administration of drugs and solutions is essential for safe, quality patient care in the operative and invasive procedure suite. The nurse ensures that the administration of drugs and solutions is performed correctly and does not harm the patient. Although the nurse may administer medications and solutions orally or by inhalation, most medications and solutions given during the procedure are administered by injection, topical application to the skin or mucous membranes, or irrigation to the operative site.

The focus of this chapter is on medications and solutions administered in the operative and invasive procedure suite by the registered nurse functioning as the circulating nurse. For discussion of drugs and solutions usually administered by an anesthesia provider (eg, anesthetic agents, intravenous [IV] preparations, and blood products) please refer to Chapter 7.

Chapter Contents

IV
Intravenous

MEASURABLE CRITERIA

The nurse demonstrates competency to administer drugs and solutions by:

- Recognizing potential adverse drug and solution reactions
- Describing the pharmacological characteristics of drugs and solutions used during operative or invasive procedures
- Describing the human response to the administration of drugs and solutions
- Obtaining a medication history
- Identifying patients at risk for adverse outcomes related to the administration of drugs and solutions (see **Table 12.1**)
- Gathering supplies and equipment
- Preparing and administering drugs and solutions according to institutional policy, manufacturers' recommendations, federal and state regulations, and recommended nursing practices.

Table 12.1	**Administering Drugs and Solutions Does Not Result in Adverse Outcomes for the Patient**	
Outcome 1	The patient is free from evidence of infection solutions related to the administration of drugs and solutions.	
Diagnosis	**Risk Factors**	**Outcome Indicator**
Risk for Infection related to the administration of drugs and solutions	☐ Extremes of age ☐ Inadequate primary defense ☐ Inadequate secondary defense ☐ Malnutrition ☐ Medical conditions and treatments ☐ Type of operative procedure	☐ Are there signs of localized or systemic infection 48 hours after the operative or invasive procedure?
Outcome 2	The patient is free from evidence of hypersensitivity reaction because of improper identification of patient allergies.	
Diagnosis	**Risk Factors**	**Outcome Indicators**
Risk for Injury related to hypersensitivity reaction because of improper identification of patient allergies	☐ Drugs commonly used during the operative or invasive procedure period that may produce an allergic reaction to include penicillin and penicillin analogs, cephalosporins, tetracyclines, streptomycin, salicylates, morphine, codeine, procaine, lidocaine, cocaine, thiopental, succinylcholine, tubocurarine, benzene, and phenol ☐ History of a past reaction to specific or related agent ☐ Inability of the patient or family members to provide an accurate drug history ☐ Use of antimicrobial drugs for self-treatment of minor infections	☐ Is the patient uneasy, apprehensive, weak, or expressing feelings of impending doom? ☐ Does the patient demonstrate a generalized pruritus or urticaria? ☐ Is erythema and angioedema of the eyes, lips, or tongue present? ☐ Is there evidence of discrete cutaneous wheals or urticarial eruptions? ☐ Does the patient have congestion, rhinorrhea, dyspnea, or an increasing respiratory distress with audible wheezing? ☐ Are rales, wheezing, and diminished breath sounds present? ☐ Is the patient hypotensive? What is the status of the pulse? Rapid? Weak? ☐ Does the patient have abdominal cramping, diarrhea, or vomiting?

Outcome 3   The patient is free from evidence of deficit fluid volume related to the use of heparin.

Diagnosis

Risk for Deficit Fluid Volume (blood loss) related to the use of heparin

Risk Factors

☐ Alteration in vitamin K absorption

☐ Cardiovascular disease

☐ Central nervous system trauma

☐ Gastrointestinal disorders

☐ Gender (women older than 60 years of age)

☐ Hematological conditions

☐ Operative intervention

☐ Other medications/substances

Outcome Indicator

☐ Is the patient's hemodynamic status (blood pressure, pulse, and central pressures) maintained within normal limits?

Outcome 4   The patient is free from evidence of deficit fluid volume related to the administration of hyperosmotic agents.

Diagnosis

Risk for Deficit fluid Volume related to the administration of hyperosmotic agents

Risk Factors

☐ Extremes in age and weight. Osmotic agents may precipitate dehydration in the elderly

☐ History of a past reaction to specific or related agent

☐ History of cardiac disease (osmotic agents may precipitate congestive heart failure)

☐ Osmotic agents which may cause hyperglycemia and glycosuria in diabetic patients

☐ Inability of the client or family members to provide an accurate drug history

☐ Nausea and vomiting related to the pain of acute angle-closure glaucoma may cause further dehydration and fluid loss

☐ Presence of other diuretics in the system

Outcome Indicators

☐ Did the client experience an unintentional increase in intraocular pressure?

☐ Was the client's fluid volume during the procedure maintained?

Outcome 5   The patient is free from evidence of injury related to an allergic or adverse reaction to a local anesthetic.

Diagnosis

Risk for Injury related to an allergic reaction to local anesthetic

Risk Factors

☐ History of a past reaction to specific or related agent

☐ Inability of the patient or family members to provide an accurate drug history

☐ Patients at risk for malignant hyperthermia

☐ Patient conditions that slow the metabolism of the local anesthetic agent (hepatic dysfunction, congestive heart failure, and cardiogenic shock)

Outcome Indicators

☐ Does the patient show signs of redness, rash, or urticaria?

☐ Are there signs of bronchoconstriction?

Outcome 6   The patient is free from evidence of injury related to allergic or adverse reaction to otic medication.

Diagnosis	Risk Factors	Outcome Indicators
Risk for Injury related to an allergic or adverse reaction because of patient sensitivity to otic medication	☐ History of a past reaction to specific or related agent ☐ Hypersensitivity to any of the components of antibiotics ☐ Inability of the patient or family members to provide an accurate drug history ☐ Presence of secondary infections in chronic dermatoses ☐ Use of antimicrobial drugs for self-treatment of minor ear infections	☐ Does the patient complain of pruritus? ☐ Is swelling or inflammation evident? ☐ Are there other clinical manifestations of allergic reaction or secondary infection?

Outcome 7   The patient is free from evidence of injury related to allergic or adverse reaction to contrast media.

Diagnosis	Risk Factors	Outcome Indicator
Risk for Injury related to an allergic reaction to contrast media	☐ Bronchial asthma ☐ Food allergies such as shellfish allergy ☐ Hay fever ☐ History of allergy to contrast media or a related compound ☐ Hypersensitivity to iodine ☐ Inability of the patient or family members to provide an accurate drug history	☐ Does the patient manifest respiratory, central nervous system, cardiovascular, renal, and local reactions to contrast media?

Outcome 8   The patient is free from evidence of injury related to toxicity from a local anesthetic.

Diagnosis	Risk Factors	Outcome Indicators
Risk for Injury related to toxicity from local anesthetic agents	☐ History of a past reaction to specific or related agent ☐ Inability of the patient or family members to provide an accurate drug history ☐ Systemic diseases that slow the metabolism of the local anesthetic agent	☐ Is the patient apprehensive? ☐ Does the patient complain of blurred vision, tinnitus, or dizziness? ☐ Does the patient experience convulsions? ☐ Are there signs of central nervous system depression such as drowsiness or unconsciousness? ☐ Does the patient exhibit signs of respiratory depression?

Outcome 9   The patient is free from evidence of decreased cardiac output related to toxicity from a local anesthetic.

Diagnosis	Risk Factors	Outcome Indicators
Risk for Decreased Cardiac Output related to toxicity from a local anesthetic	☐ History of a past reaction to specific or related agent ☐ Inability of the patient or family members to provide an accurate drug history	☐ Does the patient exhibit signs of local anesthetic-induced hypotension? ☐ Is the patient tachycardic?

☐ Local anesthetics containing epinephrine can precipitate arrhythmias

☐ The presence of cardiac depressants (can increase the effect of local anesthetics)

☐ Are cardiac arrhythmias present?

Outcome 10 The patient is free from evidence of injury related to mydriatic agent administration causing an acute angle-closure glaucoma episode.

Diagnosis

Risk for Injury related to mydriatic agent administration causing an acute angle-closure glaucoma episode

Risk Factors

☐ Age 40 years or older

☐ History of a past reaction to specific or related agent

☐ History of angle-closure glaucoma

☐ Inability of the patient or family members to provide an accurate drug history

Outcome Indicator

☐ Did the patient experience an episode of acute angle-closure glaucoma?

Outcome 11 The patient is free from evidence of impaired skin integrity related to the administration of skin medication.

Diagnosis

Risk for Impaired Skin Integrity related to the administration of skin medications

Risk Factors

☐ Existing impaired skin integrity

☐ History of a past reaction to specific or related agent

☐ History of sensitivity to the specific agent or a related compound

☐ Inability of the client or family members to provide an accurate drug history

☐ Presence of irritating secretions, blood, pus, or infected drainage

☐ Use of drugs for self-treatment of minor skin infections

Outcome Indicators

☐ Is the client's skin red after application of skin medication?

☐ Is swelling present?

☐ Does the skin have drainage?

☐ Are there other signs of local irritation?

Outcome 12 The patient is free from evidence of excess fluid volume related to the absorption of large amounts of irrigating fluid into the systemic circulation.

Diagnosis

Risk for Fluid Volume Excess related to the absorption of large amounts of endoscopic irrigating fluid into the systemic circulation

Risk Factors

☐ History of a past reaction to specific or related agent

☐ History of cardiopulmonary disease

☐ History of renal dysfunction

☐ Inability of the patient or family members to provide an accurate drug history

Outcome Indicators

☐ Does the patient have edema?

☐ Is hypotension or tachycardia present?

☐ Does the patient complain of angina-like pains?

☐ Does the patient have signs and symptoms of pulmonary congestion?

Carpentino-Moyet, L. J. (2008). *Handbook of nursing diagnosis* (12th ed.) Philadelphia: Lippincott Williams & Wilkins; Petersen, C. (2007). *Perioperative nursing data set, the perioperative nursing vocabulary.* (Revised 2nd ed.). Denver: AORN, Inc.

RESPONSIBILITY FOR DRUG AND SOLUTION ADMINISTRATION

The circulating nurse, first assistant, scrub person, and physician share in the responsibility for preparing and administering drugs and solutions during the procedure. Each team member is responsible for patient safety as it relates to identifying the patient and to verifying the name, dosage, route, time, and frequency of the medication to be administered.

MEDICATION ORDERS

The circulating nurse receives a standing, written, or verbal order from the physician and is responsible for preparing the drug or solution. Before administering the medication or placing the medication on the sterile field, the order is verified with the physician. After the medication is placed on the sterile field, the scrub person labels the receptacle and identifies the medication each time he or she passes it to the physician.

FEDERAL DRUG LAWS AND REGULATIONS

The Harrison Narcotic Act of 1914 was the first attempt to prevent drug abuse in the medical and nursing communities. Later regulations were enacted to control the use of marijuana and to make certain drugs available only by prescription (the Durham-Humphrey Amendment of 1951). Continued abuse of potentially dangerous drugs led to the passage of the Drug Abuse Amendments of 1965. With the continued spread of drug abuse in the 1960s, Congress enacted the Controlled Substance Act of 1970, which identified five schedules on controlled substances (**Table 12.2**).

Another regulation intended for patient safety is the U.S. Food and Drug Administration Pregnancy Categories (**Table 12.3**). These categories provide a method of determining drug safety for pregnant women. The categories are based on the degree to which available information has ruled out risk to the fetus, balanced against the drug's potential benefit to the patient.

In addition to being familiar with federal laws and regulations it is important to know the details of the state's Nurse Practice Act. This act, which is a collection of

Table 12.2	Controlled Substance Categories
I	High potential for abuse and of no currently accepted medical use. Examples: heroin, LSD, mescaline, and peyote. Not obtainable by prescription but may be legally procured for research, study, or instructional use.
II	High abuse potential and high liability for severe psychic or physical dependency. Prescription required and cannot be renewed.
III	Some potential for abuse. Use may lead to low-to-moderate physical dependence and high psychological dependency.
IV	Low potential for abuse. Use may lead to limited physical or psychological dependency.
V	Subject to state and local regulations. Abuse potential is low.

Department of Health and Human Services (2009). The Controlled Substance Schedule. Retrieved from http://www.dhhs.state.nh.us/DHHS/ATOD/controlled-substance.htm, accessed January 23, 2009.

Table 12.3	**Food and Drug Administration Pregnancy Categories**
A	Controlled studies show no risk. Adequate, well-controlled studies in pregnant women have failed to demonstrate risk to the fetus.
B	No evidence of risk in humans. Either animal findings show risk, but human findings do not; or if no adequate human studies have been done, animal findings are negative.
C	Fetal risk cannot be ruled out. Human studies are lacking, and animal studies are either positive for fetal risk or lacking as well. Potential benefits, however, may justify the potential risks.
D	Positive evidence of risk. Investigational or postmarketing data show risk to the fetus. Nevertheless, potential benefits may outweigh the potential risk.
X	Contraindicated in pregnancy. Studies in animals or humans, or investigational or postmarketing reports, have shown fetal risks that clearly outweigh any possible benefit to the patient.

Federal Drug Administration (2006). FDA Drug Category Ratings. Retrieved from http://www.americanpregnancy.org/pregnancyhealth/fdadrugratings.html, accessed January 22, 2009.

laws that regulate nursing, is included in the code of all 50 states, the District of Columbia, Puerto Rico, Guam, and the Virgin Islands.

RECOGNIZING POTENTIAL ADVERSE DRUG REACTIONS

Pharmacological Toxicity

Toxicity is usually the result of the patient receiving an excessive dose of a drug. If the dose is large enough, toxic effects can occur in any patient. Even with small doses, toxicity is possible if the patient is hyper-susceptible to one or another of the drug's primary or secondary pharmacological effects. Adjustment of the dose to the individual patient and vigilant monitoring on the part of the nurse will prevent the majority of toxic events.

If excessive amounts of a drug are given during the procedure, the patient can potentially experience a toxicity reaction. Even commonly used drugs such as lidocaine (Xylocaine) for local anesthesia, heparin solutions for anticoagulation, and antibacterial irrigation for prevention of infection pose a risk if given in excess. Consequently, the circulating nurse and first assistant should know about the type and dose of drugs and solutions used during the procedure.

Drug Allergy and Idiosyncrasy

Drug allergy and idiosyncrasy result because of a patient's sensitivity to a specific chemical. These conditions differ from toxicity in that they are not related to the drug's pharmacology. A reaction due to drug allergy does not occur at the first time of administration but only after the individual becomes sensitized. In an immediate, or anaphylactic, reaction, signs and symptoms develop within minutes after exposure. These reactions result from the release of active chemical mediators during the antigen-antibody reactions. The degree of severity does not depend on the drug but on how strongly sensitized the individual was when he or she received the drug at an earlier time.

In a delayed reaction, the appearance of signs and symptoms may not appear until several hours or days after exposure to the chemical. These reactions often result in a variety of signs and symptoms such as contact dermatitis, hemolytic anemia, fever, swollen lymph nodes, and edema of the face and limbs. For example, a patient may not react to a penicillin compound or mafenide acetate cream (Sulfamylon), which is applied to treat burns, until after the procedure.

Patients who are abnormally sensitive to small doses of a drug the first time it is administered may experience an idiosyncratic reaction. Malignant hyperthermia is an example of the type of reaction (see Chapter 7). This uncommon response may occur in patients who receive inhalation anesthetics such as halothane or the skeletal muscle relaxant succinylcholine.

Potential Interaction of Drugs or Solutions with Other Substances

The presence of another chemical in the body may alter the desired effect of the drug or solution. Combinations of chemicals can result in a number of reactions. The most common reaction is a change in drug metabolism that can alter absorption, distribution, biotransformation, excretion, and concentration of one or more substances. Knowing the types of medications the patient is taking and the potential interactions associated with these medications helps prevent an adverse outcome.

Patient Weight

The patient's body weight is usually the primary consideration when determining medication dosage. In general, weight affects the amount of administered dose that arrives at the reactive target tissues. In a lightweight patient, the reactive target tissue receives a greater portion of the dose. Consequently, the effect of the drug on the lightweight patient is greater than that on a heavier patient. Conversely, the reactive target tissue of a heavy patient receives a smaller portion of the dose, and the effect of the drug is less potent. The patient's weight is usually recorded in kilograms (2.2 pounds is equal to 1 kg). The kilogram weight is used when calculating dosage because dosage is often prescribed and administered on the basis of the ratio of milligrams of the drug to kilograms of body weight.

Patient Age

A patient's age can influence the response to medication. In most cases, neonates, premature infants, and the elderly are more likely to experience intense effects produced by a drug. These individuals are at risk because of an age-related inability to transform drugs to inactive metabolites or a decreased capability to excrete drugs and their remaining active metabolites.

Presence of Disease

Preexisting disease states can alter drug metabolism and excretion and cause an unexpected drug response. For example, a patient with severe liver disease is a poor candidate for general anesthesia with halothane because metabolites formed during reductive metabolism of halothane may produce further damage to the liver. In patients with renal dysfunction, administration of gentamicin can cause further renal damage. Dosage of drugs such as Vancomycin may be based on the patient's creatinine clearance rate to prevent toxicity. Diabetes, cancer, cardiovascular disease, and arthritis are common coexisting conditions that must be considered before, during, and after the procedure.

Drug Tolerance

Drug tolerance to a particular substance can result in a decreased ability to break down the drug by means of hepatic or other enzymatic metabolism. Tolerance to a drug may also develop when a patient continues to take the drug for a long time. Cross tolerance can develop with different drugs that act at the same cellular site to produce similar effects. The drug or alcohol-addicted patient, for example, may prove resistant to a general anesthetic that depresses the central nervous system (CNS) in much the same way the alcohol does.

CNS
Central Nervous System

Cumulative Effects

Cumulative effects can occur when drugs are ingested at a greater rate than the rate at which they can be eliminated by the patient. This is often seen in elderly patients with reduced liver and renal function. If a drug is taken at regular intervals, over time with decreased elimination, accumulation and overdose may result.

PHARMACOLOGICAL CHARACTERISTICS OF DRUGS AND SOLUTIONS USED DURING OPERATIVE OR INVASIVE PROCEDURES

Antimicrobial Agents

Antimicrobial agents are used to prevent an infection or control an existing infection. It has been common practice to use the terms *antibiotic* and *antimicrobial* interchangeably. **Table 12.4** describes common terms used in relation to antimicrobial therapy. An *antibiotic* is a chemical that is produced by one microorganism that has the ability to inhibit other microbes. An *antimicrobial drug* is a natural or synthetic agent that has the ability to kill or suppress microorganisms. From a therapeutic perspective there is no benefit gained from distinguishing between the two terms. Hence, in this discussion, the terms *antibiotic* and *antimicrobial* will be used interchangeably.

An antimicrobial agent can be classified by susceptible organism. Such classifications include antibacterial, antiviral, and antifungal. Antimicrobial drugs can be either narrow spectrum or broad spectrum. Narrow-spectrum drugs are active against only a few microorganisms. In contrast, broad-spectrum antimicrobial agents are active against a wide range of microbes. Another method of classifying an antimicrobial agent is by mechanism of action. This classification scheme is summarized in **Table 12.5**.

Drug Selection

Ideally, specimens for bacterial culture and sensitivity are obtained before beginning treatment. On occasion, when an emergency procedure is indicated, it is unrealistic to wait for the results of bacterial analysis. With such cases, the patient's history and presenting signs and symptoms are used as indicators of the treatment of choice until sensitivity testing is completed.

Dose and Route Selection

The dose and route of administration often depend on the severity of the infection. The most common routes during the operative and invasive procedure are IV

Table 12.4	Key Terms for Antimicrobial Drugs
Anaphylactic	Pertaining to anaphylaxis
Anaphylactoid	A clinical syndrome resembling anaphylaxis but in which no allergic reaction can be demonstrated
Anaphylaxis	A severe allergic reaction manifested by cardiovascular and respiratory collapse, laryngeal edema, hives, and urticaria. Mediated by IgE antibodies
Antibiotic	A chemical compound produced by microorganisms, which can inhibit the growth of, or kill, other organisms
Antimicrobial	A natural or synthetic agent that can kill or suppress microorganisms
Bactericidal	A compound having direct action on bacteria that results in their destruction or death
Bacteriostatic	A compound that inhibits the growth or multiplication of bacteria
Gram stain	A method of staining bacteria that is used to identify various types of bacteria
Gram-negative	A characteristic of certain microorganisms whereby they lose their initial stain when treated with a decolorizing solution used in the Gram stain procedure
Gram-positive	A characteristic whereby certain microorganisms stained with crystal violet and iodine retain their stain after decolorizing
Active immunity	Immunity that is attained by prior exposure to a pathogen or to its antigen, which stimulated production of specific antibodies; also known as acquired immunity
Passive immunity	Protection against a pathogen and its toxins by transfer of antibodies produced in the body of another individual or animal that has been actively immunized
Acquired resistance	A state in which an organism that was once sensitive to an anti-infective drug has developed the ability to remain unaffected by that drug
Congenital resistance	An inborn ability to remain unaffected by certain anti-infective drugs
Microbial resistance	The ability of a microorganism to withstand the effects of anti-infective drugs

administration, topical antibiotic irrigation, vaginal administration, and inunction (rubbing into the skin).

Length of Treatment

The length of treatment is important in avoiding relapse or the development of resistance or adverse reactions. After an antimicrobial drug is selected and administered, its administration should be continued until signs of infection are absent for several days. Documentation of antimicrobial drug administration started during

Table 12.5	Mechanism of Action for Antimicrobials
Inhibition of bacterial cell wall synthesis or active enzymes that disrupt the cell wall	Drugs such as penicillin or cephalosporins weaken the cell wall and thereby promote bacterial lysis and death
Increase cell membrane permeability	Drugs such as Amphotericin B increase the cell wall permeability, causing leakage of intracellular material
Lethal inhibition of bacterial protein synthesis	The aminoglycosides (eg, gentamicin) are the only drugs in this group. It is unknown why inhibition of protein synthesis by these agents results in cell death.
Nonlethal inhibition of protein synthesis	Like the aminoglycosides, these drugs (eg, tetracyclines) inhibit bacterial protein synthesis. These agents only slow microbial growth rather than kill bacteria at clinically achievable concentrations.
Inhibition of nucleic acid synthesis	These drugs inhibit synthesis of DNA or RNA by binding directly to nucleic acid or by interfering with the enzymes required for nucleic acid synthesis (eg, ciprofloxacin).
Antimetabolite disruption of specific biochemical reactions	The result is either a decrease in the synthesis of essential cell constituents or synthesis of nonfunctional analogs of normal metabolites (eg, sulfonamides).
Inhibition of viral DNA synthesis	These drugs (eg, acyclovir, zidovudine) inhibit viral enzymes responsible for DNA synthesis, thereby preventing viral replication

the procedure must be accurate in case the physician decides to use the agent for antimicrobial therapy after the procedure.

Drug Combinations

Emergency treatment of infections before the causative agent is known is often with a combination of two broad-spectrum drugs. If culture and sensitivity testing indicates that the pathogenic strain is fully susceptible to one of the drugs, the other antimicrobial drug may be discontinued.

Adverse Reactions

Antimicrobial agents may cause direct tissue damage when administered topically or in irrigation solutions. Although IV injection may result in phlebitis, some of the more serious forms of toxicity occur when absorbed antibiotics are poorly eliminated and accumulate in the tissue.

Allergic Reactions

Allergies have been reported with almost every kind of antimicrobial drug. Reactions are most common with penicillin-type antibiotics.

Chemoprophylaxis

Antibiotic prophylaxis before and during the procedure can decrease the incidence of infection in certain kinds of procedures. Such therapy is successful when

CMS
Centers for Medicare
and Medicaid Services

CDC
Centers for Disease
Control

SIP
Surgical Infection
Prevention

SCIP
Surgical Care
Improvement Project

SSI
Surgical Site Infections

the goal is to prevent implantation and invasion by a specific pathogen that is known to be sensitive to the antimicrobial agent. The use of antimicrobial agents to prevent or eliminate pathogens, however, should never take the place of strict adherence to aseptic technique during the procedure.

In 2002, the Centers for Medicare and Medicaid Services (CMS) and the Centers for Disease Control (CDC) implemented a Surgical Infection Prevention (SIP) project. This project eventually involved the Quality Improvement Organizations from each state and other national organizations and evolved to become the Surgical Care Improvement Project (SCIP). Because many surgical site infections (SSI) may be directly related to the improper timing, underuse or misuse of antibiotics, SCIP has developed guidelines for the timing of administration and discontinuation of antibiotics and the type of antibiotic ideally used for various types of surgery. Information contained in **Table 12.6** is available in pocket card or poster form for widespread distribution throughout healthcare facilities. The national goal for SCIP is to reduce the number of surgical complications by 25% by 2010.

Individuals with congenital or valvular heart disease and those with prosthetic heart valves are usually susceptible to bacterial endocarditis. Theses individuals can develop endocarditis after operative, dental, and other procedures that may dislodge bacteria into the bloodstream. Therefore, these patients should receive prophylactic antimicrobial therapy before such procedures.

Use During Implantation of Prosthetic Devices

Antimicrobial medications used for soaking prosthetic devices are prepared and delivered to the sterile field by the nurse. Prostheses, such as penile, testicular, breast, and orthopedic implants, are commonly soaked in an antibiotic solution before being implanted. One method is to dispense a solution of 500–1000 mL of 0.9% sodium chloride onto the field. To this, one or a combination of antibiotics is added. Commonly used antibiotics include bacitracin, polymyxin B, and gentamicin.

Anticoagulants

The process of hemostasis involves the interplay of four phases. The first three—vascular response, platelet formation, and coagulation—promote blood clotting and prevent blood loss. The fourth, the fibrinolytic phase, helps maintain blood fluidity and prevents propagation of clotting beyond the site of injury. This phase is also involved in clot dissolution. For a thorough discussion on the process of hemostasis, see Chapter 17.

Medications that prevent the coagulation of blood can be classified into three groups: anticoagulant, antiplatelet, and fibrinolytic. Anticoagulants prevent clot formation or, if they have already formed, keep clots from completely closing off a portion of the blood vessel (**Table 12.7**). Anticoagulants prevent the extension of clots but do not dissolve existing clots. Anticoagulant drugs used for this purpose include heparin and warfarin.

Heparin exerts an effect on blood coagulation by potentiating the action of antithrombin III, which subsequently acts on several kinds of circulating clotting factors to exert an immediate effect in preventing blood coagulation. Low doses (prophylactic) prevent the conversion of prothrombin to thrombin; high doses (therapeutic) prevent the conversion of fibrinogen to fibrin.

Table 12.6	Surgical Care Improvement Project Approved Antibiotics*
Surgical Procedure	**Approved Antibiotics**
CABG, Other Cardiac or Vascular	Cefazolin, Cefuroxime or Vancomycin* If β-lactam allergy: Vancomycin** or Clindamycin*
Hysterectomy	Cefotetan, Cefazolin, Cefoxitin, Cefuroxime, or Ampicillin/Sulbactam If β-lactam allergy: Clindamycin + Aminoglycoside, or Clindamycin + Quinolone, or Clindamycin + Aztreonam OR Metronidazole + Aminoglycoside, or Metronidazole + Quinolone OR Clindamycin monotherapy
Hip/Knee Arthroplasty	Cefazolin or Cefuroxime or Vancomycin* If β-lactam allergy: Vancomycin** or Clindamycin**
Colon	Cefotetan, Cefoxitin, Ampicillin/Sulbactam, or Ertapenem† OR Cefazolin or Cefuroxime + Metronidazole If β-lactam allergy: Clindamycin + Aminoglycoside, or Clindamycin + Quinolone, or Clindamycin + Aztreonam OR Metronidazole with Aminoglycoside, or Metronidazole + Quinolone
Special Considerations	*Vancomycin is acceptable with a physician-documented justification for its use (see data element *Vancomycin*) **For cardiac, orthopedic, and vascular surgery, if the patient is allergic to β-lactam antibiotics, Vancomycin or Clindamycin are acceptable substitutes. †A single dose of Ertapenem is recommended for colon procedures.

The antibiotic regimens described in this table reflect the combined, published recommendations of the American Society of Health-System Pharmacists, the Medical Letter, the Infectious Diseases Society of America, the Sanford Guide to Antimicrobial Therapy, and the Surgical Infection Society. The material was prepared by FMQAI, the Medicare Quality Improvement Organization for Florida, under contract with the Centers for Medicare & Medicaid Services (CMS), an agency of the US Department of Health and Human Services http://www.medqic.org/dcs.

* Updated Prophylactic Antibiotic Regimen Selection for Surgery

Table 12.7	Key Terms for Anticoagulant Therapy
Ecchymosis	A small spot caused by bleeding in the skin or mucous membranes, forming a round or irregular purple patch
Embolus	A clot carried by the blood from a larger vessel to a smaller vessel, which becomes blocked
Hematoma	A localized collection of blood in a space, organ, or tissue
Hemostasis	The process designed to minimize blood loss, including blood coagulation and the formation of platelets
Petechia	A tiny red spot caused by the escape of a small amount of blood
Phlebothrombosis	The presence of blood clots in a vein without inflammation
Thrombophlebitis	Inflammation and clotting within a vein
Thrombus	A solid mass of clotted blood in a vessel or in the heart

IU
International Units

Heparin is measured in standard US Pharmacopeia units, not in milligrams or International Units (IU), neither of which is equivalent to 1 U of heparin. One unit of heparin is defined as the amount of heparin required to anticoagulate 1 mL of blood. Strict adherence to heparin dosage and dilution instructions is essential in the prevention of excessive bleeding. Protamine sulfate 1% (heparin antidote) should be available for use when administering heparin. Do not mix heparin in the same solution as antibiotics. Moreover, heparin interacts with several commonly ingested drugs. Heparin must be used with caution for patients who are receiving concurrent oral anticoagulants, thrombolytic enzymes, or drugs that affect platelet function (eg, salicylates, clopidogrel, dipyridamole, nonsteroidal anti-inflammatory agents).

Warfarin, in contrast, acts indirectly. Warfarin acts in the liver to prevent the synthesis of vitamin K-dependent clotting factors and thereby preventing blood coagulation. It does not dissolve existing clots.

Antiplatelet drugs, such as aspirin, dipyridamole (Persantine), clopidogrel (Plavix), and dextran 40 injection (Rheomacrodex) interfere with the reaction that causes platelets to aggregate at arterial wall sites and in the veins.

The nurse should be careful not to confuse dextran 40 injection with dextran 70 or other dextran solutions. Dextran 40 injection is used only if the seal is intact and the solution is absolutely clear. To dissolve crystals, the unopened bottle is placed in a warm water bath until the solution clears. Any unused portion is discarded, because dextral 40 injection does not contain preservatives. A baseline hematocrit is obtained before the initiation of dextran 40 injection and after administration. The nurse should notify the physician if the patient's hematocrit is depressed below 30% by volume.

Dipyridamole acts by dilating small resistant vessels of the coronary vascular bed, possibly by causing accumulation of adenosine diphosphate, which produces vasodilatation and reduces platelet adherence. Dipyridamole can prevent thrombus formation or transient ischemic attacks.

Clopidogrel acts by irreversibly inhibiting the binding of adenosine triphosphate to platelet receptors, thereby inhibiting platelet aggregation. Clopidogrel should be discontinued five to seven days prior to elective surgical procedure.

Fibrinolytic agents, such as streptokinase, urokinase, and tissue plasminogen activator, speed the rate of the natural clot-resolving process. These thrombolytic enzymes directly dissolve thrombi by binding to the fibrin in the clot and converting plasminogen to plasmin, the clot enzyme that degrades fibrin. As the fibrin matrix dissolves, the clot is fragmented into soluble products and gradually resolves. Although dissolving thrombi in vessels that supply vital organs is beneficial, these enzymes can also dissolve clots that are necessary to prevent bleeding. Because of the risk of hemorrhage, these enzymes are used for specific situations and patients.

Hemostatic Agents

Chemical agents to control bleeding may be dispensed in sponge-type (Gelfoam), woven-type (Surgicel), powder (Avitene) or a two-part fibrin sealant (Tisseel VH) that may be mixed on the sterile field. A complete discussion of these products is found in Chapter 17.

Local Anesthetics

Local anesthetics are used during minor procedures and as an adjunct to general or regional anesthesia (**Table 12.8**). These drugs provide a loss of feeling without the loss of consciousness associated with general anesthesia. Local anesthetics act by temporarily interrupting the production and conduction of nerve impulses. This reversible block in conduction is brought about by a drug-induced reduction in the

Table 12.8	Key Terms for Local Anesthetics
Anesthesia	The loss of feeling or sensation, particularly the sensation of pain
Anesthetic	An agent that produces a loss of feeling or sensation
Topical analgesia	Application of a cream, ointment, or fluid for the purpose of anesthetizing the skin or mucous membrane
Infiltration anesthesia	Injection of solutions of local anesthetic into tissue to bring the anesthetic into contact with nerve endings in the intracutaneous, subcutaneous, and deeper structure and keep these sensitive nerve terminals from transmitting pain impulses
Field block	A form of infiltration anesthesia in which the sensory nerve pathways from the operative field are blocked off by a circular ring of subcutaneously injected solution
Central nerve block	Block that affects the roots of nerves at various points close to their origin in the spinal cord
Peripheral nerve block	Block affecting the trunks of specific nerves such as the sciatic-femoral, ulnar, or intercostal nerves, or the brachial plexus
Intravenous regional block	Local anesthesia of an arm or a leg by injection of local anesthetic into a vein after exsanguinations and application of a pneumatic tourniquet

permeability of the nerve cell membrane to sodium and potassium ions. This then interferes with the ability of the neuronal membrane to depolarize in response to stimuli.

Administration of Local Anesthetics

The nurse prepares local anesthetics used on the sterile field. Precautions are taken to prevent rapid systemic absorption from the skin, subcutaneous tissue, fascia, and muscles, as well as accidental IV injection. The physician should not inject local anesthetics into infected tissue or apply them to traumatized mucous membranes.

Aspiration is performed in several planes to ensure that the needle has not entered a vessel. Injections are made systematically by first entering the cutaneous, then the subcutaneous, and lastly the interfascicular and intramuscular planes.

The physician allows enough time for the drug's action to take effect before the procedure is initiated or before administering additional anesthetic. Knowledge of the time it takes to achieve anesthesia is essential because there is great variation between local anesthetic actions.

Lidocaine injection and commercially prepared solutions containing the drug in 5% dextrose are stored preferably at 15–30°C (59–86°F) unless otherwise directed by the manufacturer. Solutions are inspected for particulate matter and discoloration before administration and discarded if either is present.

Drug, Dose, and Route Selection

The selection of local anesthetic depends on the type of procedure, the complexity and length of the procedure, the location of the operative and invasive procedure site, and the overall condition and acuity of the patient. Drugs commonly used for local anesthetics are listed in **Table 12.9**. When administering such agents, the physician should only inject the minimal amount of medication effective for producing anesthesia. A record is kept of the total amount of solution injected and the actual number of milligrams administered is calculated. The method for calculation of a dose of injected anesthetic agent is as follows: percentage of concentration X 10 = mg/mL. For example, a 2% solution contains 20 mg/mL.

For solutions containing epinephrine, a 1:1000 concentration has 1 mg of epinephrine per 1 mL. All variations of concentration are proportions of this equation. For example, a solution containing epinephrine 1:100,000 has 1 mg of epinephrine per 100 mL of solution.

Vasoconstrictors

Epinephrine is often added to local anesthetic solutions to slow down the absorption of the drug and to keep the anesthetic at the desired site. This prolongs its blocking effect. In addition, epinephrine diminishes blood loss because of its vasoconstrictive action. High concentrations of epinephrine (1:100,000) are used in vascular areas such as the scalp and face. Lower concentrations (1:200,000) are used for areas such as the skin of the back or the extremities. Vasoconstrictors are not added to anesthetic solutions that are used in areas of restricted circulation such as the fingers, toes, tip of the nose, ears, or penis. Local anesthetic solutions are commonly referred

Table 12.9	Frequently Used Local Anesthetics	
	Trade Name	**Duration of Action (min)**
Lidocaine 2.5% and prilocaine 2.5%	Emla Cream	60–120
Mepivacaine hydrochloride	Carbocaine	60–120
Prilocaine hydrochloride	Citanest hydrochloride	30–120
Bupivacaine hydrochloride	Marcaine hydrochloride, Sensorcaine	120–240
Chloroprocaine hydrochloride	Nesacaine, Nesacaine CE	15–30
Procaine hydrochloride	Novocain	15–30
Tetracaine	Pontocaine	120–240
Lidocaine	Xylocaine	30–120
Benzocaine 14% or 20%	Cetacaine spray, Hurricane spray, Topex Spray	5–60

to as *plain* or *with epi* to distinguish between the solutions containing epinephrine. Local anesthetic solutions should be identified with the name of the solution, the concentration, and the concentration of the epinephrine when dispensed to the sterile field and should be labeled immediately. Each time the syringe is passed to the physician, the scrub person should verbally identify the solution. Under no circumstances should an anesthetic solution be prepared by mixing with epinephrine on the sterile field.

Products containing oxymetazoline hydrochloride (Afrin) may be used prior to nasal or sinus surgery. Oxymetazoline hydrochloride is delivered as a spray into the nares, usually in the preprocedure holding area.

Topical Anesthesia

Cocaine produces local anesthesia of mucous membranes such as the nose, the throat and the tracheobronchial tree. Cocaine hydrochloride topical solution (4% per 4 mL and 10% per 4 mL) may be applied into the nares with cotton pledgets before septorhinoplasty or sprayed into the throat before endotracheal intubation. Ophthalmological application produces surface anesthesia, vasoconstriction, and mydriasis. Cocaine is not administered by injection as systemic absorption can result in life-threatening side-effects. Due to the high risk for physical and psychological dependence, the use of cocaine as a topical anesthetic is becoming less widespread.

Xylocaine Viscous may be used for anesthetizing the oropharynx prior to endoscopic procedures or for local anesthesia of the urethra prior to cystoscopy. Xylocaine in combination with prilocaine (EMLA cream) may be used to anesthetize the skin prior to initiating an intravenous line, especially in pediatric patients. The cream should be applied with an occlusive dressing 30 minutes prior to needlestick.

Hurricaine Spray, Cetacaine Spray, and Topex Spray, all solutions containing benzocaine, are often used to anesthetize the nasopharynx, oropharynx, and laryngotracheal region in preparation for endoscopic examinations. These sprays have a rapid onset when delivered to the mucous membranes and are effective for up to 60 minutes. Because these products, along with Xylocaine Viscous, suppress the gag reflex, patients should be evaluated carefully in the recovery area prior to administering ice chips or liquids.

A potentially serious side effect, acquired methemoglobinemia, has been reported after use of sprays containing benzocaine or Xylocaine. Methemoglobinemia is a disorder in which the hemoglobin is unable to bind and transport oxygen effectively. Symptoms include cyanosis of the skin and mucous membranes, headache, anxiety, tachycardia, and shortness of breath. Oxygen saturation and blood gas levels may appear normal but methemoglobinemia should be considered when cyanosis appears after administration of benzocaine or Xylocaine containing sprays. Treatment is the immediate intravenous injection of 1 to 2 mg/kg of methylene blue. When not diagnosed and treated early, methemoglobinemia can cause disability or death.

Physiological Monitoring of the Patient under Local Anesthetics

Patient monitoring during operative or invasive procedures involving the use of local anesthesia is often the responsibility of the nurse. For additional information about local anesthesia and patient monitoring, see Chapter 13.

Ophthalmic Agents

The nurse prepares and administers a variety of ophthalmic medications for use during eye examinations and ophthalmological procedures (**Table 12.10**). Ophthalmic medications and solutions are used during procedures such as cataract extraction, intraocular lens implantation, glaucoma filtration, correction of muscle disorders, corneal transplant, and detached retina surgery.

Mydriatic or Cycloplegic Agents

The autonomic drugs that produce mydriasis (pupil dilation) and cycloplegia (paralysis of accommodation) are the most frequently used topical medications in ophthalmic practice. Phenylephrine hydrochloride (Neo-Synephrine) is used alone or, more commonly, in combination with a cycloplegic agent for refraction or papillary dilation. Other drugs include atropine sulfate, cyclopentolate hydrochloride, homatropine hydrobromide (Homatrocel), and tropicamide (Mydriacyl). The parasympatholytic action of cycloplegia agents causes the smooth muscle of the ciliary body and iris to relax, resulting in pupillary dilatation and paralysis of the ciliary muscles. Cycloplegic agents are contraindicated in persons with primary glaucoma or a tendency toward glaucoma.

Cycloplegic agents are administered at least one hour before refraction and/or the operative procedure. When drops are being instilled pressure is applied to the inner canthus to lessen systemic absorption of the drug. The solution may otherwise run into the respiratory tract via the lacrimal duct and be absorbed into the bloodstream. The lids should be kept open for several seconds after application to retain the solution

Table 12.10	Key Terms for Ophthalmic Drugs
Adrenergic agents	Medications that constrict the vessels of the eye, thereby reducing the rate at which aqueous fluid is formed within the eye. In addition, the outflow of fluid may be increased. This mechanism, which is not clearly understood, helps to lower the intraocular pressure.
Aphakia	Absence of the lens of the eye, which may be congenital or occur after injury or an operative procedure
Cholinergic agents	Medications that directly or indirectly cause the sphincter muscles of the iris and of the ciliary body to contract
Cycloplegic agent	Medication that causes paralysis of accommodation by relaxing the ciliary muscles of the eye
Gonioscopy	Examination of the filtration angle of the anterior eye chamber with an optical instrument designed to visualize the area and determine anterior chamber width
Hyperosmotic agents	Medications that increase the osmotic pressure of the blood plasma to a point above that of the aqueous humor and the vitreous body of the eye. Intraocular fluid then follows the osmotic gradient into the hyperosmotic plasma. The loss of fluid leads to a reduction in intraocular pressure.
Inner canthus	The angle at the nasal end of the opening between the eyelids
Miotic agent	Medication that causes constriction of the pupil
Mydriatic agent	Medication that causes dilatation of the pupil of the eye
Tonometry	The process of using a tonometer to measure intraocular pressure
Trabecula	Supporting fibers of connecting tissue

on the surface of the eye. This prolongs ocular action. After administration, the nurse should wash his or her hands and instruct the patient to do so because these drugs may be absorbed by the mucosa of the nose and mouth when fingers contaminated with the drug come in contact with these areas. The effects of these drugs can depend on the age, race and eye color of the patient. For example, the mydriatics and cycloplegics tend to be less effective in dark-eyed individuals than in blue-eyed ones.

Dapiprazole hydrochloride (Rev-Eyes) can be used to reverse the effects of phenylephrine and, to a lesser extent, tropicamide. The use of Rev-Eyes does not exclude instructing the patient to use sunglasses and avoid driving or operating dangerous machinery.

Topical Agents

Topical anesthetic agents, such as proparacaine hydrochloride (Ophthaine) and tetracaine hydrochloride (Pontocaine), act by stabilizing the neuronal membrane and preventing the initiation and transmission of nerve impulses. The onset on anesthesia begins within 20 minutes and lasts up to 15 minutes. Topical anesthetics are used in conjunction with retrobulbar infiltrative anesthesia for operative procedures.

Topical anesthetics are used before the removal of foreign bodies and sutures and during tonometry and gonioscopy to promote comfort. Topical anesthetics can also retard wound healing. Subsequent corneal infection and/or opacity with accompanying permanent visual loss or corneal perforation may occur.

Hyperosmotic Agents

Agents such as mannitol (Osmitrol) and glycerin (Osmoglyn, Glyrol) act by increasing the osmotic pressure of the blood plasma to a point above that of the aqueous humor and the vitreous body of the eye. Fluid within the eye then follows the osmotic gradient into the hyperosmotic plasma. This loss of pressure leads to a reduction of intraocular pressure so the procedure can safely be performed on a softened eye.

Miotic Agents

Parasympathomimetics (Miotics) are used primarily as topical therapy for glaucoma. This class is subdivided into direct-acting (cholinergic) agents such as pilocarpine hydrochloride and indirect-acting (anticholinesterase) agents such as physostigmine (Eserine). Both cause the sphincter muscles of the iris and the ciliary body to contract. Constriction of the pupil tends to thin the iris and pull its folds and roots out of the anterior chamber angle. This leads to a reduction of intraocular pressure in acute angle-closure glaucoma, also known as closed-angle and narrow-angle glaucoma. In open-angle glaucoma, these drugs act by opening the closed or narrowed trabecular channel and allowing the fluid to escape.

Miotic solutions should be stored in a cool place and protected from light to reduce the rate of deterioration. The solution must be checked before use. Discolored or cloudy solutions should be discarded. Physostigmine tends to turn pink or red. Epinephrine turns brown. Phenylephrine becomes cloudy. Miotic drugs such as acetylcholine chloride (Miochol) and a solution of carbachol (Miostat) are available for use during the procedure.

Acetylcholine chloride is an unstable solution and must be reconstituted immediately before use. To administer acetylcholine chloride, press the rubber stopper of the vial down sufficiently to dislodge the center rubber plug seal. This releases the solvent (sterile water) from the upper chamber. Shake the vial gently to dissolve and mix the drug in the lower chamber. If the center rubber plug seal does not move down, or is in the down position, do not use the medication. After mixing, clean the stopper with 70% alcohol and aspirate the desired dose into a dry sterile syringe with a sterile 18 to 22 gauge needle. Discard the unused portion of the drug.

Sympathomimetic Drugs

Sympathomimetic drugs work by improving aqueous outflow and, to a lesser extent, improving uveoscleral output. Dipivefrin hydrochloride (Propine) causes fewer systemic side effects than epinephrine hydrochloride (Epifrin) and can sometimes be used in patients who have developed sensitivity to epinephrine. Although used to treat some types of glaucoma, use of these agents is contraindicated in acute angle-closure glaucoma.

Accidental administration of a mydriatic instead of a miotic to a patient with angle-closure glaucoma may precipitate an acute attack, which could lead to blindness. Mydriatics should not be routinely administered for eye examinations. The physician should be asked for specific instructions for each patient.

Chymotrypsin

Chymotrypsin (Zolyse) is a proteolytic enzyme that is instilled into the posterior chamber of the eye to cause dissolution of zonular fibers attached to the lens, thereby facilitating the removal of the lens during cataract extraction. This drug is reconstituted immediately before the operative procedure. It should not be used if it is cloudy or if it contains a precipitate, and it should not be resterilized. Excessive heat, alcohol, and other chemicals inactivate the enzyme. Chymotrypsin should be stored at 8–24°C (46.4–75.2°F).

Sodium Hyaluronate

Sodium hyaluronate (Healon) is used as a surgical aid in cataract extraction, intraocular lens implantation, corneal transplant, glaucoma filtration, and a retinal reattachment procedure. Instillation of sodium hyaluronate maintains a deep anterior chamber during the procedure and allows for effective manipulation with less trauma to the cornea and surrounding tissue.

The physician should express a small amount of sodium hyaluronate from the syringe before use and carefully examine the remainder as it is injected. The literature reports an occasional release of minute rubber particles, presumably formed when the diaphragm is punctured. Reuse of cannulas should be avoided. If reuse becomes necessary, the cannula is rinsed with sterile distilled water. Sodium hyaluronate is stored at 2–8°C (35.6–46.4°F) and protected from freezing and light. Refrigerated sodium hyaluronate should be allowed to attain room temperature for approximately 30 minutes before use.

Anti-Infective Steroids

Anti-infective steroid combination agents, such as dexamethasone 0.1%, neomycin sulfate, and polymyxin B sulfate, are used for steroid-responsive inflammatory ocular conditions for which a corticosteroid is indicated. Such drugs may also be administered when bacterial infection or the risk of bacterial ocular infection exists.

Glucocorticoids

Glucocorticoids, such as sterile methylprednisolone acetate suspension (Depo-Medrol) and sterile betamethasone sodium phosphate and betamethasone acetate suspension (Celestone Soluspan) are used for their potent anti-inflammatory effects. Glucocorticoids are injected during or immediately after ocular procedures to prevent the inflammatory process. They are also used to treat severe acute and chronic allergic and inflammatory processes involving the eye, such as herpes zoster ophthalmicus, iritis, diffuse posterior uveitis and choroiditis, sympathetic ophthalmia, anterior segment inflammation, and keratitis.

Hyaluronidase

Hyaluronidase, 150U (Wydase), is a mucolytic enzyme that is added to the retrobulbar injection of local anesthetic to promote diffusion and absorption of the anesthetic agent. Injection of hyaluronidase is contraindicated in or around inflamed, infected, or cancerous areas. Because absorption of an accompanying drug is enhanced, the nurse should watch for adverse reactions and expect a shortened duration of drug action. Hyaluronidase for injection is reported to be stable for up to 3 months when stored at 2–8°C (35.6–46.4°F).

Hyperosmolar Agents

Hyperosmolar (hypertonic) agents are used to reduce corneal edema therapeutically or for diagnostic purposes (Ophthalgan). They act through osmotic attraction of water through the semipermeable corneal epithelium.

Otic Agents

The nurse prepares and administers a variety of otic medications for use during ear examinations and otolaryngologic procedures (**Table 12.11**).

Asepsis

The ear canal is cleaned and dried before instillation of medication. Strict asepsis is observed when the ear has been opened surgically or opened because of trauma. Infection is especially hazardous because of the ear's close proximity to the brain.

Table 12.11	Key Terms for Otic Medications
Auricle or pinna	External part of the ear composed of cartilage and covered by skin
Cochlea	Winding cone-shaped tube forming a portion of the inner ear
Eustachian tube	Tube that brings air to the middle ear, thus equalizing pressure on both sides of the tympanic membrane
External auditory canal	Includes the outer portion of the ear, the canal, and the tympanic membrane
Inner ear or labyrinth	A system of tubes and spaces within a hollowed-out temporal bone, collectively called the bony labyrinth
Mastoid air cells	Air-filled spaces in the temporal bone. The middle ear communicates posteriorly with the mastoid ear cells.
Ossicles	Three bones of the ear: malleolus, incus, and stapes
Tragus	Cartilaginous projection in front of the exterior meatus of the ear
Tympanic membrane	The eardrum, which divides the meatus and the middle ear cavity

Administration of Drugs

Straighten the ear canal for optimal visualization and to allow the medication to flow into the canal. In adults, pull the auricle upward and backward and pull the tragus forward. In infants and children, pull the auricle downward. Warm solutions or suspensions used for irrigation and eardrops to body temperature before they are instilled. Hot or cold solutions can cause vertigo, nausea, and vomiting. Never obstruct the ear canal when instilling drops. Obstruction may result in a pressure increase against the tympanic membrane. Examine glass-tipped medication droppers to ensure that the tip of the dropper is not chipped.

Medication Contraindications

Preparations of polymyxin B, neomycin, and hydrocortisone used for the prevention and treatment of inflammation and superficial bacterial infections of the external auditory canal are contraindicated in patients who have shown hypersensitivity to any of their components. These drugs are also contraindicated for patients with herpes simplex, vaccinia, and varicella.

Nasal Medications

Vasoconstrictors such as oxymetazoline hydrochloride (Afrin) may be sprayed into the nares prior to endoscopic sinus procedures or other nasal procedures. During nasal procedures, a topical anesthetic such as cocaine or vasoconstrictors such as epinephrine or oxymetazoline may be introduced into the nares on a cotton pledget. **Table 12.12** lists key terms for nasal medications.

Administration of drugs

After instructing the patient to blow his or her nose, the patient should be positioned in the supine position with the head tilted back. Sprays are then delivered into the nares while the patient inhales.

Medication Contraindications

Vasoconstrictors are contraindicated in patients with uncontrolled hypertension.

Table 12.12	Key Terms for Nasal Medications
Naris	The nostril
Paranasal sinus	One of the air cavities in the frontal, maxillary, sphenoid, or ethmoid bones
Septum	The structure dividing the two nostrils
Turbinate	Scroll like bone on the lateral wall of the nasal cavity
Vestibule	Floor of the nose

Skin Medications

The nurse selects, prepares, and administers a variety of topical skin preparations (**Table 12.13**). To achieve the intended therapeutic result, each preparation, whether ointment, solution, cream, lotion, or impregnated dressing should be applied to ensure the desired penetration and absorption.

Medication Administration

Avoid applying ointments, creams, and lotions in copious amounts. Not only is this practice messy, it may result in excessive absorption of this product, especially when using corticosteroids. Apply liquids and other fluids sparingly to the scalp area to prevent fluids from running into the patient's eyes. Remove blood, pus, cellular debris, or other drainage because some topical applications are inactivated by these substances.

Commonly Used Skin Preparations

Acetone. When using acetone, avoid contact with open wounds and mucous membranes, especially the eyes. Do not use acetone in the presence of an ignition source such as electrosurgery or a laser beam.

Alcohol (Ethyl and Isopropyl). Do not apply alcohol to open wounds, mucous membranes, and the eyes. Do not use alcohol in the presence of an ignition source such as electrosurgery or a laser beam.

Antibacterial Sulfonamides. When sulfonamides are applied to extensive areas, serum sulfa concentrations, urinalysis, and kidney function tests should be monitored because significant quantities of the drug may be absorbed. Sulfonamides are incompatible with silver preparations.

Table 12.13	Key Terms for Skin Medications
Antihistaminic	Antagonizes the effect of free histamine on the skin and its blood vessels and thus relieves the cutaneous signs and symptoms of allergy
Anti-infective	Used to treat or prevent skin or mucous membrane infection by pathogenic microbes (eg, antimicrobials, antifungals, antiseptics, antibacterials)
Anti-inflammatory	Used to reduce skin inflammation and relieve its signs and symptoms
Antiseptic	Chemical substance that kills microorganisms and prevents their growth
Demulcent	Used to coat the skin and mucous membranes, thereby providing mechanical protection against irritation of these surfaces
Depilatory	Chemical used to remove hair
Detergent	Used to clean the skin; usually has some antiseptic properties
Dusting powder	Inert substance applied to the skin to protect the irritated surface or to absorb excessive moisture
Emollient	Oily or fatty substance used to prevent the evaporation of water and drying of the skin
Proteolytic enzymes	Chemical substance applied to the skin to speed the breakdown of necrotic tissue in ulcerated or burned skin areas (eg, for chemical debridement of dead tissue)

12

Antibiotics. Topical antibiotic therapy most commonly makes use of combinations of several antibiotics such as bacitracin, polymyxin B, neomycin, and sometimes tyrothricin and gramicidin.

Benzoin Compound Tincture. Clean the skin thoroughly before applying benzoin because it forms an occlusive coating and may promote the retention of moisture and bacterial growth. Do not use benzoin in the presence of an ignition source such as electrosurgery or a laser beam.

Collodion (Flexible). Clean and dry the skin before application. Do not use collodion in the presence of an ignition source such as electrosurgery or a laser beam.

Glycerin. Undiluted glycerin (95%–99%) absorbs moisture and therefore may result in dehydration and irritation when applied to mucous membranes.

Occlusive Dressings for Topical Corticosteroids. Penetration of a steroid can be increased about tenfold by covering the areas of application with an impermeable plastic. The plastic covering is kept in place for several hours and then removed to prevent prickly heat lesions and maceration. Systemic toxicity, such as cushingoid signs or suppression of adrenal function, is possible but is rarely associated with topical application. The risk of adrenal suppression is increased, however, when a large occlusive dressing is used.

Oxidizing Agents (Hydrogen Peroxide). Never instill oxidizing agents into closed body cavities or into abscesses that do not allow the free oxygen to escape. Deep wound irrigation can result in systemic oxygen microemboli by passage of oxygen into the vascular system. Additionally, the release of oxygen will create an oxygen-enriched environment, thus creating a fire hazard, particularly in the presence of an ignition source such as electrosurgery or a laser beam.

Petrolatum (Hydrophilic). Avoid the use of excessive amounts of hydrophilic petrolatum. As the petrolatum warms from contact with the skin, the product may liquefy and run from the desired application location. This may cause discomfort to the patient. Do not use petrolatum in the presence of an ignition source such as electrosurgery and a laser beam.

Silver Nitrate. Silver nitrate is used for wound cauterization. Before use, clean the area to remove organic material that may inhibit drug action. If a silver nitrate pencil is used, it should be dipped in water and applied to the areas for the time that promotes the desired action. If healthy tissue is accidentally treated, it may be washed with a saline solution because the chloride in the saline forms insoluble precipitates of the silver nitrate and thus inhibits its action.

Starch/Talc. Dry skin surfaces before applying powder. If the powder cakes, it can cause further irritation to the skin. Ensure that powdered substances such as starch do not come in contact with open stomas or wounds.

Topical Dyes (Gentian Violet). Wear protective gloves to avoid staining the hands with gentian violet. Avoid accidental spilling onto the patient's skin.

Xeroform Petroleum Dressing. Do not use xeroform petroleum dressings on patients with hypersensitivity to bismuth tribromophenate. Do not use this dressing in the presence of an ignition source such as electrosurgery or a laser beam.

Zinc Oxide. Zinc, like other metals, may cause an alteration of x-ray films or x-ray therapy.

Contrast Media

Contrast media are administered to highlight a body structure during radiographic examination (**Table 12.14**). Media intended for intravascular and intrathecal use include metrizamide (Amipaque) and iohexol (Omnipaque). Agents used for intravascular injection alone include diatrizoate meglumine and diatrizoate sodium injection (Angiovist), iothalamate meglumine (Conray), and diatrizoate sodium (Hypaque). Diatrizoate meglumine (Renografin) can be used for intraureteral studies as well as IV studies. Ethiodol, a brand of ethiodized oil, is used for hysterosalpingography and lymphography. The dosage, concentration, and route of administration vary depending on the patient and the procedure being performed. Always refer to the manufacturer's recommendations and consult with the physician before preparing contrast media for administration.

Contrast media may interfere with some chemical determinations made on urine specimens. A urine sample needed for study should be collected before the administration of the contrast media or 2 days or more after the radiographic study.

A scout film is recommended before administration of the contrast media. This helps set the limits for the study and reduces the patient's exposure to contrast media.

Vials should be protected from direct exposure to sunlight. contrast media should not be frozen and should be stored at 15–30°C (59–86°). Products should be inspected for particulate matter and discoloration before administration.

Irrigating Fluids for Endoscopic Procedures

The nurse may administer a variety of endoscopic fluids. Glycine (1.5% glycine irrigation) or other suitable nonelectrolyte solutions are commonly used for transurethral operative procedures. Glycine is an amino acid that is hypotonic in relation to extracellular fluid. Because it does not contain electrolytes, it is nonconductive and suitable for urologic irrigation during electrosurgical procedures. A 1.5%

Table 12.14	Key Terms for Contrast Media
Arteriogram	Radiographic study of an artery to determine arterial perfusion, size, and shape
Arthrogram	Radiographic study of a joint cavity to outline the contour of the joint
Cholangiogram	Radiographic study of the bile ducts
Cystogram	Radiographic study of the bladder
Cystourethrogram	Radiographic study of the bladder and ureters
Discogram	Radiographic study of intervertebral disks
Hysterosalpingogram	Study of the uterus and fallopian tubes after injection of radiopaque material into those structures
Pyelogram	Radiographic study of the ureter and renal pelvis. For an intravenous pyelogram, the contrast medium is given intravenously and an x-ray film of the urinary tract is taken while the material is excreted. This provides important information about the structure and function of the kidney, ureter, and bladder.

concentration of glycine in water is sufficient to minimize the risk of intravascular hemolysis, which can occur from absorption of plain water throughout open prostatic veins during transurethral resection. Solution that is absorbed intravascularly during transurethral resection or bladder procedures is normally excreted by the kidneys.

Hyskon hysteroscopy fluid is a clear, viscid, sterile, non-pyrogenic solution of dextran 70. The fluid is also electrolyte-free and nonconductive.

The amount of fluid that is instilled into and recovered from the patient should be monitored closely. Patients undergoing lengthy procedures, receiving large amounts of irrigation fluids, or retaining excess fluid are at risk for development of dilutional hyponatremia and pulmonary edema.

Irrigation fluids should be warmed to prevent hypothermia, preferably with an automatic warming device, and should be warmed to body temperature (98.6°F [37°C]) (AORN, 2008). Using a warming device can prevent inadvertent overwarming of fluids, and the temperature of fluids should be verified before use. Patient injury can occur with irrigation of hot solutions. The solution is administered only if it is clear, the seal is intact, and the container is undamaged. It is not injected parenterally. Any unused portion should be discarded. Most solutions are intended for use as a single-dose irrigation and do not contain bacteriostatic agents, anti-infective agents, or an acid buffer.

THE HUMAN RESPONSE TO THE ADMINISTRATION OF DRUGS AND SOLUTIONS

Psychological factors influence the patient's willingness to take a medication and the degree of effectiveness of the drug. If a patient does not believe that the medication will be effective, it is possible that the desired effect will not be achieved. In the case of the placebo effect, a patient who is unaware of the inactive properties of the placebo finds the substance effective for its intended use. There have been clinical studies in such therapies as guided imagery, hypnosis, therapeutic touch, and meditation for patient care. The nurse can use these techniques alone or in combination with medications administered during the procedure.

Religious beliefs and practices play an important role in the patient's perception of health, reaction to illness, and response to medications. By assessing the patient's values and beliefs, the nurse obtains data that can influence medication administration and patient compliance. For example, a Seventh-Day Adventist may refuse to ingest narcotics or stimulants because he or she believes that his or her body is a temple of the Holy Spirit and should be protected from such substances. Jehovah's Witnesses are generally opposed to blood transfusion, although individuals may be persuaded in emergencies to accept blood. Christian Scientists believe that their religion has a healing function and although they may seek healthcare for childbirth and fracture, they generally refuse medications, vaccinations, and inoculations.

Like religious practices, culture and ethnicity may affect a patient's health beliefs. Many cultures employ folk beliefs and remedies in the treatment of illness. Some of these practices have a scientific basis. One common example is the use of the plants *Digitalis lanata* (yellow foxglove) and *Digitalis purpurea* (purple foxglove) to ameliorate the symptoms of congestive heart failure. Other folk practices and herbal treatments, although lacking in scientific basis, have significant value to those who use them. Understanding and respecting these beliefs fosters holistic care and promotes an awareness and use of many nontraditional resources.

OBTAINING A MEDICATION HISTORY

Assessment is an essential component of drug and solution administration. **Table 12.15** provides a list of potential questions to ask the patient or significant other before the administration of drugs and solutions. Responses to these questions will assist in identifying patients at risk for adverse outcomes related to the administration of drugs and solutions.

IDENTIFYING PATIENTS AT RISK FOR ADVERSE OUTCOMES RELATED TO THE ADMINISTRATION OF DRUGS AND SOLUTIONS

Table 12.1 delineates potential adverse outcomes related to the administration of drugs and solutions.

Risk for infection related to the administration of drugs and solutions. The operative or invasive procedure patient is at increased risk for nosocomial infection if aseptic technique is breached during medication preparation and administration. This breach allows microorganisms access to the body. Because the medication is often dispensed directly into the wound, strict measures must be taken to prevent the development of local, regional, and systemic infection. Faulty operative and aseptic technique, as well as the presence of infection before the procedure, increases the risk of nosocomial infection.

Risk for injury related to hypersensitivity reaction related to improper identification of patient allergies. Drug allergies can range from very mild reactions (eg, hives or urticaria), with no need to discontinue the drug, to very severe reactions, such as an anaphylactic shock reaction. Drug allergies are classified into four types.

Type I is an anaphylactic or atopic reaction that is a common type of drug allergy. Anaphylaxis is an acute reaction in the skin, lungs, and cardiovascular system that results in cardiovascular/respiratory collapse. An atopic reaction is a chronic reaction within the lung or the skin that is dependent on the antigen, the frequency of contact, the route of contact, and the sensitivity of the organ system to the antigen.

A type II (cytotoxic) reaction occurs when the foreign antigen adheres to the surface of the host's cells (target cells). Antibodies are then formed by the host, which attack the target cells. Enzymatic proteins (complement) surround the target cells and cause destruction of the target cells, either through phagocytosis or lysis.

Type III is an autoimmune reaction that is associated with an increased amount of immunoglobulin G. Anaphylatoxins and neutrophils release necrotizing enzymes that produce local ischemia and necrosis as a consequence of complement activation.

Type IV is a cell-mediated hypersensitivity reaction that is mediated through T lymphocytes rather than antibodies. This reaction may be due to a cell-mediated response that occurs as a result of T-cell contact and destruction of antigens or a delayed hypersensitivity response due to a specific interaction of T cells with the antigen.

| Table 12.15 | **Medication History** |

Demographic Data

Age _____ Weight _____ Height _____

Abnormal laboratory values or test results _____

On a scale of 1 to 10, rate your compliance with (how well you stick to) your medication regimen.

Poor Compliance ① ② ③ ④ ⑤ ⑥ ⑦ ⑧ ⑨ ⑩ Excellent Compliance

Present Condition

Do you have any allergies to drugs, foods, chemicals, or other materials such as tape or iodine? _____

Do you use alcohol, tobacco, or over-the-counter drugs? _____

Are you able to take your medications or do you need assistance or use of equipment or devices? _____

If need be, is there someone at home who can help you with your medications? _____

What medications are you presently taking? _____

What do these medications do for you? _____

Do they seem to work? _____

Do you take any special foods with, before, or after your medications? _____

Do you have any problems associated with your medications? _____

Skin problems? _____ Dental or gum problems? _____ Difficulty healing? _____

Have your medications caused any problems with elimination? (eg, constipation, polyuria, diarrhea)? _____

Do you use over-the-counter laxatives? _____

Do you use any medications, herbs, folk remedies, or alcohol to help you cope with stress? _____

Are these methods effective? _____

Do you presently use or have a history of using recreational drugs? _____

Does taking your medication interfere with your religious, cultural, or ethnic beliefs or values? _____

If so, how? _____

Past Conditions

What medications have you taken in the past? _____

Did they seem to work for you? _____

Changes related to medications. Any changes in the following:

Sensory changes? (Explain)

Vision _____

Smell _____

Taste _____

Balance or coordination _____

Hearing _____

Memory or decision making _____

Pain, discomfort, or touch _____

Level of energy? _____

Sleep habits? _____

    Do you have any nightmares or dreams associated with your medications? _____

    Do you use any aids to sleep (eg, alcohol, medications, foods)? _____

Change in how you feel about yourself since you have been taking your medications? _____

Change in your body such as weight gain or loss, enlarged breasts, or fluid retention? _____

Attitude changes such as anger, depression, and fear? _____

Ability to perform your life roles (family member, parent, employee, and so on)? _____

Sexual drive or change in you sexual relationship? _____

If appropriate: Do you use contraception? _____ When was your last menstrual period? _____

Do you have any menstrual problems related to medications? _____

Risk for deficit fluid volume (blood loss) related to the use of heparin. Heparin is often used to prevent thromboembolism during or after an operative or invasive procedure. When heparin is being given to prevent thromboembolism, it is given in such doses that bleeding associated with heparin during or after the procedure is not usually a problem. This does not negate the fact that certain patients may be at risk for bleeding during the procedure period.

The disruption of tissue and vascular integrity because of the procedure puts the patient at increased risk for bleeding. Bleeding may occur during and immediately after a spinal tap or spinal anesthesia or a major operative procedure, especially involving the brain, spinal cord, or eye. Patients receiving prophylactic therapy to prevent deep venous thrombosis after the procedure are also at risk for bleeding.

Patients who have had a recent operative procedure on the brain or spinal cord, CNS trauma, or suspected intracranial bleeding are at increased risk for bleeding. Also patients with subacute bacterial endocarditis or severe hypertension can be at increased risk for hemorrhage.

A higher incidence of bleeding has been reported in women older than 60 years of age. Ovarian (corpus luteum) hemorrhage has developed in a number of women of reproductive age receiving short- or long-term heparin therapy. If unrecognized, this complication may be fatal.

Patients with ulceration of the gastrointestinal tract, or other gastrointestinal disorders (eg, visceral carcinoma, diverticulitis), or with continuous drainage from the gastrointestinal tract are at increased risk for bleeding.

Patients with severe liver or biliary tract disease may have interference in using vitamin K and a subsequent decrease in the production of vitamin K-dependent clotting factors, which in turn may lead to a bleeding tendency. Bleeding can occur when heparin is administered to patients with hemophilia, thrombocytopenia, and some vascular purpuras. The use of drugs such as aspirin, antihistamines, digitalis, nicotine, cough preparations containing guaifenesin, and other over-the-counter medications may alter the effects of heparin.

Risk for injury related to hypersensitivity or an adverse reaction to an anticoagulant (heparin) or antiplatelet agent (Dextran). Hypersensitivity to heparin is marked by chills, rash, urticaria, pruritus, fever, occasional respiratory allergic symptoms, and anaphylactic or anaphylactoid reactions. Adverse effects from Dextran 40 include urticaria, generalized itching, headache, hypotension, nausea and vomiting, and fatal anaphylactic reaction. Hypersensitivity with dextran is most likely to occur during the first few minutes of administration. A small percentage of individuals who never received dextran experience an allergic reaction because of previous sensitization by the dextrans present in commercial sugars and dextran-producing organisms found in the human gastrointestinal tract.

Risk for injury related to an allergic reaction to local anesthetic. A variety of allergic reactions, ranging from allergic dermatitis to anaphylaxis, have occurred in response to local anesthetics. These reactions, which are relatively uncommon, are more likely to occur with the ester-type anesthetics (eg, procaine) than with the amides. Patients allergic to one ester-type anesthetic are likely to be allergic to other ester-type anesthetics. The amino esters (procaine, chloroprocaine, tetracaine) are metabolized by pseudocholinesterase. An end product of this metabolism is para-aminobenzoic acid (PABA). A small percentage of the patients receiving local anesthesia are allergic to PABA. Cross-sensitivity between the ester and amides has not be observed. Therefore, the amides can be used when the patient is allergic to ester-type anesthetics (Franco, 2007) It is unclear whether lidocaine triggers a malignant hyperthermia episode in patients genetically prone to this disorder. Unexplained signs that may precede temperature elevation such as tachycardia, rapid respirations, changes in blood pressure, metabolic acidosis, and muscle rigidity should be noted.

PABA
Para-Aminobenzoic Acid

Risk for injury related to toxicity from local anesthetic. Toxicity can occur when blood concentration of the local anesthetic reaches a level that affects the CNS. When absorbed in sufficient amounts, local anesthetics can cause CNS excitation, followed by depression. During the excitatory phase, convulsions may occur. These can be controlled by intravenous diazepam or, if necessary, a neuromuscular blocking agent (eg, succinylcholine). Convulsions may be followed by a loss of reflexes, coma, respiratory depression, and respiratory arrest. Depressant effects range from drowsiness to unconsciousness. Death can result from respiratory depression (Zamanian et al., 2008) A pseudocholinesterase deficiency increases the chance of toxic responses with an amino ester agent.

Risk for decreased cardiac output related to toxicity from a local anesthetic. The patient with cardio-depression may appear pale and complain of feeling weak, dizzy, or faint. Tachycardia may occur as the heart tries to compensate for the hypotension. The patient may become sleepy and then unconscious as the blood pressure falls to shock levels. If the condition progresses, the heart rate may decrease with a coexisting reduction in pulse pressure. Cardiac arrest or ventricular fibrillation may suddenly occur.

Risk for injury related to mydriatic agent administration causing an acute angle-closure glaucoma episode. Acute angle-closure glaucoma is a medical emergency that can result form the administration of a mydriatic such as atropine to a patient with a history of angle-closure glaucoma. Unlike the case with an asymptomatic patient with open-angle glaucoma, when an acute episode of angle-closure occurs, definite symptoms are present. Clinical signs include a moderately dilated pupil that does not react to light, complaints of blurred vision, halos around lights or a rapid loss of vision, excruciating eye and facial pain, nausea, and vomiting.

Risk for deficit fluid volume related to the administration of hyperosmotic agents. Osmotic diuretics are administered intravenously or orally for short-term reduction in intraocular pressure and vitreous volume. Administration of hyperosmotic agents such as mannitol and glycerin, may reduce intraocular pressure by increasing the osmotic pressure of glomerular filtration, thereby inhibiting tubular reabsorption of water and solutes. Elevated intraocular pressure is lowered within 30 to 60 minutes for a period of 4 to 6 hours. High oral doses of glycerin raise plasma osmotic pressure by withdrawing fluid from the extravascular spaces. Ocular pressure is then decreased by the reduction in volume of intraocular fluid.

Risk for injury related to an allergic or adverse reaction because of patient sensitivity to otic medication. Allergic cross-reactions may occur, which could prevent the use of any or all of the following antibiotics: Kanamycin, paromomycin, streptomycin, and possibly gentamicin. Neomycin is a common cutaneous sensitizer. When using neomycin-containing products to control secondary skin infections, such as chronic otitis externa, note that the skin in these conditions is more liable than normal skin to become sensitized to many substances, including neomycin.

Risk for impaired skin integrity related to the administration of skin medications. Allergic contact dermatitis may result from the exposure of the skin to a product that causes an inflammatory reaction. Contact dermatitis is caused by sensitizers and can result from the application of almost any skin product. Irritant contact dermatitis can be caused by any skin irritant. If body secretions are not properly removed before application of a skin product, the secretions, alone or in combination with the product, can cause skin breakdown. Local allergic reaction is the most common adverse effect associated with topical preparations. Skin sensitivity may develop after brief or prolonged exposure. The clinical picture may appear hours or weeks after the sensitized skin has been exposed. Clinical features may include itching, burning, erythema, vesiculation, and edema, followed by weeping, crusting, and drying and peeling of the skin.

Risk for injury related to an allergic reaction to contrast media. Many minor reactions to the opaque media require no treatment. Patients may complain of a flush and a warm feeling. Other symptoms include urticaria, pain at the injection site, nausea, and excessive salivation. Major reactions, however, can occur in almost any system. Respiratory reactions include respiratory arrest, severe asthmatic attacks, laryngospasm, and laryngeal edema. CNS reactions include syncope, convulsions, aphasia, paraplegia, and coma. Cardiovascular reactions include shock, cardiac arrest, congestive heart failure, and arrhythmias. Renal reactions include flank pain, oliguria or anuria, hematuria, and renal failure.

Risk for fluid volume excess related to the absorption of large amounts of endoscopic irrigating fluid into the systemic circulation. Fluid absorbed into the systemic circulation through open vessels may increase the volume of extracellular fluid and lead to congestive heart failure. Care should be taken to accurately measure the amount of fluid instilled into the patient and the amount of fluid that is recovered. Additionally, caution should be exercised regarding intravascular volume expansion when the patient receives an abnormal volume of fluid for the given procedure or if the procedure lasts an unusually long time.

GATHERING SUPPLIES AND EQUIPMENT

Basic Supplies and Equipment of Medication Administration

Syringes

Syringes with needles or blunt tips are commonly used in the process of reconstituting powders with a diluent and for aspirating a solution or suspension from a vial or an ampule. Syringe selection (size and type) usually depends on the medication being prepared and dispensed.

Because the amount of medication varies depending on its type and function, the nurse must use judgment in selecting the syringe's size. Generally, a 10-mL syringe is used for injection of local anesthetics and for reconstituting powders with diluent. Larger syringes are usually more difficult to control than smaller ones because greater force is needed for aspiration and injection.

When preparing small doses of potentially dangerous medications such as heparin or epinephrine, it is best to use a 1-mL tuberculin syringe to ensure accurate dosage.

Luer-Loc-tipped syringes have a tip that locks over the needle hub. They are used whenever pressure is exerted to inject or aspirate fluid. Sizes range from 2 to 60 mL.

Luer slip-tipped syringes have a plain tip that may not provide a secure connection on a needle hub. They are not recommended for preparing medications but may be needed when administering medications through catheters and ports. Sizes range from 1 to 60 mL.

Ring control syringes have Luer-Lok tips with a finger hold and thumb hold. They are ideal for injection of local anesthetics. The syringe allows firm control when injecting with only one hand. Sizes range from 3 to 10 mL.

Bulb syringes with barrels have a rubber or plastic bulb attached to the neck of the barrel. They are used for irrigation in many types of procedures and have a solution capacity ranging from ¼ to 4 ounces (7.5 to 120 mL). A bulb syringe without a barrel is also known as an ear syringe. It is a one-piece bulb that tapers to a blunt end and is used for irrigating the ear, the eye, or other small structures.

Regardless of the type of syringe used, there must be a method used to label the syringe. Labels may come pre-packaged with disposable drape packs or may be packaged individually. Several types of labels are available for inclusion in packs or as a sterile stock pack with a marking pen included. Syringes are now also manufactured with a write-on stripe that eliminates the need for pre-printed or individual labels. Solutions must be identified by both the scrub person and the circulating nurse before they are drawn up or introduced to the sterile field and each syringe must be labeled with medication and concentration. The scrub person must identify the solution to the physician each time the syringe is passed to that physician.

Needles

The size of a needle is designated by length and gauge. Gauge is the outside diameter of the needle. The bevel of a needle is its sloped edge. Commonly used sizes include ½ inch (12.7 mm) × 30—for local anesthesia in a plastic procedure; ¾ inch (19.1 mm) × 25 gauge—for local anesthesia or conjunctival injection; 1½ inches (38.1mm) × 22 gauge for subcutaneous or intramuscular injection; 2 inches (50.8 mm) × 16 or 18 gauge—for preparation of medications and solutions; and 4 inches (101.6 mm) × 20 or 22 gauge—spinal needles used for deep injection of local anesthetic. Blunt tip needles or blunt cannulas are used to draw up medications.

Diluent

0.9% Sodium Chloride is designed for parenteral use only after the addition of drugs that require dilution or must be dissolved in an aqueous vehicle before injection. It should not be used unless the solution is clear and the container is undamaged. When diluting or dissolving drugs, it is important to mix thoroughly and use the solution promptly.

Bacteriostatic Water for Injection is used as a diluting or dissolving agent according to the drug manufacturer's recommendation.

Specific Supplies and Equipment for Pharmacological Agents

Antimicrobial Agents

The selection of the size and type of syringe is determined by the type and amount of medication being prepared. For example, when administering a dose of less than 1 mL, the use of a tuberculin syringe reduces the risk of medication error. When diluting a powder with sterile water or normal saline, a 5- or 10-mL syringe can be used. After the antibiotic has been reconstituted and transferred onto the sterile field, the scrub person hands it to the physician in an irrigation syringe.

Needle selection is determined by the type of antibiotic being mixed and the route of administration. By using a 16- or 18-gauge, 2-inch needle or a blunt-tip needle or cannula, the nurse ensures a quick and easy injection, aspiration, and transfer of solution from the ampule or from one vial to another.

Whatever the size of the syringe and needle, strict aseptic technique must be maintained. The sterility of the syringe barrel, the part of the plunger that enters the barrel, the tip of the barrel, and the needle should not be compromised.

Local Anesthetics

Syringes. The size and type of syringe is determined by the amount of local anesthetic to be delivered. Ring syringes are preferred because they provide added control over the injection and allow for aspiration and injection with one hand.

Needles. A short ½-inch, 25-gauge needle is often used for the initial infiltration. For deeper injection, a longer 23- or 25-gauge or 2½-inch spinal needle is used. Syringes with needles attached should be passed using a no-touch technique.

Topical Agents

Cotton pledgets, usually ½ × 3 inches (12.7 × 76.2 mm), may be soaked in a topical solution and passed to the physician with bayonet forceps.

Ophthalmic Agents

In addition to the medication to be administered, the nurse needs cotton balls, gauze, and cotton-tipped applicators to roll the upper eyelid. A sterile dropper should come with the vial of medication. All equipment for administration of ophthalmic medications, including droppers, tubes, and plastic containers, must be sterile and never allowed to touch the eye. This helps prevent nosocomial infection in the eye and surrounding structures.

Otic Agents

Administration of otic agents requires a medication with a sterile dropper, cotton ball or ear wick, and gauze or tissue to remove excessive solution from the skin.

Nasal Medications

Administration of nasal medications usually requires that the tip of the medication bottle be inserted into the nares. Any unused solution should be discarded. The nurse should provide tissues for the patient.

Skin Medications

Depending on the type of application, the following should be available: sterile gloves; dry sterile dressings; occlusive dressing; sterile elastic (Ace) wrap, bandage (Kling), or other roll of gauze to secure the dressing; and cotton-tipped applicators or tongue blades.

Contrast Media

Administration of contrast media requires syringes, needles or blunt cannulas, IV tubing with a three-way adaptor (for intraoperative cholangiogram), and if needed, 0.9% sodium chloride for injection to dilute the media.

Endoscopic Irrigating Solutions

Large amounts of fluid are usually used. If fluids are used from a warming cabinet, several containers of fluid should be warm and ready for use. Fluids should not be stored for long periods of time in a warming cabinet. If a fluid warmer is used, it is not necessary to pre-warm the fluids. Sterile irrigation tubing should be included in the setup.

Emergency Drugs

Whenever local anesthetics are used, oxygen, a laryngoscope, endotracheal tubes, a face mask, self-inflating bag, emergency drugs, and suction should be available.

PREPARING MEDICATIONS AND SOLUTIONS FROM AMPULES AND VIALS

Gather the required supplies and equipment to include an appropriate-sized syringe and needle, protective pad for opening ampule, sharps container, and diluent (0.9% sodium chloride injection or bacteriostatic water for injection).

When removing medication or solution from the ampule, identify the type, dose, and expiration date of the medication. Tap the ampule lightly and quickly until the fluid leaves the neck of the ampule and flows to the lower chamber. Place a gauze or alcohol pad around the neck of the ampule. This helps protect the fingers when breaking the ampule. Do not remove the alcohol pad from its wrapper. Alcohol may leak into the ampule. Snap the neck of the ampule along the prescored line. Direct the snapping motion away from the body. While snapping the top off, avoid shattering the glass. If it is suspected that glass has entered the ampule, discard it and start again. Hold the ampule upside down or place it on a flat surface. You may hold the ampule upside down without danger of spillage as long as the needle tip or shaft does not touch the ampule. After the needle touches the ampule, surface tension breaks down and fluid leaks out. Insert the needle into the ampule without touching the rim. Keep the needle tip below the surface of the liquid and quickly draw up the medication without injecting air into the ampule. Injection of air forces the fluid out of the ampule. Because the fluid in the ampule is immediately displaced by air, there is no resistance to its withdrawal. Confirm the type, dose, and expiration date of the medication with the scrub person. Dispense the medication onto the sterile field. Have the scrub person position the medication receptacle at the edge of the field or hold it so that the solution can be released without contamination. The scrub person should immediately label the syringe or receptacle with the name and concentration of the medication. Dispose of the needle, syringe, and gauze or alcohol pad. This protects other personnel from inadvertent injury from the needle or glass slivers. Discard unused medication.

When removing medication or solution from a vial, identify the type, dose, and expiration date of the medication. Remove the plastic or metal cap covering the top of the unused vial. If the vial is a multiple-dose vial and has been used previously, wipe the rubber seal with alcohol before and after each use. This removes surface bacteria, dust, and dried solution from the stopper. Prepare the syringe with as much air as solution to be removed from the vial. As medication is removed, replacement with air is required to prevent build-up of negative pressure. Insert the needle, with the bevel pointing up, through the center of the vial. The center of the vial is thinner and is designed for penetration. Keep the bevel up to prevent cutting a rubber core from the seal. Inject air into the vial. While injecting air, hold onto the plunger. The plunger may be forced backward by air pressure within the vial. For vials with dry medication, diluent is used to replace air, thereby creating positive pressure in the vial. Invert the vial with the nondominant hand while grasping the syringe barrel and plunger with the thumb and forefinger of the dominant hand. Inverting the vial allows fluid to settle in the lower section of the vial. Allow air pressure to fill the syringe; pull back slightly on the plunger if necessary. Positive pressure in the vial causes the syringe to fill. After the correct volume is obtained, withdraw the needle from the vial. For multiple-dose vials, prepare a label that includes the date and time of mixing and concentration per milliliter. Confirm the type, dose, and expiration date of the medication with the scrub person. Dispense the medication onto the sterile field. Have the scrub person position the medication receptacle at the edge of the field or hold it so that the solution can be released without contamination. The scrub person should immediately label the receptacle with the name and concentration of the medication. Dispose of the needle and syringe in a sharps container.

APPLYING SKIN MEDICATIONS

Gather required supplies and equipment to include the desired cream, ointment, or solution; sterile gloves; tongue blade or cotton-tipped applicators; dry sterile dressing; and tape (paper or plastic). Inspect the site of application for lesions, reddened areas, signs of infection, and breaks in skin or membranes. Don sterile gloves to apply the topical ointment or cream. Wash the application site to remove microorganisms, blood, debris, and fluids. Dry the application site. Moisture can interfere with application of the medication and hinder absorption of the medication. Apply the medication as follows: (1) place the desired amount of medication on the sterile gauze, and (2) apply the medication with a sterile tongue blade onto the suture line or desired skin surface. If a gloved finger is used for application, put on a new sterile glove and remove glove powder. Avoid rubbing the skin, which may cause irritation, disruption of the suture line, or bleeding. Apply a dry sterile gauze or dressing as desired and secure with paper or plastic tape.

When applying an aerosol spray, shake the can vigorously, which mixes the contents and propellant to ensure a fine and even spray. Protect the patient's eyes and face from the spray by having the patient turn his or her head or by covering the patient's face with a towel. Hold the can the recommended distance from the skin (usually 6–12 inches [15–30 cm]). Spray the desired area and allow it to dry before applying a dressing or tape. This prevents the product from being removed by the dressing or tape. Cover the area with dressing as desired by the physician. Covering the area may help maintain the application on the skin.

ADMINISTERING OPTHALMIC MEDICATIONS

Gather the required supplies and equipment to include the desired ointment or drops; gloves to protect the hands from purulent drainage or blood; cotton ball, gauze, or tissue; and if needed, an eye pad and tape for dressing. Inspect the site of application for drainage, reddened areas, and encrusted areas. Position the patient in a supine or semi-Fowler position. These positions provide access to the eye and minimize drainage of medication through the lacrimal duct. If the eyelids are covered with crust or drainage, clean with sterile water or saline solution. Soak crust with warm solution if it is dry and difficult to remove. Soaking allows easy removal of crust and drainage that may harbor microorganisms. Always wipe from the inner to the outer canthus. This prevents carrying debris to the lacrimal duct. Place the thumb and index finger near the margin of the lower eyelid immediately below the eyelashes, and exert downward pressure over the bony prominence of the cheek. Ask the patient to look upward while this is being done. This maneuver provides exposure of the lower conjunctival sac while retraction against the bony orbit prevents pressure and trauma to the eyeball. Upward eye motion retracts the cornea up and away from the conjunctival sac and reduces the stimulation of the blink reflex.

To instill eyedrops, hold the dropper in the dominant hand 1–2 cm above the conjunctival sac. This prevents dropper contact with the eyeball. Instill the prescribed number of drops into the eye. If the patient blinks and drops do not enter the eye, repeat the procedure. The conjunctival sac normally holds 1–2 drops. When administering drops that cause a systemic effect protect the fingers with gloves or a tissue and apply gentle pressure to the patient's nasolacrimal duct for 30–60 seconds. This prevents absorption of the medication into the systemic circulation and prevents overflow of the drops into the nasopharyngeal passage.

When instilling eye ointment, have the patient look down to reduce the blinking reflex during ointment instillation. Hold the applicator above the lid margin and apply a thin stream of ointment evenly along the inside of the lower lid on the conjunctiva. Evenly distribute the ointment. Have the patient close the eye and gently rub the lid in a circular motion with a cotton ball. This helps distribute the ointment without causing injury to the eye. Remove excessive solution or ointment from the lids or face. This promotes comfort and prevents undesired absorption of the medication. If ordered by the physician, apply a clean eye patch.

ADMINISTERING OTIC MEDICATIONS

Gather required supplies and equipment, including the desired otic solution or suspension, cotton ball or wick, and cotton-tipped applicator. Inspect the site of application for reddened areas, signs of infection, breaks in the skin, and cerumen build-up. Position the patient in a comfortable sitting or side-lying position so that the affected ear is facing up. An infant or child can be held by the parent or another adult. If cerumen or drainage occludes the outer ear canal, clean the canal with a cotton-tipped applicator. Do not force the cerumen inward or occlude the canal in any way. Straighten the patient's ear by pulling the pinna upward and outward for adults. For children, pull the pinna down and back. Straightening the canal provides direct access to deeper ear structures.

Ensure that the medication is warmed to body temperature and instill the medication by holding the dropper 1 cm above the ear canal. Do not force the drops into the canal under pressure. Have the patient maintain the body position for 2 to 3 minutes while applying gentle pressure to the tragus. This allows complete distribution of the solution. Gentle pressure moves the medication inward. Insert a cotton ball or wick into the ear (optional). This prevents the solution from running out of the ear when the patient moves the head. Remember to remove the cotton ball.

ADMINISTERING NASAL MEDICATIONS

Gather required supplies including the nasal medication or spray, gloves, and tissues. Instruct the patient to blow his or her nose to clear the nose of mucous. Position the patient in the supine position with the head tilted back. Instruct the patient to inhale as the spray enters the nasal passage. A nasal spray may be administered as one or two sprays to each nostril or to the operative side. Position a child in an upright position to prevent swallowing of excess spray. Instruct the patient to breathe through the mouth to prevent aspiration into the trachea and bronchi, to remain in the supine position for at least one minute and to avoid blowing the nose for several minutes. Provide a tissue for any medication that may leak from the nares after the patient returns to a sitting position.

NURSING IMPLICATIONS OF ADMINISTERING PHARMACOLOGICAL AGENTS

Before the Procedure

Interview the patient and family members before the procedure and obtain a health and medication history. Assess vital signs and mental status. Document an accurate weight for the patient for calculation of safe maximal dosages. Check the patient identification or drug-alert bracelet for allergies. Have pertinent laboratory results available. The patient may be taking medications that may contraindicate the use of a medication that will be used prior to or during the surgical procedure. Note a patient or family history of bleeding disorders, glaucoma, malignant hyperthermia, or any past reaction to anesthesia. Note past history of surgical procedures and the presence of abrasions, healing incisions, open wounds, breakdown or drainage from eyes, nose, or ears. Assess the patient's need for transfusion and know the availability of whole blood, plasma, or other blood products for transfusion.

Note a history of past reactions to contrast media or a history of asthma, hay fever, or food allergies. Note a history of multiple myeloma or other para-proteinemia. Using radiopaque agents with such conditions may cause anuria, resulting in progressive uremia, renal failure, and eventually death. Note the presence of sickle cell disease. Contrast media promote the phenomenon of sickling in individuals who are homozygous for sickle cell disease when the material is injected intravenously or intra-arterially.

Because of the SCIP initiative by CMS and CDC, the appropriate anti-infective should be initiated an hour prior to the incision time. Initiation time may be crucial to the risk for development of surgical site infection. Accurate documentation is essential.

During the Procedure

Anti-Infective Agents

Prepare and administer drugs and solutions according to recommended methods. Monitor physiological changes when administering agents that are known to cause alterations in health patterns (eg, Vancomycin). Report changes in the patient's pulse, blood pressure, temperature, and respirations. Observe and report signs and symptoms of allergic response, such as urticaria, itching, and wheezing. Have standard equipment available (see **Table 12.16**). Apply ointments and dressings as indicated. Document nursing actions in the patient's record.

Anticoagulants

Have standard equipment and supplies available (**Table 12.16**). If needed, prepare and administer heparin. Heparin flush solution is commonly used to maintain the patency of central venous, femoral, or dialysis catheters. It is considered standard practice to flush a central catheter with 1 to 2 mL of normal saline before and after medication administration to avoid the possibility of drug interaction. Because heparin is strongly acidic, it is incompatible with any drugs. Avoid mixing any drug with heparin unless specifically advised by the physician or the pharmacist. Heparin is stable at room temperature of 15–30°C (59–86°F). Inspect all preparations for

Table 12.16	Equipment and Supplies Required for Administering Pharmacological Agents	
Airway maintenance	Oxygen	
	Suction	
	Face mask	
	Self-inflating bag	
	Oral and nasopharyngeal airways	
	Laryngoscope with assorted endotracheal tubes	
Monitoring	Sphygmomanometer or noninvasive blood pressure cuff	
	Electrocardiograph	
	Pulse oximeter	
Intravenous access	Assorted intravenous cannulae	
	Intravenous tubing	
	Intravenous fluids such as lactated Ringer's and 0.9% normal saline	
Medications	Atropine sulfate	
	Cortisone	
	Diphenhydramine (Benadryl)	
	Epinephrine	
	Flumazenil	
	Lidocaine (Xylocaine)	
	Naloxone (Narcan)	

discoloration and particulate matter before administration. Heparin administration in bolus form can cause a significant transient decrease in blood pressure that may necessitate intervention. When heparin is added to a solution of IV 0.9% sodium chloride for injection, invert the container at least six times to ensure adequate mixing and to prevent pooling of the heparin. A common mix is 10,000 U of heparin in 1000 mL of 0.9% sodium chloride.

Apply a pressure dressing to the IV and other puncture sites. Monitor vital signs for indications of hemorrhage or other adverse reactions. Report changes in the patient's pulse, blood pressure, temperature, and respirations. Observe and report indications of allergic response such as urticaria, itching, and wheezing. Pad and position the patient to avoid trauma to the skin and underlying tissue. Monitor blood loss and urinary output. Document nursing actions in the patient's record. Report any changes in physiological status.

Local Anesthetics

Calculate the maximal dose that can be safely administered. Prepare the local anesthetic according to recommended methods. Warn the patient before the physician injects the local anesthetic that the medication may sting or burn. Provide emotional support by reassuring the patient with conversation and touch. The scrub person should identify the local anesthetic by name and concentration when passing the syringe to the physician. The syringe should be passed using the no-touch method.

Assess for local and systemic signs of adverse reactions. Monitor the patient at scheduled intervals for allergic or toxic effects of the local anesthetic. Note the patient's blood pressure, oxygen saturation, skin condition, mental status, and emotional response. The application of topical medication may cause local reaction of itching, burning, redness, or other skin reaction. Systemic reactions include bronchoconstriction, hypotension, syncope, and ultimately, respiratory arrest.

Record and report the total amount of solution injected and the actual numbers of milligrams administered. If an adverse reaction is suspected, communicate this to the physician at once. Document the signs and symptoms of local or systemic reactions as they occur. Report any change in physiological status.

Ophthalmic Agents

Position the patient to ensure the proper administration of ophthalmic medications. Many patients undergo ocular procedures under local anesthesia. A pillow under the knees may increase patient comfort by relieving strain in the lower back. Use warm blankets to provide comfort and prevent shivering. Provide emotional support during the administration of medications. If the patient is awake, placing your hand on the patient's shoulder, brow, arm, or hand can decrease anxiety and ensure proper instillation of the medication. Alert the patient before instillation of drops, ointments, and injections. Some medications can cause temporary burning and/or irritation. Monitor the patient's pulse, blood pressure, and respirations because systemic absorption of medications can occur. Report changes in physiological status and take necessary actions. Record the type and dose of all ocular medications and the time and route of administration. Document nursing actions in the patient's records.

Otic Agents

Position the patient on his or her side with the affected ear up. A pillow under the head and between the knees may promote comfort. Instill otic solution or suspension as ordered.

Insert and remove ear wicks. Wicks of small pieces of cotton or commercially made wicks may be used as drains in the ear to remove exudates or excessive eardrops. Gently insert the wick into the canal only as far as it is possible to see. Leave the end of the wick extending out of the canal. Keep the wick moist by adding solution if the patient is in the operating room for an extended period of time. Change the wick as needed to prevent hardening and/or obstruction of drainage flow.

Provide emotional support during the procedure. If the patient is awake, placing a hand on the face or brow can offer support and remind the patient to remain in the proper position. Record the type, amount, and time of administration of medications.

Skin Medications

Prepare and administer skin medications according to recommended methods. Observe and report signs and symptoms of allergic response such as urticaria, itching, and burning. Apply lotions and ointments with a firm touch. Light dabbing can increase the sensation of itching. Record the type, amount, time and location of skin medication application. Document nursing actions in the patient's record and report any changes in physiological status.

Contrast Media

Aseptically withdraw contrast media from the vial using a sterile syringe and needle. Inject contrast media warmed to body temperature. Avoid contaminating catheters, syringes, needles, and contrast media with glove powder or draping material fibers. If nondisposable equipment is used, take care to prevent residual contamination with traces of cleansing agents. Monitor the patient for a reaction to the contrast media. Report physiologic or psychological changes and take appropriate actions if necessary. Have standard equipment available (see **Table 12.16**).

Provide emotional support during the procedure. Patients are sometimes awake during radiographic procedures. Use conversation and touch to offer support and reassurance. Diversional techniques such as listening to the radio, using audio headphones, or reading may help decrease anxiety and facilitate the patient's cooperation. Record the type, amount, route, and time of administration of media.

Endoscopic Procedures

Aseptically prepare the solution for administration. Use the appropriate administration set and attach the tubing promptly after protective seals are removed. Do not elevate the container more than 60 cm (about 2 feet) above the procedure bed. Excessive elevation can increase intravascular absorption of the irrigating fluid. Monitor the physiologic status, and note and report adverse reactions. In the event of an adverse reaction, alert the physician and, as directed by the physician, discontinue the irrigation and institute appropriate treatment. Save the remainder of the fluid for examination. Patients are often awake for endoscopic procedures. Use conversation and therapeutic touch to provide reassurance and decrease anxiety. Record intake and output, noting the amount of irrigation fluid used and the amount of fluid removed from the body cavity. Record the amount, type, and time of administration of fluid. Document nursing actions in the patient's record.

After the Procedure

PACU
Postanesthesia Care
Unit

Communicate to the postanesthesia care unit (PACU) nurse the type, amount, and route of drugs or solutions administered during the procedure along with the time of administration. Report known allergies to the PACU staff. Note any adverse effects related to the administration of drugs or solutions.

Patients who have undergone procedures as outpatients should have a followup phone call the next day to evaluate the outcome of the procedure and note any reactions to drugs or solutions administered during the operative or invasive procedure. At this time, preprocedure teaching regarding drugs that the patient may be taking after discharge may be reinforced.

CONCLUSION

The nurse is responsible for the preparation and administration of many medications and solutions in the surgical setting. Most importantly, the nurse must remember the "rights" involved in medication administration: right patient, drug, dose, route, time, and documentation. The nurse should always read accompanying drug literature and refer to the package insert and other suitable reference before administering an unfamiliar product.

COMPETENCY ASSESSMENT
Administer Drugs and Solutions

Name: _____ Title: _____ Unit: _____ Date of Validation: _____

Type of Validation: ☐ Initial   ☐ Annual   ☐ Bi-annual

COMPETENCY STATEMENT: The nurse demonstrates competency to administer drugs and solutions.

Performance Criteria	Met	Not Met
1. Recognizes potential adverse drug and solution reactions	☐	☐
2. Describes the pharmacological characteristics of drugs and solutions used during operative or invasive procedures	☐	☐
3. Describes the human response to the administration of drugs and solutions	☐	☐
4. Obtains a medication history	☐	☐
5. Identifies patients at risk for adverse outcomes related to the administration of drugs and solutions	☐	☐
6. Gathers supplies and equipment	☐	☐
7. Prepares and administers drugs and solutions according to institutional policy, manufacturers' recommendations, federal and state regulations, and recommended nursing practices	☐	☐

_____   _____

Validator's Signature   Employee's Signature

_____

Validator's Printed Name

REFERENCES

1. AORN (2009). Recommended Practices for the Prevention of Unplanned Perioperative Hypothermia. *Perioperative standards and recommended practices.* Denver, CO: AORN Inc., pp. 407–420.

2. Barclay, L. (2004). Methemoglobinemia Linked to Topical Benzocaine Use. Medscape Medical News. http://www.medscape.com/viewarticle/481037?rss, accessed March 21, 2008.

3. Berman, A., Snyder, S.J., Kozier, B., & Erb, G. (2008). *Kozier & Erb's Fundamentals of Nursing: Concepts, Process, and Practice,* 8th Ed. Upper Saddle River, NJ: Pearson Prentice Hall.

4. Deglin, J.H., & Vallerand, A.H. (2007). *Davis's Drug Guide for Nurses,* 10th Edition. Philadelphia: F.A. Davis.

5. Department of Health and Human Services (2009). The Controlled Substance Schedule. Retrieved from http://www.dhhs.state.nh.us/DHHS/ATOD/controlled-substance.htm, accessed January 23, 2009.

6. Federal Drug Administration (2006). FDA Drug Category Ratings. Retrieved from http://www.americanpregnancy.org/pregnancyhealth/fdadrugratings.html, accessed January 22, 2009.

7. Franco, C.D. (2007). Manual of Regional Anesthesia, 2nd ed, Chicago, IL, www.CookCountyRegional.com, accessed April 2, 2008.

8. Inviro Medical Devices Introduces InviroSNAP® with InviroSTRIPE®. Patient Safety and Quality Healthcare: Product News (2008). http://www.psqu.com/enews/0707o.html, accessed Jan. 13, 2008.

9. Jennings, J., & Foster, J. (2007). Medication Safety: Just a Label Away. *AORN Journal,* 86(4), p. 618–625.

10. Methemoglobinemia (2008). www.nlm.nih.gov/medlineplus/ency/article/000562.htm, accessed March 21, 2008.

11. Peterson, C. (2002). Surgical-grade stainless steel; when to administer antibiotics; medication labels; mixing medications; bioburden. *AORN Journal,* (6), p. 1078–1083.

12. Peterson, C. (2007). Perioperative nursing data set, the perioperative nursing vocabulary. (Revised 2nd ed.). Denver: AORN. Inc.

13. Shamrock Labeling Systems. http://www.sharmocklabels.com/central01.htm, accessed Jan 13, 2008.

14. Surgical Care Improvement Project (2007). http://www.medqic.org, accessed Jan. 1, 2008.

15. Tisseel, V.H. (2008). http://www.baxterbio-surgery.com/us/products/tisseel/, accessed March 2, 2008.

16. Topical Benzocaine Sprays (2006). https:.decs.nhgl.med.navy.mil/ANNOUNCHEMNTS/benzocaine.htm, accessed March 21, 2008.

17. Venes, D. (2005). *Taber's Cyclopedic Medical Dictionary,* 20th Ed. Philadelphia: F.A. Davis.

18. Zamanian, R.T., Su, M., Kapitanyan, R., Olsson, J., Local Anesthetics Toxicity, eMedicine, (2008). http://www.emedicine.com/emerg/topic761.htm, accessed April 2, 2008.

CHAPTER 13

Physiologically Monitor the Patient

Cecil King

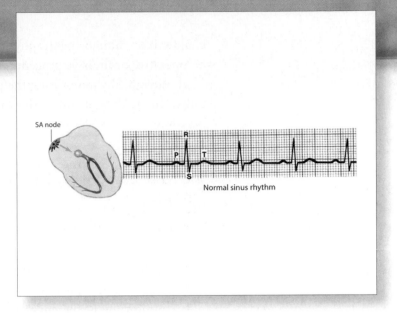

SA node

Normal sinus rhythm

INTRODUCTION

This chapter describes the patient care activities performed by the registered professional nurse in monitoring the patient's physiological status during operative and invasive procedures. The nurse monitors the patient to prevent ineffective airway clearance and an ineffective breathing pattern, air embolus from intravenous (IV) catheters, local infiltration of IV fluid, fluid volume excess or deficit, hyperthermia or hypothermia, extravasation of IV medication, and cardiodepression related to the administration of local anesthetics.

Begin the process to physiologically monitor the patient by assessing the patient's risk for potential adverse outcomes related to the physiological stressors associated with the operative or invasive procedure. After the assessment, identify nursing diagnoses that describe the patient's degree of risk. Next, delineate expected outcomes and outcome indicators for determining if the patient maintained physiological status during the procedure. After identifying the desired outcomes, identify the appropriate interventions to maintain patient's physiological status. During and at the completion of the procedure, evaluate to determine if the patient met the criteria delineated in the expected outcomes (AORN, 2008a).

During many procedures the nurse assists the anesthesia provider in monitoring the patient. However, when assigned as the monitoring nurse during procedures using moderate sedation/analgesia or local anesthesia, the nurse assumes total responsibility for monitoring duties. Consequently, every circulating nurse should demonstrate competencies related to assessment, diagnosis, implementation, and evaluation of treatments and procedures that contribute to the physiological stability of the patient (AORN, 2007). Emphasis in this

Chapter Contents

IV
Intravenous

chapter is on monitoring the physiological stressors that can affect the patient during an operative or invasive procedure (**Table 13.1**).

Physiologically monitoring the patient is always a professional nursing responsibility. Do not delegate this activity to licensed practical nurses or unlicensed assistive personnel.

MEASURABLE CRITERIA

The nurse demonstrates competency to monitor the physiological status of the patient by:

- Identifying the patient's risk for adverse outcomes related to physiological status
- Managing the patient's airway and breathing pattern
- Managing the patient's fluid intake
- Monitoring the patient's fluid loss
- Maintaining the patient's body temperature
- Monitoring the patient during the administration of moderate sedation/analgesia and local anesthesia

Table 13.1	Methods of Monitoring Physiological Stressors

Airway Clearance and Breathing Pattern
- ☐ Use pulse oximetry
- ☐ Inspect the skin and nails for color arid capillary refill
- ☐ Inspect the operative field for the color of tissue and blood
- ☐ Listen to lung sounds and ventilatory rate
- ☐ Monitor arterial blood gas values as needed

Fluid Intake
- ☐ Inspect mucous membranes and conjunctiva for color, moisture, and edema
- ☐ Monitor intake of intravenous fluids
- ☐ Note the amount and type of surgical irrigation used

Fluid Loss
- ☐ Assess blood loss, urine output, and other drainage
- ☐ Assess for third-space fluid loss and insensible fluid loss
- ☐ Assess blood pressure and pulse (rate, rhythm, and quality)
- ☐ Note the amount and rate of blood loss

Body Temperature
- ☐ Assess skin temperature and core temperature as needed

Effects of IV Sedation and Local Anesthesia
- ☐ Inspect the skin for rash, edema, or pruritus
- ☐ Check IV site for possible extravasation of IV medication into the surrounding tissues
- ☐ Monitor for changes in hemodynamic status, respiratory function, and mental and neurologic status

IDENTIFYING THE PATIENT'S RISK FOR ADVERSE OUTCOMES RELATED TO PHYSIOLOGICAL STATUS

Table 13.2 identifies the desired outcomes for the patient care event of physiologically monitoring the patient. The table shows outcomes, nursing diagnoses, risk factors, and outcome indicators specific to each nursing diagnosis.

Table 13.2	Outcomes Related to Physiologically Monitoring the Patient

Managing the Patient's Airway and Breathing Pattern

Outcome 1   The patient is free from airway obstruction or ineffective breathing during the procedure.

Diagnosis	Risk Factors	Outcome Indicators
Risk for Ineffective Airway Clearance and Ineffective Breathing Pattern during the operative or invasive procedure	☐ Alteration in level of consciousness caused by IV sedation ☐ History of sleep apnea or obstruction because of the position of the tongue ☐ Excessive salivation or the presence of viscous secretions ☐ Ineffective coughing or an inability to cough due to the nature of the procedure (cataract or other ocular procedure) ☐ Lack of understanding of how and when to deep breathe and cough ☐ Pain or fear of pain that may discourage coughing and breathing ☐ Fatigue, weakness, or drowsiness ☐ Coexisting respiratory, cardiovascular, or neurological diseas ☐ Obesity ☐ Neuromuscular or musculoskeletal impairment	☐ Is the patient's respiratory rate within normal limits (16–20 breaths/minute)? Is bradypnea or tachypnea present? ☐ Does the patient show signs of labored breathing, such as dyspnea or shortness of breath? Are there episodes of apnea? ☐ What is the patient's skin color? Is cyanosis present? ☐ Is the patient's oxygen saturation rate at least 95%? ☐ Does the patient make statements indicating respiratory difficulty? ☐ Is the pulse rate within normal limits (60–80 beats/minute)?

Monitoring Fluid Intake

Outcome 2   The patient's tissue integrity is maintained at the site of the IV infusion.

Diagnosis	Risk Factors	Outcome Indicators
Risk for Impaired Tissue Integrity related to local infiltration of IV fluid	☐ Fragile veins due to age, physical debilitation, or coexisting disease ☐ Disoriented, confused, or agitated patient who may inadvertently dislodge the catheter	☐ Does the IV site have redness, swelling, edema, or other signs of irritation? ☐ Does the patient complain of pain or tenderness at the IV rite?

Outcome 3   The patient's fluid volume is maintained.

Diagnosis	Risk Factors	Outcome Indicators
Risk for Fluid Volume Excess related to IV therapy	☐ Excess fluid or sodium intake ☐ Compromised regulatory system (conditions such as congestive heart failure, renal failure, or liver disease, resulting in sodium retention) ☐ Stress of the operative or invasive procedure intervention ☐ Cushing's syndrome or corticosteroid therapy	☐ Does the patient have edema or effusion? ☐ Does the patient show changes in mental status? ☐ Is the patient's intake greater than output? ☐ Does the patient have oliguria? Are there specific gravity changes in the urine? ☐ Does the patient exhibit shortness of breath, dyspnea, or orthopnea? ☐ Are breath sounds normal? ☐ Are there changes in blood pressure, venous pressure, or pulmonary arterial pressure? ☐ Is there evidence of jugular venous distention? ☐ Does the patient have a decrease in hemoglobin or hematocrit? ☐ Are electrolytes within normal limits?

Outcome 4   The patient's cardiac output is maintained during the procedure.

Diagnosis	Risk Factors	Outcome Indicators
Risk for Decreased Cardiac Output related to air embolus from IV therapy	☐ Delivery of fluid under pressure ☐ Presence of a central IV catheter	☐ Is the patient cyanotic? ☐ Is the patient hypotensive? ☐ Is the patient responsive?

Monitoring Fluid Loss

Outcome 5   The patient's fluid volume is maintained during the procedure.

Diagnosis	Risk Factors	Outcome Indicators
Risk for Fluid Volume Deficit related to bleeding during the operative or invasive procedure	☐ Type and duration of the procedure; the location and size of incision ☐ Clotting disorders or the use of anticoagulant medications such as aspirin, heparin, or warfarin sodium ☐ Extremes of age and weight ☐ Active loss of fluid related to diarrhea, vomiting, wound drainage, burns, trauma, or hemorrhage	☐ Is there a decrease in urine output during the procedure? ☐ Is output greater than intake? ☐ Does the patient have an increased pulse rate? ☐ Is there a decrease in pulse volume/pressure? ☐ Is the patient's skin dry to the touch? ☐ Does the patient have dry mucous membranes?

Monitoring Body Temperature

Outcome 6 The patient is at or returning to normothermia at the conclusion of the immediate operative and invasive procedure period.

Diagnosis	Risk Factors	Outcome Indicators
Risk of Hypothermia during the operative or invasive procedure	☐ Trauma or large open wound ☐ Exposure of internal organs and body cavities ☐ Extremes in age ☐ Malnutrition ☐ Sedation ☐ Decreased metabolism ☐ Use of cool fluids for irrigation and infusion ☐ Inadequate warmth during the operative procedure ☐ Dehydration	☐ Does the patient have a decrease in body temperature below range? ☐ Does the patient's skin feel cool? ☐ Does the patient show evidence of mental confusion? ☐ Does the patient have a decrease in pulse and respiration rates? ☐ Did the patient experience body temperature increase above the normal range?
Risk of Hyperthermia during the operative or invasive procedure	☐ Illness resulting in fever ☐ Use of warm fluids for irrigation and infusion ☐ Use of medication causing vasoconstriction or adverse reaction ☐ Endocrine disorders such as thyroid disease ☐ Intracranial infection or injury to the hypothalamus	☐ Was the patient's skin flushed? ☐ Did the patient have an increase in respiratory rate (particularly the non-ventilated patient)? ☐ Was there evidence of tachycardia? ☐ Did the patient have a seizure or convulsion?

Monitoring the Effects of Moderate Sedation/Analgesia and Local Anesthesia

Outcome 7 The patient's breathing pattern is maintained during the procedure.

Diagnosis	Risk Factors	Outcome Indicators
Risk for Ineffective Breathing Pattern related to moderate sedation/analgesia	☐ Respiratory disorders such as emphysema, asthma, pneumonia, pulmonary tumor, and chronic obstructive pulmonary disease ☐ Conditions that interfere with normal breathing patterns such as obesity, third trimester of pregnancy, and neuromuscular disorders ☐ Liver disease that interferes with the metabolism of sedatives and narcotics ☐ Elderly patients or debilitated individuals with poor venous access	☐ Does the patient show signs of wheezing, dyspnea, shallow respirations, hypoventilation, airway obstruction, apnea, or tachypnea? ☐ Are there signs indicating the presence of laryngospasm or bronchospasm? ☐ Is the patient agitated or combative?

13

Outcome 8 The patient is free from tissue damage related to subcutaneous infiltration of medications and IV fluids.

Diagnosis	Risk Factors	Outcome Indicators
Risk for Impaired Tissue Integrity related to extravasation of IV medication	☐ Elderly patients or debilitated individuals with poor venous access	☐ Does the IV site have redness, swelling, edema, or other signs of irritation? ☐ Does the patient complain of pain at the IV site?

Outcome 9 The patient's cardiac output is maintained during the procedure.

Diagnosis	Risk Factors	Expected Outcomes
Risk for Decreased Cardiac Output (cardiodepression) related to the administration of local anesthetics	☐ Local anesthetics with epinephrine given in conjunction with enflurane, halothane, and related drugs ☐ Local anesthetics with epinephrine given in conjunction with tricyclic antidepressants, monoamine oxidase inhibitors, and phenothiazines ☐ History of heart block or other cardiac disease	☐ Are there signs or reports of gradual or abrupt hypotension? ☐ Docs the patient show evidence of pallor? ☐ Does the patient complain of feeling faint or dizzy?

Adapted from Carpentino-Moyet, L. J. (2008). *Handbook of nursing diagnosis* (12th ed.) Philadelphia: Lippincott Williams & Wilkins; Petersen, C. (2007). *Perioperative nursing data set, the perioperative nursing vocabulary.* (Revised 2nd ed.). Denver: AORN, Inc.

MANAGING THE PATIENT'S AIRWAY AND BREATHING PATTERN

The nurse manages the airway and breathing pattern of patients when not monitored by an anesthesia provider. Airway obstruction or ineffective breathing may occur in patients with an impaired airway due to trauma, infection, or increased secretions. Other patients at risk for airway problems include those with a history of asthma, cerebrovascular accident, chronic obstructive pulmonary disease (COPD), spinal cord injury, and coma. Unconscious or comatose patients lose their protective reflexes as well as the tone of pharyngeal muscles; therefore, the tongue may fall back and obstruct the airway. An anesthesia provider should manage these patients during the operative and invasive procedure.

COPD
Chronic Obstructive Pulmonary Disease

Ineffective breathing and/or a compromised airway may also occur in patients receiving moderate sedation/analgesia. Sedated patients may be unable, reluctant, or forget to breathe and cough, if necessary. Nurses administering moderate sedation/analgesia must demonstrate competency in airway management. Competency includes the proficiency to asses the physical airway to identify patients with airways that may be difficult to bag-mask ventilate. Patients at risk include those older than 55 years, morbidly obese, with missing teeth or edentulous, who have a history of snoring or sleep apnea, have stridor, or the presence of a beard (ASA, 2002a; Langeron et al, 2000). If a patient scheduled for moderate sedation/analgesia and/or local anesthesia presents with any of these findings, consult with an anesthesia provider.

Factors That Affect Airway Clearance and Breathing

Unique factors predispose a patient to ineffective airway clearance and disturbance in breathing patterns during the operative or invasive procedure. These factors include the flow of blood or secretions into the airway, use of medications that produce sedation, the weight of surgical drapes, or the position of the body during the procedure.

Positioning the patient to provide optimal operative exposure may result in decreased lung expansion that interferes with normal breathing. Mechanical restriction or reduced ability of the diaphragm to push down against the abdominal contents can impair lung expansion. When this happens, lung compliance decreases, reducing the amount of alveolar volume available for gas exchange and the functional residual capacity.

Supplies and Equipment

See **Table 13.3** for recommended airway supplies and equipment.

Table 13.3	Equipment and Supplies for Managing the Patient's Airway and Breathing Pattern

Make available appropriate emergency equipment whenever sedative or analgesic drugs capable of causing cardiorespiratory depression are administered. Use the list below as a guide. Modify the list depending on the individual practice circumstances. For infants or children include the bracketed items.

Basic Airway Management Equipment

Advanced airway management equipment (for practitioners with intubation skills)	Source of compressed oxygen (tank with regulator or pipeline supply with flowmeter)
Cuffed endotracheal tubes 6.0, 7.0, 8.0 mm	Source of suction
Endotracheal tubes	Stylet (appropriately sized for endotracheal tubes)
Face masks [infant/child]	Suction catheters [pediatric suction catheters]
Laryngeal mask airways [pediatric]	Uncuffed endotracheal tubes 2.5, 3.0, 3.5, 4.0, 4.5, 5.0, 5.5, 6.0 mm
Laryngoscope blades [pediatric]	Yankauer-type suction
Laryngoscope handles (tested)	
Lubricant	
Oral and nasal airways [infant/child-sized]	
Self-inflating breathing bag-valve set [pediatric]	

Monitors

Electrocardiograph	Sphygmomanometer or noninvasive blood pressure cuff
Pulse oximeter	

Intravenous Access

Alcohol wipes	Intravenous fluid
Appropriately sized syringes [1-mL syringes]	Intravenous tubing [pediatric "micro-drip" (60 drops/mL)]
Assorted needles for drug aspiration, intramuscular injection	Sterile gauze pads
Gloves	Tape
Intravenous catheters [24–22-gauge]	Tourniquets

Medications	
Amiodarone	Glucose, 50% [10 or 25%]
Atropine	Hydrocortisone, methylprednisolone, or dexamethasone
Diazepam or midazolam	
Diphenhydramine	Lidocaine
Emergency medications	Naloxone
Ephedrine	Nitroglycerin (tablets or spray)
Epinephrine	Vasopressin
Flumazenil	

Adapted from *Practice Guidelines for Sedation and Analgesia by Non-Anesthesiologists* Anesthesiology, V 96, No 4, Apr 2002.

Potential Adverse Outcomes

See **Table 13.2**.

Risk for Ineffective Airway Clearance and Ineffective Breathing Pattern during the Operative or Invasive Procedure

A variety of irritants can cause partial or complete obstruction of the airway. Common irritants that may enter the airway include saliva, blood, vomitus, and other dry particulate matter. The patient is also at risk for ineffective breathing. Pain, anxiety, sedation, or mechanical force of drapes, retractors, or operative personnel inadvertently leaning on the patient may also cause an ineffective breathing pattern.

Before the Procedure

Assess and document the patient's respiratory status. Check the rate and rhythm. Look for the presence of a cough, dyspnea, rales, clubbing of the fingers, abnormal breath sounds, or cyanosis. Note the characteristics of cough and sputum. Interview the patient and the family to assess for a history of airway obstruction or respiratory, cardiovascular, or neurologic disease. Review results of related studies such as chest radiographs, sputum studies, pulmonary function tests, and arterial blood gas studies.

During the Procedure

SaO$_2$
Arterial Blood Oxygen Saturation

Administer oxygen as needed by nasal cannula or a facemask. Use a pulse oximeter to monitor the patient's arterial blood oxygen saturation (SaO$_2$), which is an indicator of the percentage of hemoglobin saturated with oxygen at the time of the measurement. Normal blood oxygen saturation is 95% or greater. The pulse oximetry sensor emits light into arterialized tissue and measures the amount of light reflected by that tissue (eg, oxyhemoglobin). Use this noninvasive, readily available, and relatively accurate technology to continually monitor the patient's level of oxygenation and heart rate for all general, regional, moderate sedation/analgesia, and local anesthesia cases.

Pulse oximetry assists in detecting potential problems that are not evident during visual assessment. In addition, it provides an accurate means of alerting the nurse to hypoxemia before signs and symptoms manifest. Apply the sensor of the pulse oximeter to the index, middle, or ring finger, using a disposable adhesive or reusable finger clip. Other sensors are available that may be used on the nose, earlobe, toe, or foot (eg, infants and neonates), as well as on the forehead, depending on patient size, perfusion, or movement.

Position the patient with the head slightly elevated or in a semi-sitting position, if permitted by the procedure. Provide emotional support by maintaining contact through touch and communication. Monitor the respiratory rate and the quality of chest excursion. Normal respiratory rate is between 16 and 20 breaths/minute. Note stridor, skin color change, or changes in mental alertness or personality.

Observe for signs of airway obstruction. In such cases, inspiration will cause drawing in of parts of the upper chest, the sternum, and the intercostal spaces. Exhalation is characterized by jerky protrusion and prolonged contractions of abdominal muscles. Seesaw movement of the chest and abdomen may occur. Tracheal tug or indrawing of the supra-sternal notch may occur.

Initiate corrective action if airway obstruction occurs. Open and inspect the mouth for displacement of the tongue and the presence of secretions, blood, and other substances. If necessary, suction the patient. There are three ways to open the airway: the chin lift, jaw thrust with head tilt and extension, and insertion of an oral/nasal airway. The simplest method is the chin lift. After placing the thumb under the patient's chin, pull upwards, and forward, lifting the patient's chin, this should open the airway. However, if the chin lift fails, use the jaw thrust with head tilt and extension. This maneuver increases the distance between the chin and the cervical spine, which puts the muscles that support the chin under tension and pulls the tongue forward. In addition, the maneuver puts further tension on the musculature that supports the tongue. Lift the mandible upward by exerting pressure on the ascending ramus of the mandible and at the same time tilting the patient's head backward. Place the fingers and palm of each hand on each side of the face to maintain head extension.

If the jaw thrust with the head tilt and extension fails to open the airway, consider inserting an oral or nasal airway (see **Fig. 13.1**) or have the anesthesia provider intubate the patient. If breathing difficulties persist, call for assistance immediately from an anesthesia provider. Administer supplemental oxygen and ventilate the patient with a positive pressure bag-mask device. Record findings and report as needed.

After the Procedure

While handing-off care of the patient to the postanesthesia care unit (PACU) nurse, report pertinent events that occurred during the procedure. Include information about the type of procedure and medications and IV fluids received; vital signs and patient response to procedure and medications; blood loss and urinary output;

PACU
Postanesthesia
Care Unit

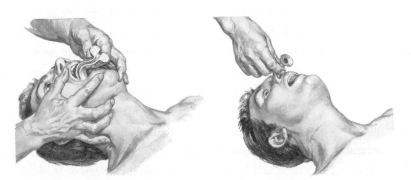

Figure 13.1

Inserting oral and nasal airways.

Source: Netter Images.

presence of drains and catheters and amount of drainage; level of consciousness; nausea or vomiting; and subjective or objective manifestations of pain, anxiety, or fear.

Consult with an anesthesia provider or respiratory therapist for assistance as needed. Make a postprocedure visit or telephone the patient to evaluate the response to measures used to maintain airway and breathing,

MANAGING THE PATIENT'S FLUID INTAKE

The nurse may administer IV fluids during the procedure. Patients undergoing an operative or invasive procedure should have IV access to administer fluids and to establish a route for IV drug administration. Most patients undergoing procedures have fluid intake restrictions before the procedure. Intravenous therapy provides water, electrolytes, and nutrients needed to meet body requirements and to replace fluid and electrolyte deficiencies. Fluid alterations during the operative or invasive procedure period can range from minimal blood loss to massive blood loss and severe alteration of electrolyte levels.

Body fluids are located within three compartments: intracellular space, extracellular/intravascular space, and extracellular/interstitial space. Maintenance of this fluid volume happens because of the interaction between intake and output through the kidney, loss of fluid from the lungs and the skin, hydrostatic pressure within the vascular compartment, and osmolarity within each compartment (Petersen, 2007).

Factors That May Affect Fluid and Electrolyte Balance

Factors that may affect fluid and electrolyte balance include fluid and food intake. During the assessment, note the last time the patient ate or drank and the type of food or fluid consumed. Other factors include excessive thirst and sources of fluid loss such as diarrhea, draining wounds, excessive urine output, and excessive perspiration. Assess the use of medications, such as diuretics and adrenocorticosteroids; these may cause fluid and electrolyte imbalances. Use of over-the-counter agents to induce urinary and bowel elimination may also contribute imbalances. Ingestion of excessive alcohol and non-prescription drugs may interfere with proper nutrition, thus leading to an imbalance. Do not overlook important contributing factors such as diabetes insipidus, diabetic ketoacidosis, adrenal insufficiency, renal failure, cancer, burns, trauma, pregnancy, and congestive heart failure.

Delivering IV Fluids

Most facilities have infusion pumps used to deliver fluids and medications. Although these devices are helpful for delivering solutions at a controlled rate and volume, they do not eliminate the need for frequent monitoring of the infusion.

Infusion pumps are commonplace in operative and invasive procedure suites, yet some nurses may find themselves in situations where they do not have access to an infusion pump, such as during a mass causality, mission work, first responder, pump malfunction, pump battery failure in conjunction with power failure, and inadequate pump inventory. In these situations, after initiating the IV, monitor the IV solutions frequently to ensure that flow remains at the desired rate. When manually monitoring the IV, flow rates can vary and not provide adequate delivery of fluid. Inadequate IV fluid flow may also contribute to a fluid and electrolyte imbalance. Height of the liquid column directly affects the flow of IV fluid. Raising the height of the infusion container improves the flow unless conditions such as an IV infiltration impede the flow. Tubing diameter also affects the flow. The clamp on the IV tubing regulates the flow by changing the tubing diameter. Large-gauge cannulas (14, 16, or 18 gauge) cause the fluid to flow faster. Tubing length and fluid viscosity will decrease flow rate. Adding tubing to provide more length decreases the flow rate. Solutions such as blood products and hyperalimentation fluids require a larger cannula than do less viscous solutions.

Calculating Intravenous Fluid Infusion Rate

The nurse monitors IV solutions frequently to ensure consistent and accurate flow rate. Patients receiving preventive IV therapy or IV infusions for drug administration have varied needs from those patients experiencing a severe depletion of fluid.

Mark the IV container with a label indicating how much fluid to infuse per hour. To calculate the flow rate, determine the number of drops per milliliter. This number varies with the type of tubing and drip chamber and is usually included with the product information. **Table 13.4** shows two formulas to calculate IV infusion drip rates.

Types of Intravenous Solutions

Fluid content and tonicity (isotonic, hypotonic, or hypertonic) determine the classification of intravenous solutions. Common constituents of IV fluids used during operative and invasive procedures include dextrose in water, sodium chloride, or multiple electrolytes. Parenteral fluid tonicity is classified in relation to the tonicity of normal blood plasma (approximately 290 mOsm/L); that is, according to whether osmolality is, respectively, the same as, less than, or greater than that of blood.

Isotonic fluids have a total osmolality close to that of intravascular fluid and do not cause red blood cells to shrink or swell. Commonly used isotonic fluids include 5% dextrose in water, normal saline (0.9% sodium chloride), and lactated Ringer's solution. Isotonic fluids increase the extracellular fluid volume, which can cause circulatory overload.

Hypotonic fluids increase the osmolality of the plasma and provide additional water needed for urinary excretion. Hypovolemic patients usually receive hypotonic fluids. Commonly used hypotonic fluids include half-normal saline (0.45% sodium chloride) and 2.5% dextrose in water.

Hypertonic fluids have a total osmolality that exceeds that of extracellular fluid. Commonly used hypertonic solutions include 5% dextrose in normal saline (0.9% sodium chloride), 10%, 20%, and 50% dextrose and water solutions, and hypertonic saline (3% sodium chloride). Excessive administration of hypertonic fluids may lead to cellular dehydration.

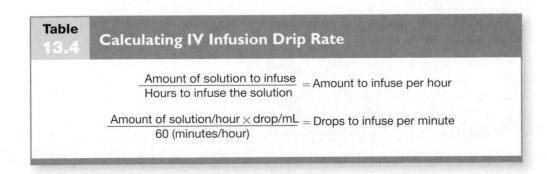

Table 13.4	Calculating IV Infusion Drip Rate

$$\frac{\text{Amount of solution to infuse}}{\text{Hours to infuse the solution}} = \text{Amount to infuse per hour}$$

$$\frac{\text{Amount of solution/hour} \times \text{drop/mL}}{60 \text{ (minutes/hour)}} = \text{Drops to infuse per minute}$$

Supplies and Equipment

The physician orders administration of intravenous fluid. Venipuncture cannulas should include indwelling plastic catheters inserted over a steel needle or indwelling plastic catheters inserted through a sterile needle and the steel scalp vein needle (butterfly set). Other supplies and equipment include IV tubing and an infusion pump.

Potential Adverse Outcomes

See **Table 13.2**.

Risk for Impaired Tissue Integrity Related to Local Infiltration of Intravenous Fluid

Local infiltration produces swelling and discomfort at the IV site. An infiltrated IV infuses slowly or may have no flow at all. If an IV infiltrates, blood will not flow into the tubing when the nurse lowers the infusion bag.

Before the Procedure

Assess for a history of IV infiltration or problems associated with IV therapy. Look for conditions that may alter vascular integrity such as diabetes mellitus and physical debilitation. Select an optimal site for IV entry. When possible, use upper extremity veins for IV access. Avoid the antecubital fossa, however, because flexion of the arm can impede the flow of the infusion. Select a site that does not impede mobility. Use of the patient's nondominant hand is preferred. Palpate the vein for elasticity and search for any hard knots, which may indicate thromboses. **Figure 13.2**

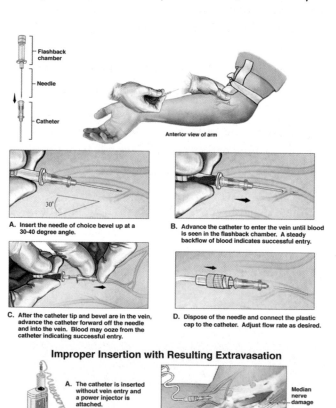

Figure 13.2

Inserting an IV catheter. Proper and improper insertion.

Source: Netter Images.

Figure 13.3

IV in the posterior forearm.

Source: Netter Images.

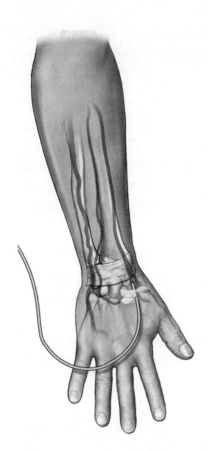

illustrates the proper technique for inserting an intravenous catheter and improper insertion with resulting extravasation. **Figure 13.3** shows an IV placed in the forearm.

During the Procedure

Frequently inspect the infusion site for infiltration, swelling, redness, or coolness. If infiltration occurs, discontinue the IV and restart it in another location. Explain to the patient what has occurred and apply a warm, moist compress to the affected area. Record and report interventions used and the patient's response to therapy.

After the Procedure

See Managing the Patient's Airway and Breathing Pattern (After the Procedure, pp. 377–378). Make a postprocedure visit or telephone the patient to evaluate the response to measures pertaining to IV fluid intake.

Risk for Fluid Volume Excess Related to Intravenous Therapy

Fluid volume excess can occur and result in generalized fluid volume overload. Excessive intake of fluid during the operative or invasive procedure occurs most frequently from over infusion of IV solutions (crystalloids) or colloids such as blood and plasma expanders. This excessive intake of fluids expands the intravascular compartment, leading to an increase in circulating blood volume.

If not corrected, hypervolemia can lead to congestive heart failure, manifested by dyspnea, neck vein distention, tachycardia, hypertension or hypotension, and cardiac ischemia. Hypervolemia can also lead to dependent edema. Laboratory findings may include a low hematocrit and low total protein count, owing to dilution. Sodium levels will decrease with over hydration secondary to dilution, and potassium levels may decrease in patients on diuretics.

Before the Procedure

Conduct a nursing history and assess for the presence of disease conditions that may predispose the patient to a risk for fluid volume overload (see Risk Factors). Assess baseline laboratory values. For high-risk patients, use micro-drip tubing and an infusion pump to assist in monitoring intake. Note the presence of edema, bounding pulse, distended neck veins, rales, dyspnea, orthopnea, elevated central venous pressure, and recent unexplained weight gain.

During the Procedure

If symptoms of fluid excess develop, slow the rate of the infusion at once and notify the physician. Monitor vital signs, electrolyte values, and report findings to the physician. Document vital signs on the operative or invasive procedure record. Measure and document the amount of IV fluid intake, urinary output, and blood loss. Position the patient to prevent or alleviate dyspnea or edema. Record and report interventions used and response to therapy.

After the Procedure

See Managing the Patient's Airway and Breathing Pattern (After the Procedure, pp. 377–378). Make a postprocedure visit or telephone the patient to evaluate the response to measures involving administration of IV fluids.

Risk for Decreased Cardiac Output Related to Air Embolus from Intravenous Therapy

Cardiac output refers to the volume of blood pumped by each heartbeat (or stroke volume) times the number of beats per minute. Normal cardiac output averages about 5 L/minute in the adult patient. Air, when introduced into the circulation in large quantity, can act as an embolus and impede the flow of blood through the circulation. Because of decreased cardiac output, the patient may become cyanotic, hypotensive, and unresponsive.

Infusions given under pressure are more likely to be associated with air embolism than are peripheral infusions delivered by gravity. In addition, infusions delivered by central catheters are more prone to air embolus formation. Although small amounts of air are not hazardous, a volume of 50 mL can be lethal when delivered as a bolus. A large air embolus in the right atrium or the right ventricle can cause an airlock that prevents returning blood from filling the right side of the heart. The result is a significant decrease in cardiac output, which can lead to hypotension and cardiac arrest.

Before the Procedure

Inspect the tubing for the presence of air. Before attaching the tubing to the catheter, prime it by letting fluid flow the length of the tubing. This will force air out of the tubing. Discontinue or replace the infusion before the IV fluid bag is empty. Secure all connections from the proximal to the distal ends of the tubing. During central line insertion, place the patient in the Trendelenburg position. This position increases central venous pressure, which decreases the risk of venous air embolus.

During the Procedure

Allow a loop of tubing to drop below the extremity as an added precaution against air embolus. Respond to a suspected air embolism by clamping the tubing, turning the patient onto the left side, and placing the bed in the Trendelenburg position. These interventions keep the air in the right atrium, where it can be absorbed or removed through a central venous catheter. Administer oxygen and support the circulation with emergency medications as ordered by the physician. Record and report the pertinent patient events that occurred during the procedure, the interventions used, and the patient's response to care.

After the Procedure

See Managing the Patient's Airway and Breathing Pattern (After the Procedure, pp. 377–378). Make a postprocedure visit or telephone the patient to evaluate the response to measures involving administration of IV fluids.

MONITORING THE PATIENT'S FLUID LOSS

During an operative or invasive procedure, the nurse monitors blood loss, irrigation fluids, and urine output. Monitoring activities include measuring blood loss from suction receptacles and sponges, amount of irrigation fluid used, and urinary output.

Factors That Affect Output

Diarrhea, vomiting, wound drainage, burns, trauma, or hemorrhage may cause an active fluid loss. Patients prone to alterations in output include those with coexisting disease such as renal failure, neurogenic bladder, urinary retention, or diabetes. Closely monitor patients with an artificial urinary drainage system (cystostomy, peritoneal or renal dialysis, and ureteral stents) so that output is accurately measured. Excessive or inadequate use of blood, blood products, IV fluids, and volume expanders may also influence output during the operative and invasive procedure period.

Supplies and Equipment

Supplies and equipment include suction tubing and containers, radiopaque sponges (size according to type of procedure), graduated measuring devices, and a scale to weigh sponges.

Potential Adverse Outcomes

See **Table 13.2**.

Risk for Fluid Volume Deficit Related to Bleeding During the Procedure

Bleeding during the procedure, if not controlled, can have dire consequences for the patient. Remain alert for possible bleeding and prepare to take actions to determine the extent of blood and other fluid loss. Patients undergoing minor procedures, even though monitored solely by the nurse, can experience excessive bleeding. Procedures such as hair transplants, facial reconstruction, and excision of scalp lesions may result in bleeding owing to the vascularity of the operative site. Additionally, the patient may lose blood when excisions of lesions thought to be small or superficial become more extensive than anticipated or involve the dissection of major blood vessels.

The type and amount of bleeding depend on the type of vessels involved. Capillary hemorrhage slowly seeps. Dark venous hemorrhage bubbles out quickly. Bright red arterial hemorrhage spurts out with each heartbeat.

Hypovolemic shock results in a decreased fluid volume owing to loss of blood, plasma, or water. A fall in venous pressure, rise in peripheral resistance, and tachycardia indicate hypovolemia. Classic signs of shock include pallor; cool, moist skin; cyanosis of the lips, eyelids, and gums; restlessness; rapid breathing; weak, thready pulse; small pulse pressure; lowering of blood pressure; and oliguria, concentrated urine, and anuria.

Before the Procedure

Assess for the presence of disease, bleeding or clotting disorders, or use of medications that may influence blood loss. Determine the presence of fluid deficit, as evidenced by such factors as poor nutritional status and skin turgor, hypotension, decreased pulse amplitude, weakness, increased temperature, and hemoconcentration. Note the presence of therapies that may alter fluid balance such as IV fluids, bowel preparations, and diuretics. Assess for a family history of bleeding or clotting disorders. Initiate an IV infusion to provide access to the circulatory system. Monitor vital signs.

During the Procedure

Prepare and administer IV fluids as needed. Insert an indwelling urinary catheter to monitor urinary output. Use of a urinary catheter depends on the patient's fluid status, the anticipated length of the procedure, and the anticipated amount of blood loss. Urine output is one of the most valuable indices of adequacy of renal perfusion. A drop in renal arterial pressure and flow produces renal arterial vasoconstriction and results in decreased glomerular filtration and decreased urine output. Normal urine flow is 50 mL/hour. An output of 0.5 mL/kg/hour is suggestive of inadequate volume replacement or cardiac failure. Monitor blood loss and the amount of irrigation solution used. Use warm, moistened sponges to prevent tissue from becoming dry and from losing heat by evaporation and convection. Keep blood-soaked sponges and soiled instruments and supplies out of the patient's visual field. Keep conversation to a minimum.

If hypotension occurs, perform the following. Place the patient in the supine or Trendelenburg position. Administer oxygen, fluids, and medications as needed. Call for emergency assistance as needed. Inspect the wound for obvious and hidden sites of bleeding. Continue to monitor vital signs. Monitor blood loss through suction and saturation of sponges. Weigh sponges as needed.

Document the type and amount of irrigation fluid used during the procedure. Record and report care given during the procedure and the patient's response to therapy.

After the Procedure

See Managing the Patient's Airway and Breathing Pattern (After the Procedure, pp. 377–378). Make a postprocedure visit or telephone the patient to evaluate the response to measures to control blood loss.

MAINTAINING THE PATIENT'S BODY TEMPERATURE

The nurse monitors body temperature to determine the extent of heat production and heat loss.

Factors That Affect Body Temperature

Temperature Control

The regulation of body temperature is a tightly controlled process. Approximately 80% of the control of autonomic responses is controlled by thermal input from core structures to the hypothalamus; in contrast, large portion of the input controlling behavioral responses is derived from the surface of the skin (Sessler & Kurz, 2006). The hypothalamus, which acts as the body's thermostat, controls body temperature. This occurs through the secretion of thyroid stimulating hormone-releasing hormone (TSH-RH), which initiates a series of actions resulting in heat production and conservation. Heat loss occurs when the hypothalamus reverses the process and shuts down the TSH-RH pathway. Illness or trauma to these centers can alter temperature control.

TSH-RH
Thyroid Stimulating
Hormone-Releasing
Hormone

Heat Production

Heat production occurs because of the chemical reactions of metabolism, thermogenesis, and skeletal muscle contractions. Increases in metabolic rate, as occurs with malignant hyperthermia, thyroid disease, or imbalances of hormonal production, may alter temperature. Heat production increases release of epinephrine, norepinephrine, and thyroxine. Stress associated with the procedure can influence the production of these hormones.

Heat Loss

In the operative and invasive procedure environment, the primary mechanisms of heat loss are radiation, conduction, convection, and evaporation of water through the lungs and the skin (Sessler, 2005). *Radiation* is the loss of heat from a warmer surface (the body) to a cooler one (the environment) and occurs through electromagnetic waves. *Conduction* occurs with the transfer of heat from a warmer surface to a cooler surface by direct contact, as occurs with the use of a cooling blanket. *Convection* is the loss of heat through circulating air currents, and is dependent upon a temperature gradient between the body and the ambient air. *Evaporation* converts liquid to vapor, as in the evaporation of perspiration; heat is transferred or lost during this conversion.

Heat Conservation

Heat conservation takes place through involuntary vasoconstriction at the periphery of the body and voluntary actions of the patient. Cutaneous vasoconstriction is the thermoregulatory defense that is consistently used to move warm blood away from the periphery to the core; in addition, behavior such as sustained shivering supplements metabolic heat production in adults by 50% to 100% (Sessler & Kurz, 2006).

Age

The very young are susceptible to temperature extremes because of immature thermal control mechanisms, underdeveloped sweat glands, less subcutaneous tissue, poor vasomotor control, and a lower metabolic rate. In addition, infants and children cool more quickly because of their high ratio of surface area to weight (Wagner, 2006), resulting in greater heat loss through convection and radiation. Temperature instability also occurs in the elderly, due to their reduced thermoregulatory efficiency (Wagner, 2006), owing to atrophied sweat glands and loss of elasticity in the blood vessels.

Body Size

Patients who are thin or small-statured, and lack of tissue mass are more predisposed to the development of hypothermia (Wagner, 2006).

Operative and Invasive Procedure Environment

Unplanned hypothermia results from anesthetic-impaired thermoregulation and exposure to the cold environment of the operative or invasive procedure suite (Sessler & Kurz, 2006). Anesthetics affect the patient's ability to regulate heat loss by decreasing metabolism and inhibiting the cold responses. With general anesthesia, the patient's ability to respond naturally, with behaviors such as shivering, is impaired; the ability to shiver is further impaired by the administration of muscle relaxants. The patient's temperature can drop 1 °C to 1.5 °C (1.8 °F to 2.7 °F) during the first hour of anesthesia (Sessler & Kurz, 2006).

Supplies and Equipment

The following are examples of the supplies and equipment needed to manage the patient's temperature: temperature-measuring device, warm blankets, fluid warmer, forced air warming device, and hyperthermia or hypothermia blanket and machine. Use reliable methods to monitor core body temperature. These methods include devices that measure the patient's temperature using the tympanic membrane, distal esophagus, nasophyarynx, and pulmonary artery. Less reliable methods include measuring core body temperature via the axillary, bladder, oral, rectal, skin, and temporal artery.

Potential Adverse Outcomes

See **Table 13.2**.

Risk for Hypothermia During the Operative or Invasive Procedure

While there are no standardized definitions of normothermia and hypothermia in the literature, the most widely accepted definitions are (ASPAN, 2002):

- Normothermia: core body temperature range of 36 °C–38 °C (96.8 °F–100.4 °F)
- Hypothermia: core body temperature less than 36 °C (96.8 °F)

Table 13.5	Factors That Predispose the Patient to Unplanned Hypothermia

☐ Chronic therapy with either antipsychotics or antidepressants

☐ Cool ambient temperature of the procedure room

☐ Decreased metabolism and free heat production

☐ Exposure of internal organs or body cavities to the external environment

☐ Heat loss due to evaporation, convection, and radiation from the open wound

☐ Infusing cool fluids, blood products

☐ Irrigating body cavities with cool fluid

☐ Loss of shivering ability

☐ Loss of temperature-sensing and temperature regulating mechanisms (hypothalamic anesthesia)

☐ Low body weight

☐ Metabolic disorders

☐ Older adults or very young children (ie. neonates)

☐ Prolonged duration of the procedure

☐ Skin vasodilatation

☐ Use of pneumatic tourniquet

☐ Ventilation with dry gases (evaporation loss)

Adapted from: AORN. (2008b). Recommended practices for the prevention of unplanned perioperative hypothermia. 2008 *Perioperative Standards and Recommended Practices.* Denver: AORN; 407–420.

While trauma patients, neonates, and patients with extensive burns have a greater risk of hypothermia, all patients share the risk of hypothermia in direct proportion to length of anesthesia. Furthermore, when the body temperature drops below 33 °C (91.4 °F), vital functions can profoundly deteriorate (Wagner, 2006). **Table 13.5** lists the factors that predispose the patient to unplanned hypothermia.

Maintaining normothermia has gained national attention with the Surgical Care Improvement Project (SCIP) with a goal of reducing surgical complications by 25% by the year 2010 (MedQIC, 2008). A subcategory of this goal is maintaining normothermia in colorectal surgery patients. With the current trends in pay-for-performance initiatives, the SCIP initiatives promote specific warming interventions known to decrease the risk of surgical site infection (SSI) (Wagner, 2006).

As shown in **Table 13.6**, patients exhibit a variety of physiological responses when experiencing hypothermia. In addition to the physiological responses, the conscious patient may respond with apathy, confusion, or drowsiness. Children younger than 3 months of age are at particular risk because hypothermia can induce reopening of fetal circulation, resulting in acidosis and hypoxemia, which becomes a circular pattern of events difficult to reverse.

Before the Procedure

Interview the patient and family members to assess the factors that may put the patient at risk for hypothermia. Institute appropriate prewarming measures in the procedure suite holding area. *Prewarming* is defined as the application of heat prior

SCIP
Surgical Care
Improvement Project

SSI
Surgical Site Infection

Table 13.6	Potential Physiological Responses Secondary to Hypothermia

☐ Alteration in acid-base balance	☐ Increased heart rate
☐ Altered metabolism of drugs	☐ Increased oxygen consumption
☐ Arrhythmias	☐ Increased stroke volume
☐ Changes in arterial blood gas values	☐ Prolonged recovery time in PACU
☐ Coagulopathy	☐ Surgical site infection
☐ Increased arterial blood pressure	☐ Ventricular irritability
☐ Increased cardiac output	☐ Ventricular tachycardia

Adapted from Soreide, E., Smith, C. E., Hypothermia in Trauma Victims-Friend or Foe? *ITACCS Winter 2005*, p. 19; AORN (2008b). Recommended practices for the prevention of unplanned perioperative hypothermia. *Perioperative Standards and Recommended Practices.* Denver: AORN; 407–420.

to procedure for the purpose of increasing the patient's temperature. Active warming of every surgical patient before the procedure is key for preventing hypothermia during the procedure. Patient should be actively warmed for at least 30 minutes in order to be effective (OR Manager, 2006).

During the Procedure

Monitor the patient's temperature and assess physiologic changes. Endocrine, liver, and kidney functions decrease as the rate of metabolism decreases. As noted, patients at extremes of ages (ie, neonates, infants, and the elderly) are the most susceptible to the development of hypothermia. Provide extra covers during the procedure to maintain a normal body temperature without using other modalities. Monitor vital signs and note changes in the electrocardiogram, blood pressure, arterial blood gas values, and blood chemistry values. Arrhythmias stemming from altered myocardial irritability vary with the degree of hypothermia and the patient's age and condition. Circulating blood volume diminishes as plasma pools in peripheral capillary beds. Temperature reduction affects the heart's neuromuscular tissue, leading to a decrease in cardiac rate, causing a reduction in oxygen consumption, a fall in respiratory rate and blood pressure.

Table 13.7 lists interventions to maintain normothermia during the procedure. Many of these devices require the use of a medical device designed for temperature control. Follow the manufacturers' written instructions when using these devices.

Monitor for behavioral changes in the conscious patient. Decreases in venous and intracranial pressure may cause hypothermia. In addition, for every degree centigrade reduction in temperature, cerebral blood flow decreases about 6% and cerebral function diminishes. If body temperature drops below the desired level, rewarm the patient as needed. For temperatures greater than 35 °C (95 °F), use passive rewarming rather than active rewarming because the latter method may result in hyperthermia. Warming methods include internal surface warming (warm saline, moist sponges, and warm IV fluids) and external surface warming (warming blanket, warm sheets, and external packs). Carefully rewarm the patient until normal functions return.

Table 13.7	Interventions to Maintain Normothermia During the Operative and Invasive Procedure Period

- ☐ Employ age-specific interventions (eg, infant warming lights, infant hats, pre-warming the room)
- ☐ Increase the room temperature as permitted according to facility policy
- ☐ Use forced-air warming devices
- ☐ Use circulating water garments
- ☐ Use energy transfer pads
- ☐ Use equipment to warm insufflation gas during laparoscopic procedures
- ☐ Use equipment to warm anesthetic gases
- ☐ Warm parenteral IV solutions to approximately 37 °C (98.6 °F) with technology designed for this purpose (eg, in-line blood and solution infusion warming units, warming cabinets)
- ☐ Warm irrigation solutions before use to near normal body core temperature 37 °C (98.6 °F) in warming cabinets
- ☐ Use supplemental patient warming measures before and after the procedure such as warm blankets and inline blood warming units

Mitchell, S. Preventing unplanned perioperative hypothermia. *AORN J*, 86:4, October 2007, pp. 660–661.

As the body temperature rises, oxygen demands increase. The cardiac output of the weakened, cold heart may not meet the body's needs.

Prepare for emergency measures, which may include cardiac massage, mechanical ventilation, infusion of IV fluids and blood products, cardioversion for ventricular fibrillation, use of antiarrhythmic drugs, and insertion of an indwelling catheter to monitor fluid status. Record and report procedure findings and care activities.

After the Procedure

See Managing the Patient's Airway and Breathing Pattern (After the Procedure, pp. 377–378). Alert the PACU or unit staff to prepare warming equipment and medications. The physician may order medications such as nondepolarizing muscle relaxants (eg, rocuronium [Zemuron], vecuronium [Norcuron]) in the intubated patient, or small doses of meperidine (Demerol) in the conscious patient, to suppress shivering. Make a postprocedure visit or telephone the patient to evaluate the response to measures to prevent hypothermia.

Risk for Hyperthermia During the Operative or Invasive Procedure

Many events affect the patient's ability to maintain normal body temperature during the operative and invasive procedure period. These events include the use of copious amounts of warm irrigating solutions, the application of impervious drapes, the use of internal or external warming techniques, and the use of medications such as vasoconstrictors. Additionally, the stress associated with the procedure may result in anxiety and concomitant increase in temperature. See Chapter 7 for information concerning malignant hyperthermia (MH) secondary to general anesthesia.

Damage to the hypothalamus or severe intracranial infection may result in hyperthermia in the patient with neurologic disease or the patient undergoing

MH
Malignant Hyperthermia

neurosurgery. If such temperature elevations are not controlled, the increased metabolic needs of the brain may make increased demands on the circulation and oxygenation of the brain. Persistent hyperthermia may indicate brain stem damage. Additionally, the presence of intraventricular blood can also cause temperature elevations.

The patient with hyperthermia may complain of headache, thirst, general malaise, and palpitations. Overt signs can include increased body temperature, flushed skin, warm skin, increased respirations, tachycardia, seizures, and convulsions.

Before the Procedure

Interview the patient and family members and assess for factors that may put the patient at risk for hyperthermia. Malignant hyperthermia is a genetic disorder, therefore, the patient should be asked if he/she has had a family member who experienced an MH episode or died during surgery (AORN, 2008c). Note the presence of fever, infection, or diseases associated with hyperthermia.

During the Procedure

Monitor the patient's temperature and assess changes as needed. Maintain the patient's comfort and normal body temperature by removing excessive drapes as needed. Apply internal/external cooling measures as needed: cool bath, hypothermia blanket, or other means. Monitor vital signs and note changes in the ECG, blood pressure, arterial blood gas values, and blood chemistry values. Measure urinary output and report if output falls below 0.5 mL/kg/hour. If body temperature increases excessively beyond normal parameters, use a cooling blanket as needed. Be prepared for emergency measures, including the use of oxygen, the infusion of cool IV fluids, the use of emergency medications, the use of anti-arrhythmic drugs, and the insertion of an indwelling urinary catheter to monitor fluid status. Record and report operative or procedure findings and care activities.

After the Procedure

See Managing the Patient's Airway and Breathing Pattern (After the Procedure, pp. 377–378). Alert PACU staff to prepare equipment or medications (eg, antibiotics and antipyretics). Make a postprocedure visit or telephone the patient to evaluate the response to measures used to prevent hyperthermia.

MONITORING THE EFFECTS OF MODERATE SEDATION/ ANALGESIA AND LOCAL ANESTHESIA

Look for reactions to external and internal stressors while monitoring the patient receiving local anesthesia, analgesia, and sedation. Nurses must have training and demonstrate competency before assuming responsibility for monitoring the patient for effects of moderate sedation/analgesia and local anesthesia.

Factors That Affect the Patient Receiving Moderate Sedation/ Analgesia and Local Anesthesia

Local anesthetic agents, analgesics, and sedatives may cause hypersensivity reactions, cardiovascular depression, respiratory depression, and central nervous system depression and toxicity.

Moderate Sedation/Analgesia

Moderate sedation/analgesia decreases the patient's anxiety and discomfort related to the procedure. An operative or invasive procedure usually results in stress manifested by fear and anxiety related to pain, loss of control, blood loss, and unfamiliar environment. Additionally, the medications, operative manipulation, conversation, or nonverbal expressions of the healthcare team can cause patient stress. Some patients, because of age or certain physiological and psychological factors, should not have a local anesthesia with monitoring by the nurse. These patients require the expertise of an anesthesia provider.

Moderate sedation/analgesia alters mood; enhances cooperation; alters perception of pain; maintains consciousness; maintains intact protective reflexes; minimizes variations in vital signs; to some degree produces amnesia; and results in a rapid, safe return to activities of daily living (AORN, 2008d). Understanding these outcomes leads to safe and effective care. Sedatives used for moderate sedation/analgesia "may cause somnolence, confusion, diminished reflexes, and depressed respiratory and cardiovascular function, and coma. Opioids may cause respiratory depression, hypotension, nausea, and vomiting" (AORN, 2008d). Overdose and adverse reaction can occur during, or after, the administration of the drug.

Local Anesthetics

Most local anesthetics fall into two categories: amino esters or amino amides. Both groups block depolarization of the nerve cell membrane by inhibiting sodium conduction across the membrane. Propagation of an action potential requires that sodium ions move from outside the axon to inside. This influx takes place through sodium channels. By blocking axonal sodium channels, local anesthetics prevent sodium entry and bring conduction to a halt (AORN, 2008e).

The enzyme pseudo-cholinesterase breaks down amino esters, resulting in para-aminobenzoic acid. About 1% of patients have an allergic reaction to this metabolite. Hepatic enzymes metabolize amino amides. Patients with hepatic disease may have ineffective metabolism, which may result in toxic responses, even with normal doses. For a discussion concerning the patient's risk of allergic and toxic reactions to local anesthetics, see Chapter 12.

Standards of Care

The nursing department, in conjunction with the departments of surgery and anesthesia, should develop standards of care for the patient receiving moderate sedation/analgesia and local anesthesia. Essential considerations when developing standards of care include the following resources or organizations published by:

- Association of periOperative Registered Nurses (AORN)
- Recommended Practices for Managing the Patient Receive Moderate Sedation/Analgesia (AORN, 2008d)
- Recommended Practices for Managing the Patient Receiving Local Anesthesia (AORN, 2008e)
- American Association of Nurse Anesthetists (AANA)
- Considerations for Policy Guidelines for Registered Nurses Engaged in the Administration of Sedation and Analgesia (AANA, 2008)

AORN
Association of periOperative Registered Nurses

AANA
American Association of Nurse Anesthetists

ASA
American Society of
Anesthesiologists

- American Society of Anesthesiologists (ASA)
- Practice Guidelines for Sedation and Analgesia by Non-Anesthesiologist (ASA, 2002b).
- The Joint Commission
- Standards for Additional Procedures: Operative or Other High-Risk Procedures and/or the Administration of Moderate or Deep Sedation or Anesthesia (The Joint Commission, 2008)
- Other considerations include the level of patient function, the presence of preexisting diseases, the type and duration of the procedure, the amount of sedation required, and the extent of monitoring required.

Supplies and Equipment

The supplies and equipment needed for monitoring the effect of local anesthesia on the patient include IV catheters and solutions, local anesthetic agents, IV medications, a marker, and labels to identify the anesthetic agent on the sterile field. See **Table 13.3** for other supplies and equipment.

Potential Adverse Outcomes

See **Table 13.2**. Allergic and toxic reactions are uncommon, but nevertheless the patient may experience serious complications when receiving local anesthesia or moderate sedation/analgesia.

Risk for Ineffective Breathing Pattern Related to Moderate Sedation/Analgesia

Some patients are given a combination of agents from a variety of chemical classes in order to achieve sedation, analgesia, relaxation, and amnesia. Moderate sedation/analgesia in combination with local anesthesia is preferred for many minor procedures. "Undesirable effects of moderate sedation/analgesia include, but are not limited to, aspiration, severely slurred sleep, hypotension or hypertension, agitation, combativeness, respirator depression, airway obstruction, and apnea" (AORN, 2008d). Furthermore, central nervous system depression caused by the depressant drugs may lead to hypoxia, hypercapnia, and respiratory failure resulting from diminished sensitivity of the respiratory center to carbon dioxide. Careful calculation and administration, as well as vigilant monitoring, are necessary. Overdose can result in laryngospasm, bronchospasm, dyspnea, hyperventilation, wheezing, shallow respirations, airway obstruction, tachypnea, or respiratory arrest.

Before the Procedure

Assess the patient for a history of sensitivity to sedatives and narcotics. Assess for signs of pulmonary dysfunction: dyspnea, tachypnea, orthopnea, skin color changes, absence or diminished breath sounds, rhonchi, wheezing, or rales. Establish physiological baseline values to assess respiratory function during the procedure. Note the patient's weight and calculate the maximum dosage of IV sedation. Note reports of respiratory status tests (chest radiographs, pulmonary function tests).

Patients receiving moderate sedation/analgesia from a nurse should have fasted 2 hours or more from intake of clear liquids and 6 hours or more from a light meal prior to the procedure to reduce the risk of aspiration (ASA, 1999). In addition, all patients will require a peripheral IV for the administration of the medications and fluid during the operative and invasive procedure period.

During the Procedure

Position the patient to facilitate breathing. Elevate the head and ensure that drapes and equipment do not interfere with breathing. Have monitoring devices in place before administering any medications. Monitor the patient's blood pressure, heart rate and rhythm, respiratory rate, oxygen saturation, skin condition, mental status, and emotional response to the procedure and anesthesia. Consult accompanying drug information and related literature before the administration of IV medication. The patient's response varies with age, physical status, and concomitant medication. When administrating IV drugs do not mix or dilute the drug with other drugs or solutions in the same syringe or container. Inject the drug slowly, taking time to assess the patient's response to the medication. Individualize and titrate the dose. Do not administer IV sedation by rapid or single-bolus IV administration. Avoid using small veins.

During the procedure, continuously monitor the patient's heart rate and rhythm, blood pressure, SaO_2, pain and level of consciousness. Record the patient's vital signs every 5 to 15 minutes during the procedure and at significant events. Communicate and record the type of medication administered, the dose, the route and time of administration, and any local reaction to IV medication. In addition to the selected sedative, have standard equipment available. See Managing the Patient's Airway and Breathing Pattern (p. 374). Document the dosage, the route, and time of administration, and the effect of medications administered, oxygen therapy, IV therapy, and the patient's response to the procedure and anesthesia. The patient will require the same level of monitoring during the acute recovery phase. The nurse should assess the patient for discharge readiness based upon specific discharge criteria established by the facility. In addition to the professional association practice guidelines and recommended practices, as well as the accrediting agency standards noted above, various state boards of nursing have also outlined standards of practice for managing the patient during moderate sedation/analgesia in their nurse practice acts.

After the Procedure

See Managing the Patient's Airway and Breathing Pattern (After the Procedure, pp. 377–378). Make a postprocedure visit or telephone the patient to evaluate the patient's response to the administration of moderate sedation/analgesia.

Risk for Impaired Tissue Integrity Related to Extravasation of Intravenous Medication

Infiltration and/or extravasation of IV medications into the subcutaneous tissue have the potential for injuring tissue. Local reactions can include tissue irritation, tissue necrosis, skin discoloration, hives, hive-like elevations, swelling, burning, warmth or coldness at the injection site, rash, and pruritus.

Before the Procedure

Assess the patient for a history of a local reaction to IV medication. Before administering medication, check for a functional IV catheter. Ensure that the patient has continuous IV access during the procedure.

During the Procedure

The nurse monitoring the patient should have no other responsibilities that could require him/her to leave the patient unattended or that would compromise continuous monitoring during the procedure (AORN, 2008d). See nursing activities under Risk for Ineffective Breathing Pattern Related to Moderate Sedation/Analgesia for guidelines for administering IV drugs. Whenever administering IV medications or local anesthetics, have standard equipment available (see Managing the Patient's Airway and Breathing Pattern, p. 374). Communicate and record the type of medication administered, the dose, the route and time of administration, and any local reaction to IV medication.

After the Procedure

See Managing the Patient's Airway and Breathing Pattern (After the Procedure, pp. 377–378). Make a postprocedure visit or telephone to evaluate the patient's response to the administration of IV medication and solutions.

Risk for Decreased Cardiac Output (Cardiodepression) Related to the Administration of Local Anesthetics

Systemic absorption of the local anesthetic can result in vasodilatation and cardiac depression. Local anesthetics can decrease the excitability in the myocardium and in the contracting system of the heart. Decreased excitability can result in bradycardia, atrioventricular heart block, reduced contractile force, and cardiac arrest.

The combination of vasodilatation and cardiac suppression can result in hypotension, which may occur gradually or abruptly. The patient may show pallor and report feeling faint and dizzy. Tachycardia may occur, followed by bradycardia, cardiovascular collapse, and cardiac arrest. In addition, cardiac arrhythmia can occur if the physician administers local anesthetics with epinephrine. Severe and sustained hypertension or hypotension can also occur with the administration of local anesthetics with epinephrine in conjunction with tricyclic antidepressants, monoamine oxidase inhibitors, and phenothiazines.

Before the Procedure

A preprocedure assessment, inclusive of but not limited to the patient's heart rate and rhythm, SaO_2, and blood pressure will provide physiological measures concerning the patient's baseline cardiac status. Note abnormal laboratory values and altered mental status. Assess for drug allergies and note use of routine medications. The assessment should include review of the electrocardiography results. A 12-lead ECG has become part of the routine pre-anesthesia evaluation for patients with a history of, suspected of, or having either cardiac disease diabetes, and/or hypertension. Patients with known cardiac disease should have a 12-lead ECG evaluate electrical impulses to the heart. The 12-lead ECG also detects the presence of arrhythmias (ie, abnormal rate and rhythm) and the effects of chemical imbalances (eg, fluid, electrolytes, acid-base imbalances) and drug therapy on cardiac function. **Figure 13.4** shows normal and abnormal sinus rhythms.

During the Procedure

Monitor the patient's blood pressure, heart rate and rhythm, respiratory rate, oxygen saturation, skin condition, mental status, emotional response to the procedure, and anesthesia. See **Table 13.3** for standard equipment and supplies that must

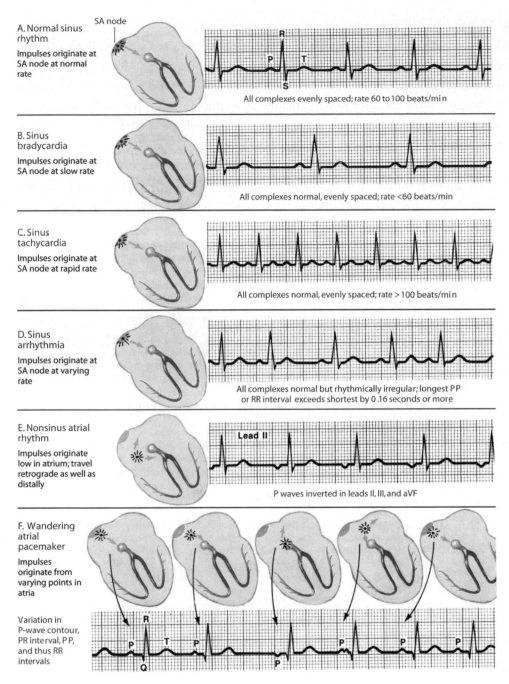

A. Normal sinus rhythm

Impulses originate at SA node at normal rate

SA node

All complexes evenly spaced; rate 60 to 100 beats/min

B. Sinus bradycardia

Impulses originate at SA node at slow rate

All complexes normal, evenly spaced; rate <60 beats/min

C. Sinus tachycardia

Impulses originate at SA node at rapid rate

All complexes normal, evenly spaced; rate >100 beats/min

D. Sinus arrhythmia

Impulses originate at SA node at varying rate

All complexes normal but rhythmically irregular; longest PP or RR interval exceeds shortest by 0.16 seconds or more

E. Nonsinus atrial rhythm

Impulses originate low in atrium; travel retrograde as well as distally

Lead II

P waves inverted in leads II, III, and aVF

F. Wandering atrial pacemaker

Impulses originate from varying points in atria

Variation in P-wave contour, PR interval, PP, and thus RR intervals

Figure 13.4

Normal and abnormal sinus rhythms.

Source: Netter Images.

be available. Document the results of monitoring activities in the patient record and report findings to the physician.

Document vital signs at 5-minute intervals and at any significant event. Document the dosage, the route and time of administration, the effect of medications administered, oxygen therapy, IV therapy, and the patient's response to the procedure and anesthesia.

After the Procedure

See Managing the Patient's Airway and Breathing Pattern (After the Procedure, pp. 377–378). Make a postprocedure visit or telephone the patient to evaluate the patient's response to the administration of IV medication and solutions.

CONCLUSION

Meeting the physiological monitoring needs of the patient during all procedures presents a challenge for the professional registered nurse providing operative or invasive procedure care. Depending on the type of procedure and anesthetic, the nurse may assist the anesthesia provider in monitoring the patient or have total responsibility for this aspect of care. Potential problems associated with airway maintenance, bleeding, fluid balance, body temperature regulation, and the use of various pharmacologic agents can develop into life-threatening events. Through conscientious monitoring of the patient's physiological status during the procedure, the nurse can prevent the development of adverse reactions, thereby promoting positive outcomes. The nurse must take prompt action to prevent problems, correct them if they occur, document the patient's responses in the record, and communicate with the appropriate caregivers.

COMPETENCY ASSESSMENT
Physiologically Monitor the Patient

Name: _____ Title: _____ Unit: _____ Date of Validation: _____

Type of Validation: ☐ Initial ☐ Annual ☐ Bi-annual

COMPETENCY STATEMENT: The nurse demonstrates competency to physiologically monitor the patient.

Performance Criteria	Met	Not Met
1. Identifies the patient's risk for adverse outcomes related to physiological status	☐	☐
2. Manages the patient's airway and breathing pattern	☐	☐
3. Manages the patient's fluid intake	☐	☐
4. Monitors the patient's fluid loss	☐	☐
5. Maintains the patient's body temperature	☐	☐
6. Monitors the patient during the administration of moderate sedation/ analgesia and local anesthesia	☐	☐

_____   _____
Validator's Signature   Employee's Signature

_____
Validator's Printed Name

REFERENCES

1. American Association of Nurse Anesthetists. (AANA). (2008). Considerations for Policy Guidelines for Registered Nurses Engaged in the Administration of Sedation and Analgesia. Retrieved August 15, 2008 from http://www.aana.com/resources.aspx?ucNavMenu_TSMenuTargetID=51&ucNavMenu_TSMenuTargetType=4&ucNavMenu_TSMenuID=6&id=706.

2. American Society of Anesthesiologists. (ASA). (2002a). Practice Advisory for Preanesthesia Evaluation. *Anesthesiology*; 96(2): pp. 485–496.

3. American Society of Anesthesiologists (ASA). (2002b). Practice guidelines for sedation and analgesia by non-anesthesiologists. *Anesthesiology*; 96(4): pp. 1004–1017.

4. American Society of Anesthesiologists. (ASA). (1999). Practice guidelines for preoperative fasting and use of pharmacologic agents to reduce the risk of pulmonary aspiration: application to healthy patients undergoing elective procedures. *Anesthesiology*; 90(3): pp. 896–905.

5. American Society of Perianesthesia Nurses. (ASPAN). (2002). Clinical guideline for the prevention of unplanned perioperative hypothermia. Retrieved August 15, 2008 from http://www.aspan.org/PDFfiles/HYPOTHERMIA_GUIDELINE10-02.pdf.

6. Association of periOperative Registered Nurses. (AORN). (2008a). Standards of perioperative clinical practice. *Perioperative Standards and Recommended Practices*; Denver, CO; AORN, Inc.: pp. 19–22.

7. Association of periOperative Registered Nurses (AORN). (2008b). Recommended practices for the prevention of unplanned perioperative hypothermia. *Perioperative Standards and Recommended Practices.* Denver, CO: AORN, Inc.: pp. 407–420.

8. Association of periOperative Registered Nurses (AORN). (2008c). AORN malignant hyperthermia guideline. *Perioperative Standards and Recommended Practices.* Denver, CO; AORN, Inc.: pp. 103–139.

9. Association of periOperative Registered Nurses (AORN). (2008d). Recommended practices for managing the patient receiving moderate sedation/analgesia. *Perioperative Standards and Recommended Practices.* Denver, CO; AORN, Inc.: pp. 461–472.

10. Association of periOperative Registered Nurses (AORN). (2008e). Recommended practices for managing the patient receiving local anesthesia. *Perioperative Standards and Recommended Practices.* Denver, CO; AORN, Inc.: pp. 453–459.

11. Association of periOperative Registered Nurses. (AORN). (2007). Perioperative competency statements. *Standards, Recommended Practices, and Guidelines*; Denver, CO; AORN, Inc.: p. 41.

12. Carpentino-Moyet, L.J. (2008). *Handbook of nursing diagnosis*, 12th ed. Philadelphia, PA: Lippincott Williams & Wilkins.

13. Langeron, O., Masso, E., Huraux, C., Guggiari, M., Bianchi, A., Coriat, P., & Riou, B. (2000). Prediction of difficult mask ventilation. *Anesthesiology*; 92(5): pp. 1229–1236.

14. MedQIC. (2008). SCIP project information. Retrieved August 15, 2008 from http://www.medqic.org/dcs/ContentServer?cid=1122904930422&pagename=Medqic%2FContent%2FParentShellTemplate&parentName=Topic&c=MQParents.

15. Mitchell, S. (2007). Preventing unplanned perioperative hypothermia. *AORN Journal*; 86 (4): pp. 660–661.

16. OR Manager. (2006). Taking steps to keep OR patients warm. *OR Manager*; 22(12): pp. 1–5.

17. Petersen, C. (2007). Perioperative *Nursing Data Set*, Revised Second Edition. Denver, CO; AORN, Inc.

18. Sessler, D.I. (2005). Temperature monitoring. In *Miller's Anesthesia*, 6th ed. RD Miller, ed. Philadelphia, PA: Elsevier; pp.: 1571–1597.

19. Sessler, D.I., & Kurz, A. (2006). Mild perioperative hypothermia. *Anesthesiology News Special Edition*; pp.: 25–31.

20. Soreide, E., & Smith, C.E., (2005). Hypothermia in trauma victims—friend or foe? *ITACCS*; Winter, 2005: pp. 18–20.

21. The Joint Commission. (2008). Standards for additional procedures: operative or other high-risk procedures and/or the administration of moderate or deep sedation or anesthesia. In *Comprehensive Accreditation Manual for Hospitals: The Official Handbook.* Oakbrook Terrace, IL; The Joint Commission on Accreditation of Healthcare Organizations; pp.: PC-41–PC-43.

22. Wagner, V.D. (2006). Unplanned perioperative hypothermia. *AORN Journal*; 83(2): pp. 470–476.

CHAPTER 14

Monitor and Control the Environment

Rose Moss

Lillian H. Nicolette

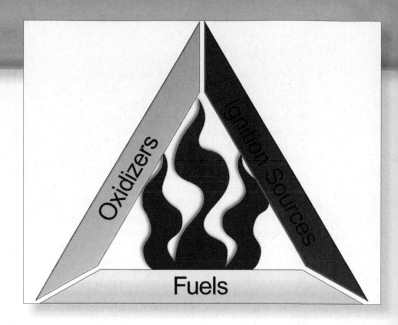

INTRODUCTION

Monitoring and controlling the operative and invasive procedure environment refers to those activities and practice-related issues performed by the nurse that promote a safe and efficacious environment during operative or minimally invasive procedures. One of the primary functions of the nurse is to protect the patient from potential hazards within the environment in order to provide an environment that promotes safety.

MEASURABLE CRITERIA

The nurse demonstrates competency to monitor and control the environment by:

- Identifying the patient's risk for adverse outcomes related to monitoring and controlling the environment
- Regulating temperature and humidity of the operating and invasive procedure room
- Protecting the patient from injury caused by extraneous objects (equipment)
- Ensuring the patient is free from chemical injury
- Ensuring electrical safety
- Ensuring fire safety
- Ensuring environmental air quality
- Monitoring the sensory environment
- Ensuring radiation and laser safety
- Maintaining suite traffic patterns
- Preventing latex exposure to sensitive patients and staff

Chapter Contents

- Performing environmental sanitation
- Providing appropriate care handling, and sterilization of instruments, supplies, and equipment

ROLE OF THE REGISTERED NURSE

The nurse implements the measurable criteria. With the appropriate supervision, the nurse may assign these tasks to qualified surgical technologists and/or assistive personnel. If assistive personnel help the nurse accomplish the measurable criteria, the professional registered nurse maintains the responsibility and accountability for all implemented patient care activities.

IDENTIFYING THE PATIENT'S RISK FOR ADVERSE OUTCOMES RELATED TO MONITORING AND CONTROLLING THE ENVIRONMENT

Failure to monitor and control the environment potentially places the patient at risk for adverse outcomes. **Table 14.1** delineates the potential adverse outcomes related to this patient care event.

REGULATING TEMPERATURE AND HUMIDITY OF THE OPERATING AND INVASIVE PROCEDURE ROOM

The nurse monitors temperature and humidity levels. A relative humidity of 30%–60% facilitates a decrease of bacterial growth and static electricity. Room temperature within the range of 68° F–73° F (20° C–22.8° C) also inhibits bacterial growth (AIA, 2006). Although temperatures within this range usually feel comfortable for the operative team members dressed in sterile attire, they nevertheless present a potential hazard for compromised patients such as those who are immunosuppressed and geriatric and pediatric patients. Consequently, the nurse must monitor and control not only the environmental temperature and humidity, but also the temperature of the patient. The supplies and equipment necessary for regulating temperature and humidity include room temperature-monitoring and humidity-monitoring devices, overhead warming units, heat conduction units, cooling or warming blankets, blood warmers, thermal body drapes, cloth blankets, warming cabinets for solutions and blankets. Patient temperature-monitoring devices include esophageal, urinary bladder, axillary, rectal, or tympanic monitors.

Before the first case of the day, take a baseline reading of the room temperature and humidity level. As noted above, maintain the room temperature within the range of 68° F–73° F (20° C–22.8° C). Keep the humidity level in the range of 30% to 60%; report temperature and humidity variations to the unit manager or according to facility policy and procedure. Except in extenuating circumstances, such as an emergency or when raising the room temperature to accommodate a patient at risk for alteration in body temperature, do not use rooms that fail to adhere to these ranges. Room temperature and humidity levels that vary from the normal criteria may contribute to alterations in patient body temperature. Additionally, an elevated room temperature or humidity level is uncomfortable, as well as stressful for the patient

Table 14.1	Monitoring and Controlling the Environment Does Not Compromise or Cause Injury to the Patient

Outcome 1 The patient is at or returning to normothermia at the conclusion of the immediate operative and invasive procedure period.

Diagnosis	Risk Factors	Outcome Indicators
Inadvertent hypothermia; risk for imbalanced body temperature; ineffective thermoregulation	☐ Extremes of age ☐ Body weight ☐ Reduced body fat for insulation ☐ Malnourishment/dehydration ☐ Debilitated or chronically ill patients ☐ Anticipated long operative time ☐ Intracranial procedure ☐ Metabolic disorders (eg, hypothyroidism or hyperthyroidism) ☐ Cold operative or invasive procedure environment ☐ Open-cavity procedure ☐ Infusions of cool fluids, blood, and blood products ☐ Cool irrigation solutions in body cavities	☐ Was the patient's core temperature greater than 36°C (96.8°F) at time of discharge from the operative or invasive procedure suite? ☐ Was the patient at or returning to normothermia at the conclusion of the immediate operative and invasive procedure period? ☐ Did the patient show signs of hypothermia, such as verbal complaint of feeling uncomfortably cold (for a conscious patient), shivering, chattering of teeth, cool skin, and decreased pulse and respiration rate?

Outcome 2 The patient is free from signs and symptoms of injury caused by extraneous objects associated with equipment use.

Diagnosis	Risk Factors	Outcome Indicators

Risk for Injury related to the use of equipment during the operative or invasive procedure	☐ Equipment used during operative/invasive procedure
	☐ Preexisting patient conditions
	   • Open wounds
	   • Skin condition
	   • Immune status
		☐ Is the patient's skin smooth, intact, warm to the touch, and free from ecchymosis, cuts, abrasions, shear injury, rash or blistering?
		☐ Is the condition of the patient's skin at the IV site free from discoloration, swelling, or induration?
		☐ Can the patient flex and extend extremities without assistance?
		☐ Does the patient deny numbness or tingling of extremities?
		☐ Are the patient's heart rate and blood pressure within expected ranges?
		☐ Are peripheral pulses present and equal bilaterally?

Outcome 3 The patient is free from signs and symptoms of chemical injury.

Diagnosis	Risk Factors	Outcome Indicators
Risk for Injury related to chemical hazards	☐ Chemicals used during operative/invasive procedure ☐ Length of exposure	☐ Is the patient's skin condition, other than the incision, unchanged between admission and discharge from the operative or invasive procedure suite?

☐ Preexisting patient conditions

- Open wounds
- Skin condition
- Immune status
- Previous chemical exposure

☐ Is the patient breathing spontaneously on room air without assistance at discharge from the operative or invasive procedure suite?

☐ Are the patient's vital signs stable at discharge from the operative or invasive procedure suite?

☐ Is the patient free from nausea, vomiting, or diarrhea following exposure to chemical agents?

Outcome 4   The patient is free from signs and symptoms of electrical injury.

Diagnosis

Risk for Injury related to the use of electrical equipment

Risk Factors

☐ Frayed or damaged power cords

☐ Damaged outlets or switch plates

☐ Use of electrical equipment adapters not approved by the manufacturer

☐ Malfunctioning line isolation monitoring systems or ground fault interrupting systems

☐ Use of extension cords

☐ Inappropriate cleaning of electrical equipment

Outcome Indicators

☐ Did the patient experience electrical-shock, cardiac fibrillation, or burns due to electrical current flowing through the patient's body to the ground?

☐ Is the patient's skin, other than incision, unchanged between admission and discharge from the operative or invasive procedure suite?

☐ Are the patient's vital signs stable at discharge from the operative or invasive procedure suite?

☐ Does the patient report comfort at the dispersive electrode site on admission to the postanesthesia unit.

☐ Is the patient's skin free of redness, blistering, or burns?

Outcome 5   The patient is free from acquired physical injury due to a fire during the operative or invasive procedure.

Diagnosis

Risk for Injury related to a fire during the operative or invasive procedure

Risk Factors

☐ Head and neck procedure

☐ Tracheostomy

☐ Oral cavity procedure

☐ Facial procedure

☐ Chest cavity procedure

☐ Use of electrosurgery, laser, or other heat source in the presence of flammable gases

☐ Use of uncuffed anesthesia tube

☐ Skin preparation with flammable agent

☐ Arcing of electrosurgical current to other metal instrument during the procedure

Outcome Indicator

☐ Did an ignition incident or fire occur?

- [ ] Accumulation of operative plume in a closed area
- [ ] Presence of oxygen or nitrous oxide
- [ ] Accumulation of eschar at the operative site or on the active electrode
- [ ] Coiling or wrapping of active or patient return electrode cords, especially around metal instrument attached to drapes

Outcome 6 The patient is free from signs and symptoms of radiation injury.

Diagnosis

Risk for Injury/Impaired Skin Integrity related to the effects of radiation

Risk Factors

- [ ] Fluoroscopy
- [ ] Multiple x-ray films during an operative or invasive procedure
- [ ] Pregnancy
- [ ] Radiation exposure to reproductive organs
- [ ] Radiation exposure to the thyroid and lymphoid tissues (upper extremities, trunk, and head x-ray films)
- [ ] Use of damaged radiation protection devices (leaded shields)
- [ ] Patients with radionuclides emitting radiation, body fluids, and tissue that are radioactive
- [ ] Implantable radioactive material

Outcome Indicators

- [ ] Did the patient's skin remain smooth, intact, free from unexplained redness, blistering, or redness in the targeted areas between admission to and discharge from the operative or invasive procedure suite?
- [ ] Radiation exposure is limited to the target site.

Outcome 7 The patient is free from signs and symptoms of laser injury.

Diagnosis

Risk for Injury/Impaired Skin Integrity related to the use of laser instruments and equipment

Risk Factors

- [ ] Unprotected eyes during laser use
- [ ] Aberrant and reflected laser beams
- [ ] Unprotected nontarget tissue
- [ ] Reflective instrumentation
- [ ] Plume and noxious fumes
- [ ] Use of flammable or combustible anesthetics, preparation solutions, drying agents, ointments, plastic resins, or plastics
- [ ] Use of flammable draping materials and/or dry sponges

Outcome Indicators

- [ ] Did the patient have contact with the laser beam other than for the intended purpose?
- [ ] Is the patient's skin smooth, intact, and free from unexplained edema, redness, or tenderness in nontargeted areas?

☐ Is the patient's vision equal to preprocedure status (nonophthalmologic patient); is the vision in the nonoperative eye unaffected (ophthalmologic patient)?

☐ Does the patient deny corneal pain or discomfort in nontargeted areas?

Outcome 8   The patient is free from injury due to latex exposure.

Diagnosis

Risk for Injury related to latex exposure; Allergic response to latex

Risk Factors

☐ Patients with risks for or latex sensitivity from exposure to natural rubber

☐ Patients with spina bifida and congenital genitourinary abnormalities

☐ Patients who work in the healthcare industry who have repeated exposure to latex (housekeepers, laboratory workers, dentists, nurses, physicians)

☐ Patients who work in the rubber industry

☐ Atopic patients (asthma, rhinitis, eczema)

☐ Patients who have undergone multiple procedures

☐ Patients with food allergies to banana, avocado, chestnut, apricot, kiwi, papaya, passion fruit, pineapple, peach, nectarine, plum, cherry, melon, fig, grape, potato, tomato, and celery

Outcome Indicators

☐ Did the patient experience contact, irritant contact dermatitis, or allergic contact dermatitis?

☐ Did the patient experience an immediate allergic reaction after exposure to a latex product?

☐ Did the patient experience an anaphylactic reaction after exposure to a latex product?

Outcome 9   The patient is free from signs and symptoms of Anxiety or Fear.

Diagnosis

Risk for Anxiety or Fear due to sensory stimuli in the operative and invasive procedure room.

Risk Factors

☐ Sights, sounds, smells inherent to the operative or invasive procedure room

☐ Inadequate preprocedure education regarding expectations

☐ Inadequate orientation to the operative/invasive procedure suite environment and care routine/practices

☐ Failure to maintain calm, supportive atmosphere

Outcome Indicators

☐ Is the patient restless or diaphoretic?

☐ Does the patient have tachypnea, tachycardia, elevated blood pressure, facial pallor, or flushing?

Outcome 10 The patient is free from signs and symptoms of infection.

Diagnosis	Risk Factors	Outcome Indicators
Risk for Infection	☐ Inadequate secondary defenses (eg, decreased hemoglobin concentration, leukopenia, suppressed inflammatory response, and immunosuppression)	☐ Is the patient afebrile?
	☐ Inadequate acquired immunity (eg, acquired immunodeficiency syndrome)	☐ Is the patient's leukocyte count within normal range 3–30 days postprocedure?
	☐ Chronic disease leading to suppressed immunity (eg, lupus erythematosus)	☐ Is the incision well-approximated and free from heat, redness, induration, swelling, or foul odor?
	☐ Malnutrition that interferes with tissue repair	☐ Are any drains present covered with sterile dressing and/or connected to continuous drainage?
	☐ Blood abnormalities such as sickle cell anemia, thrombocytopenia, and thalassemia	☐ Was the wound classification identified?
	☐ Impaired tissue perfusion	☐ Were preprocedure antibiotics given according to recommended guidelines?
	☐ High white blood cell count, low platelet count, and anemia	☐ Did the patient experience a urinary tract infection?
	☐ Impaired skin integrity	☐ Did the patient experience an upper respiratory tract infection?
	☐ Impaired tissue integrity	
	☐ Operative or invasive procedure intervention that alters tissue and skin integrity	
	☐ Invasive drains and monitors (intravenous catheters, hyperalimentation catheters, nasogastric tubes, Foley catheters, chest tubes)	
	☐ Inadequate or inappropriate surgical site preparation	
	☐ Temperature and humidity alterations within the operative or invasive procedure suite	
	☐ Hazardous environmental air quality	
	☐ Noncompliance with designated suite traffic patterns	
	☐ Failure of environmental sanitation processes	
	☐ Failure to properly clean and decontaminate instruments, supplies, or equipment	
	☐ Failure of sterilization processes	
	☐ Compromise of packaged sterile supplies	

Adapted from Carpentino-Moyet, L. J. (2008). *Handbook of nursing diagnosis* (12th ed.) Philadelphia: Lippincott Williams & Wilkins; Petersen, C. (2007). *Perioperative nursing data set, the perioperative nursing vocabulary.* (Revised 2nd ed.). Denver: AORN, Inc.

care team dressed in surgical attire. Exceptionally low temperature and humidity ranges may also cause discomfort and stress to the patient care team.

Assessing the Need for Devices to Monitor and/or Control the Patient's Temperature/Implementing Measures to Prevent Inadvertent Hypothermia

Consider the following factors when assessing the patient for the risk of the development of inadvertent hypothermia and the selection of appropriate temperature monitoring and/or control devices (AORN, 2008a):

- Patient age and physical status
- Ambient temperature of the procedure room
- Type of anesthesia that will be administered
- Type and length of the procedure
- Patient position during the procedure

Monitoring the Temperature of the Patient

Use a thermometer with an appropriate esophageal, urinary bladder, tympanic, axillary, or rectal probe to monitor the patients at risk for experiencing alterations in body temperature during the procedure. Test the thermometer before the procedure to ensure proper functioning. Usually the manufacturer provides written instructions that delineate testing procedures. After selecting the desired probe, insert it carefully into the appropriate orifice. Insert probes after the patient is anesthetized as it makes the process more comfortable for the patient and provides a dignified and comfortable approach. When placing the rectal probe in the adult patient, insert it 1–2 inches (2.5–5 cm) inside the rectum. For the infant, insert the probe no more than 1 inch (2.5 cm). Gently insert tympanic membrane probes. Aggressive insertion can cause perforation of the tympanic membrane. After insertion, tape the probe into place to avoid inadvertent removal or advancement during the procedure.

Conserving the Patient's Body Heat

Preventing heat loss through evaporation, radiation, convection, and conduction is essential to maintaining the patient's body temperature. Among these mechanisms, radiation and convection contribute most to heat loss during the operative and invasive procedure period (Sessler, 2005). When the skin becomes wet, the body looses heat through evaporation. Radiation heat loss occurs when heat is transferred from the warmer body surface to another cooler surface, such as the procedure room environment. Air currents passing over the exposed skin cause heat loss by convection. Conduction is the loss of heat from a warmer surface through direct contact with a cooler one.

Conserve the patient's body heat by covering him or her with warm blankets and exposing only the operative area or invasive procedure site. Decrease air currents by keeping the doors to the procedure room closed and limiting movement within the room. Warm skin preparation solutions, intravenous solutions, blood, and irrigating solutions; moisten sponges with warm saline before handing them to the physician. Keep the bed linens warm and dry. Blot the patient's skin dry after all skin preparation. Prevent pooling of skin preparation solutions; never allow patients to lay in the prep solution during a procedure.

Alternative Methods of Temperature Regulation

Thermoregulation systems such as warming or cooling blankets and convection warming devices provide an external source of heat to help maintain and regulate the patient's temperature. Provide these devices for patients identified as high risk for alterations in body temperature. See Chapter 11 for more information concerning the use of thermoregulation systems.

Documenting Procedures

Documentation should include the patient assessments, plan of care, implemented interventions, and evaluation of care. The following list provides examples of the activities documented by the nurse (AORN, 2008a):

- Preprocedure assessment with baseline temperature measurement;
- Plan of care for the prevention of hypothermia;
- Patient temperature measurements taken throughout the operative or invasive procedure period;
- Use of temperature-regulating devices, including the identification of the unit and temperature setting used;
- Other thermoregulation devices; and
- Postprocedure outcome evaluation.

PROTECTING THE PATIENT FROM INJURY CAUSED BY EXTRANEOUS OBJECTS (EQUIPMENT)

The performance of an operative or invasive procedure requires the use of various types of equipment, including pneumatic tourniquets, thermal blankets, and sequential compression devices; therefore, preventing injuries associated with the use of these devices requires the application of knowledge and skills regarding each item used during the procedure (Petersen, 2007). Ensure that extraneous objects do not inadvertently cause injury by coordinating the use of all types of equipment, making sure that the equipment functions properly, is used for the intended purpose, and operated according to the manufacturer's written instructions (Petersen, 2007). The interventions performed by the nurse related to the use of equipment include, but are not limited to (Petersen, 2007):

- Implementing protective measures prior to the operative or invasive procedure
- Preparing the patient, equipment, and environment prior to the procedure to ensure safety
- Applying safety devices
- Implementing protective measures to prevent skin or tissue injury due to thermal sources
- Implementing protective measures to prevent skin or tissue injury due to mechanical sources
- Using supplies and equipment within safe parameters
- Maintaining continuous surveillance
- Evaluating for signs and symptoms of physical injury to the skin and/or tissue

ENSURING THE PATIENT IS FREE FROM CHEMICAL INJURY

Hazardous chemicals used in the operative and invasive procedure practice setting include (Petersen, 2007):

- Cleaning solutions;
- Skin prep solutions;
- Irrigation solutions;
- Methylmethacrylate; and
- Tissue preservatives.

Prevention of chemical injury associated with the use of these chemicals and other chemicals not listed requires the application of knowledge and skills regarding the proper use of each chemical agent. Nursing interventions to protect the patient from chemical injury include, but are not limited to (Petersen, 2007):

- Implementing protective measures to prevent skin and tissue injury due to chemical agents;
- Verifying allergies;
- Implementing latex allergy precautions as needed;
- Applying chemical hemostatic agents (Registered Nurse First Assistant [RNFA]); and
- Evaluating for signs and symptoms of chemical injury.

RNFA
Registered Nurse
First Assistant

ENSURING ELECTRICAL SAFETY

The expanding armamentarium of electrical equipment within the operative and invasive procedure environment increases the safety risks that the patient and staff may experience related to electrical hazards. Implementation of appropriate interventions that promote a safe environment and the continuous observation for potential electrical hazards by the nurse ensures electrical safety within the operative and minimally invasive suite and ultimately promotes positive patient outcomes.

Monitoring Isolated Power Systems for Effectiveness

The National Fire Protection Agency no longer requires isolated power systems in nonflammable locations that provide anesthesia-related services (Rothrock, 2007). Isolated power systems, however, prevent accidental grounding of persons exposed to a hot wire. Each isolated power system must have an operating line monitor that is continually functioning. The operating line monitor indicates possible leakage or fault currents to ground (Rothrock, 2007).

An isolation system uses a transformer to isolate electrical circuits from the grounded circuits in the power mains. Consequently, the electrical current seeks to flow only from one isolated line to the other, thus preventing accidental grounding. A line isolation monitor measures resistance and capacitance between the two isolated lines and ground. If an inadvertent grounding of the isolated circuits occurs, the monitor sounds an alarm. A functional isolated power system sounds the alarm only when plugging faulty equipment into ungrounded circuits. In such a case, the nurse should shut off and unplug the last electrical device plugged into the electrical system. If the warning system alarm light remains illuminated, continue to search for the defective device by unplugging other connected electrical equipment. After finding the device, send it to the bioengineering and mechanical department for repair and or replacement as necessary.

Providing Safe Electrical Equipment

Ensure that all electrical equipment meets the facility's performance and safety standards. Responsibility for ensuring safe electrical equipment rests with the unit manager. Policy and procedure should specify, at a minimum, biannual routine inspections to check for defects. The bioengineering and mechanical department should inspect equipment according to the manufacturers' written recommendations. Safety checks not only prolong equipment life but also significantly enhance patient safety. Before using electrical equipment, look for malfunctioning cords, loose wires, and lack of secure connections. Test all electrical units before use for functioning audio alarms and lights. Check outlets and switch plates for damage. Do not use equipment that requires unusually high power settings to perform normal functions; send this equipment for repair. Adapters should not compromise the safety features of the equipment, therefore only use adapters approved by the manufacturer. Loose-fitting adapters can cause arcing, which may lead to shock or ignition incident. Test electrical adapters for tightness to ensure a secure connection. If necessary, replace the adapter.

Implementing Electrical Safety Practices

Minimize the potential hazards associated with the use of electrical equipment by defining safe practices for equipment use (AORN, 2008b). Electrical equipment is only as safe as the practices employed by the operator. Do not place receptacles containing liquid on top of electrical equipment. Inadvertent spills may damage the equipment and injure patients and team members. Additionally, during cleaning do not saturate electrical equipment with liquid, or spray liquid directly onto equipment; rather, clean with a damp cloth. During the procedure, equipment foot activating pedals must remain dry. Prevent heavy equipment (beds, C-Arms; fluoroscopy and x-ray machines) from rolling over electrical cords. Position the equipment to decrease stress on electrical cords and connections. When possible, avoid using extension cords. When extension cords are necessary, use only those designed for heavy-duty use and approved by the facility biomedical and mechanical engineering department. If necessary, replace short cords on high-use equipment with long cords. Maintain a safe traffic pattern by taping electrical cords securely to the floor. Remove plugs from outlets by pulling on the plug not the cord.

ENSURING FIRE SAFETY

Fire prevention and safety in the operative and invasive procedure suite are continuing concerns to nurses, physicians, anesthesia providers, and all members of the patient care team.

In 2003, The Joint Commission issued a Sentinel Event Alert on preventing surgical fires in response to the two reported cases of operating room fires, each of which resulted in serious injury to the patients (The Joint Commission, 2003). Because surgical fires are preventable, all members of the patient care team should have a thorough understanding of how fires start and how to extinguish a fire should one breakout during a procedure (ECRI, 2006). Education and training activities in fire risk reduction strategies for all members of the patient care team will promote and maintain a fire-safe operative and invasive procedure environment (AORN, 2008c). **Table 14.2** outlines examples of fires that may occur during operative or invasive procedures, heat source, fuel source, and type of oxidization involved.

The Fire Triangle

Fire is a much-dreaded incident and when one occurs in an operative or invasive procedure suite, especially during a procedure, the results can be disastrous. Before a fire can occur, the elements of the fire triangle, an ignition (heat) source, a fuel source, and an oxidizer, must converge (see **Fig. 14.1**). When the three components converge in the proper proportions, a fire can quickly result. A fire is a rapid chemical reaction of fuel with oxygen, resulting in the release of heat and light energy (ECRI, 2006). The operative and minimally invasive procedure suites have rich sources to feed each

Table 14.2	Examples of Fires During Operative or Invasive Procedures			
Type of Fire	**Heat**	**Fuel**	**Oxidizer**	**Outcome**
Bowel explosion	ESU	Bowel gas (methane) due to improper presurgery preparation	Air	Tear in colon
Fire in incision site	ESU	Gauze	100% O_2	No apparent injury
Flash fire of eyelid	ECU	Ointment	O_2 and N_2O	Minor burns
Drape fire during emergency procedure	ESU	Drapes	Air	Death (uncertain whether cause of death was the fire or the initial injuries)
Tracheal tube fire	ESU	Tracheal tube	100% O_2	Death
Throat fire	ESU; tissue ember	Gauze	O_2	Minor burns
Drape fire	ESU	Drape fibers or body hair	100% O_2	Minor burns
Drape fire during laser cauterization	Laser	Drapes	Air	Significant burns
Gown fire during an abdominal procedure with use of laser	Laser	Gown	Air	Significant burns
Facial hair fire	Bur spark	Hair	O_2 and N_2O	Significant burns

Adapted from ECRI. (1992). The patient is on fire! A surgical fires primer. Retrieved June 24, 2008 from http://www. mdsr.ecri.org/summary/detail.aspx?doc_id=8197.

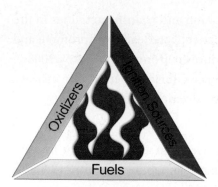

Figure 14.1
Fire Triangle.

side of the fire triangle. The primary members of the patient care team—circulating nurse, scrub person, physician, first assistant, and anesthesia provider—control different sides of the fire triangle. The physician or first assistant controls the ignition source of fires. Lasers and electrosurgical units can easily ignite fuel sources. Other physician- or RNFA-controlled devices such as drills, beat probes, fiberoptic cables, and certain coagulation devices, can produce heat with temperatures from several hundred to several thousands degrees Fahrenheit. Sparks can be created that ignite fuels. See **Table 14.3** for a list of ignition sources. Even glowing embers of charred tissue in an oxygen-rich environment can ignite some fuels. The circulating nurse and scrub person control fuel sources. A fuel is anything that will burn (see **Table 14.4** for a list of fuel

Table 14.3	Ignition Sources

☐ Electrosurgical units
 – Inadvertent activation of the active electrode when not secured in a well-insulated safety holster
 – Use of active electrodes in the presence of flammable agents and vapors
 – Direct coupling of current
 – Coiling of active or patient return electrode wires
 – Stray radiofrequency current
 – Fulguration of spray coagulation that uses higher voltage than the cut current

☐ Electrocautery units

☐ Lasers

☐ Heat-producing devices
 – High-speed drills/burrs/saws
 – Cardiac defibrillators
 – Light sources
 – Fiberoptic light cables

☐ Sparks
 – Embers of charred tissue
 – Active electrode sparking in the presence of concentrated oxygen

Adapted from: Covidien. (2008). Fire prevention and safety during surgical procedures. Retrieved June 24, 2008 from http://www.valleylabeducation.org/fire/pages/fire-12.html; AORN. (2008). Recommended practices for electrosurgery. *Perioperative Standards and Recommended Practices*. Denver, CO; AORN, Inc: pp. 315–329.

Table 14.4	Fuel Sources

☐ In or on the patient
  – Hair (facial, scalp, body)
  – Gastrointestinal gases (hydrogen, methane)
  – Gases in surgical smoke

☐ Prepping agents
  – Alcohol
  – Alcohol solutions
  – Tinctures
  – Degreasers

☐ OR attire/barrier materials
  – Scrubs, gowns, masks, hair and shoe coverings
  – Drapes, gowns

☐ OR supplies
  – Mattresses, pillows
  – Blankets, sheets, towels
  – Sponges, tape, ace bandages, steri drapes, stockinet
  – Gloves
  – Blood pressure cuffs
  – Tourniquets
  – Stethoscope tubing
  – Red rubber catheters
  – Pencil tip protectors

☐ Combustible agents
  – Oil-based ointments
  – Aerosols
  – Benzoin
  – Collodion
  – Wax

☐ Anesthesia components
  – Breathing circuits
  – Masks and airways
  – Laryngeal mask airways (LMA)
  – Endotracheal tubes

Adapted from: Covidien. (2008). Fire prevention and safety during surgical procedures. Retrieved June 24, 2008, from http://www.valleylabeducation.org/fire/pages/fire-12.html.

sources). Unfortunately, almost everything that comes into contact with the patient will burn. The patient can also provide a fuel source. Hair on the body will burn easily. Additionally, during the procedure, a portion of the tissue heated by the electrosurgery unit (ESU) turns to gas. Some of this tissue, especially those gases evolved from fatty tissue, will burn if made hot enough or if mixed with sufficient oxygen (ECRI, 2006).

ESU
Electrosurgery Unit

Many facilities use prepping agents that contain combustible fluid, such as alcohol-based products, to prepare patients. Store these liquids according to manufacturer's written instructions. Disposable and reusable linens and substances that contain wax, paraffin, or oil can burn. Aerosols may contain flammable substances, exercise care when handling these potential fuel sources. Other fuels sources include rubber, plastics, and latex components of equipment and supplies.

The anesthesia provider controls oxidizers in the operative or invasive procedure suite. During procedures under local anesthesia, the physician performing the procedure or registered nurse may control these sources. Most fuels will burn only in the gaseous state. They ignite when a sufficient amount of vapors mix with oxygen. Heat produces vapors by causing liquids to evaporate and solids to vaporize (ECRI, 2006). The oxygen and nitrous oxide delivered to the patient during a procedure are fire oxidizers (see **Table 14.5** for a list of oxidizers.) The addition of the oxidizer completes the components necessary to produce a fire.

Interventions for Preventing Fires

The patient care team can prevent most fires in the operative or invasive procedure suite by controlling ignition sources, managing fuels, and minimizing oxygen concentration. Implementation of fire-safe practices requires communication among all members of the patient care team (ECRI, 2006). Without it, the patient's risk for a fire during the procedure increases.

Interventions for the Physician and Other Members of the Scrubbed Team (ECRI, 2003; Covidien, 2008)

The physician or the assistant controls most ignition sources during the procedure. Do not use electrosurgery or other ignition sources in the presence of flammable anesthetics or other flammable gases, flammable liquids, or flammable objects. Since an oxidizer supports combustion, do not use electrosurgery or other ignition sources in oxygen-enriched atmospheres, nitrous oxide atmospheres, or in the presence of other oxidizing agents. Naturally occurring flammable gases such as methane or hydrogen, which may accumulate in body cavities such as the bowel, create a fire hazard; do not use electrosurgery or other ignition sources in the presence of these gases.

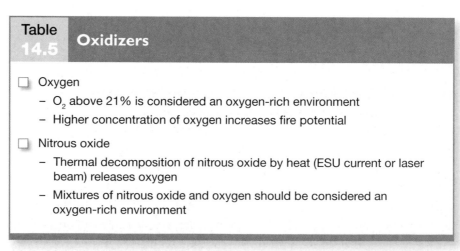

Table 14.5	Oxidizers

☐ Oxygen
- O_2 above 21% is considered an oxygen-rich environment
- Higher concentration of oxygen increases fire potential

☐ Nitrous oxide
- Thermal decomposition of nitrous oxide by heat (ESU current or laser beam) releases oxygen
- Mixtures of nitrous oxide and oxygen should be considered an oxygen-rich environment

Adapted from: Covidien. (2008). Fire prevention and safety during surgical procedures. Retrieved June 24, 2008, from http://www.valleylabeducation.org/fire/pages/fire-12.html.

The use of electrosurgery during tracheostomy to cut through tracheal rings is contraindicated. If the tip of the electrosurgery pencil or a tissue ember touches the endotracheal tube, or the tube cuff, a fire may erupt. Additionally, exercise caution during thoracic surgery cases. Oxygen may accumulate in this space if there is a leak in lung tissue of the respiratory tree. Do not place electrosurgical active electrodes and other ignition sources near, or in contact with, flammable materials such as gauze or drapes.

When not in use, place active electrodes in a nonconductive holster designed to hold electrosurgical pencils and similar accessories. Take precautions to avoid keying the active electrode in open circuit, close to, or in direct contact with a conductive object. Keep active electrode tips free of eschar buildup. As eschar builds up, resistance at the tip of the electrode increases, which can lead to arcing. Scraping the electrode on a scratch pad removes eschar buildup. Each time the tip is scratched, small grooves develop in the stainless steel surface of the electrode, which promotes further buildup at the tip. Use a coated blade such as one coated with elastomeric silicone as an alternative to using a stainless steel electrode. This allows the scrub person to remove eschar buildup by wiping the tip with a moist sponge.

Do not coil sterile active electrode cords around a metal instrument and clamp to drapes. Coiling the cord will allow stray radiofrequency current to flow through the cord to the drape or the patient's skin (if the instrument penetrates the skin), especially during open-circuit activation of the electrosurgery unit. Use the lowest possible power setting on the electrosurgery unit. Activate the active electrode for short periods; long activations increase the patient risk for an adverse outcome, particularly when using infant or neonatal patient return electrodes.

Use an integrated smoke evacuation device (active electrode combined with smoke evacuation nozzle), especially in confined spaces such as the oral cavity, tissue pockets, and cavities. This will remove the gases produced by burning tissue, thus reducing the risk for ignition to occur. Smoke produced from burning fat in an oxygen-rich environment is flammable. During the procedure, especially procedures determined to be high fire risk, place a hand or bath towel in the basin of sterile water. In the event of a fire use this fluid-soaked towel to smother the fire.

Interventions for the Circulating Nurse (ECRI, 2006; Covidien, 2008)

The circulating nurse controls the fuel sources. Use nonflammable tinctures and skin prepping agents. If flammable prepping solutions are used, avoid pooling of prepping solutions. Pooled solutions will evaporate during the procedure causing flammable vapors to accumulate under adhesive barriers and drapes. When applying the flammable prepping solution ensure that fluid does not run onto the table linen, prevent pooling, and allow the solution to dry according to manufacturer instructions before applying the drapes. The National Fire Protection Association (NFPA; 2005) advises that the implementation of *time out* prior to beginning any procedure using flammable prepping solutions. During the *time out* the patient care team verifies that the application site is dry prior to draping, and the use of electrosurgery, cautery, or laser. The team checks to ensure that solution has not pooled. If solution has pooled, the team takes corrective action and removes solution-soaked materials from the operating room prior to draping and use of electrosurgery, cautery, or laser.

NFPA
National Fire Protection Association

Do not coil, bundle, or clamp patient return electrode cords. Coiling, bundling, and clamping increases the patient's risk for an adverse outcome secondary to high frequency current leakage and capacitance. Inspect all electrical cords for frays, cuts, or loose plug connections. Apply the patient return electrode to a large muscle mass as close to the operative site as possible. The shorter the distance, the less tissue impedance encountered, thus enabling the physician to use lower power settings. Remove contaminated active electrodes from the sterile field immediately. Keep all cords clear of traffic routes.

Interventions for the Anesthesia Provider and/or Registered Nurse Providing Monitoring Services (ECRI, 2006; Covidien, 2008; Cardinal Health, 2008)

The anesthesia provider controls the oxidizers. Prevent accumulation of oxygen or nitrous oxide under drapes, especially when using ignition sources such as electrosurgery and laser. Verify all breathing circuits are leak free. Do not use oil-based endotracheal tube lubricants. Use pulse oximeter to determine oxygen saturation and need for supplemental oxygen. Inflate endotracheal tube cuff with methylene blue-tinted water or saline during airway procedures. During procedures near the head and neck, do not allow oxygen to accumulate in the patient's hair. Ensure that patients do not coat their hair with a flammable substance (hair spray, oil) before the procedure. Coat all exposed hair near the operative site with water-soluble jelly.

Management of Small Fires

Smother a small fire on the patient with a wet sponge or towel. After extinguishing the fire, remove the material that ignited from the patient. Avoid using a gloved hand to pat out the fire; doing this could cause a burn to the hand (Covidien, 2008).

Fighting Large Fires

In the event of a large fire on the patient, the anesthesia provider stops the flow of breathing gases to the patient; an unsuspected oxygen leak may be contributing to the fire. The physician and nursing staff should remove all burning material from the patient, and extinguish it away from the sterile field. If necessary, use a CO_2 fire extinguisher to put out the fire. Care of the patient then resumes. If necessary, evacuate the patient from the room. It the fire is not quickly controlled, notify the operating room control desk to secure assistance and implement the fire plan (ECRI, 2006).

Airway Fires

An airway fire is a life-threatening event. In the event of an airway fire, immediately discontinue the flow of oxygen and disconnect the breathing circuit from the endotracheal tube. Remove the burning tube in order to decrease thermal damage and attempt to remove any parts of the burned tube remaining in the airway. Reestablish the airway and ventilate the patient on room air to avoid reigniting any charred tissue; examine and treat the patient as medically necessary (Smith, 2004).

Equipment Fires

Equipment fires occur infrequently in the operative or invasive suite, most likely because of the enforcement of strict electrical safety standards, as well as to good equipment design and diligence in equipment inspection and preventative maintenance. An example of an equipment fire is one that occurred at the wall outlet. The staff handled the fire by pulling the plug from the socket. In another fire, a transformer bank ignited and required evacuation of the staff and patient from the procedure room. Most equipment fires happen because of short circuits or electrical overloads. Control these fires by stopping the flow of electricity to the device. This type of fire creates a recognizable odor and vapors (ECRI, 2006).

Fire Safety Initiatives and National Guidelines

As previously noted, in June 2003, The Joint Commission issued a Sentinel Event Alert on "Preventing Surgical Fires" that outlines the risks associated with surgical fires. Additionally they discussed strategies for reducing the risk of surgical fires. Following the alert, The Joint Commission announced that the National Patient Safety Goals for 2005 would include a goal for reducing the risk of surgical fires in ambulatory care settings as well as office based procedure units. In 2007, surgical fire prevention remained a key goal of the National Patient Safety Goals that the Joint Commission established. These goals include the education of staff and the requirements for patient care.

In May 2005, the Association of periOperative Registered Nurses, recognizing that fire is an inherent risk in operative and invasive procedure suites, published its guidance statement: Fire Prevention in the Operating Room (AORN, 2008c). In 2008, the American Society of Anesthesiologists (ASA) published its Practice Advisory for the Prevention and Management of Operating Room Fires (ASA, 2008). Both of these documents outline the various factors in an operative and invasive procedure suite that are conducive to fires; interventions to prevent and manage fires, as well as the associated adverse outcomes; and components of education and fire response protocols.

ASA
American Society
of Anesthesiologists

ENSURING ENVIRONMENTAL AIR QUALITY

Surgical smoke and aerosols, also called plume, results from the interaction of tissue and mechanical tools used to dissect tissue or achieve hemostasis (Ulmer, 2008).

Electrosurgery, the most common heat-producing device that generates plume, uses radio-frequency current to cut (vaporization) and coagulate (fulguration) tissue. The cut current heats cellular contents to the boiling point of 100°C (212°F), which explodes the cell wall. The resulting vaporization releases the cellular fluid as steam and aerosolizes cell contents, forming surgical smoke. The coagulation waveform, rather than vaporizing tissue, causes a more gradual rise in the temperature of the cellular fluid, which begins to evaporate as the temperature rises above 90°C (194°F). Next, proteins are denatured and lose structural integrity. Tissue carbonization results when the temperature reaches 200°C (392°F). The carbonized tissue contributes to the aerosolization of cellular debris (Ulmer, 2008).

Monopolar electrosurgery, the most frequently used modality, produces a greater volume of smoke than either bipolar electrosurgery or battery-operated electrocautery. Although smoke content may vary somewhat, depending on which device is used and the modality (cut or coagulation) and wattage setting of the generator, an additional variant is the type of tissue heated; however, there is very little difference in smoke content regardless of the heat source (Ulmer, 2008).

Lasers[1], the second most common heat-producing device, produce high heat (100°C [212°F] to 1,000°C [1,832°F]), which boils and explodes the cells. The resulting cellular vaporization releases steam and cell contents. The type of laser used and the type of tissue being treated determines the contents of smoke generated from laser use (Ulmer, 2006).

Comparisons of smoke generated by electrosurgery and by laser show that both are similar in content. Because of the similarities, facility policies should specify smoke evacuation when using electrosurgery and lasers (Ulmer, 2008).

Other devices that produce smoke are ultrasonic devices, high-speed electrical devices, such as bone saws, drills, and other equipment that is used to dissect and resect tissue; each type of device produces a different size particle (see **Table 14.6**) in its surgical smoke (Ulmer, 2008).

Components of Surgical Smoke

Surgical smoke is 95% water or steam and 5% cellular debris in the form of particulate matter; this particulate matter consists of chemicals, blood and tissue particles, viruses, and bacteria (Ulmer, 2008). See **Table 14.7** for the chemical contents of surgical smoke. Exposure to surgical smoke and bio-aerosols poses a hazard to patients and personnel working in the operative and invasive procedure

Table 14.6	Particle Size—Heat-Producing Devices	
Device	**Mean Aerodynamic Particle Size**	
Electrosurgical Unit	☐	0.07 micrometers
Laser	☐	0.31 micrometers
Ultrasonic Scalpel	☐	0.35–6.5 micrometers

Source: Ulmer, B.C. (2008). The hazards of surgical smoke. *AORN Journal;* 87(4): 721–734.

Table 14.7	Chemical Composition of Surgical Smoke	
Acetonitrile	1-Decene	4-Methyl phenol
Acetylene	2,3-Dihydro indene	2-Methyl propanol
Acroloin	Ethane	Methyl pyrazine
Acrylonitrile	Ethyl benzene	Phenol
Alkyl benzene	Ethylene	Propene
Benzaldehyde	Formaldehyde	2-Propylene nitrile
Benzene	Furfural	Pyridine
Benzonitrile	Hexadecanoic acid	Pyrrole
Butadiene	Hydrogen cyanide	Styrene
Butene	Indole	Toluene
3-Buteneneitrile	Methane	1-Undecene
Carbon monoxide	3-Methyl butenal	Xylene
Creosol	6-Methyl indole	

Adapted from: Barrett, W.L. & Garber, S.M. (2004). Surgical smoke—a review of the literature. *Business Briefing: Global Surgery;* 1–7.

suite (AORN, 2008d). At high concentrations, the smoke can cause ocular and upper respiratory tract irritation in healthcare personnel and creates visual problems for the surgeon. Additionally, smoke has unpleasant odors, as well as mutagenic potential (Barrett, 2004).

Heat-producing devices that generate smoke expose team members to measurable amounts of this environmental contaminant. This exposure has increased as surgical procedures have evolved and the use of various heat-producing devices has increased. In 2008, AORN published a position statement on surgical smoke and bio-aerosols. The statement recognizes hazards of surgical smoke to personnel working in the operative and invasive procedure suite and supports the use of smoke evacuation through an appropriate filtration system. The statement emphasizes the importance of education about the dangers of surgical smoke (AORN, 2008).

Protection Measures

Do not base protection solely on the wearing of masks. Even when worn correctly, with the mask fit snugly to the face, not gapping at the sides or chin, filtration efficiency of masks vary. Surgical masks usually filter particles to approximately 5 micrometers in size, whereas high-filtration masks filter particles to about 0.1 micrometers in size (Ulmer, 2008). However, approximately 77% of the particulate matter in smoke is 1.1 micrometers or smaller (Ulmer, 2008). Therefore, personnel should wear high-filtration surgical masks during procedures that generate surgical smoke (AORN, 2008b). Furthermore, do not view these masks as absolute protection from both the chemical or particulate contaminants. Avoid using masks as the first line of protection against inhalation of surgical smoke (AORN, 2008b).

Ensure protection of the patient and members of the patient care team by using a smoke evacuation system in both open and laparoscopic procedures (AORN, 2008b). Place the suction wand of the smoke evacuation system as close to the source of smoke production as possible (AORN, 2008b). The most effective smoke evacuation system is one with a triple-filter system equipped with an ultra-low particulate air (ULPA) filter. These filters are composed of a depth media material, which captures 0.12 microns of particulate matter at an efficiency rate of 99.9999% and have the capability of trapping viral and bacterial contaminants (Ulmer, 2008). When using a smoke evacuator with a triple filter system, adjust the level of vacuum to capture the amount of smoke produced. Use a vacuum source powerful enough to pull the smoke from the field, yet produces the least amount of noise.

ULPA
Ultra-Low
Particulate Air

Other smoke evacuation measures include general operating room ventilation and wall suction (Ulmer, 2008). General operating room ventilation should maintain positive pressure air exchanges through general air circulation at a minimum of 15 exchanges per hour. Wall suction provides a simple way to evacuate smoke. However, this modality has limited effectiveness. Use wall suction only on procedures that generate a small amount of smoke, and only with an inline filter.

MONITORING THE SENSORY ENVIRONMENT

Patients undergoing operative and or minimally invasive procedures frequently experience anxiety and stress due to the impending procedure. The sights, sounds, smells, and temperatures of an operative and invasive procedure suite may further increase the patient's anxiety and fear. The nurse has the ability to control and monitor the sensory environment and thus minimize the patient's anxiety and fear. The equipment and supplies needed to monitor the sensory environment include audio and video equipment, air quality devices, air filtration devices, and privacy screens.

Providing Patient Information and Education

Fear and anxiety, common emotions in patients having an operative or invasive procedure, often stem from knowledge deficit or incorrect knowledge provided from a variety of sources. Preprocedure education can provide the necessary information and thus can contribute to a positive procedure experience. Providing accurate information confirms the patient's expectations and clarifies misconceptions for the patient and family. The nurse should provide an open line of communication so proper education and knowledge assessment can occur. Providing an accurate plan with appropriate education increases the probability of a positive patient experience.

Eliminating and Modifying Sensory Stimuli

Many times, the sight, sound, or smell of a particular item or area within the operative and invasive procedure suite may cause undue stress to the patient. Witnessing an intubation or extubation, seeing tissue specimens, smelling electrosurgery or laser plume, seeing bloody instruments, or hearing the unfamiliar noises can turn a calm individual into a fearful and anxious patient. Establish traffic patterns to maximize patient privacy and safety. Protect the patient from exposure to noxious sights, sounds, and smells in order to reduce the anxiety associated with these stimuli. As an example, in addition to private cubicles, place a barrier such as a drape or a screen to prevent visualization of the procedure, blood, specimens, instruments, and equipment.

Avoid loud talking. Monitor conversations and maintain a professional environment. Conscious patients may think that a conversation applies to them and draw inaccurate conclusions about their condition and/or procedure. A quiet atmosphere should take place during the induction of general anesthesia.

Members of the patient care team should handle instruments quietly while in the presence of the patient. When testing or using noisy instruments and equipment such as drills, saws, and endoscopic equipment, tell the patient what to expect. If the procedure generates noxious odors, explain what to expect to the conscious patient.

Use music to reduce stress for the conscious patient during the procedure. A headset or MP3 player, playing a favorite selection of music may help the patient to focus on something other than the procedure. The literature confirms that listening to music during an operative or invasive procedure significantly lowered patients' anxiety levels, heart rates, and blood pressures during minor procedures with local anesthesia (Mok & Wong, 2003). Provide diversionary activities when appropriate. Activities such as music, coached breathing exercises, touch, verbal reassurance, and guided imagery may distract the patient, and help to alleviate fear, anxiety, and stress.

ENSURING RADIATION SAFETY

The use of radiation in the operative or invasive procedure suite presents significant safety concerns for both personnel and patients. The overall goal of a radiation safety program focuses on keeping the risks from ionizing radiation as low as reasonably achievable (AORN, 2008e). Excessive radiation modifies the molecular structure of cellular material in the body. The use of radiation, such as x-rays, fluoroscopy, and implantation of radioactive substances requires special handling and precautions. As with any potential hazard associated with the operative and invasive procedure suite, the implementation of safe radiation practices will protect staff members and patients against the dangerous effects of radiation exposure. Guidelines for radiation safety address the principles of time, distance, and shielding (AORN, 2008e). Supplies and equipment needed for ensuring radiation safety include radiation exposure badges or monitoring devices, lead aprons, lead gloves, lead collars and shields, x-ray cassette holding devices, and or dosimeters.

Monitoring the Amount of Radiation Exposure

The unit manager should provide radiation monitors or dosimeters for personnel frequently exposed to ionizing radiation. **Table 14.8** outlines the annual radiation occupational dose limits. When using a single monitoring device, healthcare workers should wear the device on the same area of the body. When using two monitoring devices, wear one at the neckline outside the leaded apron. This location will provide monitor exposure levels to the head, neck, and lens of the eye. Wear the second device inside the leaded apron to measure whole-body exposure levels (AORN, 2008e).

Providing Protective Devices

Protective devices decrease radiographic exposure of the patient and staff members. Before use, inspect leaded protective devices for device integrity. Biannually, the manager should have leaded protective devices radiographically inspected for

Table 14.8	Maximum Annual Radiation Occupational Dose Limits
Total effective dose equivalent	☐ 5 rems
Sum of the deep-dose equivalent and the committed dose equivalent to any individual organ or tissue other than the lens of the eye	☐ 50 rems
Shallow-dose equivalent to the skin of the whole body or to the skin of any extremity	☐ 50 rems
Lens of eye dose equivalent	☐ 15 rems
Minors	☐ 10% of the annual dose limits specified for adult workers
Dose equivalent to the embryo/fetus during the entire pregnancy, due to the occupational exposure of a declared pregnant woman	☐ 0.5 rem

Source: US Nuclear Regulatory Commission. (2007). Part 20—standards for protection against radiation. Retrieved July 7, 2008, from http://www.nrc.gov/reading-rm/doc-collections/cfr/part020/.

cracks and structural integrity. Personnel who must hold the x-ray cassette during shooting of films should protect their hands by donning lead gloves. Protect the torso and gonads by wearing lead aprons. Likewise, lead collars protect the thyroid. Minimize the risk for injury by keeping extraneous body parts out of the radiation beam. During upper torso exposure of the male patient, place a lead collar over the patient's testes. Ask female patients of childbearing age about the possibility of being pregnant. If the possibility exists, notify the physician to determine the advisability of continuing or postponing the procedure. During x-ray exposures, the patient care team should move as far away from the radiation source as possible. Staff who cannot leave the room can he protected by placing a portable lead shield on a movable stand in a convenient location in the room. Drape shields adjacent to the sterile field with sterile sheets. After use, hang the protective devices on an apron rack or store flat. Never fold these devices (AORN, 2008e). When using radiological equipment, post warning signs at entrances to operating and procedure rooms to alert personnel to potential radiation hazards, as required by state regulations (AORN, 2008e).

Implementing Radioactive Material Safety Precautions

Facilities that use therapeutic radionuclides should employ a radiation safety officer, who should determine specific organizational polices and procedures for implementation (AORN, 2008e). The radiation safety officer facilitates the radiation safety program with the ultimate goal of protecting individuals from radiation. Responsibilities include identification of individuals in frequent proximity to radiation, determining who should wear monitoring devices, and defining the requirements for monitoring and recording of occupational exposure (AORN, 2008e).

Personnel should use the principles of time, distance, and shielding when caring for patients receiving therapeutic radionuclides. Staff members who sterilize prostate seeds should receive training from the radiation safety officer that includes the handling of radioactive nuclides, minimizing exposure to radiation, and controlling and providing security for the material and emergency response to spills of radioactive materials (AORN, 2008e). During insertion, stay as far away from the source of radiation as possible. Do not touch radioactive material with bare or gloved hands, but with the instruments provided for insertion and handling when moving or touching radioactive material. After implantation of radioactive materials/devices, notify personnel on the patient care unit receiving the patient that they will receive a patient with radioactive implants.

Documentation

Document on the nursing record all interventions to protect the patient during the procedure from radiation exposure. Include the type of patient protection devices used and the areas protected. Include in the documentation the patient's skin assessment, noting the signs and symptoms of skin injury such as redness, abrasions, bruising, blistering, or edema (AORN, 2008e).

ENSURING LASER SAFETY

Lasers have dramatically increased the range of operative and invasive procedures. Yet, like other sophisticated instruments and equipment, if not used correctly, lasers may lead to an adverse outcome for the patient. The nurse ensures that only qualified personnel operate the laser, provides a safe laser unit, monitors the use of protective devices during laser procedures, and protects the patient and staff from injury.

According to the American National Standards Institute (ANSI), facilities that perform laser procedures must develop a laser safety program. Key aspects of the program include (AORN, 2008f):

ANSI
American National
Standards Institute

- Delegation of authority and responsibility for supervising laser safety to a laser safety officer;
- Establishment of use criteria and authorized procedures for all healthcare personnel working in laser nominal hazard zones;
- Identification of laser hazards and appropriate control measures;
- Education of personnel regarding assessment and control of hazards; and
- Management and reporting of accidents or incidents related to laser procedures, including associated action plans to prevent re-occurrences.

Selecting Qualified Personnel for Laser Use

Physicians, nurses, surgical technologists, and others required to work with lasers must demonstrate competency commensurate with their responsibilities. Education programs should focus on the types of laser systems used, as well as the procedures performed within the facility. A sound laser program ensures that program criteria and contents conform to applicable standards, facility policies and procedures, and federal, state, and local regulations. Criteria should delineate how often personnel demonstrate continuing competency. In addition, when the facility purchases, leases, or evaluates new laser equipment or accessories, personnel should receive competency-based training prior to use. Document and maintain on file all educational activities pertaining to laser use (AORN, 2008f).

Providing Safe Laser Units

All personnel should know the designated areas for laser use. Furthermore, policy should establish controls for access to these areas. Identify a nominal hazard zone[2] to prevent unintentional exposure to the laser beam. The laser safety officer should refer to the ANSI Z136.1 and ANSI Z136.3 standards, as well as applicable manufacturer safety information to determine the nominal hazard zone (AORN, 2008f). All team members providing care during laser procedures have responsibility to adhere to laser safety guidelines as established by the American National Standards Institute (ANSI). Developing policies and procedures should begin with a comprehensive review of the ANSI Standards (Ball, 2004).

Place regulation laser signs at all entrances to laser treatment areas when these areas are in service. In addition, doors to the nominal hazard zone should remain closed. Cover windows, including door windows, with a barrier that blocks the transmission of a beam appropriate to the type of laser in use (AORN, 2008f). All personnel in the laser treatment area should take protective measures to eliminate unintentional laser beam exposure. The laser operator managing the laser equipment should have no competing responsibilities that would require leaving the laser unattended during active use. If the nurse has responsibilities in the circulating role, it may interfere with assuming the responsibility for operating the laser. Follow the manufacturer's recommendations and instructions for laser operation, safety, and use. Evacuate the laser plume with a mechanical smoke evacuator system with a high-efficiency filter designed for this purpose.

Providing Laser Protective Devices

As a first line of defense, implement procedures to prevent accidental activation or misdirection of laser beams by restricting access to laser keys to authorized personnel skilled in operating the laser. Place lasers in the standby mode when not actively being used. Position the laser footswitch in an area convenient to the physician and identify the activation mechanism. During the procedure, the laser operator managing the laser equipment should have no competing responsibilities (AORN, 2008f).

Laser protective devices and measures shield personnel from unintentional laser beam exposure. All people in the nominal hazard zone should wear appropriate protective eyewear approved by the facilities laser safety officer (AORN, 2008f). Each laser light has a specific wavelength. Label eye protection with the appropriate wavelength and optical density for the laser in use (AORN, 2008f). Protect the eyes and eyelids of the patient from the laser beam by a method approved by the laser safety officer. Conscious patients should wear the appropriate goggles or glasses. Patients under general anesthesia should receive other appropriate protection, such as wet eye pads or laser-specific eye shields. Give patients undergoing laser treatments on or around the eyelids corneal eye shields (AORN, 2008f).

Implement measures to protect patients and healthcare workers from exposure to smoke plume generated during laser procedures. Controls to reduce smoke plume inhalation include the use of wall suction units with in-line filters for procedures with minimal plume and smoke evacuator units with a high-efficiency filter for procedures with large amounts of plume. Personnel should wear high-filtration masks designed for use during laser procedures that generate smoke plume. In addition, implement standard precautions in the laser environment (AORN, 2008f).

Implementing Laser Fire Safety Precautions

Laser beams may ignite flammable supplies, such as drapes, gowns, and clothing, as well as patient hair and tissue. Minimize patient risk by not using flammable and combustible items. Use protected or specially designed endotracheal tubes to minimize the potential for fire during laser procedures in the patient's airway or aero digestive tract. Apply moistened packs around the tube to reduce risk. Do not use alcohol-based skin preparation solutions. Use fire-retardant drapes to drape the operative site. Keep towels and sponges surrounding the target tissue wet at all times. Provide laser-appropriate fire extinguishers and water in all areas designated for laser used (AORN, 2008f).

Documentation

Documentation should include the type of laser used and the safety measures implemented during laser use (AORN, 2008f).

MAINTAINING TRAFFIC PATTERNS

Traffic patterns within the operative and invasive procedure suites should facilitate movement of patients and personnel into, through and out of defined areas. Good traffic patterns decreases the potential for cross-contamination, regulates access to the suite, and facilitates operational efficiency.

Three zones comprise the operative and invasive procedure suite. The *unrestricted zone* includes the areas of unlimited traffic where personnel interface with outside departments. Personnel may wear street clothes in the unrestricted zone. This zone includes patient reception and holding areas, and supply reception areas. In some suites, the unrestricted zone also includes communication stations, and administrative facilities. The *semi-restricted zone* may include, but is not restricted to, storage and instrument-processing areas and, depending on the design, corridors leading to restricted areas and peripheral support areas. Only authorized personnel and patients enter this zone. While in the zone personnel wear operative attire and have all head and facial hair covered. The *restricted zone* includes the operating or procedure rooms and the clean core. Personnel must wear operative attire and hair coverings. While in this zone, personnel don masks when scrubbed and in the presence of opened sterile supplies (AORN, 2008h).

Established traffic patterns reduce the potential for cross-contamination. Every operative and invasive procedure suite should have areas identified according to the level of contamination found in the area. At a minimum, the suite should have sterile, clean, and contaminated areas identified. Separate sterile and clean supplies and equipment from soiled equipment and waste by space, time, or traffic patterns. Where architectural design permits, move clean and contaminated items using separate traffic patterns. The supplies and equipment needed for maintaining traffic patterns include surgical attire, masks, hair coverings, shoe covers, solutions for cleaning, personal protective equipment (eg, eyewear, gloves, aprons), and closed or covered carts or containers to transport contaminated items.

Decreasing Potential Airborne Contamination

Keep traffic flow into, out of, and within the room and through transition zones to a minimum. When the number of personnel increases, the environmental microbial count also increases. Because corridor air may contain a higher bacterial count than the procedure room air, keep doors closed except during the movement of patients, personnel, supplies, or equipment (AORN, 2008h).

Decreasing Potential Contamination from Outside Environmental Sources

Damp dust or wipe with a germicidal solution, all equipment brought into the restricted area. Transport clean and sterile items to the procedure room in an enclosed container or via a covered cart system. Before bringing supplies and equipment into the restricted area, remove from external shipping containers. Retrieve product or equipment written instructions for use (IFU) before discarding the containers. File all IFUs for later review. Personnel should periodically access and review IFU files. Remove protective coverings before bringing supply or case carts into the room. Clean patient transport beds after each patient use (AORN, 2008i).

IFUs
Product or Equipment
Written Instructions

Confining Contamination Within Established Traffic Patterns

Contain contamination by transporting trash, soiled linen, soiled instruments, and nonsterile equipment and supplies in an enclosed cart or an impervious system. Keep contaminated objects and waste disposal operations out of patient care areas. Separate the movement of clean and sterile supplies and equipment from contaminated supplies, equipment, and waste by space, time, or traffic patterns. Never allow contaminated items to enter clean or sterile areas. Contain these items at the source or origin to decrease airborne contamination (AORN, 2008h).

Providing Clear Pathways for Traffic Flow

To maintain designated traffic patterns, store supplies as close as possible to the point of use. Keep hallways free of clutter to decrease the potential for injury and ease the flow of traffic. When hallways must contain stretchers or other equipment, isolate the equipment to one side of the hallway so there is an aisle that provides ample room to facilitate traffic flow.

PREVENTING LATEX EXPOSURE TO SENSITIVE PATIENTS AND TEAM MEMBERS

Natural rubber latex allergy presents a serious and potentially life-threatening condition to the patient in the operative and invasive procedure suite. Healthcare providers and others who experience repeated exposure to latex allergens can develop a latex sensitivity or allergy. Latex items found in the operative and invasive procedure suite include items such as airways, intravenous tubing, syringes, stethoscopes, catheters, drains, rubber bands, dressings, and bandages. Sensitivity occurs when an individual develops an immunologic memory to the specific latex proteins. Some individuals, however, remain asymptomatic. When an individual does manifest an allergy, symptoms include hives, rhinitis, conjunctivitis, and anaphylaxis. Sensitivity to natural rubber latex is more common than the actual allergy; however, any individual sensitized to natural rubber latex is at risk of a life-threatening reaction, and thus treated as an allergic individual (AORN, 2008j).

The proteins found in latex cause the allergic sensitization, predisposing to IgE-mediated reactions. Common reactions caused by latex include irritant contact dermatitis, allergic contact dermatitis, and immediate hypersensitivity (see **Table 14.9**). Chemical additives used during the processing of rubber latex may also cause some local skin reactions, such as allergic or chemical sensitivity contact dermatitis. The additives, however, usually do not cause immediate generalized allergic reactions or anaphylaxis. Unlike natural rubber latex, synthetic rubber, such as the type made with butyl or is petroleum based, is not a hazard to latex-sensitive individuals.

Identifying High-Risk Patients

Population risk groups include children with a history of frequent surgeries or the use of instrumentation, particularly if begun in early infancy, as with congenital malformations such as myelodysplasia, (spina bifida) or congenital genitourinary abnormalities. Other high-risk individuals include healthcare workers; rubber industry workers; patients with asthma, rhinitis, or eczema; and patients who have undergone multiple procedures. Patients with food or food product allergies may also have a coexisting latex allergy. Contributing foods include banana, avocado, chestnut, apricot, kiwi, papaya, passion fruit, pineapple, peach, nectarine, plum, cherry, melon, fig, grape, potato, tomato, celery, apple,

Table 14.9	**Reactions to Latex**

Type of Reaction	Description
Contact dermatitis	☐ The most common clinical reaction associated with latex and its additives (Includes both irritant and allergic responses)
Irritant contact dermatitis	☐ Not a true allergy ☐ Symptoms of non-allergic skin rash include hand erythema, dryness, cracking, scaling, and vesicle formation ☐ Caused by skin irritation from using gloves; possibly by exposure to other products and chemicals in the workplace ☐ Can result from repeated hand washing and drying, incomplete hand drying, use of cleaners and sanitizers exposure to powders added to gloves
Allergic contact dermatitis (Type VI hypersensitivity; delayed hypersensitivity; chemical sensitivity dermatitis)	☐ A specific immune response of sensitized lymphocytes to chemical additives contained in latex products ☐ Rash usually begins 24–48 hours after contact ☐ May progress to oozing skin blisters or spread away from the area of skin exposed to the latex

Immediate allergic reaction (IgE mediated hypersensitivity reaction)	☐ Can be a more serious reaction to latex than irritant contact dermatitis or allergic contact dermatitis
	☐ Certain proteins in latex may cause sensitization (positive blood or skin test, with or without symptoms); exposure at even very low levels can trigger allergic reaction sin some sensitized persons, although the amount of exposure needed to cause sensitization or symptoms is not known
	☐ Direct contact with the product is not needed for sensitization to latex; allergenic latex proteins are also adsorbed on the glove powder which, when latex gloves are snapped on and off, become airborne and can be directly inhaled
	☐ Reactions typically begin within minutes of exposure to latex, but can occur hours later
	☐ Reactions can produce various symptoms:
	  • Mild reactions involve skin redness, hives, or itching.
	  • More severe reactions may involve respiratory symptoms including runny nose, sneezing, itchy eyes, scratchy throat, and asthma.
	  • Rarely, shock may occur; a life-threatening reaction is seldom the first sign of latex allergy.

Adapted from: ACAAI. (1996). Guidelines for the Management of Latex Allergies and Safe Latex Use in Health Care Facilities. Retrieved July 7, 2008 from http://www.acaai.org/public/physicians/latex.htm.

NIOSH. (1997). NIOSH Publication No. 97–135: Preventing Allergic Reactions to Natural Rubber Latex in the Workplace. Retrieved July 7, 2008 from http://www.cdc.gov/Niosh/latexalt.html.

pear, carrot, hazelnut, wheat, and rye. During the preprocedure assessment, the nurse should determine if the patient falls into the high-risk group. If the patient does fall into this group, refer the patient for a full physical assessment, to include a nutrition assessment to determine if the patient has a food or food product allergy. When questioning the patient, ask about incidents of latex reactions. Assess for unexplained allergic or anaphylactic reactions, intraoperative events, a history of multiple operative or invasive procedures, reactions to latex cross-reacting foods, and the presence, or history of documented asthma, rhinitis, or eczema. Patients identified at risk for developing latex sensitization, follow the facility protocol for determining the need for testing for immediate hypersensitivity to natural rubber latex (AORN, 2008j).

Outcome Identification and Evaluation for Latex-Sensitive Patient

Managing and preparing the environment to care for latex-sensitive patients presents a challenge because of the complexity of the processes. In addition, costs of care and the labor to provide the care strain the system. Healthcare facilities should establish a multidisciplinary team to address these issues and develop protocols necessary to create a latex-safe environment. The American College of Allergy, Asthma, and Immunology (ACAAI) provides latex allergy guidelines for healthcare facilities (see **Table 14.10**). In operating and invasive procedure suites, use a latex-safe cart. See **Table 14.11** for suggested supplies of a latex-safe cart (AORN, 2008j).

ACAAI
American College of Allergy, Asthma, and Immunology

Table 14.10	Latex Allergy Guidelines for Health Care Facilities

☐ Latex Allergy Program

A facility-wide strategy to manage latex allergies in the healthcare environment should include the formation of latex allergy task force and the development of appropriate facility policies, awareness and educational initiatives.

☐ Latex Allergy Task Force

A multidisciplinary latex allergy task force should be a regular part of the healthcare facility employee and patient care committee.

☐ Policies

Policies should be developed to manage the latex-sensitive individual in all areas of the hospital, with particular focus in high-risk areas: emergency and X-ray departments, operating rooms, intensive care units, nurseries, and dental suites.

☐ Consultation Services

Questions regarding latex allergy should routinely be asked of presurgical patients as well as prospective hospital employees. A latex consultation service should be available for evaluation of latex allergic individuals.

☐ Review Glove Usage

A facility-wide review of glove usage should be completed to determine the appropriateness of use and thereby prevent the unnecessary use of latex gloves. Non-powdered, low-protein gloves should be the standard in a healthcare facility with powdered, low-protein gloves available only on request and their use monitored. Facilities should evaluate manufacturer information on non-latex gloves in areas of durability, barrier protection, and cost.

☐ Compendium of Products

Facilities should prepare and regularly review and update a compendium of all latex products. Ideally this compendium should include information on the content of latex protein. Lists of non-latex substitutes for medical supplies and devices should also be accessible.

14

☐ Latex-Safe Environment

A latex-safe environment should be the goal of all healthcare facilities. Latex-safe carts containing non-latex substitutes should be available in all patient care areas, particularly those with high latex usage (see Table 14.11).

Surgical or invasive procedures on latex-allergic patients should be performed in suites that are latex safe; the suites should also be monitored for airborne latex allergens, as the patient should not have any direct or indirect contact with latex. If latex-safe rooms are not available, elective patients should be scheduled as the first case of the morning in order to minimize exposure to airborne latex. If a patient has a history of a previous latex anaphylactic event, premedication with antihistamines and corticosteroids may be used in an attempt to minimize the adverse consequences of inadvertent latex exposure; however, premedication must not be considered a substitute for latex avoidance.

☐ Identification of High-Risk Patients

Patients belonging at high risk should be identified. The following should be carried out by a physician for all high risk patients:

- All historical data should be documented with written reports of all reactions to any latex exposure (medical, surgical, or dental products; household products, such as gloves, clothing, or toys). Clinical allergic responses include contact dermatitis, urticaria, angioedema, rhinitis, conjunctivitis, asthma, and anaphylaxis.

- Unexplained allergic/anaphylactic reactions, intraoperative events, a history of multiple surgical procedures, reactions to latex cross-reacting foods, and the presence or past history of documented atopic disorders (asthma, rhinitis, or eczema) should be examined and subsequently appropriately identified.

☐ Patient Testing

Patient testing should include sensitivities to rubber additives and allergic reactions to latex proteins.

Rubber Additives Patients with hand dermatitis and exposure to latex should be referred for consultation to determine and document sensitivities to rubber additives. All exposed patients with hand dermatitis should also be referred to an allergy specialist to determine if they possess IgE antibody to latex proteins.

Latex Proteins All high-risk patients in the healthcare facility should be encouraged to have latex allergy testing.

☐ Prevention and Management of Latex-Allergic Individuals

All individuals identified as latex-allergic by history or testing should be counseled by a knowledgeable physician. The following precautions should be taken:

- A medical alert bracelet should be worn to indicate their allergy.

- An epinephrine self-injection kit should be available in case of latex-allergic reactions.

- Non-latex gloves should be carried by all latex-allergic individuals, as presently, latex substitutes may not be available at all healthcare facilities

Adapted from: ACAAI. (1996). Guidelines for the management of latex allergies and safe latex use in healthcare facilities. Retrieved July 7, 2008, from http://www.acaai.org/public/physicians/latex.htm.

PERFORMING ENVIRONMENTAL SANITATION

Proper environmental sanitation of the operative and invasive procedure suite provides a clean environment for the patient and minimizes the risk for exposure to potentially infectious microorganisms. Consider every procedure as potentially infectious and apply the appropriate environmental sanitation protocols. Personnel should take precautionary measures to limit the transmission of microorganisms when performing

Table 14.11	Recommended Contents for a Latex-Safe Cart*

- ☐ 100% silicone or polyvinyl chloride (PVC) urinary catheters
- ☐ 3-way stopcocks
- ☐ Anesthesia breathing bag
- ☐ Assorted tape
- ☐ Blood pressure cuffs and connecting tubing
- ☐ Blood tubing
- ☐ Bulb syringe (60cc)
- ☐ Examination gloves
- ☐ Feeding pump bag and tubing
- ☐ Feeding tubes (5 Fr–10 Fr)
- ☐ Intravenous (IV) tubing
- ☐ Oxygen delivery supplies (eg, cannula, mask)
- ☐ Safety needles (25 g through 15 g)
- ☐ Silicone or PVC external catheters (pediatric and adult)
- ☐ Sterile gloves
- ☐ Stethoscope
- ☐ Syringes (multiple sizes)
- ☐ Tourniquets
- ☐ Underpads and small chux pads
- ☐ Urinary drainage system

* NOTE: All items must be latex-free.

Source: AORN. (2008). AORN latex guideline. *Perioperative Standards and Recommended Practices.* Denver, CO; AORN, Inc: pp. 87–102.

routine environmental cleaning and disinfection activities. While performing environmental sanitation and disinfection procedures that involve contact with blood and other potentially infectious material, comply with the OSHA Bloodborne Pathogen Standards Follow standard precautions to prevent contact with blood or other potentially infectious material. Wear appropriate personal protective equipment (PPE) when handling contaminated items and exposure to blood or other potentially infectious materials. PPE includes gloves, masks, eye protection, and face shields. Perform hand hygiene after removing gloves and as soon as possible after soiling hands. In addition, use established procedures of environmental cleaning and disinfection and wear appropriate PPE for situations that may require contact or airborne precautions (AORN, 2008i).

Perform sanitation measures before, during, and after each procedure. Nurses, surgical technologists, surgical assistants, and housekeeping personnel collaborate when performing environmental sanitation. No matter who performs environmental sanitation, however, the ultimate responsibility for a safe, clean environment remains with the nurse. Responsibility for cleaning practices that comply with established standards rests with the administration. The supplies and equipment needed to perform environmental sanitation include lint-free cloths for cleaning, Environmental Protection Agency (EPA)-registered hospital detergent/disinfectants, a wet vacuum (preferred), mop and clean mop heads, a mechanical floor scrubber, plastic

PPE
Personal Protective Equipment

EPA
Environmental Protection Agency

liners, gloves, a pistol grip sprayer, laundry bags, disposable suction tubing, suction containers, utility carts, and covered carts for linens and trash disposal.

Sanitation Prior to the Procedure

Before the first scheduled procedure, damp dust all horizontal surfaces, including furniture, operative lights, equipment booms, and equipment, with a clean, lint-free cloth moistened in a hospital-grade disinfectant. This procedure removes dust that might have settled on horizontal surfaces after terminal cleaning. Use friction while damp dusting. For subsequent procedures, inspect the room for cleanliness. Correct discrepancies before preparing the room for the next procedure. If using additional equipment from outside the restricted area for the next procedure, damp dust it before bringing it into the room (AORN, 2008i).

Sanitation During the Procedure

During the procedure, confine and contain contamination to a small area. Wear appropriate PPE, such as gloves, face shields, eyewear, and/or gowns when handling contaminated items. When organic debris falls from the sterile field, remove it with a disposable cloth and promptly disinfect the area with an EPA-registered disinfectant solution. Wipe the disinfected area with a clean cloth. Discard the contaminated cloth in an impervious container. Handle and dispose of contaminated sponges according to the OHSA Bloodborne Pathogens Standard. Leak-proof, tear-resistant containers and PPE assist in preventing environmental contamination and reduce the risk of personnel exposure to potentially infectious material (AORN, 2008k).

Occasionally, during a procedure, the scrub person inadvertently drops an instrument on the floor. When this occurs, don gloves, retrieve the instrument, and submerge it in a pan containing the cleaning agent specified by the manufacturer prior to sending the instrument for terminal decontamination and subsequent sterilization. This prevents drying of debris, which could become airborne or otherwise difficult to remove from the device. Likewise, the scrub nurse may hand off a contaminated instrument. After donning gloves, retrieve the instrument and follow the procedure describe above. Enclose nonsubmersible instruments in a clean impervious container, such as a plastic bag or case cart. If the physician requires the contaminated instrument for immediate use, prior to sterilization, decontaminate it with the type of cleaning agent specified by the manufacturer in an area separated from locations where clean activities are performed (AORN, 2008l).

Secure specimens removed from the procedural area in an impervious container that allows transfer and transport of the specimen without leaking or spilling. Label specimen containers with a biohazard sticker to warn personnel transporting or receiving the material that the container holds potentially infectious material. Additionally, protect the documents submitted with specimens from contamination (AORN, 2008m). See Chapter 15 for additional information on handling specimens and cultures.

Sanitation After the Procedure

Use a lint-free or microfiber cloth moistened with a detergent/disinfectant and water to clean and disinfect the following items after the operative or invasive procedure. The nurse may perform this task or delegate it to an unlicensed assistive person (AORN, 2008i).

- Mattresses and padded positioning device surfaces (eg, OR beds, arm boards, patient transport carts)
- Nonporous surfaces (eg, mattress covers, pneumatic tourniquet cuffs, blood pressure cuffs)
- Patient transport vehicles including straps and attachments;
- All receptacles (eg, kick buckets, bins)
- All work surfaces and tables

Ensure safety by handling contaminated disposable and reusable items according to state and federal regulations. Classification of these items include potentially infectious or noninfectious. Place disposable items caked with blood or other infectious materials in a liquid or semi-liquid state in color-coded, closable, leak-proof containers or bags. Label or tag the container or bag for easy identification as biohazard waste (AORN, 2008i).

Consider disposable items free of caked blood or other infectious materials in a liquid or semi-liquid form as noninfectious. Place these items in a separate container designated for noninfectious waste (AORN, 2008i).

When handling contaminated items wear appropriate PPE to reduce the risk of exposure to blood or other potentially infectious materials and to prevent splash or splatter when disposing of liquid waste (AORN, 2008i).

Irrigate reusable suction tips and all devices with lumens with clean water to prevent obstruction from organic debris. Disassemble all instruments with removable parts. Open the jaws of locking instruments in order to remove visible debris. Separate delicate instruments for special handling. Carefully place sharps, needles, and syringes into puncture resistant containers. Separate and place sharp instruments (eg, skin hooks, scissors, rakes, osteotomes, towel clips) in appropriate containers. Contain Instruments during transport to the designated decontamination location (AORN, 2008l).

Sanitation at the Conclusion of the Day

On a daily basis, terminally clean operative and invasive procedure rooms, as well as scrub and utility areas. Personnel who have received training and who are supervised should clean these areas after the completion of scheduled procedures and each 24-hour period during the regular workweek (AORN, 2008i). Areas cleaned include (AORN, 2008i; Nicolette, 2007):

- Floors (wet-vacuumed with an EPA-registered disinfectant)
- Surgical lights and external tracks
- Fixed and ceiling-mounted equipment
- All furniture and equipment, including wheels and casters
- All equipment that is visible within the suite
- Handles of cabinets and push plates
- Ventilation faceplates
- All horizontal surfaces inclusive of countertops, shelving and sterilizers
- Kick buckets
- Substerile areas
- Scrub/utility areas
- Sterile storage areas

Periodic Sanitation of the Operative and Invasive Procedure Suite

Management should schedule routine cleaning on a weekly and monthly basis. Areas and equipment targeted for cleaning include (AORN, 2008i):

- Heating and air-conditioning equipment
- Pneumatic tubes and carriers
- Sterilizers and their loading carts/carriages
- Clean and soiled storage areas
- Walls and ceilings
- Unrestricted areas such as lounges, locker rooms, lavatories, waiting rooms, and offices

STERILIZING INSTRUMENTS SUPPLIES, AND EQUIPMENT

Sterilization renders instruments, supplies, and equipment free from all forms of microorganisms, including spores. Several methods of sterilization are available. The type of the instrument, supply, or piece of equipment requiring sterilization dictates the use of each sterilization method. The nurse and surgical technologist need specific knowledge of all methods used in order to provide quality patient care.

Decontamination

Decontaminate all instrument trays and instruments opened during the procedure. Instrument care varies depending on the type of cleaning process required. Most general instruments can withstand washer/decontaminator processing and ultrasonic cleaning. Specialty instruments, however, frequently require special handling. Unless specified by the manufacturer, avoid using the washer/decontaminator for specialty instruments. Some instruments cannot withstand immersion in liquid; therefore, ultrasonic cleaning is also inappropriate for these instruments. Examples of specialty instruments include endoscopes, pneumatic drills, saws and hoses, dermatomes, dermabraders, cords and cables, electronic devices, silastic or silicon tubing, reusable plastic equipment, and delicate instruments. Each of these categories requires special decontamination and cleaning procedures. Decontaminate the item according to the manufacturer's written instructions.

Cleaning

During the procedure, remove gross blood and debris from instruments and devices by wiping as needed with sterile surgical sponges moistened with sterile water. Irrigate instruments with lumens with sterile water as needed throughout the procedure (AORN, 2008l).

Clean and decontaminate instruments and equipment, whether used or not, as soon as possible after use. At the conclusion of the procedure, contain all instrumentation and equipment in a manner that prevents exposure of patients or personnel to blood or other potentially infectious materials; examples include closed plastic bags, containers with lids, transport carts with doors or plastic cover. Transport soiled instruments in a timely manner to the designated decontamination area. Avoid transporting soaking instruments because of the possibility of a liquid spill, its associated cleanup problems, and the difficulty of safe disposal of the contaminated liquid unless a disposal unit is available. Open and place all instruments in water or an instrument cleaning solution recommended by the manufacturer (AORN, 2008l).

Personnel in the decontamination area must wear protective clothing, which includes a scrub uniform, a plastic apron or jump suit, hair covering, rubber or plastic gloves, and safety glasses or a face shield (AORN, 2008l). If cleaning instruments requires manual cleaning, submerge in warm water with an appropriate detergent followed by complete submersion in a rinse solution; this procedure protects personnel from aerosolization or splashing of infectious material and from injury by sharp objects (AORN, 2008l). Do not use harsh abrasive detergents for manual cleaning. Damage to the protective surfaces of instruments may occur, which contributes to corrosion, and potentially impedes sterilization. Follow manufacturer-written instructions regarding proper cleaning of instrumentation, especially for delicate instruments.

Mechanically clean general surgical instruments with an ultrasonic cleaner, washer decontaminator, washer disinfector, or washer sterilizer. This method of cleaning efficiently removes soil and provides consistent washing and rinsing parameters. When using an ultrasonic cleaner do not mix metals. Clean only instruments made of similar metals, unless otherwise specified by the manufacturer. Do not use the ultrasonic cleaner for chrome-plated instruments, power instruments, rubber, silicone, or plastic instruments, and endoscopic lenses. At the completion of the ultrasonic cycle, thoroughly rinse and then lubricate the instruments. Lubrication with a water-soluble solution such as instrument milk protects the instruments from corrosion and rust, and enhances functioning. Allow the water-soluble solutions to dry on the instruments. Theoretically, air-drying provides a protective coating. If using an automated washer-sterilizer, remove gross debris in a cold-water rinse prior to placing the instruments in the system. Minimize splashing during the rinsing process. Place instruments in perforated or meshed-bottom trays or baskets and positioned so that the cleaning portion of the washer-sterilizer cycle can reach all parts of the instrumentation (AORN, 2008l).

Obtain and evaluate the manufacturer's written, validated instructions for handling and reprocessing instrumentation and equipment. Use these instructions, which vary widely by manufacturer, to determine how to validate cleaning, processing, and the assembling of items.

After decontamination, inspect the instruments for cleanliness and proper functioning prior to assembly of the tray. This inspection provides an opportunity to identify potential problems prior to opening these devices on the sterile field. When inspecting instruments check for (AORN, 2008l):

- Cleanliness
- Alignment
- Corrosion, pitting, burs, nicks, wear, chipped inserts, and cracks
- Sharpness of cutting edges
- Missing parts
- Removal of moisture
- Proper functioning

Preparing Instruments, Equipment, and Supplies for Sterilization

Organize the instruments in a way that ensures exposure of all surfaces to the sterilizing agent. The following practices should be implemented when organizing and preparing instruments and equipment:

- Place the instruments in a container or basket large enough to distribute the metal mass in a single layer.
- Containers or baskets should provide protection and prevent puncturing of the sterilization wraps.
- Overloading trays can cause wet packs because of the increase in metal mass in the tray and may lead to condensation.
- Place broad instruments and those with concave surfaces in the side position; this will facilitate exposure of all surfaces.
- Open instruments with hinges.
- Disassemble instruments that have removable parts; use stringers, racks, or instrument peg/bars to keep instruments open and in the unlocked position.
- Place tip protectors on delicate and sharp instruments according to the manufacturers' written instructions.
- Always place heavy instrumentation on the bottom of the tray or basket.
- Use only validated containment devices to organize or segregate instruments within the sets.
- Flush suction lumens and other devices with lumens or similar channels with distilled, demineralized, or sterile water before steam sterilization.
- Remove stylets from lumens. Line the instrument basket or tray with an absorbent, lint-free surgical towel, if indicated.
- Follow manufacturers' written instructions when preparing powered equipment and attachments regarding disassembly, protection of delicate parts, loose coiling of air hoses, and packaging.
- Before wrapping the instruments and equipment, place an appropriate sterilization indicator in the center of the tray or pack (AORN, 2008l).

Wrapping Items/Packaging Systems

Packaging systems should have the following qualities (AORN, 2008n):

- Provide an adequate barrier to microorganisms, particulates and fluids
- Allow the sterilant to penetrate the barrier and contact the item and surfaces
- Permit removal of the sterilant
- Maintain sterility of the contents until opened
- Contain no toxic substances or dyes
- Allow for aseptic delivery of the contents
- Capability to have complete and secure enclosure
- Protect contents from physical damage
- Provide adequate seal integrity
- Resists tears, punctures, abrasions
- Be tamper-proof
- Allow for adequate air removal
- Be low-linting
- Allow for identification of contents
- Have a favorable cost benefit ratio associated with the packaging
- Include the manufacturer's written instructions

When packaging instruments and supplies for sterilization, use woven (cloth) or nonwoven fabrics. If using woven materials, use only freshly laundered outer wrappers. The fabric must have no holes and follow the validity characteristics as described in the manufacturer's written instructions. Use woven or non-woven material for double-thickness wrapping according to the manufacturer's written instructions. As long as the nurse can aseptically present the item, it is not necessary to wrap sequentially or use material that is bonded together (AORN, 2008n).

Use paper-plastic pouch packages for small, lightweight, low-profile items. Remove as much air as possible before sealing. The seal should ensure package integrity and not permit resealing, as well as provide an airtight seal. Double paper-plastic packaging is not routinely needed for sterilization. When used, however, assemble double plastic-paper packages in a manner that avoids folding the inner package to fit the outer package (AORN, 2008n).

Before purchasing containment devices such as rigid containers, instrument cases, and organizing trays, confirm that the device has been tested and validated for the sterilization cycles and methods used in the facility (AORN, 2008n). Choose a metal or plastic packaging system that has the following characteristics:

- Removable top that facilitates aseptic presentation of the contents
- Perforations or valves that allow for sterilant penetration and removal
- A filter or valve system that maintains the sterility of contents
- A means to identify processed or sterile containers from unprocessed or non-sterile containers
- A method of securing the top of the container to the bottom

Performing Steam Sterilization

Use saturated steam under pressure to sterilize heat- and moisture-stable devices, unless otherwise indicated by the device manufacturer. Saturated steam under pressure provides an effective, rapid, and relatively cost-effective modality for sterilizing most porous and nonporous materials (AORN, 2008o). Follow manufacturer's written instructions when using steam sterilization equipment. Steam sterilizers vary in design and performance characteristics and use a variety of cycle parameters. Examples of steam sterilization cycles include:

- Gravity displacement
- Dynamic air removal (also known as pre-vacuum)
- Steam flush pressure pulse
- Flash cycles
- Express (abbreviated steam cycles used for flash sterilization)

See **Table 14.12** for steam sterilization parameters. Certain types of equipment and implants require different exposure times and sterilization processes. According to the Association for the Advancement of Medical Instrumentation (AAMI), following steam sterilization remove the contents of the sterilizer from the chamber and leave untouched for a period of 30 to 120 minutes. The potential for the formation of condensation decreases when the contents remain untouched until the temperature differential equalizes between the chamber and outside

AAMI
Association for the Advancement of Medical Instrumentation

Table 14.12	Steam Sterilization Parameters						
Item	Exposure Time at 250°F (121°C)	Minimum Drying Time	Exposure Time at 270°F (132°C)	Minimum Drying Time	Exposure Time at 275°F (135°C)	Minimum Drying Time
Gravity Displacement						
Wrapped items	30 MIN	15–30 MIN	15 MIN	15–30 MIN	10 MIN	30 MIN
Textile packs	30 MIN	15 MIN	25 MIN	15 MIN	10 MIN	30 MIN
Wrapped utensils	30 MIN	15–30 MIN	15 MIN	15–30 MIN	10 MIN	30 MIN
Dynamic Air-Removal						
Wrapped items	—	—	4 MIN	20–30 MIN	3 MIN	16 MIN
Textile packs	—	—	4 MIN	5–20 MIN	3 MIN	3 MIN
Wrapped utensils	—	—	4 MIN	20 MIN	3 MIN	16 MIN

Adapted from: AORN. (2008). Recommended practices for sterilization in the perioperative practice setting. *Perioperative Standards and Recommended Practices.* Denver, CO; AORN, Inc: pp. 578–579.

environment. The length of cooling time depends on the contents in the processed load (AAMI, 2006). Avoid placing warm or hot items on cold or cool surfaces as moisture will condense within a packages or containers. If a sterilized package or container has formed condensation, consider the item unsterile and do not use for patient care.

Loading Items for Steam Sterilization

When loading the steam sterilizer, place items on the autoclave racks to ensure free circulation of the steam. Place items capable of holding water, such as basins and solid-bottomed trays, in the side position during the sterilization cycle. Likewise, vertically place flat packages on the shelf. Large packages should not touch. Linen packages go on the top level of the sterilizer and metal packages on the bottom when running a mixed load. To keep the packages upright, place heat-sealed plastic-paper peel-down packages on end. Lay instrument container systems and sets with perforated trays flat or in the side position during the sterilization cycle.

Operating a Steam Sterilizer

Operate the steam sterilizer according to the manufacturer's written instructions. Before removing the contents, check the sterilizer graph or printed readout to verify that sterilization parameters were met. Sterilize supplies requiring the same exposure cycle in the same load.

At completion of the sterilization cycle, before opening the door, verify that the exhaust valve reading is zero to ensure complete dissipation of steam. Stand behind the door and open it slowly to avoid the steam escaping from around the door. To prevent injury from a burn, do not touch the interior surfaces of the sterilizer. When not in use, keep the sterilizer door closed. After removing the cart from the sterilizer, place it away from air vents or fans to prevent formation of condensation. After the items have cooled, apply dust covers to designated items.

Indications for Use and Operation of a High-Speed Pressure (Flash) Sterilizer

Keep flash sterilization to a minimum. Potentially, flash sterilization increases the patient's risk for infection because of pressure on personnel to eliminate one or several steps in the decontamination, cleaning, and sterilization processes. Failure to properly clean and decontaminate instruments has resulted in transmission of infectious agents. Use flash sterilization only in selected clinical situations such as when time constraints prevent using the preferred wrapped or container method. In addition, do not use flash sterilization for implantable devices except in cases of emergency when there are no other available options (AORN, 2008o).

Do not use packaging and wrapping materials during flash sterilization cycles unless the sterilizer is specifically designed and labeled for this use. Place unwrapped items in a closed sterilization container or tray, validated for flash sterilization, in a manner that allows the steam to contact all instrument surfaces. Exercise care to prevent contamination of the items during transport and transfer to the sterile field. Use process challenge devices with routine process monitoring devices (eg, chemical indicators, biological indicators). Use items that have been flash-sterilized immediately. Do not store for later use (AORN, 2008o). See **Table 14.13** for examples of typical flash steam sterilization parameters.

Sterilizing with Ethylene Oxide

EO
Ethylene Oxide

Use ethylene oxide (EO), a low-temperature sterilization process, for heat- and moisture-sensitive devices when indicated by the device manufacturer. As an alkylating agent, at sterilizing temperatures EO kills microbes in areas typically difficult to reach. Several theories exist as to how EO kills organisms. One of the theories describes the killing rate of bacteria as relative to the rate of diffusion of the gas through cell walls and the availability or accessibility of one of the chemical groups in the bacterial cell wall to react with the EO. In addition, the killing rate depends on whether the cell is in a vegetative or spore state. Destruction takes place by alkylation and probable inactivation of the reproductive process of the cell (Nicolette, 2007). See **Table 14.14** for EO sterilization parameters.

HCFC
Hydrochlorofluoro-
carbons

CFC
Chlorofluorocarbons

Limit EO use for compatible medical devices when alternate methods of sterilization are not available. EO is typically used in 100% concentrations or with diluents of hydrochlorofluorocarbons (HCFC). Until the mid 1990s, chlorofluorocarbons (CFC) were used, but were eliminated due to the deterioration of the ozone layer and are no longer produced in the United States. Review federal, state, and local regulations before using any EO sterilizer that has HCFC components since these regulations may be in effect (AORN, 2008o).

Follow the manufacturer's written instructions for EO sterilization parameters and loading of items within the sterilizer. EO sterilizers differ in design and operational functionality. Place items in baskets or loading carts in a manner that allows free circulation and penetration of the EO. Use physical monitors and provide real-time

Table 14.13	Flash Steam Sterilization Parameters				
Type of Sterilizer	**Load Configuration**	**Time**	**Exposure Temperature**	**Drying Times**	
Gravity Displacement	☐ Metal or nonporous items only (no lumens)	3 MIN	270°F–275°F (132°C–135°C)	0–1 MIN	
	☐ Metal items with lumens and porous items (eg, rubber, plastic) sterilized together	10 MIN	270°F–275°F (132°C–135°C)	0–1 MIN	
	☐ Complex devices (ie, powered instruments that require extended exposure times)				
	☐ Refer to manufacturer's written instructions				
Dynamic Air-Removal (Pre-vacuum)	☐ Metal or nonporous items only (no lumens)	3 MIN	270°F–275°F (132°C–135°C)	N/A	
	☐ Metal items with lumens and porous items sterilized together	4 MIN	270°F (132°C)	N/A	
		3 MIN	275°F (135°C)	N/A	

Adapted from: AORN. (2008). Recommended practices for sterilization in the perioperative practice setting. *Perioperative Standards and Recommended Practices.* Denver, CO; AORN, Inc: p. 580.

assessment and documentation of the cycle parameters. Aerate EO sterilized items in a mechanical aerator to remove the gas. Aeration times depend the size and composition of the load, density, packaging, type of EO System used, and temperature (AORN, 2008o). In all situations, allow items to cool before storing packages and containers.

Implementing Safety Procedures

Operate ethylene oxide sterilizers according to both the sterilizer and equipment manufacturers' recommendations and specifications. Post signs identifying EO sterilizing areas. Isolate ethylene oxide sterilizers and aerators. Install in a well-ventilated room in order to minimize occupational exposure. Avoid exposure to EO vapor; it is extremely hazardous. Educate personnel about the health effects and potential hazards associated with exposure to EO, as well as how to implement safety procedures following exposure to EO (AORN, 2008o). Because of the occupational exposure

Table 14.14	Ethylene Oxide Sterilization Parameters	
Time	105–300 minutes	
Temperature	37°C–63°C (99°F–145°F)	
Humidity	45%–75%	
Gas Concentration	450–1,200 mg/L	

Source: Nicolette, L. (2007). Infection prevention and control in the perioperative setting. *Alexander's Care of the Patient in Surgery,* 13th ed. St. Louis, MO: Mosby; p. 69.

hazards of EO, OSHA has issued the following regulations for employers regarding personnel exposure (OSHA, 2006):

TWA
Time-Weighted Average

- Eight-hour time-weighted average (TWA)—Employers shall ensure that no employee is exposed to an airborne concentration of EO in excess of one (1) part EO per million parts of air (1 ppm) as an (8)-hour time-weighted average (8-hour TWA).
- Excursion limit—Employers shall ensure that no employee is exposed to an airborne concentration of EO in excess of five parts of EO per million parts of air (5 ppm) as averaged over a sampling period of fifteen (15) minutes.

Monitor all personnel who have potential for exposure to ethylene oxide. Use EO-monitoring devices that meet the NIOSH standards for accuracy. In addition, periodically assess employees who have potential for exposure and conduct an environmental physical assessment to determine level of compliance with defined safety parameters. Document findings according to current OSHA regulations (AORN, 2008o).

Loading Ethylene Oxide Sterilizers

Clean and dry items before sterilization. Sterilize items having common aeration times together. Unlike the procedure for steam sterilization, dry the lumina of tubing and needles. The combination of water and ethylene oxide forms ethylene glycol, a toxic substance. After packaging, place the items on metal carts or in wire baskets. Do not overcrowd the sterilizer in order to permit circulation of the sterilant to all surfaces. Items should not touch the walls of the chamber during the sterilizing cycle. Avoid stacking heavy packages. Place pouches on edge in a wire basket.

Transferring Items from Sterilizer to Aerator

Open the sterilizer door as soon as possible after completion of the sterilization cycle to decrease vapor buildup. If using a sterilizer cart when moving equipment from the sterilizer to the aerator, pull, not push, the cart to avoid inhaling ethylene oxide. Handle items sterilized with EO as little as possible before aeration in order to prevent inhalation or contact with EO gas residues. Wear butyl rubber, nitrile, or neoprene gloves that provide skin protection when handling unaerated EO-sterilized items (AORN, 2008o).

Aerating Items

Safe use of EO requires thorough aeration (AORN, 2008o). Properly aerate items by leaving approximately 1 inch (2.5 cm) between all items. Overloading the aerator decreases air circulation, which in turn prolongs the aeration cycle. Do not open the aerator until the entire cycle time has elapsed. In addition, do not remove the item from the aerator prematurely. At the completion of the cycle, allow the items to cool before storing.

Liquid Chemical Sterile Processing

Liquid peroxyacetic (peracetic) acid is a biocidal oxidizer that maintains it efficacy in the presence of high levels of organic soil. The mechanism of action of peracetic acid is not well understood; however, it is considered highly corrosive to instrumentation and must be used in combination with anticorrosive additives (Nicolette, 2007).

Use peracetic acid for immersible heat-sensitive items. Consult the device manufacturer regarding the type, monitoring, and maintenance of sterilization system used

(AORN, 2008o). Appropriate use of sterilizers should be ensured so that proper sterilization is achieved. Obtain from the manufacturer documentation concerning the types of items that can and cannot be processed using peracetic acid (AORN, 2008o).

An example of a peracetic acid sterilizer is The Steris® System 1. This sterilizer is used only for instruments that are totally immersible in liquid and able to withstand processing temperatures of up to 56°C (132.8°F) for 12 minutes. When using this sterilizer, clean and mechanically prepare instruments according to the instrument manufacturers' recommendations for liquid immersion or according to current department practices. It is not necessary to dry instruments before placing them into the processor. Place unwrapped instruments in the appropriate tray or container. For flexible endoscopes, connect the lumens to permit the liquid sterilant to reach internal and external surfaces. Insert a sealed container of sterilant into the processor. The processor automatically prepares the working concentration of sterilant and controls the exposure time (12 minutes) and temperature (50–56°C [122–132.8°F]). After sterilization, the processor rinses the instruments with sterile water to remove chemical residues without recontaminating the instruments. Upon completion of the 30-minute cycle, the instruments are available for immediate use. Before removing the instruments from the processor, observe the control panel lights and printout to verify that a successful cycle was achieved. The cycle printout is then initialed and saved for quality assurance records. A failed cycle is reported to the appropriate person for corrective action. Instruments from a failed cycle should not be used. Distribute and use instruments promptly after sterilization. The Steris® System 1 processor instrument containers are not intended for storage. Do not sterilize implants in a Steris® System 1 processor; these require sterilization in conjunction with biological monitoring.

Safety Procedures

When direct physical contact with the sterilant is a possibility, as in case of an incomplete cycle, wear protective eyewear (chemical goggles), and waterproof gloves. The diluted sterilant is nontoxic and safe for direct disposal into a sanitary sewer. No environmental or personal exposure monitoring is required; however, ensuring adequate ventilation in the work area is desirable to minimize the vinegar-like chemical odor.

Monitoring the Cycle

As with steam and EO sterilization processes, for the Steris® System 1, chemical and biological indicators provide the same level of cycle quality assurance. Run a chemical indicator with each instrument load as a secondary check of the processor's ability to monitor sterilant potency. Run a biological indicator weekly. Use the indicator systems available from the manufacturer. Interpret the results obtained according to the manufacturer's written criteria.

Low-Temperature Gas Plasma Sterile Processing

Low-temperature gas plasma (LTGP) sterilization systems effectively sterilize most items currently processed by EO, that is, moisture- and heat-sensitive items and when indicated by the manufacturer (AORN, 2008o), with the exception of linens, cellulosic materials, powders, liquids, and devices containing long, narrow, dead-end lumens. Plasma is the fourth state of matter as identified by the sequence, which is solid, liquid, gas, and plasma. In this sterilization process, microbial life is disrupted

LTGP
Low-Temperature Gas Plasma

when free radicals are created from hydrogen peroxide gas plasma interaction with microbial cell membranes, enzymes, and nucleic acids (Nicolette, 2007).

LTGP systems use a combination of hydrogen peroxide vapor and low-temperature hydrogen peroxide gas plasma (MSDS, 2003). An aqueous solution of hydrogen peroxide is injected and vaporized into the chamber surrounding the items to be sterilized. The pressure is lowered and with application of radio frequency energy, an electrical field is created that subsequently initiates the production of plasma that kills the microorganisms. At the completion of the sterilization segment of the cycle, the radiofrequency energy is turned off, the vacuum is vented, and the chamber returns to atmospheric pressure by the introduction of air through a HEPA filter. Items processed in LTGP systems require no aeration, since the end products of the system are oxygen and water in the form of humidity; at the end of the cycle, the items are dry (AORN, 2008o).

Items to be gas-plasma sterilized should be clean, dry, and packaged in nonwoven polypropylene or polyethylene wraps; cellulose-based packaging materials and liquids are not suitable; devices with lumens should comply with the lumen specifications in the written instructions. Use trays designed and validated for use with the sterilization system (AORN, 2008o).

Ozone Sterilization

Ozone sterilization is considered a strong oxidizing agent, which makes ozone sterilization an effective low-temperature sterilization process. Ozone is generated within the sterilizer using oxygen and water. When the cycle is complete, the ozone is exhausted through a catalytic converter, which in turn is converted back into the raw materials of oxygen and water. There is no aeration required, since the byproducts of the system at the end of the cycle are nontoxic (AORN, 2008o).

Follow the sterilizer manufacturer's written instructions for operating, monitoring, and maintenance. Obtain information from the device manufacturer and the ozone system manufacturer to determine the feasibility of sterilizing a device with ozone. Clean, dry, and package items for ozone according to the sterilizer manufacturer's written instructions (AORN, 2008o).

Monitoring the Sterilization Process

Evaluate sterilization conditions with mechanical, chemical, and biological monitors. Place monitors strategically side-by-side at locations that present the greatest challenge to air evacuation and sterilant penetration. Use monitors for (AORN, 2008o):

- Routine load release
- Routine sterilizer efficacy monitoring
- Sterilizer qualification testing (eg, after installation, relocation, malfunctions, major repairs, sterilization process failures)
- Periodic product quality assurance testing for all sterilization processes

Mechanical Control Measures

Monitor mechanical control monitors such as time-temperature recording devices, temperature gauges, and pressure gauges at the beginning and ending of each cycle to verify that adequate parameters have been achieved. Before removing any materials from the sterilizer, verify that adequate temperature and duration have been achieved. Report sterilizer malfunction or suspicious operation to the appropriate person. If using automated mechanical control measures, evaluate and initial the recording at the end of each cycle.

Chemical Indicators

External or internal sterilization chemical indicators may include sterilization indicating tape, labels, cards, or strips that visually identify that the package has been exposed to sterilizing conditions. Chemical indicators do not validate that sterilization has been achieved. Apply the manufacturer's criteria to interpret chemical indicator results. Use an external chemical indicator with every package as a visual check that the package has been subjected to sterilizing conditions. Place an internal chemical indicator in the most inaccessible area of every pack.

Efficacy of Vacuum System on Prevacuum Sterilizers

The presence of residual air in a prevacuum sterilizer chamber prevents steam contact with items in the load, thus hampering sterilization. Use the Bowie-Dick test to determine the efficacy of the vacuum system (assisted air removal as part of the cycle), The Bowie-Dick test does not indicate sterilization. Place a Bowie-Dick-type test sheet in the center of a 9 × 12-inch (22.5 × 30 cm) pack of folded towels that has a height of 10–11 inches (25–27.5 cm). Loosely single wrap the pack. Place the test pack horizontally on the bottom front rack of the sterilizer, near the door and over the drain of an otherwise empty chamber. Perform this test daily, in an empty chamber, in accordance with the test manufacturer's instructions before the routine biological indicator testing (AORN, 2008o).

Biological Testing of Sterilizers

Biological testing for each type of sterilizer is outlined in **Table 14.15**.

Sterilizer Performance Records

Label all processed items with lot control numbers to identify the sterilizer used, the cycle or load number, and the date of sterilization. The information recorded for each sterilization cycle should include, but not be limited to (AORN, 2008o):

- Identification of the sterilizer;
- Type of sterilizer and cycle used;
- A lot control number;
- Load contents;
- Critical parameters for the specific sterilization method;
- Operator's name; and
- Results of sterilization process monitoring (ie, biological, chemical physical).

Preventive Maintenance

Qualified personnel perform preventive maintenance and repairs, inspection, and cleaning of all sterilizers on a scheduled basis as specified by the manufacturer's written instructions in order to prevent sterilizer downtime and malfunctions (AORN, 2008o). In general, areas that need attention include filters, valves, steam traps, drainpipes, and door gaskets.

Table 14.15	**Biological Monitoring**	
Type of Sterilizer	**Biological Indicator**	**Parameters/Frequency**

Steam Sterilizers	*Geobacillus stearothermopheus*	☐ Routine load release
		☐ Routine sterilizer efficacy monitoring should be performed weekly, (preferably daily) as follows:
		  • with each load containing an implantable device; the BI should be quarantined until the results are available
		  • one BI process challenge device (PCD) should be run in three consecutive empty cycles sterilizer qualification testing
		☐ Periodic product quality assurance testing
		☐ Each sterilization mode should be tested if a steam sterilizer is intended to be used for multiple types of cycles

Ethylene Oxide	*Bacillus atropheus* (formerly *Bacillus subtilis*)	☐ Spore testing should be performed with every load
Liquid Peracetic Acid	*Geobacillus stearothermophilus*	☐ Daily for routine sterilizer efficacy monitoring ☐ The test product should be designed specifically for use with liquid peracetic acid processes ☐ The sterilizer's manufacturer's written instructions should be followed

Low-Temperature Hydrogen Peroxide Gas Plasma	*Geobacillus stearothermophilus*	☐ Routine load release
		☐ Routine sterilizer efficacy monitoring should be performed weekly, preferably daily as follows:
		  • with each load containing an implantable device; the BI should be quarantined until the results are available
		  • one BI PCD should be run in three consecutive empty cycles for sterilizer qualification testing
		☐ Periodic product quality assurance testing
		☐ The sterilizer manufacturer's written recommendations for the specific monitoring product(s) and appropriate placement of the product within the sterilizer should be followed

Ozone	*Geobacillus stearothermophilus*	☐ Routine load release
		☐ Routine sterilizer efficacy monitoring should be performed weekly, preferably daily as follows:
		  • with each load containing an implantable device; the BI should be quarantined until the results are available
		  • one BI PCD should be run in three consecutive empty cycles for sterilizer qualification testing
		☐ The sterilizer manufacturer's written recommendations for the specific monitoring product(s) and appropriate placement of the product within the sterilizer should be followed

Adapted from: AORN. (2008). Recommended practices for sterilization in the perioperative practice setting. *Perioperative Standards and Recommended Practices.* Denver, CO; AORN, Inc: pp. 591–592.

Documentation

Keep permanent sterilization records for the time specified by the facility's policies, in compliance with local, state, and federal regulations. Documentation for every sterilization cycle and modality should include (AORN, 2008o):

- Assigned lot number;
- Contents of each load; and
- Results of physical, chemical, and biological monitors.

Maintenance records should also be kept for each sterilizer; this documentation should include, but not be limited to (AORN, 2008o):

- Service date;
- Sterilizer model and serial number;
- Sterilizer location;
- Description of the problem/malfunction;
- Name of person and company performing the maintenance;
- Description of the service and parts replaced;
- Results of biological indicator testing, if completed;
- Results of Bowie-Dick testing, if completed;
- The name of the person requesting service, where appropriate; and
- The signature and title of the person acknowledging the work has been completed.

Shelf Life

Shelf life refers to the length of time a package may be considered sterile. Loss of package sterility is considered event-related rather than time-related; that is, sterilized packages should be considered sterile until an event occurs to compromise the package barrier integrity (AORN, 2008n). The length of time the package remains on the shelf prior to use does not determine its continued sterility. Several variables are used when determining shelf life, including but not limited to (AORN, 2008n):

- Multiple handling that can lead to seal breakage or compromise of package integrity;
- Compression during storage;
- Penetration of moisture;
- Exposure to airborne and other environmental contaminants;
- Conditions of the storage area (eg, type of shelving, temperature, humidity, cleanliness, traffic control);
- Consideration of the type and configuration of the packaging material used; and
- Use of impervious protective covers also known as dust covers and the method of sealing.

Policies and procedures should be established in the operative and invasive procedure practice setting related to the shelf life of sterilized packages.

COMPETENCY ASSESSMENT
Control and Monitor the Environment

Name: _____ Title: _____ Unit: _____ Date of Validation: _____

Type of Validation: ☐ Initial ☐ Annual ☐ Bi-annual

COMPETENCY STATEMENT: The nurse demonstrates competency to control and monitor the environment of the operative or invasive procedure suite.

Performance Criteria	Met	Not Met
1. Identifies the patient's risk for adverse outcomes related to monitoring and controlling the environment	☐	☐
2. Regulates temperature and humidity of the operating and invasive procedure room	☐	☐
3. Protects the patient from injury caused by extraneous objects (equipment)	☐	☐
4. Ensures the patient is free from chemical injury	☐	☐
5. Ensures electrical safety	☐	☐
6. Ensures fire safety	☐	☐
7. Ensures environmental air quality	☐	☐
8. Monitors the sensory environment	☐	☐
9. Ensures radiation and laser safety	☐	☐
10. Maintains suite traffic patterns	☐	☐
11. Prevents latex exposure to sensitive patients and staff	☐	☐
12. Performs environmental sanitation	☐	☐
13. Provides appropriate care; handling; and sterilization of instruments, supplies, and equipment	☐	☐

_____

Validator's Signature

_____

Validator's Printed Name

_____

Employee's Signature

ENDNOTES

1. Light Amplification by Stimulated Emission of Radiation.
2. "A space in which the level of direct, reflected, or scattered radiation used during normal laser operation exceeds the applicable maximum permissible exposure" (AORN, 2008f, p. 593).

REFERENCES

1. American College of Allergy, Asthma, and Immunology. (ACAAI). (1996). Guidelines for the management of latex allergies and safe latex use in health care facilities. Retrieved July 7, 2008 from http://www.acaai.org/public/physicians/latex.htm.

2. American Institute of Architects (AIA) Academy of Architecture for Health. (2006). *Guidelines for design and construction of health care facilities.* Washington, DC: AIA.

3. American National Standards Institute (ANSI), Laser Institute of America. (1996). *American National Standard for Safe Use of Lasers in Health Care Facilities.* Orlando, FL; The Laser Institute of America.

4. American Society of Anesthesiologists (ASA). (2008). Practice advisory for the prevention and management of operating room fires. Retrieved June 28, 2008 from http://www.anesthesiology.org/pt/re/anes/pdfhandler.00000542-200805000-00006.pdf;jsessionid=Lm6H18JggvQ1zLHBR3rbwKldFGM1NFJb7bF556XcG12JDvyvLD8d!832702866!181195628!8091!-1.

5. Association for the Advancement of Medical Instrumentation (AAMI). (2006). *ANSI/AAMI ST79:2006-Comprehensive Guide to Steam Sterilization and Sterility Assurance in Health Care Facilities.* Arlington, VA; AAMI.

6. Association of periOperative Registered Nurses (AORN). (2008a). Recommended practices for the prevention of unplanned perioperative hypothermia. *Perioperative Standards and Recommended Practices.* Denver, CO; AORN, Inc: pp. 407–420.

7. Association of periOperative Registered Nurses (AORN). (2008b). Recommended practices for a safe environment of care. *Perioperative Standards and Recommended Practices.* Denver, CO; AORN, Inc: pp. 351–373.

8. Association of periOperative Registered Nurses (AORN). (2008c). AORN guidance statement: fire prevention in the operating room. *Perioperative Standards and Recommended Practices.* Denver, CO; AORN, Inc: pp. 171–179.

9. Association of periOperative Registered Nurses (AORN). (2008d). AORN position statement: statement on surgical smoke and bio-aerosols. Retrieved July 2, 2008 from http://www.aorn.org/PracticeResources/AORNPositionStatements/SurgicalSmokeAndBioAerosols/.

10. Association of periOperative Registered Nurses (AORN). (2008e). Recommended practices for reducing radiological exposure in the perioperative practice setting. *Perioperative Standards and Recommended Practices.* Denver, CO; AORN, Inc: pp. 525–536.

11. Association of periOperative Registered Nurses (AORN). (2008f). Recommended practices for laser safety in practice settings. *Perioperative Standards and Recommended Practices.* Denver, CO; AORN, Inc: pp. 447–452.

12. Association of periOperative Registered Nurses (AORN). (2008g). Recommended practices for documentation of perioperative nursing care. *Perioperative Standards and Recommended Practices.* Denver, CO; AORN, Inc: pp. 311–313.

13. Association of periOperative Registered Nurses (AORN). (2008h). Recommended practices for traffic patterns in the perioperative practice setting. *Perioperative Standards and Recommended Practices.* Denver, CO; AORN, Inc: pp. 613–617.

14. Association of periOperative Registered Nurses (AORN). (2008i). Recommended practices for environmental cleaning in the perioperative setting. *Perioperative Standards and Recommended Practices.* Denver, CO; AORN, Inc: pp. 375–389.

15. Association of periOperative Registered Nurses (AORN). (2008j). AORN latex guideline. *Perioperative Standards and Recommended Practices.* Denver, CO; AORN, Inc: pp. 87–102.

16. Association of periOperative Registered Nurses (AORN). (2008k). Recommended practices for sponge, sharp, and instrument counts. *Perioperative Standards and Recommended Practices.* Denver, CO; AORN, Inc: pp. 293–302.

17. Association of periOperative Registered Nurses (AORN). (2008l). Recommended practices for cleaning and care of surgical instruments and powered equipment. *Perioperative Standards and Recommended Practices.* Denver, CO; AORN, Inc: pp. 421–445.

18. Association of periOperative Registered Nurses (AORN). (2008m). Recommended practices for care and handling of specimens in the perioperative environment. *Perioperative Standards and Recommended Practices.* Denver, CO; AORN, Inc: pp. 557–564.

19. Association of periOperative Registered Nurses (AORN). (2008n). Recommended practices for selection and use of packaging systems for sterilization. *Perioperative Standards and Recommended Practices.* Denver, CO; AORN, Inc: pp. 473–482.

20. Association of periOperative Registered Nurses (AORN). (2008o). Recommended practices for sterilization in the perioperative practice setting. *Perioperative Standards and Recommended Practices.* Denver, CO; AORN, Inc: pp. 575–598.

21. Barrett, W.L. & Garber, S.M. (2004). Surgical smoke—a review of the literature. *Business Briefing: Global Surgery;* 1–7.

22. Cardinal Health. (2008). *Surgical Fires: Keys to Awareness and Prevention*. Aurora, CO; Pfiedler Enterprises.

23. Conmed. (2008). *Reducing the Risk of Surgical Smoke*. Aurora, CO; Pfiedler Enterprises.

24. Covidien. (2008). Fire prevention and safety during surgical procedures. Retrieved June 24, 2008 from http://www.valleylabeducation.org/fire/pages/fire-12.html.

25. ECRI. (2003). A clinician's guide to surgical fires: how they occur, how to prevent them, how to put them out. Retrieved June 28, 2008 from http://www.ngc.gov/summary/summary.aspx?doc_id=3688&nbr=002914&string=surgical+AND+fire.

26. ECRI. (1996). Electrosurgical airway fires still a hot topic. Retrieved June 27, 2008 from http://www.mdsr.ecri.org/summary/detail.aspx?doc_id=8217.

27. ECRI. (1992a). The patient is on fire! A surgical fires primer. Retrieved June 24, 2008 from http://www.mdsr.ecri.org/summary/detail.aspx?doc_id=8197.

28. ECRI. (1992b). Preventing, preparing for and managing surgical fires. *ECRI Health Devices, 21(1):* pp. 24–34.

29. Material Safety Data Sheet (MSDS). (2003). *Material Safety Data Sheet 09461-0-001: Hydrogen Peroxide Solution*. Irvine, CA; Advanced Sterilization Products.

30. Mok, E. & Wong, K-Y. (2003). Effects of music on patient anxiety. *AORN Journal*; 77(2): 396–410.

31. NFPA (2005). Amendment to NFPA 99–2005 edition.

32. National Institute for Occupational Safety and Health (NIOSH). (1998). NIOSH hazard controls: control of smoke from laser/electric surgical procedures. Retrieved July 3, 2008 from http://www.cdc.gov/niosh/hc11.html.

33. National Institute for Occupational Safety and Health. (NIOSH). (1997). NIOSH Publication No. 97–135: preventing allergic reactions to natural rubber latex in the workplace. Retrieved July 7, 2008 from http://www.cdc.gov/Niosh/latexalt.html.

34. Nicolette, L. (2007). Infection prevention and control in the perioperative setting. *Alexander's Care of the Patient in Surgery*, 13th ed. St. Louis, MO: Mosby; pp. 44–99.

35. OSHA. (1992). Regulations (Standards—29 CFR) Bloodborne pathogens—1910.1030. Retrieved July 7, 2008 from http://www.osha.gov/pls/oshaweb/owadisp.show_document?p_table=STANDARDS&p_id=10051.

36. OSHA. (2006). Regulations (Standards—29 CFR) Ethylene oxide—1910.1047. Retrieved July 10, 2008 from http://www.osha.gov/pls/oshaweb/owadisp.show_document?p_table=STANDARDS&p_id=10070.

37. Petersen, C. (2007). Perioperative Nursing Data Set, The Perioperative Nursing Vocabulary, revised 2nd ed. Denver, CO; AORN, Inc.

38. Rothrock, J.C. (2007). Patient and environmental safety. *Alexander's Care of the Patient in Surgery*, 13th ed. St. Louis, MO: Mosby: pp. 15–43.

39. Sessler, D.I. (2005). Temperature monitoring. *Miller's Anesthesia*, 6th ed. RD Miller, ed. Philadelphia, PA: Elsevier: pp. 1571–1597.

40. Smith, C. (2004). Surgical fires—learn not to burn. *AORN Journal*; 80(1): 24–36.

41. The Joint Commission. (2003). Sentinel event alert: preventing surgical fires. Issue 29—June 24, 2003. Retrieved June 24, 2008 from http://www.jointcommission.org/SentinelEvents/SentinelEventAlert/sea_29.htm.

42. U.S. Nuclear Regulatory Commission. (2007). Part 20—standards for protection against radiation. Retrieved July 7, 2008 from http://www.nrc.gov/reading-rm/doc-collections/cfr/part020/.

43. Ulmer, B.C. (2008). The hazards of surgical smoke. *AORN Journal*; 87(4): 721–734.

CHAPTER 15

Handle Specimens and Cultures

Charlotte Dorsey

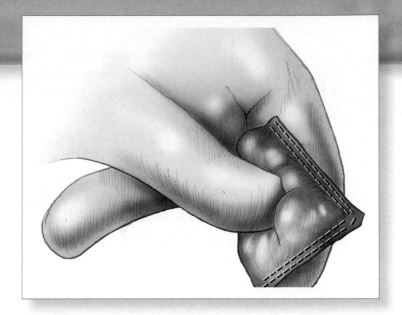

INTRODUCTION

Handle specimens and cultures describes patient care activities performed by the nurse, the surgical technologist, and other members of the patient care team to collect, process, store, preserve, and transport operative or invasive procedure tissue specimens and cultures.

MEASURABLE CRITERIA

The registered nurse, providing care as the circulator, implements the measurable criteria for safe handling of specimens and cultures. The nurse demonstrates competency to collect, identify, label, process, store, preserve, and transport specimens and cultures by:

- Identifying legal implications of handling specimens and cultures.
- Identifying the patient's risk for adverse outcomes related to the improper handling of specimens and cultures.
- Implementing infection control practices when handling specimens and cultures.
- Safely handling formalin.
- Providing supplies and equipment to collect specimens and cultures.
- Completing the laboratory requisitions.
- Documenting the collection of specimens and cultures.
- Establishing the chain of custody for specimens and cultures.
- Collecting and preparing tissue for examination.
- Collecting and preparing cultures for examination.

Chapter Contents

- Directing the transfer of specimens and cultures to the laboratory.
- Communicating pathology reports to the physician during the procedure.
- Demonstrating knowledge of storing, preserving, and maintaining tissue.

IDENTIFYING LEGAL IMPLICATIONS OF HANDLING SPECIMENS AND CULTURES

The proper care and handling of specimens and cultures ensures continuity of care for the patient. Improving the safe care of patients has recently evoked national attention. Accurate specimen identification is a challenge in all hospitals, and a mislabeled specimen can lead to devastating patient consequences including misdiagnosis and consequent inappropriate patient treatment. The circulating nurse is responsible for identifying, documenting, and properly caring for specimens and cultures in the operative and invasive procedure setting, even when some elements of this activity are delegated. Proper documentation allows tracking of the specimen from its source to its disposition. Once the testing is complete, the pathology and laboratory result documents become part of the patient's permanent record.

IDENTIFYING THE PATIENT'S RISK FOR ADVERSE OUTCOMES RELATED TO THE IMPROPER HANDLING OF SPECIMENS AND CULTURES

Handling specimens and cultures, if not done correctly, has the potential for compromising or causing injury to the patient. Incorrect handling of specimens and cultures could potentially result in the patient receiving a wrong diagnosis and subsequent treatment. **Table 15.1** identifies outcome statement, diagnosis, risk factors, and outcome indicators related to this patient care event.

IMPLEMENTING APPROPRIATE INFECTION CONTROL PRACTICES WHEN HANDLING SPECIMENS AND CULTURES

PPE
Personal Protection
Equipment

Always consider specimens and cultures as potentially infectious. When collecting and preparing specimens and cultures for examination use *Standard Precautions* and don appropriate personal protection equipment (PPE) such as gloves, gowns, masks, and eyewear or face shields. When collecting specimens from the scrub person always wear gloves and wash hands after removing the gloves. Do not contaminate the exterior surface of the specimen containers and culture tubes with blood, tissue, or other body fluids; this will reduce the risk of cross-contamination to other personnel handling the containers and tubes. If contamination does occur, clean the exterior of the specimen container or culture tube with a tuberculocidal hospital-grade chemical germicide before removing the item from the operative or invasive procedure suite. Place containers or tubes that cannot be disinfected in an impervious, clear bag for transportation to the laboratory. Label the bag, identifying the contents as contaminated. This alerts the person receiving the specimen or culture to use caution when handling the container or tube. For a specimen in a large rigid container, attach a bio-hazardous sticker to the container. Prevent contamination of

Table 15.1	Handling Cultures and Specimens Does Not Compromise or Cause Injury to the Patient

Outcome The patient is free from evidence of injury related to the handling of specimens and cultures.

Diagnosis	Risk Factors	Outcome Indicators
Risk for injury related to improper handling of cultures and specimens obtained during the operative or invasive procedure	☐ Failure to provide the correct supplies and equipment for culture and specimen collection ☐ Incorrect labeling of culture and tissue specimen containers ☐ Incorrect completion of laboratory slips ☐ Incorrect documentation of cultures and specimens on the patient's record ☐ Failure to establish chain of custody for cultures and tissue specimens ☐ Improper processing of cultures and tissue for examination ☐ Improper storage, preservation, and maintenance of tissue ☐ Failure to properly direct the transfer of cultures and specimens to the laboratory ☐ Incorrect communication of pathology reports to the physician	☐ Did the patient receive an incorrect medical diagnosis or treatment as a result of improper handling of cultures and specimens by the operative or invasive procedure nursing team? ☐ Was the culture or specimen lost? ☐ Was the culture or specimen prepared according to facility policy and procedure? ☐ Was the culture or specimen transported to the pathology department according to facility policy and procedure?

15

such documents as labels and laboratory slips. If they become contaminated, prepare fresh documents.

SAFELY HANDLING FORMALIN

Formalin is a clear aqueous solution of formaldehyde with a small amount of methanol. Formalin 10% solution is commonly used as a tissue preservative for permanent specimens.

When using formalin in the operative or invasive procedure suite, pour it directly over a specimen that has been placed in a specimen container, or pour it into a container before specimen collection. When pouring formalin over a specimen or into a container, use extreme caution to avoid splashing, contact with body surfaces, and breathing of the vapors. Always wear protective eyewear and gloves when preparing containers. Affix a hazard label to receptacles containing formalin.

Formalin is designated a hazardous material by federal law, thus a Material Safety Data Sheet (MSDS) should be maintained on file in the department and in the Occupational Health Clinic. **Table 15.2** describes precautions and handling guidelines that should be taken when using formalin.

MSDS
Material Safety Data Sheet

| Table 15.2 | Precautions and Handling Guidelines for Using Formalin |

Precautions	Handling Guidelines
Formalin is flammable.	☐ Keep formalin away from heat, sparks, and flames. Store in a well-ventilated area.
Formalin is a severe skin irritant. ☐ Repeat exposure may cause numbness and a hardening or tanning of the skin.	☐ Remove contaminated clothing immediately. Wash the affected area with soap and large amounts of water. If there are chemical burns, get medical attention. ☐ As a precaution, after handling formalin, thoroughly wash your hands with soap and water.
Formalin splashed in the eye can cause injuries ranging from discomfort to severe, permanent corneal damage and loss of vision.	☐ In the event of eye contact, immediately flush the eyes with plenty of water (at least 15 to 20 minutes). Seek medical attention.
Formalin ingestion may cause severe irritation and inflammation of the mouth, esophagus, and stomach. ☐ Severe abdominal pain, violent vomiting, headache, and diarrhea will follow ingestion. ☐ With large doses ingested there is a possibility of loss of consciousness and death.	☐ If conscious, dilute the formalin by giving water, milk or activated charcoal. Keep person warm and at rest. Seek medical attention.
Formalin vapors are toxic. ☐ Can cause difficulty breathing, burning of the nose and throat, cough, and heavy tearing of the eyes. ☐ In higher concentrations can cause severe respiratory tract injury leading to pulmonary edema, pneumonitis and death.	☐ Use formalin only in well-ventilated areas. ☐ When filling specimen containers or preparing specimens, avoid breathing the vapors. ☐ If formalin is inhaled, move the person to fresh air. ☐ If the person is breathing, oxygen can be administered. If the person is not breathing, start CPR. Seek medical attention. ☐ In the event of a formalin spill, ventilate the area and isolate the hazardous area. Shut off ignition sources and clean the area according to the facility policy and procedure.

Modified from Substance Technical Guidelines for Formalin from OSHA.

PROVIDING SUPPLIES AND EQUIPMENT TO COLLECT SPECIMENS AND CULTURES

To ensure continuity of care, facilitate the procedure and prevent any procedural delays, gather supplies and equipment needed for specimens and cultures before transferring the patient to the operative or invasive procedure suite. Determine the types of supplies and equipment needed by assessing the patient, reviewing the patient's record, checking the physician's preference card, and questioning the physician with regard to specific specimen and culture needs. If appropriate, contact laboratory personnel or the pathologist to make arrangements for special tests or procedures such as frozen sections.

Supplies and Equipment

The supplies and equipment needed for handling specimens and cultures include: an addressograph; labels and laboratory slips (histological, cytological, aerobic, anaerobic, and acid-fast studies); aerobic and anaerobic culture tubes; test tubes with caps; Petri dishes; and tissue specimen containers of assorted sizes. Transport tissue specimens to pathology in rigid containers with tight-fitting lids to prevent leakage and unnecessary exposure to personnel. Specimens should be secured in an impervious container; the size or type of container is dependent on the size of the specimen, timing of the specimen review, preservatives, and containment for transport of the specimen (AORN Perioperative Standards and Recommended Practices, 2008, p. 558). Facilities that use a computerized system may require data entry concerning the surgical specimens and cultures into the computer. If so, laboratory slips will not be needed. The computer might also generate a special computer label for the specimen container and the specimen log book.

COMPLETING LABORATORY REQUISITIONS

Specimen and Culture Labels

Correct labeling of specimen and culture containers reduces the risk of the patient receiving an incorrect diagnosis and the wrong medical treatment (Lippi, Salvagno, Montagnana, Franchini, & Guidi, 2006). Affixing the label to the container allows identification of the specimen or culture even if the laboratory slip is lost. Either a label stamped with the Addressograph card or a handwritten label is appropriate. When affixing the label attach it to the specimen container and not the lid of the container. If the label is on the lid, the specimen can easily be mixed up with other specimens, especially if more than one specimen is sent from the same patient. The label should contain at least the following information: patient's name, patient's identification number, physician's name, type of tissue specimen or source of the culture, and date and time of collection. If the labels are generated from a computer, it might contain a bar code. The computerized specimen labels furnish several labels of different sizes: one for the specimen container and a label for the specimen log book.

Specimen and Culture Requisitions

Send all specimens and cultures to the pathology or laboratory department with appropriate laboratory slips. The number and the format of laboratory slips vary from facility to facility. The purpose of the laboratory slips is to identify the type of study requested, to communicate pertinent patient information to the laboratory technologist or pathologist, and to serve as a reporting document. As with the container label, complete the laboratory slip, writing legibly and accurately. Communication failures are particularly problematic among operative or invasive procedure team members and can result in preventable morbidity, mortality, and high cost of care. In studies, communication failures have been identified as the root cause in 80% of sentinel events and other medical errors in the operating room (Makary et al, 2007). One type of communication failure that poses risks to patients is the mislabeling of a surgical specimen. The error occurs from miscommunication from the surgeon to the scrub person, then from the scrub person to the circulating nurse. For this reason some facilities are asking the scrub person, circulating nurse, and surgeon to be involved in a specimen *time out.* At that time the three would agree upon the name of the specimen, location, and type of specimen.

Use the addressograph card to stamp identifying information on the slip or write the information in the space provided on the slip. Record the following information on the laboratory slip: patient's name, patient's identification number, physician's name, tissue or culture source (be specific), date and time of collection, patient's medical diagnosis, identification of the study requested, and other pertinent information such as current antibiotic regimen. For the facilities using computer ordering, the nurse inputs the information into the computer and the appropriate labels will print.

DOCUMENTING THE COLLECTION OF SPECIMENS AND CULTURES

Accurate documentation on the patient's record of the collection, identification, and transfer of specimens and cultures to the laboratory or pathology department reduces the patient's risk for an adverse outcome related to the handling of specimens and cultures. The record should reflect the source of the type of specimen or source of the culture, the time of collection, and the studies requested (**Table 15.3**). If a specimen

Table 15.3	Types of Specimens

Tissue
- ☐ Permanent
- ☐ Frozen section
- ☐ Gross examination only
- ☐ Biopsy: tissue or fluid
- ☐ Chromosome analysis
- ☐ Hormonal receptor site
- ☐ Papanicolaou smears
- ☐ Skin sent for storage

Fluid
- ☐ Aerobic cultures
- ☐ Anaerobic cultures
- ☐ Cytology
- ☐ Gram stain
- ☐ Spinal fluid
- ☐ Urine
- ☐ Acid fast: culture or smear
- ☐ Fungus: culture or smear

Miscellaneous
- ☐ Foreign bodies (ie, bullets)
- ☐ Orthopedic hardware

is not obtained, note this information on the operative or invasive procedure record. Although they are not part of the record, place any laboratory slips with results or comments returned during the procedure on the patient's chart.

ESTABLISHING CHAIN OF CUSTODY FOR SPECIMENS AND CULTURES

Chain of custody is a mechanism to ensure accountability for tissue and culture specimens. Many facilities use log books to track the specimen from the operative or invasive procedure suite to the laboratory or pathology department. Some facilities use a dual-log book system. One log book is used to track specimens for cultures and the other log book is used to track permanent specimens and frozen sections of tissue. Each entry in the log book should include the patient's name, patient's identification number, physician's name, type of tissue specimen or object or source of culture, name of person logging the specimen, date and time logging the specimen in, name of person receiving the specimen, and date and time specimen received in the pathology or laboratory department. Diligence in the task ensures that tissue specimens, cultures, and other objects removed from the patient are not lost.

COLLECTING AND PREPARING TISSUE FOR EXAMINATION

Tissue may be taken during the procedure for a number of studies. Examples are permanent, gross examination, frozen section, biopsy, hormonal receptor site study, and Papanicolaou smear specimens.

General Guidelines

Exercise care when handling specimens and handle as little as possible. Do not shake fluid specimens, as this may rupture the cells. If using an instrument to transfer the specimen, take care not to crush, tear, or damage the tissue. This could hinder the pathologist in making a conclusive diagnosis (Philips, 2007, p. 24).

Tissue should remain in a near-natural state, especially tissue being sent for a frozen section examination. Do not allow tissue specimens to dry out. The scrub person should keep the specimen in a container, such as an emesis basin, on the back table. While the specimen is on the sterile field, the scrub person should keep the specimen damp by frequently wetting it with sterile normal saline.

Permanent Specimens

Send all tissue or other objects removed from the patient to the laboratory as permanent specimens. After removal, with permission of the physician, the scrub person passes all specimens off the sterile field as soon as possible. This helps prevent inadvertent discarding of the specimen during cleanup at the end of the procedure. The specimen is transferred to an appropriate-sized container by tipping the emesis basin, thus causing the specimen to slide from the basin into the container. Wear gloves while handling the specimen container. The scrub person can use an instrument to transfer the specimen to the container, being careful not to damage, crush or tear the tissue. During the transfer of the specimen avoid splashing the formalin. If the formalin is added after the specimen is deposited in the container, completely cover it with formalin. Avoid splashing the formalin when pouring it over the specimen. Do not immerse bladder stones or gallstones in formalin. Send these specimens dry or in saline to prevent decomposition.

When the size of a specimen makes it difficult to see, the scrub person can place the specimen on a piece of material that provides contrast. A Telfa dressing pad is suitable and can be submerged in a formalin container and sent to the laboratory.

Each container should contain only one specimen. If specimens are bilateral, such as fallopian tubes, label each specimen as left or right. Medial and lateral designations can also be made.

Place specimens too large for standard containers in an appropriate-sized basin and clear, impervious bag. Arrange to have the specimen transported immediately to the laboratory with the appropriate paperwork. Instruct the transporter to exercise care in order to avoid contaminating himself or herself and laboratory personnel. Attach a label to the outside of the basin and the outside of the bag. If specimens are transported down common halls, the transporter should cover the specimens with a towel or sheet so that visitors and hospital personnel will not see the contents. Alert pathology department personnel about the arrival of such specimens.

In most facilities, permanent specimens are collected in a central location and transported to the laboratory at designated times during the day. The transportation is either done by laboratory personnel or operative or invasive procedure suite employees.

Gross Examination Specimens

The College of American Pathologists has developed recommendations to help facilities determine the types of specimens to routinely submit to the pathology department for examination and those that need only to be submitted for gross examination. The recommendations also provide guidelines for identifying specimens that do not need to be submitted to pathology at all. Each facility should have a policy that states which specimens are submitted for gross examination only or not submitted at all (College of American Pathologists Policy, 2008).

The circulating nurse and the physician should both document the removal and disposition of any specimens or devices that are not submitted to pathology for examination. **Table 15.4** shows examples of specimens that may be chosen to exclude from routine or mandatory submission to the pathology department. **Table 15.5** shows examples of specimens that may be submitted to the pathology department for only a gross examination. However, it is at the pathologist's discretion to do any additional examinations of the tissue.

Specimens for Frozen Section

Some specimens are sent directly to the pathologist for a frozen section examination. The frozen section examination provides the physician with a quick preliminary diagnosis. Frozen sections are analyzed to determine the presence of malignancy and identify tissue during the procedure, such as parathyroid tissue and lymph nodes. When a frozen section examination is anticipated, notify the pathology department before the procedure begins. This ensures that the pathologist is available and prepared for the specimen before it arrives in the pathology department.

Table 15.4	Examples of Specimens Excluded from Routine or Mandatory Submission to the Pathology Department

- ☐ Bone donated to the bone bank
- ☐ Bone segments removed as part of corrective or reconstructive orthopedic procedures (eg, spinal fusion, rotator cuff repair)
- ☐ Cataracts removed by phacoemulsification
- ☐ Dental appliances
- ☐ Fat removed by liposuction
- ☐ Foreign bodies such as bullets or other medicalegal evidence given directly to law enforcement personnel
- ☐ Foreskin from circumcisions of newborns
- ☐ Medical devices such as catheters, gastrostomy tubes, myringotomy tubes, stents, and sutures that have not contributed to patient illness, injury, or death
- ☐ Normal toenails and fingernails that are incidentally removed (College of American Pathologists)
- ☐ Orthopedic hardware and other radio-opaque mechanical devices provided it is documented in the nursing notes
- ☐ Placentas that do not meet institutionally specified criteria for examination
- ☐ Rib segments or other tissues removed only for purposes of gaining surgical access, provided the patient does not have a history of malignancy
- ☐ Saphenous vein segments harvested for coronary artery bypass
- ☐ Skin or other normal tissue removed during a cosmetic or reconstructive procedure (eg, blepharoplasty, cleft palate repair, abdominoplasty, rhytidectomy, syndactyly repair), provided it is not contiguous with a lesion and the patient does not have a history of malignancy
- ☐ Teeth when there is no attached soft tissue
- ☐ Therapeutic radioactive sources

Table 15.5	Examples of Specimens Submitted for Only Gross Examination to the Pathology Department

- ☐ Accessory digits
- ☐ Bunions and hammertoes
- ☐ Extraocular muscle from corrective surgical procedures (eg, strabismus repair)
- ☐ Inguinal hernia sacs in adults
- ☐ Nasal bone and cartilage from rhinoplasty or septoplasty
- ☐ Tonsils and adenoids from children
- ☐ Torn meniscus
- ☐ Umbilical hernia sacs in children
- ☐ Varicose veins

College of American Pathologists (2008).

After obtaining the specimen from the patient, it is passed off the sterile field on a section of dampened Telfa dressing pad, on a towel, or in a container such as an emesis basin. Do not let the scrub person or physician pass the specimen off the field on a counted sponge. While wearing gloves, receive the specimen and transfer it to an appropriate-sized dry container. Do *not* place the specimen in fluid such as formalin or saline. During the freezing process, moisture forms ice crystals which will interfere with the examination. Attach a label and immediately have the specimen taken to the pathology department. A report of the frozen section examination may be called to the operative or invasive suite via telephone or intercom. In such cases, if the patient is awake and alert, and the physician cannot communicate directly with the pathologist via telephone, receive the report from the pathologist and communicate the information to the physician.

Depending on facility policy, the pathologist may keep the specimen or return it to the operative or invasive procedure suite. If it is returned, place the specimen in formalin and handle it as a permanent specimen.

Specimens for Fresh State

Certain specimens should be sent to the laboratory in a fresh state that is not for frozen section. An example of this would be a spleen sent for lymphoma staging. Always check the facility policy and the physician's request prior to adding formalin to the specimen.

Tissue and Fluid for Biopsy

Biopsy refers to a procedure in which tissue or fluid is removed for diagnosis. The physician obtains a biopsy to have a definitive diagnosis before scheduling further operative intervention or medical treatment. The types of biopsies include excisional, incisional, bone marrow, percutaneous, and aspiration (**Table 15.6**).

Tissue for Hormonal Receptor Site Studies

After a positive diagnosis of malignancy is made by frozen section or routine tissue examination, the physician obtains a specimen from the primary tumor site in the breast, uterus, or prostate. The test measures the amount of certain proteins in cancer tissue. Hormones can attach to these proteins. A high level of hormone receptors may mean that hormones help the cancer grow. The physician will use the results of the test to adjust the patient's treatment plan. The scrub person passes the tissue off the sterile field. While wearing gloves, place the specimen in a container. After the container is labeled, send it to the laboratory with the appropriate paperwork. Facility policy dictates whether the specimen is sent to the laboratory fresh or in formalin or normal saline.

Papanicolaou Test Specimen

The Papanicolaou test, commonly called a Pap smear, is a uterine smear for detecting cancer cells in the mucus of the uterus. The supplies needed include a speculum, spatula, an endocervical brush, and two slides with the patient's name written on the end with a No. 2 pencil. If an ink pen is used, the ink will wash off in the processing. The physician will obtain the ectocervical sample first from the external os using the spatula. Next the physician will obtain the endocervical sample using the brush. The specimen is spread quickly and evenly on the slides and fixed immediately with the facilities approved fixative. The specimen and the appropriate laboratory slip are sent to the cytology department in the laboratory.

Extraordinary Types of Specimens

Examples of extraordinary types of specimens include bullets, intrauterine devices, heart values, orthopedic hardware, and other foreign objects. Process these specimens according to the facility policy. Send these objects to the laboratory in a dry container.

Table 15.6	Tissue and Fluid for Biopsy

Type	Definition
Excisional biopsy	Removal of an entire tissue lesion through an incision in the skin or mucous membranes, or through an endoscopic instrument.
Incisional biopsy	Only a sample of tissue is cut into (incised) and removed through an incision in the skin or mucous membranes, or through an endoscopic instrument.
Bone marrow biopsy	Removal of a sample of bone marrow and a small amount of bone using a large needle. This biopsy is usually performed by a physician and a technologist from the hematology department. ☐ A skin incision or percutaneous puncture is made, and then a trocar puncture needle is inserted into the bone, usually the iliac crest or the sternum. ☐ The first sample is a bone marrow sample which is obtained by aspiration using suction with a syringe. ☐ The second sample is a core biopsy to obtain bone marrow together with bone fibers. After the needle is removed, this solid sample is pushed out of the needle with a wire. ☐ Both samples are microscopically examined to see the cells and architecture of the bone marrow.
Percutaneous needle biopsy	A sample of tissue from internal organs, such as the liver or the prostate gland, is obtained using a hollow needle. ☐ The needle is inserted through the body wall, and the tissue is removed. ☐ Unless instructed otherwise, the nurse prepares the specimen as described for permanent specimens.
Aspiration biopsy	Use of a fine-gauge needle to withdraw fluid from a cyst, abscess, or in a joint or body cavity or cells from lesions in tissue such as the breast, lymph nodes, or thyroid (a drop of blood is aspirated). Specimens sent to pathology for microscopic examination.

MedicineNet.com, http://www.medterms.com/script/main/art.asp?articlekey=30999 (accessed 20 June 2008).

In the case of a foreign object that may be used as evidence in a court case, take care to preserve the integrity of the specimen. Wrap the bullet in gauze sponge and place it in a dry container. If there is more than one bullet, use a separate container for each bullet and label the container with the location of the bullet (ie, chest, abdomen, leg, etc.) Do not allow the bullet to touch metal and take care to avoid scratching it because this can interfere with the policy ballistics test. The patient's clothes may also be used as evidence in the case. Do not cut through the hole made by the bullet when removing the clothing.

COLLECTING AND PREPARING CULTURES FOR EXAMINATION

If the physician identifies or suspects an infectious process during the procedure, a specimen for culture or other bacteriological study is obtained. Types of studies include aerobic, anaerobic, gram stain, acid-fast, and cytology examinations. Whatever the type of study, the purpose of the culture is to identify the pathogen causing the infection. The physician uses this information to order appropriate antibiotics and start a treatment regimen.

Four types of microorganisms cause most nosocomial infections: aerobic bacteria, microaerophilic bacteria, anaerobic bacteria, and nonbacterial microorganisms, such as viruses and fungi. Microaerophilic bacteria require oxygen but can survive with amounts less than are found in the atmosphere, and anaerobic bacteria grow in the absence of oxygen.

Nosocomial infections continue to be a major concern for hospitals. In US hospitals, nosocomial infections account for approximately 1.7 million infections and 99,000 related deaths annually; of these infections, the most common are (CDC, 2008):

- 32% – urinary tract infections;
- 22% – surgical site infections;
- 15% – pneumonia; and
- 14% – bloodstream infections.

MDROs
Multidrug-Resistant
Organisms

Today, all healthcare settings are affected by the emergence and transmission of *multidrug-resistant organisms* (MDROs), defined as microorganisms, predominantly bacteria, that are resistant to one or more classes of antimicrobial agents (CDC, 2006). Antibiotic resistant organisms present challenges in the management and treatment of nosocomial infections; treatment options for these patients are usually very limited and they are also associated with increased lengths of stay, costs, as well as mortality (CDC, 2006). Pathogens such as methicillin-resistant *Staphylococcus aureus* (MRSA), vancomycin-resistant *Staphylococcus aureus*, and vancomycin-resistant enterococci (VRE) are all major concerns. The widespread use of antimicrobials for prophylaxis or therapy is considered to be a major factor in antibiotic resistance (Nguyen, 2007).

General Guidelines

When obtaining fluid, tissue, or other material for culture, obtain enough of a specimen for the completion of all requested tests. Use sterile equipment and receptacles so as not to contaminate the specimen with exogenous microorganisms. Take steps to maintain the integrity of the culture. Specimen contact with chemicals, germicides, or disinfectants may compromise laboratory processing and invalidate study results. At some facilities, if multiple studies are requested the laboratory may request one culture for each test. Check with the facility laboratory manual or the laboratory department.

Aerobic Cultures

Aerobic bacteria require oxygen in order to live. To collect an aerobic culture, use a culturette composed of a sterile culture tube with a cotton swab attached to the lid. Prior to using the culturette system, check the expiration date. There are two acceptable methods of obtaining cultures using the culturette system.

The first method is to remove the sterile tube from the package. Hold the bottom of the tube with one hand while the other hand carefully removes the top of the tube and exposes the distal end of the cotton swab. The scrub person then grasps the swab between the cotton tip and the lid, being careful not to touch and contaminate the swab. The scrub person pulls the swabs out of the lid.

After the culture is taken, hold the tube and have the scrub person carefully insert the swab into the tube. Recap the tube and crush the media ampule at the of the bottom tube by gently squeezing the tube at the ampule. Next, push on the cap to ensure that the swab tip contacts the moistened pledgets. Label the tube and send it to the laboratory with the appropriate laboratory slip. If done correctly, this method is preferable because it ensures that the exterior of the culture tube is not contaminated.

For the second method, aseptically deliver the culture tube and swab to the sterile field. The scrub person removes the cotton swab and passes it to the physician. After the culture is taken, the physician or the scrub person inserts the swab into the tube. The scrub person recaps the tube and passes it off the sterile field. Wearing gloves, take the tube, decontaminate it with a tuberculocidal hospital-grade disinfectant or a 1:10 dilution of household bleach, break the media ampule, push the swab into the media, attach a label, and send it to the laboratory with the appropriate laboratory slip.

Anaerobic Cultures

Anaerobic bacteria do not require oxygen for growth and may even die in the presence of oxygen. When collecting an anaerobic culture, do not expose the specimen or cotton swabs to air for a long period of time. If using a swab to obtain the specimen, take care that it is not aerated. Send anaerobic cultures to the laboratory in an anaerobic culturette system or in a syringe with all air removed. Check the expiration date on the anaerobic culturette system before using it. Use a sterile plastic container for tissue obtained for anaerobic study. In such cases, immediately send the specimen to the laboratory.

Aseptically deliver the anaerobic culture system to the sterile field. The scrub person pulls the cap with the swab attached out of the tube and passes it to he physician. After obtaining the culture, the physician or the scrub person inserts the swab into the tube. While recapping the tube, the scrub person pushes the cap firmly onto the tube with a downward motion.

While wearing gloves, receive the anaerobic culture tube from the scrub person, decontaminate it as described for aerobic culture tubes, attach a label, and immediately send it to the laboratory with the appropriate laboratory slip.

When the physician asks for a syringe to collect fluid for an anaerobic or aerobic culture, aseptically deliver an appropriate-sized syringe to the sterile field. If a needle is needed for collection, use a large-gauge needle. If the physician uses a needle to aspirate fluid for culture, the scrub person must exercise extreme caution and must not recap the syringe. After the physician passes the syringe and needle to the scrub person, the needle should be carefully removed with a clamp and placed in a sharps container on the sterile field. Next, the syringe is capped with a Luer lock plug and passed off the sterile field.

If the physician aspirates the fluid without a needle, the scrub person caps the syringe with a lock plug and passes it off the sterile field. Preferably, the scrub person drops the syringe into an impervious container, such as a specimen transport plastic bag, for transport. Avoid decontaminating a fluid-filled syringe. During decontamination, ejection or leakage of syringe contents is possible by inadvertent pushing or pulling of the plunger.

Label the container with patient and specimen data, mark it to alert laboratory personnel that the syringe is contaminated, and send to the laboratory with the appropriate laboratory slip.

Gram Stains

A gram stain is the most commonly performed microbiology test used to identify the cause of an infection. The gram stain determines whether an infection is caused by an organism that is gram positive or gram negative. The test results guide the physician to prescribe treatment with an appropriate antibiotic. The cultures for a gram stain are collected in an aerobic culturette and immediately transported to the laboratory with the appropriate slip.

After receiving a gram stain culture in the laboratory, the technician smears a film of a culture specimen on a slide, dries and fixes the film with heat, and stains it with crystal (gentian) violet. The gram-positive bacteria retain the violet stain and the gram-negative bacteria adopt the red counterstain (Lab Tests Online, 2008; MedicineNet.com, 2008).

Cerebrospinal Fluid

Fluid removed during a spinal tap may be sent to the laboratory in sterile tubes, which are provided in the spinal tap kit. Separate samples need to be submitted for microbiology, chemistry, and hematology with the appropriate laboratory slips. Ensure that sufficient fluid is collected for each test. Guidelines for minimal amounts are 1.5 to 2 mL per tube. Immediately send the specimens to the laboratory.

Acid-Fast Cultures and Smears

Acid-fast cultures and smears are obtained to isolate Mycobacterium tuberculosis. The test can be done on respiratory secretions (sputum, bronchial washing, transtracheal aspirates, bronchoalveolar lavage, and bronchial brushings) urine, stool, CSF, body fluids, blood and tissue biopsies. The cultures and smears are sent in an aerobic culturette or a sterile specimen container. The specimen and the appropriate laboratory slips need to go immediately to the laboratory.

Fungus Cultures

Mycological studies include direct microscopic examination of a smear and culturing. Acceptable specimens include respiratory tract fluids (sputum, bronchial washings, transtracheal aspirates, bronchoalveolar lavage, and bronchial brushings), urine, CSF, exudates, abscess contents, secretions, vaginal material, skin, nails, hair, tissue, and whole blood. Swabs are acceptable for vaginal specimens but discouraged for other specimens. Send the specimen in a sterile, leak-proof container. As with other specimens, label the specimen for mycological studies, and immediately send to the laboratory with the appropriate laboratory slip.

DIRECTING THE TRANSFER OF SPECIMENS AND CULTURES TO THE LABORATORY

Correctly transporting specimens and cultures to the laboratory is essential for continuity of care. The transporter must understand where and to whom the specimen or culture is to be delivered. Assistive personnel responsible for transportation duties should receive specific training on handling specimens and cultures during transportation. Training should include log book completion, precautions, and recognition and identification of laboratory slips.

COMMUNICATING LABORATORY OR PATHOLOGY REPORTS TO THE PHYSICIAN DURING THE PROCEDURE

The nurse facilitates the communication of laboratory or pathology reports between the physician and the laboratory or the pathology department. Direct communication between the physician and the pathologist or the laboratory technician is preferred. Notify the pathologist or technician if the patient is awake for the procedure. If the circulating nurse must serve as a conduit of oral communication, the information should be written by the nurse, verified for accuracy with the pathologist or the laboratory technician, and then given to the physician. When written reports are received during the procedure, attach them to the patient's record.

STORING, PRESERVING, AND MAINTAINING TISSUE

Tissue banking should only be established in facilities where there is a need. Surgical tissue banking includes the procuring, processing, preserving, and storing of selected human tissue and cells. Human tissue includes bone, cartilage, ligaments, tendons, fascia, dura mater, sclera, corneas, heart valves, bone marrow, vessels, and skin. Each facility should establish guidelines for storing, preserving, and maintaining tissue banks according to the American Association of Tissue Banks (AATB) and the regulations and recommendation of the US Food and Drug Administration (FDA) (AORN, 2008, pp. 609–610).

Potential donors should be assessed for and be free of communicable disease agents and diseases. Exclusion criteria include: active systemic viral, bacterial, or fungal infection (eg, viral hepatitis); disease history of unknown etiology; human immunodeficiency virus (HIV); syphilis; cytomegalovirus; autoimmune diseases (eg, systemic lupus erythematosus); neurological disease of unknown cause; human-derived growth hormone; and fever associated with a possible infectious etiology (AORN, 2008, p. 602).

Policies regarding donor and recipient tissue banking vary from facility to facility. Each facility should have a tissue bank administration staff. These individuals need to remain informed of changes in the recommendations of the CDC and AATB.

AORN's *Recommended Practices for Surgical Tissue Banking* provides guidelines for recovering, processing, and transplanting tissue in a sterile environment. The tissue is removed under strict aseptic conditions and placed in a sterile container to prevent contamination of the tissue. Aerobic and anaerobic tissue cultures should be collected in conjunction with surgical tissue banking. Label the specimen container, indicating the type of tissue, recovery date and time, the type of preservation solution, and its concentration. Freeze tissue for transplantation at a later date as soon as possible to prevent microbial growth. Refrigerate skin intended for future skin grafting to minimize cellular oxygen consumption and prolong cellular life (AORN, 2008, p. 607). **Table 15.7** provides storage guidelines for various types of tissue. **Table 15.8** provides guidelines for assigning expiration dates for stored tissue.

If a tissue bank is established in the operative or invasive procedure suite, restrict access to the storage refrigeration and freezer units to authorized personnel. Access to storage units by unauthorized personnel increases the risk for tissue compromise.

AATB
American Association of Tissue Banks

FDA
US Food and Drug Administration

HIV
Human Immunodeficiency Virus

15

Table 15.7	Recommended Temperature Ranges for Refrigerators and Freezers Used for Surgical Tissue Banking	
Tissue Type and Mode	**Temperature**	
Lyophilized or dehydrated musculoskeletal tissue	Ambient temperature or cooler (but not frozen)	
Refrigerated musculoskeletal and osteoarticular tissue aseptically recovered and stored in isotonic solution containing suitable antibiotics	33.8° F (1° C) to 50° F (10° C)	
Refrigerated skin	33.8° F (1° C) to 50° F (10° C)	
Frozen musculoskeletal and osteoarticular tissue	Long term: −40° F (−40° C) or colder Short-term (fewer than six months): between −4° F (−20° C) to −40° F (−40° C)	
Frozen or cryopreserved skin	−40° F (−40° C) or colder	
Frozen, cryopreserved cardiovascular tissue	−148° F (−100° C) or colder	
Reproductive cells	Frozen and cryopreserved in a liquid nitrogen freezer Storage may be either the liquid or vapor phase	

Association of periOperative Registered Nurses (AORN) (2008). Recommended practices for surgical tissue banking. *Perioperative Standards and Recommended Practices.* Denver, CO, p. 606.

Table 15.8	Recommended Expiration Dates for Stored Tissue	
Tissue Type and Mode		**Time**
Lyophilized or dehydrated tissue	⟶	5 years
Refrigerated musculoskeletal tissue	⟶	5 days
Refrigerated skin	⟶	14 days
Frozen or cryopreserved cells and tissue −40° F (−40° C) or colder	⟶	5 years

Association of periOperative Registered Nurses (AORN) (2008). Recommended practices for surgical tissue banking. *Perioperative Standards and Recommended Practices.* Denver, CO, p. 607.

Storage units should be monitored and daily temperature checks recorded, have annual calibration checks, and have an alarm system that is continuously monitored and that sounds when the temperature is not within the acceptable range. Prepare a written contingency plan should a refrigerator or freezer malfunction. The surgical tissue bank should keep accurate records of the disuse. Develop and maintain surgical tissue banking records according to the recommendations of the AATB and in compliance with FDA rules (AORN, 2008, pp. 608–609).

COMPETENCY ASSESSMENT
Handle Specimens and Cultures

Name: _____ Title: _____ Unit: _____ Date of Validation: _____

Type of Validation: ☐ Initial   ☐ Annual   ☐ Bi-annual

COMPETENCY STATEMENT: The nurse demonstrates competency to collect, identify, document, process, store, preserve, and transport specimens and cultures.

Performance Criteria	Met	Not Met
1. Identifies legal implications of handling specimens and cultures	☐	☐
2. Identifies the patient's risk for adverse outcomes related to the improper handling of specimens and cultures	☐	☐
3. Implements infection control practices when handling specimens and cultures	☐	☐
4. Safely handles formalin	☐	☐
5. Provides supplies and equipment to collect specimens and cultures	☐	☐
6. Completes laboratory requisitions	☐	☐
7. Documents the collection of specimens and cultures	☐	☐
8. Establishes chain of custody for specimens and cultures	☐	☐
9. Collects and prepares tissue for examination	☐	☐
10. Collects and prepares cultures for examination	☐	☐
11. Directs the transfer of specimens and cultures to the laboratory	☐	☐
12. Communicates pathology reports to the physician during the procedure	☐	☐
13. Demonstrates knowledge of storing, preserving, and maintaining tissue	☐	☐

_____

Validator's Signature

_____

Employee's Signature

_____

Validator's Printed Name

REFERENCES

1. Association of periOperative Registered Nurses. (2008). *Perioperative Standards and Recommended Practices*. Denver, CO: AORN, Inc.
2. Centers for Disease Control and Prevention. (2008). Estimates of health-care associated infections. Retrieved June 3, 2008 from http://www.cdc.gov/ncidod/dhqp/hai.html.
3. Centers for Disease Control and Prevention. (2006). Management of multi-drug resistant organisms in healthcare settings, 2006. Retrieved June 3, 2008 from http://www.cdc.gov/ncidod/dhqp/pdf/ar/MDROGuideline2006.pdf.
4. College of American Pathologists. College of American Pathologists' policy on surgical specimens to be submitted to pathology for examination. Retrieved January 9, 2008 from http://www.cap.org/apps/docs/laboratory_accreditation/surgical_specimens.pdf.
5. Lab Tests Online. Gram Stain. Retrieved February 15, 2008 from http://labtestsonline.org/understanding/analytes/gram_stain/test.html.
6. Lippi, G., Salvagno, G., Montagnana, M., Franchini, M., & Guidi, G. (2006). Phlebotomy issues and quality improvement in results of laboratory testing. *Clinical Laboratory*, 52(5–6), 217–230.
7. Makary, M., Epstein, J., Pronovost, P., Millman, E., Hartmann, E., & Freischlag, J. (2007). Surgical specimen identification errors: A new measure of quality in surgical care. *Surgery*, 141(4), 450–455.
8. MedicineNet.com. Definition of gram stain. Retrieved April 21, 2008 from http://www.medterms.com/script/main/art.asp?articlekey=9583.
9. Nguyen, Q.V. (2007). Hospital-Acquired Infections. *eMedicine.* August 21, 2007. Retrieved April 21, 2008 from http://www.emedicine.com/ped/fulltopic/topic1619.htm#section~Workup.
10. Phillips, N. (2007). Foundations of perioperative patient care standards. In *Berry & Kohn's operating room technique*, 11th ed. St. Louis, MO: Mosby Elsevier.
11. US Department of Labor, Occupational Safety & Health Administration. Substance technical guidelines for formalin—1910.1048 App A. Retrieved January 2, 2008 from http://www.osha.gov/pls/oshaweb/owadisp.show_document?p_table=STANDARDS&p_id=10076.
12. Yvette, C.T. (2008) *Nosocomial Infections: Impact on Patient Care.* Pharmacy Times, March 2006 http://www.pharmacytimes.com/issues/articles/2006–03_3202.asp (accessed 21 April 2008).

CHAPTER 16

Handle Tissue with Instruments

Mary Weis

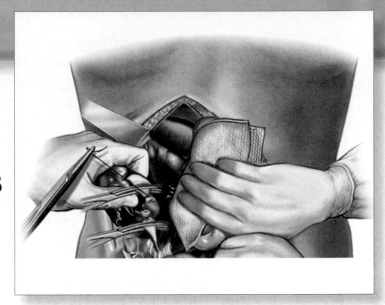

INTRODUCTION

Handle tissue with instruments refers to skills that the first assistant (FA) uses to provide exposure of the operative site and to clamp, grasp, suture, and cut tissue. Every operation, because of the mere fact that tissue is cut, causes injury to the patient. The first assistant minimizes this injury by carefully and gently handling tissues. Careful, gentle, correct handling of tissues and instruments improves the result of any operation, thus minimizing damage and accelerating healing.

HISTORICAL PERSPECTIVES

As early as 10,000 B.C., people used sharpened flint knives to perform surgery. Egyptian writings dating back to 3000 B.C. tell of tourniquets. These early writings, as well as mummies found with wounds sutured with linen, reveal the use of suture ligatures. Early Hindu physicians were even more skillful than the Egyptians. They treated fractures and also practiced a crude form of plastic surgery. Early Greek carvings depict the use of scalpels. Early Arabian physicians used cautery to control hemorrhage. Hippocrates (460–377 B.C.) recommended hot irons to control bleeding.

Ammonius (c. 247 B.C.) wrote of an instrument used to impale a bladder stone. Albucasis (d. A.D. 1013) illustrated a large number of instruments, including a trocar (for paracentesis), scissors, and a syringe. He also described the use of animal gut for sutures. Galen (A.D. 130) depicted a method of grasping a vein with a hook and twisting it to stop bleeding, and he also recommended the use of a linen ligature for an artery.

In the 14th century, instruments remained relatively crude, even though modifications were made. During this century, the bullet extractor was introduced. Riveted handles were designed in the 16th century. Ambrose

Chapter Contents

FA
First Assistant

Paré (1510–1590) used a forceps shaped like a "crow's bill." Instruments remained crude, however, because they were made by blacksmiths, armorers, and cutlers. It was not uncommon for a surgeon to use carpenter's tools, as well as kitchen knives and forks.

Hospitals began to provide appointments for surgeons in the 18th century. More surgery was being attempted, and it was evolving into a scientific discipline. Coppersmiths, silversmiths, woodcutters, and steelworkers began to produce instruments. These instruments were limited in use, however, in that only operations of dire need, such as amputations, were performed regularly. Instruments were often works of art, with intricately carved handles made of wood or ivory, and were stored in velvet-lined boxes.

The 19th century produced great changes in the design of instruments. Two important discoveries were responsible. The first was Sir Humphrey Davy's introduction of anesthesia in 1846. This enabled surgeons to work more cautiously because they no longer had to operate speedily on a struggling patient. As operative techniques were refined, a larger array of instruments was needed. The second development, in 1867, was Joseph Lister's (1827–1912) antiseptic method for the prevention of infection. Instruments needed to be sterilized, and so the ornate, hand-carved instrument handles were replaced with metal ones. This was the beginning of modern surgery.

In 1900, stainless steel was introduced and became the preferred metal for making instruments. The pivot forceps and ratchet were also developed. As surgical specialties evolved, the number of different instruments increased vastly. Today, thousands of instruments are available for every purpose and preference to fulfill the needs of all surgeons.

GENTLE HANDLING OF TISSUE

William Stewart Halsted (1852–1922) established the first school of surgery in the late 19th century at Johns Hopkins Hospital in Baltimore. Adopting Theodore Kocher's bloodless technique, Halstead emphasized the concepts of complete hemostasis, gentle manipulation of tissues, absolute asepsis, sharp dissection, and accurate reapproximation of divided tissues. He also introduced the wearing of rubber gloves during an operation. When Halsted's principles of operative technique were abused, complications such as hematoma, infection, wound disruption, and contracture often occurred. Over the years, Halsted's principles have remained intact and surgeons have learned that there are no substitutes for careful, gentle handling of tissue and accurate surgical technique.

INSTRUMENT TERMINOLOGY

Thousands of surgical instruments of varying sizes and shapes are available for use by the surgeon. Most of these instruments are categorized as sharps, clamps, graspers, and retractors (**Table 16.1**).

MEASURABLE CRITERIA

The first assistant demonstrates competency to handle tissues with instruments by:

- Identifying the patient's risk for adverse outcomes related to the handling of tissue with instruments;
- Providing exposure during surgery;

Table 16.1	**Categories of Instruments**	
Category	**Examples**	**Uses**
Cutting, grinding, and dissecting	Scalpels Scissors Bone cutters Rongeurs Chisels Osteotomes Saws Curets Dermatomes Electrosurgery active electrodes	Designed to cut or separate tissue and bone
Clamping	Hemostats (artery forceps) Vascular clamps Intestinal clamps	Designed to control bleeding and maintain hemostasis; may be used to grasp or retract tissue
Grasping and holding	Tissue forceps Tenacula Rib approximators Sponge forceps Towel clips Needle holders	Designed to grasp and hold tissue or bone during dissection, retraction, suturing
Retracting	Self-retaining Hand-held	Designed to provide exposure with minimal trauma to surrounding tissue
Probing	Probes	Designed to enter natural openings, such as the common bile duct or fistulas
Dilating or enlarging	Uterine dilators Urethral dilators	Designed to expand the size of an opening, such as the urethra or cervical os
Suctioning	Suction tubes	Designed to remove blood and other fluids from a surgical or dental operative field

Adapted from http://www.surgeryencyclopedia.com/St-Wr/Surgical-Instruments.html, 2007—Advameg Inc.

- Clamping tissue;
- Grasping tissue;
- Suturing;
- Cutting tissue; and
- Maintaining a dry field.

IDENTIFYING THE PATIENT'S RISK FOR ADVERSE OUTCOMES RELATED TO THE HANDLING OF TISSUE WITH INSTRUMENTS

Table 16.2 identifies the desired outcome for the patient care event of handle tissue with instruments. Listed in the table are criteria for this outcome with the applicable

Table 16.2	Handling Tissue with Instruments Does Not Compromise or Cause Injury to the Patient

Outcome 1 The patient is free from evidence of postprocedure wound infection.

Diagnosis

Risk for Infection related to the handling of tissue with instruments during the operative or invasive procedure

Risk Factors

- ☐ AIDS
- ☐ Alcoholism
- ☐ Altered integumentary system
- ☐ Altered or insufficient leukocytes
- ☐ Arthritis
- ☐ Bites (animal, insect, human)
- ☐ Cancer
- ☐ Diabetes mellitus
- ☐ Dialysis
- ☐ Excessive handling of tissue
- ☐ Existing infection
- ☐ Hematological disorders
- ☐ Hepatic disorders
- ☐ History of infections
- ☐ Immunodeficiency
- ☐ Immunosuppression
- ☐ Inadequate hemostasis
- ☐ Lymphedema
- ☐ Malnutrition
- ☐ Medication such as chemotherapy, immunosuppressants
- ☐ Medication therapy such as chemotherapy and immunosuppressants
- ☐ Nutritional deficiencies: proteins, carbohydrates, zinc, and vitamins A, B, C, and K
- ☐ Obesity
- ☐ Organ transplant
- ☐ Periodontal disease
- ☐ Peripheral vascular disease
- ☐ Poor approximation of tissues, resulting in the formation of dead space
- ☐ Radiation
- ☐ Renal failure
- ☐ Respiratory disorders
- ☐ Smoking
- ☐ Surgery
- ☐ Total parenteral nutrition
- ☐ Trauma
- ☐ Use of contaminated instruments

Outcome Indicators

72 hours postprocedure

- ☐ Is cellulitis present around the wound?
- ☐ Does the patient have signs and symptoms of an abscess?
- ☐ Does the patient have lymphangitis?
- ☐ Does the patient have signs and symptom of gas gangrene?
- ☐ Does the patient have signs and symptoms of Meleney's ulcer?
- ☐ Did the patient experience dehiscence?

Outcome 2   The patient is free from evidence of injury related to handling tissue with instruments.

Diagnosis

Risk for Injury related to handling of tissue with instruments during the procedure

Risk Factors

- [ ] Altered circulation
- [ ] Direct pressure on body surface from members of the surgical team
- [ ] Emaciation
- [ ] Excessive abduction or adduction of extremities during the procedure
- [ ] Excessive or improper retraction of tissue
- [ ] Exposure of the operative site with a retractor intended for use only in selected procedures or on a specific type of tissue
- [ ] Extended operative procedure
- [ ] Extremes in age, height, and body build
- [ ] Failure to evaluate the type of tissue, location of vascular or nerve structures, and the presence of organs in relation to the method used to provide exposure
- [ ] Improper clamping or grasping of tissue
- [ ] Inadequate hemostasis
- [ ] Obesity
- [ ] Presence of physical deformities or limitations
- [ ] Use of an intestinal bag

Outcome Indicators

- [ ] Does the patient show evidence of impaired physical mobility (inability to move, decreased active joint range of motion, and decreased muscle strength or control) after the procedure?
- [ ] Does the patient show evidence of impaired tissue integrity (excessive swelling at the operative site, skin discoloration on body surfaces) after the procedure?
- [ ] Does the patient show evidence of altered tissue perfusion (cold extremities diminished arterial pulses, blood pressure changes in extremities, discoloration of an extremity) after the procedure?
- [ ] Does the patient complain of excessive discomfort (excluding incisional pain) after the procedure?

Outcome 3   The patient is free from evidence of impaired tissue integrity at the wound site.

Diagnosis

Risk for Impaired Tissue Integrity related to the handling of tissue with instruments during the procedure.

Risk Factors

- [ ] Anemia
- [ ] Arteriosclerosis
- [ ] Autoimmune alterations such as lupus erythematosus and scleroderma
- [ ] Bleeding disorders
- [ ] Cancer
- [ ] Cardiopulmonary disorders
- [ ] Cirrhosis
- [ ] Dehydration
- [ ] Diabetes mellitus
- [ ] Edema
- [ ] Emaciation
- [ ] Hepatitis
- [ ] Hyperthermia
- [ ] Inadequate approximation of tissue, resulting in the formation of dead space Poor knot-tying technique; use of an inappropriate knot

Outcome Indicators

- [ ] Is the swelling at the wound site?
- [ ] Is the wound discolored? Does it have a serosanguineous discharge?
- [ ] Does the patient complain of excessive pain at the wound site?

16

- [ ] Jaundice
- [ ] Malnutrition
- [ ] Nutritional alterations
- [ ] Nutritional deficiencies
- [ ] Obesity
- [ ] Peripheral vascular alterations
- [ ] Poor intraoperative hemostasis
- [ ] Renal failure
- [ ] Thyroid dysfunction
- [ ] Venous stasis
- [ ] Wound infection

Adapted from Carpentino-Moyet, L. J. (2008). *Handbook of nursing diagnosis* (12th ed.). Philadelphia: Lippincott Williams & Wilkins, pp. 237, 340.

nursing diagnoses, risk factors, and expected outcomes specific to each nursing diagnosis.

PROVIDING EXPOSURE

Achieving operative site exposure requires adequate traction. A poorly exposed operative site because of inadequate retraction impedes the surgeon. Likewise, overly aggressive traction, although achieving good exposure, may cause injury to the patient.

When a surgeon requests exposure, the first assistant applies the principles of traction and countertraction. Countertraction creates a plane of dissection that opens the connective tissue and provides exposure. It also gives the surgeon the necessary resistance during dissection of the organ or structure.

Approach the task of providing exposure from a nursing perspective. Think about operative exposure while assessing the patient, planning and implementing patient care, and after the procedure while evaluating the patient.

Assess the patient before the procedure, and develop a plan of care that provides balanced traction to meet the exposure needs of the surgeon and protect the patient from injury. Focus the assessment on patient variables such as age, height, weight, body build, and physical deformities or limitations that affect your ability to provide exposure. Review the planned procedure to include the stages of the procedure that require exposure, the type of tissue and the location of vascular or nerve structures, the presence of organs, and the type of instruments available for exposure.

During the procedure, implement the plan and continually assess the operative site to determine the effectiveness of providing exposure. If variables change during the procedure, modify the plan accordingly. The first assistant must anticipate each step of the procedure and respond to the surgeon's moves with the appropriate follow-up move. A synergy develops and there is a synchronized movement between surgeon and first assistant. The assistant must constantly assess the operative site to ensure effective exposure and to prevent unnecessary tissue injury. After the procedure, assess the patient to determine the presence of injury related to the provision of exposure.

Stabilization of Anatomical Structures

Sponges

Use laparotomy sponges and 4 × 4 or 4 × 8 inch (10 × 10 or 10 × 20 cm) radiopaque sponges to stabilize and hold anatomical structures. Wet or dry, use sponges to hold back tissue or push it out of the way, thus providing better exposure for the surgeon. Grasp and hold tissue such as muscle, fascia, subcutaneous tissue, and skin with radiopaque 4 × 4 or 4 × 8 inch (10 × 10 or 10 × 20 cm) sponges (**Fig. 16.1**). Because of the small size of radiopaque sponges, however, do not use them in the abdominal cavity. Laparotomy sponges provide an excellent means for grasping and holding internal organs such as the large and small intestines. When using sponges to move or hold anatomical structures, handle the tissue gently but firmly; gentleness prevents bruising, tearing, and puncturing of the tissue, and firmness prevents slipping of the tissue from the assistant's hand. Organs or tissues can be packed out of the way with lap sponges to prevent obstruction of the surgeon's view. Before packing, have the scrub person moisten the sponges in warm normal saline. Keep track of the number of sponges used, and thoroughly examine the cavity for retained sponges before closure.

Intestinal Bag

An intestinal bag keeps the bowel moist, aids in retaining body heat, and protects the bowel from inadvertent abrasion during an extended procedure. When using an intestinal bag, monitor the moisture content of the bag and the tissue integrity of the bowel. Maintain moisture content with a wet towel or a large laparotomy sponge. Prevent inadvertent strangulation of the bowel by supporting the bag. A stack of towels placed between the assistant and the patient aids in this process.

Figure 16.1

Using a 4 × 4 sponge to grasp the scalp flap.

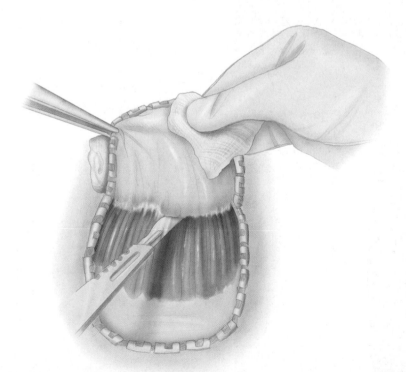

Impervious Stockinet

When isolating an extremity, use impervious stockinet to hold, reposition, or provide traction on the extremity during the procedure (**Fig. 16.2**).

Tapes and Other Devices

Use tapes, such as cotton cord ties, vessel loops, and Penrose drains to move or hold anatomical structures during the procedure and better view the operative field (**Fig. 16.3**). When using tapes, the surgeon exposes the tissue and then passes the tape around the tissue. After the tape is in place, the surgeon can gently move the structure from the operative field. Exercise care when moving or holding a structure with a tape: Too much traction may tear the tissue; likewise, insufficient traction

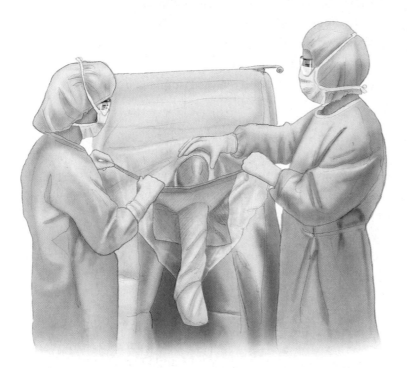

Figure 16.2

The patient is draped for an arthroscopy with an impervious stockinet which allows for manipulation of the leg during the procedure.

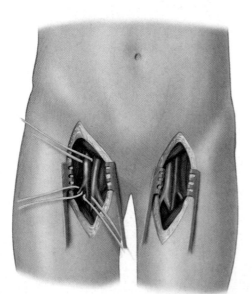

Figure 16.3

Use of vessel loops used to identify and isolate femoral arteries.

does not hold the structure steady and moves it from the operative field. A gentle, steady pull usually provides adequate traction. Learning to apply the correct amount of traction in varying situations comes with experience.

Suture Stitch

Sutures provide good retraction without the bulk of retractors. When applied correctly, they will hold tissue out of the way. Sutures are helpful in everting or fixing small mobile structures such as retracting open an arteriotomy. After the surgeon places the stitch, use it to apply the necessary traction. The amount of tension that can be exerted on the suture depends on the fragility of the tissue and the tensile strength of the suture. The surgeon may also attach the stitch to an instrument and use the weight of the instrument to apply the traction. If needed, use this stitch to lift or hold tissue out of the operative field. On very fragile tissue, the surgeon may use a pledget of Teflon felt to keep the suture from cutting the tissue.

Use of Retractors, Grasping Instruments, and Other Devices

All members of the operative team use retractors, grasping instruments, and other devices to expose the operative field. Hand-held or self-retaining retractors move and hold tissue and organs out of the operative field. Retractors come in many designs. They may be sharp or blunt; flat, round, or curved; wide or narrow; short or long; malleable, hinged, or fixed; and straight or angled. Other instruments such as clamps, stick sponges, and suction cannulas push tissue and organs away from or pull them toward the surgeon thus providing exposure of the operative field.

Before using a retractor or any other device, assess the operative site. A misplaced retractor can compress, tear, or stretch blood vessels, nerves, and organs. The wrong type of grasping instrument can puncture delicate tissue, thus causing complications during the after the procedure. Assessment factors include the size and depth of the operative site, the physiological status of the tissue, and the operative time. After placing retractors or using exposure devices, evaluate the tissue. If signs such as tissue blanching, cessation of pulse, or leaking of fluid appear, evaluate exposure methods. If the patient complains of excessive musculoskeletal pain, neuromuscular impairment, or unexplained fever after the procedure, determine whether exposure techniques were too aggressive or whether an organ was inadvertently punctured.

Self-Retaining Retractors

Available in all sizes, shapes, and forms, self-retaining retractors isolate and hold all types of tissue, from the most superficial to the deepest. Self-retaining retractors are designed to provide continuous and unchanging retraction (**Fig. 16.4**). The retractor does not need to be held, thus the assistant's hands are available to assist in other ways. This helps in preventing fatigue of the assistant normally used on muscle; smooth self-retaining retractor blades prevent tearing. Blades with sharp or dull teeth hold fasciae, subcutaneous tissue, and skin. Care must be taken when placing the self-retaining retractor to prevent injury to nerves, vascular structures, organs, or tissue by accidentally pinching the structure in the mechanism of the retractor. Moistened sponges should be used on wound edges or on organs to prevent drying of the tissue, tissue friction, and abrasion.

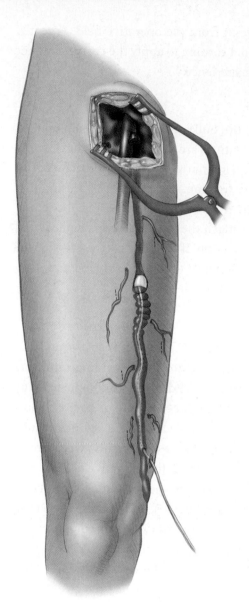

Figure 16.4

Providing exposure of the right femoral vein with a self-retaining retractor.

Handheld Retractors

Handheld retractors provide exposure by the assistant holding a retractor continuously for the duration needed (**Fig. 16.5**). The handheld retractor has many advantages as it can be quickly positioned and repositioned. The assistant can vary the pressure by pulling harder for more exposure and easing up on the pressure when less exposure is needed. The amount of traction can be altered as needed which eases the vasculature on the tissue under the retractor and allows reoxygenation to the capillary network. The handheld retractor may be necessary to prevent injury to fragile tissue. The major disadvantage of a handheld retractor is that one or both of the assistant's hands are not available to provide assistance during the procedure. There may often be the need for more than one assistant. Prolonged use of a handheld retractor may cause the assistant fatigue. The assistant should hold the retractor in a position that causes the least amount of discomfort, fatigue, or strain. The grasp should not be any harder than necessary because it will increase hand fatigue. It is important not

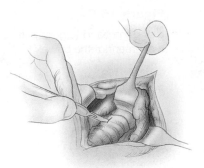

Figure 16.5

Using a handheld retractor to provide exposure during a tracheostomy.

to lean on the patient as this could cause a pressure injury to the patient. Excessive pulling on the retractor could result in tissue laceration or pressure injury to structures such as nerves. When placing the retractor, the assistant must be cognizant of anatomy to avoid injury to nerves, organs, or vascular structures.

Retractors designed with prongs are useful for retraction of shallow tissue such as skin or subcutaneous tissue. The prongs may be sharp and thus hold better, but they may cause tissue trauma. Blunt prongs are less likely to lacerate tissue. Malleable instruments are flexible and available in different lengths and widths. They are versatile and can be bent into various angles and lengths to retract when a unique angle is needed.

Stick and Peanut Sponges

Tissue is pushed aside with stick sponges and peanut sponges (Kittner dissector sponges). Stick sponges are used on straight or curved Forester sponge forceps, and peanut sponges are used on a Rochester-Pean clamp. The peanut sponge serves well as a blunt tissue dissector.

Suction Devices

Suction cannulas such as the Poole abdominal and Yankauer tonsil suction tubes are used, if needed, as exposure devices. When used in such a way, they clear fluids from the field as well as push tissue out of the way which is essential for visualization. Suction tips that have a single-end opening can cause aspiration injury to the tissue. If this occurs, force should not be used to pull tissue out of the suction tip. Instead, the suction should be broken by bending the suction tubing, then gently remove the tissue. Trauma to the tissue can occur if suction is used carelessly. Suction tips can puncture, tear, or abrade tissue.

Hands

The hands provide exposure by manually cupping, compressing, and pulling tissue and organs out of the way or into the line of sight (**Fig. 16.6**). Manual retraction allows controlled pressure, thus reducing the risk of tearing or puncturing the tissue or organ. Hands often provide better exposure than do instruments. The hand is gently padded, soft, and is responsive to the texture of tissue being retracted through tactile sensation.

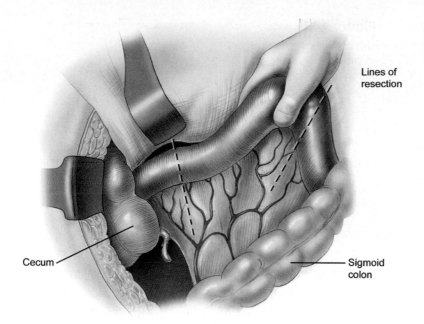

Figure 16.6

Using the hand to gently lift a segment of the bowel.

Lines of resection

Cecum

Sigmoid colon

Laparoscopic Retractors

Laparoscopic retractors and graspers come in a variety of styles (**Fig. 16.7**) and are used to retract and provide exposure during laparoscopic surgery. The first assistant needs to adapt surgical skills to endoscopic and minimally invasive procedures. The assistant needs to compensate for the loss of depth perception and a three-dimensional view. The loss of tactile sensation brings a new feel to the procedure. Care must be taken to avoid overly aggressive retraction as this may cause tissue laceration. The assistant needs to accurately judge the degree of tension being

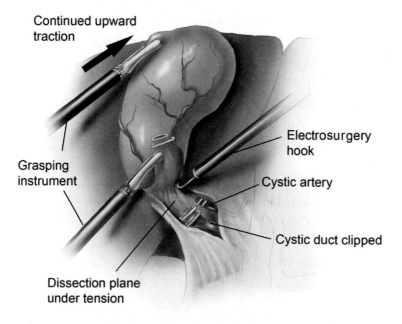

Figure 16.7

Using a laparoscopic grasping instrument to provide traction and grasp the gall bladder during a laparoscopic cholecystectomy.

Continued upward traction

Grasping instrument

Electrosurgery hook

Cystic artery

Cystic duct clipped

Dissection plane under tension

applied to tissue. Self-retaining instrumentation is also available for retraction purposes. These instruments are usually held in place by a retractor that is locked in place during the procedure.

CLAMPING TISSUE

Clamps, used to hold tissue in place, come in many sizes and shapes to accommodate the purposes of use and varieties of tissue in the body (**Fig. 16.8**). They can be small and delicate, such as those used in eye surgery, or large and heavy, such as those used for procedures on bone. Clamps also vary in length and type of serration. Some clamps have straight, curved, or angled tips; others have unusual configurations such as oval, triangular, or barrel-shaped tips.

The most widely used instrument for operative procedures is the *hemostatic artery forceps*. Also called a *hemostat*, this instrument is commonly used to grasp superficial vessels. When using a hemostat, place your thumb and middle finger inside the rings. Hold your index finger of the same hand on the handle for stabilization. Apply the hemostat so that the tip is as close as possible to the divided end of the vessel. Remove your fingers from inside the rings. Next, grasp the closed ring with your thumb and middle finger. After obtaining this position, gently and slightly lift and tilt the tip toward the surgeon. Your index finger is then free to open the ratchet by applying pressure against the ring just as the surgeon increases the tension on the first knot. Carefully release the hemostat and fully open it with a gradual, smooth motion.

Vascular clamps provide hemostasis or partial occlusion until the vessel can be sutured. These, too, are available in many sizes and shapes. Some jaws have many rows of fine teeth; others are designed to receive cushioned insets. After placing the clamp, hold it gently by the shank to avoid twisting or pulling. As with any hemostat, open the clamp widely before removing it, to prevent drag on or accidental tears of the vessel. Use *non-crushing clamps* in general surgery for intestinal operations. During transection of the small bowel, intestinal clamps that have been fitted with shods are placed on a segment of the bowel to prevent spillage of enteric contents during the procedure. Clamps are designed to be used on every organ of the body. Examples of commonly used clamps designed for specific tissue are the Heaney hysterectomy forceps, Herrick kidney pedicle clamp, Best common duct stone forceps, and Judd-DeMartel gallbladder forceps.

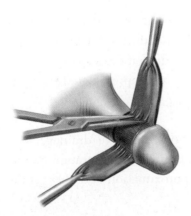

Figure 16.8

Hemostats are used to gently grasp and retract the foreskin during a circumcision.

GRASPING TISSUE

When possible, lift tissue with the gentlest of all instruments—the fingers. Because good exposure is necessary and tissue is slippery, however, use forceps as an extension of your fingers. Grasp the forceps like a pencil and squeeze together by applying pressure with your thumb and index finger.

Forceps should have light springs that enable application with the least pressure necessary to hold the tissue. Crushing of tissue can result if the grip is too tight. Check forceps before the procedure to see that they close precisely. Many varieties are available: smooth-jawed or single- or multiple-toothed and fine or bulky forceps. Most forceps are straight. The bayonet forceps, often used in small deep areas, is shaped so that the fingers do not block visibility.

Use smooth-jawed forceps on tissue that would likely bleed or easily perforate, such as bowel and liver tissue. Toothed forceps are required for skin, dense tissue, and scar tissue. Use forceps throughout the procedure to lift tissue and provide countertraction and stabilization. When selecting tissue forceps, consider tissue sensitivity and its susceptibility to crushing. Examples of dressing forceps include Cushing and Brophy dressing forceps and Cushing, Adson, and Singly tissue forceps. Smooth tissue forceps and scissors are used to open the peritoneum. When a thyroidectomy is performed, use Lahey forceps to grasp the thyroid gland.

SUTURING

Injured body tissues, whether injured from trauma or surgery, respond immediately to the injury and begin to heal. The healing process is facilitated if the operative team controls infection by (1) maintaining sterile and aseptic technique and (2) properly ligating and approximating tissues with sutures to control bleeding, bring tissues together, and hold them in place while healing. **Table 16.3** lists principles of operative technique for healing.

Wound Healing

Wound healing occurs by first, second, or third intention. The first assistant must understand these processes because each has useful applications when closing operative incisions or traumatic wounds.

First-Intention Wound Healing

First-intention healing occurs by primary union of the incised tissues. Most patients heal by first intention if tissue damage is minimal during the operation, if aseptic conditions are maintained, if tissue is gently handled, if dead space is eliminated, if hemostasis is achieved, and if tissues are accurately approximated.

Second-Intention Wound Healing

Complications such as wound dehiscence, infection, excessive drainage, and excessive scar formation impede healing by first intention. Infection, trauma resulting in excessive tissue destruction or loss, and poor approximation of tissues set the stage for healing by second intention.

Table 16.3	**Principles of Operative Technique**
Plan the incision.	Planning and designing the location, length, and depth of the incision achieves optimal exposure. Making the incision just, long enough affords sufficient operating space while reducing the amount of tissue trauma. The direction of the incision may be a factor in wound healing. Wounds heal side-to-side, not end-to-end.
Make the skin incision with one stroke of evenly applied pressure on the scalpel.	Making the skin incision with one stroke of evenly applied pressure on the scalpel aids in tissue approximation during wound closure. Sharp dissection cuts through other tissues. While cutting, watch for underlying nerves, blood vessels, and muscles to preserve as many as possible.
Handle tissue carefully and as little as possible.	Careful placement and handling of retractors prevent undue pressure on tissues. Excessive pressure and tension on tissues impair circulation of blood, slow lymph flow, alter the local physiological state of the wound, and predispose to microbial colonization. Reducing tissue trauma to a minimum aids the healing mechanisms of the body.
Provide hemostasis.	Hemostasis not only prevents loss of the patient's blood but also provides a field as bloodless as possible for accurate dissection. Bleeding may occur from transected or penetrated vessels or as a diffuse oozing from large, denuded surfaces. Mass ligation of large areas of tissue may produce necrosis and prolong healing time. Complete hemostasis before closing of the wound reduces the chance of hematoma formation. A hematoma or seroma in the incision prevents the direct approximation essential to the union of wound surfaces. Either can act as a culture medium for microbial growth, leading to wound infection.
Preserve blood supply.	Preservation of the blood supply to the wound promotes optimal healing.
Debride necrotic and devitalized tissue.	Adequate debridement of all necrotic and devitalized tissue and removal of inflicted foreign bodies promote healing, especially of traumatic wounds. Foreign bodies, such as dirt, metal, and glass, increase the probability of wound infection.
Keep tissues moist.	Periodic irrigation of the wound with warm normal saline solution or covering exposed surfaces with saline-moistened sponges or laparotomy tapes prevents drying of tissues during long procedures.
Carefully and accurately approximate tissues.	Approximation of tissues as nontraumatically as possible and with precision eliminates dead space and minimizes the potential for wound disruption. Evaluation of each patient and selection of the proper wound closure materials for the particular surgical circumstance provide maximal opportunity for healing. Accurate approximation of tissue without tension or strangulation promotes healing.
Immobilize the wound.	Adequate immobilization of the approximated wound, but not necessarily the entire anatomical part, promotes efficient healing and minimal scar formation.

Adapted from Ethicon (2008). *Wound Closure Manual.* Somerville, NJ: Ethicon, Inc., a Johnson & Johnson Company. Available at: http://www.jnjgateway.com/public/NLDUT/Wound_Closure_Manual1.pdf, pp. 4–5, accessed May 5, 2008.

When a wound heals by second intention, rather than primary union with sutures, the wound is often left open and allowed to heal from the bottom up. This is called *contraction*. During this process, granulation tissue forms in the wound defect. As the defect fills with granulation tissue, contraction begins with the secondary growth of epithelium, and the wound begins to close. Because this type of healing takes longer than first-intention healing, excessive scar tissue forms. The possibility of postoperative incisional herniation is also greater because of poor wound union.

Third-Intention Wound Healing

When the wound heals by third intention, two surfaces of granulation tissue join. A deep, wide scar usually forms. The surgeon relies on third-intention healing in an area of gross infection, after extensive tissue loss from injury, or after aggressive debridement of infected or damaged tissue (Phillips, 2007). Third-intention healing is the slowest of all the healing processes.

Needles

Suture needles must be carefully selected for a procedure. Use of inappropriate needles may prolong the operation and damage the structural integrity of tissues and may lead to necrosis of the tissue, as well as infection. In addition, approximation of the wound may fail if the wrong suture needle is used.

Sutures

Tables 16.4 and **16.5** lists many of the sutures available for a procedure. Sutures are either absorbable or nonabsorbable. However, both types are foreign bodies. Another characteristic of suture is the filament. A monofilament suture consists of a single suture strand. Because of the single strand, more knots are needed to prevent slippage. Multifilament suture consists of strands of braided suture. It is easier to tie, and the knotting is more secure. A disadvantage, however, is the possible harboring of bacteria in the braided structure of the suture strand (Ethicon, 2008).

Choose suture on the basis of the type of body tissues being sutured. To prevent suture breakage, consider the strength of the suture material. Become familiar with the nature of the suture material, the biological forces in the healing wound, and the interaction of the suture and the tissues. **Table 16.6** provides guidelines for selecting sutures.

Closure Methods
Primary Closure

When performing a primary closure, the surgeon or first assistant brings each layer of tissue into correct approximation. This means that similar tissues are brought together: fascia to fascia, muscle to muscle, subcutaneous tissue to subcutaneous tissue, and skin edges to skin edges. Approximation of similar tissues and elimination of all dead space allow each layer to heal properly.

Pulling the tissues together with the correct amount of tension is crucial for a successful closure. If sutures are too tight, the tissue blanches and then strangulates, which causes it to die for lack of adequate blood supply. Likewise, if sutures slip or become loose, dead space may form and fluid may seep into the wound, resulting in poor wound healing.

Table 16.4	Absorbable Suture Commonly Used in Surgery					
Suture	**Types**	**Frequent Uses**	**Tissue Reaction**	**Contradictions**	**Warnings**	**Tensile Strength Retention in Vivo**	**Absorption Rate**
Surgical gut	Plain	Ligate superficial vessels; suture soft tissues that heal rapidly; not used in cardiovascular OR.	Moderately high	Should not be used in tissues that heal slowly, require support, or are under stress. Should not be used in neurological tissues or patient allergic or sensitive to collagen or chromium.	Absorbs relatively quickly.	Individual patient characteristics can affect. Poor (0% at 2–3 wks).	Digested by proteolytic enzymes. Unpredictable (12 wks).
Surgical gut	Chromic	Suture or ligature for general soft tissue approximation and/or ligation, including use in ophthalmic procedures. Not for use in ophthalmic procedures and neurological tissues.	Moderate	Being absorbable, should not be used when extended approximation of tissue is required. Should not be used in patient allergic or sensitive to collagen or chromium.	Inappropriate in elderly, malnourished or debilitated patient. Absorbs relatively quickly.	Individual patient characteristics can affect rate of tensile strength. Poor (0% at 2–3 wks).	Digested by proteolytic enzymes. Unpredictable (12 wks).

16

Suture	Types	Frequent Uses	Tissue Reaction	Contradictions	Warnings	Tensile Strength Retention in Vivo	Absorption Rate
Polyglactin 910 (Coated VICRYL *RAPIDE***)	Braided	Superficial soft tissue approximation of skin and mucosa only. Not for use in ligation, ophthalmic, cardiovascular, or neurological procedures.	Minimal to moderate acute inflammatory reaction.	Should not be used where extended approximation of tissues under stress is required or where wound support beyond 7 days is required.	Risk of wound dehiscence may vary with site of application.	Approximately 50% remains at 5 days. All tensile strength lost by 10–14 days.	Absorbed by hydrolysis. Essentially complete by 42 days.
Polyglactin 910 (Polysorb*, Dexon*, Coated VICRYL**)	Braided	General soft tissue approximation and/or ligation including use in ophthalmic procedures. Not for use in cardiovascular or neurological procedures.	Minimal acute inflammatory reaction.	Being absorbable, should not be used when extended approximation of tissue is required.	Risk of wound dehiscence may vary with site of application.	Approximately 75% remains at 2 wks. Approximately 50% remains at 3 wks.	Absorbed by hydrolysis. Essentially complete between 56–70 days.
Poliglecaprone 25 (Biosyn*, Caprosyn*, Monocryl**)	Monofilament	General soft tissue approximation and/or ligation including use in ophthalmic procedures. Not for use in cardiovascular or neurological procedures.	Minimal acute inflammatory reaction.	Being absorbable, should not be used when extended approximation of tissue is required. Undyed not indicated for use in fascia.	Risk of wound dehiscence may vary with site of application.	Undyed: approximately 50–60% remains at 1 wk; 20–30% at 2 wks. Dyed: approximately 60–70% at 1 wk; 30–40% at 2 wks; lost by 28 days.	Absorbed by hydrolysis. Complete at 91–199 days.

Suture	Types	Frequent Uses	Tissue Reaction	Contradictions	Warnings	Tensile Strength Retention in Vivo	Absorption Rate
Polydioxanone (Maxon*, PDS II**)	Monofilament	All types of soft tissue approximation, including pediatric cardiovascular and ophthalmic procedures. Not for use in adult cardiovascular tissue, microsurgery, and neural tissue grafts.	Slight reaction	Being absorbable, should not be used when prolonged approximation of tissue is required. Should not be used with prosthetic devices, such as heart valves or synthetic.	The safety and effectiveness have not been established in neural tissue, adult cardiovascular tissue, or for use in microsurgery.	Approximately: 70% remains at 2 wks; 50% remains at 2 wks; 25% remains at 2 wks.	Absorbed by slow hydrolysis. Minimal until about 90th day. Essentially complete in about 6 months.
(Panacryl**)	Braided	Unique for its combined superior strength and absorbability. For use in general soft tissue and orthopedic uses including tendon and ligament repairs and reattachment to bone.	Minimal inflammatory reaction	Being absorbable, should not be used where extended approximation of tissue beyond 6 months is required.	Use may be inappropriate in patient suffering conditions which could delay wound healing beyond 6 months.	Approximately: 80% remains at 3 months; 60% remains at 6 months.	Essentially complete in 1.5–2.5 years.

Adapted from Ethicon (2008). *Wound Closure Manual.* Somerville, NJ: Ethicon, Inc., a Johnson & Johnson Company; Chapter 2 and from Syneture™ (2008). *The Thread Between Science and Healing, Wound Closure Products,* United States Surgical, Norwalk, CT.
Product Key: Syneture*; Ethicon**.

16

Table 16.5	Nonabsorbable Suture Commonly Used in Surgery						
Suture	**Types**	**Frequent Uses**	**Tissue Reaction**	**Contradictions**	**Warnings**	**Tensile Strength Retention in Vivo**	**Absorption Rate**
Silk (Sofsilk*, Perma-hand Silk**)	Braided	General soft tissue approximation and/ or ligation, including cardiovascular, ophthalmic, and neurological procedures.	Acute inflammatory reaction.	Should not be used in sensitivities or allergies to silk.	Acceptable surgical practices should be followed for the management of infected or contaminated wounds.	Progressive degradation of fiber may result in gradual loss of tensile strength over time.	Gradual encapsulation by fibrous connective tissue.
Stainless Steel (Steel*, Surgical Stainless Steel**)	Monofilament	General soft tissue approximation and/ or ligation, including cardiovascular, ophthalmic, and neurological procedures.	Minimal acute inflammatory reaction.	Should not be used in patients with known sensitivities or allergies to 316L stainless steel, or constituent metals such as chromium or nickel.	Risk of wound dehiscence may vary with site of application.	Indefinite.	Nonabsorbable.
Nylon (Monosof*, Dermalon*, Ethilon**)	Monofilament	General soft tissue approximation and/ or ligation, including cardiovascular, ophthalmic, and neurological procedures.	Minimal acute inflammatory reaction.	Should not be used permanent retention of tensile strength is required.	Risk of wound dehiscence may vary with site of application.	Progressive hydrolysis may result in gradual loss of tensile strength over time.	Gradual encapsulation by fibrous connective tissue.

Suture	Types	Frequent Uses	Tissue Reaction	Contradictions	Warnings	Tensile Strength Retention in Vivo	Absorption Rate
Nylon (Surgilon*, Nurolon**)	Braided	General soft tissue approximation and/or ligation, including cardiovascular, ophthalmic, and neurological procedures. Because of elasticity, well suited for retention and skin closure.	Minimal acute inflammatory reaction.	Should not be used permanent retention of tensile strength is required.	Acceptable surgical practices should be followed for the management of infected or contaminated wounds.	Progressive hydrolysis may result in gradual loss of tensile strength over time.	Gradual encapsulation by fibrous connective tissue.
Polyester Fiber (Surgidac** TiCon*, Mersilene**, Ethibond**)	Braided	General soft tissue approximation and/or ligation, including cardiovascular, ophthalmic, and neurological procedures.	Minimal acute inflammatory reaction.	None known.	Acceptable surgical practices should be followed for the management of infected or contaminated wounds.	No significant changes known to occur in vivo.	Gradual encapsulation by fibrous connective tissue.
Polypropylene (Surgipro*, Novafil*, Prolene**)	Monofilament	General soft tissue approximation and/or ligation, including cardiovascular, ophthalmic, and neurological procedures. Recommended for use when minimal suture reaction is desired, such as contaminated and infected wounds.	Minimal acute inflammatory reaction.	None known.	Risk of wound dehiscence may vary with site of application.	Not subject to degradation or weakening of action of tissue enzymes.	Gradual encapsulation by fibrous connective tissue.

16

Suture	Types	Frequent Uses	Tissue Reaction	Contradictions	Warnings	Tensile Strength Retention in Vivo	Absorption Rate
Poly (Vascufil*, Pronova**)	Monofilament	General soft tissue approximation and/ or ligation, including cardiovascular, ophthalmic, and neurological procedures. Resists involvement in infection and is successfully used in contaminated and infected wounds to minimize sinus formation and suture extrusion.	Minimal to mild inflammatory reaction.	None known.	Risk of wound dehiscence may vary with site of application.	Not subject to degradation or weakening of action of tissue enzymes.	Gradual encapsulation by fibrous connective tissue.

Adapted from Ethicon (2008). *Wound Closure Manual*. Somerville, NJ: Ethicon, Inc., a Johnson & Johnson Company; Chapter 2 and from Syneture™ (2008). *The Thread Between Science and Healing, Wound Closure Products*, United States Surgical, Norwalk, CT.
Product Key: Syneture*; Ethicon**.

Table 16.6	Principles of Suture Selection
When a wound has reached maximal strength, sutures are no longer needed.	☐ Tissues that ordinarily heal slowly such as skin, fasciae, and tendons should usually be closed with nonabsorbable or monofilament absorbable sutures.
	☐ Tissues that heal rapidly such as stomach, colon, and bladder may be closed with absorbable sutures.
Foreign bodies in potentially contaminated tissues may convert contamination to infection.	☐ Avoid multifilament sutures, which may convert a contaminated wound into an infected one.
	☐ Use monofilament or absorbable sutures in potentially contaminated tissues.
Where cosmetic results are important, close and prolonged apposition of wounds and avoidance of irritants will produce the best result.	☐ Use the smallest inert monofilament suture materials, such as nylon or polypropylene.
	☐ Avoid skin sutures, and close subcuticularly whenever possible.
	☐ Under certain circumstances, to secure close apposition of skin edges, skin closure tape may be used.
Foreign bodies in the presence of fluids containing high concentrations of crystalloids may act as nidi for precipitation and stone formation.	☐ In the urinary and biliary tract, use rapidly absorbed sutures.
Selecting suture size.	☐ Use the finest size, commensurate with the natural strength of the tissue.
	☐ If the postoperative course of the patient may produce sudden strains on the suture line, reinforce it with retention sutures. Remove them as soon as the patient's condition is stabilized.

Adapted from Ethicon (2008). *Wound Closure Manual.* Somerville, NJ: Ethicon, Inc., a Johnson & Johnson Company. Available at: http://www.jnjgateway.com/public/NLDUT/Wound_Closure_Manual1.pdf, pp. 27–28, accessed May 5, 2008.

COMMON TECHNIQUES

Use a continuous suture, also called a running stitch, to close a tissue layer by passing one strand of suture back and forth between the two edges of the wound (**Fig. 16.9**), the surgeon ties the suture at the end of the suture line. A continuous suture line is strong because tension is evenly distributed along the full length of the wound. If, however, the suture breaks, the whole suture line is disrupted. In addition, a continuous suture uses less suture material, thus leaving less foreign body in the wound. For a continuous suture in the presence of infection, use a monofilament suture to avoid harboring microorganisms in the interstices of a multifilament suture (Ethicon, 2008).

An interrupted suture line is a series of singly placed stitches (**Fig. 16.10**). As each suture is placed, it is tied and cut. This technique is used more often than continuous suturing, even though it takes more time, because the integrity of the suture line remains intact if a suture breaks. In addition, if infection is present, microorganisms are less likely to travel along the primary suture line of interrupted stitches (Ethicon, 2008). Commonly used stitches are described in **Table 16.7**.

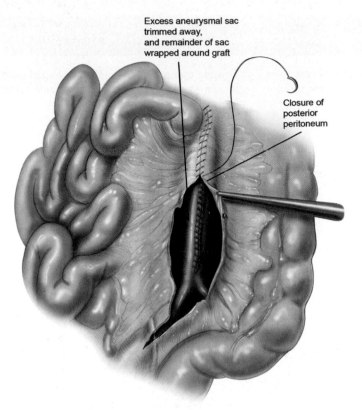

Excess aneurysmal sac
trimmed away,
and remainder of sac
wrapped around graft

Closure of
posterior
peritoneum

Figure 16.9

Using a continuous suture
to close the peritoneum.

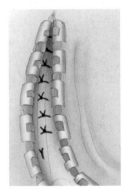

Figure 16.10

Placement of interrupted suture
during closure of a craniotomy.

Secondary Closure

The presence of an infection or gross contamination necessitates a secondary closure. This allows access to the contaminated tissue for cleaning and enables the tissue to recover from the infection before final closure. During the first stage of a secondary closure, the deep tissue, such as the peritoneum and fascia, is closed with a monofilament suture material. The next tissue layers remain open, which permits irrigation of the wound and instillation of antibiotics during dressing changes. For secondary (delayed) closure of a traumatic wound the surgeon may place suture wire to close the subcutaneous tissue and skin. These sutures are not tied; rather, they are held down with adhesive.

Some surgeons insert skin sutures during a secondary closure. This technique allows the incision edges to pull together, thus reducing the amount of tension placed

Table 16.7	**Commonly Used Stitches**
Continuous Suture	**Interrupted Sutures**
To Appose Skin and Other Tissue	
Over and over	Over and over
Subcuticular	Vertical mattress
	Horizontal mattress
To Invert Tissue	
Lembert	Lembert
Cushing	Halsted
Connell	Pursestring
To Evert Tissue	
Horizontal mattress	Horizontal mattress

Adapted from Ethicon (2008). *Wound Closure Manual.* Somerville, NJ: Ethicon, Inc., a Johnson & Johnson Company. Available at: http://www.jnjgateway.com/public/ NLDUT/Wound_Closure_Manual1.pdf, p. 24, accessed March 12, 2008.

on the incision. The amount of scar tissue that forms from this type of closure is also decreased. Skin sutures are placed far apart to facilitate the proper healing process.

Retention Sutures

In the presence of gross contamination, obesity, tissue loss, or excessive tissue damage, such as the type seen with massive trauma, retention sutures are used. Approximating the incision or damaged tissue with a large through-and-through nonabsorbable suture material reduces tension and holds incision edges together until healing is complete.

The surgeon places retention sutures about 2 inches (5 cm) away from each edge of the wound. When placing the retention suture, one of the following closure techniques is used: through-and-through retention sutures or buried coaptation-retention sutures (Ethicon, 2008).

Through-and-through retention sutures are inserted before the peritoneum is closed. When using this type of suture, the surgeon places the suture from inside the peritoneal cavity. The suture is inserted through the peritoneum, all abdominal layers, and the skin, using a simple interrupted or a figure-of-eight stitch. The wound is then closed in layers for a distance of about three-fourths the length of the wound. Next, the retention sutures are drawn and tied together and the surgeon places a finger in the abdominal cavity to prevent strangulation of the viscera during closure. Closure of the remainder of the wound continues in a similar manner (Ethicon, 2008).

Buried coaptation-retention sutures are inserted after closing the peritoneum. The sutures are placed through the fascia and then the skin. For retention, the surgeon places the sutures "approximately two centimeters apart in the posterior rectus sheath and peritoneum in the so-called 'far-and-near' or 'far-near-near-far' fashion" (Ethicon, 2008). After inserting the retention sutures, the wound is closed in layers and then the retention sutures are tied. Bolsters are used to prevent the heavy suture materials from cutting into the skin (Ethicon, 2008).

Use of the Needle Holder

Learning correct use of a needle holder takes coordination and time to get the feel of the instrument. When passing a needle holder, the scrub person should place it firmly in the palm of the assistant's hand (**Fig. 16.11**). Note that the first assistant receives the needle holder with the needlepoint toward the thumb. This prevents unnecessary wrist motion. To prevent dragging of the suture across the sterile field, the scrub person holds the suture (Ethicon, 2008). After receiving the needle holder from the scrub person, the first assistant grasps it firmly and inserts the thumb and fourth finger (ring finger) through the rings of the instrument. This technique enables the index and middle fingers to control and push the needle through the tissue. When inserting the needle, the first assistant rotates the wrist, thus pushing the needle through the tissue with one smooth easy motion.

Palming is another way to handle a needle holder. With this technique, the first assistant places only the fourth finger through the ring of the instrument, which permits opening and closing of the needle holder without having to place the thumb into the ring. Many nurses prefer this technique because it allows the assistant to handle the needle holder more quickly.

Loading of the Needle Holder

Correct loading of the needle in the needle holder prevents it from turning when entering the tissue during suturing (**Fig. 16.12**). Place the needle in the jaws just below the point where it flattens out.

Placement of Sutures

When inserting the needle, place the point at a right angle to the tissue (**Fig. 16.13**). This technique allows the needle a clean and smooth entry through the tissue. After inserting the needle, release it, grasp down away from the point, and pull it through.

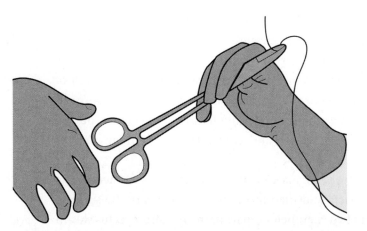

Figure 16.11

Passing a needle holder.

Source: Adapted from Ethicon (2008). *Wound Closure Manual.* Somerville, NJ: Ethicon, Inc.

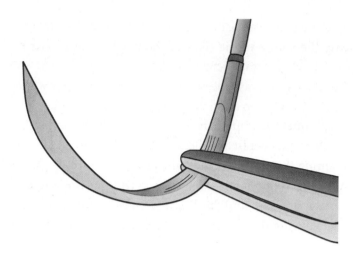

Figure 16.12

Correct loading of a needle holder.

Source: Adapted from Ethicon (2008). *Wound Closure Manual.* Somerville, NJ: Ethicon, Inc.

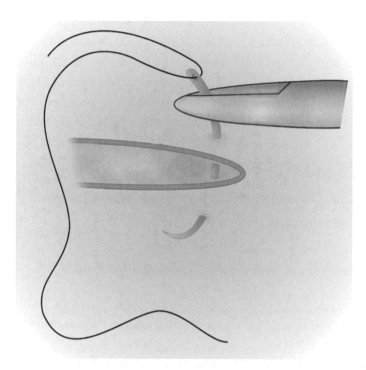

Figure 16.13

Inserting a needle through tissue.

Source: Adapted from Ethicon (2008). *Wound Closure Manual.* Somerville, NJ: Ethicon, Inc.

16

Unless there is no other way to pull the needle through the tissue, avoid grasping the point. Grasping the needle at the point dulls it and bends it out of shape. A dull or damaged needle point not only makes suturing more difficult but also causes unnecessary trauma to the tissue.

Getting the needle and suture through both sides of the incision usually requires two motions. After pulling the needle through one side, reposition it in the needle holder and place the point in the tissue so that it exits the tissue at a right angle. To bring the incision edges properly together, keep the suture at the same level in the tissue. Next, advance the suture through the tissue by using a smooth, uninterrupted, and gentle pulling motion. When suturing, bring like tissues together; peritoneum to peritoneum, muscle to muscle, fascia to fascia, subcutaneous tissue to subcutaneous tissue, and skin to skin. Many surgeons use the Smead-Jones stitch when closing the abdomen. This stitch approximates peritoneum, muscle, and fascia simultaneously.

During suturing, the free end of the suture is easily contaminated if not controlled. Control the free end by placing the suture to the right of the needle holder when using the right hand and to the left when using the left hand.

When using a straight needle for closure, grasp the skin edges gently but firmly with a tissue forceps. Lifting the edge of the incision aids in placing the needle point in the tissue. After the needle is through one side, repeat the procedure with the opposite incision edge. Place the suture at an equal depth and distance from the skin edges.

If you are not actually performing the closure, handle the ends of the suture during closure. This prevents knots and redundant suture from getting in the way of the surgeon by keeping the suture taut and straight. Placing tension on the suture also aids in controlling the tissue during the closure by holding the tissue edges up or apart. This maneuver not only makes placement of the next suture easier but also provides the necessary exposure for the procedure to proceed smoothly.

Surgical Knots

Knots keep vessels closed and hold tissues together (**Table 16.8**). When suturing, use the simple or overhand knot, square knot, or surgeon's knot. The simple knot is the first step of basic knot tying, whereas the square knot is a complete and true knot. Unless requested by the surgeon avoid the granny knot. This slip knot does not provide the security necessary to ensure that tissue holds together and vessels remain

Table 16.8	General Principles of Knot Tying

1. Tie the knot firmly to minimize slippage.

2. Use a simple knot.

3. Tie a small knot and cut the ends as short as possible to minimize foreign body tissue reaction.

4. Avoid sawing one strand of suture down over another strand when tying the knot. This may weaken the suture and result in breakage when the second throw is made.

5. Avoid excessive tension when using finer-gauge suture materials. To tie the knot securely and avoid breakage, pull the two ends of the suture in opposite directions with uniform rate and tension.

6. Do not attach clamps or hemostats to suture that will remain in situ. Avoid the crushing or crimping application of surgical instruments, such as needle holders and forceps, to the strand, except when grasping the free end of the suture during an instrument tie.

7. Do not tie suture for tissue approximation too tightly, as this causes tissue strangulation.

8. To avoid loosening of the knot, after tying the first loop maintain traction on one end of the strand for control.

9. Avoid extra throws when tying the knot. They do not add to the strength of the knot; they only contribute to its bulk.

Adapted from Ethicon (2008). *Wound Closure Manual*. Somerville, NJ: Ethicon, Inc., a Johnson & Johnson Company. Available at: http://www.jnjgateway.com/public/NLDUT/Wound_Closure_Manual1.pdf, p. 24, accessed May 5, 2008.

closed. Maintain tension or traction on the tissue with the surgeon's knot. This knot does not slip after the first throw is in place.

Most assistants use the square knot because it provides a secure and competent knot in or around the tissue. Although it is possible to tie a square knot by using the one-handed technique. Many surgeons and assistants prefer to tie by using the two-handed technique. This technique gives the assistant better control over knot placement and aids in maintaining proper knot tension.

Because it usually stays in place after the first throw is made, the surgeon's knot is used to maintain the proper position of the tissue, particularly in deep tissue. In addition, the surgeon's knot helps control the tissue. After making the double wrap, ensure proper placement and tension of the knot on the tissue by following the knot down with the tip of the finger. The square knot is another knot of choice if the surgeon's knot is not required. In an area in which a deep tie is required, a suture ligature may also be needed. After the surgeon places a suture ligature, the nurse ties the knot, using the same process as described earlier. After insertion of the suture ligature, the suture is brought back to the opposite side of the hemostat, and the knot is completed.

When making a deep tie, use a needle holder to complete the tie. Loop the suture around the end of the holder, grasp the other end of the suture, and pull it through the loop; this starts the knot. To complete the knot, wrap in the opposite direction to form a square knot.

Applying Knot Tension

Securing the knot prevents it from falling out of the tissue. Use of the correct amount of tension when the knot is tied prevents slipping when the final knot is in place. The knot tension holds the tissue together and keeps the vessel closed. This tension should approximate, not strangulate or tear the tissue.

Maintain firm and steady tension during knot tying by holding one end of the suture still while tying the knot. Steady tension prevents the suture material from breaking during the tic. Jerking, sawing, or snapping the suture may cause it to break during the procedure. Because tissues swell when knots are placed, use only the necessary number of throws to complete the knot. This reduces the bulk of the suture left in the patient. When tying deep knots, always carry the suture down to the tissue with the tip of the finger, to ensure proper placement of the tie on the tissue.

Keeping the vessel closed or the tissue in place necessitates properly placed, firmly set, and squared knots. Different types of tissue require different amounts of tension to provide the correct closure. If the tension is too loose, a gap forms in the incision. If the tension is too tight, the tissue strangulates, thus creating the potential for necrosis.

Cutting of Sutures

When cutting sutures, run the tip of the scissors down the length of the suture strand to the knot. If surgical gut has been used, cut the strand 6 mm from the knot. Cut synthetic sutures 3 mm from the knot to minimize the amount of foreign material left in the wound. Before cutting the suture, ensure that the tips of the scissors are in sight, to avoid cutting tissue. As sutures are cut, remove the ends from the operative site (Ethicon, 2008).

Laparoscopic Suturing

Suturing is required for tissue approximation in many laparoscopic procedures. A variety of tools and devices have been developed to assist surgeons in performing these minimally invasive procedures. Most surgeons use standard suture material and needles for laparoscopic sewing, but newer laparoscopic needle graspers and suturing devices help surgeons perform both intracorporeal and extracorporeal suturing more easily and quickly.

The surgeon skilled in laparoscopic suturing techniques will be better able to help patients by offering minimally invasive options for surgical problems. Skill in suturing is gained by practice, experience, and understanding the principles of ideal port placement, proper visualization, and appropriate steps in suturing. Suturing skills are essential for a large number of laparoscopic procedures.

Laparoscopic suturing may be done by intracorporeal suturing or by extracorporeal knot tying. Suture devices such as the Endo Stitch (AutoSuture™) instrument provide a fast and efficient way for laparoscopic suturing.

Staples

Skin staples are a frequently chosen method of skin closure. They are used in many locations of surgical incisions. Skin staples reduce operating time. Tissue trauma is reduced because there is uniform tension along the suture line and less distortion from the stress of the individual suture points. When properly applied, they provide excellent cosmetic results. When apposing skin with skin staples, do the following:

1. Evert the edges of the cuticular and subcuticular layers. The edges should align and be slightly raised in an outward direction. With healing, the tissue will flatten and form an even surface.

2. Align skin edges as close to their original configuration on the horizontal plane as possible.

3. The length of time the staples stay in place is dependent on the part of body affected; they are usually removed within 5 to 7 days from chest or abdominal incisions.

Most staplers employ a similar anvil type of mechanism for forming the staple, but the applying device varies from different companies. Surgeon's choice is usually determined by the stapler's weight, handling characteristics, ease of application, and unobstructed view of the incision during application.

CUTTING TISSUE

Scalpels

The modern scalpel consists of a handle that is designed to receive a variety of disposable blades. The blade is changed as soon as it becomes dull, because the edge

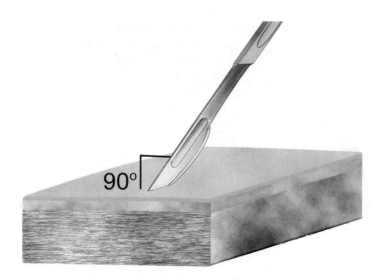

Figure 16.14
Proper scalpel angle.

must be sharp and smooth. The type of operation and the patient's size affect the choice of not only the size and location of the initial incision but also the type of blade as well. An incision must be just long enough to provide adequate space to perform the operation. For large incisions, the scalpel handle is held against the palm with the thumb and fingers gripping it from above. This is known as the power grip.

Hold the blade vertical to the skin to prevent beveling. Cut dermis and epidermis quickly with a single stroke, applying even pressure. This technique promotes precision approximation of skin, which in turn promotes wound healing. Control the depth of the incision by downward pressure of the index finger. A wide blade such as the No. 10 or 20 is commonly used.

Figure 16.14 depicts the proper scalpel angle. Note how the scalpel is at a 90-degree angle to the skin. This allows the sides of the wound to be of equal height and facilitates proper closure.

Many different sizes and shapes of blades are required for specific purposes. The No. 15 blade has a small curve and a short cutting surface. It is used for small incisions and dissecting fine tissue. The No. 15 blade can also be used with a pencil-like grip. The No. 11 blade tapers to a fine point and requires gentle, constant pressure. In the precision grip, the scalpel handle is held like a pencil and the hand is stabilized by providing light contact with the patient with the fingers. The No. 11 blade is used to make a small skin incision and is often used to puncture an abscess, cut a vessel wall, or make a sharp cut in small structures such as the fallopian tubes. The right-angled scalpel blade is used to cut tissues at the bottom of a deep hole. The crescent-shaped No. 12 blade, which has a pointed tip, can be used in a hole when the surgeon may impale tissue with the tip as she or he cuts it.

Scissors

Scissors are used for dissecting tissue, severing clamped blood vessels, and cutting suture. When using a scissors, the first assistant maintains control by inserting the thumb and fourth (ring) finger through the handle rings (**Fig. 16.15**). The index and third fingers are then used to stabilize the scissors as it cuts.

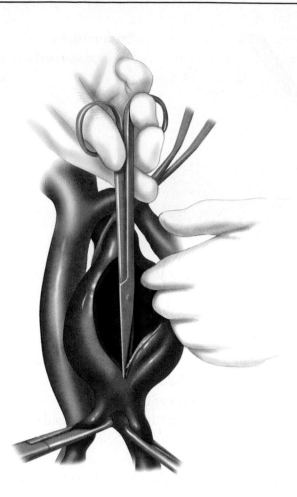

Figure 16.15
Extending the incision into an abdominal aneurysm with Mayo scissors. Note the placement of the thumb and fingers.

Electrical Cutting Devices

Several instruments can be used to cut and coagulate tissue at the same time. The electrosurgical unit uses high-frequency electrical energy to produce heat to coagulate and a more intense heat to cut tissue. Held like a pencil, it is used for both dissection and hemostasis. Care must be used to touch only the tissue to be coagulated because surrounding tissue can be damaged. This method is widely used to control bleeding. It is valuable for coagulating small vessels that are difficult to ligate because of their size or location. See Chapters 11 and 17 for more information about electrosurgery.

The Shaw scalpel is a heated blade that seals small blood vessels as it cuts. It is a slow process and is often used in delicate surgery such as infertility procedures in which bleeding must be well controlled.

Orthopedic and Other Cutting Devices

Orthopedics and specialties such as otolaryngology, plastic surgery, and neurosurgery use instruments designed for cutting bone. Some of the more common instruments are chisels, curets, bone cutters, gauges, elevators, and osteotomes. Saws and drills, reamers, and screwdrivers driven by compressed nitrogen or electricity are also widely used. Powered tools generate high heat and should be used for only short periods of time. Because this heat damages adjacent tissue, cool saline is used to drip onto the blade or drill whenever it is in use. The nurse and the assistant must take care not to obstruct the surgeon's view when the surgeon is irrigating.

Tissue Vessel Sealing, Tissue Fusion and Ultrasonic Devices

High frequency vessel sealing and tissue fusion devices, as well as, ultrasonic dissection devices are used to provide hemostasis and tissue dissection without the use of mechanical ligation devices such as suture, clips, and staples. See Chapter 17, *Providing Hemostasis,* for a description of the technology and related patient care activities.

MAINTAINING A DRY FIELD

Maintaining a dry operative site is essential in the positive outcome of surgery. The first assistant demonstrates competency in handling tissues by proper use of suctioning instruments and by using sponges to provide exposure.

Suctioning devices remove blood or fluids from the operative site. Suction tips come in a variety of shapes and sizes. While suctioning, it is essential to maintain good visualization of the suction tip. Aspiration injury or trauma to tissue can occur if the tip is used carelessly. A fine-tipped suction could puncture, tear, or abrade tissue. Aspiration injury can occur if tissue is aspirated into the end of the suction. This can be prevented by protecting the tissue with a sponge so the suction is not applied directly to the tissue. If tissue is aspirated, the tissue should not be forcibly removed from the suction tip. Instead, the suction should be broken by bending or clamping the tubing and the tissue gently removed. The suction tip should never obstruct the surgeon's vision. The first assistant coordinates moves with the surgeon's activities to anticipate the need for and the timing of suctioning.

Sponges are used to absorb blood or other fluids that collect in the operative field or as packs to provide hemostasis. During the skin incision, the first assistant may place a moistened sponge over the open ends of transected vessels. Small clots will usually form with digital pressure. In a deep cavity, a stick sponge (a sponge grasped in a forceps) may be required to apply pressure to a bleeding point. Oozing, especially in localized spaces in the retroperitoneum, can be stopped by packing moistened sponges into the area. The first assistant may also need to remove clotted blood with a sponge. Heavy rubbing movements are avoided. The sponge should be used in a gentle blotting action.

CONCLUSION

The role of the first assistant is an integral part of and can have a major effect on the outcome of the surgical procedure. By understanding essential principles, the first assistant can be of immeasurable help in promoting a favorable result. Measures of wound outcomes include wound healing without infection, relief of discomfort, and a return to normal activity and function. The first assistant works in collaboration with the surgeon in planning the surgical approach, implementing principles of tissue handling, and choosing the optimal selection of skin closure.

COMPETENCY ASSESSMENT
Handle Tissue with Instruments

Name: _____ Title: _____ Unit: _____ Date of Validation: _____

Type of Validation: ☐ Initial ☐ Annual ☐ Bi-annual

COMPETENCY STATEMENT: The first assistant demonstrates competency to handle tissue with instruments during an operative or invasive procedure.

Performance Criteria	Met	Not Met
1. Identifies the patient's risk for adverse outcomes related to the handling of tissue with instruments	☐	☐
2. Provides exposure during surgery	☐	☐
3. Clamps tissue during surgery	☐	☐
4. Grasps tissue during surgery	☐	☐
5. Sutures tissue during surgery	☐	☐
6. Cuts tissue during surgery	☐	☐
7. Maintains a dry field during surgery	☐	☐

_____   _____
Validator's Signature   Employee's Signature

_____
Validator's Printed Name

REFERENCES

1. Cameron, J.L. (2004). *Current Surgical Therapy.* Baltimore: Elsevier Mosby.
2. Ethicon (2008). *Ethicon wound closure manual.* Somerville, NJ: Ethicon, Inc. Available at: http://www.jnjgateway.com/public/NLDUT/Wound_Closure_Manual1.pdf, accessed May 5, 2008.
3. Phillips, N. (2007). *Berry & Kohn's Operating Room technique* (11th ed.). St. Louis, MO: Elsevier.
4. Soper, N.J., Swanstrom, L.L., & Eubanks, W.S. (2005). *Mastery of Endoscopic and Laparoscopic Surgery* (2nd ed.). Philadelphia, PA: J.B. Lippincott.
5. Syneture™ (2008). *The Thread Between Science and Healing,* Wound Closure Products, United States Surgical, Norwalk, CT.

CHAPTER 17

Provide Hemostasis

BJ Hoogerwerf

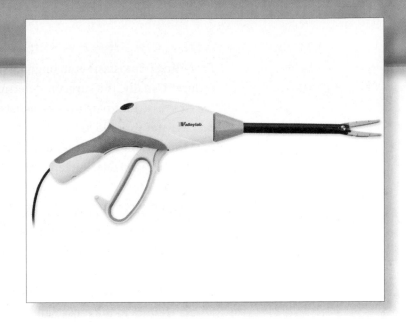

INTRODUCTION

The term *hemostasis* means prevention of blood loss (Guyton & Hall, 2006). When a blood vessel ruptures or is severed, hemostasis can occur by several different methods (Guyton & Hall, 2006):

- Vascular constriction;
- Formation of a platelet plug;
- Formation of a blood clot; or
- Growth of fibrous tissue into the clot, closing the hole.

Uncontrolled or excessive bleeding can become a life-threatening situation, has adverse physiological effects for the patient, obscures visualization of the operative site, and interferes with the healing process. Effective application of hemostatic techniques is one of the key responsibilities of the first assistant.

MEASURABLE CRITERIA

The first assistant demonstrates competency to provide hemostasis by:

- Describing the mechanism of clotting;
- Assessing the patient's clotting mechanisms;
- Describing the signs of hypovolemic shock;
- Identifying the patient's risk for adverse outcomes related to the provision of hemostasis;
- Applying mechanical methods to control bleeding;
- Applying thermal methods to control bleeding; and
- Applying chemical methods to control bleeding.

Chapter Contents

ROLE OF FIRST ASSISTANT

Providing hemostasis is an ongoing process throughout an operative or invasive procedure. Usually, the surgeon determines the appropriate hemostatic technique and the first assistant performs or assists in performing that technique. In addition, the first assistant should know the hemostatic options available in the institution, anticipate the patient's needs, request that the circulating nurse have specific supplies and equipment available, and ensure that the agents are being used in a safe manner.

MECHANISM OF CLOTTING

Understanding the mechanism of blood coagulation aids the first assistant in assessing the patient's clotting abilities and in the effective application of mechanical, thermal, and chemical hemostatic techniques. Depending on the type of trauma, a blood vessel either contracts or constricts when damaged; if cut, the vessel wall contracts. Direct trauma to the muscle in the vessel wall, however, causes it to constrict for several centimeters, resulting in vascular spasm. The greater the trauma, the greater the degree of vasospasm. For example, sharply cut vessels usually result in greater blood loss than crushed vessels.

After damage is incurred, plugging of the disrupted vessel with platelets begins. Platelets are normally oval or round disks. When platelets contact the collagen fibers of a damaged vessel wall, they swell and assume irregular shapes with protuberances. They also become sticky and secrete enzymes that activate adjacent platelets. The cumulative effect is the formation of a loose platelet plug. Next, the blood clot forms; this event occurs in three steps:

1. Prothrombin activators form in response to vessel trauma (extrinsic pathway) or damage to the blood cells (intrinsic pathway).
2. Aided by the activators, prothrombin is converted to thrombin (calcium ions are essential to this process).
3. Thrombin converts the fibrinogen to fibrin.

The fibrin threads then enmesh with the platelets in the platelet plug and the remaining blood components to form a tight, unyielding plug. Later, the clot retracts, closing the vessel even more.

After clot formation, fibroblasts invade the clot and organize into connective tissue. During this process, the proteolytic enzyme called plasmin, or fibrinolysin, is activated to digest the fibrin threads. Eventually, the clot dissolves (Guyton & Hall, 2006). Refer to the clotting cascade outlined in **Table 17.1**.

ASSESSING THE PATIENT'S CLOTTING MECHANISMS

PT
Prothrombin Time

PTT
Partial Thromboplastin Time

TT
Thrombin Time

The first assistant collaborates with the surgeon in assessing the patient's clotting mechanisms. When a patient's history or physical examination suggests bleeding or clotting difficulties, the surgeon should order platelet and coagulation studies. If no studies have been obtained on these patients, appropriate tests should be recommended, such as prothrombin time (PT), partial thromboplastin time (PTT), thrombin time (TT), or quantitative platelet counts. PT measures the extrinsic clotting mechanism and is the time required for coagulation to take place. PTT measures the activity of the intrinsic

Table 17.1	Clotting Cascade

Intrinsic Clotting Path

Internal vascular irritation or lesions initiate the intrinsic system with the mobilization of pro-proteins and pro-enzymes to stimulate the transport of kallikrein, Factors XII, XIIa, XI, XIa, IX, and Xa to the site of the irritation.

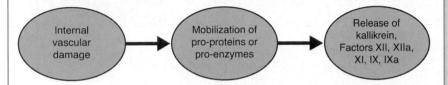

Extrinsic Clotting Path

Laceration to a blood vessel activates the extrinsic system, releasing tissue factor proteins from the damaged cells, and mobilizing Factors VII and VIIa. If the damage extends to the internal surface of the vein, the intrinsic system is also stimulated into action. United at Factors IX and IXa, the two systems continue the clotting process.

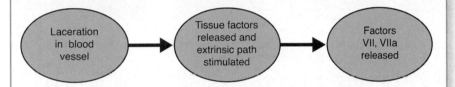

If the laceration extends to the internal vein surface, the extrinsic path unites with the intrinsic path at Factors IX and IXa.

Soft Clot Formation

Soft clot formation occurs next when Factor X and calcium phospholipids unite with prothrombin, yielding thrombin formation. Thrombin is anchored to the phospholipids, which limits thrombin to the site of the irritation or injury. Thrombin and Factor V unite in the presence of Vitamin K. This initiates the development of fibrinogen, yielding fibrin to form a mesh-like structure called a soft clot.

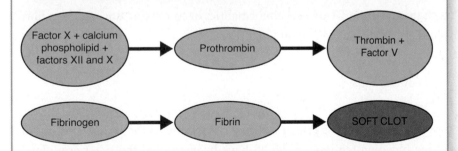

Hard Clot Formation

Next, thrombin activates Factor XII, a fibrin-stabilizing factor. Factor XII, plus the already formed fibrin-soft-clot-matrix, traps platelets, aggregating the platelets at the injury site and a hard clot is formed.

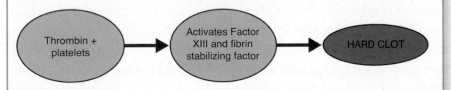

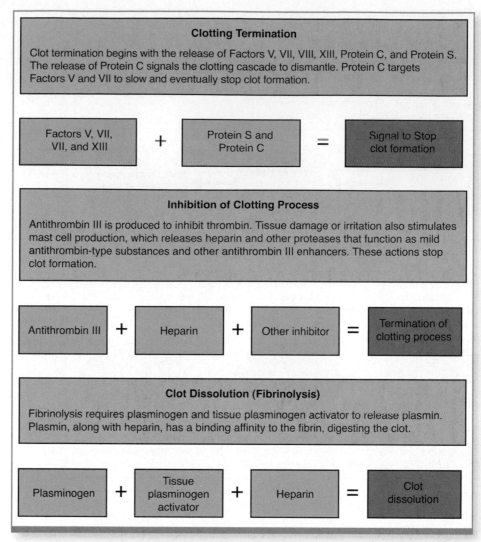

AORN. (2008a). AORN guideline for prevention of venous stasis. *Perioperative standards and recommended practices.* Denver: AORN, Inc., 141–158.

clotting mechanisms while TT detects abnormalities in converting fibrinogen to fibrin. Normal values are (Fishbach & Dunning, 2004):

- PT: 11–13 seconds
- PTT: 21–30 seconds
- TT: 7–12 seconds

Excessive bleeding can result from a deficiency of any of the blood-clotting factors. The three bleeding tendencies which have been studied the most are: platelet deficiency, hemophilia, and Vitamin K deficiency (Guyton & Hall, 2006).

1. Platelet Deficiency: Normal platelet count ranges from 150,000 to 300,000. Usually bleeding will not occur until the number of platelets in the blood falls below 50,000. Levels as low as 10,000 are often lethal. Thrombocytopenia refers to the presence of very low numbers of platelets resulting in a tendency to bleed from many small vessels or capillaries. (Unlike hemophilia in which bleeding occurs from large vessels). As a result, small hemorrhages occur throughout the body tissues and the skin may present with small purplish blotches. Most people with thrombocytopenia have the disease known as "idiopathic thrombocytopenia"

meaning unknown cause. For most of these people, specific antibodies have formed which react with their platelets, thereby destroying them. Relief from bleeding can be achieved for 1–4 days with the administration of a whole blood transfusion containing large numbers of platelets. A splenectomy sometimes may affect an almost complete cure because the spleen normally removes large numbers of platelets from the blood (Guyton & Hall, 2006).

2. Hemophilia: Hemophilia occurs almost exclusively in males; furthermore, 85% of these cases are the result of deficiency of Factor VIII. This is known as "Classic" or "Hemophilia A". In the United States, about 1 in 10,000 males have classic hemophilia. The other 15% have a deficiency in Factor IX. Both Factors VIII and IX are genetically transferred by the female chromosome. Bleeding can vary in severity but usually occurs after trauma when these individuals have experienced severe prolonged bleeding. The only effective treatment in these cases is injection of purified Factor VIII, which is expensive and has limited availability (Guyton & Hall, 2006).

3. Vitamin K: Almost all of the blood-clotting factors are formed by the liver; therefore, liver diseases such as cirrhosis, hepatitis, or yellow atrophy can depress the clotting system. Vitamin K is necessary for the liver formation of five of the important clotting factors: Factor VII, Factor IX, Factor X, Prothrombin, and Protein C. Vitamin K is continually synthesized by bacteria in the intestinal tract. Vitamin K is fat-soluble and is absorbed into the blood with fats. With gastrointestinal diseases such as ulcerative colitis or Crohn's disease, or in the presence of malnutrition or antibacterial sterilization of the gastrointestinal tract, Vitamin K absorption from the gastrointestinal tract is compromised. Another cause for Vitamin K deficiency occurs with failure of the liver to secrete bile into the GI tract as in obstruction of the bile duct or liver disease. The lack of bile prevents adequate digestion of the fat and therefore the absorption of Vitamin K. These individuals are given injectable Vitamin K 4 to 8 hours before surgical intervention. (Guyton & Hall, 2006)

Qualitative platelet defects should be suspected if the patient takes antiplatelet drugs. For example, aspirin prolongs bleeding time, an effect that can last up to 3 to 5 days. Currently, there is no available agent to reverse this action. Dipyridamole (Persantine®), sulfinpyrazone (Anturane®), nonsteroidal anti-inflammatory drugs (sulindac [Clinoril®], ibuprofen [Motrin®]), and antihistamines also have antiplatelet action, but to a lesser degree than does aspirin (Nursing Drug Handbook, 2006).

When coumarins (Coumadin,® Warfarin) are given to patients, the plasma levels of Factors VII, IX, X, and prothrombin, all found in the liver, begin to fall and the coagulative activity of the blood decreases by 50% in 12 hours and by 20% at the end of 24 hours. Normal coagulation usually returns in 1 to 3 days after discontinuing the drug. These individuals should be monitored with a PT test. For patients taking anticoagulant drugs, administering Vitamin K may restore the PT to a safe level in 12 hours (Guyton & Hall, 2006). The use of heparin in small quantities (0.5–1 mg/kg body weight) causes the blood-clotting time to increase from a normal 6 minutes to 30 or more minutes. This change occurs immediately and lasts 1.5–4 hours. Protamine sulfate can immediately reverse the effects of heparin.

HYPOVOLEMIC SHOCK

Hypovolemic shock, one of the complications of excessive blood loss, is an important concern for the first assistant. Depletion of the vascular volume caused by hemorrhage limits heart filling and decreases cardiac output. Approximately 10% of a person's total blood volume can be removed with almost no affect on arterial blood pressure or cardiac output. Greater blood loss, however, usually diminishes the cardiac output first and then the central pressure, both falling to zero with a 35%–45% blood volume loss. The decrease in arterial pressure after hemorrhage decreases the pressure in the pulmonary arteries and veins and causes a strong sympathetic reflex which stimulates vasoconstriction throughout the body; these changes result in (Guyton & Hall, 2006):

- veins and venous reservoirs constrict to maintain venous return;
- arterioles constrict to increase total peripheral resistance; and
- heart rate increases.

Hypovolemic shock can be mild to severe. The patient experiencing *mild* hypovolemic shock has lost 20% or less of blood volume. The patient's skin perfusion is poor, especially of the feet, which may be pale, cool, and clammy. The subcutaneous veins on the foot collapse. If the patient is in a supine position, the blood pressure and pulse remain normal. With sitting or standing rapidly, however, the blood pressure falls and the pulse rises. Urine output is normal. The patient may complain of being cold or thirsty.

In *moderate* shock, the patient has lost 20%–40% of circulating volume and may have pale skin and a low urine output. Many patients maintain a normal blood pressure and pulse in a supine position. A few, however, have a drop in pressure and a rise in pulse rate.

Hypotension, oliguria, and tachycardia indicate that the patient has lost 40% or more of blood volume and is experiencing *severe* shock. Skin perfusion is poor, and as the hypovolemia worsens or persists, the patient shows changes in the electrocardiogram (an indication of myocardial ischemia). As circulation decreases to the brain, the patient may become agitated, restless, or obtunded. See **Table 17.2** for the signs and symptoms of the three stages of hypovolemic shock.

Table 17.2	Signs and Symptoms of Hypovolemic Shock	
Mild	**Moderate**	**Severe**
☐ Altered level of consciousness, sometimes manifested in agitation and restlessness	☐ Tachycardia	☐ Confusion
	☐ Tachypnea	☐ Hypotension
☐ Cool, clammy skin	☐ Peripheral vasoconstriction	☐ Marked tachycardia
☐ Orthostatic hypotension	☐ Pallor	☐ Agitation
☐ Mild tachycardia	☐ Diaphoresis	☐ Anxiousness
☐ Increased vasoconstriction and myocardial contractility	☐ Restlessness	☐ Coma

Adapted from Kelley, D. M. (2005). Hypovolemic shock: An overview. *Critical Care Nursing Quarterly, 28,* 2–19; Kaplow, R., & Hardin, S. R. (2007). *Critical care nursing: Synergy for optimal outcomes.* Boston: Jones & Bartlett.

IDENTIFYING THE PATIENT'S RISK FOR ADVERSE OUTCOMES RELATED TO THE PROVISION OF HEMOSTASIS

This chapter presents potential nursing diagnoses related to alterations in the patient's clotting mechanism and the application of hemostatic techniques. **Table 17.3** identifies the desired outcome for the patient care event of provide hemostasis. Listed in the table are criteria for this outcome with the applicable nursing diagnoses, risk factors,

Table 17.3	Providing Hemostasis Does Not Compromise or Cause Injury to the Patient

Outcome 1 The patient is free from evidence of deficient fluid volume related to alterations in clotting mechanisms.

Diagnosis	Risk Factors	Outcome Indicators
Risk for Deficient Fluid Volume related to alterations in clotting mechanisms	☐ Anticoagulant drug use (coumarin [Coumadin] compounds sodium warfarin] and heparin) ☐ Aspirin, dipyridamole, sulfinpyrazone, nonsteroidal anti-inflammatory drugs (sulindac, ibuprofen, piroxicam), and antihistamine use ☐ Bone marrow replacement ☐ High doses of dextran ☐ Incompatible blood products ☐ Malnutrition, obstructive jaundice, antibiotic sterilization of the gastrointestinal tract, or malabsorption ☐ Mixed coagulation and platelet defects ☐ Myeloproliferative diseases ☐ Renal failure ☐ Retroplacental hemorrhage ☐ Severe liver disease, such as cirrhosis and hepatitis ☐ Vitamin K deficiency ☐ Widespread metastatic disease, massive trauma or burns, gram-negative or gram-positive sepsis, and some viral and malarial infections	☐ Did the patient experience uncontrollable bleeding during the procedure? ☐ After the procedure, did the patient experience bleeding, hematoma development, and excessive wound drainage? ☐ Are patient's vital signs within expected range at discharge from the OR? ☐ Are patient's blood pressure and pulse within expected range and remain stable with position change at time of transfer to PACU? ☐ Is the patient's urinary output within expected range at discharge from OR?

Outcome 2 The patient is free from evidence of injury related to mechanical hemostatic techniques used during the procedure.

Diagnosis	Risk Factors	Outcome Indicators
Risk for Injury related to the use of mechanical methods to achieve hemostasis	☐ Adhesions ☐ Application of inappropriate-sized dip ☐ Defective clip appliers ☐ Improper identification of anatomical structures before clipping ☐ Obesity (excessive tissue mass impedes exposure of the operative field, which may interfere with the use of pressure or the application of hemostatic clips) ☐ Poor operative exposure ☐ Use of packs to stop bleeding	☐ Did the patient experience hemorrhage due to the improper use of pressure or application of hemostatic clips during the procedure? ☐ Did the patient experience postprocedure infection or pain related to retained packing sponges?

17

☐ Did the patient experience postprocedure pain or neurological deficit related to inadvertent clipping of nerves surrounding the bleeding site?

☐ Did the patient experience impaired tissue integrity or damaged or destroyed integumentary and subcutaneous tissue related to inadvertent use of excessive pressure or clipping of tissue surrounding the bleeding site?

Outcome 3 **The patient is free from evidence of injury related to the use of electrical devices to achieve hemostasis used during the procedure.**

Diagnosis	Risk Factors	Outcome Indicators
Risk for Injury related to the use of electrical devices to achieve hemostasis	☐ Bony prominence at return electrode site ☐ Emaciation ☐ Excessive hair at return electrode site ☐ Exposed metal touching the patient's skin Defective return electrode ☐ Impaired skin or tissue integrity at return electrode site ☐ Impaired tissue perfusion at site of return electrode ☐ Improper identification of anatomical structure before activating active electrode ☐ Inappropriate placement of return electrode ☐ Inappropriate use of electrosurgery to stop bleeding ☐ Internal or external prosthetic device at return electrode site ☐ Laparoscopic procedure without the use of active electrode monitoring (insulation failure and capacitive coupling hazards) ☐ Obesity (excessive subcutaneous tissue does not conduct electricity as well as muscle tissue) ☐ Pacemaker or implantable cardioverter-defibrillator ☐ Poor exposure of the operative field ☐ Scar tissue at return electrode site ☐ Tension of the active and return electrode cords ☐ Use of a ground-reference generator ☐ Use of an isolated generator without return electrode monitoring ☐ Use of inflammable agents to prepare the operative site	☐ Did the patient experience impaired skin integrity at return electrode and at electrocardiographic lead sites? ☐ Did the patient experience hemorrhage during the procedure because of ineffective cauterization of blood vessels? ☐ Did the patient experience postprocedure impaired tissue integrity, hematoma formation due to ineffective desiccation or fulguration of blood vessels, and deep tissue burns? ☐ Did the patient experience postprocedure pain or neurological deficit related to inadvertent cauterization of nerves surrounding the bleeding site? ☐ Did the patient experience an ignition incident secondary to the use of electrosurgery during the procedure? ☐ Did the patient report comfort at the dispersive electrode site on admission to the postoperative care unit?

Outcome 4 The patient is free from evidence of injury related to the use of laser equipment used to achieve hemostasis during the procedure.

Diagnosis

Risk for Injury related to the use of a laser to achieve hemostasis

Risk Factors

☐ Exposed tissue around the operative field
☐ Inadequate eye protection for the patient
☐ Movement during laser operation
☐ Poor exposure of the operative field
☐ Use of dry sponges during a laser operation
☐ Use of inflammable agents to prepare the operative site
☐ Use of inflammable draping material
☐ Use of nonlaser-safe endotracheal tube during respiratory or digestive tract procedures
☐ Use of reflective instruments

Outcome Indicators

☐ Did the patient experience impaired tissue integrity surrounding the operative site or corneal burns?
☐ Did the patient experience an ignition incident secondary to the use of a laser beam during the procedure?

Outcome 5 The patient is free from evidence of injury related to the use of microfibrillar collagen hemostat, gelatin sponge, and oxidized cellulose to achieve hemostasis during the procedure.

Diagnosis

Risk for Injury related to the use of microfibrillar collagen hemostat, gelatin sponge, and oxidized cellulose

Risk Factors

☐ Allergy to bovine products
☐ Application to wound edges
☐ Failure to remove excess amounts of agent
☐ Use of a microfibrillar collagen hemostat (significantly reduces the bonding strength of methyl methacrylate)
☐ Use of blood scavenging systems

Outcome Indicators

☐ Is there evidence of abscess and hematoma formation?
☐ Was there a failure of orthopedic prosthesis due to a reduction of bonding strength of methyl methacrylate?
☐ Did the patient experience nonhealing of wound skin edges?
☐ Did the patient experience a bowel adhesion?
☐ Did the patient experience compromised urinary output due to mechanical pressure against the ureter?
☐ Was there an incident of aspiration of microfibrillar collagen hemostats?
☐ Was the patient's blood contaminated with microfibrillar collagen hemostat particles?
☐ Did the patient experience an allergic response to microfibrillar collagen hemostat?
☐ Was there a change in the patient's skin condition, other than the incision site, between admission and discharge from the OR?

Risk for Injury related to the use of collagen sponge

☐ Allergy to materials of bovine origin
☐ Use in the presence of methyl methacrylate application to wound edges
☐ Use in urological, ophthalmological, and neurological replacement procedures

☐ Did the patient experience hematoma formation due to vascular oozing from improper application or use of gelatin sponge?
☐ Was there evidence of formation of adhesions?
☐ Did the patient, have an allergic reaction?
☐ Did the patient complain of postprocedure pain or neurological deficit?

Risk for Injury related to the use of oxidized cellulose for hemostasis	☐ Hemorrhoidectomy, skin graft donor sites, and dermabrasion	☐ Did the patient experience impaired bone healing?
	☐ Nasal procedures such as polypectomy when used for packing	☐ Is there evidence of vascular stenosis?
	☐ Orthopedic procedures	☐ Does the patient complain of headaches?
	☐ Spinal cord and optic nerve procedures	☐ Did the patient experience sneezing, burning, and stinging sensations to localized application areas?
	☐ Vascular procedures	

Outcome 6 The patient is free from evidence of impaired skin integrity related to the use of gelatin sponge to achieve hemostasis during the procedure.

Diagnosis	**Risk Factors**	**Outcome Indicators**
Risk for Impaired Tissue Integrity related to the use of gelatin sponge	☐ Application to wound edges	☐ Did a hematoma form due to vascular oozing from improper application or use of gelatin sponge?
	☐ Inappropriate application of gelatin sponge, resulting in bleeding after closure	
	☐ Presence of tissue inflammation	☐ Did the patient experience postprocedure pain or neurological deficit related to inappropriate use of gelatin sponge?
	☐ Use during neurosurgery and tendon repairs	

Outcome 7 The patient is free from evidence of postprocedure infection related to thermal hemostatic techniques used during the procedure.

Diagnosis	**Risk Factors**	**Outcome Indicators**
Risk for Infection related to the use of electrical devices to achieve hemostasis	☐ Charring of tissue during the cauterization of blood vessels	☐ Does the patient have chills and fever?
	☐ Contaminated wound	☐ Is there evidence of redness, warmth, and swelling around the incision or open wounds?
	☐ Excessive use of electrosurgery resulting in large areas of tissue injury and necrosis, especially in the subcutaneous layer	☐ Does wound drainage have an unusual appearance?
	☐ Existing infection	☐ Are there abnormal white blood cell count and positive cultures from wound drainage?
	☐ Hematoma formation due to inadequate cauterization of blood vessels	
	☐ Immunosuppression secondary to blood transfusions	
	☐ Retained blood products in the subcutaneous layer (provides a growth medium for bacteria)	

Outcome 8 The patient is free from evidence of postprocedure infection related to chemical hemostatic techniques used during the procedure.

Diagnosis	**Risk Factors**	**Outcome Indicators**
Risk for Infection related to the use of microfibrillar collagen hemostat, gelatin sponge, and oxidized cellulose	Microfibrillar collagen hemostat	☐ Did the patient experience chills and fever; redness, warmth, and swelling around the incision or open wounds; and unusual wound drainage?
	☐ Retained blood products in the subcutaneous tissue (retained blood products provide an excellent growth medium for bacteria)	
	☐ Suppressed immune system secondary to blood transfusions	☐ Did the patient experience abnormal white blood cell count and positive cultures from wound drainage?

Gelatin sponge
- ☐ Allergy to gelatin products
- ☐ Application to wound edges
- ☐ Inflammation of the operative site, wound contamination, or infection

Oxidized cellulose
- ☐ Contaminated wound
- ☐ Retained blood products in the subcutaneous tissue (retained blood products provide an excellent growth medium for bacteria)
- ☐ Suppressed immune system secondary to blood transfusions

Adapted from Carpentino-Moyet, L. J. (2008). *Handbook of nursing diagnosis* (12th ed.). Philadelphia: Lippincott Williams & Wilkins; Petersen, C. (2007). *Perioperative nursing data set, the perioperative nursing vocabulary.* (Revised 2nd ed.). Denver: AORN, Inc.

and expected outcomes specific to each nursing diagnosis. Scrub nurses and circulating nurses, as well as nurses practicing as first assistants, will find the information delineated in this table useful as they assess the patient for risk factors, plan care, apply interventions to control bleeding, and evaluate the effectiveness of the interventions.

CONTROLLING BLEEDING BY MECHANICAL METHODS

The surgeon or first assistant applies pressure, hemostatic clips, clamps, staples, and sutures as mechanical methods to control bleeding. Regardless of the rate of blood flow, and whether it is from a denuded surface or a pulsatile artery, mechanical methods usually work. This discussion describes how to use pressure, clips, or staples to control bleeding.

Pressure

Pressure is the direct or indirect exertion of force on a surface to stop bleeding. Application of direct pressure with one or more fingers to the site of bleeding may be the simplest and fastest way to control bleeding. Maintaining pressure for 15–20 seconds will usually cause small clots to form at the ends of the vessels. When applying indirect pressure, use the fingers or palm to compress the area proximal to the site of active bleeding. Sponge sticks may be used to apply pressure in deep recesses. When removing the sponge, take care not to dislodge the fresh clots. The use of pressure is least traumatic to the vascular structures. When applying pressure use laparotomy sponges or other materials, such as a pack. When bleeding is extreme, pressure may be a temporary measure; suture ligatures and/or clips may be required to achieve hemostasis.

Patient Care Activities

Before using pressure, assess the need for hemostasis and determine the appropriateness of using pressure on the anatomical structure requiring hemostasis.

After the skin is incised, apply moderate pressure all along the incised surface. Control subcutaneous bleeding with a dry laparotomy sponge. Place the sponge on the bleeding surface and press with the finger tips to provide hemostasis and countertraction. The surgeon often does the same on the opposite surface. If necessary, the first assistant may use two dry laparotomy sponges, one for each side of the wound, and pull on both sides on the incised surface in opposite directions. Use a dry laparotomy sponge to apply direct digital pressure to the area of active bleeding. If the site of bleeding is hidden from view or direct pressure is unsuccessful or is impractical, apply indirect pressure to adjacent structures. For example, pressure on the scalp slows the bleeding from the dermis after an incision is made. Pressure on the femoral artery slows blood flow from a severed popliteal artery. For sudden and profuse bleeding, apply direct digital pressure. Exert only enough pressure to stop or slow the blood flow. Use pressure as a temporary measure until bleeding is controlled by other means, such as ligatures and clips. Inform the scrub person and the circulating nurse of the location and number of laparotomy sponges used as packs. Report when the sponges are removed. Use only radiopaque packing materials. Before closing the wound, recheck areas that were packed for hemostasis.

Hemostatic Clips

Hemostatic clips are used to ligate blood vessels. Quick and easy to apply, clips are efficient and effective for achieving hemostasis and also decrease the risk of foreign body reaction which can occur with suture material. Nonabsorbable clips made of stainless steel or titanium are easily seen on x-ray films. Stainless steel clips can severely interfere with a computed tomographic image. Titanium clips also interfere with computed tomographic images, but to a lesser degree than stainless steel clips. Ligating clips are available in several sizes and must be used with their respective-sized appliers. They come prepackaged and are also available in preloaded disposable appliers that can be used in either open wounds or through endoscopic cannulae. Absorbable clips are made of polydiaxanone, which are absorbed in approximately 210 days.

Patient Care Activities

Before using clips, assess the need for hemostasis and determine the appropriateness of using the clips on the anatomical structure requiring hemostasis. Check clip appliers to ensure proper functioning. Look for symmetrical jaws that securely hold the clip and close without overlapping. In the event of bleeding, isolate the severed vessel and apply direct digital pressure with a dry laparotomy sponge to control bleeding. Next, slowly roll the sponge off the incised vessel and grasp it with a nontraumatic tissue forceps. Apply the clip to a traumatized vessel (**Fig. 17.1**). The correct clip size ensures that the vessel is completely obliterated.

Apply two clips and then cut the vessel between the clips. Avoid clipping the tissue surrounding the vessel. For example, the surgeon or first assistant clips the saphenous vein distally and proximally and then cuts the vein (**Fig. 17.2**).

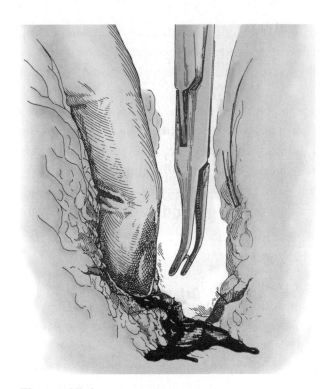

Figure 17.1

Applying a clip to a traumatic vessel.

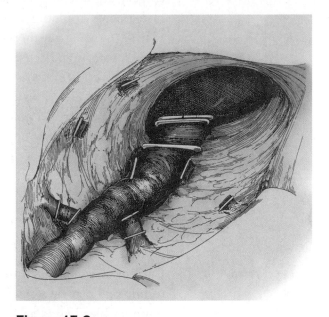

Figure 17.2

Distal and proximal application of clips to the saphenous vein.

Stapling Devices

Stapling devices place staggered rows of titanium staples and simultaneously divide the tissue between the rows. These staplers may be used in open procedures as well as endoscopic procedures in which they are placed through cannulae. Stapling devices, therefore, can be used endoscopically to achieve occlusion of vessels and tubular structures or for radiographic markings. Staplers have application in thoracic, gynecologic, pediatric and abdominal surgery for resection, transection, and creation of anastomoses. Always refer to the manufacturer's literature for proper application and use of the stapling device. Always inspect the tissue thickness and select an appropriate-sized staple cartridge. Preprocedure radiotherapy could cause changes to the tissue resulting in a tissue thickness that exceed the indicated range for staple size.

Patient Care Activities

Before using any stapling device, assess the need for hemostasis and also determine the appropriateness of the use of staples on the anatomical structure. Check the stapling device to ensure proper functioning. When positioning the stapler, ensure that there are no obstructions (ie, previously placed clips or staples) that could become incorporated in the instrument jaws (Tyco Healthcare, 2006). After firing, inspect the staple line for hemostasis. Minor bleeding can usually be controlled by electrosurgery or manual stitches.

CONTROLLING BLEEDING BY THERMAL METHODS

The surgeon or first assistant uses heat generated from low- and high-frequency electrical current, lasers, and ultrasonic devices as thermal methods to control bleeding. Depending on the method used for hemostasis, bleeding can be controlled effectively from small blood vessels and denuded surfaces, up to and including vessels 7 mm in diameter. This discussion describes the use of electrocautery, electrosurgery, argon-enhanced electrosurgery, vessel fusion, laser, and ultrasonic-powered instruments to control bleeding.

Prior to using any thermal device to control blood loss, assess the specific needs for hemostasis and determine the most appropriate energy device. Selection of the energy-based hemostasis method should be based on the location of the anatomical structure as well as overall patient requirements. Indiscriminate use of thermal energy can result in inadvertent damage to vital structures, such as nerves and delicate tissues. Use of appropriate safety precautions for the patient and the entire patient care team is essential.

Electrocautery

Electrocautery is used to coagulate small vessels. The device uses low voltage and low frequency direct current that is produced by a battery. Heat is generated as the current travels through the high impedance wire located at the tip of the device. Current does not pass through the patient as it does in electrosurgery devices. This technology may be employed in ophthalmology and other minor procedures when minimal bleeding is anticipated. Electrocautery use is limited, however, because of its inability to cut tissue, fulgurate bleeding tissue surfaces, and coagulate large bleeders. Furthermore, if care is not taken, the heated wire can stick to cauterized surfaces, which may result in rebleeding when the wire is pulled away from the tissue (Ulmer, 2007a).

Patient Care Activities

Avoid using the electrocautery device in an oxygen enriched environment. When activating the device ensure that the tip does not touch a flammable item such as a gauze sponge. Activate the unit only when the tip is in view. Deactivate the unit before the tip leaves the surgical site and gently remove it from the tissue. Before disposing of the device replace the safety cap, which will help prevent accidental activation of the unit when it is placed in the trash. Prior to disposing of the device, carefully cut or remove the cautery tip with scissors, large metal hemostats, or pliers. Do not activate the device during dismantling.

Electrosurgery

Electrosurgical generators produce a variety of high-frequency radiofrequency electrical waveforms that are delivered as bipolar or monopolar current. Electrosurgery employs alternating current, as opposed to the direct current used in electrocautery devices.

Bipolar electrosurgery is a good choice for procedures where the surgeon needs to limit thermal spread, such as on delicate tissue and/or on small anatomical structures. If there is the potential for electromagnetic interference with implanted medical devices, such as pacemakers or internal cardioverter-defibrillators, bipolar electrosurgery is a safer alternative because of the low voltages (maximum range between 300–1200 volts) used to deliver the current. With the bipolar mode there are two electrodes, an active and a return electrode; however, they are both incorporated into the same instrument. The current flows between the tips of the bipolar forceps that are grasping tissue. The tissue effect of bipolar electrosurgery, when forceps are used, is desiccation because the tines of the forceps are in direct contact with the tissue. Other instrumentation is also available that allows cutting during bipolar procedures. Bipolar current delivery can be enhanced with the use of an ammeter, which indicates when the amount of current being delivered has decreased. The ammeter signals the operator both visually and audibly that the current is flowing, confirming tissue desiccation. When the ammeter has indicated current flow has dropped, the operator can either stop bipolar activation or move the forceps to fresh or adjacent tissue to continue the process (Ulmer, 2007b).

Monopolar Electrosurgery

Monopolar is the most frequently used electrosurgical modality. This is due to its versatility and clinical effectiveness. In monopolar electrosurgery, the active electrode delivers current to the surgical site. The patient return electrode is located somewhere else on the patient's body. The current passes through the patient as it completes the circuit from the active electrode to the patient return electrode. Monopolar electrosurgery allows the surgeon or first assistant to deliver current using four different waveforms: cut, blend, fulguration, and hemostasis with division, a mode available on tissue sensing energy electrosurgery generators. When the surgeon changes from one waveform to another waveform the resulting tissue effect will change. Tissue effects will also vary according specific surgeon techniques.

The *cut* mode is designed to divide tissue with little or no hemostasis. This mode uses a continuous low voltage waveform that produces maximum current concentration, which in turn produces the greatest amount of heat over a very short period of time. The result in tissue effect is cutting, also called vaporization. Because the waveform is continuously delivered through the active electrode, the cut mode requires less voltage, with maximum voltages ranging from 1350–4000 volts. When cutting tissue, hold the active electrode tip just over the target tissue and activate the device (**Fig. 17.3**) (Ulmer, 2007a).

Most electrosurgery generators also have one or more *blend* modes. This mode is used to simultaneously cut tissue and coagulate bleeding. The blended mode uses a modified cut waveform to achieve the clinical effect. However, the difference between

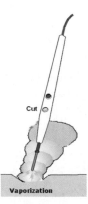

Figure 17.3

Vaporization of tissue using the cut waveform.

Source: Copyright © Covidien. All rights reserved. Reprinted with the permission of the Energy-based Devices and Surgical Devices divisions of Covidien.

the cut mode and the blended mode is the amount of time the current is on. As an example, in some units the blend waveform current is on approximately 50% of the time. Although it is not a continuous waveform like the cut waveform, the tissue is still vaporized with the added benefit of coagulation. The blended mode is a function of the cut mode. Adjusting the coagulation mode will not decrease or increase the coagulation effect of the blended mode (Massarweh, Cosgriff, & Slakey, 2006).

When the coagulation mode is activated, the generator modifies the waveform to an interrupted duty cycle of approximately 4.5–6.5%. Depending on the coagulation mode selected, the current produces spikes of voltage ranging from of 3000–9000 peak-to-peak volts of electrical current. Tissue heats when the waveform spikes and cools down between spikes of voltage, thus producing coagulation of the cells. Called *fulguration*, the sparking from the coagulation waveform coagulates the tissue over a wide area (**Fig. 17.4**). When fulgurating, hold the active electrode tip slightly above the target tissue and activate the device. The spark will jump through the air and coagulate the tissue (Ulmer, 2007b; Valleylab, 2005).

A recent innovation in electrosurgery cutting and coagulation provides a high level of hemostasis while efficiently dissecting a wide range of tissue types. Called hemostasis with division, the mode is only available on tissue sensing energy electrosurgery generators (**Fig. 17.5**) and when a special electrosurgery

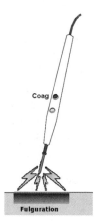

Figure 17.4

Fulguration of tissue using the coagulation waveform.

Source: Copyright © Covidien. All rights reserved. Reprinted with the permission of the Energy-based Devices and Surgical Devices divisions of Covidien.

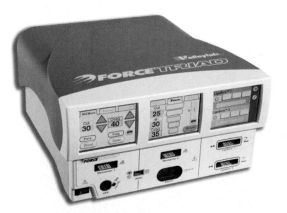

Figure 17.5

Force Triad™ Energy Platform with TissueFect Sensing Technology.

Source: Copyright © Covidien. All rights reserved. Reprinted with the permission of the Energy-based Devices and Surgical Devices divisions of Covidien.

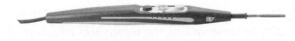

Figure 17.6

Force TriVerse™ Electrosurgical Device. The device has three buttons: cut and blend (yellow), dissection with hemostasis (clear), and blue (coagulation).

device (**Fig. 17.6**) is used. When using the hemostasis with division mode, rather than the standard coagulation waveform of conventional electrosurgery generators, the surgeon or first assistant is able to divide tissue efficiently while maintaining hemostasis and minimizing thermal injury to surrounding tissues (Valleylab, 2005). This is possible because of precise control of the electrosurgical current, called closed-loop control. The patient advantage of the tissue sensing technology is that electrosurgery energy is precisely dosed according to the patient's tissue needs.

Whether using the cut, blend, coagulation, or hemostasis with division modes, desiccation can be achieved when the active electrode is applied directly to the tissue. This technique is most efficient when the cut mode is activated because less voltage is used to achieve the desired tissue effect. Rather than cellular vaporization, cells dry out and a coagulum is formed (Ulmer, 2007a). **Figure 17.7** portrays the desiccation with the cut and coagulation mode. When using the cut mode for desiccation, activation of the device can be shorter than when using blend or coagulation modes because of the continuous delivery of the cut current.

Other variables also impact tissue effect. For example, eschar build-up on the active electrode or tissue increases resistance and causes greater sparking to surrounding tissue. Electrode size is another variable. The smaller the electrode used, the higher the current concentration. A small active electrode, such as a needle tip, can achieve the tissue effect, even though the power setting is reduced. Patient tissue also impacts the clinical efficiency of electrosurgery. High-resistance tissue, such as adipose tissue, interferes with the flow of current which results in the need for higher generator settings. Likewise, tissue that is low in resistance, such as highly vascular muscle tissue, requires lower generator settings. Distance from the patient-return electrode site to the active electrode site also impacts the flow of current. The greater

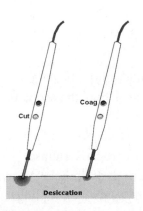

Figure 17.7

Desiccation of tissue using the cut and coagulation waveforms.

the distance, the higher the resistance; therefore, higher power settings are required. Tissue density and the amount of fluid in or surrounding the tissue also affects the amount of current and the time necessary to achieve hemostasis.

The equipment and supplies needed for electrosurgery are dry laparotomy sponges, appropriate tissue forceps, the electrosurgical generator, an active electrode, a non-conductive holster device to contain and confine the active electrode when not in use, a coated electrode tip, a scratch pad when an uncoated electrodes is used, and a patient-return electrode (when using the monopolar mode). Hemostasis with electrosurgery is less reliable on larger vessels than ties or suture ligatures; therefore, use it only on small vessels—3mm or less in size. Hemostasis of large vessels must be accomplished with ties, clips, suture ligatures, and/or vessel fusion technology.

A defective electrosurgery unit can cause burns or electrical shocks to the patient and/or members of the operative team and also increases the risk of fire and explosion hazards. Do not use electrosurgery in the presence of flammable agents such as alcohol, acetone, or prepping agents that contain alcohol. Also, do not use electrosurgery in an oxygen-enriched environment. The depth of tissue injured by the heat produced through electrosurgery is difficult to predict and to control. When using electrosurgery, injury to adjacent nerves or other anatomical structures can easily occur. Depending on the type of technology used, electrical burns can occur at the site of the patient return electrode, under electrocardiographic leads, at temperature probe entry sites, at positional pressure points, and at sites where the patient's skin comes in contact with grounded metal, such as the operative bed. Extreme caution should be exercised when using ground-reference generators and isolated generators without contact quality monitoring. Ground referenced generators are capable of causing a patient burn at alternate pathway sites and at the patient return electrode site. Likewise, use of isolated generators without return electrode monitoring technology can result in a burn at the return electrode. Manufacturer's instructions must be followed.

Burns of the skin edges may occur if a noninsulated portion of the active electrode inadvertently contacts the skin while the electrosurgery is applied to a deeper structure. A catheter or any other type of plastic tubing should not be used in an attempt to insulate exposed metal. In addition to altering a medical device, they can serve as a fuel source and could ignite during the procedure.

When using electrosurgery during laparoscopic procedures, the first assistant and the entire surgical team must be alert for potential hazards, including (Valleylab, 2005):

- Electrodes can remain hot enough to cause burns after the electrosurgical current is deactivated;
- Activation of the electrode outside the field of vision could injure the patient;
- Electrical currents can pass through conductive objects such as the scope or cannulae causing localized burns to the patient or surgeon;
- Use of hybrid trocars composed of both metal and plastic can cause capacitive coupling and unintended burns; use all metal or all plastic trocar systems;
- Activation of the electrode at high power for extended periods of time can cause burns of the abdominal wall from direct contact or from capacitive coupling;

- Compromised insulation may lead to inadvertent sparking or neuromuscular stimulation;
- Activation of the electrode while in contact with other instruments can cause unintended injury; activate the electrode only when near or touching the target tissue;
- Use the lowest power setting to achieve the desired results; and
- Use care when inserting and withdrawing the electrode to avoid possible damage to the patient.

Patient Care Activities

Follow the manufacturer's instructions and the Association of periOperative Registered Nurses' (AORN) Recommended Practices for Electrosurgery (2008). Before using electrosurgery, assess the need for hemostasis and determine the appropriateness of using the instrument on the anatomical structure requiring hemostasis by evaluating vessel size. If the vessel is large, use a ligature or clips to control the bleeding. Check the active electrode (pencil) before use. Look for frayed cords and ensure that the tip of the active electrode is securely seated. Activate the electrode by depressing and then releasing the appropriate switches. The unit should immediately activate when the switch is depressed and deactivate when the switch is released. Do not indiscriminately activate the active electrode. Identify the electrosurgery site and adjacent structures. Do not apply electrosurgery to adjacent nerves or tissue unless their destruction is intended. In the event of bleeding, isolate the severed vessel and apply direct digital pressure with a dry laparotomy sponge to control bleeding. Next, slowly roll the sponge off the severed vessel and touch the vessel with the activated electrode for as long as it takes to blanch the tissue. Charring the tissue is usually not necessary. When using tissue forceps or a hemostat, grasp the end of the vessel with the forceps or hemostat and touch the activated electrode to the instrument for as long as it takes to blanch the tissue. Avoid grasping the surrounding tissue with the instrument. Reduce the risk of electrical burn to yourself by using the lowest possible power setting, activating the cut current (it has lower voltage), not touching the patient, holding the hemostat or forceps with a full grip, and touching the active electrode tip to the instrument before activating the generator. If the scrub person operates the active electrode, verbally indicate when to begin the electrical current. Stop the flow of current by removing your finger from the active electrode (pencil) button or your foot from the foot pedal. When not in use, place the active electrode in a non-conductive safety holster. If the electrode is too large for the non-conductive safety holster place it in an area where it will not make contact with the patient or flammable materials.

AORN
Association of periOperative Registered Nurses

Argon-Enhanced Electrosurgery

Use argon-enhanced electrosurgery (**Figs. 17.8** and **17.9**) to improve the effectiveness of the electrosurgical event. This technology uses a stream of argon gas, which is inert and noncombustible, to conduct electrosurgical current. Argon gas is heavier than air and displaces nitrogen and oxygen. The electrosurgical current ionizes the argon gas, thus making it more conductive than air and creating a bridge between the electrode and tissue (Valleylab/Covidien, 2006).

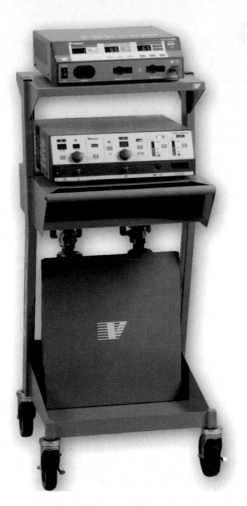

Figure 17.8

Argon-enhanced electrosurgery system.

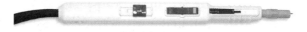

Figure 17.9

Argon-enhanced handset.

Use argon-enhanced electrosurgery for noncontact coagulation (**Fig. 17.10**), to reduce drag and tissue adhesion to the electrode in the cut mode, for less tissue damage, and to create a more flexible eschar. An additional benefit of argon-enhanced electrosurgery is less production of electrosurgery plume. The force of the gas hitting the tissue blows the blood away from the intended electrosurgery site; thus, only tissue is heated versus tissue and blood. Clinical uses for argon-enhanced electrosurgery include head and neck resection, mastectomy, thyroidectomy, liver resection, transplant procedures, trauma, open cholecystectomy, creation of skin flaps, mediastinal tumors, sternotomy, open-heart procedures, bone tumor resection, scoliosis procedures, joint replacement, bone graft, pelvic and perineal dissection, partial

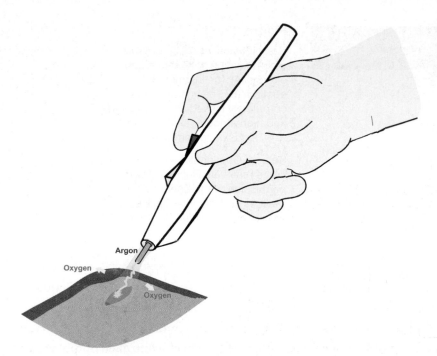

Figure 17.10

Argon-enhanced electrosurgery.

nephrectomy, retroperitoneal node dissection, gynecological oncology procedures, radical hysterectomy, and breast reconstruction. Argon-enhanced electrosurgery is also used in general, gynecologic, and thoracic laparoscopic procedures.

Patient Care Activities

Refer to the manufacturer's manual for instructions on using the hardware and disposable supplies for argon-enhanced electrosurgery. Implement electrosurgery safety precautions as listed in AORN's Recommended Practices for Electrosurgery (2008). Do not use argon-enhanced electrosurgery with right and left cardiac shunting, owing to increased risk of arterial gas emboli. Exercise extreme caution when using gas coagulation on the wall of the small intestine. Underlying tissue injury may not be readily apparent under the fine eschar produced by gas-enhanced electrosurgery. Complications such as tissue rupture may occur after the procedure. Gas coagulation may result in the formation of a venous embolism. Avoid venous gas embolism formation by not using gas coagulation for a long period of time, preventing the handset nozzle from making direct contact with an open vessel or tissue surface, setting the gas flow at the lowest level capable of producing the desired coagulation effect, and preventing activation of the gas flow from the handset for more than 5 seconds without cutting or coagulating tissue (Valleylab/Covidien, 2006).

Tissue Fusion

Tissue fusion is an advanced electrosurgical technology in which the intimal layers of the vessel wall are fused and a permanent seal is formed. Unlike other energy-based ligation methods, which shrink the vessel walls and rely on the proximal thrombus to occlude it and thus provide hemostasis, the lumen of the vessel is obliterated with this ligation method. The system works by optimizing a combination of pressure and

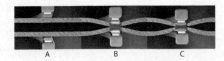

Figure 17.11

Vessel fusion works by optimizing a combination of pressure and energy. (A) The instrument is applied. (B) The instrument is completely closed and low voltage and high amperage is delivered. (C) The fusion is complete.

energy (**Fig. 17.11**). The pressure on tissue is predetermined by the ratcheting of the instrument, and the energy is supplied by the tissue fusion bipolar configured generator that delivers a very low voltage, high amperage, and a continuous electrical waveform mode. The generator delivers computer-feedback-controlled output which results in the collagen and elastin within the vessel wall liquefying and re-forming into a seal that is plastic-like in consistency and possibly translucent (**Fig. 17.12**). There is reduced sticking and charring of the tissue and minimal lateral thermal spread. Vessels 7 mm and smaller are reliably sealed with burst strengths above three times normal systolic pressure (360 mm Hg). This is statistically comparable to ligation by suture, clip, and staple. Bundles of tissues that contain one or more vessels 7 mm or smaller may be sealed, and thus the need for dissection is eliminated. Because it is a bipolar configuration, the potential for patient injury from stray current during minimally invasive procedures is eliminated. Many of the vessel fusion instruments have built-in cutting devices which eliminate the need for removing the instrument before transecting the fused tissue. **Figures 17.13**, **17.14**, and **17.15** show examples of vessel fusion instruments used for open and laparoscopic procedures (Massarweh, Cosgriff, Slakey 2006).

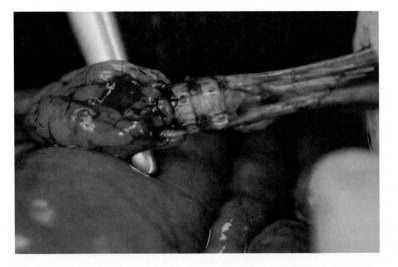

Figure 17.12

Collagen and elastin within the vessel wall liquefy and re-form into a seal that is plastic-like in consistency and possibly translucent.

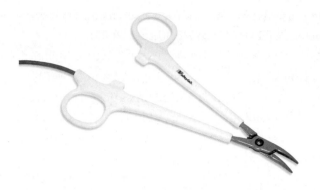

Figure 17.13

Open vessel fusion instrument without cutting mechanism (LigaSure Precise™).

Source: Copyright © Covidien. All rights reserved. Reprinted with the permission of the Energy-based Devices and Surgical Devices divisions of Covidien.

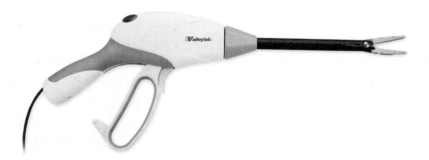

Figure 17.14

Open vessel fusion instrument with built-in cutting mechanism (LigaSure Impact™).

Source: Copyright © Covidien. All rights reserved. Reprinted with the permission of the Energy-based Devices and Surgical Devices divisions of Covidien.

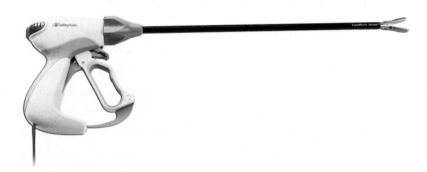

Figure 17.15

Laparoscopic vessel fusion instrument with built-in cutting mechanism (LigaSure Atlas™ Sealer/Divider).

Source: Copyright © Covidien. All rights reserved. Reprinted with the permission of the Energy-based Devices and Surgical Devices divisions of Covidien.

Patient Care Activities

To avoid incomplete sealing, do not grasp tissue beyond the electrode surface and avoid placing tissue in the jaw hinge. Prevent thermal burn by always keeping the external surface of the instrument jaws away from adjacent tissue while activating the vessel fusion device. Conductive fluids (eg, blood or saline) in direct contact with or in close proximity to the instrument may carry electrical current or heat, which may cause unintended burns to the patient; therefore remove fluid from around the instrument jaws before activating the instrument. Vessel fusion has not been shown to be effective for sterilization procedures; therefore, do not use vessel fusion devices for tubal sterilization or tubal coagulation for sterilization procedures. To ensure a complete seal, always use caution during surgical cases in which patients exhibit certain types of vascular pathology (atherosclerosis, aneurysmal vessels, etc.). For best results, apply the seal to unaffected vasculature. Do not use vessel fusion devices on vessels in excess of 7 mm in diameter (Valleylab/Tyco Healthcare, 2005).

Ultrasonic-Powered Instruments

Ultrasonic-powered surgical instruments vibrate at 55,500 times per second to cut and coagulate at the same time. This technology offers an alternative to electrosurgery for some surgical procedures. These devices have four types of action: cutting, coaptation, coagulation, and cavitation.

- Cutting: Unlike electrosurgery, which uses extreme local heat to vaporize and disrupt tissue, the ultrasonic-powered devices use a combination of tension and pressure to rapidly stretch the tissue. When the tissue reaches its elastic limit, the blade cuts easily through it.
- Coaptation: Coaptation is the adherence of tissue and is achieved by disrupting hydrogen bonds causing collagen molecules to collapse and adhere to one another at low temperature. The tissue is then transformed into a sticky coaptate.
- Coagulation: Applying the ultrasonic energy to the tissue a few seconds longer than it takes to coaptate, a rise in temperature leads to the release of water vapor and then to coagulation.
- Cavitation: A side effect of the ultrasonic energy used to cut, coaptate, and coagulate occurs when the vibration of the device is transmitted to the surrounding tissue, causing rapid volume changes of the tissue and cell fluid. Cavitation aids in tissue plane dissection and visibility of the field.

When compared to electrosurgery, the lower temperatures generated by ultrasonic devices have the potential for less charring and minimal lateral thermal tissue damage. The motion of the tip produces a vapor which, because of lower tip temperatures, could carry infectious aerosols (Barrett & Garber, 2004). The rapid mechanical motion of the devices means no electricity goes through the patient, the risk of stray–energy injuries is reduced, and dissection near vital structures is safer, however heat is produced. The risk of rebleeding with ultrasonic surgery is also reduced. This technology is being used in many open procedures such as mastectomy, axillary dissection, parotidectomy, thyroidectomy, hysterectomy, breast reduction, abdominoplasty, and harvesting of arteries. They are also used laparoscopically for colorectal, adrenalectomy, and fundoplication procedures (Ethicon Endo-Surgery, 2008).

Patient Care Activities

Follow the manufacturer's instructions when using any of the vessel-sealing or ultrasonic-powered instruments. For open procedures, the appropriate inserts are attached to the instruments and the cord is passed off to the circulating nurse. Single-use laparoscopic instruments are usually fully assembled. When not in use, they should be placed on the Mayo stand. Because the vessel fusion generator is bipolar, no return electrode is required for the system to operate. This does not replace a monopolar generator when an electrosurgical pencil will be used (a return electrode is always required for monopolar technology).

Laser

Lasers are the second most common heat-producing device used by surgeons. Laser is an acronym that describes a process in which light energy is produced—light amplification by stimulated emission of radiation. Carbon dioxide, argon, and neodymium: yttrium-aluminum-garnet (Nd-YAG) lasers are used to create beams of light. Each substance produces a different light with its own specific wavelength and depth penetration of tissue. This energy is a concentrated beam of light. It is distinguished from an ordinary light beam because it is monochromatic, collimated, and coherent. Monochromic light is composed of photons of the same wavelength or color. Collimated laser beams are waves that are parallel and can be focused through a lens. Coherent waves are orderly and travel in the same direction, providing power to the laser beam. Thermal effects vary with the wavelength, beam fluence, tissue color, consistency, and water content. This allows for selective and specific tissue effects among the various types of lasers (Youker & Ammirati, 2001). Surrounding tissue is also heated because it borders the impact site. The degree of adjacent tissue damage depends on the duration of the laser beam exposure. Lasers produce high heat—100°C to 1,000°C—which boils and explodes the cells. This cellular vaporization releases steam and cell contents (Anderson, 2004). The characteristics of the cellular matter are determined by the type of laser being used, and the type of tissue.

Patient Care Activities

Use AORN's Recommendations Practices for Laser Safety in Practice Settings (AORN, 2008c, pp. 447–452) when preparing the room, the operative team, and the patient for laser procedures. Ensure that personnel operating the equipment have been properly trained. Place warning signs at all entrances to the room and close doors. Inspect all equipment and cables. Wear eye protection appropriate to the laser being used. Use the lowest possible settings to achieve the desired effects. Have sterile water available on the field and know where the fire extinguisher is. Tape saline-moistened pads to the closed eyelids of the anesthetized patient or provide eye protection if the patient is awake. Apply damp laparotomy sponges to the tissue surrounding the operative site. Use flame-resistant or moistened drapes. For otolaryngology (ENT) procedures, laser-proof (endotracheal) ET tubes should be used and the cuff filled with a saline/methylene blue solution. Use dulled, ebonized, or nonreflective anodized finished instruments near the site of laser use. Use wet tongue blades or quartz or titanium rods as a back-stop for the beam. This prevents the beam from inadvertently hitting underlying tissue. Inform the circulating nurse when the laser is not in use so he or she may set the laser on standby. Evacuate the noxious fumes and laser plume with appropriate scavenging devices. When using a fiber through an endoscopic instrument to deliver laser energy, assure that the fiber extends to at least 1 cm past the end of the endoscope and is in view at all times during active use (AORN, 2008c, p. 448). Remember that the eye is the most vulnerable part of the body for laser injury. Corneal and/or retinal damage can occur. Fire is one of the most significant hazards associated with laser use (AORN, 2008c).

Documentation and Communication Procedures

When using *electrosurgery, argon-enhanced electrosurgery, vessel-sealing, or ultra-sound-powered instruments*, document the generator number, power settings, type of electrode and return electrode placement, if used, in the nurse's notes. In addition, document the condition of the skin at the site of the return electrode. Note any conditions of the skin that were not apparent before the procedure.

When using a *laser*, document the unit number, power setting, and safety precautions used in the nurse's notes. Include a description of the condition of the skin surrounding the operative site before and after the procedure.

CONTROLLING BLEEDING BY CHEMICAL METHODS

Direct topical applications of chemical agents such as microfibrillar collagen, hemostat gelatin sponge, collagen sponge, oxidized cellulose, thrombin, and fibrin gel (sealants) to areas of active bleeding are chemical methods to control bleeding. The surgeon or first assistant uses chemical agents as an adjunct to hemostasis when controlling bleeding by ligatures or when other conventional methods are ineffective or impractical. Successful use of chemical agents entails a slow rate of blood flow, as in denuded, oozing surfaces of the gallbladder bed or liver abrasions. The use of chemical agents on pulsating arterial bleeding is contraindicated. The surgeon or the first assistant should determine the appropriateness of using a chemical agent on the anatomical structure requiring hemostasis. In addition, the wound classification needs to be considered before using a chemical agent because the use of most agents is ill advised or contraindicated in contaminated wounds. To use chemical agents when blood or other fluids submerge the bleeding site, the bleeding must be visible. Chemical agents are not designed to act as a tampon or a plug in a bleeding site. The patient should have no known allergies to the agent being used or to the substance from which the agent was derived.

Microfibrillar Collagen Hemostat

Microfibrillar collagen hemostat (Avitene®) is a purified bovine corium (dermal) collagen. It is a fibrous, water-insoluble partial hydrochloric salt. Microfibrillar collagen hemostat is prepared in a loose fibrous form and in a compacted nonwoven web form. When microfibrillar collagen hemostat comes in contact with a bleeding surface, platelets are attracted to it and adhere to the fibrils; the platelets then aggregate, beginning the clotting phenomenon.

Because it is a foreign substance, microfibrillar collagen hemostat may potentiate wound infections and formation of abscesses. Microfibrillar collagen hemostat may significantly reduce the bonding strength of methyl methacrylate. When applied to wound edges during the closure of incisions, it interferes with the healing of the skin edges. Failure to remove excess microfibrillar collagen hemostat may result in bowel adhesion or mechanical pressure significant to compromise the ureter. Failure to remove excess microfibrillar collagen hemostat in otolaryngological procedures may result in aspiration of particles. Fragments of microfibrillar collagen hemostat may pass through filters of blood scavenging systems. Microfibrillar collagen hemostat is contraindicated in patients sensitive to materials of bovine origin. Microfibrillar collagen hemostat cannot control bleeding due to systemic disorders. The effect of microfibrillar collagen hemostat on platelet adhesion and aggregation, however, is not inhibited by heparin.

Equipment and supplies needed when using microfibrillar collagen hemostat are dry tissue forceps free of blood, dry laparotomy sponges, and suction. Microfibrillar collagen hemostat adheres to wet gloves, instruments, and tissue surfaces. Furthermore, moistening microfibrillar collagen hemostat with saline or thrombin impairs its ability to act as a hemostatic agent.

Microfibrillar collagen hemostat is inactivated by autoclaving. Sterilization by ethylene oxide is contraindicated. Ethylene oxide reacts with the bound hydrochloric acid in microfibrillar collagen hemostat to form ethylene chlorohydrin.

Patient Care Activities

Assess the need for the use of microfibrillar collagen hemostat to provide hemostasis. Ascertain if the patient has any known allergies to bovine derivatives. Determine the adequacy of primary efforts at hemostasis (clamping, electrosurgery, tying, and suturing) before using microfibrillar collagen hemostat. Evaluate the rate of blood flow. Ascertain if the bleeding site can be made visible and accessible. Determine the appropriateness of microfibrillar collagen hemostat to the anatomical structure on which it would be used. Keep microfibrillar collagen hemostat away from the skin edges when closing the incision. Do not use microfibrillar collagen hemostat on bone surfaces to which prosthetic devices are to be attached with methyl methacrylate. Determine the appropriateness of microfibrillar collagen hemostat in regards to the wound classification. Using microfibrillar collagen hemostat is ill advised in the presence of contaminated or infected wounds.

When applying or assisting in the application of microfibrillar collagen hemostat, suction or sponge the area dry. Provide additional exposure as needed. With clean dry tissue forceps, such as Mayo forceps, apply microfibrillar collagen hemostat to the bleeding site. Using moderate pressure, hold a dry laparotomy sponge on the bleeding site. Hemostasis usually occurs in about 1 minute. The time will vary, depending on the force and severity of the bleeding. Three to 5 minutes may be required for brisk bleeding such as splenic lacerations or arterial suture lines. Additional microfibrillar collagen hemostat may be used as needed. Apply the nonwoven web form of microfibrillar collagen hemostat in small squares to the bleeding site. Cover the site with a dry cottonoid strip for small areas or a laparotomy sponge for larger areas. A suction tip may be used to hold pressure on the cottonoid strip. Pack microfibrillar collagen hemostat firmly into the spongy bone surface to control oozing from cancellous bone. Avoid spilling microfibrillar collagen hemostat on nonbleeding surfaces, particularly in the abdominal or thoracic viscera. Remove excess microfibrillar collagen hemostat from all surfaces by gently teasing with blunt forceps and irrigation before closing the wound. Avoid the reintroduction of blood from operative sites treated with microfibrillar collagen hemostat. Notify the circulating nurse to discontinue the use of blood scavenging equipment once microfibrillar collagen hemostat is used. Discard unused microfibrillar collagen hemostat. Do not resterilize microfibrillar collagen hemostat.

Absorbable Gelatin Sponge

Gelatin sponge (Gelfoam®) is a pliable sponge of purified gelatin that can hold several times its weight. The sponge liquefies in 2 to 5 days after application to the bleeding mucosa of the rectum, the vagina, or the nasal passages and is absorbed in 4 to 6 weeks without excessive scar formation. The sterile gelatin sponge should not be resterilized by heat, as heating may change the absorption time (RxMed, 2008).

Because gelatin sponges absorb fluid, it expands and exerts pressure on adjacent structures. Implantation in the brain or around the spinal cord may result in compression of these structures owing to the accumulation of sterile fluid around the sponge. Gelatin sponge interferes with the healing of the skin edges when used in the closure of incisions. Use of the gelatin sponge is not recommended in the presence of infection; when gelatin sponges are used in the presence of gross contamination or infection, bacteria can become enmeshed in the sponge and thus causes the formation of an abscess (RxMed, 2008). The equipment and supplies needed are straight Mayo scissors, dry tissue forceps free from blood, dry laparotomy sponges, suction, and the gelatin sponge.

Patient Care Activities

Determine the appropriateness of using gelatin sponge on the anatomical structure requiring hemostasis. Evaluate the appropriateness of the gelatin sponge on the basis of the wound classification. Do not use during neurosurgery, for tendon repairs, and in the presence of inflammation. Before using gelatin sponge, evaluate the effectiveness of hemostasis by mechanical and thermal methods. Look at the rate of blood flow and, if possible, make the site accessible by clearing away blood with suction or a dry sponge. Provide additional exposure as needed. Cut pieces of gelatin sponges into the desired sizes. For dry application, compress each piece between the fingers and then use a clean tissue forceps to apply it to the bleeding site. Using moderate pressure, hold it with a dry laparotomy sponge to the bleeding site for 10 to 15 seconds. For wet application, the scrub person should have the sponges prepared for use by immersing the cut pieces in saline, squeezing out the air bubbles, and then placing the pieces back in the saline until used. For damp application, blot the piece of gelatin sponge on a dry laparotomy sponge. Using moderate pressure, hold the gelatin sponge in place with a dry laparotomy sponge for 10 to 15 seconds. Capillary action draws the blood into the gelatin. Wet the laparotomy sponge with saline to avoid pulling the gelatin off the site when removing the sponge. An alternative method of using wet or dry gelatin sponge is to apply suction to the laparotomy sponge while holding the gelatin in place. This technique draws blood into the gelatin and seems to hasten clotting. Pack gelatin loosely in closed spaces or cavities because it swells as it absorbs fluid. Apply light pressure in cavities or closed spaces. To prevent recurrent bleeding, leave the gelatin sponge in place. If desired, the surgeon may close the wound with the gelatin sponge left in place. Keep gelatin away from skin edges when closing the incision as gelatin interferes with wound healing. Discard unused gelatin sponges and do not resterilize.

Absorbable Collagen Sponge

The absorbable collagen sponge (Instat, Hemopad) is a purified and lyophilized (freeze-dried) bovine dermal collagen. It is prepared as a lightly cross-linked sponge-like pad. The collagen protein has a helical structure, which is preserved in the manufacturing process. Collagen's inherent hemostatic action is dependent on this helical structure. When blood comes in contact with collagen, platelets aggregate and release clotting factors. Collagen sponge is absorbed in 8 to 10 weeks.

Because collagen sponge absorbs fluid and may expand, exerting pressure on adjacent structures, it is not recommended for use in neurological, urological, and ophthalmological procedures. Collagen sponge reduces the bonding strength of methyl methacrylate and interferes with the healing of the skin edges. Formation of adhesions, foreign body reactions, and allergic reactions are among the most serious adverse effects of collagen sponges. Heating inactivates the collagen sponge. The equipment and supplies needed are straight Mayo scissors, dry tissue forceps free from blood, dry laparotomy sponges, suction, and the collagen sponge.

Patient Care Activities

Before the procedure, determine if the patient has allergies to collagen sponges or bovine derivatives. Determine the appropriateness of using collagen sponge on the anatomical structure requiring hemostasis. In addition, evaluate the appropriateness of the collagen sponge on the basis of the wound classification. Avoid the use of collagen sponges in neurological, urological, and ophthalmological procedures and in the presence of methyl methacrylate. Before using collagen sponge, evaluate the effectiveness of hemostasis by mechanical and thermal methods. Look at the rate of blood flow, and, if possible, make the site accessible by clearing away blood with suction or a dry sponge. Collagen sponge is most effective when used dry. Provide additional exposure as needed. Pack collagen loosely in closed spaces or cavities because it swells as it absorbs fluid. Compression of adjacent structures can occur as the collagen swells. Do not use collagen sponges on bone surfaces to which prosthetic devices are to be attached with methyl methacrylate. Cut pieces of collagen sponges into the desired sizes. With clean tissue forceps, apply it to the bleeding site. Hold it with a dry laparotomy sponge on the bleeding site using moderate pressure. Hemostasis usually occurs in 2 to 5 minutes. Remove excessive collagen before closing the wound. Keep the sponges away from skin edges when closing the incision. Discard unused collagen sponges and do not resterilize.

Oxidized Regenerated Cellulose

Oxidized cellulose (Surgicel, Surgicel Nu-Knit) is an absorbable, white, knitted fabric, which has a faint caramel odor. It can be sutured or cut without fraying. Oxidized cellulose is stored at room temperature. Performance is not affected by the cellulose's age, but discoloration may occur. When saturated with blood, it swells into a dark gelatinous mass, which aids in the formation of a clot. The mechanism of how oxidized cellulose works is not clearly understood; it appears to have a local physical effect, rather than altering normal clotting mechanisms.

The hemostatic effect of oxidized cellulose is unaffected by the addition of thrombin. The activity of thrombin, however, is destroyed by the low pH of oxidized cellulose. The hemostatic effect of oxidized cellulose is diminished when it is moistened with water, saline, other hemostatic agents, or anti-infective agents. Autoclaving causes physical breakdown of oxidized cellulose.

Oxidized cellulose has some bactericidal properties, but is not a substitute for antimicrobial agents (Phillips, 2007, p. 549). Because it is a foreign body, its use in contaminated wounds can potentiate infection.

Oxidized cellulose may interfere with callus formation when used in bone defects, such as fractures. Additionally, it absorbs fluid and may expand, exerting pressure on adjacent structures. This is especially true when it is used around the spinal cord in laminectomies and around the optic nerve. The rate at which it is absorbed is dependent on the amount used, the extent of blood saturation, and the tissue bed. Encapsulation and foreign body reactions can occur if oxidized cellulose is left in the wound. Stenosis of vascular structures may occur if oxidized cellulose is used to wrap a vessel tightly. The low pH of oxidized cellulose may cause burning or stinging sensations, headaches, and sneezing when it is used as a pack for epistaxis. It may also account for burning or stinging when cellulose is used after the removal of a nasal polyp, hemorrhoidectomy, and application to wound surfaces such as donor sites, venous stasis ulcerations, and dermabrasions.

Use oxidized cellulose only in the presence of whole blood. Oozing of other body fluids, such as serum, does not react with oxidized cellulose to produce satisfactory hemostasis. In addition, do not use oxidized cellulose as a wound packing material. The equipment and supplies needed are straight Mayo scissors, dry tissue forceps free from blood, dry laparotomy sponges, suction, and the oxidized cellulose.

Patient Care Activities

Determine the appropriateness of using oxidized cellulose on the anatomical structure requiring hemostasis. In addition, evaluate the appropriateness of the oxidized cellulose on the basis of the wound classification. Before using oxidized cellulose, evaluate the effectiveness of hemostasis by mechanical and thermal methods. Look at the rate of blood flow and, if possible, make the site accessible by clearing away blood with suction or a dry sponge. Provide additional exposure as needed. Avoid its use in fractured bones because it may interfere with callus formation. Avoid wrapping structures such as blood vessels and ureters. Cut pieces of oxidized cellulose into the desired size. Use only the amount necessary to achieve hemostasis. Apply it dry, with clean tissue forceps to the bleeding site. Hold it with a dry laparotomy sponge on the bleeding site, using moderate pressure until hemostasis is achieved. If possible, remove oxidized cellulose before closing the wound. It may, however, be left in place with no adverse effects if it is properly applied and is present in small amounts. Do not use it as a packing material for bleeding wounds. Discard unused oxidized cellulose and do not resterilize. Evaluate the patient after the procedure for signs of stinging and burning, sneezing, or headaches when oxidized cellulose was used for epistaxis.

Look for postprocedure burning or stinging when it is used after the removal of a nasal polyp, hemorrhoidectomy, or in application to wound surfaces such as donor sites, venous stasis ulcerations, and dermabrasions. If it is causing the patient difficulty, recommend removal.

Thrombin

Thrombin (Thrombostat,™ Thrombin-JMI®) is a protein substance produced through a conversion reaction in which prothrombin of bovine origin is activated by tissue thromboplastin in the presence of calcium chloride. Thrombin requires no intermediate physiological agent for its action; it clots the fibrinogen of the blood directly. The speed with which thrombin clots blood is dependent upon its concentration: one 5,000u vial dissolved in 5 mL saline diluent can clot an equal volume of blood in less than a second or 1,000mL in less than a minute (Rx List, 2008). Thrombin is used as an aid in hemostasis whenever oozing blood from capillaries or small vessels is accessible. Thrombin may be used in combination with an absorbable gelatin sponge. Soak the sponge and squeeze to remove any air to be more effective in promoting hemostasis. Never inject thrombin directly into a vessel or allow it to gain access to large open vessels as extensive intravascular clotting and death may result. Do not sponge area after application as the clot may become dislodged (Rx List, 2008).

Patient Care Activities

Assess the need for use of thrombin to provide hemostasis. Ascertain if the patient has any allergies to bovine derivatives. Evaluate the appropriateness of the use of thrombin. Repeated clinical applications of thrombin increase the likelihood that antibodies against thrombin and/or factor V may be formed. The use of topical thrombin has occasionally been associated with abnormalities in hemostasis ranging from asymptomatic alterations in prothrombin time (PT), and partial thromboplastin time (PTT), to mild or severe bleeding or thrombosis which rarely have been fatal (Rx List, 2008).

The intended use of thrombin determines the strength of the solution. For general use (dental extractions, skin grafting neurosurgery, and plastic surgery), solutions of 100u/mL are used. When bleeding is profuse, as in cut surfaces of the spleen and liver, higher concentrations such as 1,000 to 2,000u/mL may be required. Reconstituted solutions should be used immediately or refrigerated to use within 3 hours (Rx List, 2008). Other considerations when using thrombin include (Rx List, 2008):

- Before application, the recipient surface should be sponged (not wiped) free of blood;
- A spray may be used or the surface flooded using a syringe;
- The most effective hemostasis occurs when the thrombin mixes freely with the blood as soon as it reaches the surface;
- Avoid sponging the area after application to assure that the clot remains securely in place; and

- When thrombin is used in conjunction with an absorbable gelatin sponge, make sure the concentration is appropriate, the sponge is squeezed to remove any air, and that the sponge is held in place for 10–15 seconds with a gauze sponge.

Fibrin Gel (Glue, Sealant)

Fibrin sealants (Floseal™, Matrix, and Tisseel) recreate the natural physiological coagulation and are useful for controlling generalized oozing of blood. They are indicated for use as an adjunct to hemostasis when control of bleeding by conventional surgical methods, including suture, ligature and electrosurgery is ineffective or impractical. They do not control massive and brisk arterial or venous bleeding. All fibrin sealants are composed of two major ingredients: purified fibrinogen (a protein) and purified thrombin (an enzyme) derived from bovine or human blood. When mixed together, the resulting agent mimics the last stages of the clotting cascade to form a fibrin clot. They are used during surgery to speed the formation of a stable clot, to stop bleeding in areas difficult to reach with sutures, to reduce the amount of blood in the field, to lower postprocedure infections or inflammations, and to treat patients with blood-clotting disorders. Fibrin sealants are used in cardiovascular and thoracic surgical procedures, in trauma to the spleen or liver, in dental extractions with hemophiliacs, for hemostasis at cannula sites, in gastric ulcer surgery, on vascular grafts, and for nasal packing during endonasal surgery (Silvergleid, 2007).

Patient Care Activities

As with other chemical hemostatic agents, fibrin sealants are not intended as a substitute for meticulous surgical technique and proper application of ligatures or other conventional procedures for hemostasis. Do not use in patients with known allergies to bovine derivatives. Do not inject the sealant directly into blood vessels as extensive intravascular clotting and even death may result. Do not use for closure of skin as it may interfere with healing of the skin edges. When made from human plasma, these sealants carry a risk of transmitting infectious agents. Follow manufacturer's instructions for mixing the two components.

Documentation and Communication Procedures

Document the use of microfibrillar collagen hemostat, gelatin sponge, collagen sponge, oxidized cellulose thrombin, and fibrin sealants in the nurse's notes. Inform postoperative care unit (PACU) nurses if oxidized cellulose is used for packing or is applied to wound surfaces.

PACU
Postanesthesia
care unit

CONCLUSION

The first assistant plays an important role in providing hemostasis during an operative or invasive procedure. Knowledge of the mechanisms of clotting and how to assess the patient's clotting mechanisms will enable the first assistant to implement methods to control bleeding by mechanical, thermal, and chemical methods.

COMPETENCY ASSESSMENT
Provide Hemostasis

Name: _____ Title: _____ Unit: _____ Date of Validation: _____

Type of Validation: ☐ Initial   ☐ Annual   ☐ Bi-annual

COMPETENCY STATEMENT: The first assistant demonstrates competency to provide hemostasis during an operative or invasive procedure.

Performance Criteria	Met	Not Met
1. Describes the mechanism of clotting	☐	☐
2. Assesses the patient's clotting mechanisms	☐	☐
3. Describes the signs of hypovolemic shock	☐	☐
4. Identifies the patient's risk for adverse outcomes related to the provision of hemostasis	☐	☐
5. Applies mechanical methods to control bleeding	☐	☐
6. Applies thermal methods to control bleeding	☐	☐
7. Applies chemical methods to control bleeding	☐	☐

_____
Validator's Signature

_____
Employee's Signature

_____
Validator's Printed Name

17

REFERENCES

1. Anderson, K. (2004). Safe use of lasers in the operating room. *AORN Journal, 79*(1): 171–188.
2. AORN. (2008a). AORN guideline for prevention of venous stasis. *Perioperative standards and recommended practices.* Denver: AORN, Inc., 141–158.
3. AORN. (2008b). Recommended practices for electrosurgery. *Perioperative standards and recommended practices.* Denver: AORN, Inc., 315–329.
4. AORN. (2008c). Recommended practices for laser safety in practice settings. *Perioperative standards and recommended practices.* Denver: AORN, Inc., 447–452.
5. Barrett, W.L. & Garber, S.M. (2004). Surgical smoke—a review of the literature. *Business Briefing: Global Surgery:* 1–7.
6. Craig, J. (2006). *Valleylab™ Mode: A Comparison with Conventional Electrosurgery.* Boulder, CO: Valleylab/Covidien.
7. Ethicon Endo-Surgery. (2008). Harmonic® technology. Retrieved March 2, 2008, from http://www.harmonic.com/dtcf/pages/HarmonicTechnology.htm?pgn=1.
8. Fishbach, F.T., & Dunning, M.B. (Eds.). (2004). *A manual of laboratory and diagnostic tests.* Philadelphia: Lippincott.
9. Guyton, A.C., & Hall, J.E. (2006). *Textbook of medical physiology* (11th ed.). Elsevier: Philadelphia.
10. Kaplow, R., & Hardin, S.R. (2007). *Critical care nursing: Synergy for optimal outcomes.* Boston: Jones & Bartlett.

11. Kelley, D.M. (2005). Hypovolemic shock: An overview. *Critical Care Nursing Quarterly*, *28*, 2–19.

12. Massarweh N.N., Cosgriff, N., Slakey, D.P. (2006). Electrosurgery: history, principles, and current and future uses. *J Am Coll Surg.*; 202(3); p. 520–530.

13. *Nursing 2006 Drug Handbook* (26th ed.). (2006). Philadelphia: Lippincott, Williams, and Wilkins.

14. Phillips, N. (2007). *Berry & Kohn's operating room technique (11th ed.).* St. Louis: Mosby Elsevier.

15. Rothrock, J.C. (Ed.). (2007). *Alexander's care of the patient in surgery* (13th ed.). St. Louis: Mosby, Inc.

16. RxList. (2008). Thrombostat: Drug description. Retrieved March 2, 2008 from http://www.rxlist.com/cgi/generic/thrombin.htm.

17. RxMed. (2008). Gelfoam®. Retrieved March 2, 2008 from http://www.rxmed.com/b.main/b2.pharmaceutical/b2.1.monographs/CPS-%20Monographs/CPS-%20(General%20Mono-graphs-%20G)/GELFOAM.html.

18. Silvergleid, A.J. (2007). Fibrin Sealant. Retrieved March 2, 2008 from http://patients.uptodate.com/topic.asp?title=nasal&file=transfus%2F5850&mark=1&submit=find.

19. Tyco Healthcare. Instructions for use: Multifire endo GIA™ 30 12 mm (single use staplers with titanium staples). Retrieved March 2, 2008 from http://www.autosuture.com/AutoSuture/pagebuilder.aspx?contentID=36922&topic-ID=7398.

20. Ulmer, B.C. (2007a). *Electrosurgery self-study guide.* Boulder, CO: Valleylab/Covidien.

21. Ulmer, B.C. (2007b). Electrosurgery: History and fundamentals. *Perioperative Nursing Clinics, Vol 2, No 2,* 89–101.

22. Valleylab (2005). *Force Triad™ Electrosurgical generator user's guide.* Boulder, CO: Valleylab.

23. Valleylab (2006). *Force Argon™ II-2 user's guide.* Users Guide, Boulder, CO: Valleylab.

24. Youker, S.R., & Ammirati, C.T. (2001). Practical aspects of laser safety. *Facial Plastic Surgery, 17*(3): 155–163.

CHAPTER 18

Facilitate Care After the Procedure

Rose Moss

Carol Schramm

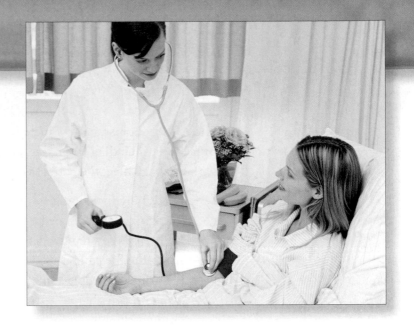

INTRODUCTION

Facilitating care after the operative or invasive procedure refers to the nursing care activities done during the postprocedure[†] period to make the patient physically and psychologically ready to begin convalescence and rehabilitation.

ROLE OF THE PERIOPERATIVE ADVANCED PRACTICE NURSE

Because practice settings vary, involvement of the advanced practice nurse (APN) in facilitating postprocedure care varies. This chapter addresses activities that advanced practice nurses, such as registered nurses, first assistants, and clinical specialists, may perform during the patient's last stages of the perioperative continuum. In the postoperative domain of patient care, the APN's role includes (CBPN, 2003):

- Evaluating and managing an individualized perioperative plan of care;
- Communicating relevant information about the procedure to postoperative care personnel;
- Collaborating with the healthcare team to manage the patient's postoperative course; and
- Serving as consultant, educator, and resource to the patient, family members, and other healthcare professionals during discharge planning.

The advance practice nurse's activities during and after the procedure should complement the nursing care the patient receives in the postanesthesia care unit (PACU), the nursing unit, the clinic,

Chapter Contents

APN
Advanced Practice Nurse

PACU
Postanesthesia Care Unit

and the home. This chapter is divided into two parts: activities of the immediate postprocedure period and discharge planning.

MEASURABLE CRITERIA

The APN demonstrates competency to facilitate care after the operative or invasive procedure, including discharge planning and teaching, by identifying the critical variables that affect the patient's convalescence. These include:

- Describing the stages of wound healing.
- Recognizing postprocedure wound complications.
- Recognizing systemic postprocedure complications.
- Assessing the patient's physiological and psychological comfort level.
- Ensuring the proper functioning of devices employed to assist recovery.
- Providing discharge instructions to the patient and family based on their individual informational needs and health literacy.
- Completing discharge followup.

POSTPROCEDURE CARE PREPARES THE PATIENT FOR CONVALESCENCE AND REHABILITATION

Table 18.1 provides guidance for preparing the patient for convalescence and rehabilitation following the operative or invasive procedure. Outcome statements, potential nursing diagnoses, and outcome indicators are identified for the postprocedure period.

Table 18.1	Postprocedure Care Prepares the Patient Physically and Psychologically for Convalescence and Rehabilitation

Recognizing Postprocedure Wound Complications

Outcome 1 The patient experiences uncomplicated wound healing.

Diagnosis	Risk Factors	Outcome Indicators
Risk for Impaired Tissue Integrity related to abscess formation	☐ Presence of pus in the wound ☐ Inadequate wound drainage ☐ Use of agents such as hydrogen peroxide, 1% povidone-iodine, 0.25% acetic acid, and 0.5% sodium hypochlorite to clean the wound ☐ Poor wound care	Does the patient show evidence of damage to integumentary or subcutaneous tissue?
Risk for Impaired Tissue Integrity related to the formation of gas gangrene	☐ Wound contamination with hemolytic streptococci or *Clostridium perfringens*	☐ Does the patient have a high fever? ☐ Does the patient complain of intense localized pain? ☐ Is a foul odor present? ☐ Is tissue crepitant, dark, and cool?

Potential for Impaired Skin Integrity: nonhealing wound	☐ Infection	☐ Are there signs and symptoms of abscess formation?
	☐ Hematomas	
	☐ Seromas	☐ Are there signs and symptoms of impending wound dehiscence?
	☐ Retained foreign substances	
	☐ Underlying diseases or conditions	☐ Are there signs and symptoms of wound infection?
	☐ Alteration in tissue perfusion due to excessive wound tension	☐ Does the patient complain of pain beyond what is normal for a healing wound?
	☐ Adjacent tissue scarring or trauma	☐ Does the wound have drainage, redness, or swelling?
	☐ Altered circulation to the affected area due to swelling	
	☐ Exudates irritating to the skin	
	☐ Use of cytotoxic substances to clean the wound	
	☐ Chemical irritation of substances used to clean an open sound	
	☐ Altered nutritional state	
	☐ Obesity	
	☐ Use of tape	
	☐ Pressure from drain tubes	

Outcome 2   The patient remains free from wound infection after the procedure.

Diagnosis	**Risk Factors**	**Outcome Indicators**
Risk for Wound Infection	☐ See Table 18.3	☐ Does the patient have chills or a fever?
		☐ Is the skin surrounding the incision or other open wound red, warm, and swollen?
		☐ Does the patient have unusual wound drainage?
		☐ Does the patient have an abnormal white blood cell count and positive cultures of wound drainage?
Risk for Infection related to seroma formation in the postprocedure wound	☐ Obesity	☐ Does the patient have chills or a fever?
	☐ Operative wound with areas of undermined skin flaps	☐ Is the skin surrounding the incision or other open wound red, warm, and swollen?
		☐ Does the patient have unusual wound drainage?
Risk for Potential Infection related to wound dehiscence or evisceration	☐ Inadequate wound closure	☐ Does the patient show evidence of wound infection?
	☐ Wounds closed under undue tension	☐ Does the patient show evidence of peritonitis?
	☐ Compromised wound healing	

18

Recognizing Fever, Tachycardia, Pulmonary Complications, Thrombophlebitis, Urinary Tract Infection, and Adynamic Ileus

Outcome 3   The patient is free from systemic postprocedure complications.

Diagnosis	Risk Factors	Outcome Indicators
Risk for Postprocedure Hyperthermia (fever)	☐ Blood administration during the procedure ☐ Removal of inflamed tissue during the procedure ☐ Decreased ambulation ☐ Wound complications ☐ Intra-abdominal abscesses or anastomotic leaks ☐ Thrombophlebitis	☐ Does the patient have an elevated temperature? ☐ Does the patient feel warm to the touch? ☐ Does the patient complain of feeling feverish?
Risk for Alteration in Postprocedure Cardiac Rate (tachycardia)	☐ Fever ☐ Lack of a medication routinely taken by the patient, such as digitalis ☐ Relative hypotension ☐ Inadequate pain relief ☐ Apprehension	☐ Is there gradual or abrupt hypotension? ☐ Does the patient have good skin color? ☐ Does the patient complain of feeling faint or dizzy? ☐ Is tachycardia present?
Risk for Ineffective Airway Clearance during the postprocedure period	☐ Bed rest ☐ Poor cough associated with narcotics, anesthesia, pain, fatigue, tenacious secretions, tracheal edema due to endotracheal intubation, procedures around the trachea such as thyroidectomy and carotid endarterectomy and abdominal distention ☐ Presence of a nasogastric tube during or after an operative or invasive procedure	☐ Are abnormal breath sounds such as rales, crackles, rhonchi, or wheezes present? ☐ Does the patient show a productive cough? ☐ Is there a change in the patient's rate or depth of respirations? ☐ Does the patient show evidence of tachypnea? ☐ Is cyanosis present?
Risk for Ineffective Breathing Patterns during the postprocedure period	☐ Ineffective airway clearance ☐ Stasis of pulmonary secretions ☐ Aspiration ☐ Smoking ☐ Hypoventilation during anesthesia (eg, deflated lung during pulmonary resection) ☐ Handling of pulmonary tissue during the procedure, leading to edema or alveolar damage	☐ Are breath sounds normal? ☐ Is there resonant percussion over the lung field? ☐ Is the pulse within normal limits? ☐ Is the patient afebrile? ☐ Is the patient's respiratory rate within normal limits (16–20 breaths/min)? ☐ Is the patient's cough productive of clear mucus only? ☐ Is there an absence of pleuritic pain? ☐ Is the white blood cell count remaining within normal limits?

☐ Are arterial blood gas values or pulse oximeter readings within normal limits?

☐ What is the patient's mental status?

☐ What is the patient's skin color?

☐ Does the patient have shortness of breath or dyspnea?

☐ Is there evidence of the use of accessory muscles to breathe, altered chest excursions, tachypnea, nasal flaring, and pursed-lip breathing or a prolonged expiration phase?

☐ Does the patient make statements indicating respiratory difficulty?

Risk for Acute Pulmonary Embolus

☐ Venous stasis from immobility

☐ Positioning during the procedure and in the PACU

☐ Abdominal distention

☐ Trauma to the pelvic veins during the procedure

☐ Does the patient show evidence of tenderness and pain in the calf?

☐ Does the patient show evidence of edema in the lower extremities?

☐ Does the patient have a fever?

Risk for Postprocedure Urinary Tract Infection

☐ Dehydration

☐ Urinary retention

☐ Indwelling urinary catheter

☐ Is the patient's urine clear?

☐ Is the patient's urine free of any unusual odor?

☐ Is there an absence of urinary frequency, urgency, or burning on urination?

☐ Is there an absence of chills or fever?

☐ Is the number of white blood cells or bacteria in the urine inconsequential?

☐ Does the patient have a negative urine culture?

Risk for Altered Postprocedure Bowel Function

☐ Manipulation of intestines during the procedure

☐ Decreased activity

☐ Administration of medications (ie, narcotics for pain relief)

☐ Peritonitis

☐ Septicemia

☐ Hypovolemia

☐ Hypokalemia

☐ Is the patient's abdomen soft and nondistended?

☐ Is there an absence of nausea and vomiting?

☐ Is there an absence of urinary frequency, urgency, or burning on urination?

☐ Does the patient have a return of bowel sounds in an appropriate amount of time, depending on the procedure?

☐ Does the patient pass flatus or stool?

18

Assessing Postprocedure Comfort Level

Outcome 4 The patient experiences physiological and psychological comfort after the operative or invasive procedure.

Diagnosis	Risk Factors	Outcome Indicators
Risk for Alteration in Comfort (postprocedure pain)	☐ Operative incision ☐ Pressure on nerve endings from edema or purulent substances ☐ Tissue necrosis from infection ☐ Chemical irritation from substances used to clean the wound ☐ Reflex muscle spasm ☐ Excessive tissue trauma ☐ Aggressive tissue retraction and manipulation	☐ Does the patient state that his or her pain is under control? ☐ Are the patient's facial expressions and body positioning relaxed? ☐ Does the patient gradually increase activity level? ☐ Is there a decreased use of pain medications?
Risk for Alteration in Comfort related to nausea and vomiting	☐ Visceral irritation ☐ Postprocedure adynamic ileus ☐ Narcotics ☐ Anesthetic agents	☐ Is the patient vomiting? ☐ Does the patient complain of nausea?
Risk for Alteration in Comfort related to inadvertent hypothermia	☐ Anesthetic-impaired thermoregulation ☐ Cold OR environment ☐ Administration of cool intravenous fluids ☐ Administration of cool, dry anesthetic gases ☐ Skin prep with cool solutions ☐ Exposure of internal organs	☐ Is the patient shivering? ☐ Does the patient complain of being cold? ☐ Is the patient normothermic (36°C–38°C [96.8°F–100.4°F])?

Ensuring the Proper Functioning of Devices to Assist Recovery

Outcome 5 The patient is free from injury related to the use of medical devices used to assist in recovery.

Diagnosis	Risk Factors	Outcome Indicators
Risk for Injury related to devices used to assist patient recovery	Malfunctioning or improperly applied: ☐ Nasogastric tube ☐ Taped pressure dressings ☐ Chest tubes ☐ Closed wound drainage devices ☐ Open wound drainage devices	☐ Are there signs of impaired skin integrity? ☐ Are there signs of damage to internal organs?

Discharge Planning

Outcome 6 **The patient and family are compliant with the rehabilitation process and the therapeutic regimen after the procedure.**

Diagnosis	Risk Factors	Outcome Indicators
Deficient knowledge related to the rehabilitation process after the procedure	☐ Demonstrate less than adequate recall of information about past procedure experiences or demonstrate misunderstanding, misinterpretation, or misconceptions ☐ Inaccurately follow through with previous instructions ☐ Inadequately perform a self-care skill ☐ Demonstrate inappropriate or exaggerated behaviors such as hysteria, hostility, or apathy ☐ Low readiness for reception of information (anxiety) ☐ Lack of interest or motivation to learn ☐ Cognitive limitations ☐ Uncompensated short-term memory loss ☐ Inability to use materials or information resources owing to factors such as cultural or language differences ☐ Unfamiliarity with information	☐ Can the patient and/or family describe in their own words the anticipated physical and psychological effects of the operative or invasive procedure? ☐ Do the patient and/or family express their feelings regarding the operative or invasive procedure and its expected outcomes? ☐ Does the patient verbalize expectations about pain relief? ☐ Can the patient and/or family member state the measures that can he taken to alleviate pain? ☐ Can the patient and family members identify family and community support systems? ☐ Is the patient able to demonstrate turning, coughing, deep breathing, incision splinting, passive leg exercising, and ambulating? ☐ Can the patient and or family describe anticipated steps in postprocedure activity resumption? ☐ Do the patient and/or family indicate that they understand verbal and written discharge instructions? Can they describe these instructions in their own words? ☐ Are the patient and/or family able to demonstrate implementation of therapeutic treatments such as dressing change and administration of medication?
Risk for ineffective therapeutic regimen management	☐ Activity intolerance: decreased strength and endurance related to age, the presence of disease, or the effect of surgery/invasive procedure ☐ Chronic pain or discomfort ☐ Acute pain or discomfort after surgery/invasive procedure ☐ Uncompensated perceptual-cognitive impairment	☐ Is the patient performing the activities of daily living (eating, bathing, toileting, dressing, and grooming)? ☐ Is the patient able to implement prescribed therapeutic regimens such as dressing changes and administration of medication?

18

☐ Uncompensated neuromuscular or musculoskeletal impairment

☐ Severe anxiety

☐ Depression

☐ Restrictive treatment modalities after surgery/invasive procedures such as immobilization (casts and traction)

☐ Operative/invasive procedure resulting in loss of limb, sight, hearing, or bowel or bladder control

☐ Lack of functional support systems in the home

☐ If the patient cannot perform self-care activities of prescribed therapeutic treatment regimens, is there a significant other present who does these activities?

Risk for Noncompliance with prescribed therapeutic regimen after the procedure.

☐ Patient history of noncompliance with prescribed therapeutic regimens

☐ For patients unable to provide self-care, a family history of noncompliance with prescribed therapeutic regimens

☐ Lack of patient support systems (family, friends)

☐ Denial of illness by the patient or the family (if the patient is unable to provide self-care)

☐ Perceived ineffectiveness of the recommended therapeutic regimens by the patient or the family

☐ Perceived lack of seriousness by the patient or the family of the health problems or risk factors

☐ Perceived lack of susceptibility to the potential complications secondary to noncompliance by the patient or the family

☐ Insufficient knowledge or skills of the patient or the family to implement the recommended therapeutic regimens

☐ Lack of a plan by the patient or the family for integrating therapeutic recommendations into daily routine

☐ Is the patient observed being noncompliant with a prescribed therapeutic treatment?

☐ Does the patient or significant other make statements describing noncompliance?

☐ Do objective tests (such as physiologic measures) reveal noncompliance?

☐ Is there evidence of the development of complications such as a wound infection?

☐ Is there evidence of exacerbation of symptoms?

☐ Does the patient fail to keep appointments?

☐ Does the patient fail to progress or resolve an identified problem?

Adapted from Carpentino-Moyet, L. J. (2008). *Handbook of nursing diagnosis* (12th ed.). Philadelphia: Lippincott Williams & Wilkins; Petersen, C. (2007). *Perioperative nursing data set, the perioperative nursing vocabulary.* (Revised 2nd ed.). Denver, CO: AORN, Inc.

CRITICAL VARIABLES THAT AFFECT THE PATIENT'S CONVALESCENCE

To facilitate postprocedure care, it is important to understand the critical variables that affect the patient's convalescence. These include preprocedure condition, procedure time, the amount of blood transfused, and the organ system(s) involved in the procedure. In addition, the expected clinical course helps predict what to anticipate during the postprocedure period. The PACU nurse must be provided with all relevant data upon admission of the patient to the unit. This includes facts about the patient's medical, surgical, social, and psychological history. For example, the PACU nurse must be informed if the patient has chronic pulmonary disease, drug allergies, or a history of smoking. Report must also include the type of procedure performed and pertinent events that may have occurred during the procedure, such as extraordinary blood loss and specimens removed. The type of drugs administered during the procedure, such as anesthetic agents, muscle relaxants, and antibiotics, are reported. Advance practice nurses and physician assistants, as well as physicians, may also write the orders after the procedure, which are necessary to direct postprocedure care. The transfer of the patient from the operative or invasive procedure suite to PACU requires reiteration of any patient care orders; postprocedure orders should address vital signs, the scope and frequency being dependent on the patient and procedure; fluid balance; respiratory care; position in bed and mobilization; administration of fluid and electrolytes; drainage tubes; medications; laboratory examinations; and imaging (Doherty, 2008). A useful rule regarding satisfactory recovery from a procedure is that some objective evidence of progress toward normal bodily function be exhibited every day. The advance practice nurse assesses for this evidence in a number of ways: by visiting the patient in the healthcare facility, through an office followup visit, telephoning the patient, and possibly even making a visit to the patient's home. During this time, evaluation should include vital signs and intake and output documentation; functioning of devices used to help the patient's recovery; auscultation of the heart, lungs, and abdomen; assessment of the legs for phlebitis; and progression toward wound healing. Observations are then recorded and referrals for additional medical treatment are made as needed. Detection of early postprocedure complications and the initiation of treatment or appropriate referral before complications are exacerbated critically affect the patient's rehabilitation course.

WOUND HEALING

Knowledge of the stages of wound healing is necessary to assess the patient for wound complications (**Table 18.2**). The healing process begins with wound inflammation. Immediately after injury, temporary vasoconstriction followed by vasodilation occurs at the wound site. During this phase, plasma and plasma proteins pass through dilated capillary walls to the site of injury. Within a few hours, the wound fills with a protein-rich exudate, containing red and white blood cells, and fibrin. Massive tissue injury or the presence of foreign material intensifies inflammation. In a clean operative wound, inflammation lasts several days.

Within a few hours of injury, the epithelial phase begins as the epidermis near the wound edge thickens. Basal cells divide and migrate across viable tissue on the wound

Table 18.2	Stages of Surgical Wound Healing		

Stage	Time	Events	
Inflammatory Stage	Immediate to 2–5 days	**Hemostasis** ☐ Vasoconstriction ☐ Platelet aggregation ☐ Thromboplastin forms a clot **Inflammation** ☐ Vasodilation ☐ Phagocytosis	
Proliferation Stage	2 days to 3 weeks	**Granulation** ☐ Fibroblasts form a bed of collagen—fills the defect and produces new capillaries **Contraction** ☐ Wound edges approximate to reduce defect **Epithelialization** ☐ Crosses moist surface ☐ Cells travel about 3 cm from point of origin in all directions	
Remodeling Stage	3 weeks to 2 years	**Collagen Remodeling** ☐ New collagen forms which increases tensile strength	

Adapted from Fishman, T. D. Phases of wound healing. Retrieved April 17, 2008 from http://www.medicaledu.com/phases.htm.

surface. Usually, within 48 hours, complete wound epithelialization has occurred. At this point, however, the wound is still weak.

By the second or third day, the cellular phase begins. The fibrin strands that filled the wound in the inflammatory phase act as a framework for fibroblast invasion. Capillaries begin to proliferate to supply nutrients to the healing wound. At 3 to 5 days, fibroplasia begins when collagen fibers replace fibroblasts. During this phase, the wound gets stronger as the collagen fibers form and organize. The collagen fibers form a thick hard ridge in the wound, which is also called the healing ridge. Eventually, the collagen fibers rearrange into an organized pattern. The healing ridge softens as the wound matures and the collagen fibers contract.

Factors that broadly affect wound healing include advanced age; hypoxemia, anemia, and hypoperfusion; use of steroids or chemotherapeutic drugs; metabolic disorders; and nutritional status. It is important to recognize abnormal wound healing in the postprocedure phase. **Table 18.3** lists the risk factors that should alert the nurse to a potential abnormal wound healing episode. Aging produces intrinsic physiologic changes that result in delayed or impaired healing of wounds, supported by clinical experience demonstrating a decrease in wound closure rates as well as

Table 18.3	Risk Factors Affecting Wound Healing

Systemic Intrinsic Factors

Aging

Diabetes

☐ Peripheral vascular disease (PVD)

☐ Immunological defects

☐ Neuropathy

Renal Disease

Jaundice

Local Intrinsic Factors

Blood supply

Changes in oxygen tension

Abnormal Scarring

☐ Hypertrophic scar formation

☐ Keloids

Extrinsic Factors

Nutrition

☐ Vitamin deficiency (Vitamins C, A, B, K)

☐ Mineral deficiency (zinc, copper, magnesium, iron)

Smoking

Radiotherapy

Infection

☐ Microbial flora of the skin

☐ Microbial colonization of the wound

☐ Pathogenic invasion

Drugs

☐ Nonsteroidal anti-inflammatory drugs (NSAIDS)

☐ Corticosteroids

☐ Immunosuppressants

☐ Chemotherapeutic agents

Wound Dressings

☐ Air exposure versus occlusion

☐ Moisture vapor transmission rates

☐ Contamination and infection

☐ Dressing choice

Adapted from Brown, J. Intrinsic and extrinsic factors affecting wound healing. Retrieved April 17, 2008 from http://judithbrowncpd.co.uk/index_files/Intrinsic%20 and%20Extrinsic%20Factors%20 Affecting%20Wound%20Healing.pdf.

tensile strength with advancing age (Barbul, 2006). Older persons tend to have more cardiovascular disease, metabolic diseases (diabetes mellitus, malnutrition, and vitamin deficiencies), and cancer, the use of medications generally increases with age, many of which impair wound healing; all of these conditions contribute to the higher incidence of wound problems in the elderly.

FIO$_2$
Fraction of
Inspired Oxygen

All aspects of wound healing are affected by oxygenation of tissues. Although healing is stimulated initially by the hypoxic wound environment, optimal collagen synthesis requires oxygen as a cofactor. Increasing subcutaneous oxygen tension levels by increasing the fraction of inspired oxygen (FIO$_2$) of inspired air for brief periods during and immediately following surgery results in enhanced collagen deposition and in decreased rates of wound infection after elective surgery (Barbul, 2006). The nurse must be aware that wound healing is affected by systemic reasons, such as low volume or cardiac failure, or local causes, such as arterial insufficiency, local vasoconstriction, or excessive tension on tissues. Addressing these factors post-procedurely can have a remarkable influence on wound outcome, particularly on decreasing wound infection rates.

Because good nutrition before the procedure helps prevent wound complications, the APN should assess the patient's nutritional status before the procedure. Protein deficiency delays almost every aspect of wound healing. Besides lowering the body's resistance to infection, protein deficiency, especially a prolonged deficiency, can cause massive tissue edema. Both of these conditions complicate wound healing. A protein deficiency should alert the APN to potential problems. Serum albumin levels provide a clue to the patient's nutritional status.

The vitamins most closely involved with wound healing are vitamin C and vitamin A. Vitamin C deficiency has been associated with an increased incidence of wound infection, and if wound infection does occur, it tends to be more severe. Vitamin A deficiency impairs wound healing, while supplemental vitamin A can reverse the inhibitory effects of corticosteroids on wound healing. Vitamin A also can restore wound healing that has been impaired by diabetes, tumor formation, cyclophosph-amide, and radiation (Barbul, 2006).

Energy is also necessary for normal wound healing. Glucose as an energy source is of little use if there is not enough insulin to use it, as in diabetes. Certain unsaturated fatty acids are essential to the inflammation response, internal cell regulatory systems, and circulation. Vitamin K is essential for the synthesis of clotting factors. Magnesium is involved in the energy-producing cycles.

Wounds that are grossly contaminated or those that occur secondary to multiple trauma place patients at risk for wound and systemic complications. Those who have had radiation to the wound site also have altered wound healing. Some medications, such as corticosteroids and chemotherapeutic agents, inhibit wound healing (see **Table 18.4**). Systemic diseases, such as diabetes, impair wound healing. Patients who have had multiple transfusions have decreased immunity. The obese and elderly are also at risk. Other factors that contribute to nonhealing of wounds and wound dehiscence include malignant growth; presence of a prior scar or radiation at the incision site; non-compliance with postprocedure instructions, such as early excessive exercise or lifting heavy objects; increased pressure within the abdomen due to ascites, inflamed bowel, severe coughing, straining, or vomiting; long-term use of corticosteroid medications; and the presence of other preexisting medical conditions, such as diabetes, kidney disease, cancer, immune problems, chemotherapy, radiation therapy (Barbul, 2006).

Table 18.4	Drugs That Delay Wound Healing

Drug	Causes of Delayed Wound Healing
Antibiotics	☐ Penicillin interferes with the tensile strength of the wound by affecting the cross-linking of collagen tetracyclines
	☐ Erythromycin demonstrates anti-inflammatory properties through the inhibition of leukocyte chemotaxis
Anti-coagulants	☐ Inhibit proper coagulation; can adversely affect wounds by increasing the risk of hematomas and seroma formation
	☐ Can cause tissue necrosis
Anti-platelet drugs/NSAIDS	☐ Inhibit prostacyclin synthesis
	☐ Inhibit inflammatory mediators derived from arachidonic acid metabolism and platelet aggregation, inflammatory response and acid mucopolysaccharide synthesis in wounds
	☐ Effect is dose dependant
Colchicine (used in the treatment of gout)	☐ Reduces granulocyte migration and cytokine release
	☐ It is vasoconstrictive, reduces fibroblast synthesis, interrupts extracellular transport of procollagen, while collagenase synthesis increases collagenolysis and inhibits wound contraction
Corticosteroids	☐ Inhibit fibroplasia and the formulation of granulation tissue
Cytotoxic drugs	☐ Decrease most red and white blood cells
	☐ Myelosuppression; neurotoxicity
	☐ Damage to basal keratinocytes leading to dermal atrophy and causing platelet-mediated inflammatory response leading to micro-thrombi formation.
Vasoconstricting drugs (eg, adrenaline, nicotine, cocaine)	☐ Can cause tissue hypoxia affecting microcirculation and tissue formation

Adapted from: Sussman, G. (2007). The impact of medicines on wound healing. *Pharmacist; 26*: pp. 874–878.

RECOGNIZING POSTPROCEDURE WOUND COMPLICATIONS

The experienced advanced practice nurse recognizes the signs of wound complications, identifies the underlying cause, and recommends and initiates appropriate treatment. The most common wound complications are infection, abscess, seroma, gas gangrene, wound dehiscence, and nonhealing wounds.

Infection

Despite increased focused on the prevention, postprocedure surgical site infections (SSI) remain a major source of illness and a less frequent cause of death in the surgical patient. As recently as 2001, these infections numbered about 500,000 per year, among an estimated 27 million surgical procedures, and accounted for a similar proportion of the estimated 2 million nosocomial infections in the United States each year (Barnard, 2002). For purposes of standardized reporting, SSIs have been defined

SSI
Surgical Site Infection

NNIS
National Nosocomial
Infections Surveillance

CDC
Centers for Disease
Control and Prevention

CAMH
Comprehensive
Accreditation Manual
for Hospitals

and classified by the CDC's National Nosocomial Infections Surveillance (NNIS) System as superficial incisional SSIs, deep incisional SSIs, and organ/space SSIs (Mangram et al, 1999). The criteria for defining SSIs are outlined in **Table 18.5**.

It is well known that infections result in longer hospitalization and higher costs (Nichols, 2001). According to information published by the Centers for Disease Control and Prevention (CDC), the incidence of infection varies from surgeon to surgeon, from hospital to hospital, from one surgical procedure to another, and—most importantly—from one patient to another (Mangram et al, 1999). The Joint Commission now devotes an entire section of the Comprehensive Accreditation Manual for Hospitals (CAMH) related to Patient Focused Functions to Surveillance, Prevention, and Control of Infection (Joint Commission, 2007).

Table 18.5 **Criteria for Defining a Surgical Site Infection (SSI)**

Superficial Incisional SSI

☐ Infection occurs within 30 days of the operation.

☐ Infection involves only skin or subcutaneous tissue.

☐ At least 1 of the following:

Purulent drainage;

Positive culture from the incision;

At least 1 symptom of infection (pain or tenderness, localized swelling, redness, heat) and incision is opened by surgeon, unless incision is culture-negative; or

Diagnosis of SSI by surgeon or attending physician.

Deep Incisional SSI

☐ Infection within 30 days of the operation if no implant is left in place or within 1 year if implant is in place and the infection appears to be related to the operation.

☐ Infection involves deep soft tissues.

☐ At least 1 of the following:

Purulent drainage from the deep incision but not from organs/spaces associated with the surgical site;

Spontaneous dehiscence of deep incision or deliberate opening by a surgeon when the patient has at least 1 symptom of infection (fever, localized pain, or tenderness), unless site is culture-negative;

Abscess or other evidence of infection involving the deep incision found on direct examination, during reoperation, or by histopathology or radiography; or

Diagnosis of SSI by surgeon or attending physician.

Organ/Space SSI

☐ Infection within 30 days of the operation if no implant is left in place or within 1 year if implant is in place and the infection appears to be related to the operation.

☐ Infection involves any part of the anatomy (eg, organs or spaces), other than the incision, which was opened or manipulated during an operation.

☐ At least 1 of the following:

Purulent drainage from drain placed into the organ/space;

Positive culture of fluid or tissue from the organ/space;

Abscess or other evidence of infection involving the deep incision found on direct examination, during reoperation, or by histopathology or radiography; or

Diagnosis of SSI by surgeon or attending physician.

Adapted from Horan, T. C., Gaynes, R. P., Martone, W. J., Jarvis, W. R., Emori, T. G. (1992). CDC definitions of nosocomial surgical site infections a modification of CDC definitions of surgical wound infections. *Infect Control Hosp Epidemiol*; 13(10):606–608.

Wound infections are a major problem that affect the outcome of surgical procedures and have an impact on the length of hospital stay and overall medical costs (Barbul, 2006). One component of the Surgical Care Improvement Project (SCIP) is perioperative prophylactic antibiotic administration, intended to reduce the overall incidence of postprocedure wound infections (MEDQIC, 2008). Studies that compare operations performed with and without antibiotic prophylaxis demonstrate that wound class II, III, and IV procedures treated with appropriate prophylactic antibiotics have only one third the wound infection rates of previously reported untreated series (Barbul, 2006) Repeat dosing of antibiotics has been shown to be essential in decreasing postprocedure wound infections in operations with durations exceeding the biochemical half-life ($t_{1/2}$) of the antibiotic, or in which there is large-volume blood loss and fluid replacement (Barbul, 2006). In lengthy cases, those in which prosthetic implants are used, or when unexpected contamination is encountered, additional doses of antibiotic may be administered for 24 hours postprocedurely (Barbul, 2006).

Infections manifest themselves in a variety of ways. However, the following signs of infection are always present; pain and tenderness due to irritation of local nerve endings, increased temperature of the area involved, redness in response to the vascularization process, and swelling due to edema and inflammatory exudate. Wound complications frequently have systemic manifestations, such as elevated temperature and tachycardia. Microbial contamination of the surgical site is a prerequisite for an SSI; the risk of an SSI increases with the dose of bacterial contamination and the virulence of the bacteria (Mangram et al, 1999). The source of microbial contamination of the surgical site may be either the endogenous microorganisms (the bacteria from the patient's own skin, mucous membranes, or hollow viscera) or exogenous microorganisms (microorganisms from healthcare personnel, the environment, surgical instruments and other materials); most SSIs are caused by the patient's own bacterial flora (Barnard, 2002). When introduced into body tissues by surgery or through medical devices such as intravenous catheters, the pathogenic potential of endogenous microorganisms increases. The most common SSI causative microorganisms are *Staphylococcus aureus*, coagulase-negative staphylococcus, and enterococcus (Barnard, 2002). Alarmingly, more SSIs are due to antibiotic-resistant microorganisms, such as methicillin-resistant *Staphylococcus aureus* (MRSA; Mangram et al, 1999).

The pathogens isolated from infections differ primarily on the type of surgical procedure. In clean surgical procedures, in which the gastrointestinal, gynecologic, and respiratory tracts have not been entered, *Staphylococcus aureus* from the exogenous environment or the patient's skin flora is the usual cause of infection; in other categories of surgical procedures, including clean-contaminated, contaminated, and dirty, the polymicrobial aerobic and anaerobic flora closely resembling the normal endogenous microflora of the surgically resected organ are the most frequently isolated pathogens (Nichols, 2001).

Streptococcus and *Staphylococcus aureus* usually cause cellulitis. This diffuse inflammatory response, without tissue necrosis or purulent exudate, exhibits all the signs of an infection and may involve a large area of skin surface. Sometimes the skin has the texture of an orange peel. The patient may also have a fever. When the inflammation

SCIP
Surgical Care
Improvement Project

$t_{1/2}$
Biochemical Half-Life

18

MRSA
Methicillin-Resistant
Staphylococcus aureus

has small focal areas of tissue necrosis and multiple tiny pockets of pus, the infection is called *phlegmon*. The inoculum is a combination of *Streptococcus* and *Staphylococcus aureus* or an aerobic gram-negative rod. If the infection has spread to the lymph system, the condition is known as *lymphangitis*. The treatment of both is the administration of a parenteral antibiotic effective against gram-positive cocci. The physician may order an antibiotic according to what typically causes this type of infection. The physician may also order cultures. If the correct antibiotics are administered, the condition of the wound improves rapidly, usually within 24 hours. If these measures do not improve the condition of the wound soon, the nurse should suspect an underlying abscess, which would necessitate drainage.

Potential Adverse Outcomes

See **Table 18.1**.

RISK OF WOUND INFECTION

Assess the wound for cellulitis, phlegmon, or lymphangitis. Look for systemic infection. Determine the patient's comfort level and assess the skin condition. Assess the wound for gas formation. The most common sites are the extremities after traumatic injury. Monitor the white blood cell count. Culture the wound if necessary. Refer for medical treatment if indicated. In the event of infection, implement measures to reduce pain such as elevating the affected area to decrease edema and applying moist heat for patient comfort. Administer antibiotics as ordered. If antibiotics have not been ordered, recommend an appropriate antibiotic to the physician. Implement patient education measures regarding the status of infection and its treatment. Reevaluate the affected area after 24 hours of antibiotic therapy. Document your findings and activities according to institutional policy.

Abscess

An abscess forms when the inflammatory process becomes suppurative, is confined within a single anatomical space, and is surrounded by granulation tissue. The abscess consists of purulent materials, necrotic host tissue, and bacteria. *Staphylococcus aureus*, gram-negative rods, and a variety of anaerobic strains working synergistically with gram-negative rods are the bacteria usually found in an abscess.

The abscessed area is usually tender to the touch. If touched in this area, the patient most likely indicates pain. The patient may have a fever. Taut skin and tissue necrosis further confirm the presence of an abscess.

The treatment of an abscess is drainage. Afterward, the physician may loosely pack the wound or insert a drain to keep it open and drained. If a drain is used, after the cavity is completely collapsed, the nurse may gradually withdraw it over several days. When packing the wound, the APN should moisten the material with normal saline. Studies have shown that hydrogen peroxide, 1% povidone-iodine, 0.25% acetic acid, and 0.5% sodium hypochlorite are toxic to human fibroblasts (Lineweaver et al, 1985; Viljanto, 1980). These agents also severely reduce a wound's ability to resist infections and thus should not be used (Rodeheaver et al, 1982). The nurse should change the packs frequently, especially if there is heavy drainage. If there is a large amount of purulent drainage, the nurse should attach a wound drainage appliance. This protects the skin surrounding the drainage site. The enterostomal therapy nurse is an extremely valuable resource in caring for problem wounds. The nurse can and should rely heavily on the enterostomal therapy nurse's expertise. The physician may order antibiotics; their role, however, is secondary to drainage and meticulous wound care.

Potential Adverse Outcomes

See **Table 18.1**.

RISK OF IMPAIRED TISSUE INTEGRITY RELATED TO ABSCESS FORMATION

Assess the patient for signs of abscess. Look for systemic signs of infection. Determine the patient's comfort level. Assess the skin condition. Monitor the white blood cell count. Culture the wound if necessary. Refer for medical treatment if indicated. Implement measures to reduce pain as described for infection. Administer antibiotics as ordered.

Implement wound care measures after the abscess has been drained. When repacking the wound, loosely pack it with material moistened in normal saline. Initiate measures to protect the skin from irritating drainage, tape, or chemicals. Daily assess the skin around the drainage site for signs of irritation or breakdown. Counsel the patient about his or her abscess, the planned treatment, and the probable clinical course. Show the patient how to care for the wound. Document your findings and activities according to institutional policy.

Seroma

Seromas are common in obese patients and in wounds with areas of undermined skin flaps. They consist of blood and protein-rich fluid. Seromas are usually sterile in the beginning but are susceptible to infections. The local swelling associated with a seroma may make the patient uncomfortable. The skin over and surrounding a seroma is usually not inflamed or compromised.

Seromas may require drainage. The physician or APN can do this at the bedside by needle aspiration. A persistent seroma, however, may necessitate the insertion of an indwelling closed drainage system, which uses suction to keep the fluid evacuated and the cavity collapsed. The APN should have these treatments prescribed by a physician or should recommend to the physician that they be done.

Potential Adverse Outcomes

See **Table 18.1**.

RISK OF INFECTION RELATED TO SEROMA FORMATION
IN THE POSTPROCEDURE WOUND

Assess the wound for signs of a seroma. Determine the patient's comfort level. Assess the skin condition. Monitor the white blood cell count. Culture the wound if necessary. Refer for medical treatment if indicated.

Implement measures to reduce pain by administering pain medication as ordered and aspirating the seroma.

Collect the supplies necessary to aspirate the seroma: 20 to 35-mL syringe, 16- or 18-gauge needle, skin preparation solution, adhesive bandage (Band-Aid), 0.5 mL of local anesthetic (optional), 3-mL syringe, and 20-gauge needle. Prepare the skin with alcohol or an antiseptic of preference. After anesthetizing the skin with 0.5 mL of local anesthetic, insert the large-gauge needle attached to the large syringe and evacuate fluid until the cavity has collapsed. After withdrawing the needle, cover the site with an adhesive bandage to keep fluid from leaking from the needle wound.

Collect the supplies necessary to insert the suction wound drainage device: skin preparation solution, wound drainage device of choice, four drape towels, No. 15 or 11 blade and No. 3 knife handle, hemostat, needle holder, suture scissors, 10-mL syringe, 18- and 25-gauge needles, 10–20 mL of local aesthetic agent, dressing sponges, tape, and sterile gloves. Prepare the skin with alcohol or an antiseptic of preference. Don sterile gloves and prepare supplies. Draw up local anesthetic agent with an 18-gauge needle. Cut the drain to the proper length and attach it to the reservoir. Square off the area with sterile drapes. Numb the skin and track site to the seroma with the 25-gauge needle and local anesthetic agent. Make an incision approximately 2 cm long well below the seroma site. With a hemostat, make a track through the subcutaneous layer to the seroma. Fluid may leak out at this point. Insert the drain through the track into the seroma cavity with a hemostat. Close the incision and secure the tubing with suture. Dress the wound. Reassess the wound daily and check the amount of drainage.

Counsel the patient about the seroma, the treatment, and the probable clinical course. Teach the patient how to care for the wound. Document your findings and activities according to institutional policy.

Gas Gangrene

Gas gangrene is often caused by a combination of two processes. One is the action of microbial enzymes in contact with healthy tissue. The other is the action of microbial enzymes indirectly by causing thrombosis of blood vessels supplying the tissue with nutrients. Destruction of tissue can be extensive, often producing visible tissue necrosis. The extent of tissue destruction and the rate at which the process spreads are functions of the resistance of the host and the species of bacteria involved.

Three types of gas gangrene exist: aerobic, anaerobic, and synergistic. Extremely virulent strains of hemolytic streptococci usually cause aerobic gangrene. The gas bacillus *Clostridium perfringens* and related species cause anaerobic gangrene. For both types, the onset is sudden, marked by high fever, intense local pain, and an incredibly foul odor. The tissue is crepitant, dark, and cool. Hemorrhagic areas may appear at the margin of the infection. The patient may also exhibit signs of jaundice, confusion, moribundity, tachycardia, and dyspnea. If untreated, gas gangrene leads to septic shock.

There are several bacterial species, usually one aerobic and one anaerobic, that cause synergistic gangrene. With the combination of bacteria, the results are more destructive than with either species alone. Meleney's ulcer is one such infection.

The physician treats gas gangrene with wide debridement of all necrotic tissue, administration of parenteral antibiotics, and delayed wound closure. The APN can assist with debridement. Hyperbaric oxygen (HBO) has been used as an adjunctive therapy along with antimicrobials and aggressive surgical debridement in the treatment of gas gangrene (Kaide & Khandelwal, 2008).

HBO
Hyperbaric oxygen

Potential Adverse Outcomes
See **Table 18.1.**

RISK OF IMPAIRED TISSUE INTEGRITY RELATED TO THE FORMATION
OF GAS GANGRENE

Assess the wound for signs of gas gangrene. Check for signs of systemic infection. Assess the patient's comfort level and skin. Check the wound for crepitus. Assess the patient's mental status. Check the white blood cell count. Culture the wound if necessary. Refer for medical treatment as indicated. Implement measures to reduce pain. Initiate safety measures if the patient is confused. Administer antibiotics as ordered. If antibiotics have not been ordered, recommend an appropriate antibiotic to the physician. Counsel the patient about the infection, the treatment plan, and the probable clinical course. Show the patient how to care for the wound. Follow institutional policies regarding the isolation of patients with gas gangrene. Assist with the debridement of the wound. Document your findings and activities according to institutional policy.

Wound Dehiscence and Evisceration

If it happens, wound dehiscence usually occurs about the fifth postprocedure day. A recent study concluded that peritonitis, wound infection, and failure to close the abdominal wall properly are most important causes of wound dehiscence (Wagar, et al, 2005). Wound edge ischemia and wound closure under extreme tension are other usual causes of wound dehiscence. Before dehiscence occurs, the patient has serosanguineous drainage. After the wound begins to separate, evisceration may occur. The patient often reports that "something gave way." The treatment of wound dehiscence or evisceration is operative closure.

Potential Adverse Outcomes

See **Table 18.1**.

RISK OF INFECTION RELATED TO WOUND DEHISCENCE OR EVISCERATION

During the first 5 to 6 days of convalescence, check the wound for signs of impending separation. Look for serosanguineous drainage. Assess the patient's level of comfort. Refer for medical treatment immediately in case of dehiscence or evisceration. If evisceration occurs, implement measures to ensure patient safety. Place the patient in a supine position. Cover the wound with sterile towels moistened with saline. Implement measures to prevent hypovolemic shock. Prepare the patient for operative closure. Counsel the patient about the wound, the treatment plan, and the probable clinical course. Assist with the closure of the wound. Document your findings and activities according to institutional policy.

Nonhealing Wounds

Infection, hematomas, seromas, retained foreign substances, underlying disease or conditions, and alteration in tissue perfusion due to excessive wound tension, adjacent scarring, or trauma may cause the patient to have a nonhealing wound. The treatment is specific to the cause.

Potential Adverse Outcomes

See **Table 18.1**.

RISK OF IMPAIRED SKIN INTEGRITY: NONHEALING WOUND

Assess the wound for signs of nonhealing. Review the patient's history before and after the procedure for risk factors. Assess the white blood cell count. Culture the wound if necessary. Refer for medical treatment if indicated. Implement measures to reduce discomfort, if present. Initiate measures to eliminate infection, hematomas, seromas, and retained foreign substances. Do not use cytotoxic substances and chemicals to clean the wound; use normal saline. Counsel the patient about the wound, the treatment plan, and the probable clinical course. Show the patient how to care for the wound. Document your findings and activities according to institutional policy.

RECOGNIZING FEVER, TACHYCARDIA, PULMONARY COMPLICATIONS, THROMBOPHLEBITIS, URINARY TRACT INFECTIONS, AND ADYNAMIC ILEUS

The APN recognizes postprocedure complications other than wound complications, identifies underlying causes, and recommends treatment. When appropriate, the APN also initiates treatment. Fever, tachycardia, thrombophlebitis, urinary tract infection, prolonged ileus, and pulmonary problems such as atelectasis, infiltration, and effusions are the most common postprocedure complications.

Fever

Elevated temperature can occur at any time after the procedure. Transient low-grade postprocedure fever, however, is considered normal. Some patients experience fever from pyrogens in blood if given blood during the procedure. If inflamed tissue was removed during the procedure, the APN should expect a constantly elevated temperature 3–5 days after the procedure. Gradually the temperature returns to normal. A spiking temperature, one that is intermittently high, may mean a more serious problem, such as bacterial seeding into the bloodstream. Determining the source of the problem is crucial. Spiking temperatures during the first 2 days after the procedure are usually pulmonary in origin. The primary treatment is increased ambulation. If fever occurs from the fourth to the seventh day, suspect wound complications. Fevers on the sixth to the ninth days are commonly attributable to intraabdominal abscesses or anastomotic leaks. Thrombophlebitis can cause a fever from the 6th to the 10th day. After the cause is determined, the appropriate treatment may be recommended.

Potential Adverse Outcomes

See **Table 18.1**.

RISK OF POSTPROCEDURE HYPERTHERMIA (FEVER)

Implement interventions to eliminate, attenuate, or modify the risk factors associated with fever. If a patient experiences a fever, evaluate its pattern and assess for the underlying cause; refer for medical treatment when indicated; and implement measures to educate the patient regarding the elevated temperature, the treatment, and the probable clinical course. Document your findings and activities according to institutional policy.

Tachycardia

Assess postprocedure tachycardia, like postprocedure fever, on the basis of its underlying cause. The most frequent causes are fever; lack of a medication routinely taken by the patient, such as digitalis; relative hypotension (eg, if the patient is ordinarily hypertensive); inadequate pain relief; and apprehension. The treatment depends on the underlying cause.

Potential Adverse Outcomes

See **Table 18.1**.

RISK OF ALTERATION IN POSTPROCEDURE CARDIAC RATE (TACHYCARDIA)

Implement interventions to eliminate, attenuate, or modify the risk factors associated with tachycardia. After it is established that the patient is tachycardiac, assess the patient for the underlying cause; refer for medical treatment if indicated; and implement measures to educate the patient regarding tachycardia, the treatment, and the probable clinical course. Document your findings and activities according to institutional policy.

Pulmonary Complications

Pulmonary complications usually appear during the first 2 days after the procedure. These can involve atelectasis, infiltrate, or effusions. They are usually accompanied by an elevated temperature, tachycardia, restlessness, elevated white blood cell count, lowered partial pressure of oxygen, increased partial pressure of carbon dioxide, dyspnea, increased respiratory rate, pallor, and shortness of breath. In severe cases, hypoxia can cause deterioration of mental status and level of consciousness and cyanosis.

Portions of the bronchial tree can become plugged with mucus if the patient cannot cough effectively. Pain and splinting are major causes of ineffective cough. Adequate pain relief can assist the patient to move the secretions; however, narcotics can depress respiratory effort. Non-narcotic methods of pain relief are encouraged and may be successful in some cases. For example, intrapleural catheters may be inserted during a thoracotomy. After the procedure, the catheter is injected with a local anesthetic agent. The patient who smokes is at especially high risk for all postprocedure pulmonary complications.

Segmental atelectasis can occur with bed rest or inadequate ventilation during an operative procedure. Bronchial obstruction, which frequently accompanies atelectasis, prevents transmission of breath and voice sounds during auscultation. The areas of atelectasis are dull when percussed.

The treatment is to increase activity, such as ambulation. In some cases, the use of the incentive spirometer, postural drainage, percussion, inspiration of humidified air, intermittent positive pressure breathing treatments with mucolytic agents, and tracheal suction may also be employed. The patient should have adequate fluid intake.

If these conditions persist, the patient may experience pneumonia. The infiltrate can be seen on radiographs. Breath sounds may be diminished, especially in the lower lobes. Crackles may also be heard. Pneumonia can develop as a result of massive or

18

subtle aspiration. Sputum cultures may be positive. Antibiotics are included in treatment measures as discussed earlier. In severe or persistent cases, the patient may require therapeutic bronchoscopy.

Postprocedure pleural effusions can be caused by pneumonia, pulmonary embolus, congestive heart failure, or subdiaphragmatic abscess. The most common cause of pleural effusion is pneumonia. Pleural effusions are often visible on chest radiographs. The diaphragmatic markings are blunted on upright films. The fluid may layer on decubital views. Pleural fluids tend to muffle all sounds when auscultated. Percussion notes are dull; breath sounds are decreased or absent, especially in the lower lobes.

Pulmonary embolus presents as sudden chest or shoulder pain, dyspnea, tachycardia, hypotension, pallor, cyanosis, restlessness, and hypoxia. The pulse oximeter readings fall significantly and suddenly. The oxygen pressure is significantly lower, even reaching dangerous levels. Sudden death can occur. Immediate resuscitative intervention may be required. Mortality is high if not treated within 24 hours. Peripheral venograms, pulmonary arteriograms, and lung scans may be ordered to confirm an embolic event. Anticoagulants may be ordered as a continuous heparin infusion or intermittent heparin injections. Long-term oral anticoagulant therapy may be desirable. Measures to prevent pulmonary embolus are directed at preventing thrombophlebitis. Pulmonary embolectomy may be necessary in cases of massive embolus, if the patient survives the initial event. Radical treatment in documented cases of recurrent pulmonary embolus entails vena caval interruption by ligating, filtering, or performing umbrella lysis of the vena cava.

Postprocedure fluid overload can lead to congestive heart failure. It is characterized by vascular congestion and the inability of the heart to pump enough blood to meet the body's metabolic needs. Careful monitoring of the patient's intake and output and daily weights is essential, especially in patients with preexisting congestive heart failure. It may be difficult to differentiate between over-hydration and third spacing of fluids. Central venous pressure monitoring is inadequate for this complication. Monitoring pulmonary wedge pressures with a Swan-Ganz catheter is more appropriate. Diuretics and inotropic drugs may be used in the treatment of over hydration.

Subdiaphragmatic abscesses irritate the diaphragm, creating a pleural effusion. The patient experiences pain on light palpation of the subcostal margin of the affected side Abscesses produce a dull sound when percussed. Arterial blood gas measurements and pulse oximeter readings gradually deteriorate. Abscesses are readily seen with ultrasonography or computed tomography. The treatment is operative or percutaneous drainage of the abscess. The effusion may be aspirated. If the effusion is severe enough, the physician may choose to insert a chest tube to drain the effusion.

Potential Adverse Outcomes

See **Table 18.1**.

RISK OF INEFFECTIVE AIRWAY CLEARANCE AND INEFFECTIVE BREATHING PATTERN DURING THE POSTPROCEDURE PERIOD

Implement interventions to eliminate, attenuate, or modify the risk factors associated with pulmonary complications. Assess for pulmonary complications. Determine the patient's activity level and ability to ambulate. Monitor arterial blood gas values, pulse oximeter readings, and pulmonary wedge pressures. Evaluate the effectiveness of cough and use of respiration depressing drugs. Monitor intake and output. Refer for medical treatment, if indicated, or immediately in the event of a pulmonary embolus. In the event of pulmonary complications, recommend appropriate diagnostic and/ or treatment modalities. Assess the effectiveness of measures to prevent pulmonary infiltrates, pneumonia, and pulmonary embolus. Implement measures to educate the patient regarding his or her role in preventing pulmonary complications. If complications occur, educate the patient regarding the treatment and the probable clinical course. Document your findings and activities according to institutional policy.

Thrombophlebitis

One component of the SCIP Project is prevention of thromboembolism, which has come to be recognized as a major source of postprocedure morbidity and mortality. The SCIP recommendations are based on guidelines developed by the American College of Chest Physicians (Hirsch et al, 2004).

Thrombophlebitis results from inactivity with venous stasis in the lower extremities or as a complication of intravenous catheters. Prolonged venous cannulation or chemical reaction from intravenous medications can cause a peripheral vein to thrombose.

By far the most serious form of thrombophlebitis occurs in the deep veins of the legs. This can be precipitated by pelvic edema resulting from operative procedures (eg, hysterectomy and hip procedures), positioning during the procedure that restricts venous return, or postprocedure bed rest. The patient may experience pain, local tenderness, swelling in the calf and foot, and transient fever. If a clot embolizes to the pulmonary circulation, sudden death can occur. Deep thrombophlebitis can be palpated: With the leg flexed at the knee and relaxed, press the calf muscles against the tibia with the fingertips and feel for increased firmness or muscle tension.

Thrombophlebitis is prevented by appropriate mechanical and pharmaceutical prophylaxis to maintain adequate venous flow. Mechanical methods of prophylaxis, which include graduated compression stockings (GCS), and the use of intermittent pneumatic compression (IPC) devices and the venous foot pump (VFP), increase venous outflow and/or reduce stasis within the leg veins. The primary attraction of mechanical prophylaxis is the lack of bleeding potential. In general, mechanical methods should be directed toward those patients in whom bleeding is a significant risk or as an adjunct to anticoagulant-based treatment. Pharmacologic approaches include low-dose unfractionated heparin (LDUH), low molecular weight heparin (LMWH), or a vitamin K antagonist. Continuous heparin infusions or intermittent heparin injections may be indicated, as appropriate. There is good evidence that appropriately used thromboprophylaxis has a desirable risk/benefit ratio and is cost-effective (Hirsch et al, 2004).

Non-mechanical and non-pharmaceutical approaches to reduce the risk of DVT formation include elevation of the legs, and muscular exercise. The patient should avoid having the legs in a dependent position unless he or she is ambulating.

Potential Adverse Outcomes

See **Table 18.1.**

GCS
Graduated Compression Stockings

IPC
Intermittent Pneumatic Compression

VFP
Venous Foot Pump

LDUH
Low-Dose Unfractionated Heparin

LMWH
Low Molecular Weight Heparin

PE
Pulmonary Embolism

SCDs
Sequential
Compression Devices

RISK OF ACUTE PULMONARY EMBOLUS

It is now recognized that the occurrence of pulmonary embolism (PE) is probably underdiagnosed. Many patients have sequential compression devices (SCDs) applied intraoperatively to their lower extremities; however, no study exists to date that proves SCDs actually decrease the incidence of PE. Nevertheless, SCDs have been shown to decrease the incidence of DVT, so it is important to implement interventions to eliminate, attenuate, or modify the risk factors associated with thrombophlebitis (Schwartz, 2006). Assess for venous thrombosis especially in higher risk populations such as neurosurgical, orthopedic, obstetric and trauma patients. Implement measures for patient comfort. Encourage early ambulation. Implement measures to educate the patient regarding his or her role in preventing thrombophlebitis. If complications occur, refer the patient for medical treatment; educate the patient regarding the treatment and the probable clinical course, and assess the effectiveness of measures to treat thrombophlebitis. Document your findings and activities according to institutional policy.

Urinary Tract Infections

Urinary tract infections can be diagnosed by the patient's description of the problem. Patients may express an urgent and frequent need to evacuate small amounts of urine. They may also verbalize bladder fullness, burning on urination, and suprapubic distention. Urine may be foul smelling or cloudy. The patient may have chills and fever. Urinalysis shows many white blood cells in the urine. A culture produces bacteria. Infections can be treated with the administration of sulfa drugs or antibiotics if necessary. Absence of urination with suprapubic distention means urinary retention. Measures to prevent urinary retention are activities that facilitate voiding, such as running water, assisting male patients in standing to void, and offering a bedpan or assistance to the bathroom every 2 to 3 hours. If these measures prove inadequate, insertion of an intermittent or indwelling catheter should be considered.

Potential Adverse Outcomes

See **Table 18.1**.

RISK OF POSTPROCEDURE URINARY TRACT INFECTION

Implement interventions to eliminate, attenuate, or modify the risk factors associated with urinary tract infection. Assess for signs of urinary tract infection. In the event of urinary tract infection, refer the patient for medical treatment; implement measures for patient comfort; educate the patient regarding the treatment and the probable clinical course; and assess the effectiveness of measures to treat urinary tract infection. Document your findings and activities according to institutional policy.

(Adynamic) Postprocedure Ileus

POI
Postoperative Ileus

GI
Gastrointestinal

"Postoperative ileus (POI) has emerged as a significant determining factor in the quality of the overall perioperative experience, from proper and adequate pain management to the optimization of recovery and discharge protocols. Although the transient cessation of normal gastrointestinal (GI) function after major surgery (ie, POI) has long been recognized, only recently have deeper insights into its pathophysiology and the true nature of its negative clinical impact been more fully appreciated" (Carter, 2006). POI is impaired bowel motility that occurs almost universally after major abdominal procedures, although it may occur with other procedures such as hysterectomy, cystectomy, thoracic procedures, and arthroplasties. Fortunately for most patients, it is transient and lasts from three to five days; however, a longer duration is not uncommon. POI results from two basic causes: the surgical procedure and pharmacologic interventions directed toward pain relief, mainly opioids (Steinbrook, 2005).

In relation to the surgical procedure, POI is a normal, response to tissue injury. The manipulation of tissue, such as incisions and physical handling of viscera, leads to three related mechanisms that contribute to POI to different degrees. *Neurogenic* causes of POI are related to sympathetic hyperactivity. *Inflammatory* causes involve cellular and humoral factors; notable among these are immune cells and endogenously produced opioid peptides. *Hormonal* causes include corticotrophin-releasing factor, thought to have a major role in the modulation of endocrine, autonomic, behavioral, and immune responses to stress. Other inflammatory mediators involved in the pathogenesis of POI include calcitonin generated peptide, prostanoids, substance P, vasoactive intestinal peptide (VIP), and nitric oxide. All these factors tend to be maximally affected, and hence lead to POI of the longest duration after surgeries involving the colon, especially open procedures. In contrast, surgical techniques that are less invasive and of shorter duration, such as laparoscopic surgery, may be expected to lead to a shorter duration of POI and, thus, improved outcomes (Saclarides, 2006).

VIP
Vasoactive Intestinal Peptide

In relation to POI and postprocedure pain management, opioids have an inhibitory effect on gastric motility and also increase tone in the antrum and the first portion of the duodenum in healthy individuals. The effects of opiates on the small intestine are slightly more complicated. Morphine sulfate has biphasic properties in humans: (1) initial effects on motility are stimulatory via activation of MMC phase III, and (2) this stimulation is followed by atony, which is responsible for the slowing of gastrointestinal transit. Morphine increases the tone and amplitude of nonpropulsive contractions and decreases propulsive waves in the colon. The additive effect of these actions is to decrease colonic motility (Luckey, 2003).

If adynamic ileus is persistent, the APN may suspect peritonitis, potassium depletion, or wound dehiscence.

Potential Adverse Outcomes
See **Table 18.1**.

RISK OF ALTERED POSTPROCEDURE BOWEL FUNCTION
Implement interventions to eliminate, attenuate, or modify the risk factors associated with adynamic ileus. Determine the patient's comfort level. Exacerbation of an ileus due to excess perioperative narcotic use may delay return of bowel function. Epidural anesthesia in abdominal surgery is becoming more popular, and the data show that pain control is improved, there is an earlier return of bowel function, and length of hospital stay is shortened. Although still not generally accepted, the limited use of mesogastric tubes and the initiation of early postprocedure feeding before the

full return of bowel function can both contribute significantly to a shorter time for postprocedure ileus. Whether bowel surgery is performed open or laparoscopically may play a role in the duration of ileus, as numerous studies have shown a decreased length of stay and improved pain control when bowel surgery is performed laparoscopically. Assess the patient for signs of prolonged ileus (Schwartz, 2006).

The nasogastric tube has long been the mainstay of treatment; however, recent randomized clinical studies have concluded that nasogastric decompression does not shorten time to first bowel movement or decrease time to adequate oral intake; in addition, these studies report that inappropriate use may contribute to postprocedure complications such as nausea, fever, pneumonia, and atelectasis (Carrère et al, 2007; Nelson et al, 2007; Akbaba et al, 2004). Although these studies do not recommend routine use of nasogastric intubation, selected patients will benefit from symptomatic relief. In the event of prolonged adynamic ileus, refer the patient for medical treatment; implement measures for patient comfort; and implement measures to educate the patient regarding the reasons for ileus and when bowel function is expected to return. Document your findings and activities according to institutional policy.

ASSESSING THE PATIENT'S PHYSIOLOGICAL AND PSYCHOLOGICAL COMFORT LEVEL

The APN assesses the patient's postprocedure comfort level, identifies causes of alterations in comfort, and then recommends and initiates appropriate treatment. Pain, nausea, and vomiting are the most common causes of alteration in comfort after the procedure.

Outcome Standard

See **Table 18.1**.

Assessing Postprocedure Comfort Level

Pain results from various types of mechanical, thermal, or chemical stimuli. Postprocedure pain is caused as a consequence of injured nerve fibers in incised, manipulated, or traumatized tissue from the procedure itself, preexisting disease or injury, complications, and insertion of tubes and drains. While acute pain usually resolves within days or weeks, it can become chronic for some patients. Over 44 million inpatient surgical procedures are performed in the United States annually (CDC, 2005). However, pain management is often less than optimal, which has significant clinical, economic, as well as human implications (Strassels, et al, 2007). Therefore, assessment and effective management of the patient's postprocedure pain and comfort levels are key nursing roles in facilitating care after an operative or invasive procedure.

The assessment of pain is an ongoing process that often begins as the patient returns to consciousness in the PACU. **Figure 18.1** presents a flow chart for the management of postprocedure pain. Pain is believed to be an interaction between physiological and psychological systems. It is a highly subjective experience and, therefore, how intense pain may be for the patient is best assessed by his or her own self-report. The use of a pain intensity scale to assess the patient's pain is very helpful (**Fig. 18.2**).

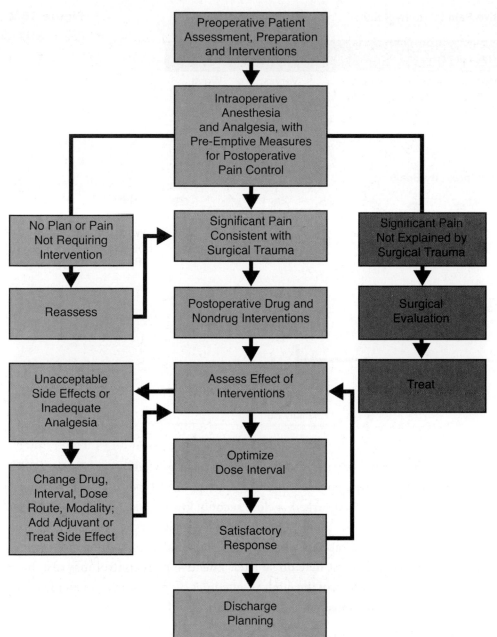

Figure 18.1

Flow chart for the management of postprocedure pain.

Several factors influence the onset, incidence, and severity of postprocedure pain, including (Feeley & Marcario, 2005):

- the very young and very old experience less pain than people in the middle years of life;
- preoperative neurotic personality traits tend to increase postprocedure pain;
- fear of the pain itself;
- the way in which the patient is prepared preoperatively for the experience of postprocedure pain; and
- the operative site.

An excellent resource for managing pain preoperatively and postprocedurely is the American Society of PeriAnesthesia Nurses' (ASPAN) Pain and Comfort Clinical Guideline© (ASPAN, 2003). See **Figure 18.1**.

ASPAN
American Society of
PeriAnesthesia Nurses

Simple Descriptive Pain Intensity Scale

Figure 18.2

Pain intensity scales.

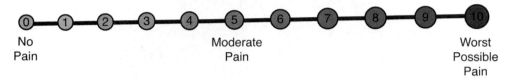

| No Pain | Mild Pain | Moderate Pain | Severe Pain | Very Severe Pain | Worst Possible Pain |

0–10 Numeric Pain Intensity Scale

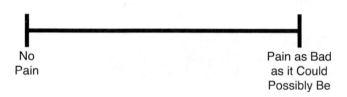

No Pain   Moderate Pain   Worst Possible Pain

Visual Analog Scale (VAS)

No Pain   Pain as Bad as it Could Possibly Be

As noted, the severity of pain is related to the type of procedure (see **Table 18.6**). In general, thoracotomy appears to be the most painful type of operative procedure, with upper abdominal surgery a close second; lower abdominal surgery is less painful (Feeley & Marcario, 2005). Severity of pain is also associated with the type of anesthetic agent used. Patients who have had regional anesthesia may not experience pain in the PACU but may do so later. Effective pain control may also have an additional benefit of improving clinical outcomes by decreasing the incidence of postprocedure complications, such as (Thompson, 2008):

- myocardial infarction or ischemia;
- risk of tachycardia and dysrhythmia;
- impaired wound healing;
- risk of atelectasis;
- thromboembolic events;
- peripheral vasoconstriction; and
- metabolic acidosis.

The nurse must become adept at recognizing the signs and symptoms of pain. The defining characteristics of acute pain include (Carpenito-Moyet, 2004) communication (verbal or coded) of pain descriptors, guarding or protective behavior, self-focusing, narrowed focus (eg, altered time perception, withdrawal from social contact, impaired thought processes), distraction behavior (eg, crying, moaning, pacing, restlessness, seeking out other people or activities), facial mask of pain (eg, lackluster eyes, grimace), altered muscle tone (spanning form listless to rigid),

Table 18.6 Severity of Pain			
Pain estimated by amount of postoperative analgesics required and time to first postoperative analgesia request.			
Surgical Procedure	Moderate Pain (%)	Severe Pain (%)	Mean Duration (Days) of Moderately Severe Pain (Range)
Intrathoracic surgery			
☐ Sternotomy	40–50	30–40	8 (5–12)
☐ Thoracotomy	25–35	45–65	4 (3–7)
Gastric surgery			
☐ Abdominal aortic aneurysm resection	20–30	50–75	4 (3–7)
Open cholecystectomy	25–35	45–65	3 (2–6)
Lower abdominal surgery	30–40	35–55	2 (1–4)
Appendectomy	35–45	20–30	1 (0.5–3)
Inguinal and femoral herniotomy	35–45	15–25	1.5 (1–3)
Head/neck/limb surgery	35–45	5–15	1 (0.5–2)
Minor chest wall (mastectomy) and scrotal surgery	35–50	10–30	1.5 (1–3)

Adapted from Polomano, R.C., Dunwoody, C. J., Krenzischek, D. A., & Rathmell, J. P. (2008). Perspective on pain management in the 21st century. *Journal of Perianesthesia Nursing; 23* (1 Suppl): S4–14.

autonomic responses not see in chronic stable pain (eg, diaphoresis, changes in blood pressure and pulse, papillary dilation, increased or decreased respiratory rate).

The APN should also know the recommended dose and effects of medication given to control or relieve pain (**Tables 18.7** and **18.8**). A common side effect of narcotics is respiratory depression. An occasional patient exhibits a previously unknown allergy to the drug being used. Those are easily recognized by patient reports of itching and a generalized rash. The patient may also report tightness in the throat. Nausea and vomiting are also common side effects of narcotics. The nurse must be aware of specific opioid related pharmacological issues beyond routine dosing and equianalgesic effects when caring for patients with postprocedure pain. If it is necessary to change the analgesic or the route of administration, patient factors such as being opioid tolerant versus opioid naive must be considered. Patient responses to a new opioid must always be monitored and doses titrated appropriately. The preoperative pain assessment will provide insight into controlling postprocedure pain, as opioid naive patients will require different amounts of medications than those who are currently taking opioids for treatment of chronic pain or those who with a history of current or past substance use. In addition to determining baseline opioid requirements, management of opioid tolerant patients should involve assessing the intervention and anticipated response, incorporating nonopioid medications into the treatment plan, and then working toward tapering down the dosage of opioids used when no longer needed. Addiction to, or psychological dependence on, opioids is quite uncommon for patients to develop when they

Table 18.7	Dosing Data for Nonopioid Analgesics			
Medication	**Usual Adult Dose**	**Maximum Adult Daily Dose**	**Usual Pediatric Dose**	**Comments**
Acetaminophen	650–975 mg orally q 4–6 hr	4,000 mg	10–15 mg/kg orally q 4–6 hr	Lacks peripheral anti-inflammatory activity of NSAIDs
Aspirin	650–975 mg orally q 4–6 hr	4,000 mg	10–15 mg/kg orally q 4–6 hr	Inhibits platelet aggregation; may cause postop bleeding
Choline magnesium trisalicylate	1,000–1,500 mg orally q 12 hr	3,000 mg	—	Effectiveness in comparison to aspirin unclear; onset of analgesia probably slower; less gastropathy and impairment of platelet function
Diclofenac potassium	50 mg orally q 8 hr	150 mg	—	Comparable to aspirin with longer duration; available with misoprostol to reduce GI toxicity
Diflunisal	1,000 mg orally initial dose followed by 500 mg q 12 hr	1,500 mg	—	500 mg superior to 650 mg of aspirin or acetaminophen, with longer duration
Etodolac	200–400 mg orally q 6–8 hr	1,200 mg	—	200 mg comparable to, and 400 mg possibly superior to, 650 mg of aspirin
Fenoprofen calcium	200–600 mg orally q 6 hr	3,200 mg	—	Comparable to aspirin; contraindicated in patients with impaired renal function
Ibuprofen	400–800 mg orally q 6–8 hr	2,400 mg	10 mg/kg orally q 6–8 hr	200 mg equal to 650 mg of aspirin and acetaminophen; 400 mg superior to 650 mg of aspirin and acetaminophen; 400 mg comparable to acetaminophen/codeine combination
Magnesium salicylate	650 mg orally q 4–6 hr	—	—	Many brands and generic forms available; does not affect platelet function
Salsalate	500 mg orally q 4 hours	3,000 mg	—	Appears to provide anti-inflammatory activity equivalent to aspirin; does not inhibit platelet aggregation
Sodium salicylate	325–650 mg orally q 3–4 hr	—	—	—
Sulindac	200 mg orally q 12 hr; after satisfactory response has been achieved, dose may be decreased accordingly	400 mg	—	Comparable to aspirin with a lower overall incidence of total adverse effects

Adapted from Krenzischek, D. A., Dunwoody, C. J., Polomano, R. C., & Rathmell, J. P. (2008). Pharmacokinetics for acute pain: Implications for practice. *Journal of Perianesthesia Nursing*; 23 (1 Suppl): S28–42.

Table 18.8	Dosing Data for Opioid Analgesics						
Drug	**Equianalgesic Oral**	**Dose Parenteral**	**Initial Adult Parenteral Dose**	**Initial Adult Oral Dose**	**Initial Pediatric Parenteral Dose**	**Initial Pediatric Oral Dose**	**Comments**
Morphine	30 mg	10 mg	1–10 mg	10–30 mg	0.1–0.2 mg/kg/dose	0.2–0.3 mg/kg/dose; 0.3–0.6 mg/kg for controlled release	Long-acting forms may be given only every 8–12 hours. Some long-acting dosage forms may be given rectally. Metabolites may cause myoclonus in patients with renal failure.
Hydromorphone	7.5 mg	1.5 mg	0.2–1 mg	1–4 mg	0.015 mg/kg/dose	0.03–0.08 mg/kg/dose q 4–6 hr	Potent opioid. Good agent for patients with renal dysfunction.
Oxycodone	20 mg	N/A	N/A	5–10 mg	N/A	0.05–0.15 mg/kg/dose q 4–6 hr	Long-acting form may be given orally/rectally every 8–12 hr.
Methadone	5 mg (Confer with pain specialist prior to parenteral use.)	N/A	(Confer with pain specialist prior to parenteral use.)	2.5–5 mg	0.1 mg/kg/dose	0.1 mg/kg/dose	Half life > 24 hr, so dosing adjustments should be made continuously. Given every 6–8 hr for pain management.
Meperidine	300 mg	75 mg	50–100 mg	Not recommended	0.75–1.5 mg/kg/dose	Not recommended	May have a role in management of neuropathic pain. Metabolized to normeperidine, a CNS stimulant, which may cause seizures in patients with renal failure.

18

Drug	Equianalgesic Oral	Dose Parenteral	Initial Adult Parenteral Dose	Initial Adult Oral Dose	Initial Pediatric Parenteral Dose	Initial Pediatric Oral Dose	Comments
Fentanyl	—	100 µg	25–100 µg	N/A	0.5–2 µg/kg/dose	N/A	Short-acting. Available as a transdermal patch.
Codeine	200 mg	130 mg	—	30–60 mg	—	0.5–1 mg/kg	5–10% of Caucasians lack the enzyme to metabolize codeine to morphine. May cause more nausea and constipation than other opioids.
Hydrocodone	30 mg	N/A	N/A	5–10 mg	N/A	—	Often combined with nonopioid analgesics, which limits the total dose per day.
Oxymorphone	N/A	1 mg	1 mg	N/A	Not recommended	Not recommended	Available as a suppository.
Nalbuphine	N/A	10 mg	10 mg	N/A	0.1 mg/kg/dose	—	May precipitate withdrawal in opioid-dependent patients.
Butorphanol	N/A	2 mg	2 mg	N/A	Not recommended	N/A	Available as a nasal spray.
Pentazocine	50 mg	30 mg	30–60 mg	50 mg	Not recommended	Not recommended	—
Buprenorphine	N/A	0.4 mg	0.4 mg	N/A	0.004 mg/kg	N/A	May precipitate withdrawal in opioid-dependent patients.
Tramadol	—	—	N/A	50 mg	N/A	Not recommended	Maximum dose 400 mg/day
Propoxyphene	—	—	N/A	65 mg	N/A	Not recommended	Metabolized to norpropoxyphene, which may cause seizures.

Adapted from: Krenzischek, D. A., Dunwoody, C. J., Polomano, R. C., & Rathmell, J. P. (2008). Pharmacokinetics for acute pain: Implications for practice. *Journal of Perianesthesia Nursing;* 23 (1 Suppl): S28–42.

are treated appropriately over a short time; concerns about it should not become an obstacle to effective control of postprocedure pain (Polomano, 2008).

As the rate of obesity increases in the general population, obstructive sleep apnea (OSA) is more prevalent. The nurse should be aware of the potential impact of OSA on the postprocedure course, especially when narcotics are being used to treat pain. Patients with disordered breathing during sleep may also be at risk for complications related to anesthesia as well as postprocedure analgesia (Meoli et al, 2003). It is important that analgesic dosing is carefully titrated to ensure that adequate pain relief is achieved without compromising upper airway muscle tone, therefore, it may be inappropriate to use patient-controlled analgesia (PCA) in this patient population without establishing dosing limits related to airway and respiratory stability (Meoli et al, 2003). The potential synergistic effects of all medication must be considered, especially in regards to central nervous system depression; sedative-hypnotics, anxiolytics, and other sedating agents should be used with caution (Meoli et al, 2003). Patient monitoring is key in evaluating medication effect; nasal CPAP can provide airway support, continuous pulse oximetry and heart rate monitoring with preset alarms should be used in the immediate postprocedure period (Meoli et al, 2003). When transferring the care of the patient, it is critical that all staff members who care for the patient after the procedure are aware of the problems associated with OSA and communicate pertinent information, such as intraoperative medication use, in order to determine the appropriate level of postprocedure monitoring (Meoli et al, 2003).

A multi-modal approach to treating pain is desirable. For example, installation of local anesthetic into the wound can be very efficacious and is easy to perform (Feeley & Marcario, 2005). The use of regional anesthesia for postprocedure pain management appears to be best suited for patients with preexisting lung disease in whom the use of narcotics would be dangerous and also when a regional technique could be effective without the adverse effects on respiration (Feeley & Marcario, 2005).

The use of narcotics in the epidural space to control postprocedure pain is an effective approach to pain management (Feeley & Marcario, 2005). The epidural route of administration is now accepted as an appropriate first-line route for the management of moderate-to-severe postprocedure pain that is expected to last for at least 24 hours (Pasero, 2005). PCEA provides more continuous pain relief with the option for more frequent bolus dosing. Small doses are required to achieve pain relief with virtually no respiratory depression. A dose of 2 to 3 mg can last from 8 to 12 hours. However, there are inherent dangers with the use of epidural catheters, such as epidural hemorrhage and infections, with resulting neurological deficits. If the medication injected drifts to higher levels on the spinal cord, respiratory arrest can result. These patients must be closely monitored for these complications while the catheter is in place. Timing of heparin, including low molecular weight heparin, administration to reduce the risk of deep venous thrombosis and pulmonary embolism usually is delayed until after the epidural catheter has been removed to lower the risk of serious complications.

It is common practice to keep the patient in a monitored care unit until the catheter is removed. Intrapleural catheters may be inserted during a thoracotomy. A 20-gauge epidural catheter is placed percutaneously through the intrapleural space immediately below the incision. After the procedure, the catheter is injected with a local anesthetic agent. A 20- to 30-mL dose of 0.5% bupivacaine with 1:200,000 epinephrine can be

OSA
Obstructive Sleep Apnea

PCA
Patient-Controlled Analgesia

18

injected every 4 to 6 hours with no respiratory depression. After injection of the bupivacaine, blood pressure, respiratory depression, and heart rate are assessed, along with the patient's comfort level. The APN can discuss the implementation of such pain control methods with the anesthesia provider and the physician during the procedure.

Intrathecal anesthesia also provides postprocedure analgesia, especially if long acting analgesic agents (eg, bupivacaine) are used; if opioid agents are administered before the block wears off, very good pain relief is possible (Thompson, 2008).

PCEA
Patient-Controlled
Epidural Analgesia

IV
Intravenous

Intravenous patient-controlled analgesia (PCA) and patient-controlled epidural analgesia (PCEA) provide consistent control of pain by allowing the self-administration of doses of an opioid by patients who are physically capable of doing so and who can understand how to use the pump. Intravenous (IV) PCA has been used successfully for about 25 years, PCEAs having come into use within the past decade and are now commonplace. These pumps help the patient overcome the analgesic gap that may occur when there are lapses in effectiveness of analgesics, delays in administration, and unanticipated episodes of severe pain (Carr et al, 2005). The most concerning adverse effect of IV PCA is respiratory depression, a risk that is markedly increased with the use of basal or continuous infusions along with demand dosing and is generally not recommended. Despite their advantages, these treatment modalities are associated with errors, some fatal. The United States Pharmacopeia (USP) has identified the three most common IV PCA errors to be improper dose/quantity, unauthorized/wrong drug, and dose omission errors (USP, 2004). Patients tend to use the medicine at increasingly longer intervals (taper off) after the first 24 hours. See **Table 18.9** for a complete list of the types of PCA errors.

USP
United States
Pharmacopeia

The APN should also know non-narcotic methods to relieve pain. These may be used in conjunction with narcotics or alone if the patient finds the level of pain control acceptable. Deep breathing relaxation have been shown repeatedly to be effective,

Table 18.9	Types of PCA Errors	
Types of Error	**Count**	**Percent**
Improper dose/quantity	1,873	38.9%
Unauthorized drug	887	18.4%
Omission error	846	17.6%
Prescribing error	443	9.2%
Wrong administration technique	230	4.8%
Extra dose	227	4.7%
Wrong drug preparation	203	4.2%
Wrong time	160	3.3%
Wrong patient	118	2.5%
Wrong dosage form	79	1.6%
Wrong route	29	0.6%
Deteriorated/Expired product	15	0.3%
Total	**5,110**	

From: USP Quality Review: Data Analysis, No. 81, 2004.

with the added advantage of improving respiratory effort. Transcutaneous electrical nerve stimulation has been helpful in some patients. Another method is teaching the patient how to splint the wound with a pillow when moving or coughing. Position changes can relieve discomfort. Diversional techniques such as back rubs, quiet conversation, aromatherapy, and distractions can assist the patient in becoming more comfortable. The patient should have a restful environment.

Potential Adverse Outcomes

See **Table 18.1**.

RISK OF ALTERATION IN COMFORT RELATED TO POSTPROCEDURE PAIN

Implement interventions to eliminate, attenuate, or modify the risk factors associated with postprocedure pain. Determine the patient's level of pain relief (**Fig. 18.2**). Assess how the patient responds to pain. In the event of inadequately controlled postprocedure pain, refer the patient for medical treatment if indicated: implement measures to educate the patient regarding his or her role in pain control; and implement nonpharmacological measures for pain relief. Document your findings and activities according to institutional policy.

Assessing Nausea and Vomiting

The APN assesses the patient's comfort level relative to nausea and vomiting. Postprocedure nausea and vomiting (PONV) are common complications that result in patient discomfort, prolonged PACU stay, and patient dissatisfaction (Feeley & Marcario, 2005; White & Freire, 2005). Common factors associated with nausea and vomiting during the operative or invasive period are outlined in **Table 18.10**.

Assessment skills include the ability to differentiate between nausea and vomiting that are narcotic induced and nausea and vomiting caused by postprocedure adynamic ileus and postprocedure complications. Narcotic induced nausea and vomiting usually

PONV
Postprocedure Nausea and Vomiting

Table 18.10	Factors Associated with Nausea and Vomiting During the Operative or Invasive Period		
Patient-Related Factors	**Anesthesia-Related Factors**	**Surgery-Related Factors**
Age	Premedication	Operative procedure
Gender	Inadequate hydration	Length of the procedure
Preexisting medical conditions (eg, diabetes)	Opioid analgesics	Blood in the gastrointestinal tract
History of PONV or motion sickness	Induction and maintenance anesthetics	Forcing oral intake
Smoking history	Reversal agents	Premature ambulation (postural hypotension)
Anxiety level	Gastric distention	Pain
Intercurrent illnesses (eg, pancreatic disease, viral infection)	Residual sympathectomy	

Adapted from White, P. F. & Freire, A. R. (2005). Ambulatory (outpatient) anesthesia. In *Miller's Anesthesia*, 6th ed., R. D. Miller, Ed. Philadelphia, PA: Elsevier, Churchill, Livingston; pp. 2589–2635.

occur shortly after the medication has been administered. The patient may state that he or she thinks the pain medicine is making him or her sick. The treatment is to administer an antiemetic and change the type of or eliminate the narcotic. A nasogastric tube is rarely necessary for narcotic induced nausea and vomiting. An excellent resource for managing PONV is the American Society of Perianesthesia Nurses' Evidence-Based Clinical Practice Guideline for the Prevention and/or Management of PONV/Post Discharge Nausea and Vomiting (PDNV; ASPAN, 2006).

PDNV
Post Discharge Nausea
and Vomiting

Potential Adverse Outcomes
See **Table 18.1**.

RISK OF ALTERATION IN COMFORT RELATED TO NAUSEA AND VOMITING

Implement pharmacologic and non-pharmacologic interventions to eliminate, attenuate, or modify the risk factors associated with postprocedure nausea and vomiting. Assess the patient for the causes of nausea and vomiting. Complementary techniques to consider include acupuncture, aromatherapy, and music therapy (Mamaril et al, 2006). Refer for medical treatment if indicated. Document your findings and activities according to institutional policy.

Assessing Inadvertent Hypothermia

Surgical patients may be admitted to the PACU with inadvertent hypothermia, defined as a core temperature <96.8° F (36° C) (Feeley & Marcario, 2005). Fourteen million surgical patients suffer from inadvertent hypothermia annually (Cuming & Nemec, 2002). Inadvertent hypothermia, which commonly occurs during anesthesia, results from anesthetic-impaired thermoregulation and exposure to the cold OR environment (Sessler & Kurz, 2006). It is important for the nurse to keep in mind that hypothermia may be present, regardless of temperature, if the patient describes feeling cold or has common signs and symptoms of hypothermia, such as, shivering, peripheral vasoconstriction, or piloerection (Frank et al, 1999). Shivering increases the metabolic rate and therefore the need to increase cardiac output and minute ventilation (Feeley & Marcario, 2005).

Potential Adverse Outcomes
See **Table 18.1**.

RISK FOR ALTERATION IN COMFORT RELATED TO INADVERTENT HYPOTHERMIA

Assess the patient's temperature and implement appropriate interventions to return the patient to a normothermic state. Once in the PACU, hypothermic patients should have supplemental oxygen, warm intravenous fluids and blood, and external warming (Feeley & Marcario, 2005). Document your findings and activities according to institutional policy. Two excellent resources for preventing and managing unplanned perioperative hypothermia are the Association of periOperative Registered Nurses' (AORN) Recommended Practices for the Prevention of Unplanned Hypothermia (AORN, 2008) and the American Society of PeriAnesthesia Nurses' (ASPAN) Clinical Guideline for the Prevention of Unplanned Perioperative Hypothermia (ASPAN, 2001).

AORN
Association of
periOperative
Registered Nurses

ENSURING THE PROPER FUNCTIONING OF DEVICES TO ASSIST RECOVERY

Several devices are commonly used to assist the patient in recovering from an operative or invasive procedure. These include nasogastric tubes, dressings, chest tubes, closed drainage systems, and open drains. The nurse should understand how these devices function, their purpose, how to check if they are functioning properly, and how to remove them after they have served their purpose.

Outcome Standard

Outcome standards for use of medical devices are listed in **Table 18.1**.

Nasogastric Tube

Although its benefit has become less clear in recent years, the purpose of a nasogastric tube is mainly to remove gastric secretions and swallowed air in patients with gastrointestinal obstructions (Luckey, 2003). It may be used to treat nausea and vomiting with distention from ileus. The patient with a nasogastric tube may be restricted to nothing by mouth; therefore, the output should be made up almost entirely of gastric secretions. Normally, the stomach secretes up to 500 to 1000 mL/day. After the nasogastric tube output has dropped below this level, the nurse should consider removing it; the tube is no longer therapeutic. Severe ear pain can mean acute otitis media if the nasogastric tube occludes the eustachian tube. In such cases, the nasogastric tube should be removed immediately. It may be repositioned to the other nostril if necessary.

Dressings

The purpose of dressings is to provide a clean environment for the incision, thus preventing the introduction of pathogens into the wound before the wound edges can seal. Wound edges seal to bacteria within 4 hours. Dressings wick drainage up and away from the skin, provide pressure and support the wound. Specialized dressings may also debride the wound. Although pressure dressings may offer some benefit in reducing edema, there can be risk of skin damage due to the tape. Dressings for hemostasis are inappropriate. The control of bleeding is best achieved during the procedure. Limit pressure dressings to immobilizing and supporting the wound. One appropriate use of the pressure dressing is on skin grafts. Pressure ensures that the donor skin stays in contact with the blood supply at the graft site. Wounds may be debrided by the frequent changing of dressing materials loosely packed into an open wound.

Chest Tubes

The purpose of chest tubes is to evacuate air, fluid, or pus from the pleural space so that the lung can completely inflate. Chest tubes are inserted after thoracic procedures. Chest tubes may be used in case of spontaneous pneumothorax, which can occur while the patient is being mechanically ventilated. Lactogenic pneumothorax (penetration of the pleural space with a needle while inserting a subclavian catheter) is also treated with chest tubes. Pleural effusions (causes discussed above) are drained via chest tubes. A variety of chest drainage systems are on the market. The nurse should know about the drainage systems most often used in an institution.

If the skin at the insertion site is not well closed, air may be pulled into the chest around it. A reliable method to prevent this is to place three sutures during the procedure. The first two close the incision around the tube and secure the tube in place. The third suture is placed to be tied to close the skin when the chest tube is removed. A frequently used, but less reliable, method to make the seal around the tube airtight is to apply petroleum jelly (Vaseline) impregnated gauze at the insertion site. Pursestring sutures in the skin around the tube provide an airtight seal; however, they are likely to cause necrosis of the skin.

The decision to remove the chest tube depends on its function. If its purpose is to drain fluid and superlative exudate, it may be removed when less than 200 mL/day is draining from the chest. If the purpose is to evacuate air, it may be removed when there is no evidence of an air leak. An air leak is present if, when the patient coughs, air bubbles appear in the water seal of the system.

Drainage Systems

Drains are used either to prevent or to treat an unwanted accumulation of fluid such as pus, blood, or serum (Doherty, 2008). Drains are also used to evacuate air from the pleural cavity so that the lungs can re-expand. When used prophylactically, drains are usually placed in a sterile location. Philosophies differ widely regarding the use of drains. Some physicians believe that drains are more likely to cause infections than to prevent them. These physicians usually remove drains much earlier than those who believe drains to be highly beneficial. The APN should have a working knowledge of the types of systems available to make recommendations to the surgeon. The APN should also know how to properly assemble, insert, and activate each system, as well as how to remove them when they are no longer needed. Closed drainage systems are placed to evacuate fluid that may accumulate or that has already accumulated in a wound. Closed drains are used more often in nonsuppurative wounds than in suppurative wounds. Closed systems are composed of a collection unit, extension tubing, and drainage tubing. Drainage tubing is available in a variety of sizes and styles. Most rely on some form of vacuum to facilitate the evacuation of fluid. These may be pumping devices that are stationary (wall suction with regulator), a line-powered pump (Gomco), or a manually activated device. Vacuum pressure is fixed for manually controlled systems, whereas it can be regulated with stationary or line-powered devices. The most common reasons for failure of closed drainage systems are inadequate diameter of the tube, improper placement or displacement of tube, loss of vacuum pressure, occlusion of the drain fenestration with clot or tissue, and retrograde contamination of the wound during emptying.

Open drains are used for the same reasons as closed systems. They are used more often in suppurative than in nonsuppurative wounds. Open drains ensure that the wound stays open for the drainage of thick suppurative and necrotic materials. Open drains can be soft latex or rigid plastic or Silastic tubing in a variety of styles, sizes, and lengths. These drains are secured with a safety pin or sutured to the skin. This prevents the drain from becoming dislodged and being pulled either into or out of the wound. A common practice with an open drain is to remove it gradually over several days. This allows the abscess cavity to drain and collapse as the drain is removed.

The drainage can be irritating to the skin. Frequent dressing changes with continuous assessment of the surrounding skin are necessary with open wounds. Wound drainage bags protect the skin when there is a large amount of drainage. The enterostomal therapy nurse is an extremely valuable resource in dealing with problem wounds.

Potential Adverse Outcomes
    See **Table 18.1.**

Risk of Injury Related to Devices Used to Assist Patient Recovery

NASOGASTRIC TUBE

Check proper positioning and functioning of the nasogastric tube. Inject 10 to 20 mL of air and auscultate the stomach for the sound of air bubbles. Reposition the tube if necessary and note output. Check the tube for patency by irrigating with about 30 mL of saline. Check the suction unit by placing suction tubing in water. Does it aspirate the water? Assess the skin condition where the tube is secured. Assess the patient's comfort level. Implement measures to relieve dryness of mucous membranes. Remove the tube when its use is no longer therapeutic.

DRESSINGS

Remove soiled dressings. Redress the wound only when drainage is present or if the purpose of the dressing is to debride the wound. Assess the skin condition under dressings and tape. Inspect wounds and the skin condition under splints and redress to continue support of the wound. Check that casts are intact.

CHEST TUBES

Check the proper functioning of the system. Note whether the suction regulator is properly set. Note the amount and nature of the drainage. Ask the patient to cough. Note air bubbles in the water seal, which indicate there is an air leak into the pleural space. Note if air is being pulled into the chest at the insertion site. Assess the skin condition around the insertion site. Remove when use of the tube is no longer therapeutic.

Removal of Chest Tubes   Collect the following supplies and equipment for chest tubes removal: suture scissors, sterile gloves, sponges, and 2-0 or 3-0 silk suture on a cutting needle if a suture to tie has not been placed during the procedure. The following supplies are optional: 3-mL syringe, 2 to 3 mL of 1% lidocaine (Xylocaine), and 25-gauge needle. Open supplies. Don the gloves. Remove the dressing. Cut the sutures securing the tube to the skin. Ask the patient to inhale deeply and hold his or her breath. With a sponge and the fingertips, apply slight pressure to the skin above the insertion site as the tube is removed to prevent air from being pulled into the chest. Remove the tube in one steady motion. Apply firm pressure above the insertion site until the incision is closed. Tie the remaining suture to close the incision. Tell the patient that he or she may breathe normally. Inject local anesthetic, if indicated. Close with 2-0 or 3-0 silk on a cutting needle if no suture has been placed during the procedure. Dress the wound.

CLOSED DRAINAGE SYSTEMS

Check the proper functioning of the system. Check if the vacuum is engaged. Note the amount of drainage collected in the past 24 hours. Compare daily amounts of drainage. Note the color, consistency, and odor of drainage. Check the patency of the tubing. Ensure that the tubing is properly connected and free from kinks and that the system is airtight. Note the amount of drainage around the insertion site. Assess the skin condition at the insertion site. Remove the drainage system when closed drainage is no longer therapeutic.

Removal of Closed Drainage Systems Collect the following supplies and equipment for removal of a closed drainage system: suture scissors, gloves, sponges, and tape. Open supplies. Don the gloves. Remove the dressing. Cut the suture securing the drain to the skin. Remove the drain in one steady motion. Dress the wound.

OPEN DRAINAGE SYSTEMS

Note if the drain is secured so that it does not come out or is not pulled into the wound. Check and compare the amount of drainage with that on previous days. Assess the color, consistency, and odor of drainage. Assess the skin condition around the insertion site. Gradually remove the drain.

Removal of Open Drainage Systems Collect the following supplies and equipment: suture scissors, gloves, and sponges. Optional supplies and equipment include wound drainage bag or tape, safety pin or 4-0 nylon suture, 3-mL syringe, 2 to 3 mL of 1% lidocaine, and 25-gauge needle. Open supplies. Don the gloves. Cut the suture, if any. Remove the drain about 5 cm. Reapply the safety pin, if applicable. Instill local anesthetic, if indicated. Suture the drain to the skin with nylon. Clean the skin around the wound. Apply the dressing or wound drainage bag. Remove the drain when its use is no longer therapeutic.

DISCHARGE PLANNING AND DISCHARGE INSTRUCTIONS

After the early recovery stage in the PACU, the intermediate recovery stage continues in the healthcare facility, whereas late recovery refers to the resumption of normal daily activities and occurs after discharge home (White & Freire, 2005). During the intermediate recovery stage, the patient is usually cared for in a recliner and progressively begins to ambulate, drink fluids, void, and prepare for discharge; the anesthetic technique, as well as the choice of postprocedure analgesic and antiemetic agents, have an impact on the duration of the intermediate stage (White & Freire, 2005).

Discharge criteria, outlined in policies and procedures, should be written and implemented (AORN, 2008). Discharge criteria should be based on standards or general guidelines for discharging patients established by accrediting organizations as well as anesthesia and postanesthesia provider associations (AORN, 2008). Guidelines for safe discharge for ambulatory surgery patients include stable vital signs, return to baseline orientation, ambulation without dizziness, minimal pain and PONV, and minimal bleeding at the surgical site (White & Freire, 2005). If the discharge criteria are not met, or if there are any questions about the patient's readiness for discharge, the nurse should consult with the anesthesia provider and/or surgeon prior to discharging the patient. Major accrediting bodies in the United States require that all ambulatory surgical patients have an escort to transport them home, and they must receive written postprocedure instructions, including whom to contact if a problem develops (White & Freire, 2005). Therefore, in order to promote effective continuity of care, and optimal patient outcomes, discharge planning is an essential nursing activity.

Today discharge planning is no longer a luxury; it is a necessity. The 2007 *Comprehensive Accreditation Manual for Hospitals: The Official Handbook* from the Joint Commission under the Patient-Focused Function of "Provision of Care, Treatment and Services (PC)" (PC 15.10) states there must be a process to address the needs for continuing care, treatment, and services after discharge or transfer" (The Joint Commission, 2007). The Standard furthers recognizes that for some patients, effective planning addresses how needs will be met as they move to the next level of care, treatment, and services, while for other patients, planning will consist of a clear understanding of how to access services in the future should the need arise. Discharge planning focuses on meeting patients' healthcare needs after discharge to include social support, home environment, and medical-surgical related needs.

PC
Provision of Care, Treatment and Services

The role of the nurse caring for the patient during the operative and invasive procedure period has evolved with regard to discharge planning. The greatly reduced hospital stays of today's environment means that there is less time for staff to carry out the discharge planning process. It is essential that the discharge planning process begin when the patient makes a decision to undergo an operative or invasive procedure (Burden, 2004). Successful discharge planning should include four primary elements:

1. comprehensive preprocedure assessment;
2. effective communication among caregivers, the surgeon or physician's office, the patient, and the family;
3. consideration of the patient's preprocedure status; and
4. a strong patient and family education plan.

See **Table 18.11** for a sample discharge planning checklist.

Outcome Statement for Discharge and Discharge Instructions
See **Table 18.1**.

Providing Discharge Instructions to the Patient and Family Based on Their Individual Informational Needs and Health Literacy

The nurse must assess the patient to determine potential problems and identify areas where the patient or family might need assistance. Effective planning for postprocedure care needs is patient-specific and should address physical, social, financial, cognitive, and sensory needs. It is crucial that a thorough interview be conducted with the patient prior to the day of the procedure, which can assist the nurse in identifying and planning for any issues that may adversely affect home care. Age-specific needs are very important and include identifying and addressing age-related barriers to learning and communication; incorporating the patient's existing physical and mental condition; addressing the impact of any social support challenges; and determining any environmental issues that can be improved to support recovery.

Table 18.11	Sample Discharge Planning Checklist

Social Support
- ☐ Does the patient live alone?
- ☐ Who will be staying with the patient? For how long?
- ☐ What is the ability of the caregiver?
- ☐ Who will drive the patient home?
- ☐ Is the patient the primary care provider for another family member?
- ☐ Does the patient drive?
- ☐ Who is the emergency contact when the patient is alone?

Home Environment
- ☐ Does the home have stairs?
- ☐ Is an elevator available?
- ☐ How far is the walk from the car to inside the home?
- ☐ What is the relationship of the bedroom, bathroom, and kitchen?
- ☐ Where is the telephone located?
- ☐ List of emergency contacts available by telephone.
- ☐ Remove safety hazards, e.g., throw rugs, small objects.
- ☐ Move cooking utensils to countertop as needed.
- ☐ Is there adequate food in the home?
- ☐ Entertainment sources (eg, books, puzzles, television, movies, radio, crafts).

Medical and Surgery-Related Needs
- ☐ Supply of prescription medications: ongoing and surgery-specific.
- ☐ Equipment needed for recovery (eg, wheelchair, crutches, braces, cold packs, etc.).
- ☐ Wound-care supplies.
- ☐ Followup physician appointment: Date? Transportation?

Adapted from Burden, N. (2004). Discharge planning for the elderly ambulatory surgery patient. *Journal of PeriAnesthesia Nursing*; 19(6), pp. 401–405.

Discharging patients to home after anesthesia and operative or invasive procedures is a serious responsibility, and it is the discharging nurse who must ensure that the plans developed by all care givers come together. Once the nurse has assured that the patient has achieved criteria for discharge and prior to releasing them from the facility, written and verbal instructions for home care must be provided. "Anxiety, discomfort and the amnestic effects of many medications given to patients can result in poor or absent recall of information from the day of surgery; therefore whenever possible, instructions should be given both to the patient and to the adult responsible for the patient after discharge" (Drain, 2003 p. 624).

The nurse assigned to care for the patient during the procedure has the opportunity to assess the patient's need for knowledge and skills as well as physical needs. This is an opportunity to help the patient and family members identify potential postprocedure problems sand needs. After establishing rapport with the patient and family, with their help, determine how the patient's illness has affected his or her role and function in the family. Pay special attention to age, financial support, shopping, meal preparation, transportation, and living arrangements. Look for medical diagnoses that indicate a need for increased discharge planning. These include multiple trauma, spinal cord injury, chronic conditions, abuse, psychiatric patients, joint replacements, terminal illnesses, acquired immunodeficiency syndrome, nutritional problems, and transplants. During the assessment, focus on prescribed medical treatments, mobility/activities of daily living deficits, sensory impairments, nutrition, psychosocial adjustment, home medical equipment, transportation, education, medical diagnosis, and other possible problems. Determine the patient's preprocedure routine and if the patient will be able to adhere to that routine after the procedure. Next, assess the patient's learning and comprehension ability and his or her interest in discharge planning and learning. Finally, determine if family finances are sufficient to meet the costs of equipment, supplies, and personnel that might be needed during the convalescent period.

Identifying Knowledge Deficit, Health Literacy, and Risk for Noncompliance with the Prescribed Therapeutic Regimen

The patient and/or family members who have a knowledge deficit experience a deficiency in cognitive knowledge or psychomotor skills regarding the condition or treatment plan (Carpenito-Moyet, 2004). They may verbalize a deficiency in knowledge or skill/request for information; express an inaccurate perception of their health status; or incorrectly perform a desired or prescribed health behavior (Carpenito-Moyet, 2004). Health literacy is the ability to read, understand, and use health information to make appropriate health decisions (Scudder, 2006). Low-health literacy is a broad term that describes a multidimensional problem that stems from a lack of education, breakdowns in communication, educational materials that are not appropriately written, and medical terminology that is too difficult for patients to comprehend (Monachos, 2007).

Every patient and family members must receive written postprocedure and followup care instructions that reflect their individual informational needs specific to home care, response to unexpected events, and followup by the physician (AORN, 2008). Discharge instructions should include the following (AORN, 2008; White & Friere, 2005):

- medication use, including side effects and signs and symptoms to report;
- when to contact the healthcare provider for additional assistance and the phone number to call;
- appropriate activities after discharge, including diet and wound care; and
- not to operate machinery, drive a car, or make important decisions for up to 24 hours.

Strategies to address the health literacy of the patient and family and increase the effectiveness of postprocedure teaching include (Monachos, 2007):

- use simple sentences and plain language;
- communicate with patients at eye level;
- limit points to two or three at a time; repeat and summarize;

- create a shame-free environment; encourage questions;
- use teach-back or show-back techniques to assess and ensure patient understanding;
- use drawings, diagrams, or models to illustrate what is being taught; and
- use the mediation reconciliation process; provide patients with a medication card listing their medications.

Effective discharge teaching is one measure to increase the patient's and family's compliance with the therapeutic regimen. The success of the postprocedure treatment regimen depends on the patient's or the family's physical, mental, and emotional ability to cooperate with the healthcare team. Identification of a patient or families at risk for noncompliance provides the nurse with the opportunity to implement interventions designed to ensure successful rehabilitation after discharge from the healthcare facility. A thorough assessment before the procedure is the key to planning interventions to eliminate the risk of noncompliance. During the assessment, open-ended questions can be asked to determine if the patient or family members have had difficulty complying with prescribed therapeutic regimens in the past. These questions should determine if the patient or the family.

Perceived ineffectiveness of recommended practices, perceived lack of seriousness of problems or risk factors, and perceived lack of susceptibility to postprocedure complications often stem from insufficient knowledge or skills on the part of the patient or family members. The nurse can intervene by implementing patient and family teaching strategies, especially concerning postprocedure care routines. Helping the patient and the family plan for the integration of the therapeutic recommendations into daily routines may also prove effective in ensuring compliance. Postprocedure home visits or telephone calls enable the nurse to verify compliance, provide motivation when needed, and identify problems.

As noted, the patient must be discharged to a responsible adult who will accompany him/her home and also be responsible for reporting any postprocedure complications or problems. At this time, the nurse should also verify the correct phone number for the patient to conduct the follow up phone call.

COMPLETING DISCHARGE FOLLOW-UP

The nurse conducts a postprocedure follow-up phone call to assess and evaluate the patient's status either within 24 hours or according to facility policy. The follow-up phone call provides an invaluable opportunity to evaluate patient education, identify trends that may require improvement in practice, determine compliance with discharge instructions, and assess overall impressions of performance; this process supports efforts to essentially *close the loop* on patient contact (Barnes, 2000).

Most organizations, especially those performing surgical and/or invasive procedures on an outpatient basis, find the postprocedure follow-up phone call to be helpful from both a timeliness, as well as patient-focused perspective (ASPAN, 2008). One recent study concluded that postprocedure follow-up via telephone using a structured protocol is a safe alternative to routine clinic follow-up for patients undergoing selected procedures and is also preferred by patients' families (McVay et al, 2008). Organizations that have chosen to adopt the phone call reassessment must also consider how it will be accomplished for patients requiring follow-up on weekends or at other times when staffing is an issue (ASPAN, 2008).

Some of the questions the nurse asks the patient and/or family member during the follow-up phone call include (Ontiveros & Schick, 2004):

- Is your pain adequately controlled?
- What level of pain are you experiencing (on the pain scale of 0 to 10)?
- Have you taken pain medication?
- Do you have any problems related to your procedure?
- Did you receive verbal and written instructions?
- How did you find your stay in the department/unit?
- How could we improve the service we provide?
- Is there anything we could have done to make your experience better?

The data collected should include specific individual needs and expectations, how well the facility met those needs, surgical site infections, and how the facility can improve patient safety (AORN, 2008). Document the results of the follow-up phone call in the patient's record. Policies and procedures for completing discharge follow-up with the patient to assess and evaluate his/her status should be written (AORN, 2008).

CONCLUSION

The APN plays important roles in facilitating the care of the patient after the procedure. Recognizing postprocedure wound complications, the signs of fever, tachycardia, pulmonary complications, thrombophlebitis, urinary tract infections, and adynamic ileus; assessing the patient's postprocedure comfort level; and ensuring the proper functioning of devices employed to assist recovery are skills that facilitate the recovery of the patient.

Through proper discharge planning the nurse will ensure that the patient and family/caregiver understand the self-care management plan for wound care, dietary restrictions, medication administration, signs and symptoms of infection and complications, and when to notify the healthcare provider. The nurse will assist the patient and the family/caregiver to obtain medications, medical equipment, and medical supplies. Care must be taken to be certain that the patient and family/caregiver know how to obtain these resources. Assistance will be provided to the patient or family/caregiver to arrange for the next postprocedure physician visit. Effective discharge instructions and postprocedure follow-up will help to promote patient compliance with the therapeutic regimen and ultimately positive outcomes. The nurse must assess the needs of the patient and family, as well as their knowledge deficit and health literacy.

Whereas home visits have not historically been an area of the postprocedure care of the patient performed by nurses, this practice, like so much else of healthcare, is changing. Today, nurses are performing home visits in some settings. These nurses consider the home visit an excellent opportunity to not only assist with the direct care of the patient but also meet the patient's educational needs and assist him or her to achieve an optimal level of health. The nurse can assist the patient if the nurse sees the patient's living conditions and knows what obstacles the patient has to overcome. Truly, home visits have evolved into an integral part of nursing.

18

COMPETENCY ASSESSMENT
Facilitate Care After the Procedure

Name: _____ Title: _____ Unit: _____ Date of Validation: _____

Type of Validation: ☐ Initial ☐ Annual ☐ Bi-annual

COMPETENCY STATEMENT: The advance practice nurse demonstrates competency to facilitate care after the operative or invasive procedure.

Performance Criteria	Met	Not Met
1. Describes the stages of wound healing	☐	☐
2. Recognizes postprocedure wound complications	☐	☐
3. Recognizes systemic postprocedure complications	☐	☐
4. Assesses the patient's physiological and psychological comfort level	☐	☐
5. Ensures the proper functioning of devices employed to assist recovery	☐	☐
6. Provides discharge instructions to the patient and family based on the their individual informational needs and health literacy	☐	☐
7. Competes discharge follow-up		

_____   _____

Validator's Signature   Employee's Signature

_____

Validator's Printed Name

REFERENCES

1. Agency for Health Care Policy and Research. (1992). Acute pain management: Operative or medical procedures and trauma. Clinical Practice Guideline No. 1. *AHCPR Publication* No. 92-0032. Rockville, MD: Agency for Health Care Policy and Research.
2. Akbaba, S., Kayaalp, C., & Savkilioglu, M. (2004). Nasogastric decompression after total gastrectomy. *Hepatogastroenterology*; 51(60): pp. 1881–1885.
3. American Society of PeriAnesthesia Nursing. (2003). ASPAN pain and comfort guideline©. Retrieved April 24, 2008 from http://www.aspan.org/PDFfiles/pain&comfort.pdf.
4. American Society of PeriAnesthesia Nursing. (2001). Clinical guideline for the prevention and treatment of unplanned perioperative hypothermia. Retrieved April 29, 2008 from http://www.aspan.org/PDFfiles/HYPOTHERMIA_GUIDELINE10-02.pdf.
5. American Society of PeriAnesthesia Nursing. (2008). Clinical practice: Frequently asked questions. Retrieved April 30, 2008 from http://www.aspan.org/clinicalpracticeFAQ.htm#Q2.
6. American Society of PeriAnesthesia Nursing. (2006). Evidence-based clinical practice guideline for the prevention and/or management of PONV/PDNV. Retrieved April 29, 2008 from http://www.aspan.org/PDFfiles/yjpan_aip.pdf.
7. Association of periOperative Registered Nurses. (2008a). AORN guidance statement: Postoperative patient care in the ambulatory surgery setting. *Perioperative Standards and Recommended Practices.* Denver, CO: AORN, Inc: 219–232.
8. Association of periOperative Registered Nurses. (2008b). Recommended practices for prevention of unplanned perioperative hypothermia. *Perioperative Standards and Recommended Practices.* Denver, CO: AORN, Inc: 407–420.
9. Barbul, A. (2006). Wound healing. In *Schwartz's Manual of Surgery*, 8th ed. Retrieved April 24, 2008

from http://books.google.com/books?id=yDhVYz6B
ovkC&pg=PT195&lpg=PT195&dq=studies+that+
compare+operations+performed+with+and+with
out+antibiotic+prophylaxis+demonstrate+that+w
ound+class+ii+iii+and+iv+procedures+treated+
with+appropriate+prophylactic+antibiotics+have
+only+one+third+the+wound+infection+rates+
of+previously+reported+untreated+series&source
=web&ots=XGzW_TbwVh&sig=M2C12jJN47AhK
qewLCKKi8v5Qmo&hl=en#PPT8,M1.

10. Barnard, B.M. (2002). Fighting surgical site infections. *Infection Control Today* [serial online]. Retrieved April 23, 2008 from http://www.infectioncontroltoday.com/articles/241feat1.html.

11. Barnes, S. (2000). Not a social event: The followup phone call. *Journal of Perianesthesia Nursing*; 15(4): 253–255.

12. Brown, J. (2008). Intrinsic and extrinsic factors affecting wound healing. Retrieved April 17, 2008 from http://judithbrowncpd.co.uk/index_files/Intrinsic%20and%20Extrinsic%20Factors%20Affecting%20Wound%20Healing.pdf.

13. Burden, N. (2004). Discharge planning for the elderly ambulatory surgery patient. *Journal of PeriAnesthesia Nursing*; 19(6), pp. 401–405.

14. Carpenito-Moyet, L.J. (2004). *Nursing diagnosis: Application to clinical practice.* Philadelphia, PA: Lippincott Williams & Wilkins.

15. Carr, D.B., Reines, H.D., Schaffer, J., et al. (2005). The impact of technology on the analgesic gap and quality of acute pain management. *Reg Anesth Pain Med*; 30: pp. 286–291.

16. Carrère, N., Seulin, P., Julio, C.J., Bloom, E., Gouzi, J.L, Pradère, B. (2007). Is nasogastric or nasojejunal decompression necessary after gastrectomy? A prospective randomized trial. *World J Surg.*; 31(1): pp. 122–127.

17. Carter S. (2006). The surgical team and outcomes management: focus on postoperative ileus. *Journal of PeriAnesthesia Nursing*; 21(2), pp. S1–S2.

18. Centers for Disease Control and Prevention. (2005). National Center for Health Statistics. Inpatient procedures, 2005 National Hospital Discharge Survey. Retrieved April 24, 2008 from http://www.cdc.gov/nchs/fastats/insurg.htm.

19. Certification Board Perioperative Nursing. (2003). *Job analysis for certified RN first assistant (CRNFA).* Denver, CO: CBPN.

20. Cuming, R. & Nemec, J. (2002). Perioperative hypothermia: complications and consequences. *Vital Signs Magazine* XII; No. 22.

21. Doherty, G.M. (2008). The immediate postoperative period. In Current Surgical Diagnosis and Treatment, 12th ed. Retrieved April 24, 2008 from http://www.accesssurgery.com/content.aspx?aID=30180.

22. Drain, C.B. (2003). Care of the ambulatory surgery patient. In *Perianesthesia Nursing; A Critical Care Approach.* Philadelphia, PA: Elsevier; p. 624.

23. Feeley, T.W. & Marcario, A. (2005). The postanesthesia care unit. In *Miller's Anesthesia*, 6th ed., R.D. Miller, (Ed.). Philadelphia, PA: Elsevier, Churchill, Livingston; pp. 2703–2727.

24. Fishman, T.D. (2008). Phases of wound healing. Retrieved April 17, 2008 from http://www.medicaledu.com/phases.htm.

25. Frank, S.M., Raja, S.N., Bulaco, C., et al. (1999). Relative contributions of core and cutaneous temperature to thermal comfort and autonomic responses in humans. *J Appl Physiol*; 86:1588–93.

26. Hirsh, J., Guyatt, G., Albers, G.W., & Schünemann, H.J. (2004). The seventh ACCP conference on antithrombotic and thrombolytic therapy: Evidence-based guidelines. *Chest*; 126:172S–173S. Retrieved April 24, 2008 from http://www.chestjournal.org/cgi/content/full/126/3_suppl/172S.

27. Horan, T.C., Gaynes, R. P., Martone, W. J., Jarvis, W. R., & Emori, T.G. (1992). CDC definitions of nosocomial surgical site infections a modification of CDC definitions of surgical wound infections. *Infect Control Hosp Epidemiol*; 13(10): pp. 606–608.

28. Kaide, C.G. & Khandelwal, S. (2008). Hyperbaric oxygen: applications in infectious disease. *Emerg Med Clin North Am*; 26(2): pp. 571–595.

29. Krenzischek, D. A., Dunwoody, C.J., Polomano, R.C., & Rathmell, J.P. (2008). Pharmacokinetics for acute pain: Implications for practice. *Journal of Perianesthesia Nursing*; 23 (1 Suppl): S28–42.

30. Lineweaver, W., Howard, R., Soucy, D., et al. (1985). Topical antimicrobial toxicity. *Archives of Surgery*; 120: pp. 267–270.

31. Luckey, A., Livingston, E., & Tache, Y. (2003). Mechanisms and treatment of postprocedure ileus. *Arch Surg*; 138(2); pp. 206–214.

32. Mamaril, M.E., Windle, P.E., & Burkhard, J.F. (2006). Prevention and management of postprocedure nausea and vomiting: a look at complementary techniques. *Journal of PeriAnesthesia Nursing*; 21(6): pp. 404–110.

33. Mangram, A.J., Horan, T.C., Pearson, M.L., Silver, L.C., & Jarvis, W.R. (1999). Guideline for prevention of surgical site infection. *Infect Control Hosp Epidemiol*; 20(4): pp. 247–278.

34. MEDQIC. (2008). SCIP process and outcome measures. Retrieved April 24, 2008 from http://www.medqic.org/dcs/ContentServer?cid=1136495755695&pagename=Medqic%2FOtherResource%2FOtherResourcesTemplate&c=OtherResource.

35. McVay, M.R., Kelley, K.R., Mathews, D.L., Jackson, R.J., Kokoska, E.R., & Smith, S.D. (2008). Postoperative followup: is a phone call enough? *Journal of Pediatric Surgery*; 43(1): 83–86.

36. Meoli, A.L., Rosen, C.L., Kristo, D. Kohrman, M., Gooneratne, N., Aguillard, R.N., Fayle, R., Troell, R., Kramer, R., Casey, K.R., & Coleman, J. (2003). Report of the AASM clinical practice review committee: Upper airway management of the adult patient with obstructive sleep apnea in the perioperative period—avoiding complications. Retrieved April 24, 2008 from http://www.aasmnet.org/Resources/PracticeReviews/cpr_260820.pdf.

37. Monachos, C.L. (2007). Assessing and addressing low health literacy among surgical outpatients. *AORN Journal*; 86(3): pp. 373–383.

38. Nelson, R., Edwards, S., & Tse, B. (2007). Prophylactic nasogastric decompression after abdominal surgery. *Cochrane Database Syst Rev*; 18(3):P. CD004929.

39. Nichols, R.L. (2001). Preventing surgical site infections: A surgeon's perspective. Retrieved April 30, 2008 from http://www.cdc.gov/ncidod/eid/vol7no2/nichols.htm.

40. Ontiveros, J.E. & Schick, L. (2004). Postprocedure follow up. In *Perianesthesia Core Curriculum*. Philadelphia, PA: Saunders.

41. Pasero, C. (2005) Improving postoperativepostprocedure outcomes with epidural analgesia. *Journal of PeriAnesthesia Nursing*; 20(1): pp. 51–55.

42. Petersen, C. (2007). *Perioperative nursing data set, the perioperative nursing vocabulary.* (Revised 2nd ed.). Denver, CO: AORN. Inc.

43. Polomano, R. (2008). Perioperative pain management: assessment and monitoring for patient safety. *Journal of PeriAnesthesia Nursing*; 23(1), pp. S1–S58.

44. Polomano, R.C., Dunwoody, C.J., Krenzischek, D.A., & Rathmell, J.P. (2008). Perspective on pain management in the 21st century. *Journal of Perianesthesia Nursing*; 23 (1 Suppl): S4–14.

45. Rodeheaver, G., Bellamy, W., Kody, M., et al. (1982). Bactericidal activity and toxicity of iodine-containing solutions in wounds. *Archives of Surgery*; 117: pp. 181–185.

46. Saclarides, T.J. (2006). Current choices— good or bad—for the proactive management of postoperative ileus: a surgeon's view, Journal *of PeriAnesthesia Nursing*; 21(2A), pp. S7–S15.

47. Schwartz, S.I. (2006). *Schwartz's Manual of Surgery*, 8th ed. Retrieved April 8, 2008 from http://www.accesssurgery.com/content.aspx?aID=3017.

48. Scudder, L. (2006). Words and well-being: how literacy affects patient health. *The Journal for Nurse Practitioners*; 2(1): pp. 28–35.

49. Sessler, D.I. & Kurz, A. (2006). Mild perioperative hypothermia. *Anesthesiology News Special Edition*: pp. 25–31.

50. Steinbrook, R.A. (2005). Postoperative ileus: Why we should treat. *Contemporary Surgery*; (supplemental issue): 4–7.

51. Strassels, S.A., McNicol, E., & Suleman, R. (2007). Acute pain pharmacotherapy. Retrieved April 24, 2008 from http://www.uspharmacist.com/index.asp?show=article&page=8_2025.htm.

52. Sussman, G. (2007) The impact of medicines on wound healing. *Pharmacist, 26*: pp. 874–878.

53. The Joint Commission. (2007). Standards frequently asked questions: Comprehensive accreditation manual for hospitals (CAMH). Retrieved April 17, 2008 from http://www.jointcommission.org/AccreditationPrograms/Hospitals/Standards/FAQs/default.htm.

54. Thompson, C. (2008). Post-operative pain. *The Virtual Anaesthesia Textbook*. Retrieved April 29, 2008 from http://www.virtual-anaesthesia-textbook.com/vat/pain.html.

55. United States Pharmacopeia. (2004). Patient-controlled analgesia pumps can lead to medication errors. Retrieved April 24, 2008 from http://vocuspr.vocus.com/VocusPR30/Newsroom/Query.aspx?SiteName=uspharm&Entity=PRAsset&SF_PRAsset_PRAssetID_EQ=92336&XSL=PressRelease&Cache=False.

56. United States Pharmacopeia. (2004). USP quality review: Data analysis. No. 81. Retrieved April 29, 2008 from http://www.usp.org/hqi/practitionerPrograms/newsletters/qualityReview/qr812004-09-01a.html.

57. Viljanto, J. (1980). Disinfection of surgical wounds without inhibition of normal wound healing. *Archives of Surgery*; 115: pp. 253–256.

58. Wagar, S.H., Malik, Z.I., Razzaq, A., Abdullah, M.T., Shaima, A., & Zahid, M.A. (2005). Frequency and risk factors for wound dehiscence/burst abdomen in midline laparotomies. *J Ayub Med Coll Abbottabad*; 17(4): 70–3.

59. White, P.F. & Freire, A.R. (2005). Ambulatory (outpatient) anesthesia. In *Miller's Anesthesia*, 6th ed., R.D. Miller, (Ed.). Philadelphia, PA: Elsevier, Churchill, Livingston; pp. 2589–2635.

Section 3
Operative and Invasive Procedures

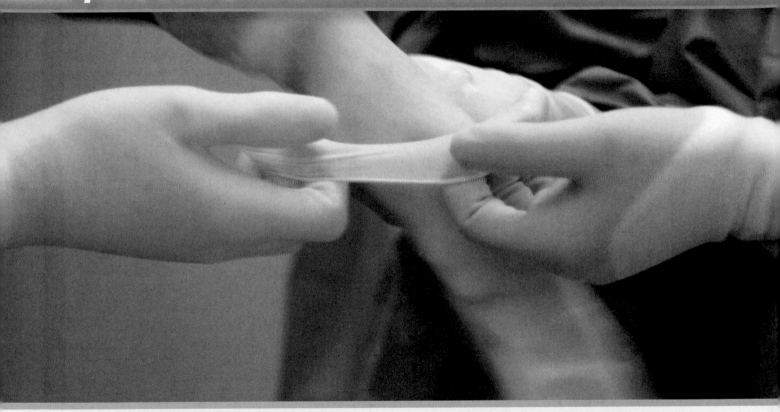

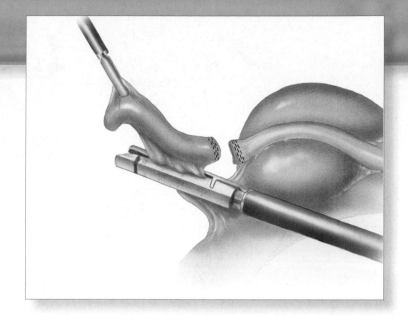

CHAPTER 19

General Surgery

Joyce M. Stengel

Noel Williams

INTRODUCTION

General surgery has long been the hallmark of surgeries for the operative and invasive procedure suite. The common procedures linked to general surgery focuses on the gastrointestinal tract and the breast. The procedure areas involve the stomach, the liver, the pancreas, the intestines, the gallbladder, the appendix, and the breast. Historically these procedures were performed with open incisions, but with the advent of minimally invasive procedures (MIP) many operations are now performed through a small incision. Once all of the criteria are met, MIP seems to be the more effective treatment option for the patient. Compared to open surgical procedures, the benefits of MIP for the patient include decreased pain, less trauma to the tissues, shorter recovery period, decreased hospital stay and potentially a lower risk for infection. The only downside for the moment seems to be a high operative expense. As new methods and practices emerge, less invasive procedures will be a more common choice for patients than previous open and invasive procedures.

ANATOMY

The stomach is a curved muscular organ that receives food from the esophagus (**Fig. 19.1**). It is divided into four areas: the cardia, the fundus, the body, and the pylorus. Each of these portions secretes fluids that aid in the digestion of food. The stomach both mixes and initiates peristalsis of food and secretions so that they are driven into the small intestine. The small intestine joins the stomach at the pylorus, which is the lower opening. In the small intestine, digestion of all ingested foods is completed. The small intestine is about 16 feet

Chapter Contents

MIP
Minimally Invasive Procedures

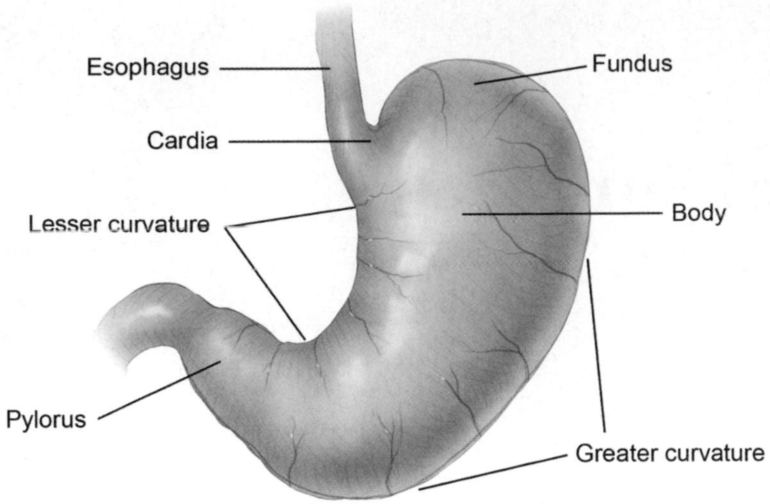

Figure 19.1

Anatomy of the stomach.

(500 cm) long and consists of the duodenum, the jejunum, and the ileum. The duodenum houses the pancreatic and common bile ducts, which provide the digestive fluids. The jejunum is supplied with blood from the mesentery, which contains fat, blood vessels, lymph vessels, lymph nodes, and nerves. The mesentery also supplies blood to the ileum, or last portion of the small bowel.

The large intestine or colon extends from the end of the ileum to the rectum. The large intestine is about 5 feet (1.5 m) long and is divided into the right and left sides of the colon. The right side of the colon consists of the cecum, the ascending colon, the hepatic flexure, and the proximal transverse colon. The left side of the colon consists of the distal transverse colon, the splenic flexure, the descending colon, the sigmoid, and the rectosigmoid colon. The large intestine is responsible for maintaining the patency of the gastrointestinal tract by eliminating and removing all indigestible materials.

The liver is one of the largest organs in the body, representing 2% of the total body weight. It is located in the upper right portion of the abdomen just beneath the diaphragm and consists of two principal lobes, the left and the right, separated by the falciform ligament (**Fig. 19.2**). The liver stores and filtrates blood, secretes bile, converts sugars into glycogen, and performs many other metabolic activities.

The gallbladder is a pear-shaped organ measuring 3 to 4 inches (7.5–10 cm) long. It is located below the liver and actually divides the liver into the right and left lobes (**Fig. 19.3**). The gallbladder's main function is the storage of bile; it can hold about 45 mL of bile when fully distended. It is divided into four portions: the fundus, the body (which serves as the storage area), the infundibulum, and the neck, which connects with the cystic duct. The cystic duct continues and is joined with the common duct.

The pancreas is a soft, finely lobulated gland that extends retroperitoneally across the posterior abdominal wall from the second part of the duodenum on the right to the spleen on the left (see **Fig. 19.3**). It consists of five named parts, which include the head, the uncinate process, the neck, the body, and the tail. The main pancreatic duct traverses the gland and passes through the duodenal wall as the ampulla of Vater and

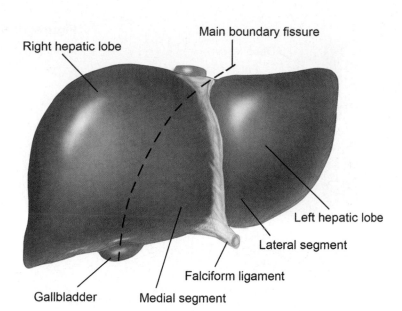

Figure 19.2

Anatomical division of the liver.

Right hepatic lobe

Main boundary fissure

Left hepatic lobe

Lateral segment

Falciform ligament

Gallbladder

Medial segment

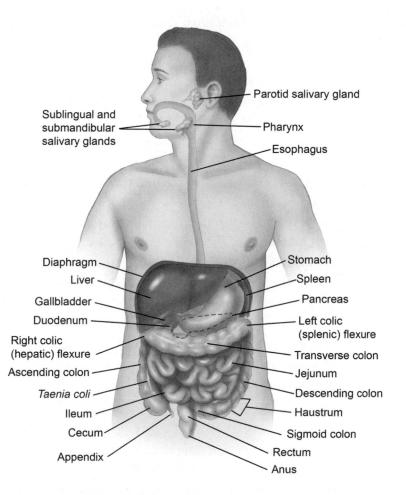

Figure 19.3

Major structures of the gastrointestinal tract.

Parotid salivary gland

Sublingual and submandibular salivary glands

Pharynx

Esophagus

Diaphragm

Liver

Gallbladder

Duodenum

Right colic (hepatic) flexure

Ascending colon

Taenia coli

Ileum

Cecum

Appendix

Stomach

Spleen

Pancreas

Left colic (splenic) flexure

Transverse colon

Jejunum

Descending colon

Haustrum

Sigmoid colon

Rectum

Anus

then into the duodenum. The pancreas has two functioning components, namely, the endocrine (insulin and glucagon) and exocrine cells, which secrete gastrointestinal hormones and enzymes. The main blood supply to the pancreas originates from branches of the celiac trunk superiorly and from the superior mesenteric artery inferiorly.

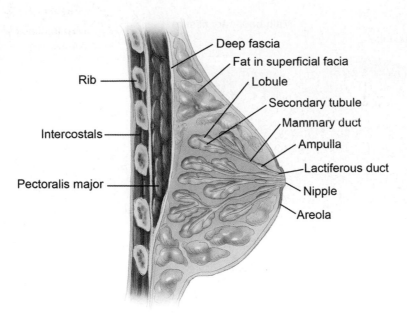

Figure 19.4

Mammary gland.

The anatomical structure of the gastrointestinal tract is complex. The previous discussion describes briefly the anatomical features of the organs involved in the operative procedures considered next. The breast is also described in this chapter because it is a major focus of general surgery.

In operative procedures for inguinal hernias, an understanding of the anatomy of the region is of paramount importance. Most hernias of the abdominal wall are made up of a sac of peritoneum that protrudes through a weakness in the muscular layers of the abdominal wall. A weakness in the transversalis fascia is the major source of groin hernias. An indirect inguinal hernia passes through the internal inguinal ring, a defect in transversalis fascia between the anterior iliac spine and the pubic tubercle. The sac is in the spermatic cord and on occasion can go all the way into the scrotum. Direct inguinal hernias occur as a result of a weakness in the transversalis fascia in the middle of the posterior part of the inguinal canal.

The mammary glands lie in the front of the chest over the pectoral muscles (**Fig. 19.4**). Each mammary gland consists of multiple lobes, which are separated by adipose tissue. Adipose tissue contributes to the size of the breasts. At the tip of each breast is an area called the areola. At the center of the areola is the nipple. Breasts have multiple ducts, which empty into the nipple. The breast produces milk after childbirth as well as functioning as a secondary sex organ.

SPECIAL INSTRUMENTS, SUPPLIES, AND EQUIPMENT

General surgery uses basic instruments and supplies. A laparotomy set is the major instrument set used for general procedures within the abdominal cavity. The instruments incorporated in a major instrument set include various scissors, forceps, and clamps, both crushing and noncrushing. Noncrushing clamps are used when less damage to tissue is warranted, whereas crushing clamps execute the opposite. Dozens of clamps are available for general surgery, and many are physician-specific. Exposure is an important aspect of general surgery and is provided with the use of retractors. There are multiple handheld retractors (eg, Deaver and malleable retractors). Self-retaining table-mounted retractors may also be employed and allow optimal exposure for the procedure (Bookwalter).

A nurse's experience in general surgery would not be complete without the use of stapling devices. Intestinal staplers have a wide range of applications, especially in general surgery, facilitating resection, anastomosis, and fascia and skin closure. Equipment for general surgery is specific for each procedure planned. Hepatic resections sometimes employ the use of a cavitational ultrasonic surgical aspirator, which aspirates diseased liver tissue through an ultrasonic handpiece. Other technologies that are also used in general surgery include argon-enhanced electrosurgery, ultrasonic dissection, and tissue fusion devices. See Chapter 17 for a discussion of these technologies.

GASTRECTOMY

Gastrectomy refers to the removal of the stomach (total gastrectomy) or a part of it (subtotal gastrectomy).

Indications

A gastrectomy is performed for the treatment of malignant disease or for chronic ulcers that do not respond to a medical regimen. If a partial gastrectomy is performed, 70%–80% of the stomach is removed and an anastomosis is made from the remaining stomach to a loop of intestine, usually the jejunum. A total gastrectomy involves an anastomosis of the end of the esophagus to the jejunum. The goal of both types of procedures is to maintain the patency and continuity of the gastrointestinal tract.

Nursing Implications

Anesthesia

The choice for an abdominal procedure is usually a general anesthetic. General anesthesia enables the surgeon to have complete relaxation of the organs and muscles involved. An epidural anesthetic (regional block) may also be used. The epidural catheter is placed before the procedure, and anesthetics can be infused at intervals or at the end of the operation. The block also aids in decreasing postprocedure pain. With narcotics, the cough reflex is depressed. Regional anesthetics do not depress the cough reflex; therefore postprocedure complications may be decreased. The patient is usually given an antibiotic before the procedure for control of infection and promotion of wound healing. Other drugs such as sedatives and smooth muscle relaxants may also be given before the procedure.

Patient monitoring is of the utmost importance during an operative procedure. The proper equipment for pulse oximetry, blood pressure management, electrocardiography, and capnography should be available. At each anesthesia work station, equipment for measuring temperature, a peripheral nerve stimulator, a stethoscope, and appropriate lighting must be immediately available. A spirometer must be available without undue delay (Backman, 2005). The anesthesia provider also monitors the patient hemodynamically. Fluid input and output is constantly assessed. Many patients undergoing an abdominal procedure require adjuvant blood therapy. If this is the case the blood products that are to be infused are checked and validated according to hospital protocol. A temperature-regulated Foley catheter may be used to aid in assessing the body temperature. Because the operative procedure may require a large exposure, a warming blanket can be used to aid in regulating body temperature.

Position

The patient is placed in a supine position. An egg-crate or soft mattress is placed under the patient before the procedure for comfort and prevention of pressure ulcers. These mattresses are used when a procedure may take a long time. The arms are placed at the patient's sides or extended on padded arm boards. The decision of arm position is determined by the surgeon or the anesthesia provider.

Pneumatic compression stockings are applied to both legs for the prevention of emboli and venous thrombosis. A pillow may be placed under the patient's knees for comfort and also to decrease any back pressure.

Establishing and Maintaining the Sterile Field

All members of the operative team are responsible for maintaining the integrity of the sterile field during the procedure. The patient is prepared from the clavicle to the groin. The operative area is cleansed with povidone iodine (Betadine) or a soap solution. This is done immediately before the procedure. The patient is covered with sterile drapes. The only area left undraped should be the operative site. The scrub person establishes the sterile field, checking sterilization indicators to ensure that all instruments are sterile. Instrument tables are positioned close to the operative field to minimize contamination. The team should constantly be alerted to breaks in technique that create an unsterile environment.

Equipment and Supplies

A major instrument set is used for a gastrectomy, along with retractors (Deaver, Army-Navy, Bookwalter), gastric and bowel staplers, and surgeon-specific instruments. These may include gastric clamps and long instruments, such as Judd Allis forceps, Babcock tissue forceps, and Mixter forceps. Surgeon-specific sutures are used. The nurse also needs culture tubes, drains, a Foley catheter, suction equipment, electrosurgery equipment, sponges and blades. All instruments and supplies should be functional. The nurse should be alerted to any problems with the equipment during the procedure.

Physiological Monitoring

A Foley catheter is placed for constant bladder drainage to monitor urine output. A nasogastric tube, usually a Levin 12 to 18 Fr., is placed for decompression of the gastrointestinal tract. A nasopharyngeal tube is placed to monitor the temperature of the patient. Hemodynamic monitoring may be used if there is a chance of marked blood loss. Arterial catheterization, usually of the radial artery, is done for monitoring blood pressure and obtaining blood gas measurements during and after the operation.

Drugs and Solutions

Normal saline and antibiotics are commonly used for irrigation.

Physician Orders and Laboratory and Diagnostic Studies

Preprocedure studies for the patient undergoing a gastrectomy sometimes include a gastric analysis, gastrointestinal radiographic series such as a barium test, and gastrointestinal radiographs. The physician's orders may also include a chest radiograph, complete blood cell count, electrocardiogram, and skin and bowel preparation. The patient is instructed to take nothing by mouth after midnight. Prophylactic antibiotics may be ordered, along with the administration of all other medications that the patient is taking, unless contraindicated.

Procedure
Incision and Exposure

An upper midline incision is made with a No. 10 blade. Electrosurgery is used for dissection and control of bleeding sites. The peritoneum is grasped by the surgeon and the assistant to facilitate entering the abdomen. After the abdomen is fully opened, a general exploration is initiated. Exposure is attained by the use of retractors.

Details

The stomach is mobilized by ligating and dividing the omental vessels. Scissors, suture ties, and hemoclips aid in mobilization. Hemoclips are titanium or stainless steel clips that are used for ligating vessels. Two hemoclips ligate the vessel, and a scissors or a knife blade divides the vessel between the clips. Suture ties enhance ligation. An intestinal stapling instrument is used to close the duodenum. Before removing the instrument, a gastric clamp (Glassman) is placed on the specimen side to prevent oozing when the duodenum is transected. Another intestinal stapling instrument is used to close the gastric pouch. The surgeon places the stapling instrument around the stomach at the level of the transection. Again, a gastric clamp is used on the specimen side before firing the stapling instrument. The remaining gastric pouch is anastomosed to the proximal jejunum.

The gastrojejunostomy is created by using another stapling instrument. The gastrointestinal anastomosis (GIA) instrument has two cartridge forks containing staples (**Fig. 19.5**). Two double rows of staples join the tissue, and a knife blade cuts between the two, creating a stoma. The surgeon inspects all areas of anastomosis for hemostasis.

GIA
Gastrointestinal
Anastomosis

Figure 19.5

Gastrojejunostomy with the use of the GIA instrument.

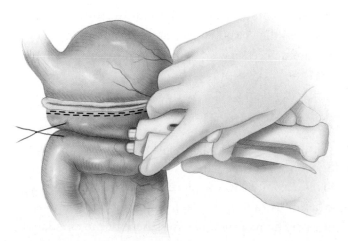

The procedure described is also called a Billroth II gastric resection. In a Billroth I resection, the remaining gastric pouch is anastomosed to the duodenum; a total gastrectomy entails anastomosis of the esophagus and the jejunum.

Closure

When hemostasis is achieved, all retractors and sponges are removed. A final inspection of the abdomen is made, ensuring that no abnormalities have been overlooked. The abdomen is irrigated with a warm normal saline solution, and drains are placed. The peritoneum, fascia, subcutaneous fat, and skin are then reapproximated and closed using surgeon-specific suture. A sterile dressing is applied.

Postprocedure Care

PACU
Postanesthesia Care
Unit

Patients are observed in the postanesthesia care unit (PACU) until they are conscious and vital signs are stable. Routine postprocedure orders include urine output measurements, administration of fluids and electrolytes, dressing changes, inspection and suctioning of drainage tubes, respiratory care, and administration of medications such as antibiotics, sedatives, and narcotics for pain relief.

Potential Complications

Potential complications include dumping syndrome (rapid emptying of the gastric contents into the small intestine), hemorrhage, infection, and gastric retention due to edema of the stoma or organic obstruction.

HEPATIC RESECTION

Hepatic resections are done to remove a portion of the liver. The resection is based on the surgical anatomy (eg, right hepatic lobectomy, left hepatic lobectomy, wedge resection, trisegmentectomy, and left lateral and left medial segmentectomy). Liver transplant surgery is the removal of the entire liver. The following discussion concerns hepatic resections.

Indications

Hepatic resections are done to remove primary or secondary malignant tumors, benign tumors, traumatic ruptures, cysts, and abscesses. The functional status of the liver is important. Cirrhosis is a relative contraindication for hepatectomy. Surgery and general anesthesia carry increased risks in the patient with cirrhosis. Anesthesia reduces cardiac output, induces splanchnic vasodilatation, and causes a 30–50% reduction in hepatic flow. This places the cirrhotic liver at additional risk for decompensation. Thus, unless absolutely necessary, surgery should be avoided in the patient with cirrhosis (Wolf, 2007).

Nursing Implications
Anesthesia

In addition to anesthesia implications already mentioned for gastrectomy, cell-saving equipment (autologous transfusion) and a rapid injection blood infusion pump may be needed. This is accomplished by placement of a 14- or 16-gauge intravenous catheter for rapid administration of blood, fluids, or medications. A central venous pressure monitor may be required for assessment of the circulation, and a Swan-Ganz catheter may be inserted for assessment of cardiac function and output. Blood warming units should also be available.

Position

The patient is placed in supine position. Electrocardiographic leads should be kept clear of the right chest wall and the presternal area in case a thoracoabdominal incision is necessitated by the position of the tumor or by operative hemorrhage. Preparation and draping should allow for exposure of the lower chest and the entire upper abdomen down past the umbilicus (Fong, 2006). See the earlier discussion for gastrectomy.

Establishing and Maintaining the Sterile Field

The patient is prepared from the nipples to the groin. An impervious split drape is used to cover the operative site. The nurse anticipates blood loss during the procedure and has available multiple drapes and bath blankets, which may he placed under the operating bed.

Equipment and Supplies

Hypothermia can be a problem and must be constantly assessed. The anesthesia provider may place a warming blanket on the patient's upper and lower body to facilitate warmth. Additional suctioning equipment should be available. In addition to a laparotomy set, a vascular set should be on the instrument table. The patient care team must be prepared for any hemorrhagic complication during the procedure. The nurse should be aware of specific clamps that are preferred by the surgeon. A large hepatic clamp should be available to occlude the segment of the liver that is being transected. The surgeon may perform a cholecystectomy at the time of resection, and gallbladder instruments should be on the surgical field. Chest instruments should also be available if the incision needs to be extended. The argon electrosurgery unit and cavitational ultrasonic surgical aspirator should be available (see earlier). In addition to suture used for a gastrectomy, sutures on large needles may be used to repair bleeding hepatic vessels.

Physiological Monitoring

See the discussion of gastrectomy and the previous section on anesthesia.

Drugs and Solutions

The following may be needed:

> Normal saline
>
> Gelatin sponge (Gelfoam)
>
> Oxidized regenerated cellulose (Surgicel)
>
> Topical thrombin
>
> Antibiotics

Physician Orders

In addition to typical admission orders for patients having an abdominal procedure, serum albumin levels should be monitored as well as those of aspartate aminotransferase and alanine aminotransferase. These levels are normally elevated in patients with hepatic disease.

Laboratory and Diagnostic Studies

Laboratory and diagnostic studies include liver biopsy, arteriography, liver function studies, hepatic angiography, and computed tomography.

Procedure

Incision and Exposure

Most hepatic lobectomies are performed through an abdominal incision, however, some surgeons prefer a thoracoabdominal approach for right lobectomies.

After the abdomen is entered, a Bookwalter retractor is placed for optimal exposure. The surgeon may use an extension of the Bookwalter retractor for retraction of the rib cage. Exposure is maintained for the procedure. Abdominal packs may be placed for retraction of other organs.

Details

Dissection begins on the vessels and ducts surrounding the liver and the gallbladder. These hilar vessels are divided and ligated. Scissors, hemoclips, and suture ties are used for the dissection. An automatic, reloadable hemoclip applier is also used for ligation. It enables the surgeon to have better visualization and control hemostasis. The scrub person prepares the cavitational ultrasonic surgical aspirator and has it ready for the transection. A hepatic clamp is placed on the lobe to be resected. The clamp occludes the blood flow and marks the line of resection. The aspirator or electrosurgery is used to transect the lobe. During the resection, hemostasis is achieved with hemoclips and suture ligatures of hepatic vessels. After the specimen has been removed, it is sent to the pathology department for diagnosis and study.

Hemostasis is controlled by electrosurgery, thrombin, gelatin sponge, or oxidized regenerated cellulose. Often, all of these agents are used. Massive hemorrhage can be a complication after resection of the liver. The surgeon may also temporarily pack the abdomen with laparotomy sponges to provide compression.

Closure

When hemostasis is attained, the abdomen is irrigated with warm saline, drains are placed, and the abdomen is closed. Surgeon-specific suture is used. Dressings are applied, and the patient is transferred to the surgical intensive care unit.

Postprocedure Care

The patient requires close monitoring and metabolic support after the procedure. Blood glucose levels are checked frequently. Vitamin K and fresh frozen plasma are administered to supply clotting factors. If hypoalbuminemia occurs, albumin is given and the serum bilirubin level is assessed daily.

Potential Complications

Potential complications include wound and pulmonary infections, fever of unknown origin, abscess formation, residual liver failure, stress ulcers, ascites, coma, varices, and hepatic encephalopathy,

PANCREATICODUODENECTOMY (WHIPPLE PROCEDURE)

Pancreaticoduodenectomy is a complex operation involving the removal of the entire duodenum, distal common bile duct, gallbladder, head, uncinate process, and neck of the pancreas.

Indications

This procedure is performed for periampullary malignant disease. Periampullary tumors consist of adenocarcinomas that arise in the head of the pancreas, distal common bile duct, and duodenum. In addition, this procedure is also performed in selective cases of chronic pancreatitis primarily involving the head of the pancreas.

Nursing Implications

Refer to the section on gastrectomy for implications concerning anesthesia, positioning, establishing and maintaining the sterile field, equipment and supplies, drugs and solutions, and physiological monitoring. Instruments include those in major instruments sets and specific instruments for gallbladder and intestinal procedures.

Physician Orders and Laboratory and Diagnostic Studies

In addition to routine admission orders, preprocedure studies for a patient undergoing a pancreaticoduodenectomy include endoscopic retrograde cholangiopancreatography (ERCP), endoscopic ultrasonography, and computed tomography of the abdomen. As in most major abdominal procedures, prophylactic antibiotics are administered before the incision.

ERCP
Endoscopic Retrograde Cholangiopancreatography

Procedure

Incision and Exposure

Laparoscopy is first performed to ensure that there is no metastatic disease that would preclude the resection of the tumor. Once this has been determined, a bilateral subcostal or an upper midline incision is made. The dissection is taken down to the peritoneum through the rectus muscles using electrosurgery. Once the cavity is opened, a full exploration is carried out, after which wide exposure is attained using a self-retaining retractor.

Details

Once the possibility of metastatic spread has been ruled out the duodenum is mobilized (kocherization) in its entirety. This enables the tumor to be examined further to ensure that it does not involve the portal vein or superior mesenteric artery. Attention is then turned to identification of the portal vein above the duodenum. The portal vein lies behind the common bile duct and the common hepatic artery. The superior mesenteric vein is then identified at the lower border of the pancreas. A finger is then placed above and below the pancreas anterior to the portal vein and superior to the mesenteric vein confluence to finally ensure resectability. Once this has been achieved, attention is then turned to dividing the duodenum just beyond the pylorus of the stomach using a GIA stapler. The gallbladder is then removed, and the common bile duct and gastroduodenal artery are divided and ligated. The neck of the pancreas is then divided using a TA-55 stapling device, following which the uncinate process of the pancreas is dissected free of the mesenteric vein. The proximal jejunum is then divided using a GIA stapler. This completes the resection of the specimen.

Attention is then turned to reconstructing the intestinal continuity. The transected proximal portion of the jejunum is brought retrocolic and to the right of the middle colic artery. The first anastomosis is the pancreaticojejunal anastomosis and is done in an end-pancreas-to-side of jejunum fashion using a monofilament absorbable 5-0 suture. This anastomosis is done with or without an internal or external anastomotic stent. The second anastomosis is the choledochojejunal anastomosis with the proximal common hepatic duct being anastomosed to a more distal portion of the side of the jejunal loop. This anastomosis is done using a 3-0 absorbable monofilament suture. The final anastomosis is the gastrojejunal anastomosis, which is done in an antecolic fashion by anastomosing the post pyloric portion of the stomach to the side of the jejunum approximately 30 cm from the choledochojejunal anastomosis. Routinely, in these cases a gastrostomy tube and a feeding jejunostomy tube are placed in their appropriate places.

Closure

Once hemostasis is achieved, two suction drains are placed in the upper abdomen in relation to the pancreatic and biliary anastomoses. After this, the abdominal cavity is irrigated with warm saline and the abdomen is closed with surgeon-specific suture. The patient is then transferred to the intensive care unit for postprocedure management.

Potential Complications

Wound and pulmonary complications and anastomotic leakage may occur.

RIGHT-SIDED COLECTOMY

A right-sided colectomy, or hemicolectomy, refers to a removal of a segment or whole portion of the right side of the colon.

Indications

A right-sided colon resection is performed for patients with an obstruction, cancer, polyps, diverticular disease, volvulus, ulcerative colitis, and Crohn's disease.

Nursing Implications

Refer to the section on gastrectomy for implications concerning anesthesia, positioning, establishing and maintaining the sterile field, equipment and supplies, and physiological monitoring. Instruments include major and intestinal instruments.

Drugs and Solutions

Normal saline and antibiotic solution are needed for irrigation.

Physician Orders

In addition to orders for all patients having abdominal procedures, a patient having a colectomy may have a bowel preparation to facilitate bowel cleansing. The patient receives clear liquids usually 48 hours before the procedure. Cathartics and enemas can be also ordered.

Laboratory and Diagnostic Studies

Laboratory and diagnostic studies include abdominal radiographs, fiberoptic colonoscopy and sigmoidoscopy, barium enema examination, and determination of baseline carcinoembryonic antigen levels. Carcinoembryonic antigen is a protein found in cell membranes of many tissues, including colorectal cancer. A blood hemoglobin determination is done for anemia, and a stool examination can be useful.

Procedure

Incision and Exposure

The patient is prepared from the nipples to the pubis, and drapes are placed, leaving only the operative area exposed. The abdomen is opened using a midline incision. Wound hemostasis is established using hemostats or electrosurgery. Suture ties and ligatures are used to ligate any bleeding vessels. The peritoneum is grasped with two hemostats to facilitate entering the abdomen, and retractors are placed.

Details

The abdomen is explored by the surgeon for metastatic lesions, abnormalities, and other disease. Biopsy is performed of any suspicious areas. The surgeon inspects and palpates the small bowel along its length. The right half of the omentum is separated from the left and is included in the resected specimen. Sometimes, an umbilical tape is tied on the transverse colon proximal to the area of resection to lessen the spread of malignant cells.

The major branches of the superior mesenteric artery are ligated and divided using hemoclips, scissors, and suture ties. The large and small intestines (ileum) are grasped on the specimen side with crushing clamps (eg, Allen intestinal clamps or Kocher intestinal forceps) and with noncrushing clamps (eg, Glassman gastrointestinal clamps) on the anastomotic side. The intestines are divided, and the specimen is removed. The right-sided colon specimen is sent to the pathology department for diagnosis and study.

Towels or laparotomy sponges are placed to isolate the areas to be anastomosed, restricting contamination by bowel contents. The G1A stapler is used to perform the ileocolostomy. A fork of the instrument is inserted into each bowel lumen. The instrument is closed and fired. The knife in the instrument is used to create the stoma between both lumina. A stapling instrument is then used to close the opening of the two ends of lumina. A row of sutures is placed for reinforcement of the anastomosis.

Closure

The abdomen is irrigated with warm saline and closed as described earlier.

Postprocedure Care

In addition to routine postprocedure care, the patient receives parenteral therapy until gastric motility is resumed. Adjuvant therapy may be started (eg, radiation and/or chemotherapy).

Potential Complications

Complications may include obstruction, perforation, bleeding, and infection.

INGUINAL HERNIA

This is one of the most commonly performed operations and consists first of identification of the hernial sac and later repair of the defect in the posterior inguinal wall.

Indications

The presence of an inguinal hernia is believed to be an indication for operative repair. Indefinite delay leads to the continued enlargement of the hernia and the possibility of strangulation.

Nursing Implications

Refer to the section on gastrectomy for positioning, establishing and maintaining the sterile field, drugs and solutions, and physiological monitoring. A dissecting instrument set is used for this procedure.

Anesthesia

Local anesthesia with monitored anesthesia care can be used for elective inguinal hernioplasty, but general, spinal, or epidural anesthesia is necessary in a patient who is unable to cooperate and for all patients with irreducible or strangulated hernias. A commonly used mixture of local anesthesia is a 50:50 mixture of 1% lidocaine and 0.50% bupivacaine, usually with epinephrine. The only contraindication for local anesthesia is a history of adverse reactions to the anesthetic agent.

Procedure

Incision and Exposure

The essential elements of any hernia repair are the elimination of the sac, the definition of normal and abnormal anatomy, and the reconstruction or strengthening of the posterior wall of the inguinal canal. There are a number of different ways to repair a hernia, but for descriptive purposes the classic Bassini repair and the newer mesh plug repair are described.

Any hernia repair is divided into parts consisting of dissection, a repair, and a closure. The operation begins with a small oblique groin incision, taking into consideration the anterior superior iliac spine and the pubic tubercle. Dissection involved in the repair of a hernia consists of opening the inguinal canal, preservation of the ilioinguinal nerve, exposure of the deep ring, mobilization of the spermatic cord, excision of the peritoneal sac and removal of the lipomas of the cord.

The Bassini repair consists of suturing the transversalis fascia, the transverse abdominal muscle, and the internal oblique muscle to the base of the inguinal ligament using a nonabsorbable suture material. More recently, a mesh plug repair has been introduced for the repair of both new and recurrent hernia. This procedure consists of the dissection as previously described followed by the insertion of a polypropylene mesh plug shaped like a shuttlecock into the defect in the posterior layer of the inguinal canal. The plug is sutured in place using a nonabsorbable suture material. Over this is placed a second flattened piece of mesh that is sutured to the base of the inguinal ligament below and the conjoint tendon above.

Closure

Care is taken to close the external oblique aponeurosis with a suture so as not to damage the ilioinguinal nerve. The skin is closed using a subcuticular suture.

Postprocedure Care

Most hernia operations are now done on an outpatient basis requiring pain medications to be administered orally for 5–10 days.

Potential Complications

The hernia may recur, or meralgia paresthetica (traumatization of the lateral femoral cutaneous nerve, which passes through the inguinal ligament) may occur.

MASTECTOMY (PARTIAL OR MODIFIED RADICAL)

A partial mastectomy is an excision of a segment of the breast that is malignant or suspicious for tumor. A modified radical mastectomy is a total removal of the breast plus axillary dissection.

Indications

Indications include a presence of a dominant mass, abnormal mammogram with a suspicious lesion, nipple discharge, and a red, indurated breast.

Nursing Implications
Anesthesia

A patient who is having a partial or modified radical mastectomy is usually admitted the day of the procedure. An anesthesia provider interviews the patient by telephone the night before or the day of the procedure. General anesthesia is preferred for patients having a partial and modified radical mastectomy. The nurse assists the anesthesia provider with placing an intravenous catheter on the affected side and then the blood pressure cuff can be placed on the unaffected breast. All laboratory values should be within normal limits. Preprocedure medications and antibiotics may be given.

Position

The patient is positioned supine on the bed. The arm on the affected side is extended laterally; one should be careful not to adduct it more than 90 degrees (to avoid brachial plexus injury). The unaffected arm can be placed along the side of the patient or extended laterally.

Establishing and Maintaining the Sterile Field

The affected breast and axilla are cleansed with povidone iodine solution or soap. The arm should be prepared to the elbow, and a sterile stockinet is used to isolate the hand and the forearm. Sterile drapes are used to cover the patient, leaving only the breast and axilla exposed.

Equipment and Supplies

A dissecting set is used for a partial mastectomy. Instruments include hemostats, Allis tissue forceps, Kocher forceps, and Kelly forceps; scissors, and tissue (thumb) forceps. A dissecting instrument set is also used for a modified radical mastectomy.

19

Suture is surgeon-specific. A therapeutic breast support or coverlet is used for dressing the operative site.

Physiological Monitoring

See discussion for gastrectomy.

Drugs and Solutions

Normal saline and antibiotics for irrigation are needed.

Physician Orders

The physician's orders include a chest radiograph, electrocardiogram, and complete blood cell count. The patient is instructed to have nothing by mouth after midnight. Preprocedure antibiotics can be ordered.

Laboratory and Diagnostic Studies

Mammography, chest radiography, a bone scan, a cytological examination of nipple discharge if evident, and a complete physical examination are done.

Procedure for Partial Mastectomy

Incision and Exposure

An incision is made with a No. 10 or 15 blade. Because accurate assessment of margins is of central importance in a partial mastectomy, it is critical that the incision be long enough to allow removal of the specimen in one piece rather than several (Lind, 2005). The fat is retracted with an Allis tissue forceps or a self-retaining retractor (eg, Weitlaner).

Details

The tissue surrounding the abnormality is freed by using scissors, knife, or electrosurgery. The suspicious tissue is then excised widely. If the lesion is suspicious for carcinoma, more breast tissue is removed. The tissue is sent to the pathology department for diagnosis.

Closure

After hemostasis is attained, the subcutaneous fat layer is closed with surgeon-specific suture. The skin incision is closed with a subcuticular suture material.

Procedure for Modified Radical Mastectomy

Incision and Exposure

An elliptical (oval) incision is made, including the areola and the nipple. Skin flaps are retracted with Allis tissue forceps or towel clips, and the breast tissue is dissected with Metzenbaum scissors or electrosurgery.

Details

The dissection continues to the smaller pectoral minor muscle, which is ligated and excised. Removal of the pectoral muscle allows axillary exposure. The axillary vein is located. Surrounding vessels and nerves are dissected free. Further dissection is along the serratus muscle, and the axillary contents are then excised along with the breast (**Fig. 19.6**). A skin-sparing mastectomy may be performed for

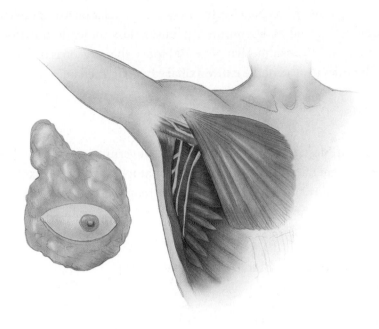

Figure 19.6
Modified radical mastectomy.

optimal cosmetic appearance. Indications for total skin sparing mastectomy include prophylaxis, invasive carcinoma, and ductal carcinoma (Wijayanayagam, 2008). This procedure involves cutting around the alveola to create an opening so that the breast tissue can be removed.

Closure

The chest is irrigated with warm saline, and suction drains are placed in the axilla and over the pectoral muscle. Closure is attained by approximating the skin flaps with suture. The skin is closed with a subcuticular stitch.

Postprocedure Care

Postprocedure care includes mobilization of the arm to prevent limitation of motion and the avoidance of intravenous fluid and medication administration and treatment on the affected side. Followup care should be done for life to detect local and distant recurrences.

Potential Complications

Complications may include hematoma, infection, brachial plexus injury from over abduction of the arm, and lymphedema.

SENTINEL LYMPH NODE BIOPSY

The sentinel lymph node is the first lymph node from the draining tumor site. If there is breast metastasis then the sentinel lymph node would be the first lymph node that is affected.

Indications

A sentinel lymph node biopsy is performed to stage the breast cancer disease. An axillary lymph node procedure provides information about the presence of lymph node metastasis and to provide regional disease control (James, 2006). Sentinel lymph node biopsy has become an accepted treatment of care. In relation to a complete axillary lymph node dissection, there is less morbidity, sensory loss, motor dysfunction, discomfort and lymphedema. In a sentinel lymph node biopsy, the surgeon is in search of one or more lymph nodes instead of the entire axillary lymphatic chain.

Nursing Implications
Anesthesia

Refer to the section on Mastectomy for implications concerning anesthesia. The anesthetic of choice is a general anesthetic. Due to the manipulation of the axillary contents, optimum pain control is necessary. The patient may also be having a combined procedure such as a partial mastectomy with the sentinel lymph node biopsy. General anesthesia is usually preferred.

Establishing and Maintaining the Sterile Field/Positioning

Refer to the section on Mastectomy.

Equipment and Supplies

A dissecting set is used for a sentinel lymph node biopsy. Hemoclips and suture ties are used for the dissection. Suture for an axillary procedure is surgeon-specific. A 4 × 8 gauze dressing is used for dressing the operative incision.

Physiologically Monitoring

The patient's vital signs are monitored. Electrocardiograph pads are placed to monitor the patient's cardiac status. A nasal temperature probe may be used to monitor the patient's body temperature. An Accutech is taken if the patient is a diabetic. An anesthesia twitch monitor may be used if the surgeon requests paralysis.

Physician Orders

Refer to the section on Mastectomy.

Laboratory and Diagnostic Studies

See the discussion for Mastectomy.

Procedure for Sentinel Lymph Node Biopsy

Prior to the procedure, the patient visits nuclear medicine where the breast is injected with a colloidal material. This material drains from the breast tissue via the lymphatic channels and is trapped and concentrated in the first draining lymph nodes (James, 2006). The surgeon may also inject isosulfan blue prior to incision. This contrast agent helps to identify the sentinel lymph node by staining it blue. The lymph nodes that have the concentrated colloid material in them will be identified during the procedure by a hand held radiation probe. Both the colloidal material and the isosulfan blue aid the surgeon in finding the node.

Incision and Exposure

The area is injected with a local anesthetic and an incision is made with a No. 10 or No. 15 blade. The skin incision descends through the fat layer to the pectoralis fascia. The fat is retracted with a self-retaining retractor. The tissue surrounding the axillary contents are freed by using scissors or electrosurgery. Then the fascia is opened and searched for the blue channel or a lymph node with radioactivity. This is done by using a handheld Geiger counter. The lymph node is excised and sent to pathology for examination.

Closure

After hemostasis is attained the incision is closed using surgeon-specific suture. A 4×4 dressing is applied.

Postprocedure Care

Most sentinel lymph node biopsies are performed as an outpatient. Postprocedure pain medications are given.

Potential Complications

Complications may include a hematoma, infection, lymphedema or an allergic reaction. If an allergic reaction occurs it could be acute leading to anaphylaxis.

LAPAROSCOPIC PROCEDURES

General surgery open procedures tend to remain classic and timeless. Currently, most all of open procedures can be done laparoscopically. For the purpose of this textbook, the most common minimally invasive procedures will be highlighted. Those include minimally invasive procedures for the gallbladder, appendix, and hernia.

Minimally invasive procedures have been practiced for many years by urologists, orthopedists, otolaryngologists, and gynecologists. More recently, high-resolution video equipment using low-heat fiberoptic lighting sources ushered in the new era of minimally invasive operative procedures. This technology overcame the problems of potential thermal tissue injury to internal organs as well as enabled the physician to have a detailed image with good color differential of the abdominal cavity.

The turning point in minimally invasive procedures occurred in 1986 when the first laparoscopic cholecystectomy was performed in Lyon, France, by Dr. Philippe Mouret. Before this, general laparoscopic procedures were limited to diagnostic visualization and an occasional liver or mesenteric biopsy. What followed the advent of laparoscopic cholecystectomy changed the practice of general surgery as never before. Patients undergoing this procedure had a shorter hospital stay, less pain after the procedure, and a quicker recovery period, and they were able to return to their normal activities, including work, in about a week. Physicians began to see the advantages of minimally invasive procedures and the positive effects they had on their patients, which led the way for research into incorporating these techniques into many other procedures.

Patient Positioning

For all of the described procedures, one or both arms are tucked at the patient's side. When tucking an arm, prevent skin-to-skin contact by padding the patient's arm and hand with at least 2 to 3 inches of dry gauze, towels, or linen. Electrosurgical current passing through small skin-to-skin contact points such as between the arm and side of the body or the tip of a finger and the leg, is concentrated and may cause a burn.

Basic Instruments, Equipment, and Supplies

A basic laparotomy set is set up in the event that it becomes necessary to convert to an open procedure. Should this need arise, time is of the essence for patient safety. In addition to the laparotomy set, a general endoscopy set is used. This set should contain the laparoscope, light cord, CO_2 tubing, electrosurgical cord, and laparoscopic instruments. All reusable instruments must be checked to ensure proper working condition. Reusable active electrodes should be closely inspected for possible holes or cracks in insulation. Defects in insulation may cause a burn to adjacent tissue. The instrument should not be used if such defects are found. Disposable instruments must be presented to the field by means of sterile technique.

Laparoscopic Cholecystectomy

Laparoscopic cholecystectomy is the removal of the gallbladder through the use of video technology and specialized endoscopic instrumentation for the treatment of gallbladder disease. Indications for the procedure are symptomatic cholelithiasis and cholecystitis.

Procedure

INSUFFLATION AND TROCAR POSITIONS

Once pneumoperitoneum is established (**Fig. 19.7**), the trocars are placed. Each trocar is inserted through a small skin incision large enough for the size of the trocar to be used. With the exception of the umbilical trocar, all subsequent trocars should be inserted under direct vision after the 10-mm laparoscope is inserted. A 10-mm trocar is placed one third of the distance between the xiphoid and the umbilicus and just to the right of the midline. One 5-mm trocar is placed two finger breadths

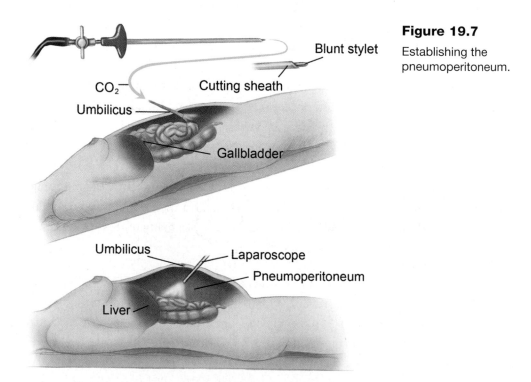

Figure 19.7

Establishing the pneumoperitoneum.

below the right subcostal margin, and a second 5-mm trocar is placed over the right midaxillary line (**Fig. 19.8**).

DETAILS

Grasping forceps are inserted, grasping the gallbladder. The gallbladder is then retracted superiorly. The peritoneal reflection is dissected from the gallbladder, exposing the cystic artery and the cystic duct (**Fig. 19.9**). It is important to recognize that the cephalad traction of the gallbladder often distorts the normal anatomy of the common bile duct, sometimes causing it to become "tented" at its junction with the cystic duct. Such distortion may result in inadvertent injury to the common bile duct if the operator is not aware of this potential abnormal appearance. An

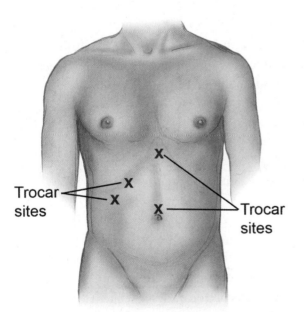

Figure 19.8

Trocar placement for laparoscopic cholecystectomy.

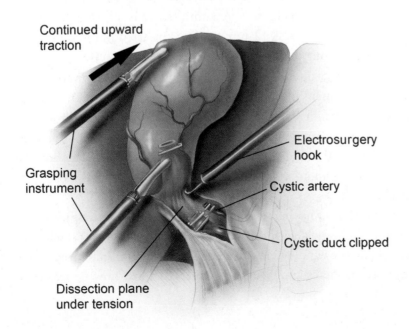

Figure 19.9

Once the cystic artery and cystic duct are clipped and cut the gallbladder can then be dissected off the liver.

endoscopic clip applier is then introduced through the 10-mm trocar to ligate both the cystic duct and the artery. Four clips are applied to each structure, three distal and one proximal to the gallbladder, and scissors or a laser is then used to transect the cystic duct and artery.

If there is evidence of gallstones, operative cholangiography may be done. A small hole may be cut into the cystic duct and a cholangiocatheter inserted, by various techniques depending on the physician's preference, and held in place with a loosely placed clip.

The gallbladder is dissected from the liver bed by means of laser or electrosurgery. The area is irrigated and checked for hemostasis. The laparoscope is removed from the umbilical site and placed in the midline trocar. The gallbladder is then removed intact from the umbilical site with a 10-mm claw forceps. If the gallbladder cannot fit through the incision, bile can be drained and the stones removed, or the incision can be made larger.

Potential Complications

Potential complications include common bile duct injury, hepatic artery injury, bile leak, retained common bile duct stones, wound infection, hernia at trocar site, and shoulder pain related to direct irritation of the diaphragm by CO_2.

Laparoscopic Appendectomy

Laparoscopic appendectomy is the removal of the appendix with the use of video technology and specialized endoscopic instrumentation for the treatment of appendicitis. The indication for the procedure is acute appendicitis.

Procedure

INSUFFLATION AND TROCAR POSITIONS

Once pneumoperitoneum is established, the trocars are placed. Each trocar is inserted through a small skin incision large enough for the size of the trocar to be used. With the exception of the 12-mm umbilical trocar, all subsequent trocars should be inserted under direct vision after the 10-mm laparoscope is inserted. A 12-mm trocar is used for the umbilical site to enable the physician to switch the laparoscope and the endoscopic GIA stapler if necessary. A 5-mm trocar is inserted at the midline just above the symphysis pubis. A 12-mm trocar is inserted in the right lateral abdomen above the cecum along the anterior axillary line (**Fig. 19.10**).

Alter all trocars are placed, the cecum is grasped and retracted upward toward the liver by using an instrument placed in the 12-mm lateral trocar. This maneuver allows the appendix to be identified. Once the appendix is grasped through the 5-mm trocar, tension is placed on the mesoappendix. This tension facilitates the creation of a mesenteric window and dissection of the vessels. The window should be at the base of the appendix, and dissection of the vessels should be as close to the appendix as possible.

Once the mesenteric window has been established, the appendix may be transected in a number of ways. One way is with the 12-mm endoscopic GIA 30 stapler. The instrument is placed into the window, closed around the appendix, and fired, amputating the appendix from the cecum. The mesoappendix must now be transected

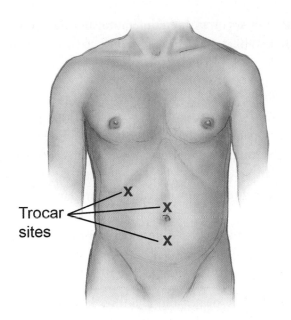

Figure 19.10

Trocar placement for laparoscopic appendectomy.

Trocar sites

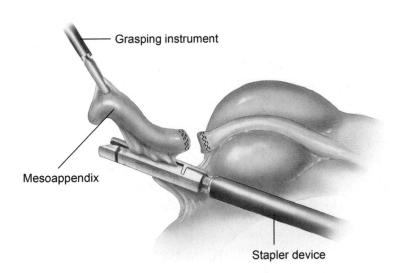

Grasping instrument

Mesoappendix

Stapler device

Figure 19.11

Once the appendix has been transected at its based from the gastrointestinal tract, the mesoappendix can then be transected with a GIA instrument.

with another endoscopic GIA stapler or by using clips and cut slowly from base to tip (**Fig. 19.11**).

The freed appendix is then pulled into the 12-mm trocar and removed. If the appendix is too large for this method, it may be placed in a bag retrieval system and removed through the trocar site. Once the appendix is removed, the abdominal cavity is irrigated and suctioned. All trocars are then removed, and the abdomen is desufflated.

Potential Complications

Potential complications of laparoscopic appendectomy are bowel obstruction, wound infection, and incomplete closure of staples.

Laparoscopic Herniorrhaphy

Laparoscopic herniorrhaphy is the repair of an inguinofemoral hernia. Indications for the procedure are right, left, and bilateral inguinal hernias.

Procedure

INSUFFLATION AND TROCAR POSITIONS

The pneumoperitoneum is established as discussed in the section Principles of Abdominal Insufflation. Once pneumoperitoneum is established, the trocars are placed. Each trocar is inserted through a small skin incision large enough for the size of the trocar to be used. With the exception of the 12-mm umbilical trocar, all subsequent trocars should be inserted under direct vision after the 10-mm laparoscope is inserted. A 10-mm trocar is used for the umbilical site to enable the physician to switch the laparoscope and the endoscopic stapler if necessary. The two 12-mm trocars are inserted below and on each side of the umbilicus (**Fig. 19.12**).

DETAILS

Once the trocars are placed, the physician locates and identifies key anatomical landmarks. The hernia defect is identified. The assistant should then apply pressure on the abdominal wall over the inguinal canal so that the physician can identify the appropriate area on the screen. The pubic tubercle is then identified in the same manner. Next, the epigastric vessels and spermatic cord structures are delineated.

After all anatomical features are identified, the peritoneal covering of the inguinal canal is opened with an endoscopic shears. The incision is made as high as possible above Hesselhach's triangle, superior to the umbilical ligament, creating a peritoneal flap. This flap is used later to close the peritoneum over the repair. Once the structures are stripped from the peritoneal covering, they are redefined and the defect is reassessed.

A spermatic window is dissected behind the spermatic cord at the level of the internal ring and is enlarged to 1.5–2 cm. With the window dissected, the physician is ready to place the mesh. A 3 × 5-inch crystalline polypropylene (Marlex) or polypropylene (Prolene) mesh is usually used for this purpose. The mesh must be cut to the size bigger

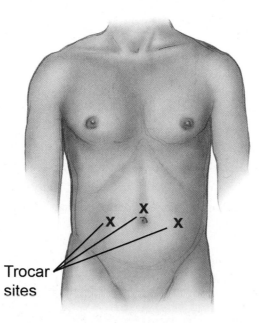

Figure 19.12

Trocar placement for laparoscopic herniorrhaphy.

Trocar sites

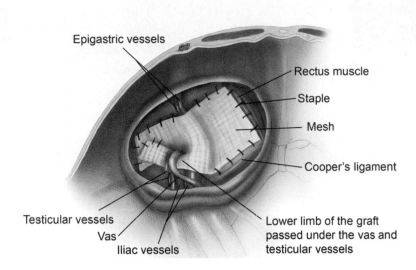

Figure 19.13

Inguinal hernia repair with mesh stapled over the defect.

Labels on figure:
Epigastric vessels
Rectus muscle
Staple
Mesh
Cooper's ligament
Testicular vessels
Vas
Iliac vessels
Lower limb of the graft passed under the vas and testicular vessels

than the repair area. The 3-inch side is cut to create two limbs that will be placed around the spermatic cord. With the mesh placed in the defect and the two limbs around the spermatic cord, the mesh is then stapled to the abdominal wall with an endoscopic stapler designed for this purpose (**Fig. 19.13**). Care should be taken when stapling Cooper's ligament. After the mesh has been stapled, the peritoneal flap is approximated and stapled closed. The trocars are then removed, and the abdomen is desufflated.

Potential Complications

Potential complications of laparoscopic herniorrhaphy are recurrence of hernia and meralgia paresthetica (traumatization of the lateral femoral cutaneous nerve, which passes through the inguinal ligament).

REFERENCES

1. Backman, S., Bondy, R., & Deschamps, A. (2006). Perioperative Considerations for Anesthesia. ACS Surgery: Principles and Practices, 6–8. Retrieved March 9, 2008 from http://www.acssurgery.com/abstracts/acs/acs0103.htm.

2. Bedi, A.S., Bhatti, T., Amin, A., & Zuberi, J. (2007). Laparoscopic Incisional and Ventral Hernia Repair. *J Min Access Surg, 3:* 83–90.

3. Bhandarkar, D.S., Shankar, M., & Udwadia, T.E. (2006). Laparoscopic Surgery for Inguinal Hernia: Current status and controversies. *J Min Access Surg, 2:* 178–86.

4. Cameron, J. (2004). *Current Surgical Therapy.* (8th ed.). Philadelphia: Elsevier Mosby.

5. Fong, Y. & Blumgart, L. (2006). Gastrointestinal Tract and Abdomen, Hepatic Resection: Introduction. *ACS Surgery: Principles and Practices.* Retrieved March 6, 2008 from http://www.acssurgery.com.

6. James, T.A. & Edge, S.B. (2006). Sentinel lymph node in breast cancer. *Current Opinion in Obstetrics and Gynecology, 18,* 53–58.

7. Jani, K., Rajan, P.S., Sendhi Kumar, K., & Palanivelu, C. (2006). Twenty years after Erich Muhe: Persisting controversies with the gold standard of laparoscopic cholecystectomy. *J Min Access Surg, 2:* 49–58.

8. Lind, D., Smith, B., & Souba, W. (2005). Breast Procedures. *ACS Surgery Principles and Practices.* Retrieved February 18, 2007 from http://medscape.com/viewarticle/503006.

9. Mahmoud, N. & Karmacharya, J. (2005). Surgical Approach to Colorectal Neoplasia and High-Risk Conditions. In Kochman, M. *The Clinicians Guide to Gastrointestinal Oncology* (pp. 157–170). Thorofare, New Jersey: Slack Incorporated.

10. Moore, K. & Dalley, A. (2006). *Clinical Oriented Anatomy* (5th ed.). Baltimore: Lippincott Willians & Wilkins.

11. Morton. P., Fontaine. D., Hudak, C., & Gallo, B. (2005). *Critical Care Nursing, A Holistic Approach* (8th ed.). Philadelphia: Lippincott Williams & Wilkins.

12. Wells, M. (2005). *Surgical Instruments: A Pocket Guide.* Philadelphia: W.B. Saunders.

13. Wetter, P.A., Kavic, M.S., Levinson, C.J., Kelley, W.E., McDougall, E.M., & Nezhat, C. (2005). *Prevention and management of Laparoendoscopic Surgical Complications.* (2nd ed.). Miami, Florida.

14. Wijayanayagam, A., Kumar, A.S., Foster, R.D., & Esserman, L.J. (2008). Optimizing the Total Skin-Sparing Mastectomy. *Arch. Surg. 143*(1), 38–45.

15. Wolf, D. (2007). *Cirrhosis. eMedicine.* 1–10. Retrieved Feb 29, 2008 from http://emedicine.com/med/Topic3183.htm.

CHAPTER 20

Bariatric Surgery

Rebecca M. Blades

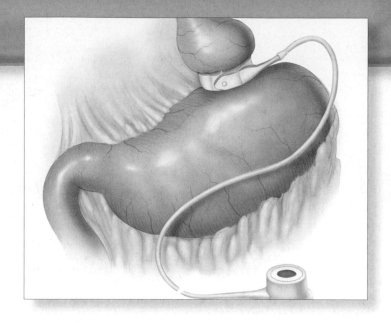

INTRODUCTION

Bariatric surgery, recognized as the most effective long-term treatment for morbid obesity, refers to the surgical modification of the gastrointestinal tract to reduce nutrient intake and/or absorption (Wikipedia, 2008a). This surgery is an option for people with a body mass index (BMI) of 40 or above. For people with life-altering comorbidities, such as depression, type 2 diabetes, arthritis, hypertension, some types of cancer, and skin infections, bariatric surgery provides an option if they have a BMI of 35–39.9.

ANATOMY

The stomach is a curved muscular organ that receives food from the esophagus following mastication. Within the highly acidic environment of the stomach, and in conjunction with the gastric digestive enzymes, large molecules, such as those from food, are broken down into smaller ones, thus allowing eventual absorption from the small intestine (Wikipedia, 2008b).

Lying between the esophagus and the duodenum, the stomach is oriented on the left side of the abdominal cavity (see **Fig. 20.1**). Divided into four parts, the cardia refers to the section where contents of the esophagus empty into the stomach. The next section, which is formed by the upper curvature, is called the fundus. The corpus, the third section of the stomach, forms the central region. The fourth section is called the pylorus or antrum. This area of the stomach facilitates emptying of the contents into the duodenum, the first section of the small intestine (Wikipedia, 2008b).

Chapter Contents

BMI
Body Mass Index

Figure 20.1

Stomach and abdominal cavity.

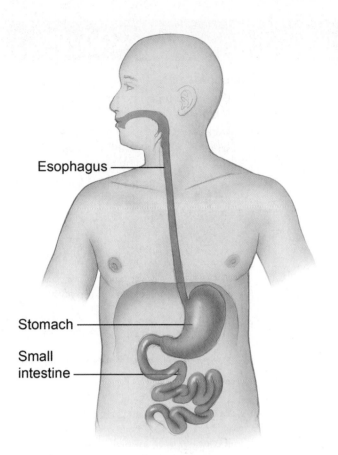

Esophagus

Stomach

Small intestine

The esophageal sphincter is found at the proximal end of the stomach in the cardiac region. At the distal end is found the pyloric sphincter. These smooth muscle valves keep the contents of the stomach contained (Wikipedia, 2008b).

The right and left gastric arteries supply the lesser curvature of the stomach. The left gastric artery also supplies the cardiac region of the stomach. The right and left gastroepiploic arteries supply the greater curvature. The short gastric artery supplies the fundus and the upper portion of the greater curvature (Wikipedia, 2008b).

Surrounding the stomach are the parasympathetic and orthosympathetic plexuses, which regulate the secretory activity and motor activity of the stomach muscles (Wikipedia, 2008b).

The small intestine is about 16 feet (500 cm) long and consists of the duodenum, jejunum, and ileum. The duodenum connects to the pancreatic and common bile ducts, which provide the pancreatic enzymes and bile. The jejunum and ileum secrete a juice called succus entericus, which also aides in digestion (Wikipedia, 2008c). **Table 20.1** outlines the digestive enzymes.

SPECIAL INSTRUMENTS, SUPPLIES, AND EQUIPMENT

Bariatric surgery is a sub-specialty of general surgery and can be done by either open or laparoscopic technique. Instruments for the open technique consist of a general surgery laparotomy set with major instruments, to include large retractors

20

Table 20.1	**Digestive Enzymes**

Gastric Enzymes	**Function**
Pepsin	☐ Breaks proteins into smaller peptide fragments
Gelatinase	☐ Degrades types I and V gelatin and types IV and V collagens
Gastric amylase	☐ Degrades starch into sugar
Gastric lipase	☐ Catalyzes the hydrolysis of lipids; aiding in their digestion, transport and processing

Pancreatic Enzymes	**Function**
Trypsin	☐ Breaks down peptides in the small intestine
Chymotrypsin	☐ Breaks down peptides in the small intestine
Steapsin	☐ Degrades triglycerides into fatty acids and glycerol
Carboxypeptidase	☐ Splits peptide fragments into individual amino acids
Pancreatic amylase	☐ Degrades most other carbohydrates (besides starch, glycogen, and cellulose)
Bile	☐ (From the liver) emulsifies fat, allowing more efficient use of lipases in the duodenum, in converting lipids to their component fatty acid and glycerol molecules

Small Intestine Enzymes	**Function**
Succus entericus—contain enzymes that degrade disaccharides into monosaccharides:	
☐ Sucrase	☐ Breaks down sucrose into glucose and fructose
☐ Maltase	☐ Breaks down maltose into glucose
☐ Isomaltase	☐ Breaks down maltose and isomaltose
☐ Lactase	☐ Breaks down lactose into glucose and galactose
☐ Intestinal lipase	☐ Breaks down fatty acids

Source: Wikipedia. (2008b). Digestive enzyme. Retrieved July 15, 2008 from: http://en.wikipedia.org/wiki/Digestive_enzyme.

and long instrumentation for grasping, handling, and suturing tissue. When done as a laparoscopic procedure, add laparoscopic instrumentation to the setup. This instrumentation includes laparoscopic graspers, dissectors, suturing devices, dilators, and a gastric band passer. Instrument manufacturers can serve as a resource for compiling the needed instrumentation based on the needs of the bariatric patient and surgeon.

In addition to the instrument sets, include an assortment of various sizes of reusable or disposable laparoscopic trocars and ports. Include laparoscopic staplers with multiple refill loads to the setup. Other equipment includes the endoscopy equipment (see Chapter 11), electrosurgery generator, and ultrasonic scalpel, depending on the surgeon's preference.

ESTABLISHING AND MAINTAINING THE STERILE FIELD

Bariatric patients, because of their obesity and possible comorbidity conditions, are at risk for wound infection related to establishing and maintaining the sterile field, particularly patients undergoing open procedures. Attention to detail while implementing aseptic technique is crucial to ensure a good outcome (Carpentino-Moyet, 2008).

Prep bariatric patients for open and laparoscopic procedures from the mid-nipple line to the pubis using the facility approved prepping agent. While preparing the operative site, prevent the accumulation of prepping agent along the sides of the patient. Seeping of the prepping agent under the patient places him or her at risk for a preparation solution-related chemical burn. In addition, if the prepping solution contains alcohol use caution when applying the solution due to the risk for fire secondary to the accumulation of vapors under the drapes. Before applying the drapes the nurse and scrub person confirm that evaporation is complete and vapors have dissipated. Follow the manufacturer's IFU, which will delineate appropriate drying times for the agent used.

The scrub person applies the sterile drapes according to the type of procedure. During the procedure the scrub person and nurse monitor the sterile field for breaks in technique and take corrective action as necessary. The instrument table and Mayo stand are arranged in a position close to the operative field.

BARIATRIC SURGERY OPTIONS[1]

Bariatric procedures are recognized as having three common categories that can have either restrictive features, that is, reducing the size of the gastric reservoir; malabsorptive features (ie, causing food to be poorly digested and absorbed); or a combination of both.

Restrictive Procedures

Procedures that are solely restrictive by design produce a small gastric pouch with a small outlet and include the vertical banded gastroplasty (**Fig. 20.2**), adjustable gastric banding (**Fig. 20.3**), and proximal gastric bypass (**Fig. 20.4**). The creation of a small stomach pouch is intended to produce early and prolonged feelings of satiety by limiting intake and delaying gastric emptying. Restrictive procedures alter the basic anatomical structure and capacity of the stomach without affecting normal digestive processes, so they do not affect caloric or nutrient absorption. Proximal gastric bypass is primarily a restrictive procedure, although it does have a minimal absorptive component. Restrictive procedures are successful in promoting weight loss in a majority of patients. However, patients must fully cooperate with a highly structured and mandatory postprocedure dietary regimen. Common problems with restrictive

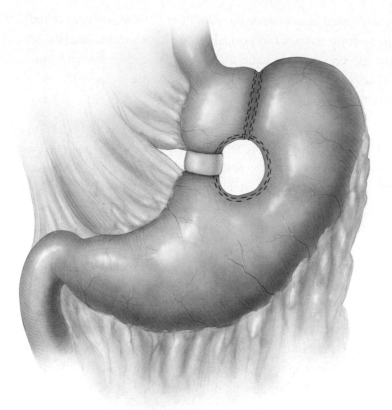

Figure 20.2

Vertical banded gastroplasty.

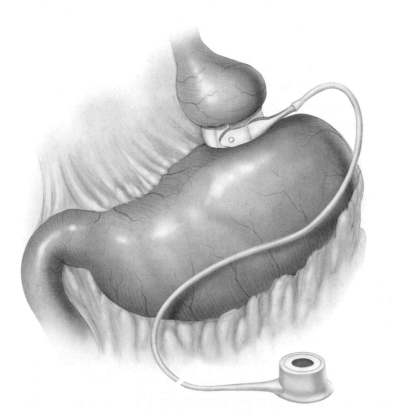

Figure 20.3

Adjustable gastric banding system.

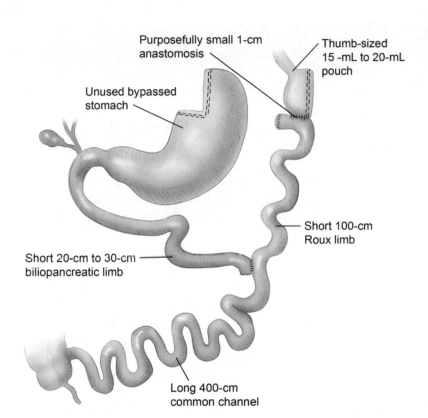

Figure 20.4

Proximal gastric bypass.

Labels on figure:
Purposefully small 1-cm anastomosis
Thumb-sized 15-mL to 20-mL pouch
Unused bypassed stomach
Short 100-cm Roux limb
Short 20-cm to 30-cm biliopancreatic limb
Long 400-cm common channel

approaches include gastric pouch dilation, meat or solid-food intolerance, and outlet obstruction resulting in gastroesophageal reflux and vomiting. Problems may surface or worsen as patients are faced with pressures and temptations that lead them to deviate from known food and quantity restrictions or otherwise overeat. Particularly challenging are those social and family functions that may center on eating, such as holidays and special celebrations when patients need to be cautious to avoid potential risks of pain, nausea, vomiting, obstruction, and possible intervention. **Table 20.2** outlines some of the identified benefits and risks of restrictive bariatric procedures.

Malabsorptive Procedures

Malabsorptive procedures are more technically complex and are geared toward passing various lengths of the small intestine to produce malabsorption. These procedures result in an incomplete digestion process and diminish the amount of calories and nutrients the body can effectively absorb. Biliopancreatic diversion (BPD) is a common malabsorptive procedure (**Fig. 20.5**). In BPD, approximately three-quarters of the stomach is removed; however, enough of the upper stomach is left to maintain proper nutrition. The remaining small pouch connects directly to the final segment of the small intestine, completely bypassing the duodenum and jejunum. Food will move through the pouch with minimal absorption. In addition, diversion of bile and pancreatic juices occurs so that they meet the ingested food closer to the middle or end of the small intestine.

The malabsorptive procedures generally produce greater sustained weight loss than restrictive procedures alone, but also place the patient at increased risk for malnutrition and vitamin deficiencies following the procedure. Daily nutritional

BPD
Biliopancreatic
Diversion

20

Table 20.2	Benefits and Risks of Restrictive Bariatric Procedures	
Procedure	**Benefits**	**Risks**

Vertical Banded Gastroplasty

Procedure	Benefits	Risks
☐ Stomach is partitioned vertically, pylorus and small intestines remain intact	☐ Lower complication rates ☐ Technically easier to perform ☐ Low mortality rate	☐ Rare staple line leaks ☐ Vertical line disruption due to vomiting or overeating ☐ Risk of infection ☐ Possible incisional hernia ☐ Risk of band erosion

Adjustable Gastric Banding

Procedure	Benefits	Risks
☐ Inflatable silicone band placed completely around the upper portion of the stomach ☐ No anatomical removals or anastomosis ☐ Inflatable band connected to small reservoir and placed under the skin (typically in the upper abdomen) ☐ Adjustments of gastric restriction occurs via injection & withdrawal from the reservoir	☐ Use of minimally invasive approach ☐ Shorter length of stay (usually 24 hours) ☐ Faster recover period (usually 2 weeks) ☐ No staple line ☐ Band is adjustable ☐ Procedure is reversible with normal stomach restoration ☐ The band is easily deflated if necessary	☐ Risk of foreign body reaction ☐ Band position can slip and lead to subsequent tissue erosion ☐ Potential for leakage and infection at the injection port site ☐ Not always covered by third-party payers ☐ Potential cost to the patient for the band can be in excess of $3,000

Proximal Gastric Bypass

Procedure	Benefits	Risks
☐ Creation of a small pouch at the top of the stomach (remainder of stomach remains intact) ☐ The Roux limb of the intestine is attached to the created pouch with a small anastomosis to slow emptying ☐ The Roux limb is relatively short before being joined by the short biliopancreatic limb to create a long common channel ☐ The long channel allows for absorption of nutrients	☐ Minimized dumping syndrome ☐ Absence or minimal occurrence of acid reflux	☐ Possibility of anastomotic stricture ☐ Possibility of anastomotic ulceration

D'Alfonso, J. & Carol, R.R. (2007). *Care of the bariatric patient*, Competency and Credentialing Institute: Denver, CO.

supplements and close postprocedure monitoring can reduce some of the potential malabsorptive complications. Although complications, such as diarrhea and steatorrhea, are less severe than those that were previously associated with jejunocolonic anastomosis, the risk of these symptoms alone can be enough to make the procedure undesirable to patients. **Table 20.3** outlines the benefits and risks associated with malabsorptive bariatric procedures.

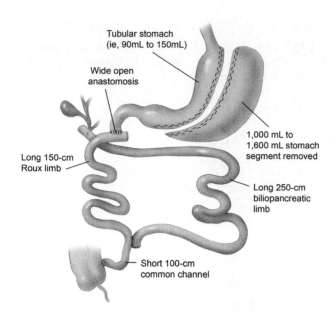

Figure 20.5

Biliopancreatic diversion.

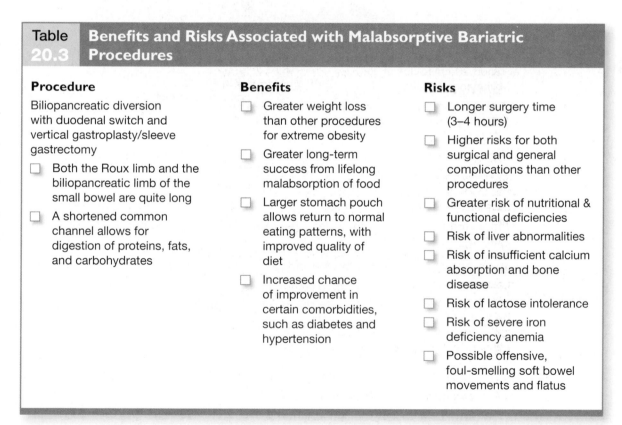

Table 20.3	Benefits and Risks Associated with Malabsorptive Bariatric Procedures		
Procedure	**Benefits**	**Risks**	
Biliopancreatic diversion with duodenal switch and vertical gastroplasty/sleeve gastrectomy ☐ Both the Roux limb and the biliopancreatic limb of the small bowel are quite long ☐ A shortened common channel allows for digestion of proteins, fats, and carbohydrates	☐ Greater weight loss than other procedures for extreme obesity ☐ Greater long-term success from lifelong malabsorption of food ☐ Larger stomach pouch allows return to normal eating patterns, with improved quality of diet ☐ Increased chance of improvement in certain comorbidities, such as diabetes and hypertension	☐ Longer surgery time (3–4 hours) ☐ Higher risks for both surgical and general complications than other procedures ☐ Greater risk of nutritional & functional deficiencies ☐ Risk of liver abnormalities ☐ Risk of insufficient calcium absorption and bone disease ☐ Risk of lactose intolerance ☐ Risk of severe iron deficiency anemia ☐ Possible offensive, foul-smelling soft bowel movements and flatus	

D'Alfonso, J. & Carol, R.R. (2007). *Care of the bariatric patient,* Competency and Credentialing Institute: Denver, CO.

Combination Restrictive and Malabsorptive Procedures

The Roux-en-Y gastric bypass is an example of a combined restrictive and malabsorptive procedure (**Fig. 20.6**). This procedure involves severely restricting the capacity of the stomach by placing staples across it to create a 15–20 cc gastric pouch. The remainder of the stomach is completely stapled shut and separated from the small pouch. The outlet from the newly formed pouch empties directly into the

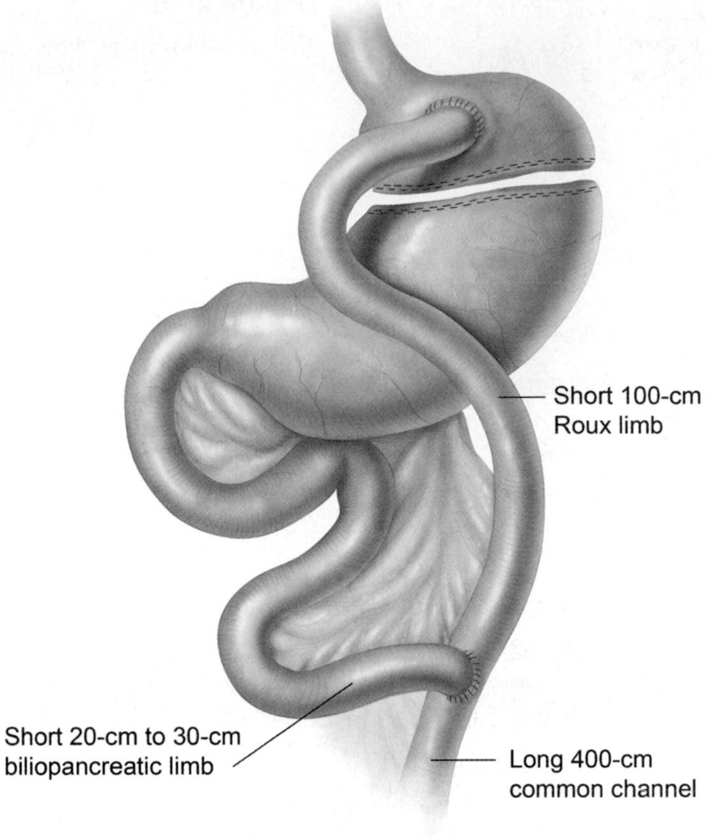

Figure 20.6
Roux-en-Y gastric bypass.

Short 100-cm
Roux limb

Short 20-cm to 30-cm
biliopancreatic limb

Long 400-cm
common channel

lower portion of the jejunum, bypassing calorie absorption. The surgeon does this by dividing the small intestine just beyond the duodenum for the purpose of bringing it up and constructing a connection with the new stomach pouch. The other side is connected to the side of the Roux limb of the intestine, creating the "Y" shape that gives the technique its name. As noted, it is a combination procedure—the small upper pouch restricts food intake and the bypass interferes with absorption, resulting in more consistent, sustained weight loss.

Combination procedures may also result in improvement of comorbidities, especially type II diabetes. The disadvantages include the development of painful dumping syndrome that occurs with sugar consumption and risks for:

- Nutritional complications, such as vitamin (A, B-12, D, E) and mineral (calcium, iron, folic acid) deficiencies
- Stomal stenosis, requiring dilation
- Y-limb obstruction, requiring surgical intervention
- Anastomosis leakage

See **Table 20.4** for the benefits and risks associated with combination procedures.

Open Versus Laparoscopic Gastric Bypass Surgery

The differences between laparoscopic and open bariatric surgery are the method of access and exposure, not the type of surgery being performed. Each type of weight loss surgery may be performed as either an open or a laparoscopic procedure. Laparoscopic approaches are termed minimally invasive because of reducing the size of the

Table 20.4	Benefits and Risks of Combined Restrictive and Malabsorptive Bariatric Procedures		
Procedure	**Benefits**		**Risks**
Roux-en-Y Gastric Bypass (Proximal Gastric Bypass and Distal Gastric Bypass Approaches)	☐ Both restrictive and malabsorption benefits ☐ Optimal weight loss results ☐ Documented improvement in comorbidities, especially Type II diabetes		☐ Risk of dumping syndrome with sugar consumption ☐ Risk of vitamin and mineral deficiencies ☐ Risk of stomal stenosis/stricture ☐ Risk of obstruction ☐ Risk of anastomotic leak

D'Alfonso, J. & Carol, R.R. (2007). *Care of the bariatric patient*, Competency and Credentialing Institute: Denver, CO.

surgical incision and minimizing the trauma associated with open operative exposure. The result should be less tissue injury after laparoscopic compared to open techniques. The important clinical advantages of laparoscopic gastric bypass surgery may not be the reduced length of hospitalization but the reduction in postprocedure pain, lower rate of wound-related complications, and faster recovery. Laparoscopic approaches may carry a slightly higher risk of anastomosis leakage and bleeding; however, cardiopulmonary and wound infection complications are known to be higher with open procedures.

In open surgery, a single-incision approach is typically used to open the abdomen for access and exposure. The incision for open procedures is typically 4½ to 6 inches long for women and can be 5½ to 7 inches in length for men.

Laparoscopic approaches involve multiple, smaller incisions in the abdominal wall to accommodate a laparoscope, video camera, and various laparoscopic surgical instruments. The surgeon views the entire procedure on a video monitor(s) placed strategically in the operating room. Most laparoscopic surgeons believe the magnification and quality of video imaging gives them a better view and improves their access to key anatomical structures. **Table 20.5** outlines the benefits of laparoscopic gastric bypass surgery.

Table 20.5	Benefits of Laparoscopic Gastric Bypass Surgery
	☐ Decreased postprocedure pain and requirements for pain medication ☐ Improved breathing with fewer pulmonary complications ☐ Decreased wound complications, such as infection and incisional hernia ☐ Quicker return to mobility and activity, including early ambulation, exercise and daily life routines, including work

D'Alfonso, J. & Carol, R.R. (2007). *Care of the bariatric patient*, Competency and Credentialing Institute: Denver, CO.

20

NURSING IMPLICATIONS FOR THE CARE OF THE BARIATRIC PATIENT

Preprocedure Preparation

Assessing the risk of both perioperative and long-term complications is critical to the success of bariatric surgery; therefore, a thorough preprocedure assessment is vital. A psychological assessment is often performed for these patients. Patients who have a history of severe psychiatric disturbance or who are currently under the care of a psychologist or psychiatrist, and those under the age of 18 years, should be required to either to have written psychiatric clearance or to undergo psychiatric evaluation before surgery. Other patients who wish to have the benefit of psychological counseling before surgery should be encouraged to do so. Other preprocedure assessment factors include:

- Potential airway problems—these patients may require an awake intubation—they also desaturate quickly
- Circulatory problems
- Skin integrity/areas of breakdown
- Medical comorbidities, including diabetes, hypertension, sleep apnea, hypercholesterolemia, and stress incontinence

See **Table 20.6** for a list of preprocedure testing and assessment parameters.

Before transfer to the operative and invasive procedure suite, administer medications, such as antibiotics and anticoagulants, per physician orders and according to facility protocols. These medications may be administered by the anesthesia provider prior to the induction of anesthesia. The patient should have been instructed to shower and not apply body lotions or oil. These substances will make it difficult

Table 20.6	Preprocedure Testing and Assessment for the Bariatric Patient

☐ Panels:
    ☐ Cardiovascular—total cholesterol, HDL, LDL, triglycerides
    ☐ Comprehensive Metabolic—Albumin, Alkaline Phosphatase, BUN, Carbon Dioxide (bicarbonate), Calcium, Chloride, Creatinine, Glucose, SGOT (AST), Sodium, Total Bilirubin, Total Protein
    ☐ Specialty—TSH, T4, PTH (parathyroid), Hepatitis B & C screening panel (Hep Bs Ag, Hep BS Ab, Hep Bc Ab, Anti HCV or total HCV), H-Pylori (all positives require treatment)
    ☐ Hematology—CBC (includes diff), Platelet Count, PT, PTT, INR, Hgb A1C, Ferritin
    ☐ Vitamins—B-1, B-12, D
    ☐ Urine—Urinary Analysis, Urine C&S
    ☐ Optional—pregnancy, drug screen

☐ Radiology:
    ☐ Ultrasound Liver and Gallbladder
    ☐ Chest X-ray
    ☐ Upper GI Swallow Study

- [ ] Cardiology:
  - [ ] Electrocardiogram
- [ ] DVT Screening:
  - [ ] Evaluation and prophylaxis according to DVT protocols
- [ ] Autologous Blood Donation:
  - [ ] At patient request; according to blood bank protocols
- [ ] Specialist Consultations, Teaching, and Testing:
  - [ ] Dietary and Nutrition Evaluation and Teaching
    - Screening for possible eating disorders
    - Failure to control weight with non-surgical measures documented
    - Dietary concerns and required changes addressed
    - Teaching on "Last Supper Syndrome," a risk of excessive eating in the weeks or months leading up to bariatric surgery, which is often controlled by prescribing a very low-calorie liquid diet one to four weeks prior to surgery. This preprocedure nutrition therapy often helps decrease weight, improve nutritional status, improve exposure and decrease surgical risks.
    - Diabetes education and information
  - [ ] Psychological Evaluation and Teaching
    - Documented patient understanding and additional informed consent
  - [ ] Cardiology
    - Stress testing
    - Echocardiogram (required if prior Fen-Phen use)
    - Medication adjustments
    - Cardiac clearance
  - [ ] Gynecology (Female patients)
    - Rule/Out Tumors
    - Pregnancy testing
    - Birth control teaching/adjustments
    - Pap Smear
    - Mammogram
  - [ ] Pulmonology
    - Consultation
    - Pulmonary function tests
    - Sleep apnea evaluation
    - Asthma evaluation
    - All smokers must quit smoking 8 weeks prior to surgery and remain a non-smoker post-op
  - [ ] Gastroenterology
    - Endoscopy (ulcers, esophageal disorders)
    - Treatment of any positive H-Pylori
    - Rule/Out Crohn's disease and Irritable Bowel Syndrome
  - [ ] Endocrine
    - Diabetes evaluation and management
    - Rule/Out thyroid disorder

20

to apply the patient return electrode, and may result in insufficient pad-to-patient interface, resulting in a return electrode contact monitoring alarm. Place anti-embolism stockings on the patient's lower legs; these will remain on the patient during hospitalization. See **Table 20.7** for the equipment, instruments, and supplies needed for intraoperative care of the bariatric surgery patient.

Anesthesia

General anesthesia is used during bariatric procedures. Consequently, airway management in many morbidly obese patients presents a challenge, particularly during intubation. Often the anesthesia provider will place blankets or towels between the patient's scapulae, thus elevating the patient and providing better visualization of the vocal cords. Have a difficult intubation cart available before the start of induction of the anesthetic agents. Be prepared to assist the anesthesia provider should the patient experience a difficult intubation. After the patient is intubated, the anesthesia provider will insert an oral gastric tube. This tube is removed before the patient leaves

Table 20.7	Equipment, Supplies, and Instruments Needed for the Intraoperative Care of the Bariatric Patient
☐	Patient transfer device, such as a Hover Mat
☐	Bariatric grade operating room table, X-ray compatible, and capable of supporting super obese weight ranges
☐	Table parts and positioning devices, such as arm boards, padding, foot board, extensions, and 2 safety straps
☐	Access to difficult intubation cart and airway management supplies
☐	Integrated Video Systems, high-definition or 3-D systems where available, and including a secondary "slave" monitor (if required)
☐	Camera Head
☐	Laparoscope(s)
☐	Camera Box
☐	Light Source
☐	Light Cord
☐	Video/Multi-media Image Recorder
☐	Bariatric grade insufflator device and tubing with CO_2 filter and warming capabilities
☐	Robotic equipment, accessories, instrumentation, and supplies (if required)
☐	Special bariatric instrumentation, retractors, endomechanical—stapling devices and laparoscopic disposable supplies—as indicated
☐	Bariatric custom drape packs
☐	Electrosurgical unit (ESU) or ultrasonic scalpel
☐	Suction—Irrigation Device
☐	Pressure Bag for Irrigation
☐	Implants (Adjustable Lap Band) and Accessories
☐	Medications—irrigation, antibiotic and local anesthetic agents
☐	Blood Products (autologous or blood-bank) accessible and verified
☐	Major Abdominal Tray and appropriate open instruments, supplies or special instrumentation, if conversion from laparoscopic approach to open laparotomy is required at anytime

the procedure room. The anesthesia provider will initiate hemodynamic monitoring depending on anesthesia, the patient's physiological status, and facility protocols.

Position

Place the patient in the supine position. Use padding devices such as egg crates to protect the patient's heels and elbows from injury. Place gel pads under the trunk of the body. Extend the patient's arms on padded arm boards and apply safety straps. Place a pillow at the knees under the lower legs. Place anti-embolism stockings on the patient's lower legs before the start of surgery; these will remain on the patient during hospitalization. Apply pneumatic compression stockings to both lower legs. Apply and secure two safety belts, one over the thighs and one over the lower legs. Attach a footboard to the OR bed; this will prevent the patient from slipping towards the foot of the OR table and reduce the risk for impaired skin integrity related to shearing force should the surgeon decide to place the OR bed in the reverse Trendelenburg position during the procedure. See Chapter 8 for more information on positioning the patient.

Physiological Monitoring

Per physician orders, insert a Foley catheter after the induction of anesthesia. The catheter will usually be removed the next morning. The anesthesia provider inserts an oral gastric tube before the procedure and removes it before patient leaves the operating room. In addition to monitoring blood pressure, EKG and SPO_2 throughout the procedure, the anesthesia provider may initiate hemodynamic monitoring if warranted by the patient's condition. Assist the anesthesia provider by monitoring blood loss during the procedure according to facility protocols.

Electrosurgery

Always use electrosurgery generators equipped with Return Electrode Contact Quality Monitoring (RECQM) circuitry and a compatible dual-section patient return electrode. Bariatric patients may present a challenge when trying to use electrosurgery. Because of their body mass, it may difficult to silence the RECQM alarm when placing them in circuit. In some situations, the alarm may intermittently activate during the procedure. In such cases, always follow the manufacturer's Instructions for Use (IFU) for silencing the alarm, which may include the application of a second patient return electrode that is attached to the electrosurgery generator using a special adapter. Under no circumstances should a non-RECQM patient return electrode be applied when using a RECQM equipped electrosurgery generator.

RECQM
Return Electrode Contact Quality Monitoring

IFU
Instructions for Use

ROUX-EN-Y PROXIMAL GASTRIC BYPASS
Establishing Access

When done as an open procedure, the **Roux-en-Y proximal gastric bypass** uses a single upper midline incision from the xiphoid process to the supraumbilical area. After the abdominal cavity is opened a self-retaining retractor is placed.

If done as a laparoscopic procedure, after establishing the pneumoperitoneum, five to six small ½- to 1-inch incisions are made over the abdomen for laparoscopic port placement. One additional puncture is made in the right upper quadrant for the Nathanson liver retractor to hold the liver up and out of the way during the surgical procedure.

Once access to the abdominal cavity is made, whether open of laparoscopic, the procedure follows the same course.

Details—Laparoscopic Roux-en-Y

The surgeon creates an ante-gastric enterotomy, then places a ¼" Penrose drain behind the stomach. After locating the ligament of Trites, a retrocolic enterotomy is created above the ligament of Trites. The ¼" Penrose drain is then pulled through the enterotomy. Next, the surgeon measures 50–70 cm from the ligament of Trites and then divides the jejunum with a stapling device. The Roux Limb is measured according to the patient's BMI, usually 150–200 cm. Enterotomies are created, and the jejunojejunotomy is then done using a stapling device, and then closed using the stapling device. Next, the surgeon tacks the bowel together with a suture to close the mesenteric defect. The drain is attached to the roux limb by a suture. By pulling the other end of the Penrose drain the roux limb is brought up behind the stomach and through the ante-gastric enterotomy. The surgeon then dissects the gastrohepatic ligament. The anesthesia provider inserts a Baker tube, inflates the balloon with 15 mL of air, and pulls back until snug. This maneuver sizes the pouch. Using a stapling device with several loads of staples, the surgeon creates the gastric pouch. Once the pouch is completed, the anesthesia provider passes an oro-gastric anvil into the pouch. The surgeon creates a gastrotomy using an ultrasonic scalpel at the intended exit site for the anvil. As the anvil is pushed through the opening, the first assistant grasps the anvil and pulls it out through the trocar incision. The assistant pulls until the stapling device anvil is in position. The surgeon steadies it with an anvil grasper and then uses the laparoscopic Metzenbaum to cut only one suture from the anvil. The anvil is now pulled completely out through the trocar incision and is discarded. After extending the trocar incision, the assistant uses dilators to stretch the fascia, making the incision large enough to accommodate the stapling device. A large enterotomy is also made in the roux limb. The stapler will be inserted through this opening and the anastomosis will be completed. The excess roux limb is excised using a stapling devise and removed. The gastrojejunostomy anastomosis is reinforced with either sutures or u-clips. The next step is to check for anastomosis leak. This is done by distally applying a bowel clamp on the roux limb to occlude the bowel. The surgeon then goes to the head of bed and performs an esophageal gastroduodenoscopy. The first assistant covers the anastomosis with saline and the surgeon visualizes the anastomosis and fills the bowel with air. The first assistant watches for signs of leakage, confirmed by air bubbles around the anastomosis. The scrub person checks the stapler for two complete rings of tissue, to assure the anastomosis is complete. When it is determined that the anastomosis has no leaks the surgeon re-gowns and gloves and returns to the sterile field to complete the procedure.

The surgeon checks to ensure that the roux limb moves freely without kinks. Next, the jejunum is tacked to the mesentery with either sutures or u-clips. The Peterson's hernia[2] is closed with either sutures or u-clips. The surgeon checks for hemostasis, suctions excess irrigation and places a 19 Fr Blake drain over the pouch anastomosis. After removing the cannulas, the fascia is closed at each cannula site, the drain is sutured into place, the skin incisions are closed, and dressings are applied.

LAPAROSCOPIC GASTRIC BANDING
Establishing Access

After establishing the pneumoperitoneum, cannulas are place as described for the laparoscopic **Roux-en-Y proximal gastric bypass**; typical placement includes a:

- 10 mm cannula for a 30-degree optical system, inserted below the xiphoid
- 10 mm cannula for the grasping forceps, inserted in the right upper quadrant
- 5 mm cannula for laparoscopic instruments, inserted in the left upper quadrant
- 10 mm cannula for the grasping forceps, band introduction, and drain placement, which is inserted on the left anterior axillary line below the costal margin

A final puncture is made in the right upper quadrant for the Nathanson liver retractor.

Details: Laparoscopic Gastric Banding

The gastric banding system can be inserted using three different dissection techniques. All of these techniques use an oral-gastric calibration tube with an inflatable balloon, which is inserted into the stomach. The calibration tube facilitates selection of the initial dissection starting point (Ferraro, 2003).

When using the *perigastric technique*, dissection is done exactly on the lesser curve at the equator of the calibration-tube balloon. The surgeon completes the dissection behind the stomach toward the angle of His, taking care to avoid the lesser sac. Next, the gastrogastric sutures are placed anteriorly to secure the band (Ferraro, 2003).

If the *pars flaccida technique* is used, the surgeon starts dissecting in the avascular space of the pars flaccida, exactly lateral to the equator of the calibration-tube balloon. After seeing the caudate lobe of the liver, blunt dissection is continued until the right crus muscle is seen, followed immediately by the left crus muscle over the angle of His (Ferraro, 2003).

The *two-step technique* starts with the *pars flaccida technique*. A second dissection follows at the equator of the balloon near the stomach. The dissection continues until the perigastric dissection intercepts the pars flaccida dissection. Next, the gastric band is placed from the angle of His through to the perigastric opening (Ferraro, 2003).

Once the gastric band is in place using one of the techniques previously described, the surgeon pulls the band around the stomach, and then locks into place. The access port is connected externally to the banding system tubing and implanted in the left rectus muscle or a similar location, which allows the device to be inconspicuous to the patient, yet provide easy percutaneous access to modify the fill volume of the band (Ferraro, 2003).

LAPAROSCOPIC BILIOPANCREATIC DIVERSION WITH DUODENAL SWITCH
Establishing Access

The patient is placed in the supine position. After the administration of general anesthesia, the patient's legs are separated. Six trocars/cannulas are inserted to gain access to the abdominal cavity. One is placed in the supraumbilical area for the camera. A 10-mm trocar is placed at the sub-xiphoid midline; this allows liver separation and access to the hiatus. Next, a 10-mm trocar is inserted at the right of the subcostal margins and a 5-mm trocar is placed on the left. The last two, a 15-mm and a 5-mm trocar, are inserted at the lateral borders of the anterior rectus muscles, above the umbilicus. The 15-mm trocar is inserted on the right and a 5-mm trocar is inserted on the left (Baltasar et al, 2002).

Details

Using vessel fusion or an ultrasonic scalpel, the greater curvature of the stomach and the descending portion of the duodenum are completely devascularized followed by division of the duodenum with a linear cutter. Next, the vertical subtotal gastrectomy is done, starting 7 cm proximal to the pylorus at the greater curvature. This is done by sequentially applying two linear cartridges parallel to the lesser curvature. A nasogastric tube stent is not used. The remainder of the stomach is then divided sequentially using the linear stapler as far as the cardia. Thus, a gastric tube is created, built on the lesser curvature of the stomach. As for the greater curvature, 70–80% is resected. Leaks along the suture-line are tested by filling the gastric remnant with methylene blue. The resected portion of stomach is extracted through the 15-mm cannula. Argon-enhanced electrosurgery or hemostatic clips are used to achieve hemostasis along the suture-line (Baltasar et al, 2002).

Next, the operative team moves to the head of the patient. The circulating nurse positions the video monitor to the right side of the patient. Measurement of the *common limb* starts at the ileocecal junction. During the measurement the bowel is not stretched. The surgeon places a suture marker at 75 cm, which indicates what is to become the *common limb*. A linear cutter is used to divide the bowel 250 cm proximal of the ileocecal valve, thus forming the *alimentary limb*. The mesentery is partially divided with vessel fusion or the ultrasonic scalpel. A side-to-end anastomosis at the 75 cm marker joins the *biliopancreatic limb* and *alimentary limb*. Narrowing of this small-sized, small bowel lumen is prevented by hand suturing. A continuous suture of 2-0 polypropylene is used to do the duodeno-ileal end-to-end anastomosis. Another alternative for the anastomosis is to use a circular stapling device, with the anvils passed by mouth. At the completion of the procedure, mesenteric defects are left open and hemostasis along the suture lines is verified. The integrity of the suture lines is verified by intraluminal irrigation with methylene blue. Only the fascia of the 15-mm trocar site is closed (Baltasar et al, 2002).

POSTPROCEDURE CONSIDERATIONS, COMPLICATIONS, AND CARE

The bariatric patient's arrival in the PACU marks the beginning of their personal journey toward weight loss. The patient has been prepared before the procedure with structured counseling concerning diet, nutrition, behavior modification, and lifestyle changes, which are imperative for sustainable success. After the procedure and transfer to the PACU or SICU, the patient remains under close observation and assessment. Evaluation of desired outcomes is closely monitored by the perianesthesia nurses, patient, family, and members of the patient care team.

Complications can occur in the immediate postprocedure phase because of preexisting behavioral and physiological comorbidities, as well as the procedure itself. In the short-term postprocedure phase, specific alterations in the GI tract and subsequent weight loss may increase risks. Long-term complications are most often related to the direct nutritional and metabolic deficiencies resulting from surgical alteration of the GI tract. Short- and long-term complications are further categorized and quantified according to the specific surgical intervention (eg, restrictive, malabsorptive, or gastric bypass) and approach (eg, open versus laparoscopic approach; Doolen & Miller, 2005; Barth & Jensen, 2006; Brethauer et al, 2006).

Vigilance is essential to circumvent potential complications in the immediate postprocedure phase. Close attention to minor changes in status are required by the entire patient care team in order to recognize and respond swiftly to any early warning signs or changes in the patient's status. Experienced perianesthesia nurses caring for bariatric patients must possess the knowledge, skills, and affect to ensure efficient, safe, and quality-oriented interventions and evaluation throughout the immediate postprocedure period.

Before the procedure tell patients and families to anticipate a minimum of one hour in the PACU. Some patients, because of pre-existing comorbidities, including those patients who experience difficulties during the procedure, may require transfer from the operating room directly to the SICU. While in the SICU, they receive ventilator support and monitoring for potential postprocedure complications. Those bariatric patients not requiring SICU care may transfer directly from the PACU to a designated Bariatric Patient Care Unit or appropriate Medical-Surgical Unit for further postprocedure care and management prior to discharge. Low-risk patients who undergo laparoscopic or less invasive approaches, such as adjustable banding procedures, may be appropriate candidates for recovery in the PACU and transfer to a short-term Recovery Care Center (RCC) for overnight stay and discharge within 24 to 72 hours. Postprocedure care must be highly individualized in close collaboration with the entire patient care team and offer the most appropriate level of care required by the patient to facilitate their safe recovery and appropriate discharge.

RCC
Recovery Care Center

The perianesthesia nurse provides care based upon the identified risks and is able to anticipate potential complications based on an individualized and thorough patient assessment. As described, prompt recognition, clear communication, education, and targeted interventions can minimize the impact of potential postprocedure complications for the bariatric patient.

COMPLICATIONS FOLLOWING BARIATRIC SURGERY

The bariatric surgical intervention, regardless of the specific approach or surgical technique, changes the basic structure and physiology of the GI tract and the consequences of this change can have far-reaching effects. The alteration in the GI tract does not correct the inherent and underlying cause of the individual's eating and/or metabolic disorders that resulted in obesity; therefore, a program of short-term and lifelong follow up and behavior modification is imperative. There are clear risks and potential complications that can arise in the postprocedure phases that must be considered and closely observed for in order to ensure optimal outcomes.

The Bariatric patient is at risk for a combination of physiologic, psychological, and metabolic challenges and potential complications. It is important to classify further complications according to phases of the patient's experience. This particular method of categorization, identified according to immediate postprocedure, early postprocedure (occurring within 30 days), and late complications, establishes a comprehensive view of potential concerns, which can assist the team in establishing goals and direction in planning perioperative patient care (Barth & Jensen, 2006).

Complications in the Immediate Postprocedure Phase
Airway Management

Airway management is a primary concern during the transition from the intraoperative phase to the immediate postprocedure phase. Obstructive sleep apnea, severe deconditioning (becoming short of breath on minimal exertion), obesity hypoventilation syndrome (Pickwickian Syndrome) and asthma are a few of the pre-existing comorbidities which may cue the team to guard closely for potential difficulties in airway management, either during initial intubation or in the immediate post-extubation/postprocedure period. Obese patients often have limited neck extension, short thick necks, and their excess weight inhibits normal chest expansion or respiration. Buildup of carbon dioxide (hypercapnia) can occur due to the patient's excess weight on the chest walls and the combined sedative affects of anesthetic agents, which may in-turn lead to hypoventilation. Reduction of abdominal pressure and ease of respirations can be aided by elevating the head of the bed at least 35° and/ or placing the patient in the reverse Trendelenburg position.

The patient may easily become hypoxic due to the numerous factors affecting respirations, therefore diligent airway assessment and continuous monitoring of oxygen saturation levels is critical (Brethauer et al, 2006; Mulligan et al, 2005). The anesthesiologist and perianesthesia team must maintain the patient's normal ventilation and remain prepared for potential difficulties in postprocedure extubation or airway emergency, including bronchospasm or laryngospasm (Doolen & Miller, 2005; Mulligan et al, 2005).

Reintubation of the patient requires that the patient be repositioned for access and clear visualization. The usual anatomical landmarks that help guide intubation may be difficult to visualize or locate on the morbidly obese patient. The reverse Trendelenburg position shifts abdominal contents away from the diaphragm and chest cavity, which may aid reintubation. Difficult intubation equipment and supplies, mechanical ventilators, and emergency tracheostomy trays, should be readily available at all times. Emergency intubation and airway management supplies should include a fiber-optic laryngoscope, a laryngeal mask specifically designed for urgent and emergent intubations, and tracheostomy tubes of adequate length to accommodate excess adiposity surrounding the neck. Some bariatric patients may require prolonged extubation with mechanical ventilation in the immediate postprocedure phase due potential airway issues. Patients requiring mechanical ventilation may require transfer to the SICU and will need to be weaned according to oxygenation, blood gas results, tidal volumes, and cardiac output results (Barth & Jensen, 2006).

Aggressive pulmonary toileting is imperative for the prevention of postprocedure atelectasis and aspiration pneumonia, which requires preprocedure teaching and postprocedure encouragement for coughing, deep breathing, the use of incentive spirometry, and early ambulation. Pulmonary toileting is an expected intervention in the plan of care for all bariatric patients regardless of their specific procedure.

Venous Thromboembolism, Pulmonary Embolism and Respiratory Failure

A serious complication that can occur in the immediate and early postprocedure phases is venous thromboembolism. Though infrequent, thromboembolism can lead to life-threatening pulmonary embolism (PE) and respiratory failure. Pulmonary embolism and respiratory failure are the most commonly cited causes of death following gastric bypass surgery. Extreme obesity increases the known risks of PE and respiratory failure, but those with a BMI ≥ 60, with chronic lower extremity edema, obstructive sleep apnea, and a previous history of pulmonary embolism are at an elevated risk. Additionally, numerous clotting factors are known to be elevated in patients with morbid obesity and surgery further exacerbates the risk of hemostatic shifts, venous stasis, and immobility. All bariatric surgery patients should receive pharmacologic prophylaxis according to institutional and program guidelines. Additional preventative measures include pneumatic compression devices that fit properly to prevent deep vein thrombosis (DVT) and a comprehensive team approach to monitor the patient closely and facilitate early ambulation (Barth & Jensen, 2006; et al, 2006; Abell & Minocha, 2006; Pannala et al, 2006; Nguyen & Wilson, 2007).

PE
Pulmonary Embolism

DVT
Deep Vein Thrombosis

Hemorrhage

Hemorrhage is another serious complication of bariatric procedures. Prevention of hemorrhage by the perianesthesia team includes management of blood pressure, control of vomiting and careful patient transfer and transport to avoid any sudden or extreme movements. The intraoperative procedure, which may include stapling, suturing and alterations in the structure of the GI tract, may pose direct and indirect risks of acute hemorrhage in the bariatric patient. Vascular injury or splenic injury related to traction or stress tears during gastric manipulation, the edges of staple lines, and at anastomosis sites are potential sources of intra and postprocedure bleeding. Therefore, maintaining hemostasis during the surgical procedure, followed by close patient observation postprocedurely is critical (Herron & Bloomberg, 2006).

Signs and symptoms of hemorrhage in the bariatric surgical patient include hematemesis, rectal bleeding, and gradual and sudden changes in vital signs and hematocrit values. Drains can reveal evidence of active bleeding and help assess the severity of blood loss. Management of hemorrhage may include the administration of crystalloid fluids and/or blood products, based upon appropriate and ongoing lab values. An unplanned return to surgery would need to be considered based upon the relative stability of the patient and the suspected location of continued bleeding.

Several endomechanical staplers are now available to help prevent possible staple line failure and the associated risks of hemorrhage or leakage. Products with shorter staple height, as well as those designed for reinforcement, may help prevent or minimize the risks of hemorrhage. Hemorrhage may also develop later into the course of weight loss and manifest as a secondary result of actual tissue healing, separation, retraction, or stress (over distention) on staple lines or at suture sites. Delayed bleeding can also arise if there is progressive ulceration, inflammation, or a malignancy in the gastrointestinal tract. This condition can be difficult to diagnose, locate, and treat (Herron & Bloomberg, 2006).

Pain

Pain management is a vital component of all nursing care in the immediate postprocedure phase. A patient-controlled analgesia (PCA) pump may be initiated in the perianesthesia area or upon arrival to the postprocedure nursing unit and will be used typically for up to a 48-hour period. Pain management is critical in supporting the patient's primary goals for early ambulation combined with consistent deep breathing, coughing, and incentive spirometry. These goals may be further enhanced through defined postprocedure pain protocols, appropriate pharmacologic selection/support and a collaborative team approach that engages the patient and family, as well as the surgeon, anesthesiologist, bariatric nurse practitioner, primary care nurse, pain nurse, respiratory therapist, physical therapist, and the entire patient care team (Beauchamp-Johnson, 2006).

Hyperglycemia

Recent advances in glucose monitoring and insulin administration have been implemented in many bariatric surgery programs as a result of emerging evidence-based knowledge and the linkages between hyperglycemia and increased postprocedure surgical site infections. Diabetes is one of the more common comorbidities found in obese and morbidly obese patients. A computerized insulin pump may be used to help regulate blood glucose through a continuous insulin infusion. Blood glucose levels are measured according to defined protocols and a computerized insulin pump may then be used to adjust insulin dosages, maintain desirable blood glucose levels, as well as cue the patient care team when the next blood glucose level should be drawn. The combination of technology and best practices is useful in preventing undesirable spikes (elevations) in postprocedure blood glucose levels. The goal of the patient care team is to maintain the patient's blood glucose level at or below 90mg/dl during and after surgery to help reduce the identified risks of hyperglycemia on postprocedure surgical site infections. Ongoing research and clinical trials on computerized insulin pump technology and blood glucose protocols will enhance the team's ability to effectively manage blood glucose levels and promote best practices in the care of the bariatric patient.

Short Term—Early Complications (≤30 Days)
Anastomotic Leak

Bariatric surgery carries a mortality risk of less than 1% and a serious complication risk of up to 10%, with pulmonary embolism, anastomotic leak, and respiratory failure identified as the leading causes of death. Together, pulmonary emboli, anastomotic leaks, and respiratory failure account for 80% of all deaths in the first 30 days following bariatric surgery (Brethauer et al, 2006). Patients usually present with signs and symptoms of an anastomotic leak very early on in the immediate postop recovery period or within 7 to 14 days following surgery. Numerous signs and symptoms can indicate leakage at the connection sites made between the stomach pouch and small intestine, but they can often be subtle and difficult to identify. Signs of anastomotic leakage may include shoulder, abdominal, and pelvic pain, vague changes in heart rate or sustained tachycardia, hypotension, and unexplained changes in urine output. (Nguyen & Wilson, 2007) Anastomotic leakage remains an unusual complication, but one that in turn leads to re-operation(s), prolonged hospitalization, and up to a 30% increased mortality rate. The patient care team can help prevent deaths from these major complications providing appropriate prophylaxis for possible thromboembolic events, identifying symptoms early, and by teaching patients/families the importance of early reporting of possible symptoms or complications.

Wound Infection

Infection can arise due to any number of risk factors commonly associated with any surgical intervention and generally occur early on in the postprocedure phase. The rate of infection in bariatric patients compared to all other complications is quite high, approximately 7% for open bariatric procedures, and 2.9% for laparoscopic procedures (Abell & Minocha, 2006). Signs and symptoms may include purulent drainage, pain, redness, and swelling at or near the incision site(s). Rate of wound infection is higher for bariatric patients because of the accumulation of bacteria and excessive moisture in skin folds and poor blood supply to the incisional areas (Barth & Jensen, 2006). Strict adherence to Surgical Care Improvement Project (SCIP) protocols and practices for perioperative antibiotic administration may help decrease the risks, but due to the higher associated risks with obese patients, there is no guarantee SCIP or routine antibiotic administration will prevent wound infections from developing. Data from studies comparing open and laparoscopic procedures have shown that patients have a lower rate of infection for laparoscopic procedures and decreased incidence of postprocedure incisional hernia. Specific wound and skin care protocols that include glucose monitoring and patient/family teaching prior to discharge are an important part of decreasing the risks and associated complications that may accompany a postprocedure wound infection (Herron & Bloomberg, 2006).

SCIP
Surgical Care Improvement Project

Dumping Syndrome

Nearly 70% of all bariatric patients experience some form of dumping syndrome that is typically due to a loss of normal pyloric valve function (bypass) or the direct result of eating too much sugar, which in turn results in food moving too quickly from the stomach to the intestine with a subsequent drop in blood pressure, abdominal cramping, sweating, and dizziness. Mild to severe symptoms may occur with gastric bypass patients after eating sweets, dairy products, or foods high in starch. Dumping syndrome is an effective result of bariatric surgery that is often referred to as the "postop police officer," since it alerts the body to inappropriate eating, discourages sweet eating, and encourages weight loss. Vasomotor changes such as flushing and dizziness may also occur, but dumping syndrome symptoms usually resolve within 30 to 60 minutes. Dietary modifications and drug therapy can help alleviate or diminish both the incidence and associated symptoms of dumping syndrome (Lynch et al, 2006).

Pressure Ulcers and Skin Breakdown

Decreased blood supply to adipose tissue further contributes to the patient's risk of skin and wound problems. Moisture and bacteria may contribute to infection, as mentioned earlier, but may also contribute to skin breakdown. Skin folds around the back, breasts, abdomen, and perineum are particularly at risk because these areas are difficult to access and cleanse, are prone to moisture buildup, and the patient typically has difficulty reaching and cleaning the areas themselves.

Frequent repositioning and ambulation is imperative for proper assessment of skin integrity, as well as proper cleansing and routine provision of skin care.

Long Term—Later Complications (>30 days)

Long-term or later complications for the postprocedure bariatric patient include a diverse list of metabolic, neurological, integumentary, gastrointestinal, and nutritional problems. Dumping syndrome, persistent vomiting and nausea, stenosis, bowel obstruction, and pressure ulcers are all part of lengthy list of long-term complications frequently associated with bariatric surgery.

Patients need to be fully informed of what they will most likely encounter as a part of the lifelong changes and potential risks of bariatric surgery. The options all bariatric patients must weigh include: enduring continued obesity with its associated comorbidities; seeking out and committing to losing weight through traditional diet and other non-invasive methods; or whether they will risk facing the potential, recognized, and documented complications related to bariatric surgery. Despite the challenges and potential risks, most patients find the "risk-reward ratio" acceptable. Some of the long-term complications and potential problems facing bariatric surgical patients include:

Incisional Hernia

Morbidly obese patients often suffer from various forms of malnourishment. Therefore, their risk for skin breakdown, wound dehiscence, and incisional hernia are heightened further by any surgical intervention. The risks become much greater after the procedure because of the inherent nutritional deficiencies from the resultant malabsorption and restrictive procedures themselves. Incisional hernias are characterized by discomfort and protrusion of abdominal contents through the abdominal wall or at the incision site. The hernia can also become incarcerated, requiring immediate surgical treatment and possible mesh repair to reinforce the incisions (Nguyen & Wilson, 2007).

Strictures and Risks of Obstruction

Partial or complete obstruction may occur at anytime during the postprocedure course, but are more common 4–6 weeks after surgery. The gastric pouch may scar down and result in increased or progressive difficulty swallowing, drinking, or eating. Gastroscopy with gradual dilation may prove successful and provide immediate relief. Surgery is rare and only used as a last resort. Ulcers and adhesions may also complicate functionality of the gastric pouch. Acid-blockers, such as famotidine (Pepcid), omeprazole (Prilosec), esomeprazole (Nexium), or lansoprazole (Prevacid), are routinely prescribed for the first two months following surgery to reduce the risks of ulcer formation. Patients are cautioned to avoid any medications that may increase the risk of bleeding, such as aspirin, acetaminophen (Tylenol), or ibuprofen (Advil) for up to two months. Cardiac and stroke prevention dosages may be permitted in consultation with the surgeon and based upon defined patient risks.

Nutritional Deficiencies

The complex metabolic derangement existing in the morbidly obese patient is a primary contributing factor in the development of obesity. The patient is unable to mobilize existing fat stores and protein is then used for energy. Most obese patients are already at risk for malnutrition, as outlined, and these risks are further aggravated because of bariatric surgery (Barth & Jensen, 2006).

Nutritional deficiencies are reported in the majority of patients following bariatric surgery. The combination of intentional malabsorption and a significantly reduction in dietary intake results in deficiencies of key nutrients. Protein, iron, fat-soluble vitamins (A, D, E and K), and the B vitamins are among those in which most of the deficiencies are reported (Herron & Bloomberg, 2006).

Nearly 70% of patients have a reported deficiency of B12 due to two possible contributing factors, including the fact that B12 may be poorly absorbed due to decreased gastric acidity and that B12 is further destroyed by bacterial overgrowth within a portion of the gastric segment. Regardless of the etiology, bariatric patients will require guided and essential supplementation in order to promote appropriate healing and to prevent or alleviate potential imbalances that may result in anemia or other neurologic complications (Herron & Bloomberg, 2006).

Risks of Pregnancy

Women of childbearing age should avoid becoming pregnant immediately following gastric bypass surgery, due to risks associated with rapid weight loss and potential nutritional deficiencies that may harm the fetus. Patients may consider pregnancy usually at 12 to 18 months post surgery, once they have reached a stable lower weight. Primary care physicians may be consulted to provide additional education and to explore possible birth control options with the patient.

Neurologic Complications

Neurologic complications are not uncommon and have been reported as a result of metabolic and nutritional deficiencies, including B1, B12, Folic Acid, Niacin, and Copper, to name a few. Additionally, neurologic complications from bariatric surgery can manifest in virtually any area of the nervous system and such complications have been identified in as many as many as 5 to 10% of patients undergoing surgery for obesity. Any part of the neuraxis, including the brain, cerebellum, spinal cord, peripheral nerve, and muscles, may be involved. Neurological complications may appear early or at any time during the extended postprocedure course, a potential consequence of micronutrient deficiency.

Patients must be assessed for and receive nutritional supplementation to circumvent the anticipated nutritional and metabolic derangements resulting from bariatric surgical procedures. The starvation state following bariatric surgery warrants close attention to all patients for any signs and symptoms of nutritional and/or neurological deficiencies.

Cholelithiasis

Gall stone development after bariatric surgery is so common that many surgeons perform a prophylactic cholecystectomy at the time of the primary bariatric procedure. It is expected that nearly half of all bariatric surgery patients will eventually develop cholelithiasis. Additionally, within three years of bariatric surgery, up to one third of all patients will require a cholecystectomy if there gallbladder is left in place (Nguyen & Wilson, 2007). Both the obese and bariatric surgery patients have a greater rate of gall stone formation related to a presumed increase in cholesterol excretion. This increase in cholesterol, the chief substance of gallstones, increases further after bariatric surgery, as does the level of a biliary protein, which promotes crystal or stone formation (Herron & Bloomberg, 2006).

Emotional Changes

The provision of support for psychological, emotional, and behavioral needs begins when the patient arrives in the physician's office for consultation and continues throughout the course of weight loss and beyond. As identified previously, the surgical intervention does not address the behavioral eating disorders that originally led to obesity. Obese patients seeking surgical interventions have undoubtedly encountered stigmatization, discrimination, and prejudice, leading a cycle of low-self esteem and overeating, as well as other types of compulsive and dysfunctional behaviors (Barth & Jensen, 2006; Voelker, 2004). Patients may present with histories that include anxiety, problems with relationships, mood disorders, high levels of stress, and report being victims of abuse (McMahon et al, 2006). Improvement in psychosocial functioning is a notable benefit of weight loss after bariatric surgery. Patients frequently report improvement in their overall quality of life, reduction in stress, and improvement in their relationships (McMahon et al, 2006).

Support groups, education, behavioral therapy, and counseling comprise the interventions for emotional and psychological care and healing throughout the pre-procedure and postprocedure phases. The multidisciplinary approach is imperative for management of the bariatric patient's experience before and after surgery. The team should be comprised of professionals from all disciplines and be involved in all phases of the patient's journey. Improved outcomes and decreased mortality and morbidity are linked with multidisciplinary and programmatic approaches. These approaches are the cornerstone to establishing an appropriate, realistic, and practical patient plan of care (Voelker, 2004).

Direct nursing care providing dignity, safety, and attention to personal needs is critical to patient comfort and support for the holistic healing process. Elements supporting dignified care include provision of adequate and appropriate equipment and supplies to accommodate the patient and by ensuring consistency in actual care-givers assigned to the patient and family. Privacy, trust, and continuity of care can contribute to improved communication, collaboration and outcomes throughout the hospitalization and in preparation for discharge (McGlinch et al, 2006).

Direct care nurses and ancillary staff members should not only have a particular desire to care for this patient population, but must also receive comprehensive education and sensitivity training. Competencies should include communication, safety, complication detection and treatment, nutrition, and targeted short- and long-term care with measurable outcomes (AORN, 2008; Barth & Jensen, 2006).

Additionally, all professionals involved in bariatric patient care should strive to increase their awareness of potential personal biases or prejudices surrounding obesity, as well as the appropriate affect, tone of voice, specific words and phrases to use or avoid, and communication styles that enhance and support the psychological and behavioral healing processes (AORN, 2008; Barth & Jensen, 2006). The humanistic component of caring and the caregiver's direct influence on creating healing environments and relationships that foster both physical and psychological well-being cannot be overemphasized.

Death

The risk of death is typically reported as less than 1% for initial procedures and approaching 2% for reoperative gastric bypass surgery. Previous abdominal or gastric surgery adds to the complexity of the procedure and risks associated with reoperation. Mortality rates reflect average bariatric patients in otherwise good health or for those who have had thorough workups and whose comorbidities are otherwise well controlled. The risk of death may increase significantly for those patients with super obesity (BMI > 50) or for those with serious or poorly controlled comorbidities.

BODY CONTOURING PROCEDURES

The surgical procedure is just the beginning of the journey for patients seeking major weight loss. After loss of significant excess weight, patients are usually left with the issue of significant redundant skin that can be discouraging, disfiguring, and problematic. The excess skin can present numerous health-related problems and can only be remedied by secondary plastic surgery, frequently called "body contouring."

As the number of bariatric procedures has increased, so has the number of plastic surgery procedures that attend to the residual effects of profound weight loss and the resultant laxity or excess skin. According to the American Society of Plastic Surgeons (ASPS), more than 68,000 patients sought out plastic surgery after significant weight loss in 2005, which represents over 48% of the 140,000 patients who underwent bariatric surgery, and demonstrates a 22% increase in these procedures over the previous year (ASBS, 2005; ASPS, 2008; Chandler, 2006).

ASPS
American Society of Plastic Surgeons

The patient's substantial weight loss may be the catalyst to a completely new life with a significant reduction in or complete resolution of previous comorbidities. However, the patient must also cope with the potential for physical disfigurement resulting from significant skin laxity that is difficult or impossible to conceal under clothing. As a result, patients may not feel they can truly enjoy or experience the full benefits of their weight loss success. Clothing options remain limited and excess skin can further restrict movement, as well as hinder their ability to express their newfound sense of being and becoming. Coping with these changes and challenges in body image can serve as a constant reminder of the patient's previous pain, depression, struggles with morbid obesity, and may actually undermine the more positive and dramatic physical benefits that bariatric surgery offer. Because of this secondary emotional turmoil, the patient may actually experience further psychological and psychosocial dysfunction (McGohan, 2007).

Skin elasticity is affected by damaged elastin fibers and the long-term stress on the tissues of the body. However, genetics, amount of sun exposure, smoking, the number and degree of weight changes, and overall nutritional status also influence skin elasticity (McGohan, 2007).

20

Following the massive weight loss, redundant tissue can be distorted, deformed, and often asymmetrical. The patient may suffer with recurrent skin infections, fungal infestations, and chafing between the thighs and under the arms, leading to skin breakdown. Additionally, significant weight loss can leave the patient with a panniculus. The result of significant weight loss, a panniculus is a large "apron" of loose or redundant layers of abdominal tissue or skin that can interfere with normal activity, cause lower back pain, increase the risk of skin breakdown, and can ultimately lead to further psychological problems for the post bariatric patient (Chandler, 2006; McGohan, 2007).

Bariatric surgery places increased demands on the patient both physically and psychologically (Chandler, 2006). Serotonin, the body's natural antidepressant, may fluctuate in the postprocedure phase because of pain, fear, and nutritional changes, and these changes can lead to both euphoria and/or bouts of depression. Psychological screening and interventions are often necessary to prevent or minimize emotional difficulties or potential depression postprocedurely (Chandler, 2006).

Plastic and Reconstructive Interventions

Body contouring procedures have developed from and in harmony with more traditional plastic surgery procedures. It is noted that many plastic surgeons are also purposefully specializing in this specialized area of plastic surgery resulting from the large number of patients who have experienced successful weight loss, and are now seeking out these types of contouring procedures. Patients seek complete fulfillment from their successful weight loss efforts. As a result, body contouring options will be tailored to the patient's weight loss, personal concerns, priorities, and needs (see **Table 20.8** for body contouring options).

The most common body contouring procedures include abdominoplasty, brachioplasty, breast lift, breast reduction, medial and lateral thigh lifts, and circumferential lower and upper body lifts. Liposuction alone is not adequate for

Table 20.8 **Body Contouring Options**		
Patient Concerns	**Procedural Option**	**Variations**
Sagging abdomen with a possible "apron" or panniculus; no waistline; abdominal wall laxity	Abdominoplasty	Mini-abdominoplasty, traditional with placation of rectus muscle and possible hernia repair, panniculectomy
"Batwing" skin and tissue along the upper arm	Brachioplasty (upper arm lift)	
Drooping breasts	Breast lift, reduction	Mastopexy, liposuction
"Saddle bags"; overly large or distorted thighs	Lower body lift, belt lipectomy	
Excess skin on upper back or bra line, chest	Upper body lift	

the extent of fat and tissue that needs to be removed. However, most contouring procedures will include some form of liposuction.

Preprocedure Planning and Preparation for Body Contouring

Patients seeking plastic surgery following bariatric weight loss are encouraged to meet certain criteria before undergoing body contouring procedures. There are weight loss requirements, psychological concerns, and physical elements that must be addressed prior to plastic surgery. Patients may be referred to a plastic surgeon during the course of the weight loss program to begin the discussions and planning that eventually lead up to the day of surgery.

Weight loss requirements may differ between surgeons. However, most plastic surgeons will usually wait for 15 to 24 months, preferring the patient to have encountered a weight loss plateau for at least three months, to have lost more than 100 pounds, and be close to their ideal body weight. Psychological concerns should have been addressed during the course of the patient's weight loss by the multidisciplinary team. Additionally, plastic surgeons will want to counsel the patient regarding the expectations, outcomes, risks, and potential complications. Patients may be told they will have removal of a significant amount of excess skin but should expect to have scars. Photographs taken before the procedure assist the surgeon in the planning phase. The photographs also can be helpful for the patient to see, thereby helping to establish realistic expectations. The preprocedure images will be compared with postprocedure photographs. Some plastic surgeons have digital capabilities allowing the images to be altered or morphed, thereby giving the patient a glimpse of how they may look postprocedurely. Regardless, patients and surgeons both should have rational expectations of outcomes. Patient's misconceptions or differing perceptions of what can be accomplished can result in serious patient dissatisfaction and potential litigation (Zuelzer & Baugh, 2007).

Thorough assessment of the patient's physical status is imperative for good outcomes from plastic surgery. Patients have been in a starvation state for one to two years. Resulting protein, vitamin, and mineral deficiencies could have a serious consequences on wound healing and increase the risk of other complications. The patient should have a complete history and physical, a metabolic panel, and be screened by an anesthesiologist. Comorbidities, such as asthma, diabetes, or heart conditions, should have been addressed throughout the weight loss continuum. Additionally, smoking should be stopped and is often a contraindication for surgery because of its detrimental effect on tissue oxygenation and subsequent postprocedure wound healing. The patient should also be free of any yeast, fungal, or bacterial infections (Zuelzer & Baugh, 2007; Heddens, 2004).

Complications

Complications and risks following body contouring are similar to those encountered after any type of lengthy or complex procedure. Venous thromboembolism, including pulmonary embolism and deep vein thrombosis, can be life threatening and need to be addressed with prophylactic treatment in all phases of care. Surgeons will usually order the application of pneumatic compression devices alone or in conjunction with subcutaneously administered anticoagulants. Postprocedure care includes the addition of early ambulation, pulmonary toileting, and appropriate hydration as preventative measures.

Wound healing is a significant concern in post weight-loss surgical patients undergoing body contouring. Nutritional status is always a concern and should be thoroughly assessed prior to surgery. The patient is at risk of dehiscence, necrosis, and flap failure, as well as infection. Optimal intake and dietary supplementation of protein, specific vitamins, and minerals can decrease the risk of wound complications. Additionally, patient education should include proper positioning and movement to reduce the potential strain on incision lines.

Seromas and hematomas may happen with body contouring procedures. Large amounts of tissue removed inevitably results in persistent drainage. Drains are placed prior to wound closure and may be in place for days and even weeks. Compression garments also are used to provide hemostasis, reduce edema, and promote evacuation of serous and capillary drainage. Thorough patient and family education on caring for incisions and drains at home is imperative. However, drains may not always relieve all of the drainage produced after complex and extensive procedures. Seromas or hematomas may develop and require an unplanned return to the operating room for evacuation and treatment.

Nursing Implications

Intraoperative nursing challenges abound in body contouring procedures. Many surgical cases may include two or more procedures independent of one another. There may be several position changes. This is expected in body lift and liposuction procedures. Monitor and frequently check patient alignment during and after positioning. Adequate padding and support of all vulnerable pressure points is a constant focus of the perioperative team.

Frequent position changes require rechecking and possible replacement of the electrosurgical dispersive pad. Extensive body contouring may require the perioperative nurse to seek unusual or infrequently used application sites for the electrosurgical dispersive pad, such as the upper or lower arm.

Maintaining normothermia is another constant focus of the perioperative nurse done in collaboration with the anesthesiologist. Two forced-air warming devices, one at the head of the bed and one at the foot of the bed, should be available. Warming blankets may be used at either location, depending upon the section of the body to be exposed during specific procedures or throughout the case.

One particular challenge for the perioperative nurse and the scrub personnel can be the sponge and needle counts. Multiple staged procedures are the norm, standardized counting procedures between procedures and during relief are imperative. It is not unusual to have over 100 needles used on a body contouring procedure. Counting tools such as needle boxes or magnets should be a standard protocol to ensure accurate and correct counts.

The nurse also must calculate input and output during the case and provide regular and continual communication with the anesthesiologist. Irrigation, tumescent subcutaneous liposuction solution, and local anesthetic medications may all be used during the case. Six to 12 hours of surgery for body contouring is not unusual and the team must continually monitor the patient's physiological status.

CONCLUSION

The journey of the bariatric surgery patient is truly a lifelong pursuit of health, wellness, and healing. The statistics identify the seriousness of obesity trends from a global and local perspective, but the most complex and challenging aspect of obesity is evidenced in the profound consequence of morbid obesity on the over-all quality and life expectancy for the individual. There are measurable benefits of bariatric surgery for the morbidly obese, especially for those unsuccessful in their struggles with more traditional approaches to sustainable weight loss. The risks of bariatric surgery are potentially serious, but the rates of morbidity and mortality are considered acceptable for those patients who meet the defined selection criteria and commit to lifestyle changes that are important to ensure optimal short- and long-term outcomes.

For further information and a thorough discussion on the care of the bariatric patient the reader is referred to the Competency and Credentialing Institute's Competency Assessment Module, *Care of the Bariatric Patient*, on which this chapter was based.

ENDNOTES

1. This section used with permission from D'Alfonso, J. & Ritchie, C.R. (2008). *Care of the Bariatric Patient: Competency Assessment Module*. Denver, CO: Competency and Credentialing Institute.
2. Peterson's hernia—herniation of the small bowel posterior to the Roux-en-Y loop. (Blachar et al, 2002).

Gastrointestinal complications of laparoscopic Roux-en-Y gastric bypass surgery: clinical and imaging findings. Retrieved July 14, 2008 from http://radiology.rsnajnls.org/cgi/content/full/223/3/625?ijkey=08494a326fe7f691ca69fbfa9a963746e35fac01.).

REFERENCES

1. Abell, T.L. & Minocha, A. (2006). Gastrointestinal complications of bariatric surgery: Diagnosis and therapy, *The American Journal of the Medical Sciences*; 331(4): pp. 214–218.
2. American Society for Bariatric Surgery (ASBS). (2005). Brief history and summary of bariatric surgery. Retrieved July 20, 2008 from http://www.asbs.org/html/patients/bypass.html.
3. American Society of Plastic Surgeons (ASPS). (2008). Body contouring after massive weight loss. Retrieved July 15, 2008 from: http://www.plasticsurgery.org/news_room/Body-Contouring-After-Massive-Weight-Loss.cfm.
4. Association of periOperative Registered Nurses (AORN). (2008). Bariatric surgery guideline. *Standards and Recommended Practices*. Denver, CO: AORN, Inc; pp. 67–85.
5. Baltasar, A., Bou, R., Miró, J., Bengochea, M., Serra, C., & Pérez, N. (2002). Laparoscopic iliopancreatic diversion with duodenal switch: technique and initial experience. *Obesity Surgery*;12(2): pp. 245–248.
6. Barth, M.M. & Jensen, C.E. (2006). Postoperative nursing care of gastric bypass patients. *American Journal of Critical Care*;15(4): pp. 378–387.
7. Beauchamp-Johnson, B.M. (2006). Scale down bariatric surgery's risks. *Nursing Management*; 37(9): pp. 27–32.
8. Blachar, A., Federle, M.P., Pealer, K.M., Ikramuddin, S., & Schauer, P.R. (2002). Gastrointestinal complications of laparoscopic Roux-en-Y gastric bypass surgery: clinical and imaging findings. Retrieved July 14, 2008 from http://radiology.rsnajnls.org/cgi/content/full/223/3/625?ijkey=08494a326fe7f691ca69fbfa9a963746e35fac01.
9. Brethauer, S.A., Chand, B., & Schauer, P.R. (2006). Risks and benefits of bariatric surgery: Current evidence. *Cleveland Clinic Journal of Medicine* 73(11): pp. 993–1007.
10. Carpentino-Moyet, L.J. (2008). *Handbook of nursing diagnosis*, 12th ed. Philadelphia, PA: Lippincott Williams & Wilkins.
11. Chandler, S.K. (2006). Considerations for body contouring after massive weight loss. *Bariatric Nursing and Surgical Patient Care*; 1(4): pp. 283–286.
12. D'Alfonso, J. & Ritchie, C.R. (2008). *Care of the Bariatric Patient: Competency Assessment Module*. Denver, CO: CCI.
13. Doolen, J.L. & Miller, S.K. (2005). Primary care management of patients following bariatric surgery. *Journal of the American Academy of Nurse Practitioners*; 17(11): pp. 446–450.
14. Ferraro, D. (2003). Laparoscopic adjustable gastric banding for morbid obesity. *AORN Journal*; 77(5): pp. 923–940.

20

15. Heddens, C.J. (2004). Body contouring after massive weight loss. *Plastic Surgical Nursing*; 24(3); pp. 107–115.

16. Herron, D.M. & Bloomberg, R. (2006). Complications of bariatric surgery. *Minerva Chirurgica*; 61(2): pp. 125–139.

17. Lynch, R.J., Eisenberg, D., & Bell, R.L. (2006). Metabolic consequences of bariatric surgery. *Journal of Clinical Gastroenterology*; 40 (8): pp. 659–668.

18. McGlinch, B.P., Que, F.G., Nelson, J.L., Wroblcski, D.M., Grant, J.E., & Collazo-Clavell, M.L. (2006). Perioperative care of patients undergoing bariatric surgery. *Mayo Clinic Proceedings*; 81(10 suppl): pp. S25–S33.

19. McGohan, L.D. (2007). Body contouring following massive weight loss. *Journal of Continuing Education in Nursing*; 38 (3): pp. 103–104.

20. McMahon, M.M., Sarr, M.G., Clark, M.M., Gall, M.M., Knoetgen, J., Service, F.J., Laskowski, E.R., & Hurley, D.L. (2006). Clinical management after bariatric surgery: Value of a multidisciplinary approach. *Mayo Clinic Proceedings*; 81(10 suppl): pp. S34–S35.

21. Mulligan, A., Young, L.S., Randall, S., Raiano, C., Velardo, P., Breen, C., & Bushee, L. (2005). Best practices for perioperative nursing care for weight loss surgery patients. *Obesity Research*; 13(2); pp. 267–273.

22. Nguyen, N.T. & Wilson S.E. (2007). Complications of antiobesity surgery. *Nature Clinical Practice Gastroenterology & Hepatology*; 4(3):138–147.

23. Pannala, R., Kidd, M., & Modlin, I.M. (2006). Surgery for obesity: Panacea or Pandora's box? *Digestive Surgery*; 23(1–2): pp. 1–11.

24. Voelker, M. (2004). Assessing quality of life in gastric bypass clients. *Journal of Perianesthesia Nursing*;19(2): pp. 89–101.

25. Wikipedia. (2008a). Bariatric surgery. Retrieved May 27, 2008 from: http://en.wikipedia.org/wiki/Bariatric_surgery.

26. Wikipedia. (2008b). Stomach. Retrieved May 27, 2008 from: http://en.wikipedia.org/wiki/Stomach.

30. Wikipedia. (2008c). Digestive enzyme. Retrieved May 27, 2008 from: http://en.wikipedia.org/wiki/Digestive_enzyme.

31. Zuelzer, H.B. & Baugh, N.G. (2007). Bariatric and body contouring surgery: A continuum of care for excess and lax skin. *Plastic Surgical Nursing*; 27(1): pp. 3–13.

CHAPTER 21

Vascular Surgery

Donna S. Watson

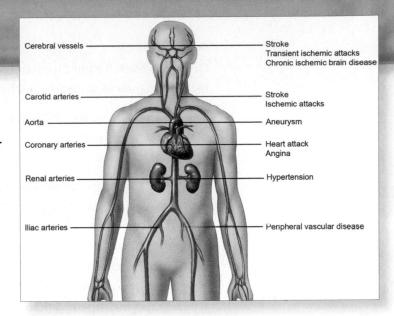

INTRODUCTION

The history of surgery goes back thousands of years. The Edwin Smith papyrus documents operative procedures from 3,000 years ago and efforts to control bleeding from the vascular system. Hot rocks and heated metal were used to cauterize vessels. Uncontrolled bleeding was, however, a major limitation in the early days of surgery. In the 16th century Ambroise Pare, a French surgeon, gained his experience by treating battlefield wounds. Pare promoted the use of ligature over cautery because it was less destructive than burning the flesh with tools available at that time. Since Pare's time, technology has evolved and improved, reducing the morbidity and improving the outcomes for operative patients (Ulmer, 2007).

Vascular surgery involves invasive procedures on the vessels of the body aimed at treating disease or correcting a deformity. Problems within the vascular system create quality of life issues for patients so anxiety is not uncommon. Successful vascular procedures preserve and restore proper function. Less favorable outcomes can result in loss of one or both limbs, stroke, or death resulting from uncontrolled bleeding. An important component of a successful outcome is a skilled and knowledgeable operative team. Each team member is responsible for understanding the procedure and anticipating the expected course of action. Knowing key facts about the procedure contributes to positive patient outcomes.

Chapter Contents

ANATOMY

Diseased vessels within the arterial system of the human reduce blood flow and thus the oxygenation of structures and tissues. Impairment of blood flow may be related to:

- the total or partial obstruction of the vessel lumen caused by plaque
- the structure of the vessel lumen (ie, narrow vessel lumen)
- trauma to the vessel

Obstruction of the vessel lumen by plaque is called *atherosclerosis*. This is often a silent disorder that progresses for years before producing symptoms. Clinical manifestations result from chronic ischemia great enough to reduce blood flow, acute ischemia due to arterial embolism or atheromatous debris, and/or acute ischemia produced by thrombosis of arteries. Common sites for the development of atherosclerotic plaque are the coronary arteries, the carotid bifurcation, the abdominal aorta, the iliac arteries, and the superficial femoral artery (Zwolak, 1990). **Figure 21.1** illustrates

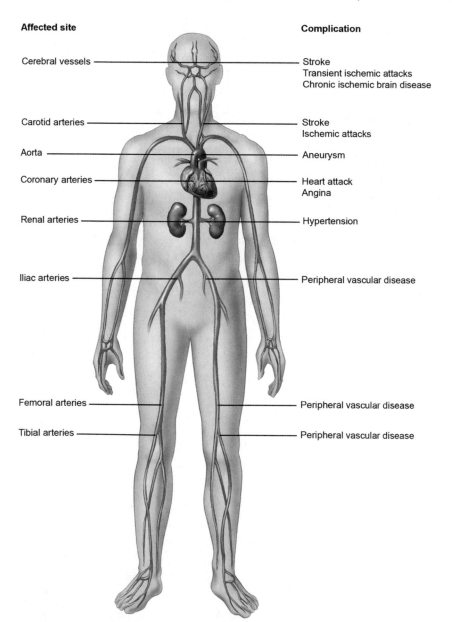

Affected site

Cerebral vessels

Carotid arteries

Aorta

Coronary arteries

Renal arteries

Iliac arteries

Femoral arteries

Tibial arteries

Complication

Stroke
Transient ischemic attacks
Chronic ischemic brain disease

Stroke
Ischemic attacks

Aneurysm

Heart attack
Angina

Hypertension

Peripheral vascular disease

Peripheral vascular disease

Peripheral vascular disease

Figure 21.1

Effect of atherosclerosis on major vessels and possible complications.

the effect of atherosclerosis on major vessels and the subsequent complications. Operative interventions include carotid endarterectomy, resection of an abdominal aortic aneurysm, femoropopliteal bypass graft, and amputation.

The major artery in the body, the aorta, originates at the aortic valve of the heart, arches away from the heart, and flows downward through the body. In the pelvis, it bifurcates into the iliac arteries, which develop branches through which blood flows to the legs (**Fig. 21.1**). The venous system mirrors the arterial system, with the major vessel in the body being the vena cava.

SPECIAL INSTRUMENTS, SUPPLIES, AND EQUIPMENT

Vascular instruments are designed to be non-crushing and minimize trauma to the vessel. The instruments are delicate and require processing care to avoid damage. A complication of vascular surgery can occur in short period of time by the absence of pedal pulses or the inability of the patient to move an extremity. For this reason, instruments should remain sterile until the patient leaves the operating room.

Special supplies include peanut dissectors, Fogarty inserts, vessel loops, suture boots, and an assortment of vascular suture. Hemostatic agents such as topical thrombin, gelfoam and hemolytics help to control oozing from the anastomosis site and must be readily available. Anticoagulation during the procedure is achieved using heparin sulfate, which is with protamine sulfate.

Diseased vessels are often replaced using manufactured fabric graft made of polyester or polytetrafluoroethylene, human allograft such as an umbilical cord vein graft, a saphenous or mammary graft, or a vessel harvested from the patient. Grafts in different sizes and shapes and should be immediately available, along with one backup. Availability should be confirmed before the beginning of the procedure during the Universal Protocol. Synthetic grafts include woven, which do not leak blood through the walls and do not need to be preclotted, and knitted, which require preclotting with the patient's blood before heparin is administered to prevent the graft from leaking. It is important to follow the manufacturer's guidelines appropriately for all supplies and equipment being used.

CAROTID ENDARTERECTOMY

Carotid endarterectomy (CEA) is the removal of atherosclerotic plaque or emboli from the carotid artery. Carotid endarectomy is conducted in patients who are at risk for a cerebrovascular accident (CVA) that may arise from atherosclerotic plaque or emboli. The indications for a CEA include two different groups of patients. These include a symptomatic patient who experiences symptoms consistent with a transient ischemic attack (TIA) with reversible neurological deficits or a cerebrovascular accident with irreversible neurological impairment. The second group includes the asymptomatic patient with demonstrable cerebrovascular disease located at the carotid bifurcation with no current or past history of sympotmatology suggestive of TIA or CVA. The main goal of carotid endarterectomy is prevention of a cerebrovascular accident, which is the major complication.

CEA
Carotid Endarterectomy

CVA
Cerebrovascular Accident

TIA
Transient Ischemic Attack

21

Indications

The incidence of stroke prevention is key for the indication for operative intervention. The World Stroke Congress developed an aggressive agenda that resulted in the World Stroke Day starting on October 29, 2008 and subsequently, annually thereafter. The message is simple: "Stroke is a treatable and preventable castrophe" (Hachinski, 2008). In the United States it is estimated the incidences of cerebrovascular accident range from 760,000 to 780,000 annually (Leary, 2003). Specific risk factors are associated for individuals at risk for an ischemic cerebrovascular accident to include: age, gender, African-American ethnicity, tobacco abuse, hypertension, diabetes, coronary artery disease, excessive alcohol intake, large body mass index, and low socioeconomic status (Biller, 2000). Common risk factors as well as potential predictors of stoke listed in **Table 21.1** include history of transient ischemic attacks, prior CVA, asymtomatic carotid bruit or stenosis, polycythemia, increased fibrinogen level, high plasma homocysteine level, microalbuminuria and oral contraceptive use (Biller, 2000).

Since stroke is a potential complication during the procedure, the risk of operative intervention versus conservative treatment must be considered. The symptomatic patient may have a *transient ischemic attack*, which is a temporary disturbance of blood flow to a part of the brain, also referred to as a mini stroke (Wikipedia, 2008). Other symptoms may include dysphasia, aphasia, hemiplegia, sensory or motor deficit, ataxia, dizziness, diplopia, dysarthria, weakness, or amaurosis fugax. If the patient has a cerebrovascular accident that includes irreversible neurological

Table 21.1	Risk Factors for Ischemic Stroke
Non-Modifiable Risk Factors	**Modifiable or Treatable Risk Factors**
Age	Arterial hypertension
Race or ethnicity	Transient ischemic attacks
Gender	Previous stroke
Family History	Asymptomatic carotid bruit or stenosis
Genetics	Cardiac disease
	Aortic arch atheromatosis
	Diabetes mellitus
	Hyperlipidemia
	Cigarette smoking
	Alcohol consumption
	Increased fibrinogen level
	Low serum folate level
	Elevated anticardiolipin antibody levels
	Use of oral contraceptives
	Microalbuminuria
	Obesity

Biller, J., & Thies, W. H. (2000). When to operate in carotid artery disease. *American Family Physician 61*(2); 400–406.

impairment, the decision for operative intervention versus conservative management must be determined. These include assessing the patient's remaining neurological function and determining that the benefits of operative intervention are greater than the potential risks. The goal is to preserve any remaining neurological function.

Recommendations for operative intervention for the symptomatic patient is based on two large landmark studies, the North American Symptomatic Endarterectomy Trial (NASCET) and the Europeon Carotid Surgery Trial (ECST). The NASCET trial is a multicenter, randomized trial of 2,226 patients at 106 centers with criteria of hemispheric, retinal transient ischemic attack or nondisabling CVA within 4 months of the study. Patients with a carotid stenosis of 70–99% who underwent a CEA, reduced the risk of stroke from 26% to 9% at 2 years (<0.001). The Europeon Trial demonstrated a benefit from CEA for stenosis greater than 69% and little or no benefit in patients with less than 30% stenosis. In 1995, the Asymptomatic Carotid Artherosclerosis Study (ACAS) a large, randomized study of 1,662 patients with asymptomatic carotid disease and carotid stenosis of 60% or greater. The study demonstrated that the operative group had a 5% risk of CVA compared to the medical management group of 11%. For women, the sample did not reach any statistical significance. In summary, multiple factors are taken into consideration for any patient undergoing operative repair for cerebrovascular disease and the trials demonstrate that surgery in select groups of patients can result in a significant reduction of CVA from a carotid lesion.

NASCET
North American Symptomatic Endarterectomy Trial

ECST
European Carotid Surgery Trial

ACAS
Asymptomatic Carotid Artherosclerosis Study

Related Procedures

Coronary artery bypass grafting may be necessary.

Nursing Implications

Anesthesia

Anesthesia for the carotid endarterectomy patient is critical as it relates to selection of anesthesia type. There is a 5% to 7% risk of perioperative stroke associated with carotid endarterectomy (Bond, 2003). A thorough assessment prior to procedure includes a cardiac, pulmonary, and neurological history. Cardiac and neurological risks are explained to the patient by the anesthesia provider and surgeon. The procedure can be performed under regional or general anesthesia. Although there is much controversy about the advantages of the local or regional technique, the main advantage is the ability to monitor the patient's neurological status during the procedure and decreased hemodynamic lability. A deep cervical plexus block is most often used. This technique varies from a single-injection interscalene approach to multiple injections of the transverse processes of C2, C3, and C4. The amount of local anesthetic agent administered is determined by patient size and the desired effect.

There is no clear evidence that the use of one anesthetic agent for general anesthesia is recommended over another for carotid endarterectomy. The choice of anesthetic agent is based on the patient's preexisting medical conditions and the best outcome. Monitoring for carotid endarterectomy generally includes direct arterial pressure, five-lead ECG monitoring, precordial heart beat, and temperature. There are a variety of neurological monitoring technology that may be applied that include, but

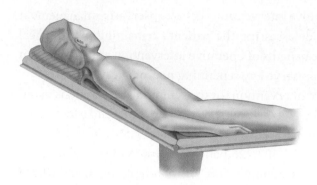

Figure 21.2

Position of patient for carotid endarterectomy.

not limited to: electroencephalography (EEG) signals, somatosensory evoked potentials (SSEPs), near infrared spectroscopy (NIRS) and transcarnial doppler.

Position

Place the patient in supine position with the arms tucked at the sides. Rotate the patient's head toward the unaffected side approximately 60 degrees to expose the operative site (**Fig. 21.2**). Support the patient's head with a dense foam or a gel headrest. To hold the patient's position, apply wide adhesive tape from one side of the bed, across the patient's forehead, over the bi-spectral index monitoring strip and secure on the opposite bed side. Place a gel bolster under the patient's shoulders to hyperextend the neck.

Establishing and Maintaining the Sterile Field

The skin preparation is conducted with solution of the surgeon's choice. Adequate time must be allowed for any product that contains alcohol to dry to reduce fire hazard potential. Place a cotton ball in the ear canal to prevent entrance of the preparation solution. Prep the neck at the incision site then work down to the clavicle level to the chest midline, continuing from the incision site up to the bottom of the ear, and including all areas of the posterior neck. The incision is draped with disposable towels and covered with impregnated adhesive drape. A full-length laparotomy drape is placed over the incision area. The right or the left lower leg may be prepped in case a saphenous vein patch is necessary.

Equipment and Supplies

In addition to major and minor instrument sets, vascular procedures will require specially designed, delicate instruments. Specialty instruments commonly contained in a vascular set are listed in **Table 21.2**.

Physiological Monitoring

Basic monitoring for endarterectomy patients includes electrocardiography. intra-arterial catheters, monitoring of cerebral perfusion, and pulse oximetry. Continuous monitoring of blood pressure is essential because sudden changes in the blood pressure can occur during the procedure. A central venous pressure and pulmonary arterial catheters are generally not indicated unless warranted by the patient's condition.

Table 21.2	**Vascular Specialty Instruments**
Beck clamps	Coronary dilators
Berkowitz clamps	Fine vascular forceps
Carotid clamps	Fogarty clamps
Castroviejo needle holders	Potts scissors 7.5"
Church scissors	Small iris scissors
Cooley clamps	Vascular bulldogs
Coronary bulldogs	Vascular clamps

Specimens and Cultures

Plaque removed from the carotid artery is collected and sent to the pathology laboratory for examination or per institution policy. Cultures are not routinely taken.

Physician Orders

Typical admission orders include a medical examination with emphasis on cardiovascular and neurological assessment, arteriography, and evaluation of the extent of carotid artery disease (eg, cerebrovacular duplex, cerebral arteriogram, computed tomography and/or magnetic resonance imaging). The patient has nothing by mouth (NPO) for at least four hours prior to the procedure or per institution protocol. Hair may be clipped on the operative side to the level of the earlobe prior to entrance into the OR. Male patients should be reminded during preadmission visit or phone call not to shave themselves. Patients should remain on antihypertensive agent(s) and aspirin throughout the perioperative course. When possible, Plavix is discontinued 7 days prior to a scheduled CEA per direction of surgeon.

NPO
Nothing by Mouth

Laboratory and Diagnostic Studies

Recommended tests include electrocardiography, chest radiography, electrolyte determinations, coagulation studies including a PT, PTT, and hematology study. Patient on anticoagulation with warfarin require an INR. A type and cross-match for two units of whole blood may be ordered. If the patient is receiving a continuous infusion of heparin sulfate before the procedure, an activated partial prothrombin time is ordered.

Procedure

Incision and Exposure

Based on surgeon preference a transverse or longitudinal (vertical) incision will be conducted. A vertical incision is made along the anterior border of the sternocleidomastoid muscle (**Fig. 21.3**). An arteriogram may be used to determine the incision site, and the length of the incision is based on its location and the size of the plaque. Electrosurgery is used to provide hemostasis and divide the platysma muscle. Blunt-edged, self-retaining retractors, such as Weitlaners, are used to provide exposure. The facial vein, which lies across the carotid bifurcation, is divided and ligated with suture. Identification and exposure of the vagus nerve, the internal

21

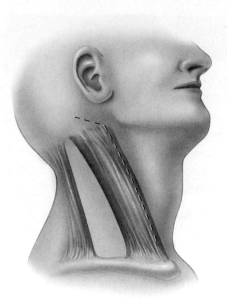

Figure 21.3
Carotid endarterectomy incision.

jugular vein, the common carotid artery, the internal carotid artery, the external carotid artery, the hypoglossal nerve, and the superficial thyroid arteries is accomplished. The internal and external carotid arteries are carefully dissected with minimal manipulation to prevent dislodging the plaque.

Details

The common carotid artery is dissected, exposing the artery and its branches. The assistant should be prepared to assist with the application of vessel loops and carotid clamps. After the artery is dissected and before the artery is clamped, anticoagulation therapy is initiated with the administration of heparin sulfate. Instruments that should be readily available include carotid clamps, knife handles with a No. 11 and No. 15 blade, vascular scissors, vascular forceps, an angled vascular clamp, an elevator, and a carotid shunt. Controversy exists regarding the routine versus selective use of carotid artery shunting for CEA. A carotid shunt is the placement of a silicon tube that functions as a temporary bypass shunting blood from the common carotid to the internal carotid artery during the procedure. The use of a carotid shunt is not without associated risk that may include hematoma, nerve injury, infection, and late carotid restenosis (Howell, 2007). Variations in practice exist among surgeons who may use routinely and others selectively. Suggested indications for selective shunting include the use of carotid artery stump pressure and abnormal EEG. The carotid artery stump pressure is the measurement of the pressure in the Circle of Willis. A carotid artery stump pressure of <50 mm Hg and abnormal EEG is suggestive for selective shunting for scheduled CEA under general anesthesia (Calligaro & Doughtery, 2005). There remains controversy over the use for routine or selective shunting with no research supporting an improvement in patient outcome (Bond, Rerkasem, & Rothwell, 2002).

The carotid artery is clamped, and an arteriotomy is made with a No. 11 blade then extended with Potts scissors. Pressure may be taken of the carotid before deciding if a shunt is to be used. A pressure line with an 18-gauge needle is used. The line is

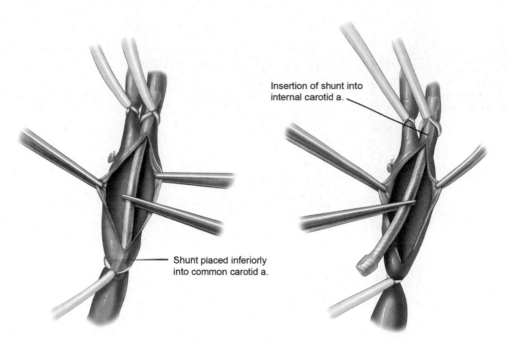

Insertion of shunt into
internal carotid a.

Shunt placed inferiorly
into common carotid a.

Figure 21.4

(A) Insertion of
carotid shunt placed
inferiorly into the
common carotid
artery. (B) Insertion
of shunt into the
internal carotid
artery.

fed to the anesthesia provider over the sterile drape who will connect it to a pressure line. If a shunt is to be used, it is inserted into the internal carotid artery and then inferiorly into the common carotid artery (**Figs. 21.4 A & B**) allowing for cerebral circulation. The extent of the plaque can be identified by the color of the atherosclerotic artery. Where plaque is present, it appears yellowish, compared with a bluish color where no plaque exists. Plaque may be removed with a Penfield endarterectomy blade. The plaque is removed first at the proximal end of the common carotid artery and then at the distal end. Special care is taken to irrigate with heparinized saline to remove any loose remnants of plaque and identify any plaque that remains. If any plaque remains that cannot be removed, it is carefully tacked down with a 7-0 nonabsorbable suture.

Closure

The arteriotomy is closed with nonabsorbable, 6-0 polypropylene suture. Closure is done with a continuous running stitch. If a patch is needed for closure, a synthetic graft or saphenous vein may be used (**Fig. 21.5**). Before complete closure, the carotid shunt, if inserted, is removed. Unclamping proceeds with the distal clamp first, allowing back bleeding and flushing, followed by removal of the proximal clamp. The suture lines are examined for leaks. To aid in controlling bleeding, leaks may be repaired with suture patches and/or oxidized regenerated cellulose such as Surgicel or Oxycel.

The sternocleidomastoid fascia and the platysma muscle are closed with either a continuous or an interrupted suture. To facilitate drainage, a temporary drain may be inserted. Skin is closed with a continuous absorbable suture or staples, Gauze is applied over the incision and secured with tape. A bulky dressing is avoided because of the possibility of concealing a hematoma.

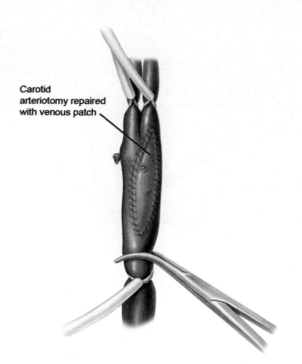

Figure 21.5
Carotid arteriotomy repaired with
venous patch.

Carotid
arteriotomy repaired
with venous patch

Postprocedure Care

The patient is transferred to the postanesthesia recovery area for routine monitoring. Depending on the cardiopulmonary status, the patient may be transferred to the nursing floor or the intensive care unit. To decrease the incidence of complications of bleeding, and thrombosis, avoid flexing and turning of the patient's neck. Elevate the patient's head 20 degrees and maintain it in straight alignment. Use towel rolls or sandbags to prevent flexion and turning of the patient's head for 12 hours after the procedure. The patient's blood pressure is frequently monitored and should not exceed 160 mm Hg to reduce the possibility of intracerebral hemorrhage. Notify the surgeon of a systolic blood pressure greater than 160 mm Hg or less than 120 mm Hg. Neurological status should be assessed every hour, including assessment of the vagus (cranial nerve X) and hypoglossal (cranial nerve XII) nerves. Closely monitor the patient for signs of hematoma. The patient is usually discharged in 1–2 days following the procedure. Some institutions perform this procedure on an outpatient basis on select low-risk patients.

Potential Complications

Potential complications include infection, stroke, emboli, nerve injury, myocardial infarction, and neck hematoma.

RESECTION OF ABDOMINAL AORTIC ANEURYSM, AORTIC BIFURCATION GRAFT

AAA
Abdominal Aortic
Aneurysm

In general, most abdominal aortic aneurysms are asymptomatic and are often discovered as an incidental finding secondary to radiology imaging or abdominal ultrasound ordered for other reasons. Abdominal aortic aneurysm (AAA) is defined as a dilation of the aorta that is 1.5 times the normal diameter (Upchurch & Schaub, 2006). The risk of an AAA is related to rupture which requires emergency intervention for survival. Treatment options include conventional open operative repair or endovascular repair.

Clinical manifestations of an abdominal aneurysm depend on the size, location, and rate of growth. Most AAA patients are asymptomatic. Patients at risk include men between 65–75 years of age with a history of smoking, and/or a strong family history of AAA (Upchurch & Schaub, 2006). Physical examination may reveal a pulsating abdominal mass. Emergent evaluation is indicated for any patient with a known history of aneurymal disease presenting with sudden severe abdominal pain, back pain, buttocks, groin, or leg pain.

Controversy exists about when to operate electively on a patient with an aortic abdominal aneurysm. The debate concerns the likelihood of rupture of an aneurysm 6 cm or larger. Most surgeons choose to operate only if the aneurysm is greater than 5 cm; the average diameter of an abdominal aorta is approximately 2 cm. The risk of rupture increases with each dilation of the aortic aneurysm. The risk for rupture for a 5.5 to 6.0 cm AAA is 9%, 6.0 to 6.9 cm is 10%; and 7.0 cm or greater is 33% (US Preventive Services Task Force, 2005). Mortality from a ruptured abdominal aortic aneurysm varies, with estimates ranging between 50% and 90%. The patient's overall health status and time to the procedure are the greatest influencing factors.

Related Procedures

Related procedures include carotid endarterectomy and coronary artery bypass grafting.

Nursing Implications

Anesthesia

General anesthesia is the most common type, although epidural and regional techniques have been used. If the patient has cardiovascular compromise, the drug of choice is etomidate because of its mild effect on the cardiovascular system.

The abdominal aortic aneurysm patient is at risk for blood loss and significant variations in blood pressure. Monitoring methods include arterial and central venous pressure catheters and the insertion of a urinary catheter. Although blood is cross-matched, the patient should be protected from multiple blood transfusions. The cell saver is a device that collects all suctioned blood, washes the cells in a heparinized saline solution, separates the plasma, and collects the cells to be re-administered intravenously as autologous packed cells. The cell saver should be used on all AAA procedures unless the patient has religious beliefs against the administration of blood or blood products.

Position

Place the patient in the supine position. To allow more room at the operative site, secure each arm on a padded armboard and positioned at a less than 90-degree angle. Place a pillow under the knees to maintain a slight frog-legged position, with padding under bilateral heels. Use a forced-air warmer to maintain normothermia.

Establishing and Maintaining the Sterile Field

Hair may be clipped from the operative site as ordered by the surgeon. Prep the patient from the sternoclavical notch to midthigh and to the table on each side. If using an alcohol-based prepping agent follow manufacturers written instructions for drying times. For emergency procedures, *do not* use a prepping agent containing alcohol because of the necessity to immediately drape the patient and begin the procedure before adequate drying and evaporation of the alcohol. If the disease process extends to the renal or mesenteric arteries, prep a portion of the ankle over the saphenous vein in case a vein graft is needed. Drape the patient, leaving the abdomen and midthigh areas exposed. Sometimes the incision is extended into the femoral areas; therefore, prevent contamination of the field by isolating the genitalia with adhesive drapes.

Equipment and Supplies

In addition to major dissection instruments, provide specialty vascular instruments. Other items to have immediately available include: a selection of aortic vascular grafts in multiple sizes, aortic bifurcated vascular grafts in multiple sizes, vessel loops, vascular clamps, vascular suture, a cell saver, the surgeon's choice of abdominal retractor, nasogastric tubes of various sizes and suction, and a beanbag to aid in positioning the patient.

Ensure availability of all types and sizes of grafts. If the disease extends past the bifurcation of the aorta, the patient will need a bifurcated vascular graft. If not, a tubular vascular graft is used. The types of grafts include woven, which do not leak blood through the walls and do not need to be preclotted, and knitted, which necessitate preclotting with the patient's blood before heparin is administered to prevent the graft from leaking.

If the aortic aneurysm ruptures during the procedure, it is considered an emergency; and every effort must be made to control the bleeding as quickly as possible. The aorta is quickly clamped. When the bleeding is controlled, the procedure can proceed as usual.

Physiological Monitoring

Because the patient is at risk for unexpected blood loss, variations in blood pressure, and possible pulmonary dysfunction, monitoring is critical to the successful outcome of the procedure. Routine monitoring includes the insertion of a pulmonary arterial catheter to monitor left ventricular pressure, cardiac output, and systemic vascular resistance. An arterial catheter is inserted to monitor arterial blood pressure and allow direct access to arterial blood for blood gas monitoring.

Specimens and Cultures

Specimens which may include plaque, aorta or femoral artery are collected and sent after the procedure. Label the specimen, place it in formalin, and send it to the pathology laboratory for examination. Cultures are not routinely taken.

Drugs and Solutions

Drugs and solutions used in the procedure may include mannitol, furosemide, heparin sulfate solution, and protamine sulfate.

Physician Orders

The complexity of AAA resection requires a number of admission orders which may include:

- a complete blood cell count and electrolyte panel
- platelet count
- prothrombin time
- INR
- partial thromboplastin time
- creatinine level
- blood urea nitrogen
- pulse status evaluation
- urinalysis
- resting electrocardiogram
- aortic angiography/magnetic resonance imaging/magnetic resonance angiography
- cross-sectional ultrasonography
- posteroanterior and lateral chest radiographs
- potassium level (if patient is on diuretics)
- blood sample for cross-matching (6 U of packed cells ordered)
- creatinine and serum potassium levels (for angiogram patients)

Patients are admitted on a same-day basis but are required to do some preprocedure preparation at home. The night before the procedure a depilatory may be ordered to be used from the nipples to the knees. The patient is often instructed to shower with chlorhexidine gluconate (Hibiclens) after the depilatory. Bowel preparation of magnesium citrate, one bottle orally at 8 P.M., or polyethylene glycolelectrolyte solution (GoLYTELY), 4 L to start at 6 P.M. the night before the procedure is routinely ordered. This is followed by a Fleet enema. The patient is to be NPO after midnight.

Laboratory and Diagnostic Studies

The results of laboratory and diagnostic studies are reviewed prior to the procedure. Ensure that all results are placed in the chart before the procedure. Report any abnormal values or results to the surgeon and anesthesia provider.

Procedure

Incision and Exposure

An abdominal midline incision is made from the xiphoid to the pubis. Electrosurgery is used to dissect to the fascia. The fascia and the peritoneum are opened with scissors. The abdomen is carefully checked for any other disease process that might cause the procedure to be aborted. A bowel nodule, diverticulitis, and accidental entry into the bowel are causes of possible contamination of a graft and reasons to abort the procedure. The small bowel is lifted from the abdominal cavity and placed into a plastic intestinal bag. The surface of the aneurysm is carefully exposed.

Details

After exposure of the aorta, vessel loops are used to identify the renal and mesenteric arteries. Exposure of the iliac or femoral arteries is accomplished and vessel loops are used to isolate/identify the vessels.

Heparin sulfate is administered before clamping of the aorta. After heparinization, the aorta is clamped with a vascular clamp such as a DeBakey aortic clamp, Fogarty, or Satinsky. To prevent back-bleeding, the femoral and iliac arteries are also clamped with smaller vascular clamps such as Fogarty vascular clamps. The aneurysm is incised longitudinally with a No. 10 or a No. 11 blade on an extended handle. The incision is extended with long, straight, Mayo scissors (**Fig. 21.6**). The thrombus and the plaque are carefully removed from the aneurysm lumen (**Fig. 21.7**).

The graft chosen by the surgeon is sewn into place at the proximal end with either 3-0 or 4-0 nonabsorbable suture (**Fig. 21.8**). A clamp is placed on the graft itself to test the suture line for leaks. Leaks are repaired with the same suture used for the anastomosis. Tension is then placed on the graft, and the graft is cut and sutured to the aortic bifurcation.

If the aneurysm extends below the bifurcation and involves the common iliac arteries, punctures are made in the artery with a No. 11 blade and extended with small vascular scissors. In rare cases, an endarterectomy is necessary to clear the

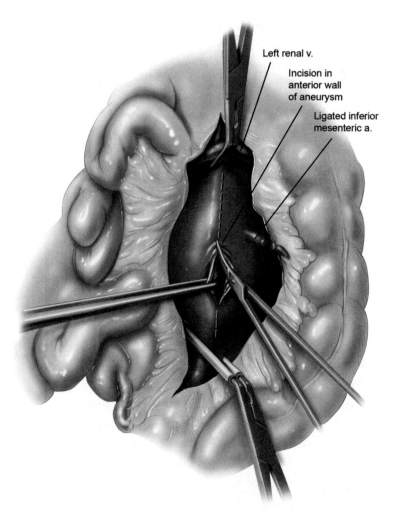

Left renal v.

Incision in anterior wall of aneurysm

Ligated inferior mesenteric a.

Figure 21.6

An incision is made in the mid portion of the abdominal aortic aneurysm. The lumen of the aneurysm is opened and aspirated. Any thrombus present in the aneurysm is removed.

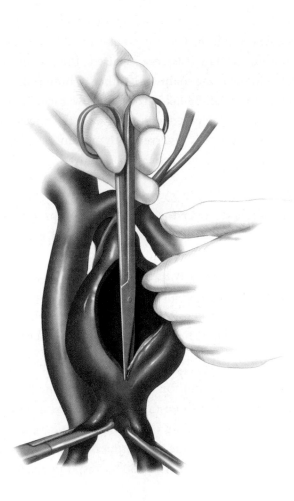

Figure 21.7

Extending the incision of the aneurysm with Mayo scissors.

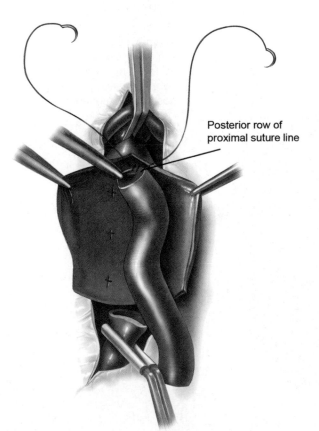

Posterior row of proximal suture line

Figure 21.8

Suturing of the graft begins proximally at the 6 o'clock posterior position, extending on each side to the 12 o'clock position with sutures of 2-0 polypropylene on large needles.

21

vessel completely. A bifurcation graft is used and the graft is trimmed to ensure a proper fit. The anastomosis is completed with 4-0 or 5-0 nonabsorbable vascular sutures. The vascular clamp is removed, and any leaks are repaired. The procedure for the other bifurcation is completed in the same manner. If either or both renal or mesenteric arteries are diseased, a vein graft can be taken from the lower leg. This is sewn into place with a 5-0 or 6-0 nonabsorbable vascular suture. After the release of all vascular clamps, the action of heparin sulfate is reversed with protamine sulfate. All suture anastomoses are checked for bleeding and repaired as needed.

Closure

The aneurysmal sac is trimmed and closed over the graft for added protection from the duodenum and jejunum (**Fig. 21.9**). The peritoneum is closed with 2-0 or other nonabsorbable suture. Typically, a drain is not used to decrease the risk of infection. A visceral retainer may he used temporarily during the closure. The skin is stapled. The genital incisions are closed in the same manner, without a drain. Pedal pulses are assessed and marked with a skin marker. If no pulses are present and no improvement in the color or warmth of the legs is noted, the incision is reopened.

Postprocedure Care

The patient is admitted to the intensive care unit for 1 or 2 days after the procedure. The patient's hemodynamic profile is monitored (arterial blood gases, blood pressure, pulmonary artery wedge pressures, cardiac output, systematic vascular resistance, cardiac index, arrhythmias). Urinary intake and output is monitored; and if it is less than 30 mL/hour, the surgeon is notified. The patient respiratory status

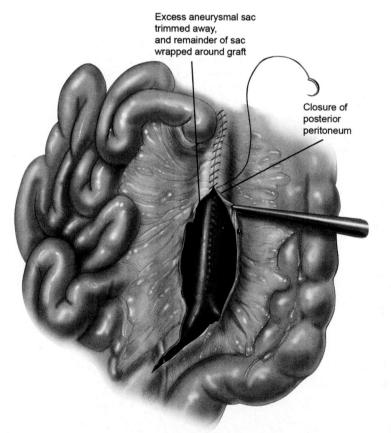

Excess aneurysmal sac trimmed away, and remainder of sac wrapped around graft

Closure of posterior peritoneum

Figure 21.9

The excess aneurysm sac is trimmed away and the remaining sac is closed over the graft to protect it from contact with the duodenum and jejunum. The posterior peritoneum is closed.

is assessed every 2–4 hours, and a chest radiograph may be ordered to detect signs of respiratory failure, adult respiratory distress syndrome, atelectasis, or effusions. Peripheral pulses are assessed every 2–4 hours. Antibiotics and pain medication are ordered. Extensive laboratory data are collected during the patient's stay in the intensive care unit. Ambulation is allowed on the first postprocedure day. If there are no complications, the patient is transferred to the nursing unit on the first or second postprocedure day. The patient is discharged 3–5 days after the procedure.

Potential Complications

Complications that may occur include arrhythmias, bleeding, bowel ischemia, congestive heart failure, infection, irreversible renal failure, myocardial infarction, paraplegia, sexual impairment, suture failure, and trash foot syndrome.

FEMOROPOPLITEAL BYPASS GRAFT

A *femoropopliteal bypass graft* bypasses atherosclerotic arterial occlusion of the femoral artery with a graft. The procedure planned may not necessarily be the procedure performed, because of the unpredictable condition of the patient's donor veins. Since the patency rate is higher with the autologous saphenous vein, it is generally the surgeon's first choice. The saphenous vein in either the same leg or the opposite leg might be unavailable because of occlusion, size, or varicosity. This may necessitate the use of other graft materials, which include other autologous veins (eg, arm veins, human umbilical cord vein), polyester, or expanded polytetrafluoroethylene.

Indications

Patients having a femoropopliteal bypass graft are at risk for loss of a limb with atherosclerotic occlusion of the femoral artery. The patient may have claudication, calf tenderness, mottling, discoloration, and even gangrene of the affected leg. Other therapeutic alternatives include:

- noninvasive, nonoperative medical treatment
- invasive, nonoperative percutaneous transluminal angioplasty
- invasive, laser-assisted angioplasty

The decision on treatment is based on the severity of symptoms and extent of arterial occlusion. The degree of ischemia and severity include ischemic chest pain, ischemic ulceration, and cutaneous gangrene.

Related Procedures

Aortic bifurcation grafting may be necessary.

Nursing Implications
Anesthesia

Anesthesia choices for patients undergoing peripheral vascular procedures include general anesthesia, regional nerve blocks, and epidural or spinal blocks. There is little research that supports one technique over the other. The choice of anesthesia depends on the cardiopulmonary status of the patient. The one that has the least compromise for the patient's physical status is the treatment of choice.

21

General anesthesia is the most frequently used, particularly if the patient has any cardiac compromise. In this case, monitoring methods include pulmonary and arterial catheters to closely monitor hemodynamic status. Anesthetic agents that minimize the effects on the cardiovascular system are best.

A regional block may be administered to the sciatic, femoral, or obturator nerves. This technique depends on the expected length of the procedure and the patient's condition.

Spinal and epidural techniques are used if the patient's condition permits. Advantages include an awake patient and greater pain control and patient management in the postprocedure recovery period.

Position

Place the patient in the supine position with legs in the frog-legged position. Secure each arm on a padded armboard and position at a less than 90-degree angle.

Establishing and Maintaining the Sterile Field

Hair may be clipped from the operative site in the preprocedure area if ordered. Prep the patient from the lower rib cage to the toes on the operative side including circumferentially on the leg, and from the midline to the bed line on the abdomen. Prep any other site that may be used as a potential vein donor site (eg, arms, unaffected leg). Prevent contamination of the field by isolating the genitalia with adhesive drapes.

Drape the patient, leaving the lower abdominal quadrant on the operative side and the entire leg exposed. If the foot is gangrenous wrap it in a sterile towel or place it in a sterile plastic bag at the time of draping to prevent contamination of the operative site.

Equipment and Supplies

In addition to general dissection instruments, special vascular items are commonly used (**Table 21.2**). In addition, grafts of all sizes and types, hemoclips and applicators, silastic vessel loops, Fogarty catheters, vascular suture, and umbilical tape are available.

Physiological Monitoring

Peripheral vascular procedures do not generally include risks related to significant blood pressure variations, large blood loss, and fluid shifts. Monitoring depends on the patient's condition, the anesthesia technique, and the surgeon's preference. Routine monitoring includes electrocardiography, pulse oximetry, and monitoring of blood pressure, respiratory rate and pattern, and temperature. A urinary catheter may be inserted to monitor urine output throughout the procedure.

Specimens and Cultures

Cultures and specimens are not routinely taken during this procedure.

Drugs and Solutions

Drugs and solutions used in the procedure include heparin sulfate solution, protamine sulfate, injectable normal saline, and antibiotic solution.

Physician Orders

Blood is typed and cross-matched for 2 units of packed cells. The patient is requested to shower with chlorhoxidine gluconate, and a depilatory is applied from the umbilicus to the toes. Aspirin may be ordered the night before the procedure. Aspirin may be administered long term for the anticoagulation effects and is found to maintain a better patency rate for polytetrafluoroethylene grafts. The patient is kept NPO after midnight. If an ischemic ulcer is present, an orthopedic bed frame with trapeze and sheepskin is ordered. To prevent decubital ulcers of the heel, protective padding is ordered.

Laboratory and Diagnostic Studies

Routine laboratory tests include urinalysis, a complete blood cell count, chemistry panel, prothrombin time, INR, partial thromboplastin time, platelet count, resting electrocardiogram, posteroanterior and lateral chest films, and blood bank sample. Pulses are assessed and recorded; an ultrasonic flow detector—Doppler—is used to assess patency of vessel and ankle pressures. An arteriogram is ordered. The results of all laboratory and diagnostic studies ordered, reviewed, and placed in the chart before the procedure. Any abnormal values are reported to the surgeon and/or anesthesia.

Procedure

Incision and Exposure

Incisions are made over the skin of the femoral and popliteal arteries proximally and distally to the obstruction. The incisions may be medial, lateral, or posterior approaches. Tissue is dissected down to the vessels, which are held with umbilical tape or vessel loops for identification and isolation.

Details

The patient is heparinized to prevent clotting of clamped vessels. The femoral artery is clamped and punctured with a No. 11 blade and the puncture is extended with Potts vascular scissors. The distal end of the vein graft is anastomosed to the femoral artery using 5-0 or 6-0 nonabsorbable suture. The clamp is removed for a few seconds, with a clamp placed distal to the anastomosis, to test for leaks. Leaks are repaired with the same suture used for the anastomosis.

A tunnel is made to feed the graft down to the popliteal artery. It is important not to twist or kink the graft. The graft should be positioned so that normal leg motion does not twist or kink the graft. Careful measuring ensures that the graft is proper size.

The popliteal artery is clamped distal to the expected graft site, and a puncture is made with a No. 11 blade. The puncture wound is extended with small, Potts vascular scissors. The anastomosis is made with 6-0 or 7-0 nonabsorbable vascular suture. When the entire graft is opened to allow blood to flow from the femoral artery, it is inspected for leaks at both anastomosis sites. The patency of the graft can be documented with an intraoperative arteriogram. Contrast material is injected into the artery, and the radiograph demonstrates its travel to the foot. A doppler monitor with a sterile probe tip is placed directly on the vessel to assess bruits. Pedal pulses are also assessed.

Closure

Subcutaneous tissue is closed with absorbable suture, and the skin is sutured. Sterile 4 × 4 gauze dressings are applied and taped lengthwise.

Postprocedure Care

The cardiopulmonary status of the patient dictates whether transfer is to the intensive care unit or to a step-down nursing unit. The legs are maintained in straight alignment for 24 hours. The patient is usually maintained on NPO status for several hours after the procedure to ensure that the graft is patent and reexploration is not indicated. Routine vital signs are assessed. Femoral and popliteal pulses are palpated every hour. A foot cradle and heel protectors are applied to decrease the potential for pressure ulcers. The patient ambulates on the second postprocedure day. Low-dose heparin administration is discontinued when the patient is ambulatory and aspirin, 325 mg, is continued daily. If there are no complications, the patient is discharged 3–5 days after the procedure.

Potential Complications

Complications may include hemorrhage, thrombosis, infection, graft stenosis, and graft occlusion.

FEMOROFEMORAL BYPASS

The *femorofemoral bypass* procedure is done to bypass an occlusion below the bifurcation of the aorta but above the femoral artery. The graft shunts blood from one femoral artery to the other, establishing complete blood flow to both legs.

Indications

The primary indications for this procedure are limb ischemia and claudication. Several factors should be considered when choosing operative intervention:

1. the extent of arterial runoff
2. the adequacy of the arterial runoff
3. the type of graft material to be used
4. patient comorbidities

Nursing Implications
Anesthesia

See the discussion of femoropopliteal bypass graft.

Position

Place the patient in the supine position. Secure each arm on a padded arm board and position at a less than 90-degree angle. Place the legs in a slight frog-legged position with a pillow as support and foam under the heels.

Establishing and Maintaining the Sterile Field

Prior to the procedure, hair may be clipped from the operative site. Prep the patient from the umbilicus to the groin and extend to the knees. When prepping groin area, take extra time for prepping and drying as these areas are considered wet prep areas with higher bacteria contamination. Prevent contamination of the field by isolating the genitalia with a cloth.

Equipment and Supplies

General dissection instruments along with specialty vascular items are needed for the procedure. Grafts of all sizes and types, hemoclips and applicators, Silastic vessel loops, vascular suture, and umbilical tapes must be readily available.

Physiological Monitoring

Peripheral vascular procedures generally do not include risks related to blood pressure variations, large blood loss, and fluid shifts. Monitoring depends on the patient's condition, the anesthesia technique, and the surgeon's preference. Routine monitoring includes electrocardiography, pulse oximetry, and monitoring of blood pressure, respiratory rate and pattern, and temperature. A urinary catheter may be inserted to monitor output throughout the procedure.

Specimens and Cultures

Cultures and specimens are not routinely taken during this procedure.

Drugs and Solutions

Heparin sulfate solution and Injectable normal saline are part of the drug administration during the procedure with protamine available to reverse the heparin.

Physician Orders

Blood is typed and cross-matched for 2 units of blood. The patient is requested to shower with chlorhexidine gluconate and use a depilatory from the umbilicus to the toes the night before the procedure. If an ischemic ulcer is present, an orthopedic bed frame with a trapeze and sheepskin is ordered. To prevent decubitus ulcers of the heel, protective padding is ordered.

Laboratory and Diagnostic Studies

Routine laboratory tests include urinalysis, a complete blood cell count, chemistry panel, prothrombin time, INR, partial thromboplastin time, platelet count, resting electrocardiogram, posteroanterior and lateral chest radiographs, and blood bank sample. Pulses are assessed and recorded. An ultrasonic flow detector—doppler—is used to assess patency of vessel and ankle pressures. An arteriogram is ordered. The results of all laboratory and diagnostic studies ordered are reviewed prior to the procedure. All results are available and placed in the chart before the procedure. Any abnormal values that would affect the outcome of the procedure should be reported to the surgeon.

Procedure

Incision and Exposure

Inguinal incisions are made over the deep and superficial femoral arteries. Vessel loops are used to identify and isolate the femoral arteries on the distal and proximal ends (**Fig. 21.10**). After the donor femoral artery is located, heparin sulfate is administered to prevent clotting while the vessels are clamped.

Details

A vascular clamp is placed on the unaffected femoral artery proximal to the proposed anastomosis site. The vessel is punctured with a No. 11 blade, and the puncture is extended with small vascular scissors. The graft is sutured to the femoral artery using 5-0 or 6-0 nonabsorbable vascular suture. The graft can be clamped and the femoral clamp removed to test for leaks. Leaks are repaired using the same suture used for the anastomosis.

A tunnel should be made across the pubis through which the graft is fed, using care not to twist or kink the graft (**Fig. 21.11**). The graft should be cut at exactly the length

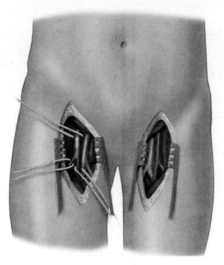

Figure 21.10

Inguinal incisions.

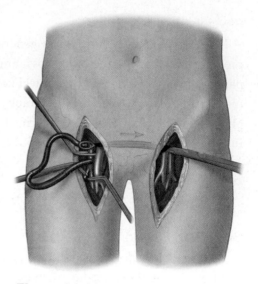

Figure 21.11

Tunneling of the graft.

needed to ensure proper placement. A vascular clamp is placed on the femoral artery on the affected side to prevent back bleeding. The vessel is punctured with a No. 11 blade and extended with small vascular scissors. The anastomosis is completed and sutured in the same manner as the other side. When all clamps are removed, leaks are identified and fixed (**Fig. 21.12**). A doppler is used to document patency of the graft.

Closure

Subcutaneous tissue is closed with 3-0 absorbable suture. Skin is closed with suture and Dermabond is applied. Popliteal and pedal pulses are noted and marked with a skin marker on the affected leg. Sterile 4×4 gauze dressings are applied and taped in place.

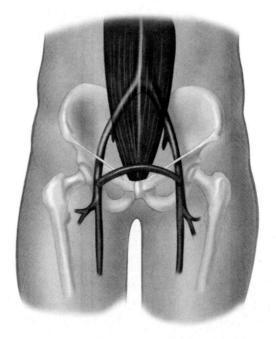

Figure 21.12

Completed anastomosis.

Postprocedure Care

The cardiopulmonary status of the patient determines if transfer is to the intensive care unit or to the step-down nursing unit. The legs are maintained in straight alignment for 24 hours. The patient is usually maintained NPO several hours after the procedure to ensure that the graft is patent and reexploration is not indicated. Routine vital signs are assessed. Femoral and popliteal pulses are palpated every hour. A foot cradle and heel protectors are generally used. The patient ambulates on the second postprocedure day. The administration of low-dose heparin is discontinued and aspirin, 325 mg, is continued daily.

Potential Complications

Hemorrhage, thrombosis, infection, graft stenosis, and graft occlusion are potential complications of femorofemoral bypass.

ABOVE-KNEE AMPUTATION

Amputation is the removal of a limb that cannot be salvaged due to a disease process or pain. Historically, amputations were primarily performed by orthopedic surgeons. Currently, nearly two thirds of all lower limb amputations are performed by general and vascular surgeons.

Indications

Amputation is a procedure of last resort for the patient. Indications for amputation include:

- continuous pain at rest
- previous bypass surgery
- gangrene
- complications from diabetes mellitus
- infection unresponsive to conservative therapy such as
  - administration of antibiotics
  - debridement
  - vascularization surgery

Trauma, burns, and frostbite are additional reasons that necessitate amputation.

Related Procedures

Below-knee and through-the-knee amputation is a related procedure.

Nursing Implications
Anesthesia

The choice of anesthesia for the patient undergoing amputation include general, regional block, epidural, and spinal. General anesthesia is the preferred method. If the patient has comorbidities that do not permit general anesthesia, other methods may be used.

Position

Place the patient in the supine position. Secure each arm on a padded armboard and position at a less than a 90-degree angle. Place the affected extremity on a positioning wedge for access.

Establishing and Maintaining the Sterile Field

Before the procedure, hair may be clipped from the operative site. Prep the affected leg from the groin to the calf. Prevent contamination of the field by isolating the genitalia with a towel. If the foot is infected or gangrenous, wrap it in a plastic isolation bag prior to prep.

Equipment and Supplies

General dissection instruments along with vascular specialty instruments are needed for this procedure. A bone cutter, elevators, rongeurs, and a bone file will also be needed. The surgeon's preference of saw should be available (eg, hand saw, Gigli saw, power saw). The type of power equipment used is dependent upon the type of anesthesia used.

Physiological Monitoring

Amputation generally does not include risks related to significant blood pressure variation, large blood loss, and fluid shifts. Monitoring depends on the patient's condition, the anesthesia technique, and the surgeon's preference. Routine monitoring includes electrocardiography, pulse oximetry, and monitoring of blood pressure, respiratory rate and pattern, and temperature.

Specimens and Cultures

Following the amputation, the assistant places the limb on an isolated sterile draped table for the circulating nurse. The limb is wrapped in plastic, labeled, and sent to the pathology department for analysis. If infection is present, cultures have usually been completed and are not taken again during the procedure.

Drugs and Solutions

Normal saline and antibiotic irrigation solution is used.

Physician Orders

Routine laboratory tests include urinalysis, a complete blood cell count, chemistry panel, prothrombin time, INR, partial thromboplastin time, platelet count, resting electrocardiogram, posteroanterior and lateral chest radiographs, and blood bank sample. An arteriogram is ordered. The results of all laboratory and diagnostic studies ordered are reviewed prior to the procedure. Place the results in the chart before the procedure, and report any abnormal values to the surgeon and anesthesia provider.

Laboratory and Diagnostic Studies

Diagnostic studies assist in determining the level of amputation. Included in the choices are angiography, ankle, and popliteal systolic pressure assessment with a doppler monitor, and transcutaneous oximetry.

Procedure

Incision and Exposure

The level of the above-knee amputation is 4–6 inches (10–15 cm) above the knee joint. A stump of this type will allow for later rehabilitation and application of a prosthesis. The incision is made circumferentially around the leg, leaving a

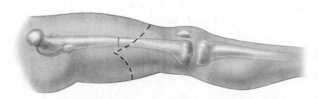

Figure 21.13

Above-the-knee amputation, outline of skin flap incisions, and level of bone division.

longer posterior portion of skin and fatty tissue to be used as a flap, bringing the postoperative suture line to the anterior surface of the leg or the thigh and providing a cushion for the bone stump if a prosthesis is used (**Fig. 21.13**). Tissue and the fascia femoris are dissected, followed by dissection of the muscles down to the bone using electrosurgery.

Details

The nerves and vessels are ligated and allowed to retract upward between the muscles. The bone is severed with a hand or power saw. The exposed bone is rounded with a fine bone rasp. Flap tissue is brought forward and secured with absorbable suture.

Closure

The fascia is closed with interrupted sutures because of the possibility of healing complications. A suction drain or a Penrose drain is inserted deep into the wound. The subcutaneous layer and skin are closed with interrupted sutures with minimal tension. The stump is dressed with a fluffed gauze dressing and wrapped with an elastic bandage or bias stockinette.

Postprocedure Care

Following recovery in the postanesthesia care area, the patient is transferred to the nursing unit. The patient is assessed for pain and drainage from the dressing. Low molecular weight subcutaneous heparin is ordered until the patient is out of bed. Drains are removed on the second or third postprocedure day. Physical therapy is started on postprocedure day 2. The patient is generally discharged in 4–7 days.

Potential Complications

Amputation complications may include failure to heal, residual limb infection, pain, flexion contractures, pulmonary complications, and thromboembolic complications. It is possible that future stump revision may also be necessary.

BELOW-KNEE AMPUTATION

Definition

A below-knee amputation has major advantages over above-knee amputation in the rehabilitation process. If 4–5 cm of the tibia is left intact, it provides sufficient knee motion and facilitates easier use of a prosthesis.

Indications

See the discussion of above-knee amputation.

Related Procedures

Above-knee amputation is a related procedure.

Nursing Implications

Anesthesia

The choice of anesthesia for the patient undergoing amputation include general, regional block, epidural, and spinal. General anesthesia is preferred. If the patient's comorbidities do not allow general anesthesia, other options may be used.

Position

Place the patient in the supine position. Secure each arm on a padded armboard and position at a less than 90-degree angle. Prop the affected leg on a positioning wedge for access.

Establishing and Maintaining the Sterile Field

See the discussion of above-knee amputation.

Equipment and Supplies

See the discussion of above-knee amputation.

Physiological Monitoring

See the discussion of above-knee amputation.

Specimens and Cultures

See the discussion of above-knee amputation.

Drugs and Solutions

Normal saline and antibiotic irrigation solution are used.

Physician Orders

See the discussion of above-knee amputation.

Laboratory and Diagnostic Studies

See the discussion of above-knee amputation.

Procedure

Incision and Exposure

In a long posterior flap technique, the level of the anterior incision is 8–12 cm below the tibial tubercle and extends circumferentially for two thirds of the leg. This area is the base for the posterior flap. The lateral incision is extended distally 5 inches (12.5 cm) posterior to the line of the fibula and directed distally—this area is the flap. The anterior incision is made to the tibia. Vessels are ligated with suture. The nerves and vessels are ligated and allowed to retract upward between the muscles. The tibial and fibular periosteums are cut gently and retracted, and the tibia and fibula are transected. Each bone is smoothed with a bone rasp. The posterior muscle mass is cut along the incision lines, completing the amputation. Care is taken to ligate all nerves and vessels. If posterior muscle mass is muscular, the gastronemius-soleus group of muscles may be trimmed to reduce excessive muscle bulk. The posterior muscle mass is sutured to the anterior tibial fascia and tibial and fibular periosteum.

Details

The nerves and vessels are ligated and allowed to retract upward between the muscles. The bone is severed with a hand or power saw. The exposed bone is rounded with a fine bone rasp. Flap tissue is brought forward and secured with absorbable suture.

Closure

The fascia and skin are closed with interrupted nonabsorbable monofilament sutures due to the possibility of healing complications. A suction drain or a Penrose drain is inserted deep into the wound. The stump is dressed with fluffed gauze dressing and wrapped with an elastic bandage or bias stockinette. On occasion, after dressings are applied, the prosthetist is brought into the operating room and a prosthesis is applied to the stump, preventing deformities of knee flexion and providing comfort on movement. Some surgeons prefer to wait for complete healing—three to four weeks—before the prosthesis is fitted.

Postprocedure Care

Following recovery in the postanesthesia recovery area, the patient is transferred to the nursing unit. The patient is assessed for pain and drainage from the dressing. Low molecular weight subcutaneous heparin is ordered until the patient is out of bed. If drains are inserted, they are removed on the second or third postprocedure day. Physical therapy starts on postprocedure day two. The patient is discharged in 3–6 days.

Potential Complications

Complications that may occur include failure to heal, residual limb infection, pain, flexion contractures, pulmonary complications, thromboembolic complications, and stump revision.

LIGATION AND STRIPPING OF VARICOSE VEINS

Ligation and stripping of varicose veins entails operative removal of varicose veins of the leg.

Indications

The patient with varicose veins will often have physical as well as cosmetic concerns. Deformities of the vein valves and weakness within the vessel walls cause the veins to bulge, discolor, or even rupture beneath the skin. Varicose veins can also cause swelling and night cramps. The patient may also experience pain, fatigue, or aching of the legs, which worsens with prolonged periods of standing.

Related Procedures

There are no related procedures.

Nursing Implications

Anesthesia

Anesthesia choices for the patient undergoing ligation and stripping of varicose veins include general, regional block, epidural, and spinal.

Position

Place the patient in the supine position. Secure each arm on a padded armboard and position at a less than 90-degree angle.

Establishing and Maintaining the Sterile Field

Hair may be clipped from the operative site in the preprocedure area if ordered by the physician. Prep the patient from the groin to the toes on the affected side. Prevent contamination of the field by isolating the genitalia with a towel.

Equipment and Supplies

General minor dissecting instruments along with specialty vascular instruments will be needed. A tourniquet may be used depending on the location and type of varicose veins. See Chapter 11 for information on tourniquet use.

Physiological Monitoring

See the discussion of above-knee amputation.

Specimens and Cultures

Specimens are collected and sent in formalin to the pathology department for examination. Cultures are not routinely taken.

Drugs and Solutions

Normal saline is needed.

Physician Orders

See the discussion of above-knee amputation.

Laboratory and Diagnostic Studies

In addition to the laboratory studies ordered by the physician, the patient is assessed with doppler ultrasound examination and often phlebography.

Procedure

Incision and Exposure

Before the procedure begins the varices are marked with an indelible marker while the patient is standing. Bergan (1990) identified the following basic principles to increase the success of the procedure:

1. transverse ankle and groin incisions/leg and thigh incisions are vertical
2. obliteration of all varicosities with careful subcutaneous closure and approximation of skin edges
3. avoid cutaneous nerves at anteromedial and posterolateral ankle incisions

While adhering to these principles, several incisions are made along the path of the affected vein. The fascia is dissected and a small self-retaining retractor is applied. Blunt dissection using nontoothed dissecting forceps and a peanut forceps is used to dissect tissue around the affected vein.

Details

The steps in a saphenous vein stripping are diagrammed in **Figure 21.14**. The stripping and ligation of any vein include mobilization of the vein. The proximal end of the vein is ligated and divided. A stripper is introduced and fed through the vein as far as possible. An incision is made over the distal portion of the stripper, exposing the vein, which is ligated, cut, and tied to the end of the stripper. When gentle traction is applied to the stripper, the vein should dislodge and come out with the stripper. If it cannot be passed the entire length of the affected vessel, the stripper should be cleaned off by removing the tie at the distal end and peeling the vein from it. It is reinserted after further mobilization of the vessel until the entire length of the affected vein has been removed. This may be necessary on the tributaries of the vein that are distended from pooled blood.

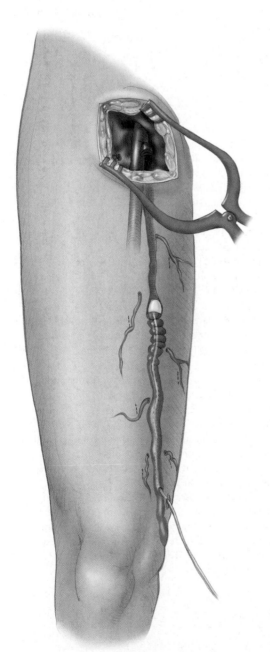

Figure 21.14

Saphenous vein stripping.

Closure

The incisions are closed with 3-0 absorbable suture with Steri-strips used on the skin. Soft dressings are applied, and the leg is wrapped in an elastic bandage.

Postprocedure Care

The procedure is done on an outpatient basis unless contraindicated by the patient's condition. After recovery in the postanesthesia care area, the patient is transferred to phase II recovery. Written instructions specific to wound care, monitoring of infection, administration of pain medication, ambulation, and activity are reviewed with patient and family prior to discharge.

Potential Complications

Complications that may occur include saphenous nerve damage, sural nerve damage, patches of numbness, lateral popliteal nerve palsy, damage to the femoral vein, arterial stripping, hemorrhage, superficial thrombosis, deep venous thrombosis, unsightly scar(s), lymphatic leak, and infection.

REFERENCES

1. AORN. (2008). *Perioperative Standards and Recommended Practices.* Denver: AORN.
2. Bergan, J. (1990). Surgery of the veins of the lower extremity. In Nora, P. (Ed.): *Operative surgery: Principles and techniques* (3rd ed.). Philadelphia: W. B. Sanders.
3. Biller, J., and Thies, W.H. (2000). When to operate in carotid artery disease. *American Family Physician.* 61(2) (January 15, 2000); 400–406.
4. Bond, R., Rerkasem, K., and Rothwell, P.M. (2002). Routine or selective carotid artery shunting for carotid endarterectomy (and different methods of monitoring in selective shunting). Cochrane *Database of Systematic Reviews 2002. Issue 1.* Art. No: CD000190. DOI: 10.1002/14651858.CD000190.
5. Calligaro, K. & Dougherty, M. (2005). Correlation of carotid artery stump pressure and neurologic changes during 474 carotid endarterectomies performed in awake patients. *Journal of Vascular Surgery,* 42(4); 684–689.
6. Dorland, N. (Ed.). (2007). *Dorland's Illustrated Medical Dictionary* (31st ed) Philadelphia: W.B. Saunders.
7. Europeon Carotid Surgery Trialists' Collaborative Group (1991). Randomized trial of endarterectomy for recently symptomatic carotid stenosis: final results of the MRC Europeon Carotid Surgery Trial (ECST). *Lancet,* 351; 1379–1387.
8. Hachinski, V. (2008) World stroke day 2008. "Little strokes, big trouble. *Stroke,* 39; 2407–2408.
9. Howell, S.J. (2007). Carotid endarterectomy. *British Journal of Anesthesia,* 99(1); 119–131.
10. Leary, M.C., and Saver, J.L. (2003). Annual incidence of first silent stroke in the United States. A preliminary estimate. *Cerebrovascular Disease,* 16(3); 288–285.
11. North American Symptomatic Carotid Endarterectomy Trial Collaborators (1991). Beneficial effect of carotid endarterectomy in symptomatic patients with high-grade carotid stenosis. *New England Journal Medicine* 325; 445–453.
12. No author. (2008). Aortic aneurysm. Wikipedia, The Free Encyclopedia. Accessed May 31, 2008 at http://en.wikipedia.org/wiki/Aortic_aneurysm.
13. Rothrock, J. (2005). *Alexander's care of the patient in surgery* (13th ed.), St. Louis: Mosby.
14. Sandmann, W. (1992). Carotid endarterectomy. In Bell, P., Jamieson, C., & Vaughan, R. (Eds). Surgical Management of Vascular Disease. Philadelphia: W.B. Sanders.
15. Smeltzer, S., Bare, B., Henkle, J., and Cheever, K. (2006). *Brunner & Suddarth's Textbook of Medical-surgical Nursing* (11th ed.). Philadelphia: J. B. Lippincott.
16. Ulmer, B.C. (2007). Electrosurgery: history and fundamentals. *Perioperative Nursing Clinics,* 2(2); 89–101.
17. US Preventive Services Task Force (2005). Screening to abdominal aortic aneurysm: recommendation statement. *Ann Intern Med,* 142; 198–202.
18. Zarins, C. & Glagov, S. (1996). Pathophysiology of vascular disease. In White, R. & Fogarty, T. (Eds.): *Peripheral Endovascular Interventions.* St. Louis: Mosby Year Book.
19. Zwolak, R. & Cronenwett, J. (1990). Pathophysiology of vascular disease. In Yeager, M. & Glass, D. (Eds): *Anesthesiology and Vascular Surgery.* Norwalk, CT: Appleton & Lange.

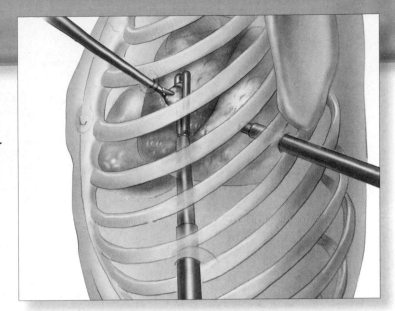

CHAPTER 22

Thoracic Surgery

Jeff Reichardt

INTRODUCTION

Thoracic surgery involves operative and invasive procedures within the limits of the thoracic cavity, with the exception of cardiac surgery which is covered separately. Thoracic surgery covers many types of procedures. Included in this chapter are procedures involving the lungs, pleura, and the mediastinum. Some thoracic procedures have been done in the same way for many years. Others, however, have changed and evolved as surgical instrumentation has changed and improved. The advent of minimally invasive techniques and robotic surgery and the impact they have had on the thoracic surgery is also discussed.

ANATOMY

The thorax is defined anteriorly by the sternum and costal cartilages, laterally by the 12 pair of ribs, and posteriorly by the 12 thoracic vertebrae. The superior extent of the thorax is at the root of the neck at Sibson's fascia. The inferior extent of the thorax is at the diaphragm.

The sternum is divided into three parts: (1) the superior portion, or manubrium; (2) the midportion, or gladiolus; and (3) the most inferior portion, or xiphoid process. The manubrium is connected to the clavicles and the first two pairs of ribs. The gladiolus is the point of attachment for rib pairs three to seven (the remaining true ribs). The 8th, 9th, and 10th rib pairs articulate with the costal cartilages of the rib above; the 11th and 12th rib pairs are not attached to the costal arch. Each pair of ribs articulates with the corresponding thoracic vertebrae posteriorly (**Fig. 22.1**).

Chapter Contents

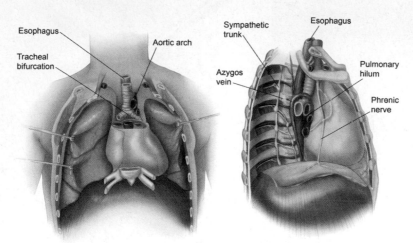

Figure 22.1

Frontal and right lateral view of the mediastinum illustrating major normal structures.

There are 11 pairs of intercostal muscles. Each pair has an internal and an external muscle. An intercostal artery, vein, and nerve are found with each muscle. The origin of the arterial blood supply is the internal thoracic artery anteriorly and the aorta posteriorly. The venous system empties into the mammary veins anteriorly and into the azygos and hemiazygos veins posteriorly. Great care must be taken to avoid damage to the intercostal nerve in each space. When necessary to disturb an intercostal nerve, some form of anesthetic agent should be used to prevent postprocedure pain.

A discussion of thoracic anatomy would be incomplete without the mention of thoracic outlet syndrome, which is the compression of the great vessels of the head, neck, and arm against the borders of the thoracic outlet. Those borders are (1) the manubrium, anteriorly; (2) the first ribs, anterolaterally; (3) the first thoracic vertebrae, posteriorly; and, (4) the posterior angle of the first vertebrae.

The thorax is further subdivided into the right and left pleural cavities. These cavities contain the lungs. The cavities are separated by the mediastinum. The lining of each hemithorax is called the parietal pleura. The parietal pleura is adjacent to the inner surfaces of the ribs posteriorly and the mediastinum medially, and it covers most of the surface of the diaphragm. The central portion of the diaphragm remains uncovered. Arising from the root of each lung is the reflection of the parietal pleura. At this reflection the visceral pleura begin and cover each lung. Between the two pleurae is pleural fluid that provides lubrication to reduce friction. Normal amounts of pleural fluid range from 0.1 to 0.2 mL/kg of body weight.

The lungs are the primary organs of respiration. Each lung extends from the apices, above the first ribs superiorly and to the diaphragm inferiorly. The hilum, or root of the lung, is where the origins of the bronchus, great vessels, lymphatic vessels, and nerves enter and leave the lung, near the mediastinum. Each lung is divided into lobes by deep fissures. Each lobe has a primary bronchus; this bronchus further subdivides into each lobe, the last subdivision being bronchioles. The right lung is divided into three lobes: upper, middle, and lower. The left lung is divided into two lobes: upper and lower. Interestingly, each lung is composed of segments. Each segment functions by expanding from the center out. Each segment has its own bronchus, artery, and vein.

The blood supply that feeds the lungs originates from the aorta and passes through the bronchial arteries. The numbers and courses of these arteries vary. In general, there're at least one, and sometimes two, to each lung. The pulmonary arteries carry the blood to the pulmonary parenchyma. The pulmonary veins are responsible for delivery of oxygenated blood back to the left atrium of the heart. Innervation of the lungs is part of the autonomic nervous system. The nerves regulate constriction and relaxation of the pulmonary tissues within the lungs.

The main function of the lungs is to exchange gases (oxygen and carbon dioxide) for the body. Movement of these gases is accomplished by expansion of the thorax, causing negative pressure in the lungs and allowing air to move into the lungs. Upon relaxation of the thorax, positive pressure in the lungs passively forces the air out of the lungs. Normal intrapleural pressure ranges are -9 to $-12\,cm\ H_2O$ at inspiration and -3 to $-6\,cm\ H_2O$ at expiration.

SPECIAL INSTRUMENTS, SUPPLIES, AND EQUIPMENT

Basic instruments and supplies, as well as specialty items, are used for thoracic procedures. Customized sets may or may not be preset in a particular institution. The basic instruments are various scissors, forceps, and both crushing and noncrushing clamps. Nonrushing clamps are used when less damage to tissue is warranted, whereas crushing clamps are used when more force is necessary. Dozens of clamps are available for thoracic procedures, and many are specific for the surgeon.

Exposure is an important aspect of thoracic procedure and is provided with the use of retractors. There are multiple hand-held retractors, such as the Deaver, scapula, and malleable retractors. Self-retaining retractors are almost always employed. A notable exception to self-retaining retractor use is thoracoscopy.

Stapling devices are other instruments commonly used during thoracic procedures. Pulmonary staplers have a wide range of applications, especially in thoracic procedures, facilitating resection, hemostasis, and fascia and skin closure. Equipment for a thoracic procedure is specific for each procedure planned. The prepared nurse has the following items close at hand for each thoracic case: chest tubes of various sizes and types, usually surgeon-specific, and some form of closed drainage system, usually agreed upon by surgeon per institutional needs.

BRONCHOSCOPY

Bronchoscopy and a *bronchoplastic procedure* refer to the visualization and manipulation of the bronchi and surrounding tissues.

Indications

A bronchoscopy and a bronchoplastic procedure are ideal for excisional therapy of low-grade and benign endobronchial upper airway tumors.

Nursing Implications
Anesthesia

General anesthetic is usually preferred for bronchoscopy or a bronchoplastic procedure. General anesthesia enables the physician to have complete confidence in the safe management of the patient's airway. It also allows for the manipulation and deflation/reinflation of lung tissue, which expedites the procedure. The patient may be given an antibiotic before the procedure for control of infection and promotion of wound healing. Sedatives and smooth muscle relaxants may be given before the procedure begins.

From anesthesia induction throughout the procedure, the anesthesia provider must constantly monitor:

- setting of the flow meters and vaporizers of the anesthesia machine
- movements of the reservoir bag or ventilator
- the sounds of air movement in the respiratory passages
- the quality of the pulse
- heart sounds
- blood pressure
- tissue color and perfusion
- overt movements
- pupil size and reactivity
- tear flow

The anesthesia provider also monitors the patient hemodynamically. Many patients undergoing a thoracic procedure require adjuvant hemodynamic therapy.

Position

The patient is placed in the supine position. An egg crate or gel mattress is placed under the patient before the procedure for comfort and prevention of pressure ulcers. The mattresses are used when a procedure is estimated to be lengthy. The arms are placed at the patient's sides or extended on arm boards. The decision of arm position is determined by the surgeon or the anesthesia provider. See Chapter 8 for additional information on positioning the patient.

Pneumatic compression stockings may be applied to both legs for the prevention of emboli and venous thrombosis, per the surgeon's direction. Thermal drapes can be used for warmth and temperature control.

Establishing and Maintaining the Sterile Field

Every member of the operative team is responsible for maintaining the integrity of the sterile field throughout the procedure. The bronchoscopic procedure is inherently not sterile; however, because the procedure is done through the oronasopharynx, attention to aseptic technique is needed to decrease the potential for infection by limiting the colony counts entering the body. The patient is covered with sterile drapes. The only area left undraped should be the operative site. The scrub person establishes the sterile field by making sure that all instruments are sterile. Instrument tables are positioned close to the operative field to minimize contamination. The team should continuously be alerted to any breaks in technique that compromise the sterile environment.

Equipment and Supplies

A specialty instrument set is used for a bronchoscopy, along with specialized light sources and a stool for the surgeon. Other items include an adapter for the endotracheal tube, which allows passage of the bronchoscope; suction tubing; suction device; a Luki-type trap; and a bronchial brush. Microscope slides, fixative, multiple specimen containers, sponges, and lubricant are also needed. Fluoroscopy equipment should be available per the surgeon's preference. Radiology safety precautions for all staff, as well as the patient, should be implemented when fluoroscopy is used. Instruments and supplies should be tested before the procedure to ensure that they are functional. The nurse should be alerted to any problems with the equipment during the procedure.

Physiological Monitoring

A nasopharyngeal tube may be placed to monitor the temperature of the patient. Hemodynamic monitoring is usually limited to noninvasive techniques unless otherwise indicated.

Drugs and Solutions

Normal saline for irrigation and antibiotics are commonly used per the surgeon's choice.

Physician Orders and Laboratory and Diagnostic Studies

Preprocedure studies for the patient undergoing bronchoscopy or a bronchoplastic procedure usually include a complete blood cell count (CBC) and renal panel, anteroposterior (AP) and lateral chest radiographs, and, when indicated, computed tomography (CT) or magnetic resonance imaging (MRI). An electrocardiogram is standard as well. The patient is instructed to take nothing by mouth after midnight. Prophylactic antibiotics may be ordered, and the administration of all other medications that the patients taking should be continued unless otherwise indicated.

Procedure

Exposure

While the patient is under general anesthesia with a large endotracheal tube in place, the flexible bronchoscope is passed to visualize the bronchus and subsequent lobes. Biopsy samples can be obtained after complete visualization of all suspected areas. Fluoroscopy may be used as well to guide the surgeon to the desired area of biopsy. When indicated, bronchial washings are obtained through the bronchoscope. A bronchial brushing to obtain tissue for analysis is generally performed during a bronchial washing.

Details

The bronchial tree is visualized by use of the flexible bronchoscope with appropriate light sources. Graspers, cup biopsy forceps, aspiration needle, and brush are used to manipulate the tissues to view and aspirate tissues and obtain biopsy specimens as appropriate. Proper suction and irrigation are essential to the smooth completion of the procedure.

Closure

There is no closure.

Postprocedure Care

Patients are observed in the postanesthesia care unit (PACU) until they are conscious and vital signs are stable. Attention to the airway is the primary focus. Routine orders include oxygen saturation measurements, respiratory care, urine

CBC
Complete Blood Cell
Count

AP
Anteroposterior

CT
Computed Tomography

MRI
Magnetic Resonance
Imaging

PACU
Postanesthesia
Care Unit

output measurements, administration of fluids and electrolytes, and administration of medications such as antibiotics.

Potential Complications

Potential complications are respiratory distress and atelectasis.

PNEUMONECTOMY

Pneumonectomy is resection of the lung. The resection is based on the operative anatomy (eg, right or left). Bilateral pneumonectomy involves removal of both lungs and is performed for lung transplantation with the consequent implantation of donor lungs. The following discussion concerns only unilateral pneumonectomy.

Indications

Lung resections are performed to remove primary or secondary malignant tumors, benign tumors, traumatic ruptures, cysts, and abscesses. The functional status of the lungs is important in assessing the operative intervention required. Previous lobe resection, on the current nonoperative side, is a relative contraindication for pneumonectomy because the limited reserve of the remaining lung tissue is usually insufficient to meet essential metabolic demands.

Nursing Implications
Anesthesia

In addition to anesthesia equipment already mentioned for bronchoscopy and a bronchoplastic procedure, a double-lumen endotracheal tube is used to allow the operative lung to deflate when necessary. A central venous pressure monitor may be required for assessment of the circulation, and a Swan-Ganz catheter may be inserted for assessment of cardiac function and output. Blood warming units should also be available.

Position

For most elective lung resections, the nurse should have positioning devices available to facilitate the lateral position. The patient's arms need special positioning attention to prevent nerve damage and to maximize exposure of the operative field. See Chapter 8 for additional information on placing the patient in lateral position.

Establishing and Maintaining the Sterile Field

The patient is prepared from the shoulder to the hips and from side to side. An impervious split drape is used to cover the operative site.

Equipment and Supplies

In major operative procedures, hypothermia can be a problem. The nurse prepares for hypothermia by placing a thermal blanket on the operating bed. Additional suctioning equipment should be available. In addition to a thoracotomy set, the nurse has a vascular set on the instrument table. Vascular control is necessary in any pneumonectomy to provide a bloodless field and decrease the risk of hemorrhage. The nurse should be aware of specific clamps that are preferred by the surgeon. A large bronchial clamp, as well as a vascular clamp, should be available to occlude the bronchus and great vessels of the lung that is being resected. In addition, long instruments of a wide variety are needed because of the depth of the operative field. A wide variety of automatic stapling devices are generally used to resect and seal the bronchus and some great vessels. Suture used for a pneumonectomy, generally is silk, used for the ligation of vessels to control hemostasis. Ligaclips of some variety are also generally used for the same reasons. Other sutures are available at the surgeon's direction.

Physiological Monitoring

See the earlier section on anesthesia.

Drugs and Solutions

Normal saline, gelatin sponge (Gelfoam), oxidized regenerated cellulose (Surgicel), topical thrombin, and antibiotics are used.

Physician Orders

In addition to typical admission orders for patients undergoing a major procedure, monitoring of the patient's respiratory function is required. Ventilation and extubation of the patient are based on physiological need and response to treatment. Oxygen saturation and blood gas measurements must be monitored closely after thoracic operative procedures. Chest tube drainage must be monitored for amount and type, as well as for pleural leakage.

Laboratory and Diagnostic Studies

Laboratory and diagnostic studies include chest radiographs, MRI, CT, pulmonary function tests, blood gases, CBC, and renal panels.

Procedure

Incision and Exposure

A posterior lateral thoracotomy incision is widely used to facilitate exposure of the structures necessary to view for a pneumonectomy. Most pneumonectomies are performed by resecting at least a portion of either the fifth or sixth rib on the operative side. After the thorax is entered, a self-retaining retractor is placed for optimal exposure. Exposure is maintained for the procedure. Sponge sticks and Kitner dissectors are useful as retraction devices for short periods of time.

Details

Dissection begins at the hilum of the involved lung. These hilar vessels are divided and ligated. Scissors, hemoclips, and suture silk ties are used for the dissection. An automatic, reloadable hemoclip applier is also used for ligation. It enables the surgeon to have better visualization and better control of hemostasis. A bronchial clamp is placed on the bronchus to be resected. The clamp occludes the upper margin of the resected airway. An automatic stapling device is generally used to ligate and divide the bronchus (**Fig. 22.2**). During the resection, hemostasis is achieved with hemoclips and suture ligatures of pulmonary vessels. After the specimen has been removed, it is sent to the pathology department for diagnosis and study.

Hemostasis is controlled by electrosurgery. During a thoracic procedure, there is an inherent risk for an ignition incident when electrosurgery or another heat source, such as a laser, is used. Using electrosurgery to resect respiratory structures such as a lung, a lobe of the lung, or the bronchial tree releases oxygen into the operative field, resulting in an oxygen-enriched environment. In such a case, oxygen can rapidly permeate a dry sponge or seep into or around drapes. Activation of the heat source in this oxygen-enriched environment may result in a fire. Sponges should he kept moist

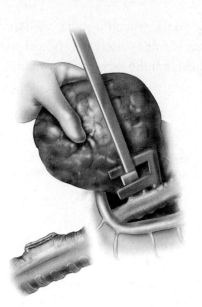

Figure 22.2
Technique of bronchial closure using the stapling device.

in an oxygen-enriched environment, and the electrosurgery unit or laser should be used with extreme caution (ECRI, 2003). Other hemostatic agents include thrombin, gelatin sponge, or oxidized regenerated cellulose. Any or all of these may be used. Massive hemorrhage can be a complication after resection of the lung. Careful attention to hemostasis is extremely important partly because of the need for chest tube drainage after the procedure.

Closure

When hemostasis is achieved, the thorax is irrigated with warm saline. Air leaks are sealed, drains placed, and the thorax closed with suture of the surgeon's preference, such as Vicryl and Prolene suture. Dressings are applied, and the patient is transferred to the intensive care unit.

Postprocedure Care

The patient requires close monitoring and respiratory support following the procedure. Blood gases and oxygen saturation levels should be checked frequently. Careful monitoring of chest tube drainage is needed to maintain hemodynamic stability. Pain control and aggressive respiratory therapy helps to decrease postprocedure mortality and morbidity.

Potential Complications

Potential complications include wound and pulmonary infections, fever of unknown origin, hemorrhage, acute respiratory distress syndrome, and pneumothorax.

INSERTION OF PERMANENT PACEMAKER

Permanent pacemaker insertion refers to the placement of a pacemaker device to restore and maintain proper electrocardiac function.

Indications

A permanent pacemaker is inserted for patients with a variety of cardiac disturbances. One of the most common reasons for placement is third-degree heart block.

Nursing Implications

Anesthesia

The most common form of anesthetic is a local one, at times with some sedation. The local anesthetic of choice is generally lidocaine. Sedation is at the discretion of the provider.

Position

The position of choice is supine, with some form of support between the shoulder blades. The table is generally placed in the Trendelenburg position, at least until venous access has been achieved.

Establishing and Maintaining the Sterile Field

The patient is prepped from chin to nipples and side to side. An impervious drape may or may not be used.

Equipment and Supplies

Manufacturers of pacemaking devices package these devices so as to facilitate their insertion. Sometimes a representative of the pacemaker manufacturer is present during a pacemaker insertion. Their role during a procedure should be clearly defined by institutional policy. Fluoroscopy is needed to advance the wires in this procedure. Therefore, radiology safety precautions need to be implemented. See Chapter 23 for more information concerning pacemakers.

Physiological Monitoring

Cardiac monitoring is critical for this procedure. Any other hemodynamic monitoring is performed at the discretion of the surgeon and the anesthesia provider.

Instruments

Most institutions have developed a specialty instrument set for this procedure. Items included are a knife, hemostats, forceps, self-retaining retractors, Metzenbaum scissors, and pacing wires. All other required items are generally included in the manufacturer's packaging. Most institutions also have a crash cart nearby.

Drugs and Solutions

Antibiotic of the surgeon's preference, lidocaine (1% or 2%), and normal saline are required

Physician Orders

Patients undergoing primary insertion of a permanent pacemaker require telemetry monitoring before and after the procedure. If their condition warrants, the intensive care unit may be chosen through mutual collaboration between the surgeon and the anesthesia provider. If the nurse monitors the patient, institutional policy must clearly state the nurse's responsibility to the patient.

Laboratory and Diagnostic Studies

Laboratory and diagnostic studies include chest radiographs, electrocardiogram, baseline CBC, and chemistry profile.

22

Procedure

Incision and Exposure

The patient is prepared as stated earlier. Upon successful completion of local infiltration, the surgeon uses one of two basic techniques to isolate and cannulate the venous system: either a venous cut down or a Seldinger approach.

Details

Once the venous system is cannulated, a guide wire is inserted under fluoroscopy to enter the heart chamber, or chambers, to be paced. When successfully placed, the surgeon then inserts and tests the lead, or leads. After successful lead testing, the surgeon develops a pocket at the insertion site of the wires to place the generator. This is accomplished by incising the skin and opening the subcutaneous tissue to the level of the fascia. The generator is placed after hemostasis is achieved with a bipolar unit. Because of lower voltages, bipolar electrosurgery is preferred over monopolar electrosurgery. If monopolar electrosurgery is used, the return electrode is placed so that current flow from the operative site is directed away (opposite direction) from the pacemaker. Likewise, because of radiofrequency current leakage, monopolar or bipolar electrodes or cords must not be allowed to lie across the pacemaker. Radiofrequency leakage from the cord or from the electrode itself can cause interference and inadvertent reprogramming of pacemaker. Bipolar electrodes greatly reduce interference. It is best to keep electrosurgery to a minimum. During monopolar electrosurgery, use low power settings and the low voltage waveform (cut current) in addition to the previous recommendations (Ulmer, 2006). Once hemostasis is achieved, the pacemaker generator and wires are secured with 2-0 or 3-0 silk.

Closure

The wound is closed with, in general, 3-0 and 4-0 Vicryl suture. An occlusive dressing is applied, and the programming is checked to coincide with the surgeon's orders.

Postprocedure Care

In addition to routine postprocedure care, telemetry monitoring is indicated until otherwise changed by the surgeon's order. It is also important to get a chest radiograph immediately after the procedure.

Potential Complications

Potential complications include pneumothorax, perforation of the ventricle or atrium, failure to sense or pace, bleeding, and infection.

LOBECTOMY

Lobectomy is the operative removal of one of the lobes of the lung.

Indication

Lobectomy is most frequently accomplished for the presence of bronchogenic carcinomas that do not invade the hilar nodes and are peripherally located.

Nursing Implications

Anesthesia, position, establishing and maintaining the sterile field, equipment and supplies, physiological monitoring, instruments, drugs and solutions, the physician's orders, and laboratory and diagnostic studies are all the same as those for pneumonectomy.

Procedure

Incision and Exposure

Incision and exposure are generally similar to those of pneumonectomy. A rib is usually partially excised. Placement of incision is somewhat dependent on the location of the lobe to be resected. See the section on pneumonectomy.

Details

The primary difference between a lobectomy and a pneumonectomy is the extent of the dissection and the amount of tissue removed. Beginning at the hilar structures, as in a pneumonectomy, the lobe to be resected is identified and its corresponding structures are located. The key to a lobectomy is to resect only that lobe and its blood supply. Careful identification and ligation of the lobular blood supply follows the same course as that of pneumonectomy with the exception that it leaves intact the blood supply to the remaining globe or lobes.

Closure

After hemostasis is achieved, the closure procedure is identical to that of other major thoracic procedures. Air leaks are identified and properly closed. Chest tubes are placed as appropriate, and the lungs are re-expanded before closure to assess function.

Postprocedure Care

See the discussion in the section on pneumonectomy.

Potential Complications

See the discussion under pneumonectomy.

SEGMENTECTOMY

Segmentectomy is the removal of 1 of the 10 segments of the lung.

Indications

The primary indication for segmental resection is bronchiectasis. A secondary indication is removal of benign disease tissue.

Nursing Implications

Anesthesia, position, establishing and maintaining the sterile field, equipment and supplies, physiological monitoring, instruments, drugs and solutions, physician's orders, and laboratory and diagnostic studies are all the same as for pneumonectomy.

Procedure

Incision and Exposure

The incision is made in the usual manner as in all other thoracic lung cases. The primary difference is that the segmentectomy incision can, at times, be limited according to the location of the segment to be excised.

Details

Upon entry into the thoracic cavity, the segment to be resected is identified and then, for the most part, is bluntly dissected manually. Any tissues that extend between the dissected tissues are most likely either vascular or bronchial and in need of ligation. This ligation can be achieved by the many means previously discussed. Once all segmental tissue is ligated and divided, the segment is removed.

Closure

See the discussion on closure for lobectomy.

Postprocedure Care

Follow the same as those for pneumonectomy, although attention should be given to the placement of chest tubes and the reinflation of the lung to ascertain whether the remaining segments have rotated to a poor position.

Potential Complications

See the discussion on pneumonectomy.

WEDGE RESECTION

Wedge resection is defined simply as a smaller area of lung tissue being removed.

Indication

This procedure is performed for localized and isolated disease processes.

Nursing Implications

Anesthesia, position, establishing and maintenance of the sterile field, equipment and supplies, physiological monitoring, instruments, drugs and solutions, the physician's orders, and laboratory and diagnostic studies are all the same as those for pneumonectomy.

Procedure

Incision and Exposure

In general, a smaller anterolateral incision can be made for a wedge resection. Often, a wedge resection can be accomplished with the assistance of VAT.

Details

Once the wedge to be resected is identified, there are two primary ways to perform the procedure. The first involves double-clamping the area around the diseased tissue, in the form of a wedge—hence the name—and excising the tissue. The area behind the clamps is closed with a basting stitch of an absorbable suture. The area of crushed tissue is over sewn with an over-and-over stitch of a nonabsorbable suture, usually silk. The second method involves the use of automatic staplers to achieve the same effect (**Fig. 22.3**).

Closure

See the discussion on closure for lobectomy.

Postprocedure Care

These aspects are the same as those for pneumonectomy.

Potential Complications

See the discussion on pneumonectomy.

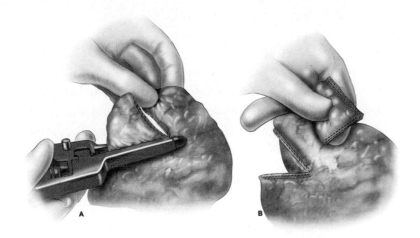

Figure 22.3
Open wedge resection with GIA stapler.

MEDIASTINOSCOPY

Mediastinoscopy is the operative access of the mediastinum through an endoscopy instrument called a *mediastinoscope.*

Indication

Mediastinoscopy is a method used to clinically stage lung tumors. It is also useful in the diagnosis of sarcoidosis. Hiiaradenopathy of unknown origin is another indication for this procedure.

Nursing Implications

Anesthesia

A general anesthetic is the anesthetic of choice for mediastinoscopy.

Position

The patient is placed supine with the neck hyperextended slightly. Positioning aides include rolled towels and a sandbag.

Establishing and Maintaining the Sterile Field

The patient is prepped from chin to abdomen and side to side. An impervious drape may be used. The Mayo and back tables are placed to facilitate overall functionality.

Equipment and Supplies

Along with the general or basic set of instruments commonly used in most operations, a specialty set for mediastinoscopy is employed for this procedure. Similar to a bronchoscopy set, the mediastinoscopy set will include a rigid mediastinoscope to view the mediastinum. A light source is also required.

Physiological Monitoring

General monitoring guidelines are the same as those for pneumonectomy. Patients in these cases usually do not require invasive monitoring. Invasive monitoring equipment, however, should be readily available.

22

Procedure

Incision and Exposure

Incision and exposure is carried out through a 2- to 3-cm incision just above the sternal notch and perpendicular to the line of the sternum. Methods differ on whether to split or divide the muscles to gain entry into the mediastinum. Once in the mediastinum, the surgeon places the mediastinoscope into the area and manipulates the tissues necessary to complete the diagnosis. It is quite easy to damage the azygous vein, innominate artery and vein, or other major vascular structure. The recourse for this is an emergency open sternotomy; therefore, the nurse should have *all* emergency supplies readily available. Once the lymph nodes or other tissues are excised, the mediastinoscope is withdrawn.

Closure

Closure is carried out in the usual manner; care is taken to gently reapproximate the platysma and the strap muscles. The wound is usually covered with an occlusive dressing, and the patient is transported to the PACU.

Postprocedure Care

The patient is closely monitored for subcutaneous emphysema and pneumothorax.

Potential Complications

Potential complications include emphysema and pneumothorax.

VIDEO-ASSISTED THORACOSCOPY

VAT
Video-Assisted
Thoracoscopy

Video-assisted thoracoscopy (VAT) is the use of minimally invasive video technology to manipulate or remove lung tissue.

Indications

This procedure is performed most often for excision of primary carcinomas and secondary site carcinomas. In addition, VAT is useful in the diagnosis and staging of lung disease. It is indicated when the size of tumor, the site of tumor, the patient's condition, and expected outcomes warrant.

Nursing Implications

Refer to the section on pneumonectomy for implications concerning anesthesia, positioning, establishing and maintaining the sterile field, equipment and supplies, drugs and solutions, and physiological monitoring. Equipment includes a video cabinet, with appropriate camera, light source, two monitors, and recording equipment of choice; thoracoscopy instruments; an electrosurgical unit; and specialty instruments per the surgeon's preference (**Fig. 22.4**).

Physician Orders and Laboratory and Diagnostic Studies

In addition to routine admission orders, studies for patient undergoing VAT include chest radiograph, CT scan, and possibly MRI. As with most major procedures, prophylactic antibiotics are administered before the incision is made.

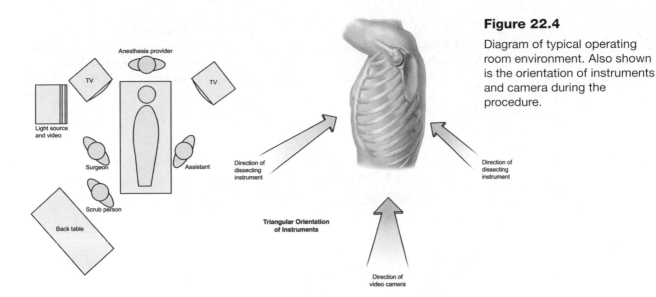

Figure 22.4

Diagram of typical operating room environment. Also shown is the orientation of instruments and camera during the procedure.

Procedure

Incision and Exposure

The first incision usually depends on the proposed operative site after diagnosis. In general, the incision is at the midaxillary line, in the fourth, fifth, or sixth intercostal space (**Fig. 22.5**). If open thoracotomy is needed, the incision can then be incorporated into the thoracotomy incision. If only a VAT procedure is done, the first site is used for the camera. Additional ports are created under direct vision of the hemithorax and are placed to best maximize the work in the field (**Figs. 22.6** and **22.7**).

Details

The primary incision is done to facilitate a 10- to 12-mm thoracic port. Great care is taken to avoid nerve damage in the intercostal space, as well as damage to the lung upon entry into the hemithorax.

Closure

Once hemostasis is achieved, a chest tube can be inserted under direct vision into one of the port sites, Proper placement of the chest tube is ensured by direct vision.

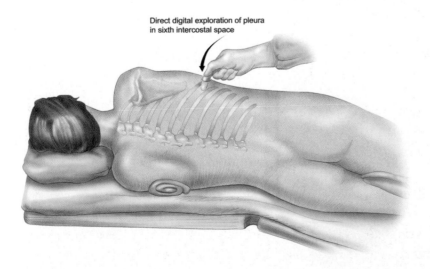

Figure 22.5

Lateral decubitus position for video assisted thoracoscopy.

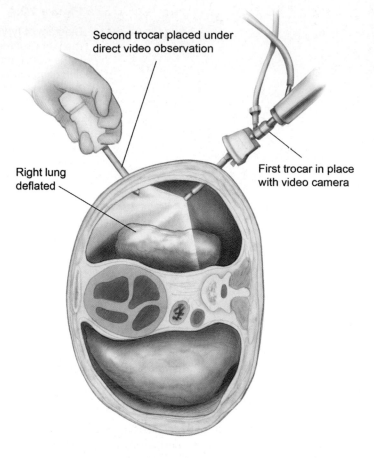

Second trocar placed under
direct video observation

Right lung
deflated

First trocar in place
with video camera

Figure 22.6

Cross section shows deflated
lung with trocars placed
for insertion of camera and
instruments.

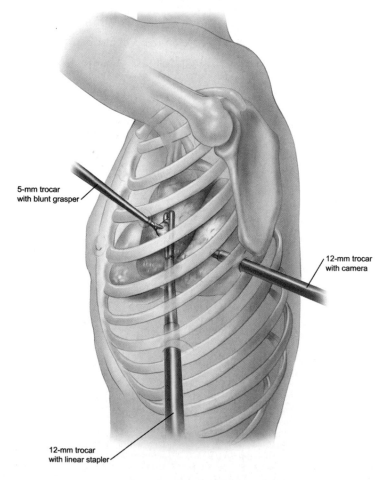

5-mm trocar
with blunt grasper

12-mm trocar
with camera

12-mm trocar
with linear stapler

Figure 22.7

Three 12 mm trocars inserted
through ports for introduction of
instruments and camera in the
collapsed lung for biopsy.

The tube is secured with 2-0 or larger silk suture. Other port sites are closed with Vicryl suture as directed by the surgeon. The patient is then transferred to the PACU for post procedure management.

Potential Complications

Potential complications include wound and pulmonary complications, air leak, and acute respiratory distress syndrome.

THE ROLE OF ROBOTICS IN THORACIC SURGERY

Robotic surgery refers to the use of a robot (such as the daVinci Surgical System®, **Fig. 22.8**) under the command of a surgeon, to manipulate instruments and tissue in the performance of many types of surgical techniques. The techniques vary in nature from diagnostics to tertiary treatments. The use of the daVinci Surgical System® is indicated when there is a need for a minimally invasive procedure, or if the procedure has the need for extreme precision, or both.

Robotic procedures range from the removal of benign schwannoma or other posterior mediastinal masses, to full pneumonectomies. In the case of one such patient, a benign schwannoma was removed by a team of surgeons at the University of Southern California using the daVinci® system (USC Robotic Surgery Institute, 2008). Using the robotic system allowed the team to operate on the patient using a much smaller incision and to delicately remove all of the benign mass. Consequently, the patient had a much shorter length of stay due to less pain and other morbidity issues.

Robot-assisted surgery allows the thoracic surgeon to accomplish the same goal as the comparable open procedure but with less pain, less morbidity and a shorter hospital stay for the patients (**Fig. 22.9**).

Endoscopic Lung Volume Reduction
Indications

The primary indication for endoscopic lung volume reduction (ELVR) surgery is a significant history of bulbous emphysema. The technique is not new. It was first described over 50 years ago by Brantigan and associates (Brantigan, 1959). The last 10 years has seen renewed interest in this concept. However, as stated in Brenner,

ELVR
Endoscopic Lung Volume Reduction

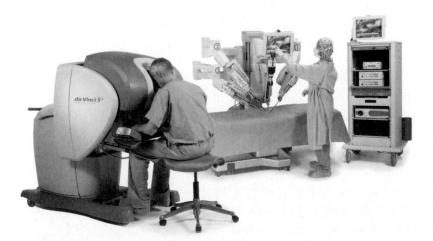

Figure 22.8

da Vinci® Surgical System.

Source: Image courtesy of Intuitive Surgical®, 2008.

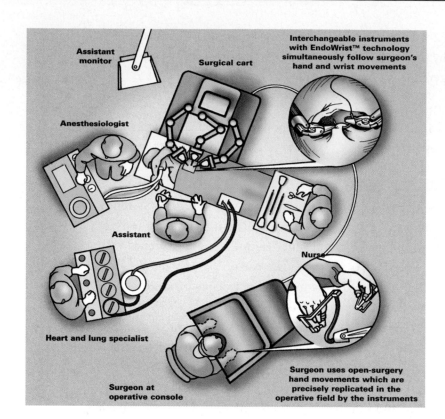

Figure 22.9

Robot-assisted surgery.

Source: Image courtesy of Intuitive Surgical®, 2008.

et al. (2004). "Many aspects of LVRS for the treatment of emphysema symptoms remain controversial. However, extensive literature has demonstrated that carefully selected patients receive benefit in terms of symptomatic improvement and physiologic response." As with any surgical procedure, careful determination of the best procedure for the patient is of utmost importance.

Nursing Implications

ANESTHESIA

A general anesthetic is the anesthetic of choice for the ELVR procedure.

POSITION

The patient is placed per physician preference owing to the specific surgical site. Expect a lateral position if only one lung is involved and a supine position for a procedure involving both lungs. Positioning aides may include rolled towels, gel pads, and possibly sandbags.

ESTABLISHING AND MAINTAINING THE STERILE FIELD

The patient is prepped from chin to the level of the iliac crests and side to side. An impervious drape may be used. The Mayo and back tables are placed to facilitate overall functionality.

PHYSIOLOGICAL MONITORING

General monitoring guidelines are the same as those for pneumonectomy. Patients in these cases usually do not require invasive monitoring. Invasive monitoring equipment, however, should be readily available.

EQUIPMENT AND SUPPLIES

Along with the general or basic set of instruments commonly used in most thoracic operations, a specialty set for endoscopy is employed for this procedure. Likewise, specific specialty items will be employed related to how the lung volume is reduced. The devices used may include: surgical resection with compression/banding devices, endobronchial blockers, sealants, obstructing devices and valves, and bronchial bypass methods. Additionally, the nurse needs to have requisite video and robotic equipment as needed.

Procedure

INCISION AND EXPOSURE

Incision and exposure can be varied. Muscle sparing anterior thoracotomy can be used for this procedure as well as ports for video/robotic access. The literature supports muscle-sparing approaches in most cases of thoracic surgery with the greatest advantage being earlier recovery due to less pain and other co-morbidities. However, there are significant pitfalls to this type of surgical approach. First among those is longer time under anesthesia and the concomitant risk involved therein.

Placement of ports and/or incisions can vary as well, though they are usually placed at easily recognizable anatomic landmarks (midclavicular and midaxillary lines are the norm). If ports are used, the incisions are only wide enough to allow their placement.

Methods differ on whether to split or divide the muscles to gain entry into the thoracic cavity. Once entry has been made into the thoracic cavity, the surgeon can either place an endoscope and other ports for a VATS/Robotic approach, or the surgeon can open the incision further, for a more traditional approach.

DETAILS

As with nearly all other thoracic procedures, there is a risk to damage to major vascular and bronchial structures. The recourse for this is an emergency open thoracotomy; therefore, the nurse should have all emergency supplies readily available. Once the lung volume is reduced and tested, the instruments are withdrawn and closure can begin.

CLOSURE

Closure is carried out in the usual manner; care is taken to gently reapproximate the tissues and to avoid further damage. The nurse should expect to have a variety of chest tubes on hand to facilitate surgeon preference. The wound is usually covered with an occlusive dressing, (as are any chest tubes), and the patient is transported to the PACU.

Postprocedure Care

The patient is closely monitored for subcutaneous emphysema and pneumothorax.

Potential Complications

Potential complications include subcutaneous emphysema, pneumothorax, hemorrhage, and infection.

Thoracoscopic Drainage of Empyema and Decortication

Indications

The primary indications for endoscopic drainage of empyema and decortication are that there has been a wealth of data to support this approach over the open procedure. Substantial decreases in mortality and morbidity have been demonstrated. However, the primary limitation of this procedure is that a lung with chronic empyema may require a decortication. Such a procedure can be accomplished through a VATS/Robotic procedure; however, there is a high rate of conversion to an open procedure.

Nursing Implications

ANESTHESIA

A general anesthetic is the anesthetic of choice for the empyema/decortication procedure.

POSITION

The patient is placed per physician preference owing to the specific surgical site. Expect a lateral position with the affected side up. Positioning aides may include rolled towels, gel pads, and possibly sandbags.

ESTABLISHING AND MAINTAINING THE STERILE FIELD

The patient is prepped from chin to the level of the iliac crests and side to side. An impervious drape may be used. The Mayo and back tables are placed to facilitate overall functionality.

PHYSIOLOGICAL MONITORING

General monitoring guidelines are the same as those for pneumonectomy. Patients in these cases usually do not require invasive monitoring. Invasive monitoring equipment, however, should be readily available.

EQUIPMENT AND SUPPLIES

Along with the general or basic set of instruments commonly used in most thoracic operations, a specialty set for endoscopy is employed for this procedure. Likewise, specific specialty items will be employed related to large bore suction and endoscopic retraction. The nurse needs to have the requisite video and robotic equipment as needed.

Procedure

INCISION AND EXPOSURE

Incision and exposure can be varied. When using a Vats/Robotics ports for access are generally established along the midclavicular and midaxillary line. Muscle sparing lateral thoracotomy can be used for this procedure as well if the need to convert occurs. Generally, at least two ports can be connected to facilitate access this access.

DETAILS

As with nearly all other thoracic procedures, there is a risk to damage to major vascular and bronchial structures. The recourse for this is an emergency open thoracotomy; therefore, the nurse should have all emergency supplies readily available. Once the empyema has been sufficiently drained and the decortication is complete, the lung/lungs are checked for air leaks, the instruments are withdrawn and closure can begin. It is not uncommon for an irritant to be used to stimulate pleural adherence after the procedure. (Typically, sterile talc, though other agents have been employed.)

CLOSURE

Closure is carried out in the usual manner; care is taken to gently reapproximate the tissues and to avoid further damage. The nurse should expect to have a variety of chest tubes on hand to facilitate surgeon preference. The wound is usually covered with an occlusive dressing, (as are any chest tubes), and the patient is transported to the PACU.

Postprocedure Care

The patient is closely monitored for subcutaneous emphysema and pneumothorax.

Potential Complications

Potential complications include subcutaneous emphysema, pneumothorax, hemorrhage, and infection.

REFERENCES

1. AORN. (2008). Recommended practices for electrosurgery. *Perioperative Standards and Recommended Practices and Guidelines.* Denver: AORN.
2. Brantigan, O.E., Mueller, E., & Kress, M.D. (1959). A surgical approach to bullous emphysema. *Am Rev Respir Dis,* 80, 194–206.
3. Brenner, M., et al. (2004). Innovative approaches to long volume reduction for emphysema. *Chest, 1(26):* 238–248.
4. ECRI. (2003). A clinician's guide to surgical fires: How they occur, how to prevent them, how to put them out. *Health Devices, 32*(1); 5.24.
5. Ulmer, BC (2007). *Electrosurgery Self Study Guide.* Boulder: Valleylab/Covidien, August 2007.
6. USC Robotic Surgery Institute. (2008). USC surgeon performs surgical "first" with robotic assistance. *USC Cardiothoracic Surgery* (On-line). Available: http://www.cts.usc.edu/rsi-article-surgicalfirstwithroboticassistance.html. Date accessed: March 11, 2008.

CHAPTER 23

Cardiac Surgery

Patricia C. Seifert

Jill Collins

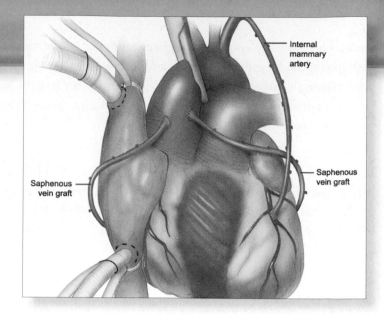

INTRODUCTION

The treatment of acquired and congenital cardiac disease affecting the heart and proximal great vessels has undergone profound changes both at the microscopic and the macroscopic levels. At the cellular level, researchers are investigating the processes of cardiac cellular regeneration and death, genetic sequencing, and the effects of atrial natriuretic peptide hormones, homocysteine, and other biomarkers. This new knowledge about the function of cardiac myocytes has affected the treatment of patients with heart disease by the application of new knowledge to the macroscopic level with innovative and improved operative techniques. Refinements in anesthetic management, preprocedure and postprocedure care, operative procedures for heart failure, and technological advances have expanded patients' choices and provided new learning opportunities for perioperative nurses. Understanding the geometry in valvular dysfunction, the long-term patency of grafted vessels, and approaches to operating on life-threatening dissections and aneurysms of the aorta also has stimulated new surgical procedures. Procurement techniques and the availability of cryopreserved grafts such as aortic conduits and heart valves have greatly improved the survival of individuals afflicted with congenital and acquired valve disease. Mechanical ventricular assist devices have expanded beyond serving only as a bridge to heart transplantation by also serving as end-destination therapy in selected patients. The growing demand for minimally invasive, endovascular techniques—developed in the interventional laboratories—is increasingly reflected in traditional operating rooms (ORs) where previously "open" procedures are currently often

Chapter Contents

ORs
Operating Rooms

performed via a percutaneous, endovascular route. Early discharge, streamlining of services, and an emphasis on financial considerations have also challenged nurses to design and deliver care in innovative ways that positively affect patient outcomes. This chapter addresses the trends and illustrates evidence to assist the perioperative nurse in providing optimal care for the patient undergoing cardiac operative and other invasive procedures.

ANATOMY AND PHYSIOLOGY

The heart (**Fig. 23.1**) is a four-chambered muscular organ about the size of a fist located in the mediastinal cavity between the lungs, posterior to the sternum, and anterior to the esophagus and the descending aorta. The heart's inferior surface comes in contact with the diaphragm. Enclosed in a pericardial sac, the cardiac muscle is composed of three layers: the epicardium, the myocardium, and the endocardium. Any one or all three layers may suffer ischemic injury, depending on the severity of myocardial infarction. The heart is oriented toward the left side of the chest and rotated toward the left side. The right ventricular surface and the apex of the left ventricle are immediately visible upon entry of the chest and incision of the pericardium. Two concepts are important for understanding the orientation of the heart and cardiac anatomy and physiology: (1) the preponderance of electrical activity of the heart travels in a line from the right shoulder to the left foot, and (2) the point of maximal intensity is the fourth intercostals space, mid-clavicular line, which is the position of the left ventricle.

The heart is divided into right and left halves, separated by a septal wall. Each half is made up of two cavities. The upper, atrial cavities empty into their respective ventricles on each side. Thus the right atrium (RA) empties into the right ventricle (RV) and the left atrium (LA) empties into the left ventricle (LV). The right atrium receives oxygen-desaturated blood from the venous system by way of the inferior and superior vena cavae (IVC, SVC) and from the heart's venous system by way of the

RA
Right Atrium

RV
Right Ventricle

LA
Left Atrium

LV
Left Ventricle

IVC
Inferior vena cavae

SVC
Superior vena cavae

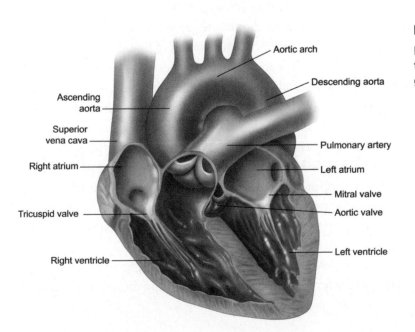

Figure 23.1

Illustration of the heart depicting the 4 cardiac chambers and the great vessels.

Aortic arch

Descending aorta

Ascending aorta

Superior vena cava

Right atrium

Tricuspid valve

Right ventricle

Pulmonary artery

Left atrium

Mitral valve

Aortic valve

Left ventricle

PA
Pulmonary artery

PV
Pulmonary veins

AV
Atrioventricular

coronary sinus (located in the right atrium). From the RA, blood goes through the tricuspid valve into the RV. This blood is ejected by the RV through the pulmonary valve into the pulmonary artery (PA) and the lungs and the pulmonary circulation. In the lungs, blood becomes saturated with oxygen and returns to the left side of the heart via the pulmonary veins (PV). The PVs empty blood into the LA. From the LA, blood travels through the mitral valve into the LV, from where it is ejected through the aortic valve into the systemic circulation (Rubertone, 2008).

The atrioventricular (AV) valves permit one-way blood flow from each atrium into the ventricle. The tricuspid valve on the right side has three leaflets; the mitral valve with two leaflets is in the left heart. The pulmonary and aortic valves (the "semilunar" valves) each contain three leaflets. The function of the valves is to maintain one-way, forward blood flow during the cardiac cycle of contraction and relaxation.

The heart maintains a cardiac output of approximately 5 to 7.5 Liters per minute (L/min) throughout the circulation. As blood enters the atria, intra-atrial pressure increases, forcing the AV valves to open and fill their respective ventricles. The last 20% of volume entering the ventricle is a result of the "atrial kick." This late muscular ejection of atrial blood is absent during atrial fibrillation, resulting in the loss of cardiac efficiency and optimal volume (Seeley et al, 2008).

The strength of ventricular contraction depends on how far the ventricle is stretched when filled with blood. The higher the intraventricular pressure, the more forceful the subsequent ventricular contraction. The rate of contraction (heart rate, beats-per-minute) multiplied by the stroke volume of each stroke constitutes the cardiac output (HR $\times$ SV $=$ CO).

The right and left ventricular outlet valves are much less complex and open and close passively with changes in blood pressure during systole (contraction) and diastole (relaxation). Valvular abnormalities may be corrected surgically or with a growing array of interventional techniques (commonly performed in the cardiac catheterization laboratory). Stenotic valves restrict the blood flow and can cause the heart to enlarge, a condition that reduces the output and efficiency of the heart. Over time, this condition leads to cardiac failure. Incompetent or insufficient valves are a result of leaflet degeneration, vegetation growth, ruptured chordate tendineae, or changes in intraventricular geometry. These changes can produce regurgitation of blood into the chamber from which it originated. This condition increases the workload of the heart, subjecting the myocardium to failure if surgical replacement or repair is not performed.

The left ventricle pumps blood through the aorta into the systemic circulation, supplying all the tissues with oxygen-rich blood. The aorta divides at the arch into several branches, supplying the head and upper extremities, while the descending aorta continues inferiorly, supplying the trunk, abdominal organs, and finally the lower extremities via the iliac bifurcation. Saturated blood travels to the arteries and arterioles of the circulatory system, where respiration takes place, giving off oxygen to the tissues and receiving metabolic waste products which flow into the venous system that returns blood to the right heart.

The right ventricle pumps blood through the lungs via the right and left branches of the pulmonary artery to the level of the alveoli, where carbon dioxide is exchanged for oxygen.

The right and left coronary arteries originate in the sinuses of Valsalva behind the right and left cusps of the aortic valve within the proximal aorta. These vessels initiate the coronary arterial system, which provides nutrients to the myocardium (**Fig. 23.2**). The left main coronary artery, which supplies the left ventricle, quickly divides to form the left anterior descending and circumflex branches. The right coronary artery serves the right ventricle and often terminates in the posterior descending artery. The location and degree of atherosclerotic plaque within coronary arteries coincide with ischemic changes in the heart muscle as evidenced by angina or electrocardiographic changes. If this ischemia is not corrected, irreversible damage can occur to the myocardium. Initial pharmacologic management is often implemented to temporarily dilate coronary arteries or prevent thrombus formation that could result in a myocardial infarction (Fuster, 2007).

The main coronary arteries are visible on the surface of the heart in the epicardium. Along the epicardial surface, points are identified distal to coronary arterial narrowings

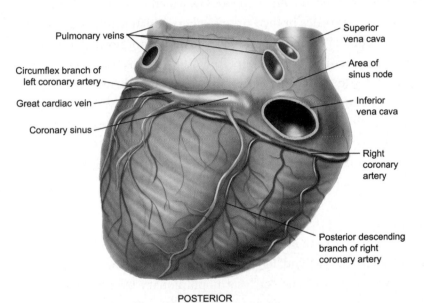

POSTERIOR

Figure 23.2

Coronary arteries and veins.

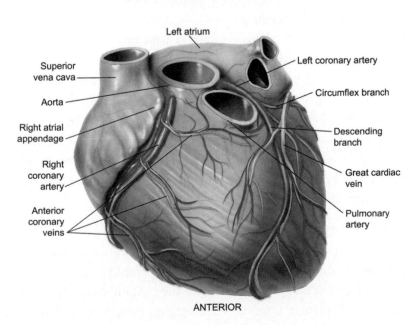

ANTERIOR

for the insertion of bypass grafts (eg, harvested greater saphenous vein or internal mammary artery). Septal perforators are coronary arterial braches of the left anterior descending coronary artery that dive into the septum. Transmural perforators penetrate the full thickness of muscle. The heart's venous system terminates in the right atrium via the coronary sinus; thebesian veins open directly into the right atrial and ventricular chambers.

The heart's conduction system coordinates pumping action. Cardiac muscle cells depolarize independently. Cells with the fastest rate control the depolarization rate of the remaining cardiac cells. In a normal heart, the impulse originates in the pacemaker cells of the sinoatrial node, located in the right atrial wall near the entry of the SVC. From the sinoatrial node, the wave of excitation passes from cell to cell until it encounters a second mass of specialized cells called the AV node. The AV node delays the action potential for 0.1 second, which allows the atria to contract and empty blood into the ventricles before ventricular contraction occurs. From the AV node, the action potential travels through fibers called the bundle of His which divides into right and left bundle branches and terminates in the Purkinje fibers which produce a coordinated ventricular contraction (Wagner, 2008). If conduction is not normal, the heart will initiate rescue maneuvers and initiate impulses from various areas within the conduction system. The rate and character of impulses can clearly identify the initiating site. Abnormal conduction sites or tissue can be ablated (ie, destroyed) in an effort to stem aberrant and multiple foci that may cause dysrhythmias. These dysrhythmic periods may cause the heart to fail as an effective pump. Conduction tissue is also subject to blunt or penetrating injury as a result of trauma or surgical procedures in which conduction tissue within the myocardium is incised or otherwise injured.

NURSING IMPLICATIONS

Procedures in the OR have become increasingly complex and varied. Patients also tend to have more advanced disease and higher acuity levels. Nurses must be familiar with resuscitation equipment, "on" and "off" cardiopulmonary bypass techniques, equipment trouble-shooting, and knowledge of new technologies such as endoscopic, robotic, and/or minimally invasive procedures.

These trends in cardiac procedures challenge nurses who provide care during operative and invasive procedures to expand their knowledge into new areas. Moving patients safely and expeditiously through the perioperative period requires a working knowledge of critical concepts, pharmacology, mechanical ventilation, cardiac assist devices, and hemodynamic monitoring, as well as basic perioperative nursing skills such as infection control, asepsis, positioning, and anxiety reduction (AORN, 2008). Nurses play a critical role in coordinating patient care and, consequently, regularly employ their skills in communicating and collaborating with all members of the surgical team (Seifert, 2008).

Environmental Considerations

The physical environment is a critical factor in the provision of safe care for patients and staff. The OR should be free of physical hazards such as faulty equipment or frayed electrical cords and should have a mechanism for the containment of biohazards. Ambient temperature control is important for keeping the patient warm on entry to the OR (to reduce myocardial oxygen consumption) and during post-bypass rewarming, and cool during periods of bypass when a lower body (and myocardial) temperature facilitates myocardial protection. There should be adequate space for emergency equipment such as defibrillators, bypass machines, intra-aortic balloon pumps, and ventricular assist devices so that these devices can be placed in close proximity to the patient.

General preparation of the cardiac procedure room should be a consistent for both elective and emergent operations. Changes in supplies and equipment specific to the procedure and the patient are instituted as necessary. Special conditions (eg, diabetes, obesity, anatomic anomalies, and repeat sternotomy) may require some alteration of the standard procedures. Diabetic patients may require additional glycemic control; obese patients may need additional table extenders and protective padding; patients with anomalies may require special prostheses; and patients undergoing reoperation may need additional blood available and special saws to incise sternal adhesions. A consistent routine along with case- and patient-specific questions will guide the nurse in comprehensive preparation.

Clinical Pathways and Practice Guidelines

Lengths of stay for many cardiac procedures have been reduced from more than one week to 4 to 6 days. Admission to the hospital often occurs on the morning of the procedure unless the patient is at high risk or requires special preprocedure evaluation or testing. Same-day admission procedures for these patients challenge the cardiac team members to review results of testing and diagnostic data, reevaluate individual needs, reinforce patient teaching, and determine the need for further teaching. This is accomplished within a small window of opportunity along with preparing the environment, instruments, and supplies needed for the procedure. When nurses visit patients later in the day, patients may have already been extubated, weaned of vasoactive infusions, and transferred to the step-down unit.

There are many new and innovative techniques that support these efforts to "fast-track" patients. Fast tracking of patients having operative or invasive procedures is driven by several mechanisms. Improved perfusion techniques and operative approaches to cardiac problems have decreased morbidity and mortality for many patients. As surgical and nursing knowledge has improved, so have interventions used by cardiac anesthesia providers. Anesthetic techniques and careful titration of postprocedure analgesics have fostered early extubation and facilitation of the recovery of cardiac patients.

To further achieve these goals, clinical pathways are used in many cardiac care centers to guide inter-disciplinary teams by outlining the timing and sequencing of interventions for patients with a particular diagnosis or operative therapy. Pathways are designed to minimize delays, decrease duplication of services, and maximize the quality of patient care. Pathways are used for the care of patients who have a predictable course of illness and are useful for standardizing high-volume, high-cost, or high-risk diagnoses and procedures (eg, coronary artery bypass or valve replacement). Pathway packets may be included in the informational materials provided to patients and families. These packets inform patients and family members what to expect during the course of care. Family members and patients as well as clinicians

PNDS
Perioperative Nursing
Data Set

can use the pathway to measure progress throughout the operative or invasive procedure stay. When the identified patient outcomes are not met, variances are identified and evaluated to see whether a change in the plan of care should be made. Nurses can develop pathways that incorporate elements of the perioperative nursing data set (PNDS): patient outcomes, nursing diagnoses and nursing interventions (Beyea, 2002; Kleinbeck, 2004). It is important to maintain sufficient flexibility within a guideline because individuals respond differently to physiological, pharmacological, and emotional stressors.

Clinical practice guidelines are useful for developing pathways in that they are written at a global level and identify the critical elements required for the care of a patient with a specific diagnosis or procedure (Kleinbeck, 2004). Guidelines are based on expert panels, governmental agencies, and/or published research that provides supporting evidence for practice.

Assessment

The trend to standardize cardiac care should not be interpreted to mean that an individual's special needs are unimportant or unmet. In fact, standardizing setups (eg, Mayo tray arrangement of instruments, location of supplies and accessories) enables team members to focus better on the patient's unique needs because staff does not need to create an entirely new process for each patient. There is a wide variation in pathology and functional health patterns among cardiac patients. Some patients may have been diagnosed after routine physical examination and may be relatively "healthy," whereas others may have suffered severe myocardial damage or have co-morbid conditions, and are expected to be physiologically unstable. In collaboration with the other members of the cardiac team, the nurse should formulate a dynamic plan of care that can be revised promptly as indicated by the patient's status.

History and Preprocedure Evaluation

Many cardiac patients are admitted on the day of the procedure. Laboratory and diagnostic studies are commonly performed before admission to the hospital. The nurse should review the patient's laboratory tests, including but not limited to arterial blood gases, electrolytes, blood chemistry, cardiac enzymes, coagulation profile, and complete blood count. Deviations from normal should be noted and discussed with anesthesia and surgical colleagues. Diagnostic images (eg, chest x-ray films, angiograms) should be available and reviewed. A complete list of the patient's medications also should be available.

Patients also must be assessed for the presence of coexisting health problems and risk factors for heart disease that may impede the recovery and rehabilitation process following operative intervention. Irreversible risk factors (eg, aging, male sex, genetic factors), risk factors that can be reversed (eg, tobacco use, hypertension, obesity, sedentary lifestyle, stress), and others receiving increased scrutiny (eg, hyperlipidemia, hyperglycemia, diabetes mellitus, and behavior patterns) should be assessed (Stewart, 2008).

Physical Examination

The nurse reviews the patient's documented physical examination and also performs a brief review of systems, noting skin integrity, color and turgor; sensory disturbances such as impaired vision or hearing; and level of pain (if any). Patients may be subject to neurovascular compromise and skin breakdown as a result of pressure, low cardiac output states, and immobility of areas that are hidden by the surgical drapes during the operation. Applying the ABCs of basic life support—airway, breathing, circulation—can be useful assessment tool for the nurse. Level of consciousness, mentation, restlessness, sensory changes, and paralysis may all be indicators of perfusion status and should be reported to the anesthesia provider and/or the surgeon. A respiratory assessment can be obtained quickly and with general observation of the effort, pattern, and rate of breathing. If indicated, oxygen can be delivered to the patient.

Hemodynamic monitoring is established in the preprocedure area with electrocardiographic (ECG) leads, an intra-arterial blood pressure catheter, and a pulse oximetry finger cot. Patients with greater acuity may come to the procedure area with indwelling central pressure lines such as a central venous pressure (CVP) line and a pulmonary artery pressure (PAP) line. The patient's status may change rapidly and the nurse needs to be vigilant and have a working knowledge of ECGs, hemodynamic monitoring, and pharmacological therapy instituted in these cases (Seifert, 2008).

ECG
Electrocardiographic

CVP
Central Venous Pressure

PAP
Pulmonary Artery Pressure

Diagnostic Studies

Included in the routine preprocedure tests is a 12-lead ECG or Holter monitor test that displays electrical changes of either acute or chronic nature and points to areas of the heart that are ischemic. The 23-hour Holter monitor correlates ECG changes with activities. Patients will often have had a stress test on a treadmill.

Physiological parameters such as blood pressure, heart rate and ECG are continuously monitored. In some patients who are physically unable to perform a treadmill test, various drugs can be used to simulate exercise conditions.

Anteroposterior and lateral view chest radiographs are routine, and should be available at the time of the procedure. The films (which may be digitized) can provide valuable information about pulmonary status, cardiac size, plaque in the aorta, sternal adhesions in patients undergoing reoperation, and the position of previously placed stents and prosthetics. Other imaging studies such as computed tomography (CT) scans and magnetic resonance imaging (MRI) may be employed. CT and MRI studies are generally used to image the aorta for dissections and aneurysms. Arteriography and angiography also may provide valuable information about the extent of vascular disease.

Transthoracic echocardiography is a noninvasive study that uses ultrasound technology to assess valve function for flow characteristics and quantitate the efficiency of the heart's cardiac output, reported as an ejection fraction (EF). The echo probe is placed on the chest to image the heart. Transesophageal echocardiography (TEE) uses ultrasonography and is used during the procedure. After endotracheal intubation the probe is inserted into the esophagus and the tip positioned behind to the

CT
Computed Tomography

MRI
Magnetic Resonance Imaging

EF
Ejection Fraction

TEE
Transesophageal Echocardiography

heart. TEE not only measures cardiac/ventricular function but also evaluates native and prosthetic valve function, assesses perivalvular leaks, and identifies areas of plaque in the aorta. It can be used also for detecting air in the intracardiac chambers, positioning intra-aortic balloon catheters, pressure catheters, and indwelling cannulas placed for minimally invasive techniques.

Nuclear studies, using thallium or other isotopes, may be performed to illustrate wall motion and perfusion of the heart. These studies also enable clinicians to quantify myocardial function.

Cardiac catheterization is commonly performed to provide information about the extent and location of atherosclerotic obstructive coronary lesions, valve function, ejection fraction (the percentage of blood ejected with each systolic contraction—an indicator of ventricular function), global wall motion, and hemodynamic pressure measurements within the cardiac chambers (see Chapter 33). Radiopaque dye is injected into the coronary arteries to outline areas of narrowing as well as to illustrate the anatomy of the coronary system. Intracardiac pressures are measured in the various cardiac chambers as well as in the systemic and pulmonary circulation. Pressure gradients above and below cardiac valves can indicate the degree of severity of valvular stenosis; valvular regurgitation (reverse flow) is reported on relative scale ranging from +1 to +4.

In addition to diagnostic imaging studies, many therapeutic interventional procedures are performed in the cardiac catheterization laboratory and the electrophysiology (EP) laboratory. Coronary angioplasty with stent insertion is a common procedure performed in the cardiac catheterization laboratory for patients with significant coronary artery disease (CAD). Implantation of pacemakers and implantable cardioverter defibrillators—once almost exclusively performed in the OR, are now performed routinely in EP laboratories. Occasionally, it is necessary to do these procedures concurrently with another cardiac procedure, and perioperative nurses need to maintain competency in these procedures.

Planning and Implementation

Before the patient enters the OR, the nurse will have ensured that the room where the procedure is to be performed is ready to receive the patient. Planning and implementing safe patient care requires checking the perioperative inventory of equipment, instruments, and numerous supplies.

Equipment

Numerous types of equipment are employed in the cardiac OR. **Table 23.1** lists some of the more common devices. Of special importance are items such as the sternal saw, the defibrillator, headlights, warming/cooling devices, suction devices, external pacemaker generators, and energy sources (eg, electrosurgical unit/ESU, cryo or radiofrequency energy sources for atrial fibrillation surgery). Because cardiac patients are at risk for sudden hemodynamic decompensation, all equipment should undergo routine preventive maintenance and be checked for functionality before each procedure. Additionally, there should be back-up devices in the event that a piece of equipment does not work. This is especially important for sternal saws, defibrillators, and external pacer generators, but most equipment should be immediately replaceable.

EP
Electrophysiology

CAD
Coronary Artery
Disease

Table 23.1	**Cardiac Surgery Equipment**	
Equipment	**General Uses/Considerations**	**Safety Considerations**
Electrosurgical Unit (ESU) Defibrillator and pads	See Chapters 11 and 17 Internal and external defibrillation, synchronized cardioversion, pacing, or ECG monitoring Keep internal and external paddles sterile until patient leaves OR Check defibrillator for proper equipment daily (pads, synchronizing cable, cables, gel, EKG leads)	See Chapters 11 and 17 Perform a user test defibrillator each day Check defibrillator batteries and for sufficient printer paper daily If a patient comes to the OR with an internal defibrillator or pacemaker, contact the manufacturer representative to disable the device Do not use pediatric pads on adults, there may be a weight limit for pediatric pads Avoid placement of pads over pacemaker generator or internal defibrillator
Sternal saw	Determine the type of saw to be used on each case (eg, electric saw, portable battery charged saw, pneumatic saw) Determine the type of saw blade to be used (eg, oscillating, size) Ensure all attachments are damage free prior to use and connections are attached properly Determine how surgeon uses a sternal saw blade (eg, facing up or down) Load properly	Saw should be turned off, have "safety" on, or not be plugged in until use When passing the saw to another person, ensure that it is in a position that will not cause injury to the person receiving the saw Turn saw off or on stand-by after and before use Dispose of saw blade after use in sharps container Include saw blade in sharps count
Endoscopes and video router	Used for endoscopic vein harvest Ensure necessary attachments are functional (fiber optic light cable insufflation tubing, endoscope camera, bipolar cable) Turn video router on to monitor for endoscopic vein harvest White balance to adjust camera to light Place video monitor in front of staff member harvesting vein	Fibers in light cable can easily break, check after each use If using de-fogging solution, add to count in miscellaneous items Dispose of endoscopic dissecting scissors in sharps Turn light source off to prevent burns
Cryo-energy and radiofrequency energy (RF) sources	Used for atrial fibrillation surgery Ensure correct energy source per surgeon Cryo-energy probes come in different shapes/sizes Ensure cryo-energy nitrous tanks are opened and turned on prior to use Attach sterile cryo-energy probes to cryo-energy machine Keep nitrous oxide tanks Warm via Bair Hugger	Check nitrous tank levels prior to start of use Bleed nitrous tanks at completion of the procedure, ensuring there is no pressure in the tank prior to removing probes Do not turn cryo-energy probes on between freezes, may cause damage to tissue of patient or staff Keep warm saline available to defrost cryo-energy probes between freezes Cryo-probes need to be sterilized between cases Place RF foot pedal where it cannot be inadvertently activated (fire potential)

	Attach insufflation tubing to suction	
	RF manufacturers use different pre-packaged probes	
	For RF probes requiring irrigation, connect sterile tubing to sterile 09% normal saline 1,000 cc bag and test flow to tips of probe	
	Provide foot peddle for surgeon to use with RF machine	
	Wipe tips of RF probe between activations with moistened sponge	
	Connect RF probe to proper energy source (eg, bipolar or monopolar or isolator site)	
Cardiopulmonary bypass machine (CPB) and cell saver autotransfusion	Operated by perfusion staff	Maintain sterility of all lines throughout procedure
	Encompasses a complete artificial heart circuit, providing oxygenation, pressure, a pumping mechanism, heating and cooling system, and a means to maintain homeostasis through ongoing lab value analysis	Provide correct connectors (perfusion adapters) to connect to aortic and/or venous cannulation
		Prevent air from entering into aortic cannula
	May cannulate for arterial inflow through aorta, femoral artery, subclavian artery, or internal jugular artery	Clamp all pump tubing at maximal fill level
		Keep all cannulas sterile throughout case as there is a possibility of going back on bypass
	May cannulate for venous drainage through right atrium or femoral vein	
	Cell saver is a sterile suction that leads to a complex filter, in which a patient's suctioned blood is recycled into autologous packs of red blood cells that are in re-infused into the patient	
Fibrillator and pacer generator, pacing wires and cables	Provides means to controlling the heart's electrical function during the procedure	Correctly attach venous and atrial pacing cables to external pacer generator
	Fibrillator box requires attachment of ventricular pacing cables to patient	Set ECG rate according to surgeon Discontinue only with surgeon order
	Allows for surgeon to operate on heart without using cardioplegia	Disconnect pacing cables from fibrillator box and turn off once operation completed and under surgeon instruction
	Pacer Maker box used to control patient rhythm post-CPB as patient may have ventricle and or atrium paced	Prevent metal tips of pacing cords from touching; may cause arrhythmia
	Provide alligator pacing cables	

Other Necessary Equipment

"Slush" machine	Heating/cooling machine for saline irrigation, ice	Turn off machine once case completes Check sterile
		Slush drape for holes

Light Sources	Attach surgeon headlight to light source	Replace light bulbs in overhead operative lights as needed
Thermal Devices	Turn operative lights on throughout procedure, unless otherwise instructed	Cover light handles with sterile handle covers, change covers when contaminated and between cases
	Warming devices (eg, Bair Hugger) may be applied to the lower body, upper body, underbody, or around the sides (tube shaped)	Monitor warming device temperature; patients may burn
		Note skin condition if burn suspected; notify surgeon
	Warm blankets	Do not turn on warming devices until directed to re-warm patient
	Warm saline	Human tissue requires less oxygen when in hypothermic state; patients are kept cold on CPB, and are warmed when heart is required to function independently
Transesophageal Echocardiography (TEE)	Required for surgery opening chambers of heart (eg, valve surgery, septal defects as well as procedures where surgeon wants to assess cardiac function, residual air, thoracic aneurysm, heart transplant)	Clean TEE probe before and after case
		Label TEE video tape, and keep with patient records
	Requires TEE probe and TEE monitor	Do not unplug TEE monitor until monitor is properly shut down as patient study may erase
	Used to check efficiency of surgical intervention and detect air inside chambers of heart	Check TEE probe for broken tip and handle with care
		Check TEE monitor cord for frays or non-patent plug adapter
Discard Suction tubing	Used for discard suctioning of saline, or pericardial fluid, or other wasted liquids	Filter all blood through cell savor not discard suction
		Change suction tip after suctioning hazardous liquid (eg, hemostatic glues)

Additional Needed Supplies and Equipment

Foot peddles, safety straps, foam or gel padding, drape supports, batwing, sliding boards, blankets, documentation, computers, printers, hand/foot control electrosurgical units, case/surgeon specific instrumentation, typed and crossed patient red blood cells, and medication box.

Equipment and Supplies to Have Available as Needed During the Procedure

Intra-aortic balloon pump, Ventricular assist devices (VADs), femoral arterial lines, high pressure tubing, sleds, over-arm boards, TED therapeutic stockings, sand bag for positioning, fresh frozen plasma, platelets, cryoprecipitate.

Adapted from Ball, K. (2007). Surgical modalities. In Rothrock, J.C. (Ed.). *Alexander's Care of the Patient in Surgery,* (13th ed.). St Louis: Mosby, 183–227; Seifert, P.C., Collins, J.U., & Ad, N. (2007, July). Surgery for Atrial Fibrillation. *AORN Journal 86* (1): 23–40. Beating Heart Surgery: "Medtronic Octopus® Evolution Tissue Stabilizer" http://www.medtronic.com/cardsurgery/products/mics_octopus_evolution.html. Accessed: February 10, 2008. Medtronic Inc, 2007.

Of critical importance is the cardiopulmonary bypass equipment. Generally this is managed by the perfusionists of a dedicated heart-lung team. However, the nurse should have a basic understanding of this equipment and the principles of cardiopulmonary bypass. Moreover, close communication and collaboration between nurses and perfusionists is important for patient safety.

IABP
Intra-Aortic Balloon
Pump

VADs
Ventricular Assist
Devices

Other types of equipment are devices to support a compromised or failing heart. The intra-aortic balloon pump (IABP) is a counterpulsation device used to improve myocardial perfusion and reduce the workload of the heart. Patients may have this inserted before the procedure following an acute myocardial event or other form of cardiac decompensation in the catheterization laboratory. Mechanical ventricular assist devices (VADs) may also be part of the cardiac inventory (Seifert, 2007).

Instruments

Table 23.2 lists typical sets of instruments for the most common procedures and consist of sternal, vascular, and general (ie, dissecting) surgical instruments. Of particular importance are the vascular clamps. These instruments are created with special atraumatic jaws that minimize injury to the delicate blood vessels that must be clamped. The scrub person in particular should ensure that the jaws of the vascular clamps are properly aligned and free of burrs or other imperfections that could damage the vessel. Vascular clamps are designed to totally or partially occlude a blood vessel. Common vascular clamps include cross-clamps that totally occlude a vessel (usually the aorta or femoral artery) and partial occlusion clamps that isolate a portion of the blood vessel or cardiac chamber (eg, the aorta, the right atrial appendage).

Self-retaining retractors are used to open the sternum (or the thorax). Special retractors for exposing the mitral valve are employed to facilitate viewing this valve (which is often difficult to visualize). A retractor for elevating the left and/or right sternal border is valuable for exposing the internal mammary artery (IMA), one of the most commonly used conduits for coronary bypass surgery. Hand-held retractors are also useful for temporarily visualizing blood vessels or for protecting blood

IMA
Internal Mammary
Artery

Table 23.2	Cardiothoracic Instruments Sets		
Basic Sternotomy Set	**Valve Set**	**Coronary Set**	**Thoracic Aneurysm Set**
Dissecting instruments	Atrial retractors	Delicate instruments	Thoracotomy instruments (for descending aorta)
Sternal retractors	Aortic root retractors	Fine forceps	Rib cutters
Handheld retractors	Handheld retractors	Bulldogs	Rib approximators
Needle holders	Valve hooks and probes	Fine needle holders	Endovascular instruments and accessories
Wire needle holders	Hemostats to tag suture	Coronary probes	
Sternal wire cutter	Long instruments (eg, Allis, Crile)	Webster cannula	
Vascular forceps and clamps	Long needle holders	Micro knife handle	
Aortic dilators	Dental mirror	Coronary scissors	
Tubing clamps	Small curettes		
	Valve sizers, handles, holders		

vessels (eg, the innominate vein, located in the area of the sternal notch, which may be lacerated during opening of the sternum).

For coronary artery bypass grafting (CABG), a special set may be developed containing fine forceps, delicate bulldogs, scissors, and needle holders for the coronary anastomoses. Dissecting instruments for harvesting the great saphenous vein may also be part of the set and include mini-mosquitoes to clamp venous tributaries and vein cannulas for infusing solutions to distend the vein and identify leaking areas that need to be repaired.

Operative procedures for valve disease (most commonly of the aortic or mitral valves, although the tricuspid valve may require repair) may include hand-held retractors, longer needle holders, and hooks and probes to assess the valve structures. Valve instruments expose, debride, and replace or repair the tricuspid, mitral, and/or aortic valves. Accessory instruments include valve sizers (obturators) specific to the prosthesis to be implanted and handles that attach to the sizers as well as the prosthetic valve holder.

CABG
Coronary Artery
Bypass Grafting

23

Suture Material

A variety of suture material is used in cardiac procedures. General closure suture materials such as polyglactins (braided absorbable) and polypropylenes (monofilament nonabsorbable) are used to close wounds. They range in size from 2-0 to 1 USP and come on a variety of needles, both taper and cutting. Polypropylene sutures such as 4-0 and 3-0 are often used for oversewing cannulation sites and repairing large vessels.

For instituting cardiopulmonary bypass, synthetic sutures of Teflon, Dacron, and polyester (braided nonabsorbable, 2-0) are used to create a purse string in the cannulation sites (often the proximal ascending aorta and the right atrium). A tourniquet is placed over the suture ends and tightened down onto the blood vessel. This maneuver holds the cannulas securely during bypass. After discontinuation of bypass and removal of the bypass cannulas, the surgeon removes the tourniquet and ties down the purse strings to close the cannulation sites. Occasionally, the surgeon will oversew the site for hemostasis.

Teflon, Dacron, and polyester sutures are used for insertion of valvular prostheses or annuloplasty rings (see below). The suture is double armed and is also alternately colored (eg, blue/white, green/white—depending on the manufacturer—to minimize confusion with the multiple sutures that are placed close to one another around the prosthesis.

Coronary distal anastomoses (saphenous vein to coronary artery, IMA to coronary artery) are created commonly with polypropylene in the range of 6-0 to 8-0. Proximal anastomoses (vein to aorta) are commonly created with 5-0 to 6-0.

Most cardiac sutures used for anastomoses and repair are double armed, which facilitates sewing techniques used for end-to-end and end-to-side anastomoses. The surgeon will sew first with one half of the suture to anastomose the graft to the target vessel. The other arm of the double-ended suture is tagged by the surgeon or the assistant with a clamp whose tips are covered with rubber shods so that the suture material is not injured. Both the needles and the suture are very delicate and commensurately delicate needle holders should be used on these sutures.

Other Supplies

Cotton or polyester umbilical tapes are used to isolate and retract the great vessels. Other disposable items include syringes, hypodermic needles, peanut sponges (Kittners, cherry sponges), rubber shods, vein graft cannulas, silastic tape to retract the coronary arteries, and red rubber or clear silastic catheters used for tourniquets. Strips or small squares of Teflon pledgets in a variety of sizes can be used to reinforce a suture line or serve as a buttress when sewing myocardium (which tends to rip when the suture line is not reinforced).

Prosthetics and Implantable Devices

There is a wide variety of prosthetic materials used to repair or replace cardiac structures, including patches, valve prostheses, and implantable mechanical devices. Clinicians should be aware of the Food and Drug Administration's (FDA) Safe Medical Devices Act that requires notification of a device structural failure. Nurses should follow their institutional guidelines for reporting problems to their quality improvement department for possible reporting to the FDA. Log books should be maintained within the operative suite to track implants, follow trends, and maintain inventory control (Denholm, 2008).

Patch material may be used for intracardiac repairs (eg, atrial or ventricular septal defects—ASD, VSD), reinforcing suture lines after resection of heart muscle, or oversewing bypass cannulation sites. Patches commonly are made of synthetic materials such as Teflon, Dacron, and polyester, and reflect varying stiffness and porosity. When using these prosthetic materials, the desired effect is formation of scar and healing while producing little or no inflammation. Small pieces of patch material (ie, pledgets) may be cut to the desired size from larger patches, or they may come precut from the manufacturer.

The Dacron graft is most commonly used in aortic or vascular reconstruction and comes in two types: knitted or woven. The woven graft has a lower porosity and is best suited for procedures employing full systemic anticoagulation (where hemorrhage through the graft material's tighter interstices is minimized). Knitted grafts have the advantage of faster neo-revascularization, but they are more porous. Knitted grafts are now commonly impregnated with collagen which reduces bleeding from the interstices of the graft and allows them to be used in situations where systemic heparinization is used. Grafts of two different diameters can be anastomosed to one another in situations where there is an extensive, tapering length of the vessel (eg, the aorta).

Tissue patches can be created from a patient's own pericardium (ie, autograft) or from porcine or bovine pericardium (ie, heterografts or xenografts—tissue from another species). Allograft material (ie, from another human) also may be used to repair large blood vessels. Allografts are usually cryopreserved and must be thawed prior to implantation. Both tissue and prosthetic vascular conduits come in a variety of shapes and configurations. For thoracic aortic reconstruction, sizes may range from 26 mm to 30 mm (or greater), depending on which part of the aorta is involved.

The aorta is the most common area for major arterial reconstruction, but vascular grafts are used to reconstruct other structures such as the pulmonary artery, the subclavian artery, and arteries of the upper and lower extremities. For the lower

---

FDA
Food and Drug Administration

aorta, bifurcated grafts are available and have two "legs" if disease extends into the iliac arteries beyond the aortic bifurcation.

Valve Prostheses

Prosthetic valves fall into two major categories: mechanical and biological. Mechanical valves are constructed on a frame (eg, pyrolytic carbon, titanium, or plastic) and covered with a polyester sewing ring. Commonly, the prosthetic "leaflets" are made of pyrolytic carbon mounted on pivots on either side of the carbon ring. Prosthetic valves may have one or two tilting disks (**Fig. 23.3**). The optimal prosthesis opens as close to 90 degrees as possible for maximal outflow. However, closing less than 90 degrees ensures that an aortic valve will be closed by the column of blood in the aorta at the end of ventricular systole (thereby minimizing aortic regurgitation). Another consideration for mechanical valves is thromboresistance. Prosthetic foreign material promotes thrombosis; therefore, these patients require long-term anticoagulant therapy after the procedure. Traits of the ideal prosthetic valve include: unlimited durability, ease of implantation, hemodynamic characteristics similar to that of the native valve, resistance to thrombosis, silence, and compatibility with the host tissue. Such a prosthetic device does not exist, but currently available prostheses incorporate many of these desired traits (Lehmann et al, 2007; Oakley et al, 2008). Sizers (**Fig. 23.4**) specific to the prosthetic valve should be used to measure the valve annulus.

Some patients with a combination of aortic valve and proximal (ascending) aortic vascular disease require a composite valve-graft prosthesis. The composite prosthesis may use a mechanical or a biologic valve which is attached to the vascular graft.

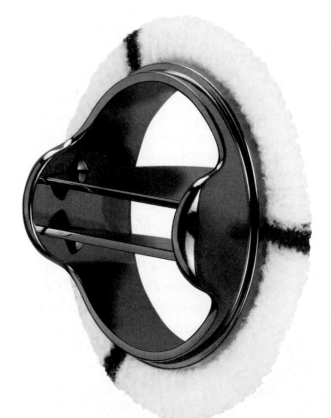

Figure 23.3

St. Jude Medical valve.

Source: Permission to reproduce granted by St. Jude Medical, Inc. Copyright St. Jude Medical.

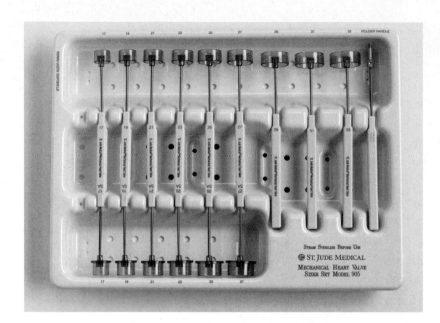

Figure 23.4

St. Jude Medical valve sizers.

Source: Permission to reproduce this image granted by St Jude Medical, Inc. "Copyright" © St. Jude Medical.

When the aortic arch or distal aorta also is involved, an additional tube graft can be anastomosed to the distal portion of the composite prosthesis.

Tissue or biological valves (**Fig. 23.5**) are valves commonly explanted from pigs (porcine) or valves that are constructed from calf (bovine) pericardium. Porcine valves are explanted and attached to struts. Bovine pericardial valves are created by cutting 3 leaflet-shaped pieces of pericardium and attaching them to struts. There are also stentless porcine valves (**Fig. 23.6**); the pig valve and tangential aortic tissue are removed and treated with glutaraldehyde (as are all tissue valves). Before implantation, biologic valves preserved in glutaraldehyde solution must be rinsed for a minimum of 2 minutes each in 3 separate basins of normal saline (total = 6 minutes). After the rinsing procedure the prosthesis should be kept moist with saline to prevent drying of the tissue.

In general, biologic valves do not require long-term anticoagulation. The exception to this occurs when a patient has a pre-existing condition (eg, chronic atrial fibrillation) that requires anticoagulation. In these patients, a mechanical valve is often implanted because the patient already requires chronic anticoagulation.

Cryopreserved allografts (tissue from cadavers) are valuable for patients with infective endocarditis, or who have a small aortic root and require maximal flow to achieve acceptable hemodynamics. Advantages include superior hemodynamic characteristics, less risk of infection, little risk of thromboembolism, and little risk

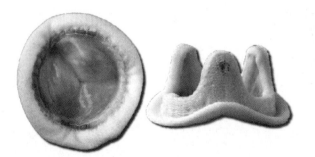

Figure 23.5

Hancock II porcine bioprosthesis.

Source: Courtesy of Medtronic Heart Valves, Minneapolis, MN.

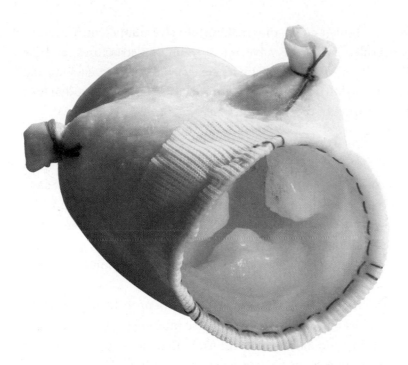

Figure 23.6

Stentless procine bioprothesis.

Source: Courtesy of Medtronic Heart Valves, Minneapolis, MN.

of mechanical failure. There are possible immune responses from cadaver valves; the Food and Drug Administration (FDA) has approved a decellularized human heart valve which has cellular debris from the donor removed. The advantage of this valve, according to the FDA, is that valves treated in this manner may have a lower risk of producing an immune response and tissue rejection (FDA, 2008).

Allografts require proper freezer storage, thawing, and preparation. Several procurement groups supply cryopreserved grafts but the supply does not meet the demand for them. Improved procurement and preservation techniques may increase the supply of allografts; the shortage has stimulated greater use of heterograft (porcine) stentless valves with attached aortic tissue.

Annuloplasty Rings

Preserving the patient's native valve has become the preferred surgical treatment for mitral (and tricuspid) valve disease. There are many reparative techniques aimed at correcting the specific valve deficiency, such as, annular dilatation, ruptured chordae tendineae, torn leaflets. Mitral valve annular dilatation—particularly of the posterior leaflet—is suitable for repair using a ring (**Figs. 23.7 A, B**) designed to reduce the dilated portion of the annulus by cinching the valve annulus and drawing it closer

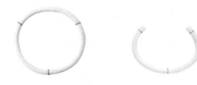

Figure 23.7 A, B

Annuloplasty rings. (A) The ring is positioned around the entire annular circumference (left).
(B) The semi-circular ring is used for repair of the posterior leaflet (right).

Source: Courtesy of Medtronic Heart Valves, Minneapolis, MN.

together to make the valve leaflets coapt, thus making the valve competent. This technique requires less debridement of the valve and surrounding structures, and the result is closer to normal valve function. Patients are evaluated before, during, and after termination of bypass with TEE to assess for proper valve flow, hemodynamic parameters, and characteristics of the valve function.

Immediate Preprocedure Care

Upon admission to the preprocedure area, the patient's identity and surgical procedure are confirmed. The Joint Commission's (TJC, 2008) National Patient Safety Goals stress the importance of patient identification and confirmation of the surgical procedures as well as goals related to assessing (and treating) pain, reconciling medications along the continuum of care, protecting patients from falls, promoting communication among care givers, and encouraging patients and families to participate actively in their care.

Providing safe care includes connecting the cardiac patient to ECG and blood pressure monitors as well as pulse oximetry. The nurse interviews the patient and completes the required documentation, and confirms that the consents (eg, for the procedure, blood, anesthesia, and postprocedure care) have been obtained. If the consents have not been documented, the nurse contacts the physician (eg, surgeon and/or anesthesiologist) to inform the patient and obtain the consent. Operative sites are noted and marked as appropriate; median sternotomy often does not require marking, but nurses should follow their institutional guidelines, policies, and procedures. The circulating nurse will visit the patient and attending family members, answer questions, confirm that consents have been obtained, review laboratory and diagnostic imaging studies, and confer with the preprocedure nurse and the physicians that will be also caring for the patient in during the procedure.

After the requisite information is obtained, the patient may be sedated. Cardiac patients may be highly anxious and may be at risk for blood pressure fluctuations and other hemodynamic changes during this period, so the preprocedure area should have available resuscitation equipment. An arterial pressure line may be inserted in the preprocedure area. Often the line is placed in the radial artery of the non-dominant arm. There may be an exception to this when the non-dominant radial artery is to be used as a coronary artery bypass graft. In this case, the arterial line may be placed in the dominant arm. More invasive, central lines (eg, central venous pressure line, pulmonary artery pressure line) are generally inserted in the OR after the induction of anesthesia.

Entry to the Operating Room

Once the preprocedure preparations are completed, the patient is transported to the operating Room (OR). After the patient's transfer to the operating bed, the nurse or the anesthesia provider places ECG pads to the patient and connects the pulse oximetry device to the OR monitor. The nurse and other team members confirm that arterial pressure and oximetry readings are accurate and within normal ranges. A pillow may be placed under the patient's head, and the hands and elbows may be padded to prevent musculoskeletal injury. The hands and arms are placed along the patient's side and the draw sheet wrapped around the arms and tucked under the patient. The nurse ensures that the patient's fingers are not malpositioned nor impinging upon the metal portions or joints of the OR bed.

During this time, the nurse should be vigilant for acute changes in the patient's hemodynamic stability. Intravascular catheter insertion, anxiety, or medications may cause the patient to deteriorate and cause severe cardiac dysfunction. Induction of anesthesia is a vulnerable period for the patient; premedications and inhalation agents may produce hypotension. In combination with preexisting ischemia, the patient may undergo a chain of events leading to cardiac decompensation. During induction, all OR team members must focus on the patient's status and hemodynamic parameters.

The patient may be anesthetized and intubated before additional procedures are performed. General endotracheal anesthesia is used for cardiac surgery requiring cardiopulmonary bypass. The patient is routinely premedicated (eg, with morphine and scopolamine or midazolam) to allow for smoother anesthesia induction. Anesthesia is induced using a combination of drugs. Inhalation agents are used for intubation and muscle relaxants are given to prevent shivering, which increases myocardial oxygen consumption. Induction of anesthesia is a vulnerable time for the cardiac patient, particularly those with critical coronary stenosis. Many of the agents used for induction have a hypotensive effect, which may produce ischemia in a compromised patient. Once induction has begun, team members should be ready to open the chest and cannulate for bypass if the patient requires resuscitation. Other drugs are used for vascular dilatation or constriction, arrhythmia and rate control, and anticoagulation and reversal (**Table 23.3**).

In some institutions, central lines—central venous pressure (CVP) and a pulmonary artery pressure (PAP) lines—may be inserted before intubation. The CVP line is inserted to measure right heart pressures and to infuse medications and replace volume directly into the heart. The PAP line measures pressures directly in the right heart, the pulmonary artery and pulmonary bed; indirect pressure measurement of the left atrium and the left ventricle also can be performed. The PAP catheter can deliver on-line real-time information such as venous oxygen saturation and continuous cardiac output. Nurses should be alert to hemodynamic changes and collaborate with the anesthesia provider to monitor the patient's status.

After the patient is anesthetized and the central lines are inserted, the nurse inserts a urinary drainage catheter (which may or may not have a thermistor to measures bladder temperature). The urinary catheter prevents bladder distension and by measuring urine output, provides an indication of ventricular function and renal perfusion. Because many cardiac procedures employing cardiopulmonary bypass require some amount of systemic cooling, temperature measurements can be obtained via a bladder catheter thermistor, the pulmonary catheter, esophageal or rectal temperature probe, or other temperature measuring systems.

The "time out" or surgical "pause" (TJC, 2008) should be performed by the operating surgeon during this period—prior to the incision. The entire team of individuals caring for the patient during surgery must agree verbally to the patient's identity, correct procedure, availability of necessary diagnostic images and lab results, and

Table 23.3	Cardiac Surgery Medications

Vasopressors

Drug Name	Drug Action	Drug Use	Infusion Dose
Dopamine	Increases cardiac output	Increase perfusion Shock Hypotension	2–5 mcg/kg/min
Dobutamine (Dobutrex)	Increases cardiac output and contractility	Cardiac decompensation Cardiogenic shock	2.5–10 mcg/kg/min
Epinephrine	Cardiac stimulation	Cardiac arrest Shock Ventricular tachycardia Ventricular fibrillation Asystole	1–8 mcg/kg/min Dilute: 1 mg/10 mL 0.9% NaCl
Norepinephrine (Levophed)	Increases cardiac contractility and heart rate Improves coronary blood flow Increases cardiac output	Acute hypotension Shock Cardiac arrest	8–12 mcg/min Titrate to patient blood pressure
Phenylephrine (Neo-Synephrine)	Contracts blood vessels	Hypotension Supra-ventricular tachycardia Shock	180 mcg/min Maintenance dose 40–60 mcg/min
Milrinone (Primacor)	Increases cardiac contractility Reduces preload and afterload	Congestive heart failure (short term treatment)	IV bolus 50 mcg/kg over 10 minutes) Infuse at 0.375–0.75 mcg/kg/min

Vasodilators

Drug Name	Drug Action	Drug Use	Infusion Dose
Nitroprusside (Nipride)	Reduces cardiac preload and afterload Anti-hypertensive	Hypertensive crisis Acute congestive heart failure Myocardial infarction Decrease operative bleeding	0.5–8 mcg/kg/min
Nitroglycerine (Tridil)	Decrease cardiac preload and afterload Dilates coronary arteries Improves blood flow through coronaries	Angina Congestive heart failure Controls hypotension	5 mcg/min

Rhythm & Heart Rate Drugs

Drug Name	Drug Action	Drug Use	Infusion Dose
Esmolol (Brevibloc)	Antidysrhythmic	Supraventricular tachycardia	Bolus dose 500 mcg/kg/1 min
	Slow AV node conduction	Hypertension	Maintenance dose 50 mcg/kg/min
	Decrease heart rate	Hypertensive crisis	
	Decrease myocardial oxygen consumption		
Verapamil (Isoptin)	Antihypertensive	Treats unstable angina	Bolus dose 5–10 mg/2 min
	Calcium channel blocker	Vasospasm	May repeat 30 min after primary bolus
	Dilates coronary arteries	Dysrhythmias	
	Decreases SA/AV node conduction	Hypertension	
		Supraventricular tachycardia	
		Atrial flutter/fibrillation	
Adenosine (Adenocard)	Antidysrhythmic	Supraventricular tachycardia	Bolus dose 6 mg
	Slows AV node conduction		May repeat 12 mg in 1–2 min
	Restores SA node conduction		
Diltiazem (Cardiazem)	Calcium channel blocker	Atrial fibrillation	Bolus 0.25 mg/kg over 2 min
	Dilates coronary arteries	Atrial flutter	Continuous infusion 5–15 mg/hr up to 24 hrs
	Slows AV/SA node conduction	Supraventricular tachycardia	

Antiarrhythmics

Drug Name	Drug Action	Drug Use	Infusion Dose
Lidocaine (Xylocaine)	Decreases automaticity	Ventricular tachycardia	20–5-mcg/kg/min
	Antidysrhythmic	Ventricular dysrhythmia	Bolus 50–100 mg over 2–3 min
		Myocardial infarction	
Procainamide	Antidysrhythmic	Left threatening ventricular dysrhythmias	Bolus 100 mg every 5 min, given 23–50 mg/min
	Slows conduction in atrium		
	Depresses cardiac muscle electrical stimulation		

Other

Drug Name	Drug Action	Drug Use	Infusion Dose
Heparin	Anticoagulant	Prevents pulmonary emboli, myocardial infarction, atrial fibrillation emboli, disseminated intravascular coagulation (DIC)	150–300 units/kg
	Anti-thrombotic		
	Prevents conversion of fibrinogen to fibrin		
Protamine sulfate	Heparin antagonist	Heparin overdose	1 mg protamine per 100 units heparin over 1–3 min
	Binds with heparin	Open heart surgery	
		Hemorrhage	

Adapted from Skidmore-Roth, L. (2007). *Mosby's Drug Reference,* New Mexico: Mosby Inc.

correct laterality (where applicable). Other components of the "time out" may include verbalization of fire safety resources and other safety considerations.

Positioning, Prepping, and Draping

After the patient has been anesthetized, central lines and urinary catheter, inserted, and the electrosurgical dispersive pads applied (commonly bilaterally to the buttocks), the patient is positioned for the surgical prep. The most common position for accessing the heart and mediastinum is the supine position. This position is used for coronary artery bypass surgery, most valve procedures, and proximal aortic lesions. A pillow or other device may be placed under the shoulder blades to elevate the chest and facilitate exposure of the chest cavity, and under the legs to raise them upward and rotate them slightly externally. This leg position allows exposure and harvest of the saphenous vein (located along the inner aspect of the leg).

When procedures on the descending aorta are planned (eg, repair of a descending thoracic aneurysm). The lateral decubitus position is used with the patient placed on his or her right side. Complex aortic reconstruction (eg, of the aortic arch and branch vessels) generally require that supine position with the modification of a small roll under the upper left torso to facilitate exposure of the distal aortic arch. When the distal thoracic aorta is involved, the lower left chest may be elevated further with a pillow or roll. In patients placed in the lateral position, the groin area should be exposed bilaterally to enable insertion of bypass cannulas, an intra-aortic balloon, or a femoral arterial pressure monitoring line.

In some re-operative procedures (in which adhesions make the sternal approach unreasonable) or minimally invasive procedures, a thoracotomy approach can be used. At other times a semi-lateral position can be obtained with the patient in the supine position and the left side slightly raised with a sandbag or rolled sheets placed under the patient along the long axis of the body.

Once the proper position has been achieved, the circulating nurse preps the patient to remove residual flora from the skin. For most patients, the anterior and lateral portions of the entire chest, abdomen, and groin, as well as the legs (to below the knees), are included in the prep. Including the groin and upper legs (to below the knees) makes the groin area available for access to the right and/or left femoral artery, and provides access to saphenous vein should emergent revascularization be required. In patients undergoing coronary artery bypass surgery, the legs are prepped circumferentially to—and including—the feet. To accomplish this, the heels of the feet can be placed on holder by the circulator. After the prep is completed, sterile personnel lift the legs (allowing the circulator to remove the leg holding device) and position the legs onto sterile drapes.

Cardiac patients frequently have an adhesive drape applied to the exposed and prepped skin. A sterile drape is placed under the legs for coronary artery bypass procedures as well as along the sides of the patient, and over the head (in a manner that allows access to the endotracheal tube by the anesthesia provider). The feet are covered with sterile boots; the perineum is covered in a manner that allows access to the groin. In some institutions, patients' legs are always circumferentially prepped—even in procedures where the use of bypass grafts is planned (eg, aortic or mitral valve procedures). The nurse should communicate with the surgeon about specific draping preferences. At times when the nurse is uncertain whether to prep "more or less," these authors recommend "more." The possibility of emergency revascularization is ever present.

Once the patient is prepped and draped, sterile team members attach the sterile electrosurgery cords (and place ESU pencils into holders), suction tubing, internal defibrillator cords, and bypass lines to the drapes. The cords and tubes that are passed off are connected to their respective sources by the circulator and perfusionist. The circulating nurse continues to direct traffic flow—moving in the tables and Mayo stand(s), attaching headlight cords and electrosurgery equipment, and engaging the sternal saw cable to the motor (for electric saws). A battery-powered saw may be used; the circulating nurse should have a back-up battery available. The internal defibrillator cords should be attached to the defibrillator only after the chest has been opened. While the chest is closed, external paddles—or patches attached to the patient's posterior right shoulder and lateral left chest—should be attached to the defibrillator.

Before the start of the procedure, blood products should be available, especially if the patient has a low preprocedure hemoglobin or hematocrit. The circulator orders blood (eg, 1–2 units of packed red blood cells) and stores it in a blood refrigerator. Autotransfusion devices may be used to salvage and process lost blood that can be reinfused into the patient. Occasionally, in patients with a normal hematocrit, a predetermined amount of the patient's blood may be removed and stored for use post-bypass; this autologous blood is not subject to the hemodilution and damage suffered on cardiopulmonary bypass. Additionally, vasoactive infusions are used to control blood pressure, heart rate, and contractility of the heart (see **Table 23.3**). Which drugs and what doses are dependent on the patient's preexisting condition, height and weight, hemodynamic goal, allergies, and other considerations.

THE CARDIAC PROCEDURE

After the patient has been draped and the equipment attached and activated, the surgeon makes an incision along the sternal midline from one finger breadth below the suprasternal notch to approximately 3 cm below the xiphoid process. The midline of the sternum, along with any bleeding sites from the incision, is cauterized. The assistant applies retraction to the upper angle of the skin incision to provide exposure. The suprasternal ligament is cut with heavy scissors or cautery, and the sub-xiphoid area is bluntly dissected to create an opening for insertion of the sternal saw. The saw is positioned either at the upper or lower portion of the incision, depending on whether the surgeon opens the sternum from top-to-bottom, or vice versa. If the patient is undergoing re-operative sternotomy, a different saw may be needed to prevent damage to the retrosternal adherent cardiac tissue. The assistant should be ready with suction. After the sternum is split, a thin layer of bone wax or electrocautery may be used to provide hemostasis. The chest retractor is inserted and opened gradually to avoid injury to underlying tissue. Residual thymus tissue is dissected to the level of the innominate vein. While the surgeon and assistant each pull upward on the pericardium with forceps, the surgeon cuts longitudinally into the pericardium, exposing the heart. The pericardium is dissected from the heart and aorta and sewn to subcutaneous tissue with stay sutures to form a cradle for the heart (Khonsari & Sinek, 2008).

For patients undergoing coronary artery bypass grafting (CABG), the surgeon and assistant harvest the bypass conduits. For valve surgery or other procedures not requiring the harvesting of conduits, the surgeon will prepare to institute cardiopulmonary bypass (CPB) after exposing the heart.

CPB
Cardiopulmonary Bypass

CARDIOPULMONARY BYPASS

Cardiopulmonary bypass is indicated for procedures on the heart or great vessels in which a motionless and bloodless field is necessary. In order to achieve this, the activity of the heart must be temporarily stopped without producing irreversible injury to the myocardium or to the other organs of the body. The goal of cardiopulmonary bypass is to provide perfusion to the body's tissues without requiring the heart itself to pump or the lungs to perform gas exchange. The bypass circuit achieves this goal by using a mechanical pump to simulate the heart's activity and an oxygenator/gas exchanger to simulate the function of the lungs.

The bypass circuit consists of several key components: pumps to propel the blood, suction, and vent control to decompress the heart of air and blood, heating and cooling exchangers, and reservoirs to hold blood and other fluid for volume control. During bypass, a venous cannula is inserted into the right atrium. Blood returning from the systemic circulation into the superior and inferior venae cavae drains by gravity into the heart-lung machine; occasionally, two venous cannulas are used. Roller pumps draw the blood through filters and an oxygenator and then propel the blood back into the patient through a cannula that has been placed in the ascending aorta (**Fig. 23.8**). Arterial and venous cannulas come in a variety of sizes and types that suit cardiopulmonary bypass demands. Patient size, coexisting vascular disease, the type of procedure, and surgeon preference dictate cannula selection. Arterial cannulas are narrower than their venous counterparts. They must provide some resistance to perfuse the arterial circuit. Venous cannulation can be performed with a single, 2-stage cannula that can return blood from two points within the one cannula, or,

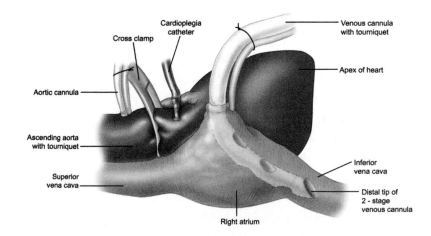

Figure 23.8

The aortic cannula is placed in the ascending aorta (with tourniquet attached with heavy silk tie). Proximal to the aortic cannula is the cross clamp. A 2-stage (single) venous cannula drains systemic venous return. Openings in the distal end of the cannula drain blood from the lower body; openings in the mid portion of the cannula (within the right atrium) drain blood returning from the upper body as well as coronary venous drainage exiting from the coronary sinus. The antegrade cardioplegia infusion catheter is inserted proximal to the aortic cross clamp and the arterial infusion cannula.

two separate cannulas can be inserted: one into the superior vena cava (SVC) and one inserted into the inferior vena cava (IVC), producing bi-caval cannulation.

Extensive adhesions or large aneurysms of the ascending aorta (that encroaches the right atrium) may make the standard right atrial-aortic cannulation technique dangerous, impractical or impossible. Entry into a chest with dense adhesions can cause laceration of the anterior right ventricular wall or rupture a dilated aneurysm. Alternative cannulation sites include the femoral vein and artery, and the subclavian artery. Insertion of the cannulas (eg, femoral vein-femoral artery cannulation) before opening the chest enables the surgeon to initiate bypass promptly if sudden, severe hemorrhage occurs on entry into the mediastinum.

Cardiopulmonary bypass can be partial or complete. With partial CPB, the single, 2-stage cannula (see **Fig. 23.7**) is inserted into the right atrial wall. The distal end is inserted into the inferior vena cava and the midportion of the cannula (containing openings) is positioned in the right atrium. Blood returning from the upper body can drain into the cannula openings in the midportion section; drainage entering the IVC largely enters the distal openings of the cannula. With partial bypass, some returning blood enters the RA, and a small amount of blood circulates through the heart and lungs. Complete CPB diverts most of the returning systemic venous blood to the pump before entering the heart. Complete bypass requires bi-caval cannulation of the SVC and the IVC. Tightening the caval tissue around the cannulas (with an umbilical tape) forces almost all of the returning blood into the cannulas.

In an effort to preserve volume and minimize the use of banked blood, bypass circuits are primed with physiological solutions. Colloid and crystalloid solutions are used to prime the pump. The average amount of crystalloid required to prime this circuit is approximately 2000 mL. Heparin, mannitol $NaHCO_3$, albumin, corticosteroids, and antifibrinolytics such as aminocaproic acid are also added, depending on institutional, perfusion and surgeon preferences. Most circuits incorporate in-line arterial and venous blood-as monitoring, line pressure manometers, anesthetic vaporizers, temperature monitoring systems, and numerous safety devices with computerized override mechanisms to be used in the event of mechanical failure or operator error (Nagelhout and Zaglaniczny, 2005). Although the crystalloid priming solution (that eventually mixes with the patient's blood) produces a drop in the hematocrit, it does not significantly reduce the oxygen carrying capacity of the pump volume to meet the cellular demands. Blood viscosity is also reduced, and this may increase perfusion to distal tissue beds during cardiopulmonary bypass flow (Kouchoukos et al, 2003).

While systemic heparinization commonly is required, there are newer heparin-bonded circuits that can reduce (but not completely obviate) the amount of heparin given to the patient. The activated clotting time (ACT) is used to evaluate the patient's response to heparin infusion and reversal with protamine sulfate. Appropriate therapy can be instituted based on the ACT. Other laboratory tests performed during the pump run include arterial blood gases, venous oxygen saturation, pH, hematocrit, and electrolyte levels.

ACT
Activated Clotting Time

Cardiopulmonary bypass protects the heart and perfuses vital organs during cardiac arrest, but CPB is not without complications. Several postcardiotomy complications are directly related to the use of CPB. There is some amount of damage and destruction to blood cells owing to the bypass circuit's foreign surface-blood cell interface. This damage leads to leaking capillaries and third spacing of fluid after bypass. Interstitial fluid leaks affects pulmonary capillary permeability, causing poor gas exchange, increasing oxygen requirements, and possibly necessitating long-term ventilator support (ie, greater than 24 hours after the procedure). Evidence of recovery in the clinical pathway includes weaning from and elimination of breathing support and reduced oxygen requirement. Organ dysfunction, such as transient kidney or liver dysfunction, may occur as a result of prolonged bypass runs (ie, greater than 6 hours) or long periods of hypotension.

Post-bypass is also a period of acid "washout," as acid accumulated during low-flow states is eliminated with the restoration of normal flows and rewarming. Acidosis, although transient, may produce some cellular derangement and is usually treated with sodium bicarbonate, active rewarming, and maintenance of an adequate cardiac output. CPB may also be associated with coagulopathies that occur secondary to the inflammatory response to cell damage, hemodilution, and unreversed heparin. Coagulation and heparin profiles are drawn after bypass and in the intensive care unit so that blood products can be administered as needed.

Initiating Cardiopulmonary Bypass

After the pericardial reflection is dissected from the aorta, heparin is given, and cannulation sutures are passed to the surgeon. Aortic cannulation suture (braided) is sewn in two concentric purse strings placed in the ascending aorta in the adventitia. Generally aortic cannulation is performed before venous cannulation so that blood can be infused directly should the patient experience sudden blood loss. The suture needles are cut and the remaining suture ends are caught and brought through a small catheter with a Rumel tourniquet. The purse string and tourniquet hold the cannulas in place. A No. 11 blade is used to create a stab wound in the middle of the aortic purse string. The aortotomy may be dilated before insertion of the aortic cannula. The purse string sutures are tightened around the cannula using the tourniquet and a hemostat. A tie of heavy silk can be used to secure the aortic cannula to the tourniquet. The aortic cannula is then connected to the arterial pump tubing. Immediately after the aortic cannula is connected to the pump tubing, the surgeon and assistant check that there is no air in the area of the connection; if air is noted, the connection must be opened, air removed, and the connection re-established. Once the connection is completed, the cannula and tourniquet may be sewn to the chest drape for further stabilization of the arterial line. Following decannulation, the purse string is tightened and tied to close the aortotomy and prevent blood loss through the cannulation site. Aortic cannulation is subject to several complications, including dissections and mobilization of plaque. Friable aortas may require repair.

For venous cannulation, the right atrial appendage is grasped with a C-shaped vascular clamp and another purse string suture is placed in the appendage. The atrial appendage is excised, the venous cannula is advanced as the clamp is removed, and the pursestring suture is tightened as described earlier. The cannula is then attached to the venous outflow line. Air at this point is not as critical as on the arterial side, but an airlock prevents venous drainage. Large airlocks must removed by manipulating the venous line in order to restore bypass flow after the previously placed tubing clamps are removed and cardiopulmonary bypass is initiated.

Femoral Vein–Femoral Artery Cannulation

When the right atrium and/or the aorta cannot be cannulated safely (eg, due to aortic aneurysm or dissection), the femoral vessels can be cannulated. For venous return, the femoral vein is exposed and opened with a knife blade and a venous cannula is inserted. Because the femoral venous cannula mainly drains the lower body, the venous line may be "Y'd" and a second venous cannulae inserted into the right atrium to drain the upper body. Insertion of this atrial cannula can be accomplished after the surgeon has controlled the aorta and minimized potential injury to tangential aneurismal vessels. For arterial perfusion, the femoral artery is exposed and cannulated with a femoral arterial cannula.

Termination of Cardiopulmonary Bypass

After the surgical repair is completed and systemic rewarming has begun, the surgeon starts to direct more of the venous return into the heart by gradually occluding the venous cannula; the perfusionist reduces arterial inflow. The response of the heart to the increasing volume load is monitored closely and inotropic medications may be required to help the heart to pump an adequate cardiac output.

When the venous cannula is totally occluded and all venous return is entering the heart, the perfusionist stops arterial inflow, and the patient is off bypass. The perfusionist may give some volume through the arterial line. Protamine sulfate is given to reverse the heparin. The surgeon confirms that the patient is hemodynamically stable before removing the cannulas. Femoral venous-arterial decannulation is achieved in a similar manner.

Suctioning and Venting

Suction keeps the field clear of excess blood. Blood conservation can be achieved with cell saver systems that collect, wash, and spin the blood to retrieve the red blood cells that can be given back to the patient. The use of blood salvaging devices in elderly patients may reduce neurocognitive dysfunction after the procedure because cell saver systems remove lipid particles (that may embolize to the brain) during reprocessing of the blood (Baumgartner WA, 2007; Djaiani et al, 2007).

A discard ("waste") suction should also be available to remove solutions (eg, topical antibiotics) that should not be salvaged or recycled into the patient's circulatory system.

Pump suctions may be used only when the patient is adequately (systemically) heparinized. Blood scavenged via the pump sucker can be added immediately into the pump volume and help to maintain an adequate hematocrit.

Venting allows both blood and air to be removed from the heart and great vessels. A common venting cannula for surgery requiring entry into the heart chambers is the right superior pulmonary venting catheter. The catheter is placed through a purse string created in the right superior pulmonary vein, manipulated into the left atrium, passed through the mitral valve, and finally positioned in the left ventricle. Blood flowing through the left ventricular vent cannula is removed by the pump, filtered, oxygenated, and combined in a reservoir with blood from the venous cannula. Both CPB and the use of vents allow the heart to remain decompressed, thereby minimizing myocardial oxygen demand. Vent lines can also be used to evacuate air from the aorta or other blood vessel before the cross-clamp is removed and bypass is discontinued.

Off Pump Procedures

More and more open and minimally invasive procedures are being performed without the use of CPB. The patient is not cooled to avoid risking ventricular fibrillation. Active warming devices help to maintain normothermia. Warming of intravenous fluids can prevent hypothermia (Jeong et al, 2008).

Motivating factors for the use of off-pump surgery include an anticipated decrease in perioperative morbidity and mortality (secondary to avoiding an inflammatory response associated with CPB) and the expectation that off-pump techniques produce better outcomes in patients with pre-existing cerebral or peripheral vascular disease. The evidence has not substantiated that one technique is significantly better than another (Lytle, 2007; Hannon et al, 2007; Raja & Berg, 2007). Nurses should be familiar with both techniques. When off pump procedures are performed, the cardiac team should always be prepared for instituting CPB if the patient deteriorates and requires resuscitation on bypass.

MYOCARDIAL PROTECTION

Although CPB provides blood flow to the organs of the body, when the aorta is cross-clamped (proximal to the aortic perfusion cannula) pump blood cannot enter the coronary circulation. In order to protect the heart itself and conserve myocardial energy resources, techniques are employed to prevent injury to the myocardium. These techniques are based on two main principles: hypothermia and diastolic cardiac arrest.

Systemic hypothermia of the body is achieved through the CPB circuit. A predetermined core temperature is achieved via the bypass heat exchanger. The desired temperature depends on the condition of the heart and the anticipated length of the procedure. Specific coronary hypothermia is also used to reduce the metabolic demands of the heart during the period when there is no coronary blood flow. Moderate hypothermia, 82.4°F (28°C), reduces oxygen consumption by approximately 50%. Every degree beyond that point further reduces myocardial oxygen demand. Temperatures as low as 59°F (15°C) may be obtained during complex operations on the aortic arch and branch vessels. This deep hypothermia and alternative perfusion techniques provide additional neurological protection.

The heart may be cooled topically or transmurally. Topical cooling of the heart is achieved through the instillation of cold saline slush directly onto the heart or into the pericardial sac. The use of ice chips in the mediastinum has been associated with phrenic nerve palsy, possibly disabling the diaphragm; saline slush is preferred. Insulating pads under the heart may prevent heat transfer from other organs. Transmural cooling of the heart is accomplished with the use of cold cardioplegia solution which also produces a prompt, diastolic arrest. Potassium is a common component of cardioplegia solution. Other components of the solution may include magnesium, procaine, glucose, oxygen, bicarbonate, phosphate, and adenosine. Together, these elements safely stop the heart, meet myocardial energy demands in the absence of coronary blood flow, provide cellular membrane stability, and act as a buffer to metabolic acidosis. Depending on the surgeon's preference, cardioplegia solution may be prepared as an asanguineous (ie, crystalloid) solution or as a blood mixture.

Cardioplegia can be delivered via the antegrade or the retrograde routes. Antegrade cardioplegia is infused through a needle inserted through a purse string into the aorta proximal to the aortic cross-clamp (see **Fig. 23.7**). The solution flows into the right and left coronary ostia and into the coronary arterial system, capillaries, venous system, and finally exits into the right atrium through the coronary sinus. Exiting cardioplegic solution mixes with returning systemic venous blood and drains into the CPB circuit.

Retrograde cardioplegia is delivered via a catheter inserted through a purse string in the right atrial wall and positioned in the coronary sinus. The solution is infused into the coronary sinus and flows into the coronary venous system, capillaries and the arterial circulation, finally exiting through the coronary ostia in the aorta. Returning retrograde effluent entering the aorta is suctioned away through the antegrade cardioplegia infusion catheter (which is "Y'd" to a suction line). The retrograde route is especially useful when coronary lesions impede transmural antegrade cardioplegia; both the antegrade and the retrograde routes are used alternatively to arrest the entire heart. And in cases where the aortic valve cannot prevent regurgitation, the retrograde route is used for arrest (antegrade solution would preferentially flow into the left ventricle and distend the heart).

Instillation of cardioplegia can be achieved also by directly infusing the solution into the coronary ostia when the aorta is opened (eg, during aortic valve replacement). Direct access to the coronary ostia risks injury to coronary arterial endothelium; this technique is generally used when neither the antegrade nor the retrograde route produces a timely arrest. Direct infusion may also be useful during minimally invasive procedures when access to the aorta or right atrium is limited.

Once the patient is on CPB, the aorta is cross clamped and the heart has been arrested with cardioplegia, the cardiac repair is performed. The following sections describe surgery for coronary artery and valvular heart disease, aneurysms and dissections of the aorta, cardiac dysrhythmias, and heart failure.

Minimally Invasive Cardiopulmonary Bypass and Myocardial Protection

Percutaneous endovascular catheters enable surgeons to institute CPB and to protect the myocardium, and anesthesia providers to monitor cardiac function. Multi-lumen catheters are inserted intravenously into the right heart; the distal tip is positioned into the coronary sinus for infusion of retrograde cardioplegia. A second lumen of the catheter allows inflation of the balloon tip to occlude the coronary sinus, and a third lumen measures pressures. Another multi-lumen catheter is inserted and floated into the pulmonary artery to measure PA pressures, infuse medications, and/or vent the pulmonary system. Complications include injury to the jugular vein, superior vena cava, right atrium, and coronary sinus. Injury to the tricuspid valve, perforation of the right ventricle, dysrhythmia, and hemorrhage also may occur.

For instituting endovascular CPB, the surgeon and sterile team members insert the endocatheters that will be used for venous drainage and arterial perfusion. The venous cannula is inserted into the femoral vein, and the arterial cannula placed into the femoral artery. A triple-lumen, endarterial clamp is inserted into the arterial (femoral artery) cannula and threaded to the ascending aorta. One lumen contains a balloon, that when inflated occludes the aorta, thereby serving as a (endovascular) cross-clamp. The lumen also contains utility ports for infusing cardioplegia fluid, monitoring proximal aortic pressures, and measuring the pressure that the balloon is exerting on the inner wall of the aorta. Femoral vein-femoral artery cannulation risks include plaque embolization, arterial thrombosis, ischemia to the distal leg, and dysrhythmias.

CORONARY ARTERY BYPASS GRAFTING (CABG)

Indications for coronary artery bypass graft (CABG) surgery include chronic stable and unstable angina with coronary artery lesions documented by cardiac catheterization. Some patients will have undergone coronary angioplasty with stent insertion (ie, percutaneous coronary intervention—PCI), but in patients with 3-vessel or 2-vessel disease there is a survival advantage with CABG versus PCI (Opie et al, 2006; Hannon et al, 2008).

PCI
Percutaneous Coronary Intervention

The goal of coronary bypass surgery is to increase perfusion to ischemic myocardial cells distal to the obstructed portion of the coronary artery. Increasing blood flow to the distal portions of the heart is achieved with bypass grafts (conduits) that are attached below the narrowed portion of the artery. Ischemia (or infarction) of various areas of the heart may give rise to other ischemic-related disorders such as valvular dysfunction, dysrhythmias, left ventricular aneurysm, and post-myocardial infarction ventricular septal defects. Generally coronary lesions demonstrating a 75% reduction in cross-sectional area (which correlates to a 50% reduction of arterial diameter)—and the coronary arteries distal to the lesion have adequate size and quality—are considered suitable for bypass grafting (Góngora & Sundt, 2008).

LAD
Left Anterior Descending

LIMA
Left Internal Mammary Artery

RIMA
Right Internal Mammary Artery

Selection of conduits depends on the target vessel and availability of bypass grafts. For lesions of the left anterior descending (LAD) coronary artery (which supplies the anterior wall of the LV), the left internal mammary artery (LIMA) is commonly used because of its long-term patency (Berger et al, 2004). The LIMA is usually prepared as a pedicle graft, leaving the proximal side attached at its take-off from the left subclavian artery. The right internal mammary artery (RIMA—branching off the right subclavian artery) can be similarly dissected from its retrosternal bed. The RIMA may be used as a pedicle graft, or, as a free graft (ie, transected both proximally and distally).

The surgeon exposes the IMA with a retractor that elevates the left (or right) sternum to expose the retrosternal target IMA. Before the IMA is clamped and divided, heparin is given systemically to prevent thrombosis of the artery. The IMA is then cut and papaverine solution is instilled into the distal end to prevent vasospasm. Bleeding from the IMA pedicle should be brisk and pulsatile in concert with the heartbeat. After the IMA is judged to be satisfactory, the distal end is clamped with a bulldog or a metal clip. The pedicle may be wrapped in a papaverine-soaked sponge and placed in the pleural cavity until needed for the coronary anastomosis.

While the surgeon is dissecting the IMA, the assistant harvests the greater saphenous vein that runs along the inner aspect of the right and left legs. Unless there are clinical contraindications for use of the vein from the right or left leg (eg, due to varicosities or previous vein stripping), laterality issues are related mainly to assistant (or surgeon) preference. The vein may be harvested in the traditional manner (ie, an incision along the length of the leg), but it is increasingly common to obtain saphenous vein conduit via video-assisted endoscopy.

After the vein is removed, a small cannula is placed into the (ankle) end of the vessel and a heparin blood solution is infused into the vein. This solution dilates the vessel and demonstrates leaking tributaries that can be tied, or tears that can be repaired with a 6-0 or 7-0 polypropylene suture. Restrictive adventitial bands on the vein are removed to avoid restricting the diameter of the vessel. The vein may be marked with a surgical marker so that twisting is avoided during the anastomosis.

Additional conduits include the radial artery, inferior epigastric artery, and the gastroepiploic artery (Haywood & Buxton, 2007). These arterial conduits may be used to supply multiple arterial grafts (eg, in younger patients with severe atherosclerotic disease); or they may be used for patients who do not have available (or suitable) IMAs or saphenous vein.

Once the conduits are prepared, the surgeon initiates CPB and assesses the heart to identify target areas for bypass grafting. Systemic cooling is achieved and cardioplegia is infused to stop the heart. The surgeon positions the heart to provide optimal exposure of the target vessel. Some surgeons employ slings to hold the heart in position; others have an assistant to hold the heart (cotton gloves on the assistant's hands provide sufficient but gentle traction). Cold, wet laparotomy pads may be placed under the apex to elevate the heart.

The distal anastomoses to the lateral or posterior coronary arteries usually are performed first. Once the target vessel is identified, a longitudinal incision is made into the coronary artery with a fine knife blade. The vessel is entered obliquely with the blade to avoid cutting into the back wall of the artery. The arteriotomy is enlarged using angled, forwards, and backwards coronary scissors. The vessel may be probed to determine size and patency. If the surgeon is using both saphenous vein and IMA grafts, the venous grafts are usually performed first. The vein conduit end is cut and beveled with fine scissors and coronary forceps to approximate the length of the arterial incision. An end-to-side anastomosis is performed with a 6-0 or 7-0 double-armed polypropylene suture. Before the suture is tied, the vein is flushed with cardioplegic, blood, or heparin solution to check for any leaks as the suture is drawn tight. If the proximal anastomoses are to be performed while the aorta is cross clamped and the heart is arrested, the vein grafts may be attached to the aorta, or, more commonly, they may be placed out of the way until all the distal anastomoses are completed. If the proximal grafts are to be attached to the aorta with a partial occlusion clamp (and the heart beating), the grafts will be clamped with a vascular bulldog. The bulldog prevents air from going into the heart after the anastomosis is complete and before the aortic clamps are removed.

After all distal free grafts are completed, the mammary graft is attached. Generally the IMA anastomosis is performed after the other grafts are completed in order to protect the IMA from inadvertent injury during vein grafting and retraction of the heart. While the IMA is being anastomosed (using 7-0 or 8-0 polypropylene), the pedicle is clamped with a bulldog to prevent blood flow from the pedicle into the coronary circulation (which would warm the heart and possibly lead to fibrillation or contraction—and cause increased myocardial oxygen consumption).

Because the IMA graft is generally the last anastomosis, systemic rewarming is usually initiated during this period. When the aorta remains cross clamped, the relatively warmer systemic blood is separated from the heart, which remains cool. This allows the larger systemic surface areas to warm before the heart is opened to warm blood.

After the distal anastomoses are completed, the proximal anastomoses are created. These anastomoses can be made either while the heart is arrested, or after the aortic cross-clamp has been removed and the heart is beating. If the surgeon works on an arrested heart, the grafts are attached to the aorta one after another (with the exception of the IMA pedicle, which is already attached proximally to the subclavian artery). The surgeon creates an aortotomy for each graft with a knife, then uses a punch to create a circular opening in the aorta. The selected saphenous vein graft is distended with solution and placed on the aorta where it is to be anastomosed. Venous return may be quickly occluded to allow the heart to fill and distend. This mimics the size of the heart in its natural state and prevents the vein graft from being cut too short. The graft is then cut to the proper length and sewn end-to-side fashion onto the aorta with 5-0 double-armed polypropylene suture.

If the proximal anastomosis is to be performed on a beating heart, each graft is clamped with a bulldog before the cross clamp is removed so that air does not enter the coronary circulation. In most cases, the heart beats spontaneously in a normal or near-normal rhythm when the cross clamp is removed. If the heart is fibrillating, internal defibrillator paddles are used to defibrillate using energy levels of 10–20 joules.

A partial occlusion clamp is placed on the aorta to isolate the section of the aorta for each proximal anastomosis. The clamp allows blood ejected by the LV to flow through the unclamped portion of the aorta into the systemic circulation. The anastomoses are performed in a manner similar to that on the arrested heart. Before the partial occlusion clamp is removed, the vein grafts are de-aired with an aspiration needle (25 Gauge) at the highest point of the vein (where air collects). Bulldogs previously placed on the grafts are then removed. Some surgeons may use a small hemoclip or other radiographically opaque device to mark the position of the grafts for future radiologic identification. After all anastomoses are completed (**Fig. 23.9**) and observed for bleeding, cardiopulmonary bypass can be terminated and the cannulas removed. Pacing wires are attached, chest tubes are inserted, hemostasis is achieved, and the patient's incision is closed.

Off-Pump CABG

CABG performed without the use of CABG necessitates working on a beating heart. One of the key technical challenges is to create an anastomosis in a small area (1–3 mm) that is moving. The ability to create such anastomoses was enhanced by the development of stabilizers and retraction devices (**Fig. 23.10**) that enable surgeons to create the bypass grafts. The stabilizer isolates the portion of the coronary artery to be bypassed and maintains a quiet field. The retractor uses a suction mechanism that attaches to the apex of the heart and allows the surgeon to access lateral and posterior coronary arteries. Because the heat is beating, there is some blood flow

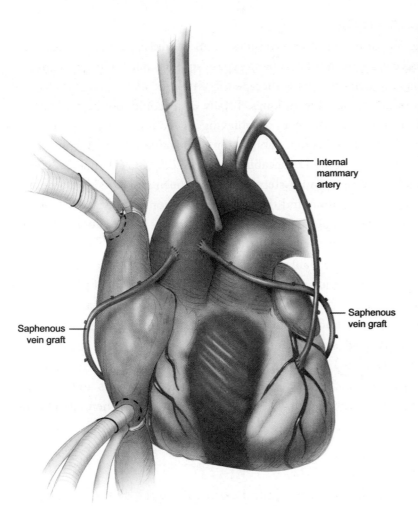

Figure 23.9

Coronary Artery Bypass Graft (CABG) showing internal mammary artery to the left anterior descending coronary artery and saphenous veins graft to distal right coronary artery and a marginal branch of the circumflex coronary artery.

Internal mammary artery

Saphenous vein graft

Saphenous vein graft

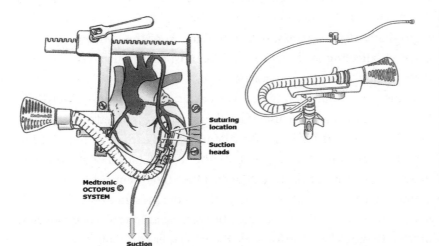

Suturing location

Suction heads

Medtronic OCTOPUS © SYSTEM

Suction

Figure 23.10

"Off pump" retractor stabilizes site of coronary anastomosis (left). Suction device attached to left ventricular apex exposes apical and lateral coronary arteries for CABG (right).

Source: Courtesy of Medtronic Heart Valves, Minneapolis, MN.

entering the arteriotomy. Silastic sutures with a blunt needle may be placed through the heart muscle around the coronary artery distal and proximal to the anastomotic site and tightened to occlude the vessel and prevent bleeding. Small suction catheters are used to remove blood that does enter the field.

Minimally Invasive CABG

The percutaneous insertion of endovascular CPB cannulas can be considered a minimally invasive component of coronary bypass surgery, but the performance of the vascular anastomoses—the main therapeutic endpoint of the surgery—is less amenable to minimally invasive techniques. Totally endoscopic robotic cardiac surgery was initially introduced as a means of achieving a safer, less invasive approach to the heart, but problems with bleeding, stabilization of the target artery, and prolonged CPB runs demonstrate the limited applicability of robotic CABG (Damiano, 2007).

The use of smaller incisions (mini-sternotomy) has been employed by some surgeons for both the chest incision and the harvesting of conduits. Smaller thoracic chest incisions have been employed in patients with single lesions (eg, of the left anterior descending coronary artery), but these are not commonly performed due to the significant postprocedure pain associated with thoracic incisions, and because thoracic incisions do not provide optimal exposure for the majority of patients who have multi-vessel disease. Various instruments have been designed to aid exposure, isolate and stabilize the anastomotic site, and create the anastomoses in the presence of smaller incisions through small openings.

Endoscopic, video-assisted harvesting of the saphenous vein and the radial artery are increasingly performed. This technique is popular with patients and referring physicians, but there is a learning curve that must be considered when introducing this technology.

VALVE REPAIR AND REPLACEMENT

The function of the 4 cardiac valves—mitral, aortic, tricuspid, and pulmonary—is to maintain 1-way flow through the heart. When a valve becomes unable to close tightly and prevent backflow (due to dilatation of the annulus, leaflet tears, or other pathology), the valve is said to be regurgitant or insufficient. When valve leaflets become stiff or otherwise act as an impediment to forward flow, the valve is said to be stenotic. Regurgitation and stenosis, or a combination of the two, are the main pathologic conditions affecting the heart valves. The most common valves requiring treatment in the adult are the mitral and aortic valves.

Causes of valve disease include rheumatic fever, bacterial endocarditis, atherosclerosis, and calcification. The decision to undertake the procedure is based on symptoms presented as well as data obtained from echocardiograms and cardiac catheterization studies. Although there are numerous causes for either regurgitation or stenosis, the amount of damage to the valve itself usually determines treatment. Although there has been a preference for biologic valves or allografts in the presence of endocarditis (Friedewald et al, 2007), mechanical valves may be suitable as long as adequate debridement of infected tissue as been performed (Baumgartner et al, 2007).

It is preferable to salvage the native valve with reparative techniques, rather than removing and replacing the valve (Fedak et al, 2008). The mitral (and tricuspid) valve is especially suited to repair because its components—annulus, leaflets, chordate tendineae, and papillary muscles—are each amenable to surgical repair. Aortic valve disease usually requires replacement due to anatomic considerations that preclude repair (Carabello, 2007). Valve replacement involves removing the patient's natural valve and substituting a prosthetic mechanical or biologic valve. Prosthetic mechanical and biological valves, allografts, and annuloplasty rings have been described (see **Figs. 23.3** to **23.6**).

Mitral Valve Repair

Cardiopulmonary bypass is established with two venous cannulas—one is inserted into the inferior vena cava and the second into the superior vena cava. After systemic cooling and placement of the aortic cross clamp, cardioplegia is delivered to arrest the heart. The heart is retracted toward the left side of the patient and a left atriotomy is made to expose the mitral valve. The surgeon makes a thorough assessment of the valve and its components and makes a final determination of the type of repair best suited to the patient. If the surgeon decides that the valve is too deteriorated to be repaired, valve replacement may be required.

Ring annuloplasty is the most common mitral valve reparative technique. Often it is the posterior leaflet (versus the anterior leaflet) of the mitral valve (**Fig. 23.11**) that has become dilated, thereby preventing the leaflets from creating a tight seal when the valve is closed (ie, during ventricular systole). Annuloplasty rings are available in a variety of sizes and types. The rings may be semi-rigid or flexible and shapes can be circular, bean-shaped, or C-shaped. These differences are related to the surgeon's functional goal of retaining the normal shape of the annular orifice, promoting annular expansion and narrowing, or selectively repairing the posterior leaflet's annular dilatation.

After determining the type of ring to use, sizing obturators (specific to the prosthetic ring selected) are used to measure the annulus and determine the appropriate ring size (**Fig. 23.12**). Stitches are inserted around the annulus of the valve (**Fig. 23.13**) and then into the ring with double-armed polyester sutures (**Fig. 23.14**). After the sutures are inserted, the ring is seated and the stitches are tied and cut (**Fig. 23.15**).

Anterior Leaflet

Posterior Leaflet

Figure 23.11

Mitral valve with anterior leaflet (top) and posterior leaflet (bottom).

Source: Courtesy of Medtronic Heart Valves, Minneapolis, MN.

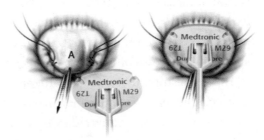

Figure 23.12

The anterior leaflet "A" is retracted and the annuloplasty sizer/obturator is placed over the leaflet to determine the correct size ring for implantation. The "M" on the sizer denotes the position for sizing the mitral valve. Turning the sizer to display the "T" enables the surgeon to properly size the tricuspid valve.

Source: Courtesy of Medtronic Heart Valves, Minneapolis, MN.

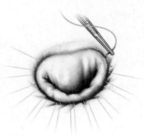

Figure 23.13

Insertion of individual stitches into mitral valve annulus.

Source: Courtesy of Medtronic Heart Valves, Minneapolis, MN.

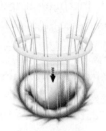

Figure 23.14

After removal from the ring holder, the annuloplasty ring is lowered down onto the annulus.

Source: Courtesy of Medtronic Heart Valves, Minneapolis, MN.

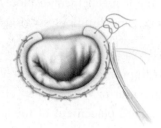

Figure 23.15

Each suture is tied around the band securely and the excess suture is trimmed.

Source: Courtesy of Medtronic Heart Valves, Minneapolis, MN.

In addition to ring annuloplasty, other reparative techniques include patching torn leaflets with a piece of the patient's pericardium, incising the fused portion of the leaflets (ie, commissurotomy), suture repair of ruptured chordate tendineae, and the suture approximation of the edges of the anterior and posterior leaflets (Fedak et al, 2008).

Mitral Valve Replacement

Valve replacement requires the same setup, preparation, and establishment of bypass as does valve repair surgery. The mitral valve is excised and calcium is debrided as needed with Rongeurs, a No. 15 blades, and/or scissors. The anterior leaflet, papillary muscle, and chordae are excised; the posterior leaflet is usually retained to maintain the geometry of the left ventricle. Sufficient annulus is retained to allow for fixation of the prosthetic valve. After the valve is resected, the surgeon irrigates the field to remove debris and other particles that could embolize to the systemic circulation after removal of the cross clamp.

The mitral annulus is sized, and the appropriate valve is opened. If a biological valve is selected, it must be rinsed in three baths of saline (for a minimum of 6 minutes total) to remove the glutaraldehyde preservation solution. Often the surgeon will size and select the valve, and then begin the placement of the annular stitches. The circulating nurse can promptly open the valve and deliver it to a sterile member of the surgical team. This person will rinse the valve while the surgeon completes the insertion of all the annular stitches. Mechanical valves do not require special preparation before insertion.

Double-armed nonabsorbable braided sutures with pledgets are commonly used. After the annular stitches are inserted, the surgeon places the stitches through the sewing cuff of the replacement mitral valve. Once all the sutures are placed, the sutures and valve are irrigated, the valve is seated into position and the stitches are tied.

The left atrium is closed with two running 3-0 polypropylene sutures, each starting from a corner of the atriotomy and meeting in the middle of the incision. Before the sutures are tied, a small venting catheter may be inserted in the suture line and the tip of the catheter placed through the mitral valve in order to allow air within the left ventricle to escape. The patient is placed in the Trendelenburg position to allow air to rise to the aorta where the air is removed through the aortic vent line. Additionally, a Valsalva maneuver is performed (by anesthesia) whereby the lungs are inflated, allowing air to evacuate the heart. A 19-gauge needle and syringe may be used to aspirate air from the apex of the left ventricle. Once it has been determined via TEE that no air remains in the LV, the atrial catheter can be removed and the left atrial closure sutures tied. The aortic cross-clamp is removed. Once the heart fills with blood and begins to beat, the surgeon prepares to terminate CPB. TEE is used to assess valve function and to look for any residual air.

Minimally Invasive Mitral Valve Surgery

Small right thoracotomy incisions can be made for access to the mitral valve. Venous drainage for CPB may employ a long femoral venous cannula with openings in the distal portion to drain venous return from the right atrium. Arterial inflow can be established in the ascending aorta through a small chest incision. Transthoracic vascular clamps can be used to occlude the aorta. The use of smaller incisions may be useful when there are extensive sterna adhesions from previous sternotomy.

A number of *percutaneous* approaches for mitral valve repair are currently under investigation. Interventional procedures performed in the cardiac catheterization laboratory have been employed to enlarge a stenotic orifice (ie, balloon angioplasty), but the percutaneous delivery of a prosthetic valve ideally will be performed in an operating room with catheterization imaging devices. These procedures should be performed with both a cardiologist and a cardiac surgeon in order to provide the requisite skills for fluoroscopic delivery and insertion as well as the ability to open the chest and perform surgery in the event of complications (Friedewald et al, 2007). Early clinical studies are looking at methods to replace the mitral valve, mitral annular realignment to improve leaflet coaptation, and the edge-to-edge procedure that approximates prolapsed segments of the mitral leaflets (Fedak et al, 2008).

Tricuspid Valve Repair

The tricuspid valve may be dysfunctional due to endocarditis or secondary to mitral valve disease. Commonly, reparative techniques are employed; rarely is the tricuspid valve replaced with a prosthetic valve. Tricuspid valve competence can be restored with an annuloplasty ring (**Fig. 23.16**) or with a suture technique that narrows a dilated annulus.

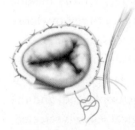

Figure 23.16

Completing the tricuspid valve repair.

Source: Courtesy of Medtronic Heart Valves, Minneapolis, MN.

Generally, a pulmonary artery pressure (PAP) catheter will not be inserted as it would obscure the right atrial operative field. The patient may have a CVP line inserted before the incision is made. If a PAP line is required after the procedure, it can be inserted at the end of the procedure. An alternative is to insert a left atrial pressure line to measure left sided pressures.

Double cannulation is performed, as with mitral valve surgery. After the heart is arrested, the right atrium is opened. The tricuspid valve is inspected and debrided as necessary. Sterile team members should be aware that the AV node (and other conduction tissue) is in close proximity to the tricuspid valve and is vulnerable to injury during surgery.

After the repair is completed, the right atrium is closed with two running polypropylene sutures. The atrium is de-aired by filling the heart with blood and allowing back-bleeding while the sutures are tied and cut. TEE is used to ensure that intracardiac air is removed, and that the valve in particular and heart in general are functioning. The patient is weaned from bypass and venous cannulas are removed.

Aortic Valve Replacement

AS
Aortic Stenosis

Aortic stenosis (AS) produces obstruction to outflow from the left ventricle (LV). As the aortic valve orifice narrows, the LV must generate greater pressure to force blood through the stenotic valve. The ventricle compensates for the increased pressure load by developing hypertrophy. The LV may generate a pressure of 150 mm Hg in order to eject enough blood to produce an aortic pressure of 100 mm Hg; thus a 50 mm Hg pressure gradient is produced. The larger the pressure gradient, the more severe the stenosis. Eventually the heart dilates and may fail without replacement of the stenotic valve. Patients may faint or have anginal pain as a result of the inadequate cardiac output that causes insufficient cerebral or coronary blood flow.

AI
Aortic Regurgitation/
Insufficiency

Aortic regurgitation/insufficiency (AI) allows backflow of blood into the ejecting chamber (LV) which increases systolic volumes that must be ejected into the aorta. Dilatation and then hypertrophy of the left ventricle eventually produce coronary insufficiency and congestive heart failure. Patients may complain of shortness of breath, hypotension, and fatigue. Cardiopulmonary bypass can be achieved with a 2-stage venous cannula (see **Fig. 23.7**) and an arterial cannula placed in the ascending aorta. When the aorta is cross clamped, retrograde cardioplegia may be given to arrest the heart. If the retrograde catheter cannot be inserted, the surgeon may open the aorta and deliver cardioplegia directly into the coronary circulation with hand-held catheters.

After the aorta is opened the surgeon assesses the aortic valve leaflets, the location of the right and left coronary ostia, and other anatomic features. Some surgeons may place a small gauze sponge into the LV in order to prevent calcium emboli and other debris from falling into the chamber. Other potential safety factors include meticulous cleaning of all instruments used during the valve surgery to remove loose debris. The valve is measured and then excised with scissors, forceps, and/or a knife. Rongeurs may be used to debride calcium from the annulus and surrounding tissue. Sutures are placed to mark the commissures and tagged with clamps. The valve is sized with the appropriate type of sizers for the prosthesis to be implanted, and the selected prosthesis is delivered promptly to the field. If a biological valve is selected, valve rinsing can be started as soon as the valve is delivered to the field. The rinsing procedure is similar to that described above for the mitral valve.

Individual double-armed nonabsorbable pledgetted sutures are placed through the annulus of the aortic valve. Each stitch is then placed through the sewing ring of the valve. The sutures are moistened and the valve is lowered and seated into the aortic root. The sutures are then tied and cut. The aorta is closed with 3-0 or 4-0 double-armed polypropylene suture. Two sutures are used—one at each corner of the incision. The aorta is sewn with a mattress stitch and the sutures are tied where they meet in the anterior aorta. A second set of sutures is used to oversew the initial suture line and provide reinforcement and hemostasis. Before the aorta is closed, the patient is placed in the Trendelenburg position, and positive pressure is applied to the lungs so that air and blood are expelled from the aorta. The cross-clamp is removed only after the surgeon is satisfied that the heart has been sufficiently de-aired. After confirming that the valve is functioning properly and hemostasis is achieved, the surgeon terminates CPB and closes the chest.

Minimally Invasive Aortic Valve Surgery

An upper, hemi-sternotomy or a right mini-thoracotomy between the 2nd or 3rd intercostal space allows a minimally invasive—but directly visible—access to the aorta for both arterial cannulation and the aortic valve replacement. In some cases, the surgeon will use femoral vein-femoral artery cannulation (see the earlier discussion of endovascular technique). In these (and other MIS) cardiac patients, access to the LV for defibrillation is difficult; the circulator will have applied external defibrillator patches that can be activated to treat ventricular fibrillation. Special long instruments that allow the shafts to be flexed out of the way are useful for excising the native valve and implanting the replacement valve.

Percutaneous treatments for aortic valve replacement were initially developed in the cardiac catheterization laboratory. Additional trials to study newer generation techniques and devices for percutaneous replacement continue to be performed by cardiologists in interventional laboratories are currently under FDA review. In one device, a balloon-expandable prosthesis is threaded through the aorta to the aortic valve. The balloon is inflated, compressing the native valve. The prosthesis is deployed and the catheter removed (Grube et al, 2007). Future percutaneous valve replacement will stress the need for greater collaboration between cardiologists and surgeons.

AORTIC ANEURYSMS AND DISSECTIONS

Lesions of the thoracic aorta may affect the ascending aorta, the aortic arch, the descending aorta, or more than one section of the aorta. Aneurysms and dissections may extend into the abdominal aorta (ie, thoracoabdominal aortic aneurysms). The operative approach and the techniques of repair will depend on the location of the lesion, the nature of the lesion and the patient's condition. Genetic and environmental factors have been associated with increased risk for the formation of both aneurysms and dissections (Kuivaniemi et al, 2008). Diagnostic imaging—such as three dimensional computed tomographic (CT) scanning—is especially effective for providing an assessment of the size, location, and extent of the lesion; selecting either open or endovascular repair; and creating a baseline for future comparison (Conrad & Cambria, 2008).

Aneurysms are a weakening of the blood vessel and affect all layers of the vascular wall: intima, media, and adventitia. Atherosclerosis is the most common cause, but trauma, infection, and degenerative changes may also produce aneurismal dilation. The weakened aortic wall commonly dilates circumferentially (*fusiform aneurysm*), but some aneurysms have a localized out-pouching (*saccular aneurysm*). Of immediate concern is the potential for rupture with subsequent exsanguination. Patients may not have specific symptoms of an aneurysm, but if an aneurysm is suspected, imaging techniques are effective in detecting the lesion (Kuivaniemi et al, 2008).

Dissections are different from aneurysms in that there are degenerative changes within the medial layer of the aorta. Etiologic factors include collagen and connective tissue disorders, and a history of hypertension. In dissection, the artery tears, blood enters the tear and dissects the aortic layers. The dissection may extend distally and proximally, thereby compromising perfusion to smaller arterial branches. Aortic dissection retrograde toward the heart can cause dilatation of the aortic valve annulus and produce aortic valve insufficiency. Dissections of the ascending aorta are prone to rupture and are true surgical emergencies.

Patients with dissections of the descending aorta may have better outcomes with medical management (versus surgical repair) that includes pharmacologic control of hypertension. The introduction of endovascular stent-grafts has provided an effective and relatively safe technique for repairing the descending thoracic aorta and their availability has expanded the therapeutic options for selected patients (Goksel et al, 2008; Conrad & Cambria, 2008; Svensson et al, 2008).

There two main classifications systems used for dissections (Kouchoukos et al, 2003). The DeBakey system is divided into three types: Type I (ascending aorta and aortic arch), Type II (ascending aorta only), and Type III (the descending thoracic aorta). The Stanford system includes the Stanford A (involving the ascending aorta and arch) and the Stanford B (only descending aorta). Dissections (and aneurysms) may not always fit neatly into one category, so the perioperative nurse should be prepared for combined lesions that require patient-specific positioning, instrumentation, and surgical technique.

Repair of the Ascending Aorta

For operations on the ascending aorta, the patient is placed in the supine position. Standard instrumentation for sternotomy is used, but the nurse should also be prepared and have available instrumentation for aortic valve replacement and coronary bypass grafts. Tube grafts of various sizes should be immediately available along with pledget material and polypropylene suture for the anastomoses. If the aortic valve is to be replaced, individual valve sutures should be available.

CPB with myocardial protection (ie, cardioplegia) is employed. Because the ascending aortic tissue would be too fragile to cannulate, arterial infusion may be accomplished with femoral artery cannulation (retrograde perfusion). Occasionally, the right atrium (RA) is not accessible due to the size of the ascending aneurysm; in this situation, femoral vein cannulation is used until the RA can be approached safely. In preparation for subsequent atrial cannulation, the femoral venous line may have a length of tubing "Y'd" to the femoral venous line. This line is clamped until the atrium can be entered; generally this occurs after the aorta is cross-clamped.

An atrial venous cannula is inserted and connected to the RA tubing; the clamp is removed and venous return is allowed to drain into the bypass machine.

After bypass is established and the patient is systemically cooled to approximately 82.4°F (28°C), the surgeon cross-clamps the aorta and opens the aneurysm. If there is an aortic dissection, the surgeon locates the site of the intimal tear and includes this portion of the aorta in the excision. (If the site of the tear were not excised, blood would continue to enter the tear and recreate the dissection.) A tube graft is inserted and sewn proximally and distally to repair the aorta.

If there is evidence of aortic dilatation with aortic valve regurgitation, the aortic valve and aorta both can be replaced with a graft-valve prosthesis (**Fig. 23.17**). The valve (proximal) end of the prosthesis is attached to the aortic annulus (see aortic valve replacement). Using such a composite graft to replace the aortic valve and the aorta obliterates the origins of the right and left coronary arteries. Consequently the surgeon must revascularize the myocardium by reimplanting the coronary ostia as "buttons" into the tube graft, or, by creating coronary artery bypass grafts. The decision of which technique to use is dependent on whether the patient has coexisting coronary artery disease, which would indicate the need for CABG. When revascularization is completed, the surgeon prepares for the distal anastomosis. The surgeon measures the length of graft needed for the distal anastomosis, cuts the graft to the correct size and completes the anastomosis. The lungs may be inflated to de-air the left ventricle. An aspirating vent or needle is used to remove air from the aorta. After assessing the anastomotic sites, the cross-clamp is removed and hemostasis is achieved. The patient is weaned from bypass, and the sternal closure is completed.

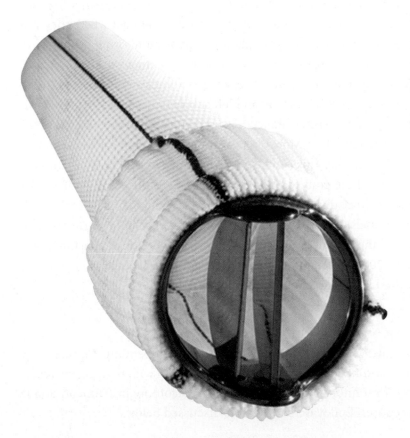

Figure 23.17

St. Jude Medical graft-valve prosthesis used to replace the aortic valve and the diseased segment of the ascending aorta.

Source: Permission to reproduce this image granted by St. Jude Medical, Inc. "Copyright" © St. Jude Medical.

Repair of the Aortic Arch

For repairs of the proximal arch, the supine position is used; repairs involving the distal arch may require a semi-lateral position to enhance access to the descending aorta. Sternotomy instruments are used with thoracotomy instruments as indicated. A supply of tube grafts should be available; grafts with "branches" are available for arch replacements requiring individual anastomoses of each aortic arch branch vessel.

Repair of the aortic arch involves the vessels to the head and neck and the potential for interruption to cerebral flow. Additional protective measures are required to protect not only the heart, but also the brain. Femoral vein-femoral artery bypass is instituted and the patient is cooled to approximately 53.6°F–59°F (12°C–15°C). A portion of venous tubing is "Y'd" to the venous line and a venous cannula is inserted and positioned in the superior vena cava.

Because of the difficulty of accessing the arch vessels and occluding them with cross clamps, the surgeon employs a technique called *hypothermic circulatory arrest* that obviates the need for clamps during part of the repair. Once the patient is cooled to the desired temperature, the bypass machine is turned off. Blood flow ceases, producing a relatively dry field (although some blood drains into the field and requires suctioning). The patient's head is packed with bags of ice to maintain cerebral cooling; the nose and ears are padded for protection. The aorta is opened and the distal arch anastomosis is performed under circulatory arrest. Although deep hypothermia offers cerebral protection, additional interventions are used. Retrograde cerebral perfusion (RCP) can be used to provide cerebral perfusion during the period of circulatory arrest. The superior vena cava cannula is connected to the arterial line within the bypass circuit; the perfusionist can slowly pump arterialized blood into the cerebral venous circuit is order to remove acid waste buildup and replenish nutrients. The retrograde flow also pushes potential emboli out into the surgical field where they can be removed. Electroencephalograms and evoked potential monitoring enable team members to detect and treat changes in brain wave activity that may indicate cerebral insult or injury. After selection of a graft, the distal anastomosis is performed. If the arch vessels (innominate artery, left carotid and left subclavian arteries) require individual anastomoses, a graft with three branches is used and each branch is anastomosed to its respective recipient artery. More often, a straight tube graft can be fashioned to connect the branches *en bloc*. This is achieved by making an oval opening into the upper (convex) portion of the graft to which is anastomosed the common origin of all three branch vessels. Once this is completed, the cross-clamp is applied to the graft proximal to the arch vessels. RCP is discontinued, femoral vein-femoral artery perfusion is reinitiated, and the patient gradually rewarmed. The proximal anastomosis is then created (Seifert, 2007). The graft and aorta are vented and air is aspirated. The cross clamp is removed, and the patient is fully rewarmed.

RCP
Retrograde Cerebral Perfusion

Repair of the Descending Aorta

When operative intervention is indicated (eg, risk of impending rupture), the patient is placed in a modified right lateral decubitus position with both groins accessible and prepped for monitoring or bypass lines. Thoracotomy instrumentation is used for open procedures. Endovascular repair is discussed below.

The heart is not arrested; it continues to beat and perfuse the upper body. Femoral vein-femoral artery bypass may be used to perfuse the kidneys and the rest of the lower body. Occasionally, the kidneys are packed in slush for additional protection, especially in patients with pre-existing renal disease. Some surgeons elect to use a "clamp and sew" technique, whereby femoral bypass is not employed; commonly, patients undergoing this type of repair have sturdy, relatively healthy tissue above and below the aneurysm.

A left thoracotomy incision is made to provide sufficient exposure of the aorta to place clamps both proximally and distally. The incision may be extended down to the abdomen and the aortic bifurcation if there is a thoracoabdominal aneurysm. After femoral bypass is initiated, the aorta is clamped and opened, and the diseased tissue is resected. A graft is selected and the proximal anastomosis is completed. "Buttons" or pedicles may be fashioned to perfuse intercostal arteries supplying the spinal cord. These arteries may be reattached to the vascular graft with cuffs of native aorta encompassing several arterial origins. This technique is easier than sewing each vessel individually and decreases bypass and surgical time. After the proximal anastomosis and the pedicle portions are completed, the distal anastomosis is performed.

Paraplegia is a serious complication and is related to the interruption of spinal cord perfusion. Regional hypothermia with the infusion of epidural iced saline may be used to protect the spinal cord during the period of cross-clamping. Other protective measures include cerebrospinal fluid drainage and the use of evoked-potential monitoring (Conrad & Cambria, 2008).

Endovascular stents. Endovascular repair is rapidly gaining popularity. There are FDA-approved stent grafts and a number of others awaiting FDA-approval. First generation stents were associated with insertion-related stroke, iatrogenic aortic dissection or penetration, leaks, kinking, and graft migration. More recent models have shown significant improvement (Svensson et al, 2008).

The patient is placed in the supine position on an OR bed that allows fluoroscopic imaging. Nothing should be placed on the patient's skin that will interfere with imaging the aorta and surrounding tissue. Translucent EKG pads and hemodynamic monitoring pads should be used to ensure endovascular visualization. The scrub person drapes the patient and the C-arm, and prepares for the femoral artery cutdown. Because the guidewires and catheters are lengthy, is important for the scrub person to protect the sterility of these devices by weighing them down with wet towels or other heavy sterile objects (the scrub person ensure that the table coverings are impermeable to fluid).

After the femoral artery is exposed, the surgeon inserts a needle into the artery. Next a guidewire is threaded through the needle and passed into the aorta; the needle is removed and dilators are then inserted over the guidewire to enlarge the arteriotomy. The last dilator is removed and a sheath is inserted over the guide wire. A marker wire (often with a "pigtail" distal tip) is inserted after which the guide wire is removed, leaving the sheath and the marker wire in place. An intravascular ultrasound probe is inserted to measure the internal dimensions of the aorta, after which the probe is removed. The furled endostent graft is inserted into the catheter, positioned in the aorta under fluoroscopy, opened and deployed (**Fig. 23.18**) (Svensson et al, 2008).

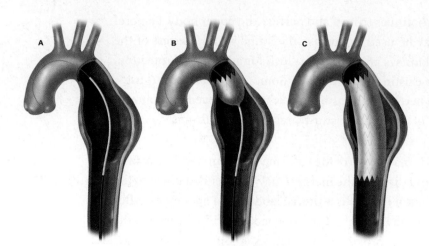

Figure 23.18
Insertion of endostent to repair aneurysm of the descending thoracic aorta. Left, the stent deployment device is positioned in the aorta. Middle, the stent is unfurled proximally, fixing it into the aortic wall. Right, the stent is fully deployed and all catheters and deployments devices are removed.

SURGERY FOR CONDUCTION ABNORMALITIES

Surgery for Atrial Fibrillation

AF
Atrial Fibrillation

Atrial fibrillation (AF) is a supraventricular rhythm abnormality characterized by rapid atrial contractions of 350 (or more) beats per minute. These contractions are uncoordinated and can lead to ventricular irregularities such as tachycardia. Because atrial contraction contributes a significant portion of blood to the left ventricle, the presence of AF can reduce the overall cardiac output. AF also leads to stasis of blood in the atrium, increasing the risk of clot formation and subsequent thromboembolism.

The growing number of patients with AF and the complications associated with AF (stroke and compromised hemodynamics secondary to a reduction in cardiac output) have prompted greater interest in surgical interventions. Successful early attempts to create an electrical maze that forced aberrant atrial impulses toward the atrioventricular (AV) node encouraged newer techniques both in the electrophysiology (EP) laboratory and in the OR. The surgical goal is to ablate specific areas of the heart that are the source of the atrial fibrillatory impulses. Often these impulses originate in the area where the pulmonary veins enter the left atrium, but other sites also may generate the aberrant impulses. By employing hypothermic, radiofrequency, or other energies to destroy the target cells within these sites, the surgeon enables a normal conduction pathway to resume. The surgery may be performed in conjunction with another surgery (eg, mitral valve surgery) or it can be performed as a standalone procedure. Depending on the patient's needs, the surgeon may employ a sternotomy or a minimally invasive thoracotomy approach (Seifert, Collins & Ad, 2008).

Pacemaker Insertion

Currently, pacemaker insertion is commonly performed in the electrophysiology (EP) laboratory. Occasionally, however, pacemaker electrodes and generators are inserted transvenously in the OR for patients with complex anatomy or severe co-morbid conditions. Pacemakers are indicated for patients with heart block or other conduction disorder producing bradycardia, which is generally defined as a heart rate of less than 60 beats per minute (Pelter, 2008; Trupp & Bubien, 2008). The diagnosis is confirmed with an EGG or ambulatory 24-hour EGG monitoring.

The patient is transported to the OR, transferred to the OR bed and placed in the supine position. Pressure areas should be padded and the patient's head may be elevated slightly; supplemental oxygen is administered if necessary. Venous access and continuous EGG monitoring are established. Local anesthesia (lidocaine 1%) with monitored intravenous sedation is commonly used for pain control and relaxation.

The fluoroscopy machine ("C-arm") is brought into the room. In order to protect themselves from harmful radiation, the sterile members of the surgical team should don lead aprons before scrubbing and gowning. X-ray screens should be available for nonsterile staff.

The circulating nurse prepares the entire neck and chest to the nipple line. The scrub person drapes the chest in a manner that exposes the skin over both the right and left subclavian vein. After draping, the scrub person passes alligator cables off the field to the individual who will be operating the pacemaker analyzer (this may be the pacer representative, the cardiologist, or another individual with knowledge of pacing analysis). The fluoroscopy machine is also draped and moved into position over the chest.

The surgeon makes an incision in the deltopectoral groove to expose the subclavian vein. Either the right or the left vein may be accessed, depending on the surgeon's preference. The vein is opened approximately 3 mm and probed for patency.

An introducer is inserted into the vein; the pacing lead is inserted into the vein and advanced under fluoroscopy to the right atrium, through the tricuspid valve, and into the right ventricle (**Fig. 23.19**). Transvenous leads usually have a coil spring which is embedded into the right ventricular endocardium. A second lead may be inserted through the same sheath and positioned in the right atrial appendage. The implanted leads are connected to the alligator pacing cables to test the leads' ability to sense electrical activity and to pace the heart muscle. The leads are secured to the fascia with nonabsorbable suture. After the leads are secured, the patient may

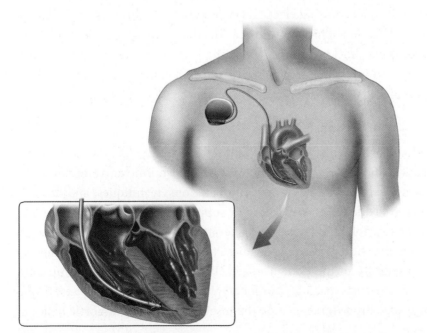

Figure 23.19

Placement of pacemaker generator and lead. *Inset* shows the flow of electrons during the pacemaker spike from distal to the electrode, through the endocardium, to the proximal electrode.

be asked to breathe deeply and cough while the lead positions are examined under fluoroscopy for possible dislodgment.

The generator pocket is then made by separating the pectoral muscle fascia from the overlying subcutaneous tissue. The leads are cleaned of blood with a moist sponge and connected to the selected generator which is placed into the skin pocket. The area is irrigated with antibiotic solution. After verification of the pacing system's functioning, the fascia and skin layers are closed with absorbable suture.

Patients receiving intravenous sedation are transported to the postanesthesia care unit for monitoring. A postprocedure chest radiograph is taken to confirm the position of the pacemaker.

Implantable Cardioverter Defibrillator

ICD
Implantable
Cardioverter
Defibrillator

The implantable cardioverter defibrillator (ICD) is an electronic device that senses lethal dysrhythmias (ventricular tachycardia, ventricular fibrillation) and shocks the heart, thereby interrupting the dysrhythmia. Insertion of the ICD leads is commonly performed in the EP laboratory via a transvenous route. In rare cases when a patient needing an ICD has severe venous disease that would preclude insertion via the transvenous route, defibrillator patches may be sewn to the heart. Whether transvenous catheters or patches are used, the leads are connected to a defibrillator generator (in a manner similar to pacemaker insertion). The operative suite may be needed for emergency repair following complications in the EP laboratory.

For insertion via the transvenous route (whether in the OR or the EP suite), the patient is prepped and draped to expose the anterior chest over the subclavian vein. A C-arm is used to image the ICD components. If patch leads are planned, the patient is placed in the supine position and prepped and draped for a midline sternotomy.

The nurse places temporary external defibrillator patches on the patient's right shoulder and left lateral chest in the event that the patient fibrillates and requires defibrillation. The transvenous leads are guided from the subclavian vein to the superior vena cava and into the right side of the heart while observing with an image intensifier. Threshold and stimulation measures are taken by the cardiologist. Ventricular fibrillation is induced using electrical current, and the heart is defibrillated with the leads connected to a temporary device. The goal is to achieve defibrillation with the lowest possible shocking energy level. The permanent device then is connected to the leads and implanted in a subcutaneous pocket. The circulating nurse should be prepared for external defibrillation and resuscitative measures.

PROCEDURES FOR HEART FAILURE

Therapeutic options for patients with heart failure have been expanded to include not only mechanical and biologic support devices, but also innovative methods to use and transform current technology. Several operations, techniques, and devices now are currently available to restore, repair, or support the failing heart. Whether failure is transient (eg, following a cardiac operative procedure) or the result of viral infection, hypertension, ischemia, or idiopathic in origin, treatments can be targeted more specifically to the patient's need. Procedures to restore pump efficiency include biventricular pacing, cardiomyoplasty, and ventricular resection. Temporizing or bridge procedures include the insertion of the intra-aortic balloon and insertion of right, left, and biventricular assist devices. These devices may support cardiac function and rest the heart, serve as a "bridge" to transplantation, or serve as "end-destination" therapy (Hunt, 2007; Lietz et al, 2007).

Bi-Ventricular Pacing

Also known as cardiac resynchronization therapy (CRT), biventricular pacing may be used in patients with dilated cardiomyopathy and congestive heart failure (Trupp & Bubien, 2008). The procedure is similar to standard pacemaker insertion except that there is a lead placed in the right atrium, a lead placed in right ventricle, and a third lead inserted into the coronary sinus and extended toward the left ventricular portion of the great cardiac vein. The goal of the procedure is to enhance the pumping function of both right and left ventricles and enhance atrioventricular synchrony (Seifert, 2008). CRT is usually performed in the EP laboratory under fluoroscopy.

CRT
Cardiac Resynchronization Therapy

Cardiomyoplasty

Cardiomyoplasty is a procedure whereby latissimus dorsi (LD) muscle is wrapped around the heart to aid in contraction. Because the LD muscle is skeletal, it must be trained to overcome fatigue and contract more like cardiac muscle. The training is achieved by electrically stimulating the LD muscle with a small implanted generator and electrodes. Once the muscle is trained and conditioned (over a period of weeks), it can function as a support to the patient's cardiac muscle. The procedure is not widely performed but may be suitable for patients who are not candidates for cardiac transplantation or mechanical assistance.

LD
Latissimus Dorsi

Left Ventricular Resection

Chronic heart failure may be the result of dilated cardiomyopathy whereby the heart muscle dilates and becomes unable to contract efficiently enough to eject an adequate cardiac output. Occasionally left ventricular dilatation is localized, enabling the surgeon to resect that portion of the wall and reapproximate the edges. The ventricular chamber is reshaped (remodeled) to form a more efficient pumping chamber. These procedures include the Batista and the Dor procedures (Seifert, 2007). Resection may also be used for repair of a left ventricular aneurysm that can develop after a myocardial infarction.

The patient is prepped and draped as for a median sternotomy. Cardiopulmonary bypass is established and the patient is cooled. After the heart is inspected, the heart is inspected the decision as to the extent of resection is made. The muscle then is resected and the ventricle is reapproximated with 0 polypropylene suture reinforced with felt strips or pledgets. Bypass is terminated, and the sternum is closed in the normal fashion.

Intra-Aortic Balloon Pump

The intra-aortic balloon pump (IABP) is the most widely used mechanical support device (Paul & Vollano, 2008). The balloon is inserted through the femoral artery by means of a percutaneous or cut-down technique. The artery is entered with a needle and a guide wire is inserted through the bore of the needle. The needle is removed and then dilating catheters of increasing size are threaded over the guidewire to enlarge the arteriotomy. The dilators are removed and the balloon catheter is threaded over the wire to a position in the descending thoracic aorta just distal to the left subclavian artery. The balloon catheter is secured to the leg with 2-0 silk sutures. Pressure monitoring lines are passed to the balloon console. Another line is passed off and connected to the pump which inflates the balloon with carbon dioxide.

The IABP reduces the workload of the heart by increasing coronary perfusion proximally and end organ perfusion distally when the balloon is inflated, and by decreasing systemic vascular resistance when the balloon is deflated. Counterpulsation is timed with the EGG or the arterial blood pressure. During left ventricular ejection, the balloon is deflated; during ventricular diastole the balloon is inflated. The IABP can be used following an acute myocardial infarction, after a cardiac procedure when left ventricular function is diminished, or as support prior to the insertion of a ventricular assist device (Paul & Vollano, 2008).

Ventricular Assist Devices

A ventricular assist devices (VAD) can provide mechanical assistance for postcardiotomy support, as a bridge to transplant, or as end-destination therapy (Grady & Shinn, 2008). Right ventricular assist devices (RVAD), left ventricular assist devices (LVAD), or biventricular assist devices (BiVAD) are available. Generally, VADs are used as a bridge to transplant until a donor heart can be found, but at least one device has been approved by the FDA for end-destination therapy (Hunt, 2007).

Left and Right Ventricular Assist Devices

Both short-term and long-term devices are available. The IABP is an example of a short-term device; other devices include a centrifugal pump or compressed air to propel flow. Long-term devices include variations of the HeartMate LVAD that provide mechanical circulatory support for irreversible left ventricular failure (ie, as a bridge to cardiac transplantation) or as destination therapy. Some patients have remained on the VAD for extended periods (eg, months, years) awaiting a donor heart (Grady & Shinn, 2008). Other VADs, such as the ABIOMED, Novacor, Thoratec, and CardioWest) can be used for RVAD and BiVAD support (as well as LVAD support). These devices may be pneumatically-, battery-, or electrically-powered.

The HeartMate LVAD is a pulsatile device that consists of an implantable blood pump, an interconnecting drive line, implant conduits, and a power source (current models are available with battery power that enables the patient to ambulate). The pump is implanted in the upper left abdominal quadrant beneath the diaphragm. Porcine xenografts incorporated in both the inflow and outflow conduits ensure unidirectional flow. Blood from the heart is directed to the pump via the inlet conduit and then propelled through an outlet tube anastomosed to the ascending aorta.

The ABIOMED can serve as a left, right, or biventricular assist device. In contrast to the HeartMate, the ABIOMED uses drive lines externalized to blood pumps that are situated outside the body. The ABIOMED is for short-term use. The device can be converted to the opposite ventricle or to biventricular mode as needed.

RVAD
Right Ventricular Assist Devices

LVAD
Left Ventricular Assist Devices

BiVAD
Biventricular Assist Devices

TRANSFER TO THE INTENSIVE CARE UNIT

Communication with the nursing staff in the intensive care unit (ICU) is important for ensuring continuity of care during the patient hand-off (TJC, 2008). Information that should be provided includes the procedure, use of bypass (or whether performed off-pump), monitoring lines, hemodynamic variables, temperature, laboratory results, electrolyte levels, medications to be set up in the ICU, blood/components given and available, pacemaker status, and any personal concerns of the patient. If a ventricular assist device is in use, this also should be reported. Generally, a phone call to the ICU receiving nurse is made approximately ½ hour before the patient's anticipated arrival to the unit. Changes affecting the patient's status should be made to update the ICU nurse.

ICU
Intensive Care Unit

Risk factors for a prolonged ICU stay and increased morbidity and mortality include female gender, increased age, previous cardiac surgery, emergency surgery, and impaired ventricular function. Other risk factors include a history of cerebrovascular disease and chronic renal failure. Strategies during the procedure that may enhance postprocedure recovery and also reduce morbidity include minimizing both bypass and cross-clamp times (Atoui et al, 2008). In addition to anesthetic and surgical interventions (eg, supporting the heart with medications and mechanical assistance), perioperative nurses can play an important role by collaborating with perfusion personnel to develop and implement an efficient plan that facilitates the extracorporeal components of the procedure, and by preparing for the surgery and having necessary supplies and equipment available so that unnecessary delays do not prolong cross-clamp time. Knowledge of the procedure, thorough preparation, and competence in the technical skills required for the surgery enable the perioperative nurse to make a positive impact on the patient's perioperative experience.

REFERENCES

1. Association of periOperative Registered Nurses. (2008). *Perioperative Standards and Recommended Practices.* Denver: AORN.
2. Atoui, R., Ma, F., Langlois, Y., & Morin, J.F. (2008). Risk factors for prolonged stay in the intensive care unit and on the ward after cardiac surgery. *Journal of Cardiac Surgery* 23: 99–106.
3. Baumgartner, F.J., Milliken, J.C., Robertson, J.M., et al. (2007). Clinical patterns of surgical endocarditis. *Journal of Cardiac Surgery* 22: 32–38.
4. Baumgartner W.A. (2007). Neurocognitive changes after coronary bypass surgery. *Circulation* 116: 1879–1881.
5. Berger, A., MacCarthy, P.A., Siebert, U., et al. (2004). Long-term patency of internal mammary artery bypass grafts: relationship with preoperative severity of the native coronary artery stenosis. *Circulation* 110 (11 Suppl 1): 14.
6. Beyea, S.C. (2002). *Perioperative Nursing Data Set,* ed 2. Denver: AORN.
7. Carabello, B.A. (2007). Aortic stenosis: Two steps forward, one step back. *Circulation* 115: 2799–2800.
8. Conrad, M.F. & Cambria, R.P. (2008). Contemporary management of descending thoracic and thoracoabdominal aortic aneurysms: Endovascular versus open. *Circulation* 117: 841–852.
9. Damiano, R.J. (2007). Robotics in cardiac surgery: The emperor's new clothes. *The Journal of Thoracic and Cardiovascular Surgery* 134 (3): 559–561.
10. Denholm B. (2008). Clinical Issues: Implant documentation. *AORN Journal* 87 (2) (February 2008): 432–435.
11. Djaiani, G., Fedorko, L., Borger, M.A., et al. (2007). Continuous-flow cell saver reduces cognitive decline in elderly patients after coronary bypass surgery. *Circulation* 116: 1888–1895.
12. Fedak, P.W.M., McCarthy, P.M., & Bonow, R.O. (2008). Evolving concepts and technologies in mitral valve repair (Review). *Circulation* 117: 963–974.
13. FDA (Food and Drug Administration). FDA clears for market first decellularized heart valve. http://www.fda.gov/bbs/topics/NEWS/2008/NEW01794.HTML. Accessed February 12, 2008.
14. Friedewald, V.E., Bonow, R.O., Borer, J.S., et al. (2007). The Editor's Roundtable: Cardiac valve surgery. *The American Journal of Cardiology* 99 (9): 1269–1278.
15. Fuster, V. (Ed.). (2007). *The Heart,* (12th ed.). New York: McGraw-Hill.

16. Goksel, O.S., Tireli, E., Kalko, Y., et al. (2008). Mid-term outcome with surgery for Type B aortic dissections: A single center experience. *Journal of Cardiac Surgery* 23: 27–30.

17. Góngora, E.I. & Sundt, T.M. (2008). Myocardial revascularization with cardiopulmonary bypass. Cohn L.H. (Ed.). *Cardiac Surgery in the Adult*. New York: McGraw-Hill, 599–632.

18. Grady, K.L. & Shinn, J. (2008). Care of patients with circulatory assist devices. In D.K. Moser & B. Riegel (Eds.), *Cardiac Nursing: A Companion to Braunwald's Heart Disease*. St Louis: Saunders Elsevier, 977–997.

19. Grube E., Schuler G., Buellesfeld L., et al. (2007). Percutaneous aortic valve replacement for severe aortic stenosis in high-risk patients using the second- and current third-generation self-expanding CoreValve prosthesis: device success and 30-day clinical outcomes. *Journal of the American College of Cardiology* 50: 69–76.

20. Hannon, E.L., Wu, C., Smith, C.R., et al. (2007). Off-pump versus on-pump coronary artery bypass graft surgery: Differences in short-term outcomes and in long-term mortality and need for subsequent revascularization. *Circulation* 116: 1145–1152.

21. Hannon, E.L., Wu, C., Walford, G., et al. (2008). Drug-eluting stents vs. Coronary-artery bypass grafting in multivessel coronary disease. *New England Journal of Medicine* 358 (4): 331–334 (January 24, 2008).

22. Haywood, P.A.R. & Buxton, B.F. (2007). Contemporary graft patency: 5-year observational data from a randomized trial of conduits. *Annals of Thoracic Surgery* 84: 795–800.

23. Hunt, S.A. (2007). Mechanical circulatory support: New data, old problems. *Circulation* 116: 461–462.

24. Jeong, S.M., Hahn, K.D., Jeong, Y.B., Yang, H.S., & Choi, I.C. (2008). Warming of intravenous fluids prevents hypothermia during off-pump coronary artery bypass graft surgery. *Journal of Cardiothoracic and Vascular Anesthesia* 22 (1): 67–70.

25. Khonsari, S. & Sintek, C.F. (2008). *Cardiac Surgery: Safeguards and pitfalls in operative technique* (4th ed.). Philadelphia: Wolters Kluwer.

26. Kleinbeck, S.V.M. (2004). *PNDS @ work: Policies, procedures, and pathways*. Denver: AORN.

27. Kouchoukos, N.T., Blackstone, E.H., & Doty, D.B., et al. (2003). *Kirklin/Barratt-Boyes Cardiac Surgery* (3rd ed). Volume 1. Philadelphia: Churchill Livingstone.

28. Kuivaniemi, H., Platsoucas, C.D., & Tilson, M.D. (2008). Aortic aneurysms: An immune disease with a strong genetic component. *Circulation* 117: 242–252.

29. Lehmann, S., Walther, T., & Kempfert, J., et al. (2007). Stentless versus conventional xenograft aortic valve replacement: Midterm results of a prospectively randomized trial. *Annals of Thoracic Surgery* 84: 467–472.

30. Lietz, K., Long, J.W., & Kfoury, A.G., et al. (2007). Outcomes of left ventricular assist device implantation as destination therapy in the Post-REMATCH era: Implications for patient Selection. *Circulation* 116: 497–505.

31. Lytle, B.W. (2007). On-pump and off-pump coronary bypass surgery (Editorial). *Circulation* 116: 1108.

32. Nagelhout, J.J., & Zaglaniczny, K.L. (2005). *Nurse Anesthesia* (3rd ed.). St Louis: Elsevier Saunders.

33. Oakley, R.E., Kleine, P., & Bach, D.S. (2008). Choice of prosthetic heart valve in today's practice. *Circulation* 117: 253–256.

34. Opie, L.H., Commerford, P.J., & Gersh, B.J. (2006). Controversies in stable coronary artery disease. *Lancet* 367: 69–78.

35. Paul, S., & Vollano, L. (2008). Care of patients with acute heart failure. In D.K. Moser & B. Riegel (Eds.), *Cardiac Nursing: A Companion to Braunwald's Heart Disease*. St Louis: Saunders Elsevier, 916–929.

36. Pelter, M.M. (2008). Electrocardiography: Normal electrocardiogram. In D.K. Moser & B. Riegel (Eds.), *Cardiac Nursing: A Companion to Braunwald's Heart Disease*. St Louis: Saunders Elsevier, 597–611.

37. Raja, S. & Berg, G.A. (2007). Impact of off-pump coronary artery bypass surgery on systemic inflammation: Current best available evidence. *Journal of Cardiac Surgery* 22: 445–455.

38. Rubertone, J.A. (2008). Anatomy of the cardiovascular system. In D.K. Moser & B. Riegel (Eds.), *Cardiac Nursing: A Companion to Braunwald's Heart Disease*. St Louis: Saunders Elsevier, 45–64.

39. Seeley, R.R., Stephens, T.D., & Tate, P. (2008). *Anatomy & Physiology*, (8th ed.). Boston: McGraw Hill.

40. Seifert, P.C. (2007). Cardiac surgery. *Alexander's care of the patient in surgery*, (13th ed.). St Louis: Mosby Elsevier.

41. Seifert, P.C. (2008). Nurses in perioperative settings. In D.K. Moser & B. Riegel (Eds.), *Cardiac Nursing: A Companion to Braunwald's Heart Disease*. St Louis: Saunders Elsevier, 286–308.

42. Seifert, P.C., Collins, J., & Ad, N. (2008). Surgery for atrial fibrillation. *AORN Journal* 86 (1): 23–40.

43. Stewart, S. (2008). Epidemiology of coronary artery disease. In D.K. Moser & B. Riegel (Eds.), *Cardiac Nursing: A Companion to Braunwald's Heart Disease*. St Louis: Saunders Elsevier, 9–30.

44. Svensson, L.G., Kouchoukos, N.T., & Miller, D.C., et al. (2008). Expert consensus document on the treatment of descending thoracic aortic disease using endovascular stent-grafts. *Annals of Thoracic Surgery* (supplement) 85: S1–S41.

45. TJC. The Joint Commission. www.jointcommission.org/PatientSafety/NationalPatientSafetyGoals. Accessed February 8, 2008.

46. Trupp, R.J. & Bubien, R.S. (2008). Care of patients with implanted cardiac rhythm management devices. In D.K. Moser & B. Riegel (Eds.), *Cardiac Nursing: A Companion to Braunwald's Heart Disease*. St Louis: Saunders Elsevier, 876–896.

47. Wagner, G.S. (2008). *Marriott's Practical Electrocardiography*, (11th ed.). Philadelphia: Lippincott Williams & Wilkins.

CHAPTER 24

Transplantation Surgery

Susan Ulmer DeWolf

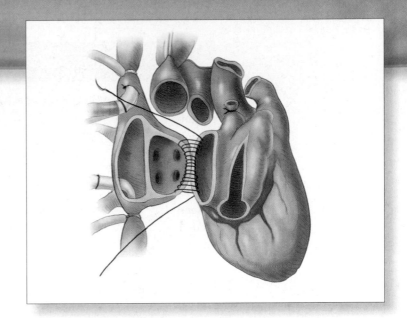

INTRODUCTION

Transplant surgery, the art and science of removing an organ or tissue from the body and surgically placing it into the body of the same or a different individual provides options for patients with organ failure or injury. Successful transplant extends and improves quality of life for these patients. Usually, only patients with end-stage disease, who have no other medical treatment options, and who meet transplant criteria become transplant surgery candidates (Encyclopedia of Surgery, 2008). As of August 2008, there were approximately 99,220 eligible recipients waiting for an organ transplant in the United States and the list continues to grow. **Table 24.1** shows US transplant statistics as reported by the United Network for Organ Sharing (UNOS).

When evaluating patients for possible transplant surgery, transplant specialists consider the patient's age, general physical state, diagnosis, and stage of disease. Patients with the following conditions generally do not meet selection criteria to become a transplant candidate (University of North Carolina, 2008; Encyclopedia of Surgery, 2008):

Chronic hepatic, pulmonary, or renal disease unless these are target organs for transplant

Compromised circulation in the lower extremities

Malignancy

Active drug or alcohol abuse

History of behavior pattern or psychiatric illness

Chronic infections

Social factors that would affect ability to follow medical regimen do not meet the criteria

Chapter Contents

UNOS
United Network for Organ Sharing

Table 24.1	United States Transplant Data	
Transplant Waiting List as of August 18, 2008		
Kidney		76,468
Pancreas		1,582
Kidney/Pancreas		2,266
Liver		16,149
Intestine		229
Heart		2,644
Lung		2,134
Heart/Lung		97
Transplants performed January–May 2008		
Deceased donor		9,089
Living donor		2,426
Donors recovered January–May 2008		
Deceased donor		3,379
Living donor		2,424

Adapted from Summary transplantation data for the entire United States as reported 18 August 2008 by United Network for Organ Sharing (UNOS), http://www.unos.org/data/default. asp?displayType=usData. Retrieved May 18, 2008.

COSTS OF TRANSPLANTS

On a yearly basis, surgeons and other physicians perform approximately 44.9 million inpatient procedures. When compared with the total number of procedures done, transplant surgery makes up a small portion of the total. However, when comparing costs, transplant surgery costs contribute significantly to total healthcare expenditures. Costs vary from region to region, and between hospitals. In addition, costs accelerate if a patient develops complications. **Table 24.2** shows examples of typical hospital and physician fees. This table does not include costs related to pre-transplant or followup treatments (CDC, 2005; National Foundation for Transplant, 2007).

TYPES OF TRANSPLANT GRAFTS

Autograft

An *autograft* is "tissue derived from an individual for implantation exclusively on or in the same individual" (AORN, 2008, p. 610). Examples of autograft tissues include skin for a skin graft, vein extraction for coronary artery bypass graft surgery, and reimplantation of a functioning kidney in a different anatomical location such as the iliac artery, iliac vein, or bladder.

Allograft

A patient given an *allograft* receives an organ or tissue taken from a living or nonliving genetically nonidentical donor of the same species. Allografts constitute the majority of human transplants. Allograft recipients must take immunosuppressive drugs for the rest of their lives in order to prevent transplant rejection (Types of Transplants, 2008).

Table 24.2	Costs of Transplants
Heart	$650,000
Lung	$400,000
Double Lung	$550,000
Heart/Lung	$875,000
Liver	$520,000
Kidney	$250,000
Pancreas	$300,000
Kidney/Pancreas	$370,000
Kidney/Heart	$760,000
Liver/Kidney	$660,000
Intestine	$900,000
Bone Marrow (autologous)	$270,000
Bone Marrow (allogeneic related)	$480,000
Bone Marrow (allogeneic unrelated)	$600,000
Cornea	$23,300

National Foundation for Transplants (2007). How much does an organ transplant cost? Retrieved 22 August 2008, http://www.transplants.org/LearnMore.php.

Isograft

An *isograft* is tissue derived from an individual for implantation in a genetically identical recipient, such as an identical twin. The recipient of an isograft does not need immunosuppressive therapy (Types of Transplants, 2008).

Xenograft

A patient given cells or tissue from a nonhuman source receives a *xenograft* (AORN, 2008, p. 610), such as transplant of porcine heart valves into a human recipient.

Split Transplants

Occasionally, two recipients share a donated organ, resulting in a *split transplant*. An example includes dividing a liver and transplanting the parts into an adult and a child (Types of Transplants, 2008).

Domino Transplant

Some patient's have a *domino transplant* when it is technically easier to replace associated organs en bloc. As an example, a patient with cystic fibrosis in need of a bilateral lung transplant receives the lungs and heart of the donor en bloc, even though he/she may have a healthy heart. Another recipient in need of a heart then receives the healthy heart taken from the cystic fibrosis patient (Types of Transplants, 2008).

ORGAN DONATION

Prior to the Uniform Anatomical Gift Act (AGA) of 1968, each state handled organ and tissue donations. Revisions of the AGA in 1972 mandated that all 50 states must recognize the Uniform Organ Donor Card as a legal document for anyone 18 or older

UAGA
Uniform Anatomical Gift Act

to donate organs upon death. In 1984, the National Organ Transplant Act (NOTA) created a national computer registry for donated organs. The UNOS operates this registry. As science advanced and the number of transplants increased, the federal government began addressing legal and ethical issues of transplantation. Congress addressed some of these issues by passing the Patient Self Determination Action of 1991, which encourages advance-care medical directives, living will, and durable powers of attorney for patients deciding to donate organs (*Encyclopedia of Everyday Law/Organ Donation*, 2008).

Types of Donors

Living Donors

People receiving an organ from a living donor receive an organ that is a related tissue match or an unrelated tissue match. When a donor gives an organ such as a kidney, the remaining kidney assumes the workload of the donated kidney. For donations such as a partial liver, the remaining portion of the liver assumes the workload until the liver regenerates.

Deceased Donors

There are two types of deceased donors.

BRAIN-STEM DEATH DONORS

Brain death donors do not have brain activity or have an absence of brain stem function necessary to support normal physiological parameters required for daily life. Ventilators or other mechanical and chemical means keep these donors viable until an organ procurement time has been set.

CARDIAC DEATH DONORS

Cardiac death donors show brain function but have injuries so severe that normal physiological activity will not return without supportive measures. After transfer to the operating room, the patient is removed from life support. Monitoring of the patient continues until death occurs, usually within an hour. The procurement teams stand by until time of death and then begin the procurement of donated organs. If death does not occur after an hour has passed, the patient is usually transported back to the Intensive Care Unit (ICU) for further evaluation and monitoring.

Types of Organs and Tissues Transplanted

Table 24.3 lists the types of organs and tissues suitable for transplant.

Allocation of Donated Organs

The UNOS implements the Health and Human Services (HHS) guidelines for organ allocation and maintains a registry of potential recipients divided by specific organ type and ABO blood types. Several factors determine organ list priority: ABO blood type compatibility, proximity of the recipient to the donor, time on the waiting list, gravity of the illness, and unique circumstances related to the recipient's medical condition. For kidneys, allocation criteria also include human leukocyte antigen (HLA) matching and antigen sensitivity via a panel reactive antibody (PRA)

Table 24.3	Types of Organs and Tissues Suitable for Transplant

Solid

Kidney (deceased donor and living donor)

Liver (deceased donor and living donor)

Pancreas (deceased donor and living donor)

Intestine (deceased donor and living donor)

Heart (deceased donor only)

Lung (deceased donor and living donor)

En bloc Heart/Lung (deceased donor and domino transplant)

Tissue, Cells, and Fluids

Tendon (deceased donor and autograft)

Bone (deceased donor, living donor, and autograft)

Bone marrow/stem cell (living donor and autograft)

Blood vessels (deceased donor and autograft)

Blood Products (living donor and autograft)

Heart valve (deceased donor, living donor, and xenograft-porcine/bovine)

Cornea (deceased donor only)

Skin (deceased donor, living donor, and autograft)

Islets of Langerhans (deceased donor and living donor)

Types of Transplants. Transplant History. (2008). Retrieved January 10, 2008, from Wikipedia Web site: http://en.wikipedia.org/wiki/organ_transplantation.

percentage. Liver and lung recipients must meet objective scoring criteria before receiving an organ. Liver recipients must meet criteria defined in the Model of End-Stage Liver Disease (MELD) and lung recipients the criteria defined in the Lung Allocation Score (LAS). The scoring systems uses defined laboratory and physiologic parameters and a point scale system to rank order the recipient's place on the allocation list. UNOC lists intestinal recipients as Status I or Status II and Cardiac recipients as Status IA, IB, or 2. Eye banks handle donor cornea tissue (Finger, 2006).

Immunology and Tissue Matching

Before transplanting solid organs, histocompatibility testing (matching of donor and recipient tissue types) is done to determine recipient potential for rejecting the transplanted organ.

Blood Type Matching

The four major blood types identify the type of glycoprotein on the surface of the blood cells in an individual. Humans naturally contain antibodies to the glycoproteins their own red blood cells lack. **Table 24.4** lists blood cell types, glycoproteins, antibodies, and compatibility with other types.

Type AB blood group people are considered universal recipients because their blood does not have antibodies on the surface of the red blood cells to react and attack the transplanted organ. Type O blood group people are considered universal

MELD
Model of End-Stage Liver Disease

LAS
Lung Allocation Score

Table 24.4	Blood Type Matching		
Recipient Blood Type	**Glycoproteins**	**Antibodies**	**Donor Blood Type Compatibility**
A	A	B	AB, O
B	B	A	AB, O
AB	A, B	None	A, B, AB, O
O	None	A, B, AB	O

DNA
Deoxyribonucleic Acid

donors because their blood does not have glycoproteins on the surface of their red blood cells to react with any other blood group. Type O people have antibodies to all other blood groups, and thus can only receive an organ from a type O donor (Friedman, 2006). Rh factor in blood has no effect on the transplanted organ and therefore is not included in the ABO matching. Before the transplant the nurse locates the ABO documentation in the recipient's medical record and verifies blood type compatibility between the donor and recipient.

Human Leukocyte Antigen Matching

Humans have a set of proteins or markers on the surface of their leukocytes known as human leukocyte antigens (HLA). These proteins are part of the body's immune recognition system that determines "self" from "non-self." Deoxyribonucleic acid (DNA) inside each cell carries the information that determines which HLA antigens are on the surface of the leukocytes. The most common HLA antigens identified in solid organ transplantation are HLA-A, HLA-B, and HLA-DR. Every human has two sets of A, B, and DR antigens, one set from each parent, thus giving each person a total of six-antigens (Twyman, 2003). In HLA testing or tissue typing, leukocytes are tested and matched from the donor and potential recipients. A six-antigen match is made when the donor and recipient share the same identical HLA antigens, the higher the number of identical antigens, the less chance of organ rejection.

Panel Reactive Antibody Testing

Another histocompatibility test is the *panel reactive antibody* (PRA) test. This test combines the recipient's blood serum with samples of cells containing known antigens from a donor panel of different individuals. PRA testing determines if the recipient has acquired antibodies from a previous blood transfusion, transplant, or pregnancy to a spectrum of antigens. The test checks for possible antibody–antigen mismatches by looking at the number of cells in the sample that react and how strongly the cells react. PRA testing is reported as a percentage of panel donors who show a positive reaction with the recipient's serum. If the recipient's serum reacts with 50% of the panel donors the test is reported as a PRA of 50%. The PRA percentage predicts the results of the final crossmatch, the higher the PRA percentage, the greater risk of organ rejection. Recipients with a high PRA score require prospective crossmatch testing.

Crossmatch Testing

Prospective or retrospective crossmatching, which is the final histocompatibility test, can take several hours to complete. Except for kidneys, most solid organs are crossmatched retrospectively because of short organ viability time from procurement to transplantation. The test mixes donor lymphocytes with recipient lymphocytes. A positive crossmatch is reported when cells bind together and clump. This indicates that the recipient has antibodies against the donor antigens and will reject the organ. Conversely, with a negative crossmatch the cells did not bind or clump together, which indicates that the lymphocytes are compatible. Most likely, this patient will not reject the transplanted organ. Kidney transplants are crossmatched before the procedure. The surgeon may proceed with the transplant before completion of the final crossmatch if the HLA antigen match is high and the PRA is a low percentage. Each hospital should have a crossmatch policy in place for nursing staff to follow. For kidney transplants, the nurse usually verifies that the final crossmatch is negative before the patient arrives in the operating room suite.

Intravenous Immunoglobulin

Recipients of kidneys from incompatible donors receive *intravenous immunoglobulin* (IVIG) before the procedure. This blood product contains immunoglobulin G (IgG) or antibodies from the plasma of over a thousand blood donors. IVIG reduces the risk of kidney rejection by suppressing the inflammatory response. In 2004 the Food and Drug Administration approved the Cedars-Sinai High Dose IVIG treatment, which allows recipients to receive a kidney from non-tissue matched donors and non-ABO compatible living donors (IVIG Intravenous, 2008). When a recipient receives IVIG before the procedure, information concerning the negative final crossmatch may not be documented in the patient's medical record. Each hospital should have a policy concerning documentation requirements.

IVIG
Intravenous
Immunoglobulin

IgG
Immunoglobulin G

TRANSPLANTED ORGAN GRAFT REJECTION

Despite preprocedure tissue matching, organ rejection can still occur. In these cases, the body of the transplant recipient fails to accept the transplanted organ as "self" and the immune system attacks. Usually, the first indicator of graft or organ rejection is an inflammatory response (Transplantation, 2004). As a preventative measure, transplant recipients take immunosuppressive agents for the rest of their lives.

Hyperacute Rejection

Hyperacute rejection occurs when the recipient has pre-existing ABO blood type antibodies to the donor. As an example, a recipient with pre-existing ABO antibodies will reject the transplanted kidney within minutes of reperfusion. In order to prevent a severe inflammatory response, the surgeon must immediately remove the kidney. Prospective crossmatching prevents this type of rejection. For other organ transplants, the use of ABO compatible grafts prevents hyperacute rejection.

Acute Rejection

Acute rejection can begin as early as one week after transplantation or can occur months to years later. The patient is at most risk for acute rejection during the first three months following transplantation. Kidneys and livers are at greatest risk for rejection because of organ vascularity. Acute rejection occurs due to mismatched HLA antigens. The recipient's T-cells cause cells in the transplanted organ to produce cytokines that lead to necrosis of the organ (Transplantation, 2004). Excluding an isograft transplant, to some degree, this response may occur in all transplanted organs. Diagnosis of acute rejection relies on recipient clinical data, laboratory testing, and a transplanted organ tissue biopsy. If recognized early and treated promptly with a short course of high-dose corticosteroids, a single episode of acute rejection rarely leads to organ failure. Other treatment options can be initiated if the corticosteroid treatment is unsuccessful. Recurrent episodes of acute rejection can lead to chronic rejection.

Chronic Rejection

Chronic rejection is a result of a slow, persistent immune response against the transplanted organ. This response is irreversible and therefore untreatable. Usually, the patient requires another organ transplant after approximately 10 years.

Immunosuppression Complications

Side effects or complications of immunosuppression therapy include short- and long-term opportunistic infections, hypertension, malignancy, and end-organ toxicities, primarily to the liver, kidneys, and the pancreas. Musculoskeletal changes secondary to steroid-induced osteopenia may occur. Other complications to steroid therapy include Cushing's disease, cataracts, and gastrointestinal bleeding. Although effective therapies exist for many of these complications, some remain significant causes of morbidity and mortality in all organ transplant recipients.

CONSIDERATIONS FOR ORGAN PROCUREMENT AND TRANSPLANTATION PROCEDURES

The following information pertains to the common elements of care for organ procurement and organ transplant patients. For deviations from these common elements of care, see procedure descriptions.

Anesthesia for Organ Procurement

The anesthesia provider hemodynamically monitors and maintains the patient with medications and fluids until cross clamping of the aorta. After cross clamping of the aorta, the anesthesia provider discontinues interventions that maintain oxygenated blood flow in the donor.

Anesthesia for Organ Transplant

The anesthesia provider will use general endotracheal anesthesia for transplant procedures. Where applicable, the patient may receive epidural anesthesia for pain control following the procedure. For some procedures, the anesthesia provider inserts a nasogastric tube to decompress the stomach. The patient receives prophylactic antibiotics prior to the incision. Anesthesia, medications, and arterial and venous monitoring lines vary for each procedure, depending on the type and severity of the recipient's disease process, the type of organ transplanted, and the current hemodynamic status of the recipient. During the procedure, the anesthesia provider may begin immunosuppressive therapy. Each hospital usually has protocols or clinical pathways for administration of immunosuppressive agents and line placement for monitoring the recipient during the procedure.

Before the Patient Arrives

The nurse circulator and scrub person usually prepare the operating room suite. Check all equipment and lighting for proper function before the procedure. Using aseptic technique, prepare the slush or ice machine. Turn it on and pour sterile saline into it; this will ensure that an adequate amount of slush is available for the donated organ.

Patient ID and Safety

After the patient arrives in the operating room, implement *Time Out* procedures according to hospital policy and procedure. While implementing the *Time Out* protocol, verify ABO compatibility. Implement additional safety measures according to hospital operating room policy and procedure. Document the patient identification process and safety measures on the medical record.

Considerations for Transplant Patients

Before the induction of anesthesia, apply sequential pressure stockings according to the manufacturers written instructions. Connect the tubing to the sequential pressure device and test it to ensure that it functions properly. After the induction of general anesthesia and prior to positioning the patient, insert a Foley catheter and connect it to a collection device.

Position

See **Table 24.5** for positioning considerations for organ procurement and organ transplant. Refer to Chapter 8 for detailed descriptions of placing the patient in the supine and lateral positions.

Equipment and Supplies

Table 24.6 lists standard operating room furniture and equipment. **Table 24.7** lists standard supplies and instrumentation.

Establishing and Maintaining the Sterile Field

Refer to Chapter 9 for detailed information concerning establishing a sterile field for patients placed in the supine and lateral positions. Hair removal protocols should conform to guidelines published by the Surgical Care Initiative Project.

Table 24.5	Positioning for Organ Procurement and Transplant

Procedure	Position
Organ Procurement	Supine with the arms tucked and secured at the sides or placed on armboards at an angle of less than 90 degrees
Living Related or Non-Related Kidney Donor	Lateral; remove the x-ray tunnels on the operating bed to allow elevation of the kidney rest if necessary; place a bean bag on the bed for adequate patient support during positioning
Living Donor Kidney Recipient Transplant	Supine with the arms place on armboards at an angle of less than 90 degrees
Deceased Donor Kidney Transplant	
Pancreas Transplant	
Liver Transplant	
Intestine Transplant	
Heart Transplant	
Lung Transplant	Supine with the arms lifted anteriorly and abducted
Heart and Lung Transplant	

Table 24.6	Standard Operating Room Equipment for Organ Transplant

Slush/ice machine	Kick buckets
Anesthesia machine	Prep table
IV poles × 2	Electrosurgery generator
Operating room bed	Suction machine/Neptune suction
Back table	Standing stools
Organ backbench table	Sequential compression device
Rolling stool	Headlight and light source
Mayo stand	Doppler box
Ring stand	

Organ Documentation

Organs received from the United Network for Organ Sharing and the regional Organ Procurement Organizations require the documentation of ischemic, and reperfusion times during transplantation procedures. The circulating nurse documents the times in the patient's medical record according to policy and procedure (**Table 24.8**). In the case of a living donor, document the cross-clamp time as the time when the surgeon removes the kidney from the donor and places it on ice on the backbench table. Additionally, before the end of the procedure request an ICU bed for patient transport to the ICU.

Table 24.7	Standard Surgical Supplies, Instruments, and Retractors for Organ Transplant	
Slush/ice machine drape	Light gloves	
Sequential compression stockings	X-ray detectable lap sponges	
Back table cover	Knife lades (surgeon preference)	
Backbench table cover	Syringe and needles	
Surgical drapes appropriate for the surgical incision (laparotomy sheet or transverse laparotomy sheet for transverse incisions or a universal pack)	Needle counter	
	Electrosurgery pencil with extended tip	
	Suction tubing and tips	
	Irrigating syringe	
Foley catheter and urimeter	Suture (surgeon and organ transplantation specific)	
Ioban Steri-drape	Sterile Doppler handpiece	
Prep solution	Vessel loops/umbilical Tape	
Gowns	Suture boots	
Gloves	Ligaclips and appliers	
Towels	Major retractor pan	
Basin set	Bookwalter, Thompson, or iron intern retractor	
Metal basin for organ preparation and storage		
Light gloves		

Table 24.8	UNOS and OPO Required Documentation for Ischemic and Reperfusion Times
A.	Time of donor aorta cross clamp time (time is usually noted on the outside of the transporter box for the organ or on the inside paperwork that arrives with the donated organ)
B.	Time the organ is removed from ice
C.	Time the venous anastomosis begins
D.	Time the arterial anastomosis ends and all clamps are removed
E.	A calculation of warm ischemic time or anastomosis time ($C - D = E$)
F.	Total preservation or cold ischemic time ($A + D = F$)

The information recorded may vary from hospital to hospital, however, critical times needed reflect how long the organ was out of the donor prior to transplantation, (known as cold ischemic time), and the length of time the organ was out of ice to reperfusion with recipient's blood (known as warm ischemic time).

Postprocedure Care

After applying the sterile dressing, transport the patient to the postanesthesia care unit (PACU) or ICU. Communicate patient information necessary for the appropriate continuation of care to the PACU or ICU nurse patient information necessary for appropriate continuation of care. See **Table 24.9**.

PACU
Postanesthesia Care Unit

Table 24.9	Nursing Report to PACU or ICU Nurse
Patient name	Drains/Tubes
Allergies	Medications given and quantity
Procedure	Urine output
Type of incision	Estimated blood loss
Foley	Pain control catheters present

ORGAN PROCUREMENT

OPO
Organ Procurement
Organization

DCD
Donation after Cardiac
Death

After identifying a potential deceased organ donor within a hospital system a collaborative team of professionals begin the donation process, to include notification of the local regional Organ Procurement Organization (OPO). The team initiates critical pathways for organ donation as well as donation after cardiac death (DCD) and manages the potential donor according to the pathway guidelines. While the family makes their decision regarding organ donation, the OPO completes the donation consent paperwork and communicates with UNOS to identify which recipients match with the donated organs. Attempts to match the donor with local and regional recipients take priority. Comprehensive donor testing and documentation determines current function and viability of the organs intended for donation. Recipient hospitals receive notification and contact potential recipients to check in for final evaluation, testing, and possible transplantation.

Several factors determine procurement time of the organs. Resuscitation of the donor must correct physiological imbalances and then maintain physiological status, which may result in a time delay for procurement. Placement of organs and the arrival of procurement teams for multiorgan donation require careful coordination. Occasionally additional preprocurement tests for specific organ function become necessary prior to a transplant surgeon accepting an organ. Procurement delays can also occur due to preprocurement histocompatibility testing to determine the best match of donor to recipient. Busy operating room schedules or case loads and staff availability may also affect procurement times.

The OPO supplies all packaging supplies for the donated organs, the organ perfusion solutions, skin prep solution, and the general sterile pack of necessary supplies for the operative procedure. See **Table 24.10** for hospital provided general equipment and other supplies necessary for the procurement of organs.

Equipment and Supplies

Table 24.6 lists standard operating room furniture and equipment. **Table 24.7** lists standard supplies and instrumentation.

Organ Donation Procedure

Prep the donor from the neck to the pubis and drape in a sterile fashion. The chest is opened via median sternotomy and the abdominal cavity is entered. Retractors are placed and the cavities are inspected by the surgical teams for signs of occult pathology and organ suitability for transplanting. Occasionally a biopsy of an organ or organs is

Table 24.10	Hospital Provided Supplies for Organ Procurement	
Equipment	**Supplies**	**Instruments**
Back table × number or organs to be recovered	Gloves	Major vascular van
Bovie × 2	Suture	Sternal saw
Ice/Slush machine	Staplers	Major retractor pan
Suction × 2 or Neptune suction	Ligaclip appliers	Chest retractor
Flexible bronchoscope (for lung donors)	Various stapling devices and reloads	Major laparotomy pan
Large basin for each back table		

necessary to determine suitability for transplanting. The right colon is mobilized, the posterior peritoneum is incised, and the pancreas and duodenum are reflected. This allows exposure of the inferior vena cava (IVC) and the aorta. The attachments of the heart, lungs, liver, kidneys, and pancreas are incised. The aortic arch, IVC, abdominal aorta, and portal vein are cannulated for the infusion of the preservation solution. The aortic arch and supraceliac abdominal aorta are cross-clamped. The cold preservation solution is infused through the inferior aortic, portal, and cardiac cannulae. Drainage of effluent is via the IVC. The thoracic and abdominal cavities are then packed with ice (Finger, 2006). Donated organs are removed by the surgical teams in the order of organ susceptibility to warm ischemic time. The heart/lung team are followed by the abdominal team. Organs are removed and initial preparation is done on the backbench table. Organs are then packaged in a sterile fashion, placed usually in a transport box filled with ice, sealed, and transported to the recipient locations.

IVC
Inferior Vena Cava

Kidney Transporter

The increasing number of people on the waiting list for a kidney transplant has lead to the development of kidney transport systems such as the LifePort® kidney transporter manufactured by Organ Recovery Systems. This machine supplies continuous perfusion to kidneys from expanded criteria donors (ECD) also known as non-optimal donors for various medical reasons. The machine delivers a low-flow, low-pressure pulsatile perfusate to the kidney. The fluid used supplies the kidney with nutrients, antibiotics, antioxidants, anti-inflammatory drugs, calcium channel blockers, and immunosuppressive agents. In the past, kidneys donated from an ECD were rejected by transplant surgeons due to poor organ transplant outcomes in the recipients. The small size of the transporter facilitates easy transport to the recipient hospital. Rechargeable batteries power the unit. Furthermore, the unit runs automatically and does not require a technician operator. When the surgeon is ready to transplant the kidney, the circulating nurse removes the outer cover. The scrub team then drapes the opened machine with the sterile plastic drape supplied with the machine. The kidney is disconnected from the machine and brought to the sterile field for final preparation and transplantation (Kidney Transporter, 2005).

ECD
Expanded Criteria Donors

Procurement Complications

Problems that may occur during the procurement phase usually relate to the patient becoming hemodynamically unstable. The circulating nurse assists the anesthesia provider by providing any additional supplies or drugs not already on hand to manage the patient.

As mentioned earlier, visualization of the organs sometimes reveals problems that are not detected during the presurgical evaluation of the donor, such as fatty liver disease. Preprocedure liver function blood testing may have revealed normal values. Occasionally a fatty liver or cirrhotic liver may make the liver unsuitable for transplantation. Inadvertent operative damage to the vasculature of a donated organ also makes the organ unsuitable for transplantation.

Postprocedure Care

After the procurement of the organs, the procurement team closes and the nursing team prepares the donor for transfer to the hospital morgue.

Organ Preparation

After flushing the organ with perfusate and minimally preparing it for transportation, the procurement team places the organ in a self-contained sterile bag or container, packs it in ice, and boxes it for transportation. Kidneys may arrive in the kidney transporter discussed in the previous section of this chapter. All organs need backbench preparation to remove excess tissue and prepare the vascular structures anastomosis. Some organs require extensive backbench preparation as they may have been procured en bloc with other organs or structures. The circulating nurse usually opens the transport box and delivers the organ in a sterile fashion to the surgeon staffing the backbench. Preparation of organs always requires a metal basin containing sterile ice/slush to maintain preservation temperatures, a backbench instrument set, suture, and clip appliers, and sometimes various stapling devices. The surgeon may complete backbench organ preparation prior to patient arrival in the operating room suite, or preparation can occur as the anesthesia provider inserts necessary lines for patient monitoring. Sometimes the kidney preparation occurs after the recipient's vascular structures have been isolated and made ready for transplantation. **Figure 24.1** is an example of the backbench preparation of a kidney with unusual anatomy containing four arteries.

ORGAN TRANSPLANTATION PROCEDURES
Living Related or Non-Related Kidney Donor

A living donated kidney usually has better survival rates in the recipient as opposed to a deceased donor kidney for six reasons.

1. The cold ischemic time on the kidney from a living donor is greatly reduced since the kidney is transplanted almost immediately after removal from the donor.
2. Donor and the recipient have a better match because they are usually relatives and share some of the same HLA markers.
3. The procedure is elective in nature and performed hopefully prior to the recipient needing dialysis.

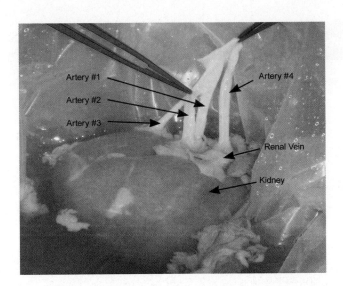

Figure 24.1
Back bench preparation of the kidney with 4 arteries.

Artery #1

Artery #2

Artery #3

Artery #4

Renal Vein

Kidney

24

4. The supply of deceased donor organs cannot keep up with the demand, which greatly increases the time waiting for a kidney transplant.

5. The donor and the recipient can usually be brought to the operating rooms at the same time.

6. One surgical team prepares the donor for the removal of the kidney while another surgical team prepares the recipient for receiving the donated kidney.

Indications

Usually, with a living related or non-related kidney donor, a healthy donor wants to donate a kidney. Occasionally preprocedure evaluation reveals a potential underlying disease process, which may result in altered or decreased renal function in the donor, which prevents the kidney donation.

Equipment and Supplies

Table 24.11 lists additional items for hand assisted laparoscopic technique.

Special Considerations

The donor-circulating nurse maintains communication with the recipient-circulating nurse during the procedure in order to establish readiness of both teams for the removal of the kidney and accepting the kidney. The recipient surgeon comes to the recipient room just before the kidney is removed to set up the perfusate solution tubing and prepare the ice-filled basin for the kidney immediately upon removal. The time the kidney is removed is documented by the circulating nurses and serves as the "cross-clamp" time on the kidney in some institutions.

Procedure: Donor Laparoscopic Hand-Assisted Nephrectomy

The donor nephrectomy historically was performed using an open retroperitoneal approach through a flank incision. Newer technology has introduced gel hand ports that allow a hand-assisted laparoscopic approach. Usually the left kidney offers the best choice for donation due to anatomical location and greater length of the renal vessels, making implantation into the recipient easier.

A midline incision is made to include the umbilicus. The incision is made large enough to accommodate the surgeon's hand. For a large patient, a paramedian incision may be

Table 24.11	Additional Items for Hand-Assisted Laparoscopic Technique				
Equipment	**Instruments**	**Supplies**	**Medications Anesthesia**	**Medications Sterile Field**	**Medications in Room**
Arteriograms	Renal laparoscopic pan	CO_2 tubing	Mannitol	Marcaine 0.5% with epinephrine	Perfusate solution $\times 2$ on ice for kidney perfusion
Light source for camera	Renal open pan and retractor (pan is available)	Sterile IV tubing without a filter	Lasix	Surgicel/Gelfoam	Papaverine
Video monitors $\times 2$	10/12 trocars $\times 2$	Extension tubing	Heparin		
CO_2 insufflator	Stapling device	Hand port	Protamine		
Pillows $\times 5$	Endoclips	Sterile KY Jelly			
Bean bag	10° & 30° scopes	Defogger			
Rolled sheets $\times 2$ for under bean bag	Camera	Cysto tubing			
Extra IV pole for kidney prep table	Hemoloc clip appliers	Hemoloc clips			

used. The incision is extended into the peritoneum and the gel port is placed, which allows insertion of a hand to assist with dissection and manipulation of tissue surrounding the kidney, and removal of the donated kidney. A mixture of sterile KY Jelly and normal saline applied to the back of the surgeon's hand allows for easier insertion into the gel port. Two 12 mm port incisions are then made to accommodate the camera and laparoscopic instrumentation. After insufflation of the abdomen with CO_2, dissection of the kidney begins at the splenic flexure of the colon and continues down over the kidney. Next, Gerota's fascia is medially incised; the ureter is identified and dissected distally. Division of the ureter with clips will occur later in the procedure. Dissection of the renal vein begins by freeing the anterior surface. The gonadal vein and the adrenal vein are identified to their origins on the renal vein, clipped, and ligated. Some surgeons prefer to dissect the gonadal vein down the length of the ureter close to the bladder and then ligate the vein distally just prior to ligation of the ureter. Circumferential control of the renal vein is then accomplished. The renal artery is identified and mobilized to the origin from the aorta. The kidney is then fully mobilized to the hilum. Usually the kidney will not be removed until the recipient transplanting surgeons have completed their dissection to prepare for placement of the kidney. After the patient is heparinized, the ureter is clipped and ligated distally. Next, the renal artery and vein are clipped, ligated, and the kidney is removed and prepared for perfusion with the perfusate solution by the transplanting surgeon. Protamine is given to reverse heparinization. The abdomen is inspected thoroughly for any bleeding points. Clips and/or electrosurgery are applied as necessary to achieve hemostasis. Surgicel or Gelfoam may be placed in the area of the adrenal gland for hemostasis. The midline wound is then closed in a single layer with interrupted braided nylon or non-interrupted absorbable monofilament sutures. Port site fascia may or may not be closed with a synthetic braided suture. Skin is usually closed with a subcuticular stitch utilizing synthetic absorbable monofilament or braided sutures. A sterile dressing is applied and the patient is usually taken to the recovery room

Robotics

If available, the surgeon may use a robotic system such as the da Vinci S Surgical System, a high-definition 3D system, during the donor nephrectomy procedures. The system uses a robot to assist the surgeon during the procedure. After inserting the robotic arms and the camera into the patient via four port incisions, the surgeon can manipulate robot via hand controls and foot pedals and remove the kidney via a three-inch Pfannenstiel incision (High-Definition, 2007).

Operative Complications

Occasionally the hand-assisted laparoscopic approach for a donor nephrectomy must convert to an open procedure. The usual causes for conversion are bleeding and/or the inability to visualize anatomical structures adequately. Conversion requires an extension of the midline incision and additional instrumentation for an open nephrectomy.

Postprocedure Care

Pre-established routine postanesthesia and postoperative guidelines are followed for management of the donor. Living donors are usually healthy and require minimal monitoring. Closely monitor urinary output. The surgeon usually discontinues the Foley catheter when the patient tolerates fluids and has adequate urinary output. The donor routinely goes home in 3–5 days.

Living-Donor Kidney Recipient Transplantation

The recipient of a living donated kidney receives the donated kidney immediately. As mentioned earlier, donor and recipient usually arrive to their operating rooms at the same time. Once removed, the surgeon places the donated kidney on ice and immediately perfuses it with a cold renal preservation solution. The kidney is then taken to the adjacent recipient room where the recipient surgeon completes any additional preparation necessary for transplantation. The surgeon then transplants the donated kidney in the retroperitoneal space, which was exposed through an oblique incision above the right inguinal ligament (**Fig. 24.2**).

Indications

Many diseases can lead to end-stage renal failure. Some of the more common disease processes include diabetes, hypertension, diabetic nephropathy, glomerulonephritis, polycystic kidney disease, Lupus, chronic pyelonephritis or glomerulonephritis, and renal vascular disease.

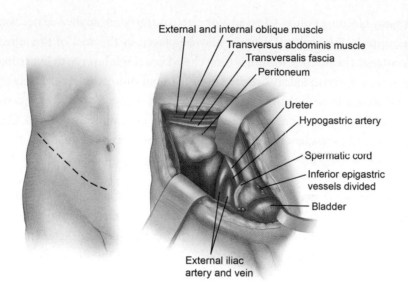

External and internal oblique muscle
Transversus abdominis muscle
Transversalis fascia
Peritoneum
Ureter
Hypogastric artery
Spermatic cord
Inferior epigastric vessels divided
Bladder
External iliac artery and vein

Figure 24.2

Oblique incision exposing the site transplantation of a donated kidney.

Equipment and Supplies

Table 24.12 lists additional items for a living-donor kidney recipient.

Procedure: Living Donor Kidney Recipient

A standard transplant right lower quadrant skin incision is made. Dissection is extended through the subcutaneous tissues, fascia, and into the retroperitoneal space exposing the iliac fossa and its contents. The external iliac artery and vein are mobilized for a suitable distance proximally and distally for the kidney implantation. The dome of the bladder is mobilized. Initial preparation of the donated kidney began immediately after removal from the donor. Excess tissue is removed. Any branches arising from the renal artery and vein that were not clipped during the donor procedure are clipped and ligated. The renal artery, vein, and ureter are prepared for implantation. The patient is usually given 3,000 to 5,000 units of IV heparin. A side-biting vascular clamp or other suitable vascular clamp is placed on the external iliac

Table 24.12	**Additional Items for Living-Donor Kidney Recipient Procedure**		
Instruments	**Supplies**	**Anesthesia Medications**	**Sterile Field Medications**
Renal recipient pan	10 mm JP drain	Solumedrol	Heparin 1:1000 1 cc in 100 normal saline
Renal recipient retractor pan	6 × 12 double J ureteral stent	Lasix	Surgicel
Goosen aortic punch		Mannitol	Papaverine 60 mg (available)
			Neosporin G.U. Irrigant 4 cc in 1,000 normal saline
			Papaverine available
			Marcaine with epinephrine

vein, a venotomy is made, and the renal vein is anastomosed end-to-side to the external iliac vein with a running synthetic nonabsorbable polypropylene suture. The external iliac artery is occluded proximally and distally or with a partial occlusion vascular clamp. An arteriotomy is made and may be enlarged using an aortic punch. The renal artery is anastomosed end-to-side to the external iliac artery with a running nonabsorbable polypropylene suture. The vascular clamps are removed; the kidney reperfuses, and assumes an appropriate color. The kidney is inspected and any bleeding sites are controlled with electrosurgery, clips, or additional synthetic nonabsorbable polypropylene suture. The ureter is shortened and spatulated. Some surgeons may fill the bladder with sterile saline at this point for expansion of the bladder surface. The ureter is taken to the bladder dome where a muscular hiatus is made. On male recipients, the ureter is taken under the spermatic cord. The bladder mucosa is opened and the spatulated ureter is anastomosed mucosa-to-mucosa over a 6 × 12 double J ureteral stent with a running absorbable monofilament suture. The bladder detrusor muscle is closed over the neocystotomy with a running or interrupted absorbable monofilament suture. Lasix and mannitol are usually given IV to encourage diuresis. The entire wound is irrigated and thoroughly inspected again for any bleeding points, which are clipped, cauterized, or sutured as necessary. A #10 JP drain may be placed. The wound is closed according to surgeon preference in either in one or two layers using #1 nonabsorbable polypropylene, #1 absorbable monofilament, or a combination of both. Staples are usually used on the skin. A sterile dressing is applied and the patient is taken to the recovery room or intensive care unit.

Complications

While uncommon, complications related to technical problems in renal transplantation, if present, may threaten survival of the allograft. Arterial thrombosis, a devastating complication, has an incidence of less than 1%. However, when it does occur, immediate diagnosis and alleviation increases the chance of salvaging the kidney. If the Foley catheter is unobstructed, suspect an arterial thrombosis if the patient has an abrupt decrease in urine output. Intervention for arterial thrombosis requires an immediate return of the patient to the operating room for thrombectomy and revision of the arterial anastomosis.

Venous thrombosis is even rarer and can usually be treated with systemic anticoagulation.

Bleeding after the procedure secondary to uremia-induced platelet dysfunction or from the anticoagulation associated with hemodialysis before the procedure can lead to hematoma formation, which can cause obstruction of the collecting system. In such a case, the patient would require operative evacuation of the hematoma.

Renal artery stenosis can cause or exacerbate hypertension. The physician uses arteriography to diagnosis this potential long-term complication. If arteriography confirms the diagnosis, the physician most likely will immediately proceed with a transluminal angioplasty.

Other possible complications include anastomotic stricture, anastomotic leak, and ureteral necrosis. Anastomotic strictures present early or late and cause hydronephrosis. Depending on the situation and the expertise available, the physician may try to correct the stricture with percutaneous nephrostomy. If unsuccessful, operative correction is necessary. A leaking anastomosis requires operative revision. Necrosis of the ureter requires resection of the nonviable tissue and an anastomosis of the transplant renal pelvis to the ipsilateral native ureter (ureteropyelostomy).

ATN
Acute Tubular Necrosis

While not a technical complication, acute tubular necrosis (ATN) may result from the organ ischemic period. The large dose of furosemide given intraoperatively may also contribute to ATN. If present, it is usually transient in transplants from living donors. Deceased donor renal transplantation has a higher incidence of ATN because of the longer obligatory ischemic time from procurement time to transplantation time. As with acute rejection, ATN becomes apparent by anuria or oliguria and a rising creatinine. Percutaneous biopsy is the most reliable means of distinguishing between ATN and acute rejection. ATN can last up to several weeks. Because there is no definitive treatment the patient usually requires dialysis until the kidney begins to function.

If the recipient experiences an episode of acute rejection, the physician intensifies the immunosuppressive regimen, and prolongs the hospital stay. The physician will treat a primary acute rejection episode by increasing the amount of daily steroids, followed by a gradual lowering of the steroid dose to baseline. Subsequent or steroid-resistant episodes may require even more aggressive immunosuppression. If chronic rejection does not respond to steroids and becomes progressive, the patient may ultimately lose the graft.

If the allograft functions promptly, and there are no signs of rejection or other medical-surgical complications, the recipient can go home within 5–7 days.

Postprocedure Care

Follow routine postanesthesia and postprocedure guidelines. However, these patients frequently have a significant number of comorbid conditions, potentially making postprocedure care more complicated than that of other surgical patients.

Strictly monitor fluid replacement to prevent hypovolemia. In the case of anuria or oliguria, until the physician makes a definitive diagnosis, restrict fluids as though the patient had renal failure. The management of each case has to be individualized.

Once established, if urine output abruptly decreases or ceases, most likely a thrombus has obstructed the Foley catheter. Usually, irrigation of the catheter with saline will restore catheter drainage. However, if the problem persists, the patient may require a cystoscopy to evacuate large clots and coagulate a bleeding site at the tip of the ureter. If catheter irrigation fails to yield any blood and re-establish diuresis, consider obstruction of the renal artery as the cause of the anuria or oliguria. Although rare, accelerated acute rejection also causes a decrease or cessation of urine output and usually results in loss of the allograft.

Assess the patient's renal function daily by checking 24-hour urine output, serum electrolytes, blood urea nitrogen, and creatinine. These laboratory values help determine if the patient requires temporary dialysis. If the patient has a shunt, protect it during and after the procedure because of the possibility for dialysis. With a functioning allograft, each day the patient will have normal urine output and a decreasing creatinine level. This patient will no longer need dialysis.

Sophisticated immunosuppressive therapy and anti-rejection medications have greatly improved the prospects of transplant patients. Patients will receive tacrolirnus or cyclosporine combined with azathioprine or mycophenolate mofetil. The physician evaluates medication doses on a daily basis and makes changes based on blood levels and/or side effects. Tacrolimus and cyclosporine are nephrotoxic therefore closely monitor the patient. Patients still receive steroids.

Usually, the physician will remove the stent placed in the donor ureter to the recipient bladder during surgery in 2 weeks to 3 months after the procedure.

Deceased Donor Kidney Transplantation

The UNOS maintains a national list of potential recipients for deceased donor kidneys. When an organ becomes available and matched to the recipient, the transplant coordinator notifies the recipient to check into the hospital for final evaluation prior to transplantation. Depending on the severity of renal failure, the recipient may or may not have had to start either hemodialysis or peritoneal dialysis. Before the procedure, a final crossmatch between the donor and recipient is completed and documented as negative on the recipients chart. When the donor and recipient have a 6-HLA antigen match and the PRA is a very low percentage the surgeon may begin the transplant without the final crossmatch results. The donated kidney arrives in the operating room in the sealed transport box or kidney transporter. Some surgeons prefer to prepare the kidney prior to the recipient arrival to the operating room. Other surgeons prepare the recipient for transplantation, deliver the donated organ to the sterile field, prepare the organ, and then begin the transplantation.

Indications

See indications for the living-donor kidney transplant.

Equipment and Supplies

See **Table 24.13** for additional items for a deceased-donor kidney recipient.

Table 24.13	Additional Items for Deceased-Donor Kidney Recipient		
Instruments	**Supplies**	**Medications Anesthesia**	**Medications Sterile Field**
Renal transplant recipient pan	10 mm JP drain	Solumedrol	Heparin 1:1,000 1 cc in 100 normal saline
Renal transplant retractor pan	6 × 12 double J ureteral stent	Lasix	Surgicel
Goosen/aortic punch		Mannitol	Papaverine 60 mg (available)
TLV vascular stapler and reloads (if right kidney)		Protamine	Neosporin G.U. irrigant 4 cc in 1,000 normal saline

Procedure: Deceased Donor Kidney Recipient

See the procedure for a living-donor kidney recipient. **Figure 24.3** shows a prepared kidney from a deceased donor. Right kidneys will require extra preparation of the vena caval conduit using a linear stapler and clips.

Complications

See the section on complications for a living-donor kidney recipient.

Postprocedure Care

See the section on postprocedure care for a living-donor kidney recipient.

Pancreas Transplant

Patients in need of a pancreas transplant usually receive a kidney at the same time. However, if necessary, a patient may have a pancreas transplant as a standalone procedure. When performed as a dual transplant, two surgeons may work as a team in order to reduce cold ischemic time of the organs. While one surgeon exposes anatomical structures in the recipient for transplantation, and prepares and transplants the kidney, the second surgeon prepares the pancreas for transplantation. As a standalone procedure, the surgeon will usually prepare the pancreas before the patient arrives in the operating room. See **Figure 24.4** for an example of a pancreas with ligated structures (Hakim, 2002).

Indications

IDDM
Insulin Dependent
Diabetes Mellitus

A pancreas transplant is the preferred treatment for patients with insulin dependent diabetes mellitus (IDDM). This procedure reduces, if not eliminates the need for insulin immediately following the transplant. For these patients, receiving a new pancreas provides them with the ability to maintain normal carbohydrate metabolism and may help stabilize the secondary complications of diabetes such as neuropathy, gastroparesis, retinopathy, nephropathy, and cardiovascular disease.

Equipment and Supplies

Table 24.14 lists additional items for a pancreas transplant.

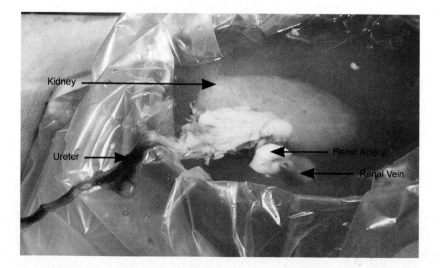

Figure 24.3

Back bench prepared kidney from a deceased donor.

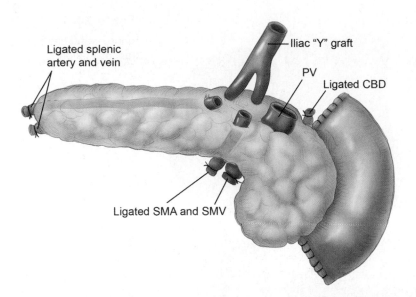

Ligated splenic artery and vein

Iliac "Y" graft

PV

Ligated CBD

Ligated SMA and SMV

Figure 24.4

Pancreas with ligated structures (splenic artery and vein, superior mesenteric artery [SMA], superior mesenteric vein [SMV], and common bile duct [CBD]). Also shown are the pulmonary vein (PV) and iliac artery "Y" graft.

Table 24.14	Additional Items Pancreas Transplant				
Equipment	**Instruments**	**Supplies**	**Medications Anesthesia**	**Medications Sterile Field**
Extra slush/ice machine if a dual procedure	GIA stapler and reloads	Extra slush/ice machine drape	Solumedrol	Heparin 1:1,000 1 cc in 100 normal saline
	Goosen/aortic punch	10 mm JP drain	Lasix (with kidney transplant)	Surgicel
			Mannitol (with kidney transplant)	Papaverine 60 mg (available)
				Neosporin G.U. irrigant 4 cc in 1,000 normal saline

Procedure: Pancreas Transplant

The abdomen is prepped and draped in a sterile fashion. The abdominal cavity is entered through a standard midline incision. Dissection is extended through the subcutaneous tissues, fascia and into the retroperitoneal space exposing the iliac fossa and its contents. The right external iliac artery and vein are mobilized for a suitable distance proximally and distally for the pancreas implantation. The patient is usually given 3,000 to 5,000 units of IV heparin. A side-biting vascular clamp or other suitable vascular clamp is placed on the external iliac vein, a venotomy is made, and the donor portal vein is anastomosed end-to-side to the external iliac vein with a running nonabsorbable polypropylene suture. The external iliac artery is occluded proximally and distally. An arteriotomy is made and may be enlarged utilizing an aortic punch. The backbench created "y" artery graft is anastomosed end-to-side to the external iliac artery with a running nonabsorbable polypropylene suture. The vascular clamps are removed; the pancreas is reperfused, and the organ assumes an

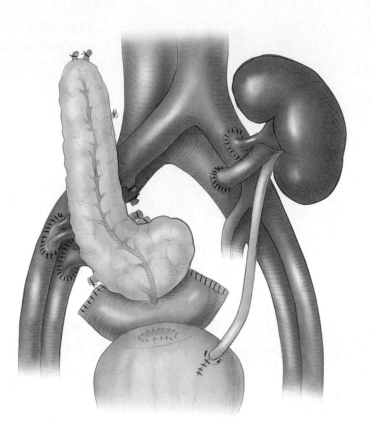

Figure 24.5

Kidney-pancreas transplantation.

appropriate color. The pancreas is inspected and any bleeding sites are controlled with electrosurgery, clips, or additional nonabsorbable polypropylene suture. The small bowel is then brought into the surgical field and clamped with bowel clamps for a side-to-side anastomosis with the duodenal cuff of the transplant graft. Usually, the anastomosis is done using a running nonabsorbable polypropylene stitch. The small bowel anastomosis can be completed either in continuity or to a Roux-en-Y limb. An alternative to anastomosing the donor duodenum to the small bowel is an anastomosis to the bladder. An example of a kidney-pancreas transplantation can be seen in **Figure 24.5** (Hakim, 2002). The surgeon irrigates, applies hemostasis, inserts a drain, and closes the wound as described for the living-donor kidney recipient.

Complications

Vascular thrombosis after pancreas transplantation rarely occurs. The absence of immediate clinical signs for vascular thrombosis makes diagnosis difficult. The patient does becomes febrile and may become systemically ill. However, by the time the physician makes the diagnosis, the patient requires a transplant pancreatectomy. Prophylactic anticoagulation during and after the procedure helps, but has not eliminated this devastating problem.

Anastomotic leak at the duodenojejunostomy or duodenocystostomy, depending on the route chosen for exocrine drainage can also occur. The usual findings for this infrequent problem are those associated with an intestinal or urine leak, respectively. A leak at either site requires operative correction but does not necessarily mean loss of the graft.

Graft pancreatitis may result from the period of ischemia or over manipulation of the pancreas during the procurement or the implantation. Fortunately, this usually resolves with appropriate management; if severe, however, the surgeon may have to remove the graft.

As with all organ transplants, acute rejection is a major concern, and an immunosuppressive regimen described for renal allograft recipients is used for its prevention. A decline in the patient's exocrine function provides the first sign of pancreatic rejection. Patients with bladder drainage will have a decreasing amount of amylase excreted in the urine. Patients who underwent simultaneous kidney-pancreas transplantation will have a rising serum creatinine may indicate renal allograft rejection. Most likely, this would be accompanied by rejection of the pancreas as well. Unless severe or untreated, pancreatic rejection does not result in hyperglycemia, making this an unreliable screening tool. Treatment of acute pancreatic rejection is similar to that described for acute rejection of a renal allograft.

Because of their comorbid conditions, these patients typically have a longer post-transplant hospitalization than those who only receive a kidney. Some patients may require several weeks of inpatient convalescence; their number of readmissions during the first 6 months after discharge is also higher. However, the majority have a successful outcome, which is associated with a tremendous improvement in their quality of life.

Postprocedure Care

Routinely, pancreatic transplant patients receive initial care in the intensive care unit because of the potential comorbid conditions associated with long-standing diabetes mellitus and the need for hourly blood glucose measurements. Optimally, the patient does not require insulin after leaving the operating room, but this is not always the case. Insulin requirement signifies graft dysfunction, but this usually disappears within the first 12 to 24 hours. On the first postprocedure day, the patient can usually transfer out of the intensive care unit. In addition to the special needs of these patients, such as urinary amylase collection and determination, frequent blood glucose measurements, and psychological support, routine postprocedure nursing considerations apply. The patient should ambulate as early as possible. Patient and family education also continues. Even though they have been prepared beforehand, patients need a lot of teaching and encouragement before they are ready for discharge. All members of the transplant team share in this responsibility.

Liver Transplantation

Usually, the surgeon transplants a donated liver in the normal anatomical location. This type of transplant, known as orthotopic transplantation, follows a total hepatectomy on the recipient. The standard surgical technique for liver transplantation includes five separate anastomoses: suprahepatic vena cava, infrahepatic vena cava, portal vein, hepatic artery, and common bile duct. Variations of the standard operation include the "piggyback technique" where the liver is dissected off the inferior vena cava and the vena cava is preserved. This technique eliminates the infrahepatic anastomosis and the donor infrahepatic cava is over sewn or tied. Another

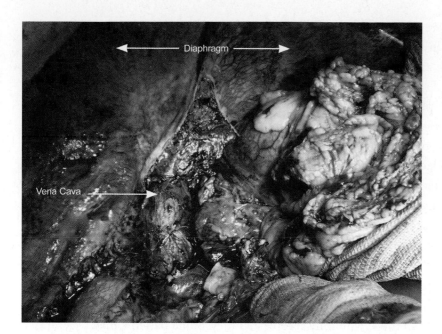

Figure 24.6

Exposed vena cava after removal of the native liver.

variation uses a vascular stapler to divide the suprahepatic left and middle veins from the suprahepatic vena cava leaving the vena cava exposed and requiring only partial occlusion for a side-to-side anastomosis between the donor vena cava and the recipient vena cava. **Figure 24.6** shows the exposed vena cava after removal of the native liver. Some surgeons will perform a portacaval shunt or use systemic bypass via cannulation into the greater saphenous vein into the common iliac vein in order to maintain venous blood flow during the implantation of the new liver.

A living donor may donate a portion of his or her liver, usually the right lobe, for transplant into a recipient. However, due to the technical difficulty of the resection and potential risk to the donor this is not a common procedure.

Indications

Patients with a disease process, which results in end-stage liver failure, may receive a liver transplant. Frequently seen diagnoses in the adult patient include chronic active hepatitis C or B, primary biliary cirrhosis, sclerosing cholangitis, cirrhosis secondary to autoimmune hepatitis, biliary atresia, Laennec's (alcoholic) cirrhosis, nonalcoholic fatty liver disease, fulminant hepatic failure, and liver cancer (Molmenti & Klintmalm, 2002).

Preprocedure Care

Usually, the surgeon prepares the liver for transplantation while the anesthesia provider places hemodynamic monitoring lines. A cell saver perfusionist will collect blood during liver transplants unless the recipient has the diagnosis of hepatic carcinoma or other contraindicated disease process. **Table 24.15** lists nursing considerations before liver transplant.

Equipment and Supplies

Table 24.16 lists additional items for a liver transplant.

Table 24.15	**Nursing Considerations Before Liver Transplant**

Have 5 units of packed cells and 5 units of fresh frozen plasma checked and ready prior to patient arrival to the OR

Have cold Lactated Ringers solution on ice for allograft perfusion during the caval anastomosis

Verify that the blood type of the donor allograft and the recipient match

Open the transportation box and deliver the liver in a sterile fashion to the backbench surgeon for preparation

Assist the anesthesia provider with intubation and line placement

Table 24.16	**Additional Items for Liver Transplant**

Equipment	Supplies	Instrumentation	Medications Anesthesia	Medications Sterile Field
Cell saver	Cell saver suction	Liver transplant pan	Dopamine	Heparin 1:1,000 5 cc in 500 cc normal saline
Argon beam coagulator	Isolation bag (for liver after preparation)	Liver retractor pan	Amicar available	Surgicel
Electrosurgery generator × 2	2nd Electrosurgery pencil with extended tip	Liver bench set		Gelfoam available
Neptune suction machine	Sterile IV extension tubing	Argon handpiece		Thrombin available
	Extra suction tubing and Tip	Surgeon specific instruments		Hemaseel available
	6 × 12 ureteral stent (for bile duct)	Micro-needle holder set		
		GIA stapler and reload		

Intraoperative Care

Table 24.17 lists nursing considerations during liver transplant.

Procedure: Deceased Donor Liver Transplantation "Piggyback"

A Mercedes or bilateral subcostal skin incision is made and carried down to the abdominal cavity using electrosurgery. The Bookwalter or retractor of surgeon choice is placed for exposure. The Falciform ligament is dissected with electrosurgery, clamped, divided, and ligated with a 0 silk tie. The supporting ligaments of the liver are divided with electrosurgery. The suprahepatic and infrahepatic inferior vena cava are dissected free from surrounding tissues for later placement of vascular clamps. The gastrohepatic ligament is divided and the right and left hepatic arteries

Table 24.17	Nursing Considerations During Liver Transplant

Every hour during the case send a blood sample for CBC and coagulation to the lab

Hang cold lactated ringers solution upon surgeon request for flushing the liver

Request additional units of blood or fresh frozen plasma if needed

Record hepatic artery ligation time

Record portal vein ligation time

Record clamp time of vena cava

Record time of liver off ice

Record anastomoses start and end times

Record unclamp times of vena cava, portal vein, hepatic artery

Record warm ischemic time (calculate time from liver off ice to portal vein unclamp time)

Notify the ICU of pending arrival of patient and ensure ICU bed is delivered prior to transporting the patient

are individually taken between clamps, divided, and ligated with silk ties. The cystic duct and common bile duct are individually taken between clamps, divided, and ligated with silk ties. The Portal vein is dissected free from surrounding tissues for later placement of a vascular clamp. A partial occlusion or suitable vascular clamp is placed across the portal vein proximally and ligated distally. The liver is removed off the inferior vena cava in a caudad to cephalad direction. Direct branches are taken between surgical clips and silk ties. At the level of the hepatic veins, a straight Potts clamp or other suitable vascular clamp is placed across the infrahepatic inferior vena cava, a curved Potts or other suitable vascular clamp is placed across the suprahepatic inferior vena cava and the liver is removed sharply. The middle and left hepatic vein orifices are ligated with a running nonabsorbable polypropylene suture. The right hepatic vein orifice is triangulated onto the inferior vena cava for a single orifice. The previously prepared allograft liver seen in **Figures 24.7, 24.8,**

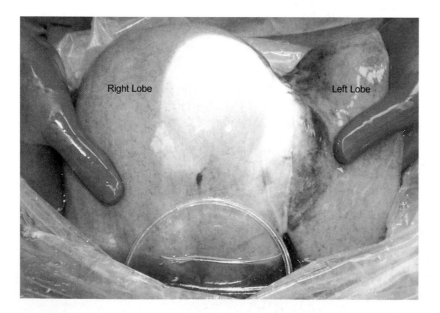

Right Lobe   Left Lobe

Figure 24.7

Anterior view of back bench prepared liver.

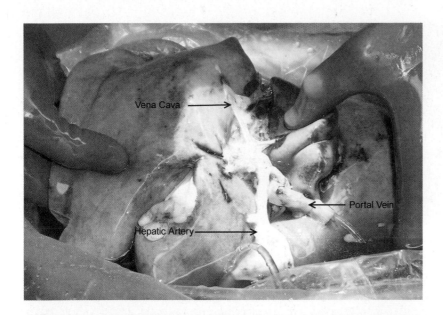

Figure 24.8
Posterior view of prepared liver.

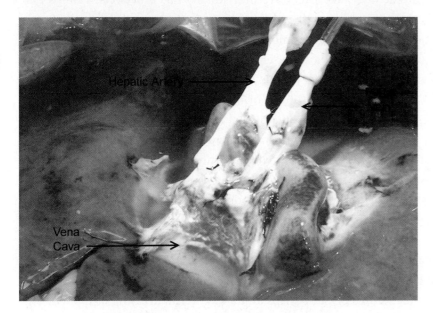

Figure 24.9
Prepared liver with hepatic artery and portal vein.

and **24.9** is then brought to the field and the infrahepatic inferior vena cava of the donor is doubly ligated with 0 silk ties. The suprahepatic portion is triangulated. The suprahepatic anastomosis is created with a running nonabsorbable polypropylene suture in a piggyback fashion. Approximately 1000 mL of cold lactated Ringer Solution is flushed through the portal vein and effluent out this anastomosis prior to completion. The portal vein anastomosis is completed in an end-to-end fashion with a running nonabsorbable polypropylene suture with the use of growth stitch or air knot for venous expansion. Venous clamps are then removed, first suprahepatic, second infrahepatic, third portal vein with good perfusion of the allograft. The hepatic artery is flushed with heparinized saline and clamped distally. The recipient hepatic artery is dissected down to the level of the gastroduodenal artery and clamped. The right and left hepatic orifices are opened to a single confluence and an end-to-end arterial anastomosis is completed with a running nonabsorbable polypropylene suture. Arterial clamps are removed with a good pulse and thrill noted

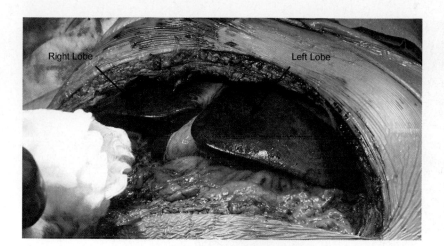

Figure 24.10
Completed orthotopic liver transplant.

through the vessels. The gallbladder is removed off the gallbladder fossa with electrosurgery. The cystic duct and artery are individually taken between clamps and ligated with silk ties. Hemostasis of the gallbladder fossa is accomplished with Argon beam coagulation. The biliary anastomosis can be an end-to-end choledochocholedochostomy (duct to duct) or a Roux-en-Y choledochojejunostomy. The anastomosis is created over a 6–8 French double-J ureteral stent or a feeding tube using running absorbable monofilament sutures or interrupted absorbable monofilament sutures. Bile production is usually noted at this time. The wound is irrigated with saline solution and inspected for hemostasis. Any bleeding points are controlled with additional nonabsorbable polypropylene sutures, clips, ties, Argon coagulation, or electrosurgery. **Figure 24.10** shows a transplanted liver just prior to wound closure. Two 10 mm Jackson-Pratt drains or drains of surgeon's choice are placed via separate stab wounds below the incision. Internal drain placement consists of one suprahepatic and one infrahepatic. The fascia is closed in two layers with running #1 absorbable monofilament sutures. The subcutaneous tissue is irrigated with saline solution and the skin is closed with surgical skin clips. The drain exit sites are secured with either sutures or Steri-strips and a dry sterile dressing is applied. The patient is then transported directly to the Intensive Care Unit (ICU) intubated.

ICU
Intensive Care Unit

Complications

Although significant improvements have been made in the technical aspects of liver transplantation, technical complications remain significant causes of morbidity. Bleeding that requires reoperation is the most common complication seen in the first 24 hours. The usual signs of hypovolemia are present. Evacuation of the hematoma or blood, usually without being able to identify a specific bleeding source, is usually definitive therapy.

HAT
Hepatic Artery
Thrombosis

Hepatic artery thrombosis (HAT) is a complication that can occur any time after transplantation and is more common in children. If it occurs early, extremely elevated hepatocellular enzymes (ALT, AST, and LDH), fever, and signs of systemic toxicity (eg, tachycardia, oliguria, and tachypnea) are potential manifestations. Late-onset HAT is usually manifested by biliary pathology. Because the biliary tree is exclusively supplied by branches of the hepatic artery, HAT results in bile duct ischemia and eventual necrosis. Bile duct strictures or a biloma, resulting in cholangitis and/or biliary sepsis, may occur. If HAT is diagnosed within a few hours of its onset, thrombectomy and revision of the arterial anastomosis may allow salvage of the graft. Otherwise, re-transplantation is usually required. Portal vein and IVC thrombosis is uncommon and usually necessitates re-transplantation.

Biliary anastomotic leaks unrelated to HAT are potential early complications and usually require reoperation for drainage and possible revision of the anastomosis. However, endoscopic approaches can be successful in selected cases.

Acute rejection has an incidence of approximately 50% and usually occurs within the first 6 months. This is usually asymptomatic but can be accompanied by fever. It is usually suspected because of rising hepatocellular enzymes and confirmed by percutaneous liver biopsy. Treatment of acute liver rejection is usually successful and follows the same strategy outlined for acute rejection of a renal allograft. Chronic liver rejection is an entirely different event and is manifested by a scarcity of bile ducts (vanishing bile duct syndrome). Nothing has proved to be effective therapy for chronic rejection, and survival of the graft is jeopardized.

Because of the impact of liver failure on extrahepatic physiological subsystems, liver transplant recipients may require long in-hospital convalescence (several weeks or more). If, however, the liver functions well from the beginning, many of these subsystems simultaneously improve, and dramatic, immediate changes from a patient's preprocedure condition are common.

Postprocedure Care

Care after the procedure can be extremely complicated and requires tremendous vigilance and thoughtful, individualized therapeutic decisions from the transplant multidisciplinary team. Acute and chronic liver adversely affects all physiological subsystems, and chronic liver failure patients are always malnourished.

All monitoring devices placed before the procedure remain and are used in the ICU setting, to include Swan-Ganz and arterial catheters. Inotropic agents are commonly needed during the procedure, but they can usually be gradually discontinued over the first few hours in the ICU.

Usually, liver transplant patients remain intubated during transport to the ICU from the operating room suite. The nurse should advise the ICU at least 30 minutes prior to arrival. This will allow ICU staff to obtain a ventilator and set up prior to patient arrival.

Upon arrival in the ICU a radiology technician immediately takes a chest radiograph, which helps the physician assess the lung fields and the position of the endotracheal tube and central venous devices. The arterial catheter allows frequent blood gas evaluations, and a pulse oximeter gives a continuous display of the arterial oxygen saturation. Initially, the ventilator provides total respiratory support, but as the patient awakens, the support gradually decreases until the patient can be extubated. Depending on the patient's condition before the procedure, this can take several hours or several days.

Renal function after the procedure varies and depends primarily on preprocedure renal function. The patient may have normal urine output, or may require temporary dialysis. The ICU staff should measure urine output hourly. These measurements provide the basis for fluid management. Some immunosuppressive agents are nephrotoxic and can contribute to renal dysfunction. Consequently, the physician must assess immunosuppressive doses daily.

Neurologically, the patient may awaken without incident within a few minutes or hours. If, however, the patient was encephalopathic (or even comatose) before the procedure, several days may elapse before this state reverses.

Prophylactic antibiotics are given, but because of the patient's liver disease and immunosuppression, the patient has an unusually high susceptibility to infection. A low threshold for obtaining blood, urine, and sputum cultures is therefore appropriate. If evidence of an infection develops, aggressive use of therapeutic antibiotics is indicated, even before the results of any cultures are known. If no cultures are positive for microbial growth, the decision to discontinue antibiotic therapy must be based on the surgeon's clinical suspicion of infection.

The immunosuppressive regimen is center-specific but is usually cyclosporine- or tacrolimus-based. However, if renal dysfunction is present, the physician may use muromonab-CD3 (OKT3) in induction therapy to avoid using these nephrotoxic agents. Initially, in addition to cyclosporine or tacrolimus (or OKT3), the patient receives high-dose steroids. The steroid dose is gradually tapered to a baseline level by the time of discharge, although further reductions are likely over the long term. Either azathioprine or mycophenolate mofetil are commonly used as a third agent. As with renal and pancreas transplantation, the doses are assessed daily and changed based on side effects and/or blood levels.

Intestine Transplantation

Intestine transplantation has evolved over the last 40 years into an accepted treatment option for individuals with intestinal failure. The introduction of tacrolimus as the primary immunosuppressive agent in 1990 greatly improved patient and graft survival. Options for intestinal transplant include an isolated procedure, a dual procedure which includes a liver and intestine transplantation, and a multivisceral (intestine, liver, stomach, pancreas, and possibly kidney) transplantation for individuals with multiple associated organ dysfunction (Gilroy, 2007). A living donor may donate a portion of bowel; however, due to potential risk to the donor this is not common practice. Operative time can range from 8–16 hours depending on the recipients anatomical variations from previous surgeries, pretransplant medical status, and the number of organs being transplanted (Park, 2003).

Indications

TPN
Total Parenteral Nutrition

Intestinal failure patients cannot maintain an adequate nutritional state with an enteric diet and depend on total parenteral nutrition (TPN) for fluid, electrolyte, and caloric intake. Diseases of another organ such as the kidney or stomach, as well as TPN induced liver disease, may require a dual transplant. Diseases affecting multiple organs may require a multivisceral transplantation. Structural or functional anatomical abnormalities can also lead to an intestinal transplant. **Table 24.18** lists examples of structural and functional abnormalities (Park, 2003).

Table 24.18	Structural and Functional Intestinal Abnormalities		
Structural and Functional	**Structural**	**Functional**
Short Gut Syndrome (aka short bowel syndrome)	Anatomical Abnormalities	Absorptive Disorders
	Resection of the Small Intestine	Secretory Disorders
		Motility Disorders

Park, B.K. (2003). Intestinal Transplantation. In *Transplantation Nursing Secrets* (p. 178). Philadelphia: Hanley & Belfus.

Table 24.19	Additional Items for Intestinal Transplantation				
Equipment	**Supplies**	**Instrumentation**	**Medications Sterile Field**	**Medications Anesthesia**
Extra ice/slush machine	Ice/slush machine drape	Intestinal transplant pan	Antibiotic irrigation solution	IV steroid
	Variety of GIA and TA staplers	Intestinal transplant retractor pan	Heparin 1:1,000 5 cc in 500 cc normal saline	
	Stapler reloads			

Equipment and Supplies

Table 24.19 list additional items for intestinal transplant.

Procedure: Isolated Intestinal Transplantation

The patient is prepped and draped in a sterile fashion. A standard midline incision is made for dissection and exposure down into the peritoneal cavity. The diseased intestine is removed from the ligament of Treitz to the ileocecal valve or ileocolic anastomosis for patients with dysmotility or dysfunctional absorption. The residual intestine is usually retained in patients with functional disorder. Vascular anastomoses may vary depending on previous surgeries and the patient's current anatomy. The most common method includes an anastomosis of the donor superior mesenteric artery (SMA) to the recipient infrarenal aorta and the donor superior mesenteric vein (SMV) to the recipient portal vein or inferior vena cava (IVC). Following graft reperfusion, the intestine is reconstructed via an anastomosis of the donor jejunum to the recipient's residual duodenum or jejunum. The ilium is connected to the native colon in an end-to-side fashion. An ileostomy is formed by exteriorizing the distal end of the graft and anastomosing the recipient's ileum or colon to the side of the graft below the stoma (Humar, Matas, & Payne, 2006; Kuo & Davis, 2005). The layers of the abdomen are closed with #1 absorbable monofilament and or #1 nonabsorbable polypropylene. The skin is closed with staples.

SMA
Superior Mesenteric Artery

SMV
Superior Mesenteric Vein

Complications

The most common complications are postoperative hemorrhage, vascular leaks, or vascular occlusions. Postoperative hemorrhage can occur at an anastomotic site and usually requires operative exploration and repair with sutures. Gastrointestinal bleeding is the most common complication and can be caused by rejection or infection. Gastrointestinal leaks, another complication, require operative exploration, as well as antibiotic or antifungal therapy. Biliary leaks or obstruction can occur in patients with combined intestine—liver transplants and usually requires operative repair.

Vascular occlusions or thromboses of the arteries may lead to necrosis of the organ or organs. Treatment may include a graft enterectomy in the case of isolated intestine transplant, or retransplantation with multi-organ transplantation.

Postprocedure Care

Immediate postprocedure care may require aggressive hydration due to third-space fluid loss. Electrolyte imbalances should be monitored and corrected aggressively. Careful frequent monitoring is employed for the first 24 hours. Sepsis syndrome may result from vascular compromise or perforation and require re-operation.

For the first 6 months, intestinal transplant recipients are prone to complications such as technical problems related to the transplant, rejection, and infection. Management of the immunosuppressive agents requires a balance between avoiding rejection and preventing infection. Acute rejection of the graft is common due to the large quantity of lymphoid tissue associated with the intestine. Monitoring includes lab studies, clinical presentation, endoscopic examination of the graft, and definitive histologic findings (Park, 2003).

The leading cause of morbidity and mortality in intestinal transplant patients is infection. Bacterial infection can be seen in over 80% of these patients; therefore, immediate postprocedure care usually requires antibiotic prophylaxis with a broad-spectrum antibiotic. Subsequent followup management includes routine surveillance for infectious complications. Several factors predispose patients for fungal infections. Treatment can include intravenous (IV) amphotericin B, oral nystatin, and or fluconazole. Cytomegalovirus (CMV) is the most common viral pathogen found after the procedure. Risk factors include donor-recipient mismatch as well as the postprocedure administration of immunosuppressive agents. Treatment at this point is hospital specific but the administration of IV ganciclovir and/or CMV-specific hyperimmunoglobulin and routine monitoring is the standard (Park, 2003).

Immunosuppressive agents administered to intestine transplant recipients can also result in Epstein-Barr viral (EBV) infection or EBV-associated lymphoproliferative disease (PTLD). Treatment requires the reduction of or discontinuation of immunosuppression, which in turn places the recipient at risk for organ rejection.

Adequate nutrition, fluid, and electrolyte homeostasis is also an important part of the postprocedure care regimen. In the early post operative period Total Parenteral Nutrition (TPN) is used for providing nutritional support. A gastrograffin study evaluates the integrity of the intestinal anastomosis prior to the start of enteral feedings.

IV
Intravenous

CMV
Cytomegalovirus

EBV
Epstein-Barr Viral

PTLD
Lymphoproliferative
Disease

TPN
Total Parenteral
Nutrition

The ileostomy created during the transplantation is temporary and during the critical first 6 months following surgery provides an excellent avenue for post transplant endoscopic examinations. Reversal or closure of the ileostomy can be performed after 3 months or up to 1-year post transplantation depending on patient physiological parameters, transplant protocols or pre-established clinical pathways (Park, 2003).

Heart Transplantation

Potential heart recipients undergo extensive evaluation using the New York Heart Association classification (**Table 24.20**) to establish the severity of their disease and prognosis. Once accepted, patients are listed with UNOS in either category 1A, 1B, or 2. If the recipient has a high PRA percentage, a prospective crossmatch is completed with each potential donor. The crossmatch must be negative in order to proceed with the transplantation.

Survival rates for heart transplantation have greatly improved since the first transplant in 1967 partly due to the discovery of the immunosuppressant cyclosporine A, the development of the endomyocardial biopsy forceps, and the categorization of the histological grading system for rejection. Early standard operative techniques consisted of four anastomoses: the left and right atrium, the pulmonary artery (PA), and the aorta. In the mid-1990s, a bicaval anastomotic technique was developed and consists of five anastomoses: the left atrium, the inferior vena cava (IVC), the superior vena cava (SVC), the PA, and the aorta. This newer technique helps preserve normal atrial anatomy with reports of improved atrial contractility, improved sinus node function, and improved atrioventricular valve function. The standard technique; however, reduces preimplantation dissection and is still used for patients with scarring from previous surgeries (Iazzetti & Rigutti, 2007).

PA
Pulmonary Artery

SVC
Superior Vena Cava

Indications

Candidates for cardiac transplantation have irreversible end-stage cardiac failure (New York Heart Association class IV). Etiologies include idiopathic cardiomyopathy,

Table 24.20	New York Heart Association Functional Classification
I	No symptoms No limitation in ordinary physical activity (eg, shortness of breath when walking, stair climbing, etc)
II	Mild symptoms (mild shortness of breath and/or angina pain) Slight limitation during ordinary activity
III	Marked limitation in activity due to symptoms, even during less-than-ordinary activity (eg, walking short distances ~20–100m) Comfortable only at rest
IV	Severe limitations Experiences symptoms even while at rest, mostly bed-bound patients

Adapted from Wikipedia (2008). New York Heart Association Functional Classification. Accessed 26 August 2008, http://en.wikipedia.org/wiki/New_York_Heart_Association_Functional_Classification.

coronary artery disease, and end-stage valvular disease. Indicators that confirm clinical decline include frequent admissions for congestive heart failure, potential fatal arrhythmias, failing renal and hepatic function, hypotension, progressive weakness, and cachexia (Cupples, 2003).

A heart transplant candidate must have a mandatory cardiac evaluation before being placed on the transplant list. The results should show an ejection fraction less than 20%, pulmonary vascular resistance less than 6 Wood units[1], and maximal oxygen consumption less than 12 mL/minute.

Equipment and Supplies

Table 24.21 lists additional items for heart transplantation.

Procedure: Orthotopic Bicaval Heart Transplantation

Under general endotracheal anesthesia, appropriate arterial and venous lines are inserted. A median sternotomy is performed and subcutaneous tissue dissection is completed down to the sternum, which is split using a sternal saw. The pericardium is then opened and the pericardial edge is suspended with sutures. Heparin is then administered systemically. Cannulation for cardiopulmonary bypass is performed by first placing a pursestring suture distally in the ascending aorta. The aortic cannula is inserted and secured with the pursestring suture. A pursestring suture is then placed in the SVC and the IVC. Right-angled cannulas are placed for venous drainage and secured with umbilical tape snares. A left ventricular vent is placed via the right superior pulmonary vein (SPV) and is secured with a pursestring suture. CO_2 tubing may be brought to the wound for flooding of the surgical field to reduce the risk of air embolism. The adventitial attachments between the aorta and pulmonary artery are divided using electrosurgery. The aorta is completely separated from the main, left, and right pulmonary arteries. The ascending aorta proximal

SPV
Superior Pulmonary Vein

Table 24.21	Additional Items for Heart Transplant			
Equipment	**Supplies**	**Instrumentation**	**Medications Anesthesia**	**Medications Sterile Field**
Cardiopulmonary bypass machine	Bypass cannulas	Sternal saw	Heparin	Antibiotic irrigation solution
Defibrillator	External paddles	Sterile internal paddles	Protamine	Heparin 1:1,000 5 cc in 500 cc normal saline
Cell Saver	CO_2 tubing	Chest retractor (Sumo retractor)		
	Pacing wires	Cardiac transplant pan		
	Pledgets	Cardiac retractor pan		
	Chest tubes			

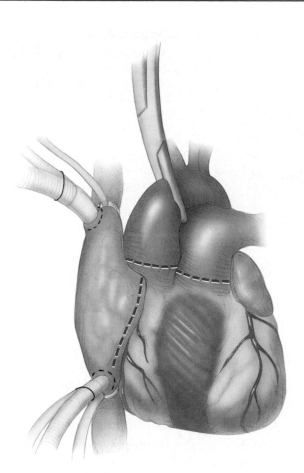

Figure 24.11

Lines of incision for the cardiectomy.

to the arterial cannula is cross-clamped. The native heart is excised at the atrioventricular groove (**Fig. 24.11**) (Kuo & Davis, 2005). Dissection of the interatrial groove and separation of the right and left atrial cuffs is completed. The left atrial cuff is trimmed and the remnants of the coronary sinus and left atrial appendage are removed. The right atrial cuff is trimmed to individual SVC and IVC cuffs. The aorta and PA are divided at the level of the commissures of their respective valves. The previously prepared donor heart is brought to the field. The recipient left atrial cuff is anastomosed at the level of the left SPV to the donor left atrial remnant with a running nonabsorbable polypropylene stitch. The recipient left atrial appendage is excised leaving the donor left atrial appendage in place. The heart is then lowered into the pericardium onto an ice-cold lap sponge. The anastomosis is continued caudally along the left side of the atrium. A second nonabsorbable polypropylene stitch is run along the dome of the left atrium and then along the interatrial septum. The excess cuff tissue is trimmed and sutures tied to complete the anastomosis. The donor IVC is anastomosed to the recipient IVC end-to-end fashion with a running nonabsorbable polypropylene suture starting on the posterior wall. The donor and recipient SVC anastomosis is then completed in an end-to-end fashion with a running nonabsorbable polypropylene suture beginning with the posterior wall. The donor and recipient pulmonary arteries are then anastomosed end-to-end with a running nonabsorbable polypropylene stitch. The donor and recipient aortas are then anastomosed end-to-end with a running nonabsorbable polypropylene stitch.

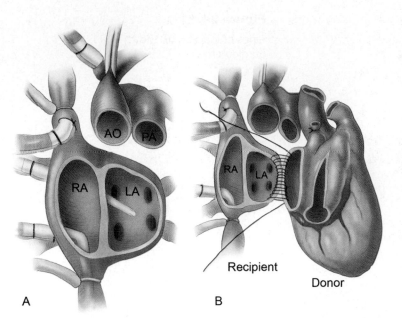

A   B

Figure 24.12

(A) Appearance of the recipient mediastinum after excision of the diseased heart. Note the position of the arterial and venous cannulas for cardiopulmonary bypass, as well as the left ventricular vent catheter passing through the right superior pulmonary vein. Posterior cuffs of left atrium (LA), right atrium (RA), aorta (AO), and pulmonary artery (PA) have been fashioned. (B) The donor heart has been lowered into the operative field, and the lateral wall of the left atrial anastomosis is being fashioned.

Figure 24.12 shows the cardiac anastomoses. Cold cardioplegia and topical cooling may be administered to reduce graft rewarming. The air is removed from the heart and the cross-clamp is removed resulting in reperfusion. Atrioventricular epicardial pacing wires may be placed and secured with nonabsorbable polypropylene stitches. Adequate hemostasis is obtained and after a reperfusion period of 30 to 60 minutes, the patient is weaned off cardiopulmonary bypass. The IVC cannula is removed. The SVC cannula is removed. The aortic cannula is removed and the heparin is reversed with protamine sulfate. Graft function may be assessed in the operating room suite with a pulmonary artery catheter and transesophageal echocardiography (TEE). The pericardium is left open. Chest tubes are inserted and hemostasis is established. The sternotomy is closed with stainless steel wires. The fascia is closed with an absorbable suture. The skin is closed with an absorbable subcuticular stitch (Kuo & Davis, 2005).

TEE
Transesophageal Echocardiography

Complications

The heart transplant patient is admitted to the ICU immediately following the procedure. It is necessary to maintain protective isolation in a positive-flow room with doors closed. Personnel entering the room must observe strict hand washing.

In the immediate postoperative period, the heart transplant recipient is at risk for problems related to the denervation of the transplanted heart and the global ischemia associated with the procedure, which may result in decreased diastolic compliance, impaired contractility, and depressed systolic function. Hemodynamic parameters, including blood pressure, heart rate, pulmonary artery pressures, and right heart pressures, are assessed and documented every 15 minutes for the first hour and every 30 minutes thereafter. Pulmonary vascular resistance is calculated every 8 hours. Right heart pressures are monitored closely, and rhythm strips are taken often (atrial arrhythmias are often the first sign of rejection). The need for analgesics and/or anxiolytics should be assessed every 4 hours and as needed. Thermodilution cardiac outputs are performed and documented, and mixed venous oxygen saturation level (SvO_2) may be monitored.

Patients are monitored for signs and symptoms of cardiac tamponade (hypotension, narrowing pulse pressure, decreased heart tones). Chest tube drainage is measured often, and the patient is monitored closely for signs of infection (fever, change in mental status, fatigue, change in secretions, and integrity of the surgical wound). An immunosuppressive protocol is followed. Patients are extubated as early as possible and allowed out of bed when stable.

Postprocedure Care

Routine followup care for the heart recipient includes frequent assessment for rejection. The endomyocardial biopsy is the gold standard for diagnosis of rejection and may be performed more frequently during the first 6 months to 1 year following transplantation (Kuo & Davis, 2005).

Other long-term followup care can vary among hospital transplant programs but usually includes routine blood analysis, chest x-ray, echocardiogram, electrocardiogram, 24-hour urine analysis, cardiac catheterization, and extensive screening for infection as it is the leading cause of morbidity and mortality after transplantation for the first year.

Other potential problems seen post-transplant can include vasculopathy, metabolic disorders, gastrointestinal disorders, renal insufficiency, reduced exercise tolerance, and malignancy.

Lung Transplantation

Lung transplantation has become a viable treatment of choice for patients with end-stage lung disease. Medical treatment for these patients is minimal and leans toward supportive care only. Usually their life expectancy is less than 24–36 months. Transplants may be either a single lung or double lung depending on the disease process.

Indications

Lung transplantation is indicated for patients with an airway disease including emphysema/chronic obstructive pulmonary disease (COPD), bronchiectasis, cystic fibrosis, or chronic bronchitis; pulmonary hypertension; or an interstitial lung disease such as pulmonary fibrosis, sarcoidosis, silicosis, scleroderma, pneumoconiosis, calcinosis cutis, Raynaud phenomenon, esophageal dysmotility, sclerodactly, telangiectasias (known as CREST), eosinophilic granuloma, idiopathic pulmonary fibrosis, hemosiderosis, and Goodpasture syndrome (Manzetti & Lee, 2003).

COPD
Chronic Obstructive Pulmonary Disease

Equipment and Supplies

Table 24.22 list additional items for lung transplantation.

Procedure: Double-Lung Transplantation

A standard transsternal bilateral anterior thoracotomy (clamshell incision) is made at the level of the fourth intercostal space. In a female patient, the incision is

Table 24.22	Additional Items for Lung Transplant				
Equipment	**Supplies**	**Instrumentation**	**Medications Anesthesia**	**Medications Sterile Field**
Bean Bag	Endoscopic GIA staplers and reloads	Sternal saw	Heparin	Antibiotic irrigation solution
Overhead armboard	Chest tubes	Chest wall retractor	Methylprednisolone	Heparin 1:1,000 5 cc in 500 cc normal saline
Pillows		Lung transplant pan		
		Lung retractor pan		

GIA
Gastrointestinal
Anastomosis

made at or below the inframammary crease. A breast flap is developed and retracted superiorly on each side and the chest is opened through the fourth intercostal space. Alternatively, a muscle sparing posterolateral thoracotomy through the fifth intercostal space can be used for a single-lung transplant or on both sides for double-lung transplant. The internal mammary artery and vein are identified and ligated on both sides. A sternal saw is used to divide the midportion of the sternum transversely. Hemostasis is accomplished via sutures, clips, and electrosurgery. The chest wall retractors are placed on each side. The pericardium is left intact unless cardiopulmonary bypass is anticipated. Intercostal muscles in the fourth intercostal space are divided to maximize overall exposure. The latissimus dorsi and serratus anterior muscles are spared laterally. Arterial and venous cannulas for cardiopulmonary bypass can be placed at this time or at any point in the operation. Intravenous heparin is administered for systemic anticoagulation prior to cannulation and before mobilization and division of hilar structures. The right lung is deflated exposing the hilum and the superior pulmonary vein and pulmonary artery. Pleural adhesions are taken down and the mediastinal pleura is divided to mobilize the hilar structures. The superior pulmonary vein, the right PA, and the inferior pulmonary vein are mobilized and divided with an endoscopic gastrointestinal anastomosis (GIA) stapler. The branches of the right pulmonary artery are mobilized. The truncus anterior, the apical and anterior branches of the right pulmonary artery are divided with an endoscopic GIA stapler. The inferior pulmonary ligament is divided and the pulmonary vein is mobilized and divided with an endoscopic GIA stapler. The right mainstem bronchus is mobilized and divided distally with an endoscopic GIA stapler. The remaining pleural adhesions are divided without injury to the phrenic nerve. The right lung is removed and hemostasis is achieved at this time. Two sets of figure-of-eight #1 monofilament polyglyconate synthetic absorbable pericostal sutures are placed in the intercostal release incisions at this point due to the excellent exposure while the lung is out of the pleural cavity. The posterior chest tube is placed in the pleural cavity through a separate skin incision. A small suction catheter is placed into the chest tube and connected to suction to facilitate drainage of fluids throughout the case. A flexible drain may be placed in the axillary space at this time. The right mainstem bronchus is cut with a No. 10 blade just proximal to the takeoff of the right upper lobe bronchus. Mucus or secretions are removed from the lumen. A retraction stitch is placed anteriorly to secure the bronchus. The remainder of the bronchial wall is sharply divided, and irrigated with an antibiotic solution. Cold laparotomy pads are placed posteriorly in the pleural cavity. The bronchial posterior wall anastomosis is completed first with a running absorbable monofilament suture. The anterior wall anastomosis is then completed. The anastomosis is tested for obvious air leaks under water while the right lung is manually inflated. The stapled recipient right pulmonary artery is clamped proximally with a vascular clamp and the staple line is trimmed. The donor pulmonary artery is cut to an appropriate length to avoid kinking. The anastomosis is completed with a running nonabsorbable polypropylene suture. A second vascular clamp is placed distal to the anastomosis and the first clamp is removed to test the anastomosis. A Pennington clamp is used to retract the stapled superior and inferior right pulmonary vein stumps laterally for placement of a vascular clamp toward the body of the left atrium. The staple lines are trimmed. The superior pulmonary vein and inferior pulmonary vein are connected sharply, creating a large recipient left atrial cuff on the right side. Anastomosis of the donor left atrial cuff to the created recipient left atrial cuff is started using a running nonabsorbable polypropylene suture. A bolus of methylprednisolone and mannitol are given prior to completion of the anastomosis. Prior to completion of the anastomosis, the vascular clamp is partially removed to allow blood flow into the implanted right lung and remove any air from the pulmonary vasculature. Controlled, low-pressure perfusion of the lung is achieved over 10 to 15 minutes by gradually releasing the pulmonary artery clamp. Ventilation with room air is begun by hand then continued with mechanical ventilation. The left lung is selectively deflated exposing the hilum. Pleural and mediastinal adhesions are taken down. The phrenic nerve is preserved. The pleura and pericardium are opened medially on the left side. The superior pulmonary vein, inferior pulmonary vein, left pulmonary artery, and left main bronchus are stapled and divided with an endoscopic GIA stapler and reloads. A silk retraction stitch is placed inferiorly on the pericardium posterior to the phrenic nerve and anterior to the inferior pulmonary vein. A Rummel tourniquet is placed to reinforce the retraction stitch, which allows the heart to be retracted upward and to the right for hilar structure exposure and dissection. The tissue connecting the left pulmonary artery and the left superior pulmonary vein is divided. Hemostasis is obtained. Posterior chest tubes and the axillary drainage tube are placed. The left mainstem bronchus is divided with a new No. 10 blade proximal to the staple line. Mucus and any secretions present are removed from the bronchus lumen. An anterior retraction stitch is placed to aid in exposure. The left bronchial anastomosis is completed with an absorbable monofilament suture in the same fashion as completed on the right side. Testing for obvious air leak is completed as was on the right. The left pulmonary artery is occluded proximally with a vascular clamp and the staple line is trimmed. The recipient and donor pulmonary arteries are trimmed to an appropriate length to avoid kinking. The anastomosis is completed with a running nonabsorbable polypropylene suture. A second vascular clamp is placed and the previous clamp is removed to test the anastomosis. The superior pulmonary vein and the inferior pulmonary vein are identified, mobilized, and divided using endoscopic GIA staples. The stumps are retracted laterally with Pennington clamps. A large vascular clamp is placed toward the body of the left atrium. The staple lines are trimmed and the orifices are connected sharply creating a large recipient left atrial cuff. A running nonabsorbable polypropylene stitch is used to anastomose the donor atrial cuff to the newly created recipient left atrial cuff. Prior to completion of the anastomosis an intravenous bolus of methylprednisolone and mannitol are given and the pulmonary vascular bed is de-aired by partially releasing the vascular clamp on the pulmonary artery allowing blood flow into the transplanted left lung. The vascular clamp is released on the recipient left atrium to force any residual air out of the left atrium just prior to tying down the suture. The pulmonary artery clamp is gradually released over a period of 10 to 15 minutes to achieve controlled reperfusion of the transplanted lung. Ventilation with room air is again initiated by hand and continued by mechanical ventilation. Two anterior chest tubes are placed underneath the medial surface of the upper lobes and brought out through separate stab wounds inferiorly. The wound is inspected for hemostasis. The incision is approximated with three sets of #5 wires. The remainder of the incision is closed with the #1 monofilament polyglyconate synthetic absorbable sutures placed earlier and additional #1 suture of the same material in a figure-of-eight fashion. The pectoral fascial layer, the subcutaneous layer, and the subdermal layer are approximated and closed. Staples are used to close the skin (Kuo & Davis, 2005).

Complications

First-degree failure occurs in 10%–15% of cases. Its etiology is unknown, which makes prevention difficult. Typically, the radiographic appearance of the allograft is dense, with diffuse "fluffy" infiltrates. The patient is considered to have first-degree graft failure if this infiltrate fails to clear within 24 hours and the patient continues to require fractional inspired oxygen in excess of 0.60. Both the clinical features and the management of graft failure are similar to those of acute respiratory distress syndrome. The patient is maximally supported (with efforts to avoid infection in the profoundly immunocompromised host) while the injured lung is allowed to heal. If the lung heals before the patient incurs a fatal infection, the patient may go on to achieve normal lung function.

The major complications that may occur include delayed bronchial healing, rejection, and infection. The bronchial anastomosis is threatened by ischemia and bronchial strictures. If an anastomotic stricture develops, it can be handled by using a short silicone stent placed endoscopically.

Signs and symptoms of rejection and infection are similar, making diagnosis difficult. In the absence of apparent sepsis, the development of a hilar infiltrate on the x-ray film or a decline in arterial oxygenation suggests the onset of rejection. If rejection is suspected, the patient is given 1,000 mg methylprednisolone IV; improvement in the hilar infiltrate is expected within 12 hours. If no improvement is seen on the radiograph, a transbronchial biopsy is performed to confirm the diagnosis of rejection and rule out infection.

The reimplantation response may develop and is evidenced by a perihilar and/or lower lobe air space beginning in the first 36 hours after transplantation. It varies in severity from a subtle perihilar haze to dense perihilar and basilar consolidation. This condition usually remains the same or worsens during the next 2–4 days and then begins to clear. Generally, the pattern of clearing involves a decrease in air space disease, with residual reticular interstitial disease that eventually clears completely. This reaction may be correlated with a prolonged ischemic time (longer than 4 hours) or more likely is related to decreased or absent lymphatics in combination with the trauma of reimplantation.

Postprocedure Care

After the patient is in the ICU, protective isolation is enforced while he or she is most susceptible to infection. Masks are worn for the first 7 days, and strict handwashing is mandatory. Aggressive use of diuretics keeps the lungs as dry as possible.

Under normal circumstances, a standard volume of cycled mechanical ventilatory support is supplied. The goals of respiratory management are to:

Maintain the lowest possible peak airway pressure.

Maintain the lowest possible fraction of inspired oxygen.

Provide adequate pulmonary toilet.

Start chest physiotherapy early because a denervated airway results in a decreased cough reflex.

After lung transplant patients are extubated and hemodynamically stable, they are transferred to the thoracic surgical floor in protective isolation. The goals of physiotherapy in the subacute stage of recovery are to ensure maximal clearance of secretions, to wean from supplemental oxygen, and to increase exercise tolerance. During exercise sessions, an increase in the work of breathing and/or an unexpected decrease in oxygen saturation may indicate the beginning of a rejection episode. Diligent and careful monitoring of temperature and oxygen saturation during rest and exercise prevents unnecessary delays in the diagnosis and treatment of rejection. Weaning from supplemental oxygen and increasing exercise tolerance take about 1–2 weeks. In patients with chronic obstructive pulmonary disease and emphysema, it is extremely important to avoid hyperventilation of the native lung.

Heart and Lung Transplantation
Indications

Heart and lung transplantation is indicated for patients with pulmonary vascular disease, specifically, primary pulmonary hypertension or Eisenmenger's syndrome[2] with cardiac repair (White-Williams, Kugler, & Widmar, 2008). Candidates undergo an extensive transplant evaluation and need to meet pre-determined objective measures of a deteriorating medical condition.

Equipment and Supplies

Table 24.23 lists additional items for a heart and lung transplantation.

Table 24.23	Additional Items for Heart-Lung Transplant				
Equipment	**Supplies**	**Instruments**	**Medications Anesthesia**	**Medications Sterile Field**
Cell saver	Cell saver suction tubing	Heart/Lung transplant pan	Isoprenaline	Antibiotic irrigation solution
Defibrillator	External paddles	Sterile internal paddles	Dopamine	Heparin 1:1,000 5 cc in 500 cc normal saline
Cardiopulmonary bypass machine	Chest tubes	Sternal saw	Heparin Protamine	

Procedure: Heart and Lung Transplantation

Under general endotracheal anesthesia, arterial and venous lines are placed. The skin is prepped and draped in a sterile fashion. A median sternotomy or bilateral thoracosternotomy (clamshell) incision is made and dissection is carried down to the pericardium to allow maximum exposure of all the mediastinal structures and access to the hilum of both lungs. Pleural adhesions are divided using electrosurgery. IV heparin is administered to achieve systemic anticoagulation. The anterior pericardium is opened with a T incision. Two stay sutures are placed on each pericardial edge to facilitate exposure of the hilar structures. The ascending aorta is separated from the pulmonary trunk and the superior vena cava (SVC) and the inferior vena cava (IVC) are dissected free. Cannulas are inserted and secured with tapes into the aorta, the SVC, and the IVC for cardiopulmonary bypass. Preservation of the phrenic nerves, vagus nerves, and left recurrent laryngeal nerve is achieved with careful dissection and excision of the recipient heart and lungs. The distal ascending aorta is cross-clamped. Cardioplegia is delivered to the aortic root for myocardial preservation and ice slurry is added to the pericardium for topical cooling if the recipient's heart is used for domino donation (discussed earlier in this chapter). After the heart is arrested, the SVC is clamped cephalad to the right atrium, the IVC tape is tightened, and the heart is then excised. The SVC is then divided close to the atrial-caval-junction for maximum length. With domino donation, the SVC is divided 1 cm cephalad to the atrial-caval-junction to avoid damaging the sinoatrial node. The heart is retracted to the left for proper exposure of the IVC. The IVC incision is made leaving 1 cm of tissue around the IVC cannula. The pulmonary veins, the distal pulmonary trunk, and the posterior pericardial reflections behind the roof of the left atrium are divided to complete the cardiectomy. The pulmonary trunk at its bifurcation is bisected. The left recurrent laryngeal nerve is identified and protected. Hemostasis is accomplished in this area with clips instead of electrosurgery. Sharp dissection is used to free the left and right PAs laterally toward the lungs. The anterior hilum of the left lung is dissected. The left lung is mobilized by dividing the pulmonary ligament with electrosurgery. The pleural reflection along the cut edge of the pericardium is opened. The pericardium is incised adjacent to the pulmonary vessels. The stumps of the pulmonary veins and stump of the left PA are then delivered to the pleural cavity. Traction on these vessels is applied to extend the incision in the pericardium to encircle the pulmonary veins. The pericardial incision is then extended inferiorly toward the diaphragm to enlarge the pericardial window for passage of the left donor lung. The posterior lung hilum is dissected. The left lung is brought out of the wound and retracted to the right of the midline to expose the posterior aspect of the left hilum. The pleural reflections overlying the left main bronchus are incised close to the lung to avoid injury to the left vagus nerve. The pleura is swept away from the surface of the bronchus toward the mediastinum. Branches of the bronchial artery are ligated then divided. The left lung is returned to the pleural cavity and the remaining soft tissue and lymph nodes on the anterior surface are divided using electrosurgery to skeletonize the left main bronchus. A transanastomotic stapler is used to seal the bronchus, which is then divided, distal to the staple line. The right is dissected free and excised repeating the same steps as for the left lung. The right phrenic nerve lies much closer to the right lung hilum so extra care is taken to avoid injury. With both lungs excised, the two-stapled bronchial stumps are visible through the central defect in the posterior pericardium. The anesthesia provider suctions out any secretions present and washes out the airway by introducing 30 mL of 10% aqueous Betadine solution directly into the endotracheal tube. Fibrofatty tissue and carinal lymph nodes surround the distal trachea and the tracheal carina. A transverse incision is made as low as possible into the pericardial tissue using electrosurgery. Tissue clamps applied to each of the bronchial stumps are retracted downward to bring the tracheal carina into the operating field. The tracheal carina and bronchial stumps are skeletonized by blunt dissection. Care is taken to avoid injury to both vagus nerves during this maneuver. At this point meticulous hemostasis of all the posterior mediastinal structures is completed. Next, the donor heart-lung bloc is inspected, oriented, and the trachea 2 cm above the carina is transected. Blood supply to the donor airways is preserved by leaving the pericardial fibrofatty envelope on the donor carina undisturbed. Secretions are aspirated from the donor airways and sent for microbiologic examination. Each donor bronchus is washed out with normal saline. The donor trachea is trimmed to one cartilage ring above the carina for implantation. The recipient trachea just above the carina is opened transversely and carried around the anterior two-thirds portion with a No. 11 blade. The peritracheal soft tissue envelope is left undisturbed to preserve blood supply to the recipient side of the tracheal anastomosis. Tracheal traction is achieved with a 2-0 Silk stitch through the anterior aspect of the trachea. The first tracheal anastomosis stitch is placed in the 3 o'clock position in the recipient trachea. This stitch aids with gentle traction on the tracheal stump. The division of the membranous part of the trachea and excision of the recipient carina is completed. The donor heart-lung bloc is partially wrapped in a cold, wet laparotomy pad and steadied in the anatomic orientation. The posterior membranous tracheal anastomosis is completed with the nonabsorbable polypropylene running stitch placed earlier. After three passes of the suture, the donor heart-lung bloc is lowered into the chest cavity. The right lung is maneuvered through the pericardial window into the right pleural cavity. The left lung is maneuvered in the same fashion to the left pleural cavity. Orientation of both lungs is checked at this point. Traction is applied to the donor aorta anteriorly and inferiorly to provide exposure. The tracheal anastomosis is continued onto the cartilaginous part of the trachea and completed. Using flexible bronchoscopy, the anesthesia provider aspirates any blood in the airways during the anastomosis. The peritracheal soft tissue surrounding the donor and recipient airways is approximated with a running nonabsorbable polypropylene suture to cover the tracheal anastomosis. The lungs are reinflated and ventilated with a tidal volume of 5 mL/kg using room air. The heart is displaced through the left pericardial window into the pleural cavity to enhance exposure for the IVC anastomosis completed with an extra-long nonabsorbable polypropylene-running suture in a posterior to anterior direction. The heart is returned to the pericardial cavity. The SVC anastomosis is completed with a nonabsorbable polypropylene running suture. The aortic anastomosis is performed with a nonabsorbable polypropylene running suture and left untied for subsequent de-airing of the right atrium prior to aortic cross-clamp release. A pulmonary artery catheter, if desired, may be advanced at this point and gradual warming of the patient to 37°C begins. The patient is placed in steep Trendelenburg for de-airing of the heart. The tapes around the venae cavae are removed and the venous circuit is partially unclamped to allow filling of the heart. The right atrium is thoroughly de-aired through the SVC anastomosis before the suture is tied. The right ventricle is de-aired through the pneumologia site in the donor pulmonary trunk. The tidal volume of the ventilator is increased to 10 mL/kg. De-airing of the left heart is accomplished through the vent opening on the tip of the left atrial appendage and the cardioplegia site on the donor aortic root. The aortic cross-clamp is removed to begin reperfusion. An isoprenaline and a dopamine infusion is started to decrease pulmonary vascular resistance and increase cardiac contractility. Further de-airing of the heart is accomplished prior to the closing of the pulmonary trunk, the left atrial appendage, and the aortic root with nonabsorbable polypropylene sutures. The aorta can be de-aired using a 21 G needle or a cardioplegia cannula attached to a suction catheter. Temporary epicardial pacing wires are secured to the donor right atrium and right ventricle and brought out through the skin below the incision. Two pleural drains are placed in the midaxillary line on each side. Two mediastinal drains are placed anteriorly, one in the posterior pericardial cavity and the other retrosternally, connected to underwater seal drain bottles and placed on suction of 7 kPa[3]. Normothermia is achieved and the patient is weaned off cardiopulmonary bypass. The venous cannulas are removed; the patient is given protamine sulfate, clotting factors, and platelets. The aortic cannula is removed and hemostasis is achieved. The sternotomy is closed with stainless steel wires. The fascia is closed with an absorbable suture. The skin is closed with a subcuticular stitch (Kuo & Davis, 2005).

Complications

Complications consist of combined information from the previous sections for lung transplantation and heart transplantation.

Postprocedure Care

Postprocedure care is a combination of care listed in the previous sections for lung transplantation and heart transplantation.

Multidisciplinary Care

All transplant recipients are followed by a multidisciplinary team of caregivers, including physicians, surgeons, advanced practice providers, anesthesia providers, nurses, social services, psychiatrists, nutritionists, pharmacologists, and financial services. The team provides extensive pre-operative evaluations for all transplant recipients, follows the patient through the surgical transplantation phase, and provides continuity of care for the rest of the recipient's lifespan. Collaboration of all team members is essential for providing the best scenario for transplantation positive outcomes.

ENDNOTES

1. The term *Woods units* refers to "a simplified system for measuring pulmonary vascular resistance that uses increments of pressure. Measurement is made by subtracting pulmonary capillary wedge pressure from the mean pulmonary arterial pressure and dividing by cardiac output in liters per minute" (Drugs.com, 2008).

2. "Eisenmenger's syndrome … is defined as the process in which a left-to-right shunt in the heart causes increased flow through the pulmonary vasculature, causing pulmonary hypertension, which in turn, causes increased pressures in the right side of the heart and reversal of the shunt into a right-to-left shunt" (Eisenmenger's Syndrome, 2008).

3. Kilopascal (kPa) is a unit of pressure measurement widely used throughout the world. Kilpascal largely replaces the pounds per square inch (psi) unit except in some countries still using the imperial measurement system (Pascal Pressure, 2008).

REFERENCES

1. AORN (2008). Recommend Practices for Tissue Banking, *2008 Perioperative Standards and Recommended Practices*. Denver, CO: AORN, pp. 609–610.

2. Center for Disease Control (CDC) (2005). Fast Stats A to Z, Inpatient Procedures. Accessed 18 August 2008, http://www.cdc.gov/nchs/fastats/insurg.htm.

3. Cupples, S.A. (2003). Heart transplantation. In S.A. Cupples & L. Ohler (Eds.), *Transplantation Nursing Secrets* (pp. 85–105). Philadelphia: Hanley & Belfus.

4. Cupples, S.A., & Ohler, L. (2003). *Transplantation Nursing Secrets*. Philadelphia: Hanley & Belfus.

5. Daniel Luke Geyser, "Organ Transplantation: New Regulations to Alter Distribution of Organs," *Journal of Law, Medicine & Ethics, 28*, no. 1(2000): pp. 95–98.

6. Eisenmenger's Syndrome (2008). Retrieved 26 August 2008 from Wikipedia Web Site: http://en.wikipedia.org/wiki/Eisenmenger%27s_syndrome.

7. Encyclopedia of Everyday Law/Organ Donation. (2008). Retrieved February 13, 2008, from enotes Web site: http://www.enotes.com/everyday-law-encyclopedia/organ-donation.

8. Encyclopedia of Surgery (2008). Transplant Surgery. Retrieved 18 August 2008, http://www.surgery-encyclopedia.com/St-Wr/Transplant-Surgery.html.

9. Finger, E.B. (2006). Organ Procurement Considerations in Trauma. Retrieved 13 February 2008, from eMedicine Web site: http://www.emedicine.com/med/topic3220.htm.

10. Friedman, A. (2006). Make Me a Perfect Match: Understanding Transplant Compatibility. *Aakprenalife, 21*(5). Retrieved 14 February 2008, from aakp Web site: http://www.aakp.org/aakp-library/Transplant-Compatiility/index.cfm.

11. Gilroy, R.K. (2007). Intestinal and Multivisceral Transplantation. Retrieved 2 March 2008, from eMedicine Web site: http://www.emedicine.com/med/topic3502.htm.

12. Hakim, N. (Ed.). (2002). Pancreas and islet transplantation. Oxford: Oxford.

13. High-Definition Robot Used During Living-Donor Kidney Transplant. (2007). Retrieved 11 February 2008, from Rush University Medical Center Web site: http://www.exaxhealth.com/24/15357.html.

14. Humar, A., Matas, A.J., & Payne, W.D. (2006). *Atlas of Organ Transplantation*. Singapore, Asia: Springer.

15. Iazzetti, G., & Rigutti, E. (2007). *Atlas of Anatomy*. Cobham, UK: TAJ Books LTD.

16. IVIG Intravenous Immunoglobulin (2008). Retrieved 16 February 2008 from Wikipedia Web site: http://en.wikipedia.org/wiki/organ_transplantation.

17. Kidney Transporter. (2005). Retrieved 11 February 2008, from www.acfnewsource.org/science/kidney_trans.htm.OsgoodFile (2005).

18. Kuo, P., & Davis, R.D. (2005). *Comprehensive Atlas of Transplantation*. Philadelphia: Lippincott Williams & Wilkins.

19. Manzetti, J.D., & Lee, A. (2003). Lung Transplantation. In S.A. Cupples & L. Ohler (Eds.), *Transplantation Nursing Secrets* (pp. 75–83). Philadelphia: Hanley & Belfus.

20. Molmenti, E.P., & Klintmalm, G.B. (2002). *Atlas of Organ Transplantation*. Philadelphia: W.B. Saunders.

21. National Foundation for Transplant (2007). How much does an organ transplant cost? Retrieved 18 August 2008, http://www.transplants.org/LearnMore.php.

22. Ohler, L., & Cupples, S. (2008). Core Curriculum for Transplant Nurses. St. Louis, MO: Mosby.

23. Park, B.K. (2003). Intestinal transplantation. In S.A. Cupples & L. Ohler (Eds.) *Transplantation Nursing Secrets* (p. 178). Philadelphia: Hanley & Belfus.

24. Pascal Pressure (2008). Retrieved 26 August 2008, from Wikipedia Web site: http://en.wikipedia.org/wiki/Pascal_(unit).

25. Stedman's Medical Dictionary (2008). Wood units. Retrieved 26 August 2008 from Drugs.com Web site: http://www.drugs.com/dict/wood-units.html.

26. Transplantation Rejection. (2004). Retrieved 10 February 2008, from http://biomed.brown.edu/Course/B1108/B1108_2004_Group04/rejection_overview.htm.

27. Twyman, R. (2003). Tissue Matching for Transplantation. Retrieved 10 February 2008, from http://genome.wellcome.ac.uk/doc_WTD020937.html.

28. Types of Transplants. Transplant History. (2008). Retrieved 10 January 2008, from Wikipedia Web site: http://en.wikipedia.org/wiki/organ_transplantation.

29. University of North Carolina Pancreas/Kidney Transplant Education Booklet. Retrieved 18 August 2008 from UNC Web site: http://surgery.med.unc.edu/AbdominalTransplant/.

30. White-Williams, C., Kugler, C., & Widmar, B. (2008). Lung and heart-lung transplantation. In L. Ohler & S. Cupples (Eds.), *Core Curriculum for Transplant Nurses* (pp. 391–420). St. Louis, MO: Mosby.

CHAPTER 25

Plastic Surgery

Susan K. Chandler

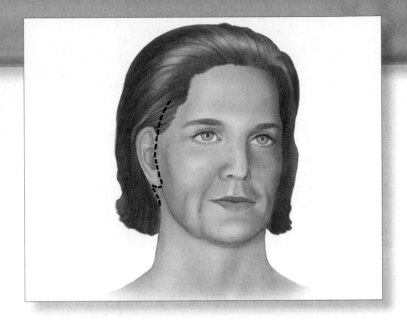

INTRODUCTION

Contrary to public and media perception, plastic surgery is much more than cosmetic procedures—facelifts, breast implants, and lip augmentations. It is not limited to one anatomical region of the body or organ system. Plastic surgery is both aesthetic and reconstructive; indeed, sometimes the arenas of aesthetics and reconstruction blend in the surgeon's efforts to restore appearance as well as function. One common thread, however, is the plastic surgeon's ability to manipulate and transfer tissue, whether it is skin, digits, muscle flaps, or microvascular structures. While based on sound surgical principles, plastic and reconstructive surgery is a specialty that is creative, innovative, and, in many respects, without boundaries.

ANATOMY

Integumentary System

The integument, or skin, is the largest organ of the human body. It forms a protective, pliable covering over the entire exterior surface. It works by acting as a crucial barrier to prevent the introduction of harmful organisms and also regulates body temperature. At the various openings of the body (the mouth, nares, anus, urethra, and vagina), the skin is continuous with mucous membrane linings. The skin contains three layers: the epidermis, dermis, and subcutaneous tissue (**Fig. 25.1**).

The epidermis is the outermost layer of the skin. It comes from the Greek word *derma*, meaning skin. It does not contain any blood vessels and relies on deeper layers of the skin for its nutrients and oxygen. The dermis contains numerous specialized structures: the

Chapter Contents

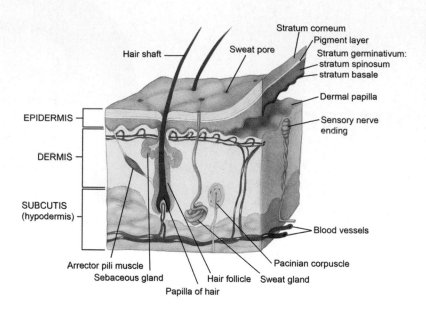

Figure 25.1

The three layers of skin.

hair, the nails, and integumentary glands. The subcutaneous layer contains fat, connective tissue, blood vessels, and nerves.

The skin of an adult has a surface area of about 1.8 cm (3000 square inches) and may weigh anywhere from 3–5 pounds. It is thickest on the palms, the soles, and the back, and thinnest on the tympanic membrane and over the eyelids. The attachment of the skin varies from loose to tight. It is separated from the underlying structures in most parts of the body by a subcutaneous tissue called the *superficial fascia* (hypodermis). The superficial fascial system provides support for the surface tissues of the body. It also allows the muscles that underlie most of the skin to move freely. At some points where the superficial fascia is minimal and no muscles underlie the skin, as on the anterior surface of the tibia, the skin attaches to the periosteum of the bone. In plastic and reconstructive procedures, it plays a major role in providing support when tissue has been rearranged.

Skin color is caused in part by the pigment carotene (yellow), which is in the surface layer and in thin skin, and by the color of the circulating blood, which shows through to give the flesh appearance. The intensity of the flesh color depends on the state of contraction or dilation of the superficial vessels and on the extent of oxygenation of the blood. The difference in color among individuals and ethnic groups is due to the concentration of the pigment *melanin*. Skin grafting takes into account the difference in thickness and coloration from various areas of the body, especially when grafted skin is placed in a visible location.

Function

The functions of the skin are many. Basically, the skin stands as a protective barrier against the ever-changing and often adverse conditions of the external environment, and adapts itself to them. Skin receptors provide an awareness of this external environment. As skin wears, it adapts by the thickening of the stratum corneum to form calluses if necessary. It prevents the body from drying. The oiled surface of the skin sheds water, and its pigment helps to protect the body from harmful ultraviolet radiation. Skin is an effective first line of defense against infectious organisms.

The skin is an important regulator of body temperature. It accomplishes this through the coordinated activity of the nerve endings, the blood vessels, and sweat gland secretions; to a limited extent, excretion is a function of the skin. The skin has a limited capacity for absorption, especially when materials such as hormones, vitamins, and drugs are placed on the skin in a proper vehicle.

Structures

EPIDERMIS

The *epidermis* is the outer and thinner layer of the skin. Five layers can be distinguished from the innermost outward: stratum basale, stratum spinosum, stratum granulosum, stratum licidum, and stratum corneum. The stratum basale contain cells shaped like columns. Here the cells divide and push upward into higher layers, where they eventually flatten and die. The cells of the *stratum spinosum* contain varying amounts of the brown pigment melanin. Only in albinos is the skin without melanin. The *stratum granulosum* consists of three to five layers of flattened cells whose cytoplasm contains many keratyhyalin granules. The *stratum lucidum* is a clear homogenous band outside the stratum granulosum. It is composed of rows of flattened cells. The *stratum corneum*, the outermost layer, consists of flat, scale-like dead and cornified cells. They contain fibrous protein called *keratin*.

There are three types of specialized cells in the epidermis layer: melanocytes (produce pigment); Langerhans' cell (acts as defense for the immune system); and Merkel's cell, whose function is not clearly understood.

DERMIS

The *dermis* is a layer of dense connective tissue. The protein collagen accounts for most of the dermis, and is arranged in bundles that run horizontally, held together by elastic fibers. It consists of an outer papillary layer, which fits intimately into the underside of the epidermis, and a deeper reticular layer. The dermis is thicker than the epidermis, ranging from 0.6 mm on the eyelids to as much as 3.0 mm on the palms and soles. It contains many nerve endings that give us sensation for temperature and pressure.

The papillary layer contains papillae, which are bumpy, fingerlike projections that extend into the epidermis. This results in the appearance of ridges, which occur in unique patterns that we know as fingerprints. The function of these ridges is to aid the hand (or foot) in grasping by increasing friction.

The deeper, reticular layer gives the dermis its strength and elasticity. This region contains hair roots, sebaceous glands, sweat glands, nerve endings, nails, and blood vessels. It is also where tattoo ink is injected.

SUBCUTANEOUS LAYER

This deep layer of the skin consists mostly of fat, and functions to insulate and cushion the body. It also contains larger blood vessels and cutaneous nerves. The subcutaneous fat is described as superficial, intermediate, or deep. In terms of liposuction, removal of excess fat takes place most often from the deep areas, although sculpting of the superficial layer is sometimes a desired technique. Throughout the body, zones of adherence of the superficial fascial system exist and encase fat, producing creases, bulges, and various contour irregularities.

GLANDS

The important glands of the skin are the sebaceous, sudoriferous (sweat), and mammary glands.

The *sebaceous glands*, with few exceptions, develop from the epithelium in the necks of hair follicles. The secreting portions of the sebaceous glands are sac-like masses of epithelial cells. They function to keep the skin lubricated, reduce water loss from the skin surface, and protect the skin from infection. The majority of sebaceous glands open into the hair follicle.

The *sudoriferous (sweat) glands* are in the form of simple coiled tubules extending down into the reticular layer of the dermis or, in some cases, into the subcutaneous tissue. They are found in most skin areas, being absent only on the margins of the lips, the concave surface of the external ear, the skin of the nipple, and skin portions of the genital organs. The secretion of the sweat glands is a thin, watery solution.

The *mammary glands* are paired glands that are rudimentary in the male and larger in the female. The adult breast is situated on the anterior chest wall, between the second and seventh ribs. It extends medially from the sternocostal junction to the midaxillary line along the lateral chest wall. The axillary tail of Spence is breast tissue that extends up into the axilla. The gland consists of multiple lobules connected by lactiferous ducts and are arranged in a radial pattern. The lactiferous ducts drain into sinuses which also serve as a reservoir for milk. The sinuses communicate with the nipple.

The gland is situated within connective tissue and fat. Fibrous bands called *Cooper's ligaments* are connective tissue support structures running from the deep muscle fascia, through the breast tissue, attaching to the dermis of the skin. The amount of fat and breast parenchyma varies widely from individual to individual and depends upon many factors, such as age, hormonal and genetic factors, and amount of body fat.

Blood is supplied from the internal mammary artery, intercostal perforators, and laterally from the thoracoacromial artery. The breast sits on the pectoralis major muscle. Medially, the breast covers portions of the rectus abdominis muscle. Inferiorly, the external oblique muscle inserts under the breast, with the serratus and latissimus dorsi muscles found laterally. The muscles carry a rich supply of blood to the breast parenchyma, fat, and skin, are important in wound healing, and provide coverage of implants.

OTHER STRUCTURES

Blood and lymphatic vessels, nerves, and nerve endings are all located within the integumentary system. Their location and patency are crucial to wound healing, nourishment, and function, especially with disruption and movement of tissue flaps and muscles, as well as grafting. When secondary procedures are performed, knowledge of blood vessel and nerve anatomy is necessary in order to prevent necrosis.

SPECIAL INSTRUMENTS, SUPPLIES, AND EQUIPMENT

Plastic and reconstructive procedures are highly specialized, and while a basic instrument set may be used, instrumentation should be prepared that take into account not only the procedure being performed, but the technique as well. There is a great degree of customization and implantable materials are frequently used with this surgical specialty. The circulating nurse should always collaborate with the plastic surgeon to determine the need for preferred and/or special equipment. Basin sets, light handles, electrosurgical pencils and units, skin marker, Raytec, and laparotomy sponges are supplies common to almost all plastic surgery procedures. If local anesthesia will be used, 5 and 10 mL syringes, and 30 and 25 gauge needles of varying lengths are the most frequently requested.

Preference for suture material is always highly individual, and the circulator needs to confirm the type and amount to be used before opening any onto the sterile field. Drainage tubes are usually sutured in place; liposuction access sites are often left open to drain.

Several different sizes and lengths of instruments should be included in the trays. Depending upon the particular tissue being handled and the size of suture material used, the instrumentation may need to be extremely delicate, sturdy, or somewhere in-between. Positioning aids are also required for the various positions required by liposuctioning and grafting procedures. Positioning equipment includes bean bags, sand bags, extra pillows, foam padding, and 3 inch tape.

The application of dressings is a crucial part of most plastic procedures. Dressing materials should be verified with the surgeon and assembled beforehand. In addition to dressings, postprocedure garments such as bras, bodysuits with or without legs, vests, and compression girdles are frequently used following many different plastic surgical procedures. When ordering garments, it is important to know what type of garment will be used, the size, and the number of garments needed, for frequently the patient will request an extra.

Implant materials that are used for plastic and reconstructive surgery may be grouped into one of four categories: Polymers, metals and alloys, ceramics, and acellular and mammalian dermis. Plastic and reconstructive surgery incorporates a wide variety of implantable products for the many different procedures. For the procedures described later in this chapter, the most common are polymers.

Examples of solid polymers are breast implants which, at the time of this publication are either saline-filled or cohesive silicone gel. Regardless, the outer shell of both is constructed of a silicone elastomer. Polymers may also be porous (Marlex, Goretex, Dacron patches) or meshed (Marlex mesh, Dacron, or Prolene). Some may be mixed and molded intraoperatively.

Skin grafts may be acellular, commercially prepared products, in addition to the more traditional autologous split or full-thickness grafts. Cultured epithelial autografting allows full-thickness small skin biopsies to be placed in a culture medium that promotes tissue growth and, over the course of 21 days, expanding the size of the sample into tissue that can cover large wounds. Bioengineered skin, utilizing bovine collagen, shark cartilage, and silicone sheeting, are combined to create a scaffolding system which is placed over damaged dermis, allowing the growth of new collagen. Once regenerated, the scaffolding is removed and split thickness grafts may be placed over the restored dermis.

BREAST AUGMENTATION

A popular aesthetic procedure, breast augmentation is routinely requested by women seeking to enlarge small, normal, or even moderately sized breasts with the use of implantable mammary prostheses. It may improve the appearance of breasts with a minimal degree of ptosis as well as improve overall contour.

Related Procedures

Breasts are paired glands, and more often than not are asymmetrical in size. When the size difference is marked then surgical correction may be desired with the use of mammary implants. Poland's syndrome involves absence of the head of the pectoralis major muscle, resulting in asymmetry of the chest and affected patients may benefit from a breast implant in conjunction with a chest wall prosthesis. Unilateral congenital absence of the breast may be corrected with augmentation. Tubular breast deformities may also be improved with the addition of implants in conjunction to release of the constricted breast.

Nursing Implications

Prior to the procedure, the circulating nurse must know the specific types and sizes of breast implants to have available, as well as if the surgeon will be using sizers during the procedure to determine the final implant size (**Table 25.1**). As a part of the pre-procedure interview, confirm which approach the patient and surgeon have decided upon (perioareolar, inframammary, or axillary, **Fig. 25.2**); whether saline or gel implants will be used; and if known, the placement of the prostheses—subglandular or submuscular (**Fig. 25.3**). Confirm that preprocedure photos have been taken, and if the surgeon will need them during the procedure. If the patient is a part of a breast implant study program, Institutional Review Board (IRB) approval is mandated,

IRB
Institutional Review Board

Table 25.1	Ordering Information for Breast Augmentation Implants
Will sizers be used?	"Sizers" are temporary implants used during the procedure to determine correct size, shape, and placement
What type of implant?	Saline or Cohesive Gel
Surface of implant	Smooth or Textured
Shape	Round or Contour
Projection	Moderate or High Profile
Size	Variety of sizes are available, ranging from 100 cc to 800 cc and over; custom implants are possible for larger sizes
How many implants should be ordered?	If bilateral: 2 implants plus 1 backup per size ordered (minimal)
	If unilateral: 1 implant plus 1 backup per size ordered (minimal)

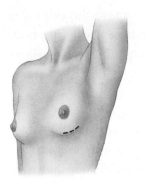
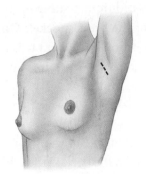
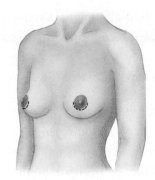

Figure 25.2

(A) Inframammary incision, (B) Axillary incision, and (C) Perioareolar incision.

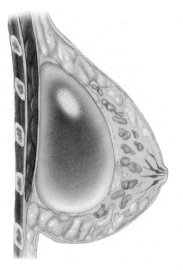
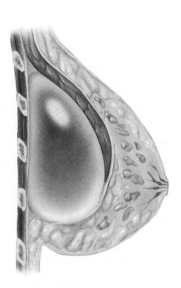

Figure 25.3

Placement of the prostheses— (A) subglandular and (B) submuscular.

along with registration and copies of the Informed Consent. If preprocedure marking is desired, it is usually done before transfer to the operating room and before any sedation is administered, since it is performed most often with the patient in a sitting or standing position. Ensure that the patient is sitting (or standing) with the shoulders even and arms at her side. The incision site is marked, as well as the existing inframammary folds and the new fold location following augmentation. Some surgeons will also mark the midline of the chest and the edges of the pectoralis muscle.

Check the fiberoptic light source to verify functioning. Have extra bulbs available in case one fails during the procedure. Assemble and place positioning aids as appropriate.

Anesthesia

Choices for anesthesia are either general anesthesia or monitored anesthesia care with use of local anesthesia infused throughout the operative site. Even with general anesthesia the surgeon may use a local anesthetic.

Position

Place the patient in the supine position, with the arms extended on armboards or tucked. Check with the surgeon before securing the arms and prepping for preferred arm position. The knees should be slightly flexed to alleviate stress on the back, and the operating table flexed at the waist. Shoulders should be even and the entire body in good alignment. During the procedure the surgeon may request the side to be rotated to optimize visualization of the breast pocket. Once the implant has been inserted, it may be necessary to reposition the patient to a sitting position to evaluate implant placement. Re-evaluate position and restraints after any changes.

Establishing and Maintaining the Sterile Field

After positioning and securing the patient, bilaterally prep the anterior chest, even if the procedure is unilateral. This will enable the surgeon to compare the contralateral breast. The field should extend from the neck to the umbilicus, include the axilla, and reach to the lateral chest wall to the back. Place impervious sterile drape material laterally. After the prep replace these drapes with dry sterile impervious drapes. Take care to prevent pooling of any prep solution under the patient. The use of implants requires vigilant attention to the maintenance of strict aseptic technique. Gloves should be changed before inserting the prostheses, and they should be handled as minimally as possible. Contamination sets the stage for infection, while increased bioburden may contribute to the incidence of capsular contracture.

Equipment and Supplies

> Major plastic surgery set
>
> Spinal needle for local anesthesia infusion (22g, 3½ inch, for example)
>
> Blunt dissector
>
> Asepto syringe
>
> DeBakey forceps
>
> Fiberoptic retractor and compatible light source
>
> Fog reduction agent
>
> Electrosurgery pencil with regular and long tip; needle tip may be requested
>
> Electrosurgical unit
>
> Suction with plastic tonsil tip
>
> Fill kit or self-filling syringe system (for saline implants)
>
> Breast sizers of various sizes
>
> Breast implants: range of sizes; backup implant for each size
>
> Drains (per surgeon preference)

Physiological Monitoring

Blood loss is usually minimal during breast augmentation; however, when developing the pocket, visualization is challenging and rapid bleeding may occur. Monitor sponges and laps for blood loss. Positional changes may result in physiological responses evidenced by changes in vital signs. Inadvertent intravascular injections may occur during local anesthesia infusion. Temporary tachycardia may result.

Specimens and Cultures

Specimens are not routinely collected as a part of augmentation mammaplasty; however, circumstances may occur where tissue may be removed for biopsy. Send any breast tissue removed during the procedure for pathological examination, even if previously unplanned.

Drugs and Solutions

Prior to the procedure, an antibiotic of the surgeon's choice should be administered intravenously. Local anesthesia drugs vary according to surgeon preference but may include lidocaine with epinephrine. Saline solution is used to irrigate the prepared breast pocket before insertion of the implant. Some surgeons may request an antibiotic irrigating solution as well.

Physician Orders

Depending upon the patient's age and surgeon preference, baseline mammography may be ordered. Verify antibiotic orders, choice of local anesthesia, and implant choice. Preprocedure preparation includes studies appropriate to the patient's health history and facility guidelines. Some physicians include pregnancy testing before any elective aesthetic procedures utilizing anesthesia. Sequential compression devices and stockings may be desired.

Procedure

Incision and Exposure

After the patient is fully anesthetized, the local anesthesia is infiltrated and the constricting properties of the epinephrine given time to be effective. The incision is placed according to the predetermined location—perioareolar, inframammary, or axillary. Exposure is provided with Senn retractors initially and, as the dissection is carried deeper through the breast parenchyma, the fiberoptic retractor is placed.

Details

Dissection continues through the breast tissue to the pectoralis major fascia. For subglandular placement of the implant, the breast is dissected from the muscle, usually with the finger or a metal sound, resulting in a pocket above the muscle. The muscle is not disturbed. For submuscular placement of the implants, the medial pectoralis major fibers are divided and the pocket is developed under the muscle. If the transaxillary approach is used, an endoscopic technique will be used to facilitate visualization and development of the pocket. After incising the skin in the axillary floor, and dissecting down to the muscle, the lateral pectoral fascia is opened and dissection continues as with the other techniques. Regardless of implant placement or incisional approach, once the pocket has been created it is irrigated with saline solution, dried, and checked for hemostasis. Antibiotic irrigation may be introduced. Some plastic surgeons will introduce a long-acting local anesthetic agent at this point to improve postprocedure pain management. The surgeon should be provided with new gloves, the implants inserted into the pocket, their position being carefully adjusted. At this point the surgeon may request the patient be repositioned to a sitting position to verify symmetry and implant placement.

Closure

The deep fat and fascial layer is closed first, followed by the subcutaneous layer. Skin closure is frequently a subcuticular running stitch. All sutures materials should be verified with the surgeon prior to opening them on the sterile field. If drains are used, they are usually a closed system, and may exit at the edge of the incision or laterally on the chest wall. The dressing is applied; a supportive bra may or may not be used.

PACU
Postanesthesia Care
Unit

Postprocedure Care

While transferring the patient to the Postanesthesia Care Unit (PACU), slightly elevate the stretcher head. During the handoff the PACU nurse reports the estimated blood loss, type, and amount of local anesthesia, drain placement, and location of implants.

Implants that are placed submuscularly as well as those inserted through the transaxillary approach may result in more postprocedure discomfort. Analgesic medicines, amount and times should also be reported. Some physicians will order ice bags to be placed over the breasts. Ensure that the ice bags are not too heavy.

Potential Complications

Hematoma is the most frequently reported complication following augmentation mammaplasty and may develop immediately postop. Attention to hemostasis is imperative, and any sudden swelling should be brought to the surgeon's attention. Asymmetry in edema is normal; however, marked asymmetry accompanied by intense pain are cardinal symptoms of hematoma development. A hematoma may develop up to 10 days after the procedure, so caution the patient to limit her activity according to postprocedure instructions. It is important to control nausea after the procedure in order to reduce its contribution to hematoma formation.

Infection, although possible, is extremely rare with augmentation mammaplasty. Administration of preprocedure antibiotics, irrigation with antibiotic solution, strict aseptic technique, and better identification of risk factors (diabetes, smokers) contribute to reduce the incidence. Should infection occur, redness, increased warmth to the breast, and increased pain are heralding signals. The incision may show signs of delayed healing or even dehisce, requiring removal of the mammary implant.

REDUCTION MAMMAPLASTY

The goal of a breast reduction procedure is to remove excessive breast tissue, eliminating or improving neck, shoulder, and back pain from the weight and discomfort of heavy, pendulous breasts. The challenge is to accomplish this with minimal scarring and maintaining or improving shape. Breast shape benefits from improved contour following excision of excess tissue, and the nipples are relocated to a more appropriate position.

Related Procedures

Mastopexy, or breast lift surgery, uses incision approaches similar to reduction mammaplasty. The difference between the two procedures is the amount of breast parenchyma that is removed. With both procedures the nipples are relocated to a higher level on the breast, and excess skin is removed. Mastopexy usually requires little to no tissue resection, however. Excision of gynecomastia in males may be accomplished through a periareolar approach using a combination of liposuction and direct excision. Following massive weight loss, males may require a modified reduction mammaplasty procedure if there is excessive skin and breast tissue.

Nursing Implications

Photographs are required by third-party payers when reimbursement is a consideration, and should be taken before marking begins. They also help document pre-existing asymmetries and other subtle differences that may have been previously unnoticed due to the size of the breasts. Preprocedure marking is a crucial component of the planning for reduction mammaplasty, and, usually, is done in the holding area. Because of the need to expose a large amount of body surface, implement interventions to maintain the patient's body temperature such as covering the patient with a forced warm air blanket throughout the procedure. During the marking process protect the patient's privacy and dignity. Apply compression stockings and sequential compression devices. After anesthesia induction, if ordered, insert a Foley catheter. Have scales for weighing the excised breast tissue in the operating room. Check the scales to assure accuracy before the case begins. Place impervious pads under the patient, one per side, before the procedure begins and remove immediately upon completion, before applying dressings.

Anesthesia

General anesthesia is used for this procedure, with the patient intubated. Local anesthesia may be injected at the incision sites.

Position

Place the patient in the supine position, taking care to assure that her body is properly aligned and shoulders are level. Reduction mammaplasty may be a lengthy procedure, and the padding and positioning of the patient should take into account all possible safety measures to prevent undue pressure or potential positioning injuries. Secure the arms on well-padded armboards after careful positioning to avoid ulnar or brachial nerve pressure. Flex the operating bed at the knees and bent at the hips, as in a modified lawnchair position. Protect the heels with additional padding.

Establishing and Maintaining the Sterile Field

Prep the patient from neck to umbilicus, to include the shoulders and the axilla, and extend the prep to the mid upper arms. Take the prep down to the level of the bed laterally. Before prepping, place a sterile impervious drape under each side of the chest; replace these drapes with sterile drapes after the prep. The breasts are then draped with towels (it may be necessary to staple them in place) and covered with a fenestrated drape that opens at the chest and covers the entire body, including the extended arms.

Equipment and Supplies

> Major plastic surgery set
>
> Nipple markers of varying sizes
>
> Multiple No. 10 blades for de-epithelialization
>
> Marking pens (or methylene blue and cotton-tipped applicators)
>
> Electrosurgery unit and pencil, regular and long tips
>
> Tonsil tip suction and tubing
>
> Liposuction cannulaes and suction machine (per surgeon preference)
>
> Fluid warmer
>
> Bair Hugger
>
> Sequential compression device
>
> Suture according to procedure and surgeon preference

Physiological Monitoring

Vessels throughout the breast tissue may be plentiful and large, and bleeding may be profuse and rapid if not well controlled. Carefully estimate blood loss, taking into account accumulated blood on drapes and any lateral pooling. The amount of irrigation used should be deducted from the fluid in the suction canister. If liposuction is used as an adjunct procedure, record totals for each breast. If a Foley catheter has been inserted, report urine output at regular intervals to the anesthesia provider.

Specimens and Cultures

Label all excised breast tissue according to the laterality, and weigh before sending the tissue to pathology.

Drugs and Solutions

Intravenous antibiotics should be administered prior to the procedure. Use warm irrigating saline. Provide additional supplies (marking pens, methylene blue, cotton-tipped applicators) to touch up preprocedure markings. Use warm intravenous fluids which will help maintain the patient's core temperature.

Physician Orders

Preprocedure laboratory evaluation typically includes complete blood count with differential and, depending upon the patient's medical and pharmacological history, serum electrolytes. If the patient has donated autologous blood, a type and cross match should also be ordered. Depending upon anesthesia guidelines, at predetermined ages a chest x-ray and EKG may also be required. Baseline mammography is often ordered prior to reduction mammaplasty.

Procedure

The choice of procedure depends upon several factors: the distance the nipple must be elevated, the amount of breast tissue and skin to be excised, and the type of pedicle to be used. Pedicles are islands of tissue supported by specific vasculature. They are identified (named) according to their geographical locations: Inferior, Central, Medial, Superior, Superiormedial, Lateral, and Combination pedicles. The distance that the nipple is to be relocated also dictates choice of procedure (**Figs. 25.4**, **25.5**, **25.6**). If the patient is a smoker, has gigantic or extremely ptotic breasts, then removing the nipples and placing them in their new location as full-thickness free nipple grafts would be a safer alternative.

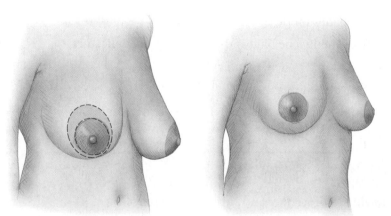

Figure 25.4

Nipple relocation.

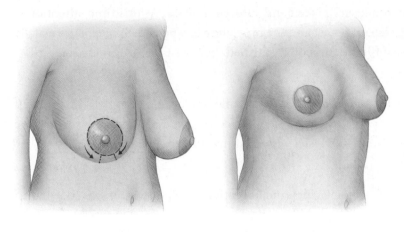

Figure 25.5

Incision and nipple relocation.

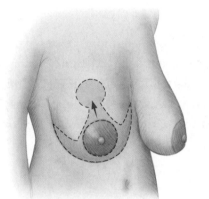
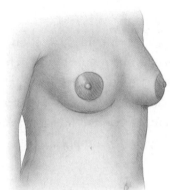

Figure 25.6

Incision and nipple relocation.

Incision and Exposure

Before the initial incisions are placed, the markings are reinforced if necessary and a local anesthetic may be instilled along the incision lines. Some surgeons may prefer to inject a tumescent anesthesia, in addition to the general anesthesia, to reduce bleeding. Depending upon the reduction procedure being performed, the incisions are made circumferentially around the nipple, from the nipple vertically to the inframammary fold and, if indicated, varying lengths along the inframammary fold or crease.

Details

Once the incisions are made, de-epithelialization of the pedicle takes place. Skin that has been removed may be kept in saline-soaked sponges until the completion of the procedure in case tissue is needed as a graft. The surgical assistant provides exposure and compression to the incised parenchyma, allowing the surgeon to fully develop the pedicle. The pedicle is then elevated off the chest wall, taking care to preserve the vascular supply. The desired amount of breast tissue is excised and passed off the sterile field to the circulating nurse to weigh. After the appropriate amount of tissue has been removed and hemostasis is obtained, the pedicle is carefully rotated into place and the nipple secured in its new position. The base of the areola is attached and the internal limbs of the parenchyma brought together. If a horizontal incision has also been indicated along the inframammary fold it is approximated at this time.

Should additional contouring along the lateral chest wall or axilla be desired, this may be accomplished with liposuction before final skin closure. After all tissue has been removed, drains are placed and sutured in place. At this time, attention is turned to the contralateral breast and the procedure is repeated. Skin closure usually does not take place until the surgeon is satisfied the breasts are symmetrical.

Closure

Edges of the newly approximated parenchymal tissue are closed with interrupted sutures. Depending upon surgeon preference, a deep and superficial layer may be placed. The skin incisions are closed with running subcuticular sutures.

Postprocedure Care

During the report to the PACU nurse include estimated blood loss, presence of drains, use of Foley and total urine output if removed before transferring to the PACU. If the nipples have been relocated as free nipple grafts this should also be communicated.

Potential Complications

Potential complications include infection, hematoma, seromas, excess and widened scars, partial or total nipple loss, flap necrosis, and delayed wound healing. Infrequent but possible complications are total or partial loss of nipple sensation, inability to breastfeed, asymmetry, and undesirable breast shape. Pseudoptosis may result from inadequate resection of inferior breast tissue. Under-resection of one or both breasts is also a potential complication.

LIPOSUCTION

Liposuction is designed to correct contour deformities and improve overall shape. Originally used for smaller body surfaces, with an improvement in technology and safety it has become a sophisticated sculpting technique used for circumferential re-shaping, spot contour correction, and superficial delineation. The choice for liposuction procedures has expanded from traditional liposuction to syringe techniques, ultrasonic-assisted, and power-assisted liposculpture. Removal of undesired fat with liposuction is not difficult; the challenge for the plastic surgeon is removing it from the correct tissue plane and establishing fluid alterations from suctioned to nonsuctioned areas.

Related Procedures

Liposuction is used as an adjunct to many surgical procedures, including but not limited to reduction mammaplasty, excision of gynecomastia, abdominoplasty, brachioplasty, thighlift, and bodylifts. Aspirated fat is often harvested to be re-injected into body areas that are lacking in volume, such as lips, cheeks, and contour deficiencies.

Nursing Implications

Confirm with the surgeon the liposuction sites and the order in which the procedure will be performed (**Fig. 25.7**). This will help facilitate planning for positioning and redraping. Gather positioning aids and devices before the patient enters the room. Prepare tumescent solution according to facility policy, and ask the surgeon the amount to be infused per site. Liposuction techniques and instrumentation vary according to surgeon preference; therefore, verify with the surgeon that the

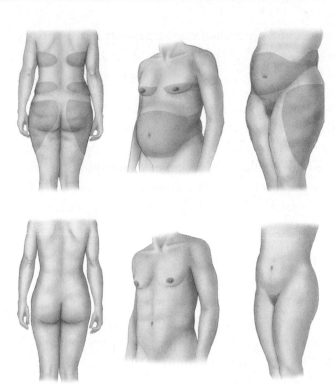

Figure 25.7
Liposuction sites (top) and results after Liposuction (bottom).

correct equipment is available. Liposuction frequently involves multiple sites and may extend for two or more hours, requiring insertion of a Foley catheter and use of sequential compression devices.

As with other aesthetic plastic procedures, verify that preprocedure photographs have been taken and are available for the surgeon during the procedure. Marking the sites takes place in the holding area before the patient has had any sedation. Maintain patient privacy and body temperature during this process.

Anesthesia

The choice of anesthesia depends upon the number of sites and total body surface to be liposuctioned. It is possible to comfortably perform liposuction under local anesthesia if limited areas are involved and the patient is not anxious. Attention should be paid to the total amounts of local anesthesia injected to prevent lidocaine toxicity (**Table 25.2**). The introduction of tumescent anesthesia opened the possibility for choices over than general anesthesia. For liposuction of lower extremities, epidural anesthesia may be a choice. Other options are deep sedation, and of course, general

Table 25.2	**Lidocaine Toxicity**
Early Symptoms	**Advanced Symptoms**
Restlessness	Shivering
Lightheadedness	Tremors
Numbness of tip of tongue	Convulsions
Slurred speech	CNS depression

anesthesia. Final anesthesia choices are also influenced by patient's health history and anesthesia assessment.

Position

The surgical position is related to the anatomical site to be liposuctioned and the surgeon's preference. Potential positions include supine, lateral, or prone. If multiple areas are involved, the patient may require repositioning, prepping, and draping during the procedure. Large body surfaces are frequently exposed during this process. Take care to maintain the patient's body temperature. In such cases consider temporarily increasing the room temperature. Assemble positioning aids necessary to prevent injuries before the patient enters the OR.

Establishing and Maintaining the Sterile Field

Because much of liposuction involves paired structures, the amount of body surface needed to be prepped and draped is often extensive. Place impervious draping material under the patient as well as "squared off" in the traditional manner to prevent contamination. During the procedure, attention should be paid by both circulator and the team members at the sterile field to the maintaining of the correct placement of the drapes due to the constant motion required by liposuction. Tubing for the tumescent infusion, ultrasonic probe cords (if used), and the aspiration machine are placed after draped is completed and secured with non-penetrating towel clips.

Equipment and Supplies

Minor plastic surgery instrument set

Tumescent infusion tip and tubing

Infusion pump

Traditional cannulas of various diameters and lengths and suction tubing

Aspirator machine

Ultrasonic probes, if applicable

Ultrasonic machine, if applicable

Skin protection ports

Extra draping materials if patient is to be repositioned

Sequential compression devices and stockings

Bair Hugger blanket and machine

Foley catheter if indicated

Asepto syringe (for unplugging cannulas)

Physiological Monitoring

Maintenance of a normal fluid and electrolyte balance is essential with the introduction of large volumes of tumescent solution and subsequent removal of the desired amount of aspirate. Preprocedure lab and testing should be performed according to the patient's health history and facility guidelines. Collaborate with the anesthesia provider to monitor input and output, including measuring ongoing aspirate totals and urine output if a Foley catheter has been inserted. Sequential compression devices are frequently indicated, and body temperature must be monitored and maintained.

Specimens and Cultures

Aspirate that is removed is not sent for pathologic diagnosis; it is held for comparison to that removed from the contralateral site and for evaluation of total aspirate removed.

Drugs and Solutions

Warmed tumescent solution (500 mg Lidocaine, Epinephrine 1:1,000, 1,000 mL Lactated Ringers Solution) volume infused is per surgeon's preference; standard is 1:1 per site. Local anesthesia may be injected at each incision site. Sodium bicarbonate is sometimes added to increase patient comfort during the introduction of local, especially if they are awake. Tumescent medication should be allowed to sit for 20–30 minutes after it has been infused before the application of ultrasonic energy or aspiration begins for its vasoconstrictive properties to take effect.

Physician Orders

Many plastic surgeons will instruct their patients to wash with antiseptic soap before the procedure. Routine labs and tests are ordered according the patient's health history and anesthesia guidelines. The surgeon will mark the operative sites with the patient in a standing position; therefore any preprocedure sedation should be given only after that has been completed. Confirm with the surgeon the total amount of tumescent solution to be prepared. Antibiotics are routinely given before the start of the procedure.

Procedure

Incision and Exposure

Multiple small stab-like incisions are made in the operative field of the planned liposuction sites in inconspicuous areas, using creases and folds whenever possible. The infusion cannula is introduced and tumescent solution infused with a pump at the correct plane for each location to be treated. Ample time is given for the tumescent anesthesia's properties to take effect.

Details

If the plastic surgeon will be using the ultrasonic machine before removal of fat occurs, the ultrasonic probe is introduced and passed back and forth throughout the deep subcutaneous plane to aid in cavitation of the fat. To prevent thermal injury, constant motion of the probe coupled with irrigation of the entrance site with saline is required. After the area has been treated with the ultrasonic energy, liposuction may begin. The deeper planes are suctioned first, moving more superficially as the desired amount of fat is removed. The motion is back and forth with the cannulae moved in a fan-like pattern. Larger cannulas are used first and replaced by ones with smaller diameters as the surgeon moves toward more superficial planes to feather the transition from deep to superficial. Many surgeons also employ a cross-tunneling technique in each plane as well. This aids in the prevention of contour irregularities. The end point is reached when the surgeon is satisfied that the desired amount of fat has been removed, unless bleeding occurs, in which case suctioning in that area must cease. The surgeon will compare skin thickness to ensure it is even, and employ the "pinch test." This involves rolling the skin between the thumb and index finger to assess smoothness and evenness.

Closure

The incisions are the size of stab wounds and may be closed with a single absorbable suture. Many surgeons prefer to leave the incisions open to facilitate drainage for the ensuing 24–48 hours. At the end of the procedure, the operative sites may be massaged to hasten drainage, cleaned and an absorbent dressing applied to prevent the garment from becoming immediately soaked.

Postprocedure Care

The patient is transferred to PACU, with garment in place. Handoff communication includes the sites treated, total amount of aspirate infused, volume of fat removed, IV fluids, and urine output if catheterized during the procedure. Report analgesia used and times given. Pain management should be addressed, and prior to discharge the dressings changed if the drainage has been profuse, which it can be. Instruct the patient to expect drainage from the entrance wounds over the following 24–48 hours. It should gradually lighten as it reduces in amount. Bright red bleeding, however, would be reason to call the surgeon.

Potential Complications

Contour irregularities—skin rippling, over correction, and under correction are the most frequently encountered complications. If ultrasound has been used before suctioning, there is a potential for burning the skin from probes kept in contact with tissue too long. As with any procedure, infection and bleeding are possible but are rare in liposuction. Bruising is to be expected and may be dramatic. Lidocaine toxicity, fat embolism, skin necrosis, perforation of adjacent structures or organs, and death has been reported, but are extremely rare.

FACELIFT

A traditional facelift includes both face and neck. The aging process results in loss of fat content of the face, atrophy of the collagen fibers of the skin, gravitational effects on the mid and lower face, and separation of the platysmal bands of the neck. Facelifts have become very individualized in their planning and execution, depending upon the specific needs of the patient. Liposuction is frequently used as an adjunct, fat injections or other fillers may be injected to correct contour deformities, and the procedure may be performed as a skin only lift, with or without midface lifting, and often is combined with other cosmetic procedures of the forehead, eyelids, and chin. The goal of a successful rhytidectomy, or facelift, is redraping and removal of excess skin, along with repositioning and support of the fascial support structures of the cheek and neck. The end result is a rested, natural appearance, without the skin being pulled tightly (**Fig. 25.8**).

Related Procedures

Partial or mini-lifts, involving only the neck, are often performed on younger patients without undesirable aging effects of the neck. Likewise, sometimes the patient may request only correction of the appearance of a sagging neck, which is called cervicoplasty. Eyelid surgery, or blepharoplasty, is frequently performed at the same time as rhytidectomy, as are forehead or brow lifts. These may be endoscopic or open. Additionally, insertion of chin implants at the time of facelift will balance the symmetry of the profile.

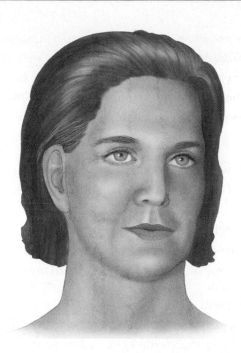

Figure 25.8
Postprocedure face lift.

Nursing Implications

The complexity and sophistication of today's facelift procedures dictate good communication between the nurse and surgeon in order to be thoroughly prepared for the correct procedure and techniques. Consequently, confirm the specifics of the procedure with the plastic surgeon. Verify the use of and amount of local anesthesia, even in the presence of general anesthesia. Suture choice, use of liposuction, injection of autologous fat or other filler material, as well as related procedures (blepharoplasty, augmentation mentoplasty, or browlift) and bandaging preferences are among the items to be discussed with the surgeon or his staff. Have preprocedure photographs available for the surgeon to refer to during the procedure, as anatomy is often distorted with the patient supine and/or intubated. Marking of the face and neck may take place with the patient awake and in a sitting position, or once they are anesthetized, prepped, and draped, according to surgeon preference.

Facelifts may be performed on adults of any age if there is a deformity to be corrected; however, the majority of procedures are performed on individuals in their mid-to-late forties and older. When indicated, check for medical or cardiac clearance and accompanying normal laboratory and test results. Because of the length of the procedure, Foley catheters are often inserted, and compression stockings and venous compression devices used. Convection warming blankets are placed to preserve body temperature.

If liposuction will be performed, ensure that the necessary cannulas and suction equipment will be available. A fiberoptic lighted retractor and accompanying light source should be functional, with extra bulbs readily available. Bipolar electrosurgery is often preferred by plastic surgeons for rhytidectomies.

Anesthesia

Deep sedation with local anesthesia or general anesthesia, with or without local anesthesia injected for better hemostasis, are the two most often used anesthesia techniques. The choice depends upon surgeon preference and health history of the patient. If general anesthesia is employed, the patient will be intubated, and it presents the added challenge for the operative team to operate around the tube as well as compensate for potential distortion of facial structures and tape used to secure tube placement. Care must be taken to protect the eyes from unintended corneal injury. Corneal shields are frequently placed, as is ophthalmic ointment.

Position

Place the patient in the supine position, with the shoulders and body properly aligned. Secure the extremities and position as to avoid compression injuries. Cushion pressure points in order to prevent injury to the skin and underlying structures. During the procedure, the head will be repositioned as the surgeon completes the first side and proceeds to the other. Exercise care when moving the patient's head and neck, and the surgeon and/or assistant should protect the airway or endotracheal tube at all times.

Establishing and Maintaining the Sterile Field

Prepping and draping the surgical field demands attention to strict aseptic technique. Include the face, neck, ears, and scalp in the sterile field. Before prepping, protect the eyes with ophthalmic ointment, and place plugs in the external ear canals to prevent pooling of prep solution. Place a sterile, impervious drape under the patient's head and tuck it under the shoulders. At this point, begin prepping one side of the face at a time, followed by the neck, and ending with the scalp. The prep should center at the site of the planned incision and extend to the central face. Once the prep is completed, remove the original drape sheet and place a new, sterile, impervious drape sheet under the head and shoulders, followed by towels and drape sheets, according to surgeon preference. It may be necessary to sew towels to the scalp; if so, local anesthesia is infiltrated at the site and a large nylon suture with a cutting needle is used to secure the towels. Standard towel clips may be used on the remaining drape material.

The scrub person should secure cords, tubing, and other equipment to the drapes at this point with non-penetrating towel plastic clips. In addition, the scrub person should place electrosurgery pencils inside non-conductive safety holster to prevent unintentional damage or injury. Attention should be directed to the placement and pull on the drapes from heavier instrumentation, such as the fiberoptic retractor and cord.

Equipment and Supplies

Major plastic surgery instrument set

Facelift scissors of various lengths

Additional x-ray detectable sponges

Handheld electrosurgery pencil with regular and long tips; may request needle tip

Bipolar electrosurgery

Calipers

Fixation forceps

Facial liposuction cannulas

Liposuction tubing

Aspirator machine

Fiberoptic retractor

Fiberoptic cord

Suction tubing

Tonsil tip suction (non-metallic)

5 mL syringe, 10 mL syringe

Fill kit or self-filling syringe system (for infiltrating local anesthesia)

3 ½ inch spinal needle

25 gauge 1 ½ inch needle

Skin marking pens

Multiple No. 15 blades

Suture, according to surgeon preference

Foley catheter

Compression stockings and sequential compression device

Bair hugger warming blanket and device

Extra towels for draping

Extra impervious drape for draping after prep

Psychological Monitoring

Due to the length of the procedure, pay attention to intake and output. Carefully monitor urinary output and blood loss. The face is extremely vascular and bleeding may be rapid. Preprocedure lab and testing should be performed according to the patient's health history and facility guidelines. Vital signs and oxygen concentration are monitored continuously. Temporary tachycardia may result from the injection of local anesthesia intravascularly. Closely monitor and maintain the patient's temperature. Apply sequential compression stockings and devices.

Specimens and Cultures

While specimens and culture are not routinely obtained during facelift procedures, preserve collection of aspirated fat upon the completion of the procedure should the surgeon elect to correct contour deformities, both anticipated and unanticipated, with the injection of the autologous fat.

Drugs and Solutions

Intravenous antibiotics should be administered before the procedure begins. Local anesthesia of surgeon's choice (eg, 0.25% Xylocaine with Epinephrine 1:100,000), recommended volume infused should not exceed 35 mg/kg. Infuse warm intravenous fluids during the procedure. Extra marking solution and materials should be available. Use saline solution for irrigation once the undermining of the skin is completed.

Physician Orders

Routine orders include preprocedure lab work and testing required by the anesthesia guidelines as well as the patient's health history. The patient will often be instructed to shampoo and wash the face, ears, and neck both the night before and the morning of the procedure. IV antibiotics are given before the procedure. A Foley catheter should be inserted, and antiembolic stockings and sequential compression devices applied. The patient is instructed to take routine cardiac and blood pressure medications as they normally would, the morning of the procedure. The exception may be diuretics. Often, anesthesia providers may be instructed to maintain the patient's blood pressure at slightly hypotensive levels to avoid undue bleeding.

Procedure

Incision and Exposure

Once the patient is prepped and draped, the surgical marking is reinforced, and the surgeon will begin to inject local anesthesia along the planned incision lines. Many surgeons consider facelifts as including 3 phases: the first half of the face, the neck, and the contralateral face. In order to stay within safe parameters of the recommended amount of local anesthesia (35 mg/kg), the local is injected in phases as well. Time is given for the epinephrine properties to take full effect before the first incisions are made.

Incision placement varies according to technique and surgeon preference. The incision extends from the temporal scalp above the ear, distally to the earlobe. In the preauricular area, the incision should follow the contours of the anterior ear or may pass along the posterior rim of the tragus. At the base of the earlobe the incision is carried up onto the posterior ear skin and may or may not take a 90° turn across the mastoid skin into the scalp. To correct midline neck and platysmal aging, an incision is placed under the chin, either in the submental crease or just below.

Details

Three compartments are elevated and flaps are raised in a facelift procedure: temporal, cheek, and neck (**Fig. 25.9**). Prior to undermining these compartments, liposuction may be used as an adjunct to improve facial and neck contours, using

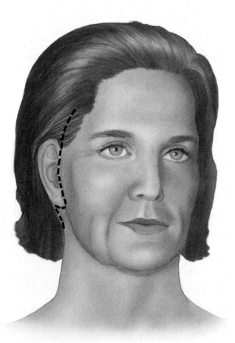

Figure 25.9

Incision areas for a face lift—temporal, cheek, and neck.

small-diameter cannulas. There are a variety of techniques used, depending upon the presenting anatomical defects, surgeon preference, and type of procedure to be performed. The three most common techniques are skin lift only, skin with sub-cutaneous musculo-aponeurosis system (SMAS) plication, and skin with SMAS elevation. In younger patients with minimal skin laxity, a skin-only facelift with or without liposuction of the lower cheeks or jowls may suffice. Here, a skin flap is ele-vated, advanced, and approximated to its new location with key sutures, and excess skin removed. Facial aging is not just a problem of the skin, however. The underly-ing support structures of the facial skin (SMAS) also sags along with the skin as the effects of aging and weight fluctuations extract their toll. Repair of muscle laxity with SMAS correction is an essential component of the facelift. Whether the SMAS is plicated or elevated, once it is repositioned it is secured with sutures. SMAS sutures may be interrupted or running, the choice of absorbable versus permanent suture material depends upon the surgeon's preference. At this point, the neck skin is dis-sected off the platysma; if bands are prominent, they may be addressed directly by incision, suturing, or excision. The neck skin is redraped towards the postauricular region, trimmed, and sutured. A drainage tube may be placed under the flap at this time, and the surgeon's efforts are directed toward the opposite side of the face, or he (she) may elect to continue closing the original side. The submental incision is usu-ally not closed until the facelift has been completed on both sides.

SMAS
Subcutaneous
Musculo-Aponeurosis
System

Closure

Prior to closure, all tissues are re-examined for hemostasis. Choice of suture mate-rial is highly variable. The skin is redraped in a superior-lateral fashion, approximated in its new location, and held in place with key interrupted sutures. Heavier sutures are placed where there is maximal tension, such as the temporal and postauricular skin. Two layers of closure are used to decrease tension and scarring. In locations where the incisions are visible, finer sutures are placed without tension to minimize the potential for widened scars. Drainage tubes usually exit in the postauricular or scalp areas and should be secured with sutures.

Postprocedure Care

At the completion of the procedure, carefully clean the patient's face, ear, and neck. Examine the ear canals for the presence of any drainage (prep solution or blood) and thoroughly clean. Remove ophthalmic shields at this point, and gently wipe eyelashes with saline solution to remove debris. The choice of dressing mate-rial and dressing type and technique is another highly individual choice made by the surgeon, so confirm his or her preference before proceeding. Typically, non-adherent dressing material is placed over the incisions and around the drainage tube sites. Fluffed gauze is placed behind both ears, 4×4 gauze sponges and thick pads, such as ABDs, are placed under the neck and across the checks, and then the head and neck are wrapped with 3 inch Kling. The dressing should be secure but not compressive in order to prevent compromise to the circulation of the flaps or the airway; leave the eyes, nose, and mouth exposed. Some surgeons prefer elastic facial compression garments in lieu of traditional bandages or may use a combina-tion of both.

Elevate the head and shoulders, and transfer the patient to the PACU. Handoff reporting should include meds received, estimated blood loss, skin integrity, IV fluids received, and urinary output.

Potential Complications

Hematoma formation is the most frequently reported complication following rhytidectomy. Prevention of hypertension is critical to avoiding this problem. Nausea, vomiting, pain, and a full bladder can contribute to episodes of hypertension, triggering bleeding and hematoma formation. If the patient is complaining of pressure and increasing pain, examine the lips and oral mucosa for evidence of ecchymosis, an indication of hematoma development.

Nerve injury is another serious potential complication. At risk nerves for transection or trauma include the facial, marginal mandibular, buccal, and greater auricular nerves. Depending upon whether the structure is a motor or sensory nerve, the patient could experience temporary or permanent loss of motion or sensation.

Infection is possible but infrequent. Flap necrosis, poor wound healing, excessive scarring, contour irregularities, pigmentation changes, and hair loss are among other potential complications following rhytidectomy.

BURNS

TBSA
Total amount of Body Surface Area

Burns are characterized according to the source of injury (thermal, chemical, or electrical); the total amount of body surface area (TBSA); and depth of the injury: superficial, superficial partial-thickness, deep partial-thickness, and full thickness (**Table 25.3**).

Table 25.3	**Burn Depth Categories in the United States**			
Burn Degree	**Cause**	**Surface Appearance**	**Color**	**Pain Level**
First (superficial)	Flash flame ultraviolet (sunburn)	Dry, no blisters, no or minimal edema	Erythematous	Painful
Second (partial thickness)	Contact with hot liquids or solids, flash flame to clothing, direct flame, chemical, ultraviolet	Moist blebs, blisters	Mottled white to pink, cherry red	Very painful
Third (full thickness)	Contact with hot liquids or solids, flame, chemical, electrical	Dry with leathery eschar until debridement, charred vessels visible under eschar	Mixed white, waxy, pearly; dark, mahogany; charred	Little or no pain, hair pulls out easily
Fourth (involves underlying structure)	Prolonged contact with flame, electrical	Same as 3rd degree, possibly with exposed bone, muscle, or tendon	Same as 3rd degree	Same as 3rd degree

Adapted from Klein, M.B. (2007). Thermal, chemical, and electrical injuries. In Thorne, C.H., Beasley, R.W., Aston, S. J., Barlett, S.P., Gurtner, G.C., & Spear, S.L. (Eds): *Grabb and Smith's Plastic Surgery* (5th ed., p 136). Philadelphia: Wolters Kluwer Lippincott Williams & Wilkins.

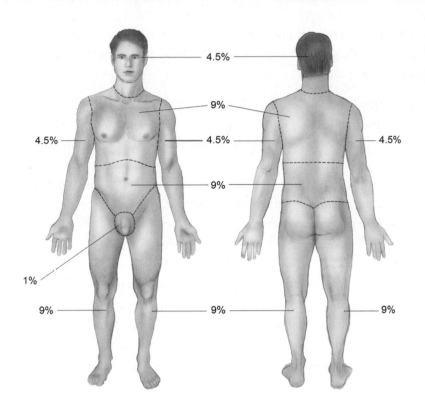

Figure 25.10

The body is divided into segments for estimating TBSA for both adults and children.

To estimate TBSA, the "rule of nines" is a frequently used method. Superficial burns are not considered when calculating TBSA. **Figure 25.10** illustrates how the body is divided into segments for estimating TBSA for both adults and children. The management of burns involves early excision and skin grafting, which has proven to improve survival, decrease infection, and decrease length of hospitalization. If autologous grafts are not a possibility, biologic dressings, cultured epithelial autografting (CEA), and cadaver allografts are among the alternatives.

Skin Grafts and Preparation of the Site

Split-thickness grafts contain the entire epidermis and varying levels of the dermis—thin, intermediate, or thick, based on the thickness of the graft. Full-thickness skin grafts retain characteristics of normal-appearing skin; specifically color and thickness, so are desirable for more visible body areas. In children, these grafts also have the ability to grow as the child grows.

Before moving the graft to its new location, the recipient site must be carefully prepared. This may entail debridement or excision of necrotic tissue, trimming wound edges, and cleaning highly contaminated wounds. Viability of the grafted tissue is related to nourishment, blood supply, and low bacterial counts.

Related Procedures

Skin grafts are indicated when there is a lack of tissue, whether from trauma, disease, or as a complication from the procedure. Skin and muscle flaps are procedures that also rely on moving tissue from one area of the body to another, and re-establishment of an effective blood supply. Grafts may be of varying thicknesses, and are identified as either split- or full-thickness. Treatment of the donor site is different for the

CEA
Cultural Epithelial Autografting

two procedures, as full-thickness requires primary closure. Implantation of a tissue expander with gradual filling of the implant and stretching of the skin is another method of gaining for skin for defect coverage.

Nursing Implications

Depending on the mechanisms of injury or tissue loss, these patients range from healthy to critically ill. Assessment of the patient and anticipation of nursing needs are essential to the care and planning for the patient undergoing skin grafting. Positioning may be challenging, and aids should be anticipated and assembled before the beginning of the case. Special attention should be paid to padding and securing the patient in the desired positioned. Repositioning is often indicated once the graft has been harvested, so the patient must be re-evaluated whenever moved. Placement of the electrosurgical patient return electrode may present a challenge, especially in the presence of extensive burns. After any repositioning, the patient return electrode must be checked by the circulator for continued contact.

Extra blades, proper functioning of the dermatome, and special dressing materials desired by the surgeon should also be verified and assembled before proceeding. Inquire if graft material not used will be saved and stored, and have the correct supplies available.

Anesthesia

Unless the patient's physiologic condition contraindicates it, general anesthesia is usually employed as the anesthetic technique of choice. Intubation is not always a requirement since muscle relaxation is not necessary and these procedures may be brief. Full-thickness donor sites are usually augmented with local anesthesia with epinephrine to minimize blood loss.

Position

Positioning is frequently a challenge in order to provide exposure and access to both donor and recipient sites. Once the graft has been harvested and the donor site covered and protected, the patient may be repositioned so that the surgeon has the access and exposure necessary to place and secure the graft. Position the patient using proper positioning aids, safety straps, and without pressure to vulnerable pressure points and nerves.

Establishing and Maintaining the Sterile Field

Verify the prepping agent of choice with the surgeon. Prep and drape donor and recipient sites. Strict attention should be paid to the prepping technique, as success of the procedure depends on prevention of infection and reducing bioburden is an important consideration. Place sterile towels and drapes on both areas, with the donor site covered until the recipient site has been prepared and harvesting of the graft is imminent.

Equipment and Supplies

Major plastic surgery instrument set or Minor set with extra clamps

Weck knife, blades, and guards of varying sizes

Dermatome and blades

Mesher (if indicated)

Tongue blades

Donor site (split-thickness) dressing of surgeon's choice: Opsite, Biobrane, etc.

Marking pen or methylene blue

Sterile container with lid (if excess skin graft material will be saved)

Sterile, unexposed x-ray film material (optional)

Physiological Monitoring

The patient is monitored during the procedure according to his or her condition and anesthesia technique. Typical monitoring includes vital signs, pulse oximetry, electrocardiography, and end tidal carbon dioxide. If the patient has a Foley catheter, output is monitored by the circulator. Blood loss is usually minimal unless extensive debridement of the recipient site is necessity. In this event, sponges are examined and estimated blood loss is calculated.

Specimens and Cultures

There are no routine specimens collected during grafting. If desired by the surgeon, excess autologous graft that remains may be stored for two weeks according to institutional policy. Cultures are rarely taken, as highly contaminated recipient sites are contraindicated for placement of graft material.

Drugs and Solutions

Mineral oil

Sterile saline solution

Antibiotic solution (optional)

Phenylephrine HCL (optional)

Physician Orders

Labs and tests necessary for preprocedure evaluation are performed prior to the procedure. These may include chest x-ray, EKG, urinalysis, complete blood counts, and electrolytes. Antibiotics may be ordered before the procedure.

Procedure

Incision and Exposure

Preparation of the recipient site is the first step. If the wound is open, then the site is debrided and wound edges are freshened by trimming.

Details

After the recipient site has been prepared, attention is turned to the donor site. The dermatome of choice is connected, blade inserted, and power source tested to verify proper functioning before the instrumentation is used on the patient. The surgeon may craft a pattern of the defect surface and mark the donor site for the amount of skin to be removed. A thin layer of mineral oil is applied to the skin surface over the area chosen to be harvested. With the surgical assistant or scrub person maintaining even skin tension, the dermatome is applied to the skin and the graft removed

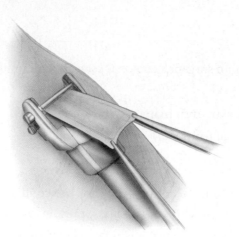

Figure 25.11

Skin graft removal using a dermatone.

(**Fig. 25.11**). If meshing is to be performed, the graft is placed on the mechanical mesher or the meshing may be performed by hand using a No. 11 blade. It is immediately placed on saline-soaked sponges, unless it has been meshed (in which case it remains on the carrier and a saline-soaked sponge placed on top), and removed to the instrument table while the donor site is cared for.

If a full-thickness graft is planned, the donor site is outlined, local anesthesia instilled to minimize bleeding, and the incision made around the pattern. The desired tissue is removed, usually in one piece, and is prepared by removing all subcutaneous tissue. Undermining of tissue edges may be necessary to aid in closure. Hemostasis is obtained and a sterile, saline-soaked sponge is placed over the site until suturing takes place.

Closure

Hemostasis of the donor site is verified before the graft is placed. The material is stapled or sutured in place and, if desired, bolster sutures are placed around the periphery of the graft site, with the tails left long enough to tie over the dressing. Clamps are attached to the individual tails until the "tie-over" takes place. For full-thickness grafts, the graft is sutured around the edges, although staples may also be used.

Postprocedure Care

Application of the dressing is a crucial step in skin grafting, and is frequently performed with the patient still anesthetized in order to protect the fragile graft and prevent complications. A non-adherent dressing is placed over the graft and saline-moistened, fluffed gauze sponges placed on top. If a bolster dressing is being used, the suture ends are draped across the dressing at this point and tied centrally. A protective soft or hard splint may be applied after the dressing is placed. The donor site dressing of the surgeon's choice is applied.

Potential Complications

Partial or complete loss of the skin graft, due to infection and excessive bleeding with hematoma formation, are the most frequently encountered complications. Others include disruption due to shearing forces, seroma, and, later, contractures, contour irregularities, and hyperpigmentation.

REFERENCES

1. Boyce, S., Kagan, R., Greenhalgh, D., Warner, P., Yakuboff, K., Palmieri, T., & Warden, G. (2006). Cultured skin substitutes reduce requirements for harvesting of skin autograph for closure of excised, full-thickness burn. *The Journal of Trauma Injury, Infection, & Critical Care, 60*(4), 821–829.

2. Chandler, S. (2007). Plastic and reconstructive surgery. In J. Rothrock (Ed.): *Alexander's Care of the Patient in Surgery* (13th ed.). St. Louis: Mosby Elsevier.

3. Davison, S.P., Mesbahi, A.N., Ducic, I., Sarvia, M., Dayan, J., & Spear, S.L. (2007). The versatility of the superomedial pedicle with various skin reduction patterns. *Plastic and Reconstructive Surgery, 120*(6), 1466–1476.

4. Donelan, M.B. (2007). Principles of burn reconstruction. In Thorne, C.H., Beasley, R.W., Aston, S.J., Barlett, S.P., Gurtner, G.C., & Spear, S.L. (Eds.): *Grabb and Smith's Plastic Surgery* (5th ed., pp. 150–161). Philadelphia: Wolters Kluwer Lippincott Williams & Wilkins.

5. Gingrass, M.K. (2007). Liposuction. In Thorne, C.H., Beasley, R.W., Aston, S.J., Barlett, S.P., Gurtner, G.C., & Spear, S.L. (Eds.): *Grabb and Smith's Plastic Surgery* (5th ed., pp. 3–14). Philadelphia: Wolters Kluwer Lippincott Williams & Wilkins.

6. Gladfelter, J. (2007). Breast augmentation 101: understanding cosmetic augmentation mammaplasty. *Plastic Surgical Nursing, 27*(3), 136–145.

7. Hall-Findlay, E.J. (2005). Reduction mammaplasty. In Nahai, F. (Ed.): *The Art of Aesthetic Surgery Principles & Techniques* (pp. 1951–2043). St. Louis: Quality Medical Publishing, Inc.

8. Hanna, M.K. & Nahai, F. (2005). Applied anatomy of the breast. In Nahai, F. (Ed.): *The Art of Aesthetic Surgery Principles & Techniques* (pp. 1790–1815). St. Louis: Quality Medical Publishing, Inc.

9. Herman, S. (2002). The history of skin grafts. *Journal of Drugs in Dermatology, 1*(3), 298–302.

10. Kenkel, J.M., Rohrich, R.J., & Janis, J.E. (2005). Liposuction: basic techniques. In Nahai, F. (Ed.): *The Art of Aesthetic Surgery Principles & Techniques* (pp. 2147–2190). St. Louis: Quality Medical Publishing, Inc.

11. Klein, M.B. (2007). Thermal, chemical, and electrical injuries. In Thorne, C.H., Beasley, R.W., Aston, S. J., Barlett, S.P., Gurtner, G.C., & Spear, S.L. (Eds.): *Grabb and Smith's Plastic Surgery* (5th ed., pp. 132–149). Philadelphia: Wolters Kluwer Lippincott Williams & Wilkins.

12. Mendez-Eastman, S. (2005). Burn injuries. *Plastic Surgical Nursing, 25*(7), 133–139.

13. Mendez-Eastman, S. (2004). Full-thickness skin grafting: a procedural review. *Plastic Surgical Nursing, 24*(2), 41–45.

14. Sattler, G. (2005). Advances in liposuction and fat transfer. *Dermatology Nursing, 133*(7), 1159–1166.

15. Spector, J. & Karp, N. (2007). Reduction mammoplasty: a significant improvement at any size. *Plastic & Reconstructive Surgery Journal, 120*(4), 854–850.

16. Thorne, C. (2007). Techniques and principles in plastic surgery. In Thorne, C.H., Beasley, R.W., Aston, S.J., Barlett, S.P., Gurtner, G.C., & Spear, S.L. (Eds.): *Grabb and Smith's Plastic Surgery* (5th ed., pp. 3–14). Philadelphia: Wolters Kluwer Lippincott Williams & Wilkins.

CHAPTER 26

Neurosurgery

Thomas Hendrickson

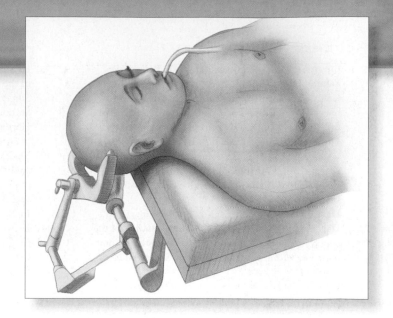

INTRODUCTION

Neurosurgery can be one of the most complex, time consuming, detail-oriented, and demanding surgeries a nurse will participate in. Providing for the needs of the team, including anesthesia, the surgeons, the scrub personnel, and ancillary staff while caring for the patient can be a challenge for the most seasoned nurse.

Neurosurgical procedures, in the crudest forms, have been performed since the sixteenth century BC. Documents on papyrus from Egypt describe treatment of head and vertebral column injuries. William Keen of Philadelphia was the first surgeon in the United States to remove a brain tumor. This was accomplished in 1888 (Phillips, 2007). The father of modern neurosurgery is Harvey Cushing (1869–1939). He reduced the mortality rate for meningiomas from 96 to 5 percent and he established the first school of neurosurgery at Harvard (Phillips, 2007).

Technology has exploded in recent years, with rapid advances seen in neurosurgery. Neuro monitoring, image-guided tumor resection, navigation systems, artificial discs, resorbable plates, robotics, and coiling for aneurysms are just a few. Keeping abreast of technology is perhaps the greatest challenge for the perioperative nurse.

Neurosurgery primarily involves the structures of the central nervous system (CNS); the brain, spinal cord, and supporting structures, and the peripheral nervous system (PNS), those structures outside the CNS. This chapter will address surgery involving the brain and spinal cord.

Chapter Contents

CNS
Central Nervous System

PNS
Peripheral Nervous System

ANATOMY

The nervous system is one of the most complex and least understood body systems (Ferrara, 2007). The nurse's ability to understand basic neuro-anatomy will help in anticipating the needs of the surgical team and the patient.

Scalp

The brain is protected by several layers of tissue. The scalp consists of a thick subcutaneous layer of fat, which is richly supplied with blood vessels, and the galea aponeurotica, a thick fibrous tissue layer. The subaponeurotic space, under the galea and subgalea space, provide the mobility of the scalp. Blood supply is from branches of the external carotid arteries.

Skull

The skull consists of twenty-eight bones, eight in the cranium, that provide protection for the brain. This rigid cavity has a volume of 1400 to 1500 mL and contains the brain, which weighs less than three pounds. The bone consists of three layers, the outer and inner are solid hard bone and the middle layer is soft, spongy cancellous bone. This provides strength with a minimum of weight. The bones forming the cranial cavity are the frontal, parietal (two), occipital, temporal (two), ethmoid, and sphenoid. The irregular bony seams that join the bones are called sutures and can be used as landmarks during surgery. The only movable bone is the mandible. The frontal, parietal, and occipital bones form the top of the cranium and the temporal bones and the wings of the sphenoid form the sides. The cranial floor is formed from the sphenoid and cribiform plate (**Fig. 26.1**).

The skull consists of three cavities called fossae; anterior, middle, and posterior. The anterior fossae contain the frontal lobes. The middle fossae contain the temporal lobes, the upper brain stem, and the sella turcica. The brain stem (pons and medulla) and the cerebellum are contained in the posterior fossa.

Figure 26.1

Bones and sutures, right side of the skull.

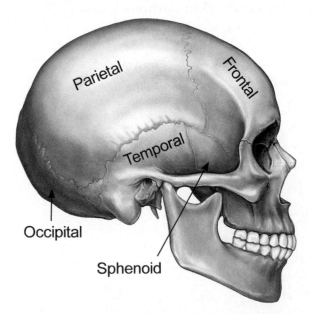

Parietal

Frontal

Temporal

Occipital

Sphenoid

Meninges

The meninges completely cover the brain and spinal cord. The meninges consist of three membranes that provide support and protection; the dura mater, arachnoid mater, and the pia mater.

The dura mater is a tough fibrous membrane lining the inner surface of the skull. The dura forms folds that divide the brain into four compartments. The falx cerebri is a midline fold that separates the hemispheres of the cerebrum; the falx cerebelli is a smaller vertical fold that separates the cerebellar hemisphere. The tentorium cerebelli is a transverse fold that folds a roof over the posterior fossa. This fold is the basis for describing areas of the brain as supratentorial or infratentorial. The brain stem and the cerebellum are infratentorial structures.

Layers of the dura separate at the folded areas to form venous sinuses. There are also several major arteries between the dura layers; the most important is the middle meningeal artery. Tearing of this artery due to trauma is often the cause of epidural hematomas but can also cause subdural hematomas.

Under the dura is a fine membrane known as the arachnoid mater. The inner surface of the arachnoid mater is separated from the layer below, the pia mater, by the subarachnoid space. This space is filled with cerebral spinal fluid (CFS) and large blood vessels. At the base of the brain, the spaces enlarge into cisterns. The arachnoid villi are projections of the arachnoid that absorb CSF into the venous system.

CFS
Cerebral Spinal Fluid

The meningeal layer closest to the brain is the pia mater. This delicate membrane follows the convolutions of the brain and contains numerous blood vessels. These vessels form part of the choroid plexus of the ventricles.

Brain

The brain is divided into several major segments: cerebrum, basal ganglia, thalamus, hypothalamus, midbrain, brain stem, and cerebellum.

The largest section of the brain is the cerebrum. It consists of two hemispheres divided longitudinally that are joined by the corpus callosum (**Fig. 26.2**). The lobes of the cerebrum are the frontal, parietal, temporal, and occipital, which correspond to the overlying bones of the skull. The surface of the cerebrum is marked by folds

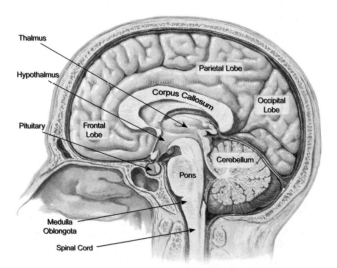

Figure 26.2

Sagittal view of the brain and spinal cord.

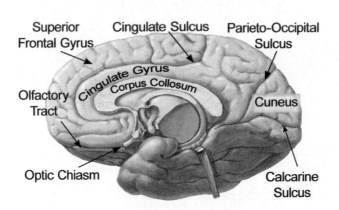

Superior Frontal Gyrus — Cingulate Sulcus — Parieto-Occipital Sulcus — Cingulate Gyrus — Corpus Collosum — Olfactory Tract — Cuneus — Optic Chiasm — Calcarine Sulcus

Figure 26.3

Major landmarks of the cerebral hemisphere.

called gyri and small furrows called sulci. These markings are used as anatomical landmarks during cranial operative procedures (**Fig. 26.3**). The outer cerebral tissue is gray matter, or cerebral cortex, and the inner tissue is the white matter.

The basal ganglia are located near the corpus callosum at the center of the cerebrum. They include the caudate nucleus, putamen, globus pallidus, claustrum, subthalamic nucleus, and substantia nigra.

The thalamus and hypothalamus are adjacent to the third ventricle. Together they are known as the diencephalons.

The midbrain lies between the cerebral hemispheres and the pons. It contains cerebral peduncles, nerve tracts, and nuclei.

The medulla oblongata and pons compose the brain stem, which lies below the midbrain. There are 12 pairs of cranial nerves that arise from the undersurface of the brain and they are named by their distribution or function.

The cerebellum is contained in the posterior fossa. It is divided in the midline to form two lobes that are marked transversely by small fissures. The tissue between the lobes is called the vermis.

The brain contains four chambers called ventricles. There are two lateral ventricles, the third ventricle, and the fourth ventricle. They are lined with a membrane called the ependyma. Inside of each ventricle is the choroids plexus, (**Fig. 26.4**) a vascular structure that produces the CSF by an osmotic filtration of fluid elements from the blood. This fluid circulates through the brain and around the spinal cord, functioning as a liquid support and flotation device for the tissues (**Fig. 26.5**). The CSF absorbs the shocks of external trauma, and allows the brain to be buoyant and lighter.

The normal adult volume of CSF is 125 to 150 mL (Ferrara, 2007). The volume of fluid can fluctuate somewhat to maintain a consistent intracranial pressure, but space-occupying lesions and mechanical obstructions of flow can elevate intracranial pressures. When the intracranial pressure elevation reaches a level for which the body cannot compensate, a herniation of the lower portions of the brain through the tentorial notch can occur.

The brain requires 20% more oxygen than any other organ. Cerebral circulation is designed to support the oxygen requirements of the brain, even if there is an interruption in one of the supplying arteries. The arteries entering the brain are the two internal carotid and two vertebral arteries. These arteries are connected by the

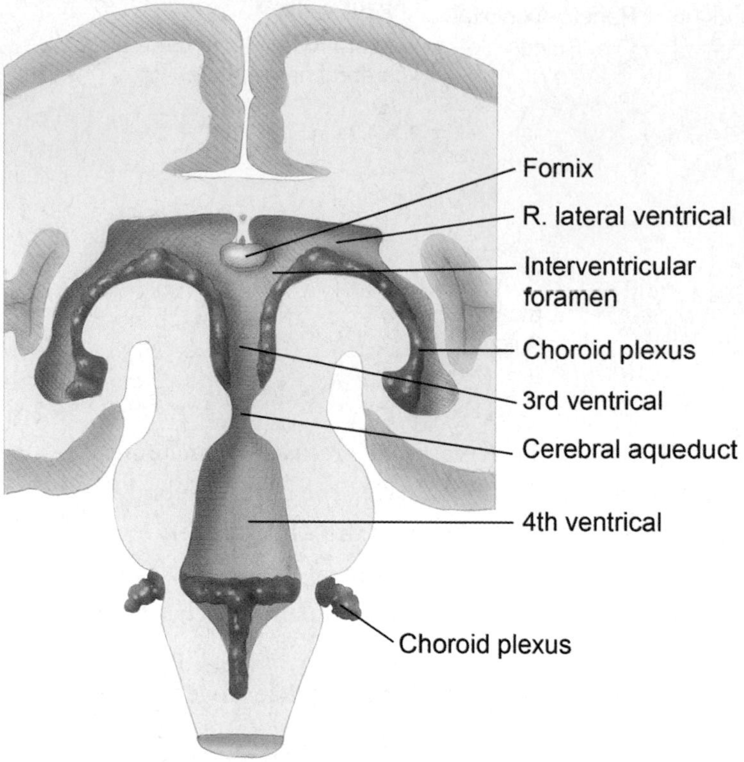

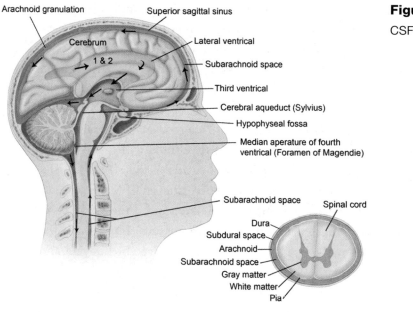

Figure 26.4

Ventricals of the brain.

Fornix

R. lateral ventrical

Interventricular foramen

Choroid plexus

3rd ventrical

Cerebral aqueduct

4th ventrical

Choroid plexus

Figure 26.5

CSF circulation.

Arachnoid granulation

Superior sagittal sinus

Cerebrum

1 & 2

Lateral ventrical

Subarachnoid space

Third ventrical

Cerebral aqueduct (Sylvius)

Hypophyseal fossa

Median aperature of fourth ventrical (Foramen of Magendie)

Subarachnoid space

Spinal cord

Dura

Subdural space

Arachnoid

Subarachnoid space

Gray matter

White matter

Pia

basilar artery and the circle of Willis (**Fig. 26.6**). Branching from the circle of Willis are the anterior, middle, and posterior cerebral arteries. The circle of Willis is located at the base of the brain in a small area, about one square inch in diameter. The circle of Willis ensures a continuous blood supply in the event of an interruption in any of the four supply vessels.

Venous drainage of the brain is effected via a network of veins that converge into the venous sinuses of the dura (**Fig. 26.7**). Blood is carried away from the brain via the jugular veins.

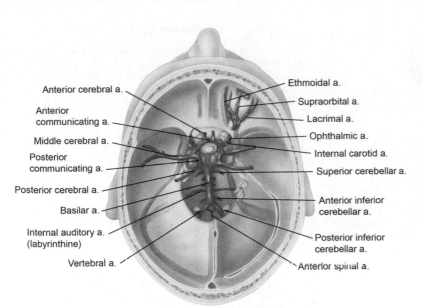

Figure 26.6

Arterial supply of the brain.

Anterior cerebral a.
Anterior communicating a.
Middle cerebral a.
Posterior communicating a.
Posterior cerebral a.
Basilar a.
Internal auditory a. (labyrinthine)
Vertebral a.

Ethmoidal a.
Supraorbital a.
Lacrimal a.
Ophthalmic a.
Internal carotid a.
Superior cerebellar a.
Anterior inferior cerebellar a.
Posterior inferior cerebellar a.
Anterior spinal a.

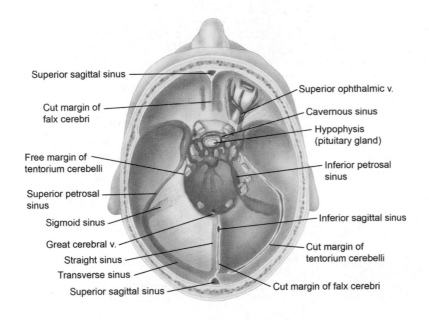

Figure 26.7

Venous drainage of the brain.

Superior sagittal sinus
Cut margin of falx cerebri
Free margin of tentorium cerebelli
Superior petrosal sinus
Sigmoid sinus
Great cerebral v.
Straight sinus
Transverse sinus
Superior sagittal sinus

Superior ophthalmic v.
Cavernous sinus
Hypophysis (pituitary gland)
Inferior petrosal sinus
Inferior sagittal sinus
Cut margin of tentorium cerebelli
Cut margin of falx cerebri

Spine and Spinal Cord

The vertebral column's role is to protect the spinal cord and maintain stability, while allowing range of motion. The vertebral column is composed of 33 vertebrae, which are referred to by number and location: 7 cervical, 12 thoracic, 5 lumbar, 5 sacral (fused), and 1 coccyx made of four small fused vertebrae. The column has four curves: cervical lordosis, thoracic kyphosis, lumbar lordosis, and sacral kyphosis. The structure of the vertebra varies somewhat with their location, but the basic elements are common to all 33 (**Fig. 26.8**). Most of the vertebrae are composed of a vertebral body, two transverse processes, two pedicles, two laminae, and the spinous process. Each vertebra has a body, which is a solid block of spongy bone lying anteriorly. The vertebral bodies are separated from one another by an intervertebral disc of fibrocartilaginous material which acts to absorb stresses between the vertebrae. The periphery of the disc is the tough annulus fibrosus, and the inner portion is a soft, gelatinous layer

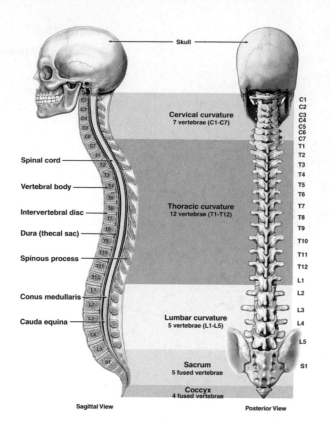

Figure 26.8

The vertebral column.

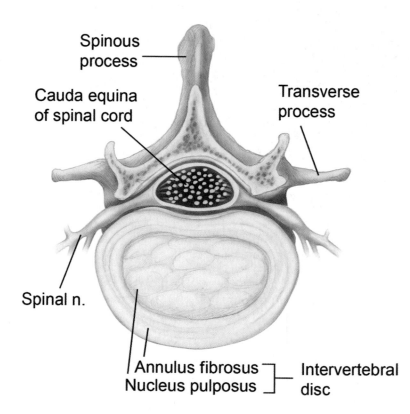

Figure 26.9

Normal relationship of the intervertebral disc to the spinal cord and nerve branches.

called the nucleus pulposus (**Fig. 26.9**). **Figure 26.10** shows a prolapsed nucleus pulposus impinging on the nerve. The vertebral arch consists of the most posterior segment, the spinous process, and the transverse processes, which are connected to the spinous process by laminae. Articular surfaces, or facets, form the joints with the vertebrae above and below. The spinal column is held together by and forms support

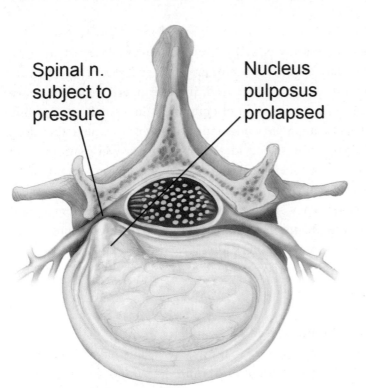

Spinal n. subject to pressure

Nucleus pulposus prolapsed

Figure 26.10

Prolapsed nucleus pulposus impinging on the nerve.

26

for muscles and ligaments. The posterior body consists of a spinous process and two transverse process project laterally for attachment of muscles and ligaments.

The spinal cord is located in the spinal foramina, collectively known as the spinal canal. The spinal cord along with arterial and venous blood supply are located in the spinal foramen where it is protected by the bony spinal column. The spinal cord is an extension of the brain stem and starts at the upper border of the second vertebra and ends at the upper border of the second lumbar vertebra as the conus medullaris. Spinal nerves exit the cord and emerge from out of the vertebral column via the intravertebral foramina at each vertebral level. There are 31 pairs of spinal nerves having their origin in the spinal cord. Each pair consists of an anterior and posterior root. The anterior root is motor in function and the posterior root is sensory in function. They have no special names but are numbered according to the level of the spinal column at which they emerge (Hickey, 2002). The spinal cord performs sensory, motor, and reflex functions.

In the lumbar area, a vertical bundle of spinal nerves forms the cauda equina. The spinal cord is covered by a dural sac that ends between the first and third sacral vertebrae. Under the dura is the arachnoid. The subarachnoid space contains the cerebral spinal fluid. Adhering to the cord is the delicate pia mater. The cord contains a central canal that is an extension of the forth ventricle and is also filled with spinal fluid. The spinal cord is a roughly shaped H composed of gray matter. White matter surrounds the gray matter and is subdivided in the midline. The spinal cord is covered by the dura mater. The dura mater does not attach directly to the bones of the vertebra, but creates a space between bone and the dura mater called the epidural space. The middle meningeal layer which is thin and lacking blood vessels, is called the arachnoid mater. The innermost layer is the pia mater and contains blood vessels and nerves.

SPECIAL INSTRUMENTS, SUPPLIES, AND EQUIPMENT

Neurosurgery requires a large array of specialized equipment and instruments. Under ideal conditions a large room with numerous electrical receptacles, vacuum outlets, and inline nitrogen should be used. In older operative and invasive procedure suites the challenge is to fit a lot of equipment in a small space, while trying to connect electrical equipment and suction lines in a manner that does not cause a tripping hazard. In less than ideal conditions proper planning and open discussion among team members helps in setting up the room for maximum use and efficiency. Diagrams on how the room should be set up assists staff members and provides consistency on how to plan, set up, and implement a good nursing care plan. Some equipment may have to be moved during the procedure (ie, microscope and x-ray equipment) and require a clear path to the surgical field without compromising the sterile setup.

Power Equipment

All powered equipment should be used safely and according to manufacturers' guidelines. Most come with a safety device that prevents accidental activation and it should always be utilized. Careful attention should determine where the powered equipment is placed in relationship to the patient. Power tools and equipment should not rest on the patient. Most are activated by a foot pedal and careful placement should be made with a review of what pedals activate which piece of equipment with the surgeon. Some policies prevent the surgeon from having more than one foot pedal at a time as a safety precaution. Powered equipment is useful because it decreases surgical time which will decrease and reduce fatigue of the surgical team, and it decreases anesthesia exposure for the patient. Power equipment can be broadly divided into two categories; air-powered and electric/battery powered.

The craniotome has multiple attachments. The perforator creates a burr hole in the skull. The perforator will automatically stop before the dura is penetrated as a safety precaution. Another attachment is a laterally cutting burr with a dural guard. It makes linear cuts in the skull between burr holes for lifting a bone flap. A wire-passing attachment permits the drilling of small holes in the bone to reattach the bone flap. There are several manufacturers of power equipment. The Midas Rex is available in either nitrogen- or electric-powered. This is a versatile high-speed drill with multiple accessories including a perforator. The Midas Rex can be used for spinal procedures and craniotomies. Handpieces are available in straight and angled with a wide variety of burrs they refer to as dissecting tools. The electric version is easier to assemble and use whereas the nitrogen-powered unit requires oil lubrication and is more cumbersome to assemble and use. Codman produces a craniotome that is used for perforation and lifting a bone flap. The Hall Surgitome Two is a high-speed nitrogen-powered drill that can be used for spinal procedures. It offers straight and angled attachments with a variety of burrs.

Manufacturers' instructions for operation, maintenance, and sterilization of all power equipment should be closely followed.

Miscellaneous Equipment

Large Mayo stands, prep tables, ring stands, instrument tables, microscope, standing stools, sitting stools, kick buckets, overbed instrument tables, sequential compression device, a hair clipper, a cooling/heating unit, blood warmer, electrosurgical unit (monopolar and bipolar), nitrogen supply (wall or portable tank) for air-powered instruments, suction units, fiberoptic headlight, and video equipment are all commonly used equipment. A video camera is often incorporated into the headlight or microscope and provides visualization of the operative field to the non-scrubbed team members. This aids in anticipating the needs of the surgeon.

Blood salvage equipment may be used during the procedure unless an infection or malignancy is present. This equipment is operated by trained hospital personnel or by contracted services. Staff should be familiar with emergency setup of the equipment to begin blood collection. However, staff are not responsible for processing the blood.

Surgical Table and Attachments

The surgical table is selected along with attachments as required by the procedure, position, and the surgeon's preference. The nurse must determine if a neurosurgical headrest is going to be used and if it will adapt to the surgical table or require a specific surgical table. Questions to be answered regarding the table include:

- What side will be operated on?
- Is the table in the correct position?
- Will it accommodate x-ray equipment?
- Will fluoroscopic x-ray equipment such as a C-arm be used?
- Will a Wilson frame be needed?
- Will a Jackson table or Andrews frame/table be required?

A basic toolbox with knowledge of how to use the tools may be required to set up the surgical table with adaptors and attachments. Comprehensive planning is the key to success. Staff must be familiar with all attachments and how they adapt to surgical tables.

Microscope

A microscope may be used for surgery on the spine or brain. The microscope provides an intense light under magnification that can be focused with hand or foot controls. Viewing structures through the microscope allows for greater surgical accuracy and precision. Results are improved through better visualization of nerves and vascular structures, smaller incisions, less retraction of brain tissues, better hemostasis, and more accurate nerve and vascular repair.

The nurse must discuss with the surgeon and assistant the position of the patient and where the surgeon and assistant will be standing in relationship to the incision to set the microscope up properly. The location of the assistant's eyepiece must be established before sterile draping of the microscope is done. The assistant may stand next to the surgeon (on the left or right) or they may stand across from them. If a video camera is incorporated into the microscope it should be tested prior to draping. Modern microscopes have self-balancing, auto focus, zoom controls, and light controls that work off of hand controls so the surgeon never removes his/her eyes from the oculars. Some microscopes can record images onto portable media, record video images onto DVDs, and print pictures, all through the hand controls of the surgeon.

Neurophysiologic Monitoring

Neurophysiologic monitoring is used to assess the functional integrity of the spinal cord, nerve roots, and other peripheral nervous system structures (Devlin & Schwartz, 2007). The principal point of neurophysiological monitoring during surgery is to avoid neurological injury resulting from surgical manipulation (Weinzeiri, Reinacher, Gilsback, & Rohde, 2007) that can result from retraction that may cause nerve damage from compression or disruption of blood flow. A number of monitoring devices are currently available and provide improved surgical results while minimizing morbidity (Sala, Manganotti, Tramontano, Bricolo, & Gerosa, 2007).

The best way to assess the functional integrity of sensory and motor pathways is to use somatosensory evoked potentials (SSEP) and muscle motor evoked potentials (MEP) (Sala, Beltramello, & Gerosa, 2007).

SSEP
Somatosensory Evoked Potentials

Somatosensory evoked potentials (SSEP) test the sensory system from the peripheral nerve to the sensory cortex of the brain. Weak electrical stimulations are applied to peripheral nerves by way of surface electrodes. The signals demonstrate whether the nerves that connect to the spinal cord are able to send and receive sensory information. Information can indicate if the spinal cord or nerves are being damaged. SSEP uses leads placed over the posterior tibial or peroneal nerve and median or ulna nerve that are stimulated. Subdermal scalp electrodes are placed to capture the signal and are recorded on a computer screen. Electrical waveforms are observed after taking baseline recording pre-positioning or before the incision is made. Changes in wavelength, a slowing of the electrical impulses, evaluate spinal cord function.

MEP
Motor Evoked Potentials

A significant change can indicate surgical invasion of the spinal cord, peripheral nerves, brainstem, or midbrain. To avoid permanent damage, the patient's position may need to be adjusted or the surgeon may need to adjust retractors or instrumentation, alter the surgical approach, or change the procedure.

Motor evoked potentials provide a means of assessing descending motor pathways during neurosurgery. MEP is performed by electrically stimulating the brain through electrodes placed on the scalp. Receptor leads are attached to muscles in the upper and lower limbs. A decrease in the MEP amplitude or increases in the stimulating thresholds are warning signs. Caution should be used in MEP monitoring in patients with a history of epilepsy or implanted metallic devices in the brain.

SSEP and MEP monitoring is often combined to reassure the surgeon that motor function is still intact and surgery can continue safely (Weinzeiri et al, 2007). It is important to ensure that anesthesia inserts a bite block to prevent damage to the tongue and lips when motor testing to prevent injury.

Electromyography

EMG
Electromyography

Electromyography (EMG) looks at the electrical activity in muscles and at the function of the nerve roots leaving the spine. This can be accomplished by looking at how well the electrical currents in the nerves are being transmitted to the muscles.

Damage to nerves or pressure on them changes the way electrical current is transmitted. This information can be captured in the muscles as they react to the information sent to them from the brain by the nerves. The EMG can detect abnormal electrical signals in the muscles. This can demonstrate a nerve is being pinched or irritated as it leaves the spine. Combinations of these tests are often performed intraoperatively to monitor the patient.

Monitoring Equipment

The neurosurgical room should be equipped with all of the standard anesthesia equipment. This should include electrocardiography, arterial pressure, central venous pressure, and pulmonary arterial pressure. A pulse oximeter and telethermometer, and capnography (measures carbon dioxide levels). Doppler ultrasonography should be available when a cranial procedure is performed when the patient is in the sitting position. Continuous electroencephalography (EEG) monitoring can be used for assessment of cerebral blood flow and depth of anesthesia throughout the procedure.

At least two fluid or blood warmers should be available. A heating blanket should be available to maintain the patient's body temperature within normal limits. Maintaining the patient's normal body temperature decreases postprocedure infections and prevents unnecessary cardiac strain.

EEG
Electroencephalography

Lighting

Overhead operative illumination is best accomplished by a two-light system, either on two tracks or swiveling from a central point. This is especially helpful when the procedure involves two sites simultaneously. It is also advantageous when light coming from two angles provides superior visualization of a small, deep operative wound, as in a craniotomy, or to a long wound as in spinal procedures.

Additional illumination is provided by headlights worn by the surgeons. The headlight is connected by a fiberoptic cable to a light source or to a battery pack worn on a belt. The headlight illuminates the exact spot that the surgeon is focusing on. The headlight may be combined with magnifying loupes, or the loupes may be attached to frames worn independently of the headlight. The microscope provides the best source of light.

Positioning Devices

The nurse uses knowledge about the procedure and the position in selecting the correct positioning devices, the surgical table, and attachments. The nurse must meticulously position the neurosurgical patient because longer procedures place the patient at unusual risk for tissue injury and skin breakdown. Protective devices should be used to the fullest possible extent. Standardized positioning devices are used to protect the patient and prevent vascular compromise and nerve damage. They include doughnuts, pillows, axillary rolls, chest rolls, gel pads, and air mattress. The use of linen and foam should be discouraged, as they do not promote the best in available material for positioning. Dry visco-elastic polymer (gel pad) should be used whenever possible.

Positioning devices specific to neurosurgery provide support of the head and the spine during the procedure. The head section of the standard surgical table is replaced by a neurosurgical headrest when a craniotomy is to be performed. An adapter may be required to attach it to the surgical table or it may fit on existing brackets. Neurosurgical headrests come in a variety of configurations, which are used according to the desired position and the surgeon's preference. One commonly used system is the Mayfield neurosurgical headrest. This consists of a basic unit that attaches to the surgical table with several different headrest attachments. The general purpose headrest has rubber cups mounted in a half circle that supports the head when the patient is supine. The horseshoe headrest is a horseshoe-shaped, sponge rubber padded unit (**Fig. 26.11**). This is typically used for patients in the prone position. The headrest also has a pulley bar that can be used when cervical traction is desired, for example during a cervical fusion procedure.

A three-pin headrest is standard for positioning the head for most craniotomies and some cervical procedures. The Mayfield is a common type of headrest (**Fig. 26.12**). Both of these types consist of a movable arc-shaped segment with places for pins on each end with a pin holder opposite. Two headpins are positioned on one side of the head and the third one is placed on the opposite side of the head. The cone-shaped pins are removable so they can be sterilized. Single-use sterile pins are also available. This device holds the head firmly and securely (**Fig. 26.13**). The device can assume multiple positions and it uses three points to secure the head into position. Some headrests also have attachments so retractors can attach to the frame.

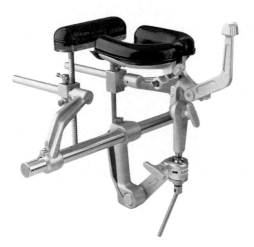

Figure 26.11

Mayfield neurosurgical headrest.

Source: Michael Molloy, Sr. Product Manager, Integra LifeSciences Corporation, Cincinnati, OH 45227.

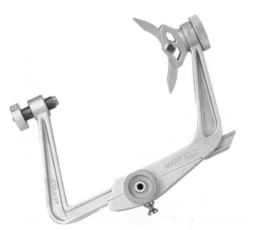

Figure 26.12

Mayfield skull clamp headrest.

Source: Michael Molloy, Sr. Product Manager, Integra LifeSciences Corporation, Cincinnati, OH 45227.

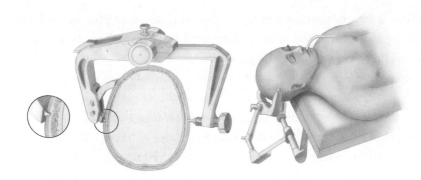

Figure 26.13

(A) Pins penetrate the scalp and are fixed to the outer table of the skull. (B) Skull clamp applied with the patient in the supine position.

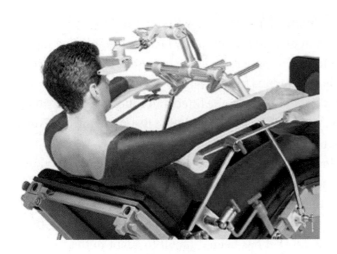

Figure 26.14

Head holder used with a crossbar attachment for a patient in the sitting position.

Source: Michael Molloy, Sr. Product Manager, Integra LifeSciences Corporation, Cincinnati, OH 45227.

The crossbar attachment connects to the rails on the surgical table and arches across it over the patient's legs. The crossbar holds the head attachment when the patient is in a sitting position (**Fig. 26.14**).

For procedures on the spine, a surgical table, the Wilson frame, the Andrews frame/table, or the Jackson table may be used.

Prone Position Devices

The prone position is considered a risk factor because it increases intraocular pressure, leading to blindness, and corneal abrasions can occur. The prone position can cause increased intraabdominal pressure which can influence blood loss, and decrease blood pressure and cardiac function. The prone position interferes with abdominal excursion, and respiratory interference can occur. There can be increases in airway pressure, and there is an increased incidence of pressure ulcers on the elbows, knees, and feet (Manna, Ibraheim, Samarkandi, Alotaibi, & Elwatidy, 2005).

The patient's trunk is supported on gel rolls or a padded frame to allow maximal chest expansion while allowing the abdomen to freely hang. Pressure on the abdomen will increase intraabdominal pressure resulting in increased bleeding. Rolls are placed on either side of the trunk from the shoulders to the iliac crest. The head should be supported on gel doughnuts or foam blocks. Care should be taken not to place any pressure on the jugular veins by turning the head too far. Care must be taken to provide padding to prevent pressure areas and nerve impingement. This can be accomplished with the use of gel pads and pillows. The anterior knees should be padded to prevent nerve damage and pressure ulcers. Pillow and/or gel rolls should be placed under the ankles to prevent plantar flexion and decrease pressure on the toes. Arms may be placed next to the patient and secured or on armboards flexed at the elbows with padding to prevent nerve damage.

There are special positioning devices/tables that are commonly used for the prone position. The Wilson frame may be placed on a conventional surgical table or the Jackson table. Two lateral tapered pads with an adjustable lordosis arch are built into the frame. The center of the frame allows the abdomen to hang freely. Care must be taken to prevent the abdomen from not being able to hang free so a sheet should not be put across the rolls or the Wilson frame. The frame is radiolucent and portable, allowing it to go from one surgical table to another.

The Jackson table allows for fluoroscopic studies without the limitations of a standard surgical table. Patients can be positioned on the table without lifting them because of the rotational capabilities. For patients with neck trauma the use of a cervical collar and the Jackson table may reduce the possibility of additional spinal cord compromise because the patient does not have to be lifted and rolled over (Bearden, Conrad, Horodyski, & Rechtine, 2007). Pads can be added to the table for the prone position or a Wilson frame can be added.

The Andrews table/frame allows patients to be placed in the knee-chest position. The positioning of the patient can be labor-intensive (Bowen, 2007) and it may lead to significantly more bleeding than other positions (Rigamonti, Gemma, Rocca, Messina, & Beretta, 2005). The frame acts as an accessory to a surgical table that has some notable disadvantages because it has been difficult to adapt to the surgical table and x-ray images are not always adequate. The Andrew's table resolves most of those disadvantages and is less labor-intensive to position the patient. When the Andrews table is broken to place the patient in a kneeling position, the knees are padded and a padded support rest is placed against the buttocks. There should be a 90-degree-angle at the hips, knees, and ankles, with all pressure points padded.

Radiology

Radiology is frequently used during spine surgery. A standard portable x-ray machine can be used to verify correct location, usually in spine surgery, or a fluoroscopic machine can be used, commonly referred to as a C-arm. Lead aprons and thyroid shields must be worn to protect the surgical team from the harmful effects of radiation. Monitoring badges should also be worn by staff to warn of overexposure to radiation.

Laser

A laser may be attached to the microscope or may be used freehand under normal vision or with magnification provided by loupes. The carbon dioxide laser is used in brain surgery to ablate a tumor. Brain tissue has a high water content. The carbon dioxide laser beam is absorbed by water and therefore the laser affects only a small area of brain tissue at a time. This provides a sharp zone of destruction and preserves normal brain tissue. The carbon dioxide laser has also been used on spinal procedures for discectomy because of the same water content properties. Appropriate safety measures must be employed: warning signs on operative suite doors, eye protection for the patient and staff, protection of surrounding tissue with moist sponges, evacuation of the laser plume, isolation of the laser foot pedal, and testing the laser before use. Some facilities designate an extra person in the room as the laser safety officer, whose sole purpose is placing the laser on standby when it is not being activated.

Ultrasonography

Ultrasound image quality has improved considerably in recent years. Ultrasound waves are generated by a unit that has a monitor for visualization of the image. A sterile probe is supplied to the scrub person; the probe is applied directly to the brain tissue. This must be accompanied by continuous irrigation to eliminate air space between the probe tip and the brain surface. Ultrasound waves can only be passed through tissue without air. The advancement of 3D ultrasound systems matched with neuronavigation has become an alternative for intraoperative imaging. Preprocedure 3D MRI or CT data is downloaded into a computer. Using an ultrasound probe during surgery allows visualization of a live ultrasound image enhanced with the MRI image. The advantage of this technology is it allows visualization of any shifting of tissue after surgery has begun. Brain tissue can move during large open craniotomies due to many factors including changes in blood and CSF pressures, and manipulation and removal of tissue (Gobbi, Comeau, & Peters, 2000).

Ultrasonic Surgical Aspirator

The ultrasonic surgical aspirator provides precise tissue removal by rapid mechanical motion (**Fig. 26.15**). It is called ultrasonic because tip vibrations are in the 23–55 kHz range and are above the sonic range of human hearing. The ultrasonic handpiece simultaneously fragments, irrigates, and aspirates tissue. The tip fragments tissue at the cellular level.

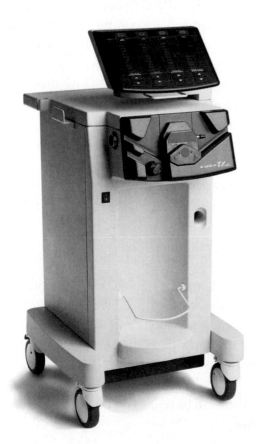

Figure 26.15

Cavatational Ultrasonic Surgical Aspirator, CUSA Excel Console.

Source: Michael Molloy, Sr. Product Manager, Integra LifeSciences Corporation, Cincinnati, OH 45227.

As the tip rapidly moves it produces a pulsating cavitational effect within the cells, whereby cavities are formed. When the surface tension of the cavity can no longer withstand the pulsating effect the cavity implodes resulting in cell destruction. During fragmentation sterile fluid is delivered through the handpiece to suspend tissue particles. The tissue debris is then aspirated through the suction tip. This technology enables the surgeon to remove tumors that are high in water content or moderately calcified, while sparing tissue that is high in collagen such as blood vessels and nerves. Some units have the ability to change frequencies to adapt to the type of tissue. Handpiece tips come in straight and curved to aid in visibility (Robinson, Sun, Bodurka-Bevers, Im, & Rosenshein, 2000).

Nerve Stimulator

Nerve stimulators are used to identify nerve tissue and to evaluate nerve responses. The device consists of a generator to which a sterile probe is connected. Sterile disposable self-contained nerve stimulators are also available.

Navigation Systems

Stereotactic and image-guided equipment is commonly used in neurosurgery. Stereotaxis pertains to precise localization of a specific point in the brain based on three-dimensional coordinates (Hickey, 2002). A navigation system is similar to an automobile navigation system. While the automobile is moving a signal is reviewed by a satellite that can locate the vehicle's position and superimpose it on a map. These systems only provide images in one plane. A neurosurgical navigation system provides the same guidance but in three different planes: axial, coronal, and sagittal. Information from a radiological study (MRI, CT scan) is downloaded into a computer. The computer creates the anatomical area on three intersecting geometric coordinates. This is used by the surgeon to assist in orientating anatomic relationships. Different views are available on a computer screen during surgery. A sterile probe is utilized which transmits its location back to the computer and its location within the brain can be viewed on the monitor. The probe can be guided to a specific location within the brain with minimal damage to normal tissue. A clear path must be maintained between the probe and the computer monitor to receive the signals from the probe.

Using three-dimensional planes the guidance system can be a frame-based or a frameless system. The frame-based system uses a head frame that provides a marker system during computer imaging. The device attaches to a headrest, typically a 3-pin headrest. Instrumentation can be attached to the frame. The frame does take up space and may limit accessibility.

A frameless system uses fiducials which are temporary markers that are placed on the scalp. A CAT scan or MRI is taken incorporating the fiducials. The fluoroscopic image becomes the "map" and the fiducials help locate you where you are on the "map" of the brain. The system can then create a three-dimensional computer graphic image of the brain. The frameless systems enable more elaborate image guidance. The fiducial markers initially are placed on the skull prior to fluoroscopic studies just prior to surgery. The fiducial makers can be removed just before the prep in the operative and invasive procedure suite.

When surgery has begun, a handheld sterile probe sends a signal to the computer and it will register on the monitor its exact location. This is useful when attempting to determine the location, depth, and size of a tumor along with improved safety and accuracy.

Navigation systems have proven to be helpful as a tool because it increases the safety of the procedure, provide a high degree of accuracy in targeting lesions, provide good anatomical orientation, and minimize brain trauma.

Hemostasis

Neurosurgery often involves small incisions through very vascular structures. A small amount of bleeding can obstruct the vision of the surgeon. Hemostasis is important for the field of vision and for hemodynamic balance of the patient. A number of items are used to achieve hemostasis.

The vascularity of the scalp necessitates special efforts to control bleeding when an incision is made. Scalp clips, such as Raney or Leroy, are utilized. These are applied over the edges of the incision on the scalp flap and remain until closing. The plastic clips apply pressure and therefore limit blood loss from the highly vascular scalp. They can be applied with a reusable instrument that holds one clip at a time or with a gun-like device that holds multiple clips. If a disposable gun is used to apply the clips, a removal device will be required at closing to remove the clips. Lidocaine with epinephrine may be infiltrated along the incision line. Local anesthesia with epinephrine is used to decrease bleeding and prolong the effect of the anesthetic.

Bone wax is used to seal cut edges of bone. This is a soft wax that is easily shaped and rubbed on in a thin layer with an instrument such as a freer elevator. Small balls are usually created the size of a pea (5 mm in diameter) and kept on a small metal tray. Bone wax is a blend of beeswax and a synthetic ester and allergies to insect stings should be considered.

Absorbable gelatin sponge (Gelfoam) is frequently used. It is water soluble, malleable, porcine gelatin. It can be cut into desired sizes and shapes according to the surgeon's preference. It can also be soaked in a solution of topical Thrombin. The gelatin sponge is then applied directly to the area of bleeding. It can be left in place or removed.

Absorbable knitted fabric of oxidized regenerated cellulose (Surgicel) is available in multiple sizes and can be cut into small sections. It is applied dry over a bleeding area and it provides a substrate for clot formation. If it is removed it should be done gently after hemostasis has been achieved.

Hemostatic matrix (FloSeal) is prepared by mixing a powdered gelatin matrix with Thrombin in two joined syringes. The end product has a paste consistency that can be applied with a syringe with a special nonmetallic tip. It should not be injected into blood vessels.

Fibrin Sealant (Tisseel, Evicel) is a complex natural agent that contains human plasma. It is used to achieve rapid hemostasis and tissue healing.

Thrombin comes as a powder and needs to be mixed with saline. Applied directly as a liquid or added to Gelfoam, it clots the fibrinogen of blood directly.

Neurosurgical patties made of compressed rayon material are available in many different sizes. They contain a radiopaque marker and they may have a string attached.

Cottonoids is the brand name of Johnson & Johnson, but the term is usually applied generically. Strips come six inches long in a variety of widths from ¼ inch to 1 inch. They also come in multiple sizes depending on the application. Patties are presented to the surgeon moist on a small metal tray and are removed by the surgeon with forceps. They are used on nerve tissue that might be injured by the coarse gauze sponge. Because numerous patties are used to protect tissue and isolate areas and to provide hemostasis, numerous patties may be in the wound at any given time. The scrub person must be attentive to the number of patties in the wound and all patties should be included in the surgical count. Patties should never be cut.

Cotton balls provide hemostasis in a deep area such as a bed of a tumor. Several moist cotton balls may be packed into the space to provide pressure. As the cotton balls are removed one by one, hemostasis is ensured. The cotton balls should have a radiopaque maker on them, such as a string, to help in recovery of them so they will be located on an x-ray in the event of an unresolved count.

ESU
Electrosurgery Units

Electrosurgery units (ESU), both monopolar and bipolar, are used routinely in neurosurgery. Care must be taken when using these devices. A protective device, such as a plastic safety holster, should be used to place the pencil and bipolar forcep in when the device is not being activated. Using a pencil, a forcep, or suction tip, coagulation takes place when contact is made in a dry field. This can be a challenge as suctioning may be necessary to provide a dry clear view. A standard monopolar unit provides both cutting and coagulation to tissue. A bipolar unit is used for coagulating fine vessels while minimizing the possibility of damage to adjacent tissue. It is safe to use the bipolar on the dura of the brain and spinal cord (Ferrara, 2007). The bipolar unit functions by passing current through one side of a forcep electrode, across the tissue, and back through the other side of the forceps electrode. A patient return electrode is not required for this device. The forceps must be kept clean of charred tissue. Scraping bipolar forceps tips with a rough or sharp device can damage them; instead they should be cleaned with a wet towel or sponge. Some bipolar units have a continuous irrigation system to the bipolar forceps tips that prevents drying out of the tissue and therefore helps to keep the tissue from adhering to the forceps. Bipolar electrosurgical units are available as an independent unit or they can be incorporated into a monopolar unit. The ESU power settings must be confirmed with the surgeon before activation. Manufacturer's recommendations for placement of the patient return electrode should always be followed. The pad should be placed on a large muscle mass as close to the surgical site as possible. Pads should never be placed over scar tissue because of de-vascularization of the area.

Ligating clips are used on larger vessels where use of the ESU would not provide adequate hemostasis. Clips can be manually loaded on a reusable instrument or come in a disposable instrument that has multiple clips pre-loaded. Specialty clips for aneurysm will be discussed later.

Lasers can be used to both coagulate and vaporize tissue. There are many types of lasers that have specific applications and also limitations. When using a foot pedal-activated laser, no other foot pedal should be available for the surgeon. This will prevent inadvertent activation of the laser.

Irrigation and Suction

Irrigation and suction go hand in hand. Irrigation is used to wash away blood and debris from the field and cool the tip of burrs and other power equipment. As irrigation is added to the field it needs to be removed quickly so vision is not impeded. Irrigation of surgical wounds is common with normal saline. A bulb syringe should always be available with room-temperature saline. Suction is necessary to remove blood and irrigation fluid. Careful attention should be taken to avoid placing the suction tip on brain tissue. Suction tips should be inspected for clean smooth edges. Often the burr from a high-speed drill will come in contact with the suction tip. A suction tip with sharp edges should be discarded. The amount of irrigation should be noted, a suction container full of red fluid can be mostly saline or a lot of blood.

Specialized suction tips of many styles are used in neurosurgery. Suction tips are employed for retracting, dissecting, evacuating smoke, picking up surgical patties, and removing blood and irrigation fluid. Suction tips that are also active electrodes with an ESU unit are used for hemostasis. The scrub person should always be prepared to switch and clean suction tips. Frequently tips become clogged with bits of bone and tissue, because of their small diameter. Clearing the suction can be done with a stylet, but irrigation with a 10 mL syringe is often quicker and more effective in dislodging the blockage. Care must be taken with how much force is used and where the tip of the suction is pointed during this cleaning maneuver. For irrigation in the operative field a 30 mL syringe filled with normal saline with a plastic IV catheter tip is helpful.

Instruments

Microsurgical instruments consisting primarily of dissectors, forceps, needle holders, and scissors enable the performance of delicate procedures, but they are useful only when they are in perfect working condition. These instruments must be maintained in exact alignment without nicks or burrs on the working areas. Proper care of microsurgical instruments consists of washing by hand, sterilizing and storing in specialized racks or trays, and careful handling of them during the procedure. The instruments should not be wiped with gauze during the procedure because the fibers might snag and bend them. Instead, use special microsurgical cleaning pads.

Several self-retaining retractors are especially designed for use during craniotomy. These are attached to the surgical table, the neurosurgical skull clamp, or the skull itself. The retractors hold brain spatulas on flexible arms and can be configured into a variety of positions. Common retractors of this type are the Leyla, Greenberg, and the halo retractors such as the Sugita or Budde (**Fig. 26.16**). The Budde and Sugita halo retractors serve a dual purpose in that the supporting ring also acts as a hand rest. This is especially useful in microsurgical procedures in which tremors caused by hand fatigue can be detrimental to the progress of the operation. Other self-retaining retractors such as the Weitlaner and the cerebellar retractor are also useful, especially for posterior fossa procedures.

Spinal procedures necessitate specialized retractors such as the Taylor and the Hibbs retractors. The Scoville retractor is a self-retaining retractor with a variety of detachable blades often used during laminectomy. Retractors made of composite fibers will stand up to the regimens of retracting while being radiolucent.

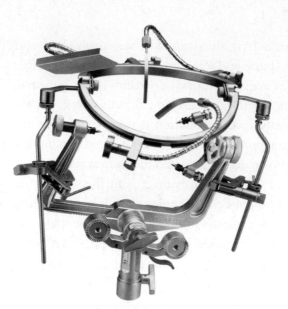

Figure 26.16

Budde-Halo System.

Source: Michael Molloy, Sr. Product Manager, Integra LifeSciences Corporation, Cincinnati, OH 45227.

Implantable Materials

Cranial operative procedures or trauma can cause defects or deformities that can be repaired for functional or cosmetic reasons with implantable materials. Defects of the dura can be covered with frozen or freeze-dried human cadaver dura or synthetic material. When a portion of the skull is missing, it can be repaired with a cranioplasty kit. This contains a slow-setting form of methyl methacrylate (bone cement) that can be molded into the correct shape and then trimmed to fit the defect exactly. The cranioplasty kit should be carefully differentiated from the aneuroplastic kit, which contains a fast setting form of methyl methacrylate used for coating cerebral aneurysms. Adequate ventilation and a source to vacuum the fumes while the methyl methacrylate cures are necessary. Burr hole covers made of silicone are sometimes used to fill the spaces left by the burr holes. Stainless steel plates are also used to both cover the burr holes and to secure the bone flap in place.

Spine procedures use allograft (cadaver) bone, and synthetic material is often used in place of a bone graft. Titanium, composite plastic, and bone matrix are used along with plates and screws.

Robotics

Robotic-assisted instrumentation make it possible for precise dissection and placement of screws and other hardware. Robots are able to accomplish some maneuvers that are not possible in the realm of the human range of motion (Phillips, 2007). Robotics coupled with radiological studies and computer advancement allow for very precise implantation of devices accurately.

GENERAL NURSING CONSIDERATIONS

Careful planning and preparation can decrease anesthesia and surgical time. This can also reduce the physical and psychological stress on the patient and the surgical team (Ferrara, 2007).

Neurosurgery patients will have had an extensive workup prior to admission to the operative and invasive suite unless it is for an emergency procedure. Diagnostic tests that should be available in the OR include radiological studies (both the report and hard copy), laboratory results, and the availability of any ordered blood products. Availability of special instruments and/or implants should be confirmed before the procedure is scheduled to begin. Often specialized trays and/or implants are delivered to Sterile Processing the day before surgery to be cleaned and sterilized. If there is an expectation that a manufacturer representative will be present, this should be confirmed. Often a surgical procedure will either be delayed or moved up in the schedule; therefore all ancillary personnel should be notified including manufacturer representatives. The surgical schedule should be reviewed to determine there are no conflicts with equipment. Too often two procedures are scheduled at the same time using the same piece of equipment, such as a C-arm or specialized positioning devices, or microscope.

Arrival in the Operative and Invasive Procedure Suite

Elective and emergency surgery patients require the same care and expertise. Emergencies tend to raise the stress level when the hemodynamic stability of the patient is in jeopardy. Time should be taken to identify the patient with at least two qualifiers, such as name and birth date. The surgeon should identify the correct surgical site and mark it per hospital policy. When the patient arrives in the OR anesthesia can be induced on the transfer stretcher (for prone position) or transferred directly to the surgical table. Anesthesia begins with the application of monitoring equipment, initiating of IV lines, and the induction of anesthesia. Correct side site surgery identification is everybody's responsibility along with a time out.

Careful role delineation helps ensure an efficient intraoperative procedure and can reduce the likelihood of errors:

- Radiological studies in the room. Designate who is responsible for placing them on the view box. Some facilities require that the operating surgeon is the only person allowed to put the x-ray studies on the view box as this reduces the chance of them being put up backwards and helps prevent wrong-site surgery.
- Hair is removed with clippers. Razors should be discouraged because of the incidence of higher surgical site infections (Tanner, Moncaster, & Woodings, 2007). Generally, the neurosurgeon prefers to perform this function. Hair removal may be done in the pre-induction area with the patient awake or inside the OR after the patient is under anesthesia. Hospital policy should be review and followed for hair removal. Some institutions consider hair the patient's personal property and require it be saved in a labeled container and others dispose of it.
- IV started and attachment of monitoring devices. Additional monitoring devices, such as arterial line, esophageal temperature probe, and triple lumen catheter may be required.
- Endotracheal intubation when initiated will require the attentiveness of the circulator assisting and suction availability. In difficult airway management, a fiberoptic intubation may be required and so the equipment should be available.

- Insertion of a urinary catheter, with a metered container for accurate measurements is necessary. This is usually done after the patient is anesthetized.
- Compression stockings should be applied before induction of anesthesia. Long immobility of the neurosurgical patient can create an environment for thrombus formation. Consequently, sequential intermittent pneumatic compression stockings should be applied to the legs to promote venous return. Sequential intermittent pneumatic compression stockings should be applied before the procedure or prior to the induction of anesthesia, and continued during and after the procedure until the patient is ambulating. Intermittent pneumatic compression stockings are effective in the prevention of deep vein thrombosis and pulmonary emboli (Epstein, 2005).
- The patient is positioned carefully with adequate help with support and padding in place. Pressure points need to be examined with appropriate padding added. Neurosurgical procedures can be lengthy with four to twelve hours being normal depending on the procedure and pathology. Special care must be taken to position the patient to avoid trauma to the skin and the underlying tissue. The surgical table should have additional padding in place using dry visco-elastic polymer (gel pad). Knowledge of pressure points and how to provide support and adequate protection is required.
- If the head is placed in a three-pin headrest, antibiotic ointment should be applied around the pin sites. The ointment provides a seal around the puncture wound to prevent infection.
- The eyes should be protected with lubricant and eye patches taped in place. Covering the eye patches with transparent adhesive wound dressing material (Op-site, Tegaderm) is a good method to ensure that the patches remain in place throughout the procedure. If the patient is in the prone position care must be taken to protect the eyes and determine pressure has been taken off them. Care must be taken to exclude antiseptic solution from the eyes and ears.
- Positioning and prepping can take considerable time, from 30 minutes to over an hour. After the patient is positioned and prepped, the surgeon should draw out the incision line.

Time Out

Prior to making the incision a Time Out is done to confirm correct patient, correct surgical procedure, correct side site, and correct surgeon.

Drugs and Solutions

The circulating nurse should obtain and dispense topical Thrombin, hemostatic agents of the surgeon's choice, antibiotics, and saline for irrigation. All of them should be clearly labeled.

Physiological Monitoring

Blood loss should be monitored both on the sponges and in the suction. The nurse should establish the availability of blood before the start of the procedure and be prepared to obtain blood and blood products at the request of the anesthesia provider. Urine output should be monitored. Small portable equipment that can provide immediate hemoglobin and hematocrit results should be in the room.

CRANIOTOMY

Indications

Craniotomy is an incision into the cranium, including the raising of scalp, bone, and dural flaps, usually to remove blood clots, a tumor, repair an aneurysm or arteriovenous malformation, or placement of a shunt or drain. A basic craniotomy will be described followed by the procedure to be accomplished based on the pathology. These will include hematoma, aneurysm, arteriovenous malformation, tumor, and shunts.

Nursing Implications

Anesthesia Awake Craniotomy

During an awake craniotomy, the patient is awake and alert during the middle of the procedure to answer questions and respond as needed. The patient may be asked to move a finger, toe, count one to ten, etc. This allows the neurosurgeon to directly and indirectly monitor and map the neurological functions that are being electrically stimulated. After the mapping is completed, the surgeon can proceed to remove a tumor while protecting the areas that surround it. This will limit or prevent some postprocedure deficits. An awake craniotomy can be conducted in one of two ways. A patient is initially fully anesthetized with general anesthesia, then awakened for the mapping part of the procedure and then anesthetized again, or the patient can initially be consciously sedated, the mapping is performed with the patient awake and then the patient is sedated for completion of the procedure (Palese, & Infami, 2006). Since the brain has no sensory receptors no pain is felt.

Nurses need to make adjustments in their practice when caring for an awake craniotomy patient. There is less verbal communication between staff members and more non-verbal than normal. This will limit the discussions in order to reduce the patient's anxiety. Because of the reduced verbal communication each staff member is more attentive to the proceeding to help anticipate needs of the team and patient, who will often ask questions. Nurses report that participating in an awake craniotomy is emotionally draining and stressful and they do not recommend inexperienced staff members participate because of the limitations placed on verbal requests. (Palese, & Infami, 2006).

Anesthesia Non-Awake Craniotomy

Craniotomy is performed with the patient under general anesthesia. The anesthesia provider uses invasive monitoring techniques for this procedure, including the placement of arterial and central venous catheters. A pulmonary arterial catheter may also be required. Brain relaxation is achieved by placement of a lumbar drainage device, administration of medications (mannitol, furosemide, dexamethasone), and/or hyperventilation. Hyperventilation decreases the partial pressure of carbon dioxide, which causes vasoconstriction. Relaxation of the brain achieves a larger space for the operation and makes retraction easier (Drummond & Patel, 2000). If the incision site is going to be infiltrated with a local anesthetic with epinephrine, it is done immediately after prepping to allow it to take its pharmacological action prior to the incision. The anesthesia provider should be consulted prior to injection for review of vital signs and notified of the amount injected.

Position

The position for a craniotomy depends on the location and type of the pathology. The supine position allows access for frontal, parietal, and temporal approaches. A three-pin headrest or a gel doughnut is used for positioning. The sitting position is used for a posterior approach. The prone position is used for access to the occipital lobe. A padded horseshoe-shaped head holder can be used, or the three-pin head holder (Phillips, 2007).

Establishing and Maintaining the Sterile Field

The head is draped with towels that are sutured or stapled in place. If staples are used a staple remover will be needed at the end of the procedure. Some craniotomy drapes incorporate a plastic pocket with a suction port that collects fluid during the procedure. Drapes are positioned to cover the patient completely while forming a tent for the anesthesia provider so that the patient can be observed without encroaching on the sterile field. The tent is formed with a combination of Mayo stands and IV poles to support the drapes. Suction and electrosurgery cords are secured and handed off the field. A safety holster, recommended by the manufacturer, should be used to hold the electrosurgery devices.

Equipment and Supplies

Cranial perforator, three-pin headrest, microscope, mono and bipolar electrosurgery unit, suction, and compression pneumatic stockings are standard items that may be required for the procedure.

Drugs and Solutions

Drugs that may be needed include antibiotics, Thrombin, Gelfoam, Flo-Seal, Decadron, and saline.

Blood loss should be monitored both on the sponges and in the suction. Urine output should be observed. Standard hemodynamic monitoring is done by the anesthesia provider.

Specimens and Cultures

A frozen section may be required for an immediate diagnosis. The specimen is sent directly to pathology without any preservative added. The tissue is frozen, and then sliced thinly, stained, and viewed microscopically (Price, 2007).

Laboratory and Diagnostic Studies

Magnetic Resonance Imaging (MRI). An MRI produces a 3-D image of the brain that can expose tumors and aneurysms.

Computed Tomography (CT). This computer-generated image is useful in diagnosing trauma and bleeding issues. Images of the brain can be with or without contrast media.

Positron Emission Tomography (PET). Useful in depicting brain activity more so than structure. PET scan can distinguish living tissue from necrotic tissue (Phillips, 2007).

Procedure
Incision and Exposure

An incision is made into the scalp over the area of the intended area of the brain. Raney or Leroy clips are applied. Soft tissue is separated from the underlying bone

MRI
Magnetic Resonance Imaging

CT
Computed Tomography

PET
Positron Emission Tomography

with a periosteal elevator. The skin flap is retracted out of the way. This can be accomplished with Allis clamps or towel clips held by rubber bands attached to the drapes. Hemostasis is accomplished with electrosurgery–monopolar or bipolar. Burr holes are created through the cranium with a perforator. Saline irrigation is used during the drilling process to reduce heat generated. A dural separator is used in each burr hole to dissect the dura away from the bone (**Fig. 26.17**). A side cutting burr with a dural protector is attached to a high-speed drill and is used to connect the burr holes. The bone flap is elevated from the underlying dura with periosteal elevators and dissectors. Small holes may be made at this time on the bone flap and the cranium in preparation of closing. A brain spatula is used under the skull edges to protect the brain from the drill bit (**Fig. 26.18**). The bone flap can remain attached to the muscle or it can be removed completely to be replaced at closure. The bone flap should be wrapped in a saline-moistened or antibiotic-moistened sponge and placed in a basin in a secure location on the back table.

Some surgeons prefer to leave some muscle attached to the bone flap. In this situation, the bone is cut on only three sides and the side under the muscle is fractured and then smoothed with a rongeur. The bone and muscle are wrapped in moist gauze and secured back in the same manner as the scalp flap. After hemostasis is achieved with sponges, bone wax, and electrosurgery, the dura mater is incised and retracted out of the way (**Fig. 26.19**). Often this is accomplished with sutures and the dura is protected with moist sponges. Vessels are coagulated with bipolar electrosurgery or ligated with clips. Exposure is made and the specific surgery proceeds. This can be for a tumor resection, aneurysm, shunt, or hematoma. These will be discussed separately.

Figure 26.17
Retraction of a scalp flap.

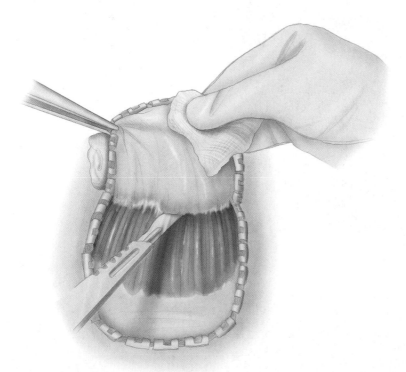

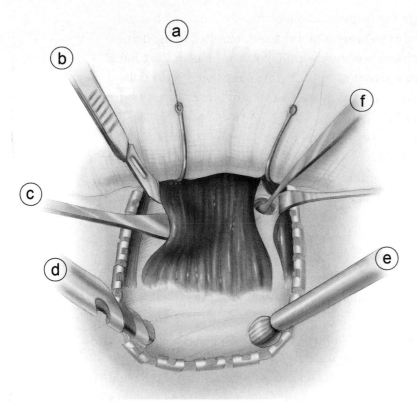

Figure 26.18

(a) retraction of scalp flap,
(b) incision of the muscle,
(c) separation of muscle, from bone with a periosteal elevator,
(d)and (e) creation of burr holes, and (f) separation of the dura from the skull.

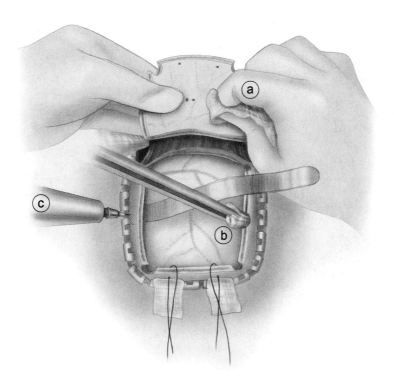

Figure 26.19

(a) and (b) waxing of the bone and (c) drilling wire holes.

Closure

When completed the dura is closed with interrupted or running sutures (**Fig. 26.20**). The dura is secured to the bone flap with a tack-up stitch. The dural suture line should be watertight and a sealing agent may be added. A synthetic and absorbable polyethylene glycol sealant (DuraSeal) can be used to make a watertight seal. For large dural defects, synthetic dura can be used.

The bone flap is replaced and secured with one of several methods—suture, wire, plates, and screws. The cranial fixation system utilizes small round plates that cover both sides of the burr hole and are connected by a thin metal shaft. Both plates are drawn together and hold the bone flap in place and they cover the burr holes. The Raney or Leroy clips are removed from the scalp. The galea is closed and the skin is closed with sutures or staples (**Fig. 26.21**). The incision is cleaned with hydrogen

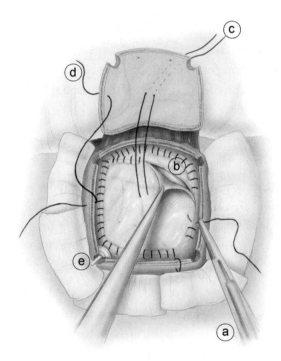

Figure 26.20

(a) suturing the dura matter, (b) dura graft, (c) central tack-up suture, (d) bone wires, and (e) silicone button.

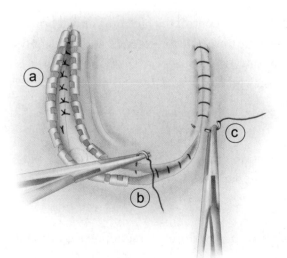

Figure 26.21

(a) sutures in the fascia, (b) suturing the galea aponeurotica, and (c) suturing the skin.

peroxide or saline and antibiotic ointment is applied. The head is supported while the neurosurgical headrest is replaced with the head of the surgical table. The dressing is applied and secured with a head wrap of elastic gauze or tubular elastic material. Ears contained within the dressing should be padded with cotton to avoid excessive pressure. The dressing may be anchored to the skin with tape.

Postprocedural Care

After a craniotomy, patients are admitted to an intensive care unit for close monitoring. The neurological condition can be assessed uniformly if a system of specific criteria such as the Glasgow Coma Scale is used. The head of the bed is kept elevated 30 degrees to decrease the intracranial pressure. The hemodynamic status is continuously assessed by electrocardiogram and arterial pressures. Arterial blood gas values indicate the adequacy of the respiratory effort, and central venous pressure and urine output indicate fluid balance.

As the patient's condition stabilizes, monitoring and supportive devices are removed. The patient is transferred to a step-down unit. Normal diet is resumed, and progressive activity is initiated. Rehabilitation for any residual neurological deficits is planned and implemented. Patients may be discharged from the hospital as early as 7 days after surgery or much later, depending on the patient's age, preexisting condition, and residual problems.

Potential Complications

The patient must be informed of the risks and hazards of craniotomy: additional loss of brain function, including memory; recurrence or continuation of the condition that necessitated the operation; stroke; blindness; deafness; inability to smell; double vision; coordination loss; seizures; pain; numbness; and paralysis.

HEMOTOMA

A head injury may result in bleeding and an accumulation of blood in the subdural or epidural space. As the space fills with blood there is an increase in intracranial pressure causing the brain tissue to shift within the cranial cavity. If left untreated it can be fatal. Epidural tears usually occur suddenly and subdural hematomas can be acute, subacute, or chronic (Price & Price, 2001). A craniotomy is performed to evacuate the hematoma, decrease the pressure, control the bleeding, and debride the area. This can be accomplished with a single burr hole for evacuation of clots only or by lifting a bone flap for further exploration. The clot is evacuated and hemostasis is achieved with electrosurgery. A drain may be utilized.

Nursing Implications
Position

The position is dependent on the location of the hematoma. The supine position with the head turned to one side is the standard position.

Equipment and Supplies

Standard equipment includes a drill with a perforator, monopolar and bipolar electrosurgery, and the 3-pin headrest.

Drugs and Solutions

Antibiotics, Thrombin, Gelfoam, and Flo-Seal may be needed.

Specimen and Culture

Clots removed are often sent to pathology for examination.

ANEURYSM

A cerebral aneurysm is a saccular outpouching of a intracranial artery that presents in a variety of sizes and shapes (Hickey, 2002).

Indications

Annually 10 to 15 million Americans are treated for cerebral aneurysms (Wagner & Stenger, 2005). A cerebral aneurysm is a vascular disorder in which weakness in the wall of a cerebral artery leads to a dilation or ballooning of the vessel. A true aneurysm is a weakness in all three layers of the vessel and a pseudoaneurysm or false aneurysm is a weakness in just the inner layer of the vessel wall. Mortality rates are between 30% and 60% and higher depending on the clinical grade of the patient at the time of presentation. When an aneurysm ruptures it causes blood under high pressure to be forced into the subarachnoid space. Intracranial pressure increases and cerebral pressure decreases. A cerebral aneurysm is usually undiagnosed until a hemorrhage occurs. The symptoms are severe headache, meningeal irritation (rigid neck, mild fever, photophobia, blurred vision, irritability, and restlessness), and alteration in the level of consciousness.

Aneurysms may result from congenital, traumatic, degenerative processes, or infectious processes, and abnormal dilations of the intracranial vessels. Congenital aneurysms are the most common and manifest themselves either by rupture, which results in subarachnoid hemorrhage, or by expansion, which causes pressure on surrounding structures (Wright, 2007).

Classification

The following categories are used to classify by size:

Small = less than 15 mm

Large = 15 to 25 mm

Giant = 25 to 50 mm

Super-giant = greater than 50 mm (Wright, 2007)

The common types are berry, saccular, and fusiform.
Classification by shape is as follows:

Berry: The most common type, it is berry-shaped with a neck or stem.

Charcot-Bouchard: A microscopic aneurysm associated with hypertension.

Dissecting: Related to atherosclerosis and inflammation. The intimal layers separate forcing blood between the layers.

Fusiform (saccular): An outpouching of the arterial wall that does not have a stem.

Mycotic: A rare type caused by septic emboli.

Traumatic: Results from head injuries, the least common type (Wright, 2007).

The symptoms of a ruptured aneurysm can be assessed by using the Hunt and Hess scale of subarachnoid hemorrhage severity:

Grade I: Asymptomatic; or minimal headache and slight nuchal (neck) rigidity. Survival rate is 70%.

Grade II: Moderate to severe headache, nuchal rigidity, no neurological deficit except cranial nerve palsy. Survival rate is 60%.

Grade III: Drowsy; minimal neurological deficit. Survival rate is 50%.

Grade IV: Stuporous; moderate to severe hemiparesis; possibly early decerebrate rigidity and vegetative disturbance. Survival rate is 20%.

Grade V: Deep coma, decerebrate rigidity, moribund. Survival rate is 10% (Hickey, 2002).

The Fischer Grade classifies the appearance of subarachnoid hemorrhage on CT scan:

Grade 1: No hemorrhage

Grade 2: Subarachnoid hemorrhage less than 1 mm thick

Grade 3: Subarachnoid hemorrhage more than 1 mm thick

Grade 4: Subarachnoid hemorrhage of any thickness with intraventricular hemorrhage

Diagnosis

Diagnosis of the aneurysm is made by detailed neurological examination, lumbar puncture, computed tomography, and cerebral arteriography.

Nursing Implications
Position

The operative approach to both cerebral aneurysms and arteriovenous malformations varies according to the location of the lesion. The following discussion assumes a standard craniotomy with an approach involving a bone flap. Suboccipital or posterior fossa craniotomy is necessary for some aneurysm procedures. Special positioning requirements for this approach are discussed as well.

Equipment and Supplies

An assortment of aneurysm clips, temporary and permanent, should be in the room or on the sterile field along with at least two clip appliers.

Drugs and Solutions

Papaverine may be needed to prevent vasospasm.

Treatment Options

Treatment options include placing an aneurysm clip across the neck of the aneurysm encasing the aneurysm in methyl methacrylate (bone cement), ligation of the feeding vessel (Price & Price, 2001) or endovascular coiling. Endovascular coiling will be discussed separately.

Aneurysm Clips

Aneurysm clips have been the choice of treatment because of their success rates and proven durability. The clips are made of titanium with a spring mechanism that forces the jaws to be closed tightly. They come in a variety of shapes and sizes. Careful attention must be given to the types of clips available. Two types of clips may be included in the set, temporary or trial clips and permanent clips. Temporary clips are used to control giant aneurysms, to establish the best position for the permanent clip, and to control bleeding without damage to the vessel. Temporary clips should be discarded after being used. Clips, after being placed in the clip applier, should only be compressed by the neurosurgeon. Once a clip has been compressed and not applied, it should be discarded, as the spring mechanism may have been sprung (Ferrara, 2007).

Methyl Methacrylate

When clipping of the aneurysm is not possible, it may be wrapped or coated with an agent such as methyl methacrylate. This is done by placing the agent in a syringe attached to a plastic angiocatheter cannula. The area around the aneurysm is isolated with moist patties before the substance is applied. Methyl methacrylate will encase the aneurysm so it can not expand. The methyl methacrylate, which is a fast-setting cement, must be specific for aneurysm.

Procedure

A craniotomy is performed and careful dissection is carried out to visualize the aneurysm. A self-retaining retractor may be used that supports the brain with spatulas attached to flexible arms that conform to a variety of positions. Common retractors are the Leyla, Greenberg, and the halo retractor such as the Sugita or Budde. The microscope should be pre-tested and draped. Microsurgical instruments will be required including scissors, forceps, and micro-bipolar forceps. Multiple suction tips must be available; vision can be obscured with sudden blood loss and small lumen suction tips become obstructed easily.

Details

The anesthesia provider may be requested to lower the patient's blood pressure to increase visibility and reduce the risk of rupture. The aneurysm clip will be applied and the blood pressure slowly increased. Bleeding will be controlled and an intraoperative angiogram may be performed to check for positioning or leakage.

Closure

The wound is closed and a dressing is applied as described for craniotomy.

Postprocedure Care

Postprocedure bleeding and intracranial pressure are monitored with attentiveness to neurological signs (Price & Price, 2001).

Potential Complications

Cerebral vasospasm and stroke is the most dreaded complication of ruptured cerebral aneurysm. Cerebral arteries may develop spasms as early as 3 days and as late as 2 weeks following the initial hemorrhage. This can result in a stroke. The etiology of the spasm is thought to be secondary to a response of the blood vessels to break down products of hemoglobin. Vasospasm alters the cerebral circulation and may cause neurological deficits and changes the level of consciousness. Preventing vasospasm is a major consideration in the care of these patients before and after the procedure. Activities that cause an increase in blood pressure or intracranial pressure must be avoided.

ENDOVASCULAR COILING

Indications

Endovascular coiling was introduced in 1991 and this minimally invasive technique is a treatment option for specific type and size aneurysms. Soft and flexible platinum coils are inserted through a catheter via the femoral artery. Using fluoroscopy the coils are fed into the aneurysm and deployed. Multiple coils may be placed in the aneurysm. The coils prevent the flow of blood into the aneurysm by filling it with coils and thrombus. Additional healing causes a membrane to form across the neck of the aneurysm (Wright, 2007). Coils offer advantages over traditional aneurysm clipping.

Nursing Implications

As a minimally invasive procedure, multiple aneurysms can be treated, including some aneurysms that could be difficult to treat using the traditional surgery technique. The hospital stay and recovery is much shorter than the traditional clipping technique. Small aneurysms with small necks have been demonstrated to have the best results. Currently, about 30% of all aneurysms are suitable for coiling.

Position

Position is supine on a surgical table that is radiolucent at the head.

Establishing and Maintaining the Sterile Field

Room preparation and setup is similar for an aneurysm clipping. Instrumentation and aneurysm clips and appliers need to be open and ready as a precaution. A second back table is prepared with angiography supplies and a femoral artery-introducing sheath.

Equipment and Supplies

Radiolucent surgical table, C-arm fluoroscopy, aneurysm coils, angiographic guide wires and catheters, aneurysm clips and clip appliers.

Drugs and Solutions

Local anesthesia, heparinized saline, contrast dye, antibiotics, and Thrombin mixed with Gelfoam.

Procedure

Incision and Exposure

A catheter is introduced into the femoral artery and advanced to the aneurysm site. An angiogram will be performed to pinpoint the location of the aneurysm. Coils are deployed into the aneurysm filling the sac. An electrical impulse is used to detach the coil from the catheter. Multiple coils may be needed to fill the aneurysm sac.

Closure

The catheter is removed and the femoral artery puncture site is treated as per institution procedure. Pressure should be applied for several minutes and the dressing applied.

Postprocedure Care

The patient's leg is secured to prevent movement. Dressings are inspected for signs of bleeding and pedal pulses are checked for evidence of occlusion. The patient may spend one night in the ICU and an additional day in a medical surgical unit before being discharged.

Potential Complications

Hemorrhage and infection are potential complications.

ARTERIOVENOUS MALFORMATION

Setup and the procedure are similar to an aneurysm clipping.

Indications

An arteriovenous malformation (AVM) is a nest of blood vessels that form an abnormal communication between arterial and venous systems. Blood from the arteries is shunted directly into the venous system without passing through the usual capillary network. The result of this shunting is inadequate cerebral perfusion. This chronic ischemia results in cerebral atrophy, scarring, and focal infarction. (Hickey, 2002). The scarring of the brain tissue that occurs is known as gliosis. The results of this process may be neurological deficit, seizures, hydrocephalus, or hemorrhage. Surgical excision of the lesion is the treatment of choice. Surgically inaccessible lesions can be treated by embolization, proton beam radiation, or stereotaxic laser therapy (Hickey, 2002).

AVM
Arteriovenous
Malformation

26

Treatment Options

Resection of an arteriovenous malformation is similar to aneurysm occlusion. Involved vessels are identified and isolated and clips applied. The vein draining the lesion is the last vessel to be ligated before the malformation is totally removed.

Endovascular embolization involves advancing tiny catheters into the cerebral vessels that feed the AVM. A sclerosing agent is then injected that occludes the vessels (Price & Price, 2001) or small silastic beads can be injected. Embolization is usually the first step followed a month later with surgical resection (Phillips, 2007).

Closure

Meticulous attention to hemostasis is given before closure.

SHUNTS

Indications

A shunt is indicated when a patient has hydrocephalus. Hydrocephalus is a progressive dilation of the cerebroventricular system because the production of cerebral spinal fluid (CSF) exceeds the absorption rate. This can be caused by congenital hydrocephalus, spinal bifida, tumors, intracranial/intraventricular hemorrhage, aqueductal stenosis, and Chiari malformations. The purpose of a shunt is to divert the excessive fluid from the cranium to another area of the body where it can reabsorb.

VP
Ventriculoperitoneal

Types of Shunts

The two most common methods to divert CSF from the ventricles are internalized ventriculoperitoneal (VP) shunt, a permanent device, and the externalized ventriculostomy catheter for temporary shunting (Hickey, 2002). Other types also include ventriculoatrial and ventriculopleural.

Nursing Implications

Anesthesia

Patients are placed under general intubated anesthesia with standard hemodynamic monitoring.

Position

The patient is normally placed in the supine position with a gel doughnut under the head. The head is slightly turned to expose the side of the head in which the shunt will be placed.

Ventriculostomy

Incision and Exposure

Placement of the ventriculostomy catheter is made through a burr hole that allows access to the lateral ventricle. The catheter is placed into the ventricle and confirmed with the flow of CSF. The distal end of the catheter is tunneled beneath the scalp. Through a small scalp incision the catheter is passed and connected to an external drainage collection bag. The height of the drainage chamber is determined and set by the neurosurgeon to maintain control of the patient's intracranial pressure.

Drugs and Solutions

Thrombin with Gelfoam, antibiotic irrigation, antibiotics, and a local anesthetic with epinephrine should be available.

Specimens and Cultures

Cerebral spinal fluid may be taken as a specimen and cultures may also be taken.

Radiology Study

An x-ray may be taken to verify proper catheter placement.

Postprocedure Care

The patency of the shunt must be verified before the patient leaves the operating room.

Potential Complications

Infection and the need for shunt revision.

Ventriculoperitoneal Shunt

The VP shunt consists of a primary catheter, a reservoir (optional), a one-way valve, and a distal catheter. The primary catheter (ventricular) is placed through a burr hole into the lateral ventricle. The catheter is tunneled under the scalp. The reservoir and one-way valve are connected in the area of the mastoid bone. Valves come in a variety of different pressures and flow settings. The valve prevents CSF backflow. Some valves are programmable and can be adjusted postprocedure. The distal catheter (peritoneal) is connected and then tunneled under the skin to the ending point. This is usually the peritoneal cavity; however, it can be placed in the subarachnoid space, pleural cavity, or vena cava. Reservoirs allow access to CSF for laboratory analysis, placement of medications and contrast dye, and to test the potency of the shunt (Ferrara, 2007).

Position

The patient is supine with the head slightly elevated and turned to the non-operative side for a shunt. A gel doughnut stabilizes the head in position. The arm on the operative side is tucked in at the patient's side. The opposite arm is placed on an armboard. Gel pads are placed under the heels. A restraint strap is placed across the thighs.

Establishing and Maintaining the Sterile Field

The patient's hair is removed from both the scalp and abdomen. The area from the scalp to the abdomen is prepped and draped.

Incision and Exposure

A U-shaped incision is made, scalp clips are applied to control hemorrhage, and the scalp flap is elevated. A burr hole is made, the dura incised, and hemostasis is accomplished with a bipolar forcep. The catheter is placed into the lateral ventricle; this may be accomplished with a stylet.

The reservoir is filled with saline and attached to the catheter. The distal tubing and valve are filled with saline and tested for proper functioning. A tunnel is created from the scalp under the skin to the distal site. Several small incisions may be made to aid in the passing of the catheter to the exit site. A uterine packing forcep or a special shunt passer is used to aid in the process. The tubing is pulled through the tunnel and a subcostal incision is made and the catheter tip is inserted into the peritoneum and secured with suture. Some hospital polices will allow the neurosurgeon to place the catheter in the peritoneum and other institutions will require a general surgeon to complete this part of the procedure.

Drugs and Solutions

Some surgeons like to soak and irrigate the reservoirs and catheters with an antibiotic solution before implantation. The circulating nurse should prepare this solution as required.

Specimen and Cultures

Cerebral spinal fluid may be taken as a specimen along with cultures.

Radiology Studies

After the shunt and reservoir are implanted, the surgeon may confirm placement with an x-ray. The circulating nurse should confirm that an x-ray technician is available along with the required equipment.

Closure

The incisions are closed and dressings applied.

Postprocedure Care

Care after the procedure consists of monitoring of vital signs, neurological assessment, and care of the incisional lines. The surgeon may order pumping of the shunt. If the size of the ventricles is reduced too rapidly, excessive traction on the meninges may cause tearing and consequent subdural bleeding. For this reason, excessive pumping of the shunt should be avoided and the head of the bed should be kept flat for 24 hours. Sutures are removed in 7–10 days. The time of discharge depends on accompanying medical problems. The neurosurgeon may also reprogram the shunt after the surgery.

Potential Complications

The potential complications of shunt insertion are displacement, shunt malfunction, and infection. Shunt revisions are not uncommon and are necessary because of shunt failure or growth of a child. One or more parts of the shunt may need to be replaced or the distal segment lengthened. Infection is treated with antibiotics. If this treatment is not effective, the shunt is removed. Interim external drainage systems can be used until the infection resolves, and then another shunt is implanted.

If the patient has a programmable shunt in place and has an MRI, then the shunt will have to be reprogrammed after the MRI. The shunt is programmed using magnets and the valve setting may have changed.

CEREBRAL TUMORS

Indications

The incidence of brain tumors in the United States is about 17,000 per year, half of them metastatic. The one-year survival rate is 50% and the five-year survival rate is approximately 25% (Hickey, 2002; Ferrara, 2007), depending on the grade of the tumor. The primary cause of brain tumors is unknown. Brain tumors are classified based on a number of criteria including primary/secondary, anatomical location, histological origin, malignant/being, neuroembryonic, and childhood/adult tumors. The World Health Organization classifies more than 120 types of brain tumors.

Brain tumors may be benign or malignant, but any lesion that occurs within the cranium has the potential to create damage through compression of brain tissue, infiltration/invasion of brain tissue, and erosion of bone. This can cause pathological changes, including edema, increased intracranial pressure, neurological deficits, seizures, alterations in pituitary function, and obstruction in flow of the CSF (Hickey, 2002). The incidence and severity of the pathological condition is related to the size and location of the tumor. Lesions in the posterior fossa are approached through a suboccipital craniotomy. Tumors in the anterior and middle fossa are resected through a craniotomy that creates a bone flap for access. That procedure is the same as described earlier.

The signs and symptoms of a brain tumor are related to the size and location of the pathophysiological changes just mentioned. Typical symptoms are headache, vomiting, papilledema, personality changes, changes in level of consciousness, seizures, ataxia, loss of coordination, visual changes, and pituitary dysfunction (Hickey, 2002).

Diagnosis of a brain tumor is established by a thorough neurological examination, and radiological studies including magnetic resonance imaging, computed tomography, angiogram, and electroencephalogram (**Fig. 26.22–26.26**). Additional preprocedure studies include chest x-ray, electrocardiogram, complete blood cell count, electrolyte studies, chemistry, clotting studies, and urinalysis.

Treatment can be narrowed to three options: surgery, irradiation, and chemotherapy. They can be used alone or in combination. The selections of modalities are based on the type of tumor, location and size, symptoms, the general condition of the patient, and age. Malignant tumors treated with surgery only have a 17-week survival rate. If surgery is combined with radiation therapy, the survival rate is approximately 37 weeks (Hickey, 2002).

Conventional surgery is used to biopsy tissue and complete or partial removal of the tumor. Surgical accessibility to the tumor will determine if the resection will be possible, total or partial. The purpose of radiation therapy is to destroy tumor cells without injuring normal cells. This is accomplished because tumor cells are more radiosensitive than non-tumor cells. Radiation can be administered over a 6–8-week period and it can include both pre- and post-surgery. Interstitial brachytherapy is high-dose focal irradiation utilizing implanted radioactive isotopes for a short period of time (Hickey, 2002). Chemotherapy uses drugs or chemicals that act as a cellular poison. These drugs, unfortunately, also affect normal tissue. Chemotherapy is offered to patients who have had surgery and have continued regrowth of the tumor or no improvement in their condition (Hickey, 2002). Glidel wafers are placed intraoperatively and chemotherapy can also be administered through implanted

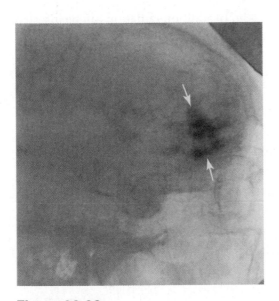

Figure 26.22
Carotid angiogram showing tumor stain.

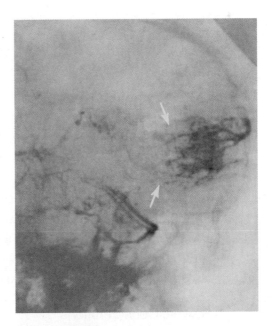

Figure 26.23
Carotid angiogram showing a halo of abnormal vessels surrounding an avascular tumor mass.

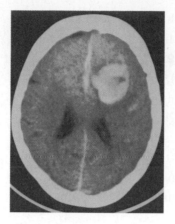

Figure 26.24

CT scan showing
a glioblastoma.

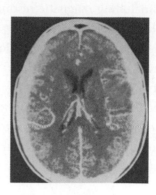

Figure 26.25

Contrast medium-enhanced CT
scan showing an astrocytoma.

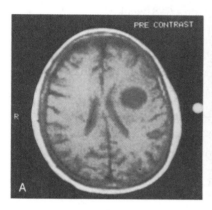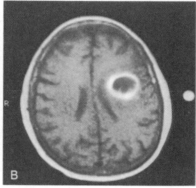

Figure 26.26 A and B

(A) MRI of a glioblastoma and
(B) the same lesion shown with
contrast medium enhancement.s

catheters with reservoirs placed under the skin. In addition radiation can be inserted
into the tumor using a gliasite radiation balloon.

Nursing Implications
Anesthesia

Anesthesia can be general with intubation or an awake craniotomy can be performed.
If the procedure is performed with the patient in the sitting position, the possibility of
air embolism must be anticipated. Air embolism occurs when there is a negative pressure
gradient between the right atrium and the venous sinuses or the diploetic veins.
Entrainment of air can also occur from the soft tissue, bone edge, or dural edge. Usually, air embolisms are detected by an ultrasonic Doppler probe placed over the heart.
A turbulent sound indicates the presence of the embolism. A right atrial catheter must
also be in place so that the embolism can be aspirated from the heart.

Special Considerations

When the patient is in the sitting position, the scrub person must be constantly
alert to the potential for air embolism. If this occurs, an Asepto syringe of irrigation
fluid and sloppy wet sponges should immediately be passed to the surgeon to occlude
the site of air entry. The scrub person should have two Asepto syringes so that at least

one can always be full of irrigation solution. If the entry site is in bone the area is closed with bone wax.

When operating on the posterior fossa the irrigation fluid should be body temperature or slightly warmer. Cold irrigation on the brain stem could cause cardiac arrest.

Position

The position of the patient is determined by the location of the lesion. The supine position is the standard position for most lesions, with the patient's head secured in the 3-pin headrest.

Equipment and Supplies

Standard craniotomy instruments are required along with microsurgical instruments, microscope, ultrasonic aspirator, navigation system, and neuro monitoring.

Establishing and Maintaining the Sterile Field

Standard craniotomy is performed as discussed previously. The lesion is located and it is resected by use of suction, bipolar electrosurgery, various dissectors, cup forceps, or the carbon dioxide laser or ultrasonic aspirator. The tumor bed is irrigated to ensure all bleeding points have been eliminated. At this time wet x-ray-detectable cotton balls may be inserted into the tumor bed to achieve hemostasis through direct pressure. During the entire procedure, the assistant should retract the brain as gently as possible to avoid unnecessary damage to normal tissue, assist with hemostasis, and irrigate as necessary.

Drugs and Solutions

Glidel wafers are a chemotherapy used intraoperatively. They are placed in the bed of a resected glioblastoma tumor. Gliadel wafers must be kept frozen until implantation time and precautions in handling the wafers must be followed. Double gloves must be worn and the wafers should only be handled with instruments. The outer gloves should be disposed of into a biohazard container.

Physiological Monitoring

A Doppler probe is indicated if the patient is in the sitting position.

Specimens and Culture

Frozen section analysis is indicated when a definitive diagnosis of the tumor is required.

Postprocedure Care

Care must be exercised when removing the head from the 3-pin headrest. This is a joint effort between the surgeon, anesthesia provider, and the circulator. The transfer to the bed must be organized with careful consideration to all the lines, catheters, and drainage bags.

Potential Complications

Potential complications include bleeding, seizures, fever, cerebral edema, hydrocephalus, neurological deficits, and infection.

THE SPINE

Conservative Care

Eighty percent of the US population will be affected by back pain some time in their life. The goal for patients with back pain is relief of pain and restoration of function; the sooner the better. Most back pain can be relieved with total bed rest, anti-inflammatory medication, physical therapy, and patient education to prevent additional injury. Conservative treatment can last up to six months (Brady & Jackson, 2005).

Indications

As a person ages, changes in the spine occur that make it more vulnerable to injury. Loss of fluid content of the nucleus pulposus and weakening of the annulus fibrosus and the posterior longitudinal ligaments produce a situation in which the disc may herniate into the spinal canal when an unusual stress is placed on the spine (Hickey, 2002). Herniations occur most commonly in the lumbar spine and cervical spine. Herniation in the less flexible thoracic spine is uncommon. Herniation may be caused by trauma (from lifting, falls, and sneezing) or degenerative diseases such as osteoarthritis and ankylosing spondylitis.

Herniation of the disc causes pain. The pain is due to pressure on the nerve root. If pain relief is not achieved by conservative therapy (rest, bracing, physical therapy, medication) the herniation is removed surgically.

Surgical Options

There are several surgical options for the treatment of lumbar disc disease. In addition to the long-standing traditional approach of lumbar laminectomy with discectomy, choices include microdiscectomy, percutaneous discectomy, and minimally invasive procedures.

Microdiscectomy involves a 1-inch (2.5 cm) incision; the microscope is used for visualization and illumination of the anatomical structures, allowing a smaller incision and more precise dissection. Less tissue disruption results in less postprocedure pain, quicker recovery, and earlier hospital discharge, usually within 2 days of surgery.

Percutaneous discectomy is done endoscopically to remove a segment of a bulging disc. The procedure is done under local anesthesia with some sedation. The patient must be alert enough to assess the radicular pain in the leg. Under fluoroscopic control a trocar is inserted into the disc capsule. A cutting probe is then advanced to excise the disc and aspirate it, relieving the pressure on the spinal nerve root (Phillips, 2007).

Lumbar laminectomy with discectomy involves a midline vertical incision over the lumbar spine (4–6 inches long) and removal of vertebral lamina, ligaments, and disc material.

The patient who is scheduled for a laminectomy has usually been through a series of conservative treatments before being scheduled for surgery. The major symptom of lumbar disc disease is pain in the lower back, which may radiate down one or both legs. Normal posture is modified to compensate for the pathological alterations: a normal lumber lordosis is absent, and lumbar scoliosis occurs with spasms of the paravertebral muscles (Hickey, 2002). Because pain is often aggravated by movement, the patient moves stiffly, slowly, and cautiously. There may be some motor weakness on the affected side, numbness and paresthesias of the leg and foot, and diminished or absent reflexes in the knee and ankle.

Lumbar disc surgery may be accompanied by spinal fusion if several levels are involved. Fusion is performed to provide stability of the area. A bone graft may be taken from the iliac crest or cadaver bone is used and placed between the vertebrae. Movement is limited to prevent injury to the spinal cord and nerve roots.

Laminectomy

Indications

If conservative treatment fails and other modalities fail to provide pain relief and function then surgery may be indicated.

Laminectomy is removal of part of the laminae, ligaments, facet joints, and any osteophytes to free up space for the nerve. The goal of this surgery is to relieve leg pain and a return to preinjury activities of daily living. This procedure does not usually provide immediate relief. (Harvey, 2005). A laminectomy can also be performed for insertion of a pain management infusion pump or a spinal cord stimulator.

Nursing Implications

ANESTHESIA

General anesthesia is induced and the patient is intubated on the transfer stretcher. When all lines are secured the patient is transferred to the surgical table in the prone position.

POSITION

The patient is placed in the prone position, prepped, and draped. One hip may be slightly elevated to position for graft procurement.

ESTABLISHING AND MAINTAINING THE STERILE FIELD

After prepping and draping an x-ray is taken to verify and mark the correct surgical level; this may be repeated after surgical exposure has been created. Discectomy is the removal of part of the disc that has herniated and is pressing on the spinal cord or a nerve root. If a microdiscectomy is done a microscope will be needed.

EQUIPMENT AND SUPPLIES

A high-speed drill such as the Midas Rex will be needed along with laminectomy instruments. Portable x-ray equipment will be utilized to identify the correct surgical level.

DRUGS AND SOLUTIONS

Antibiotics, Thrombin, Gelfoam, and Flo-seal are standard drug-related supplies.

SPECIMENS AND CULTURES

Disc material will need to be retrieved as it is removed and saved as a specimen.

CLOSURE

The wound will be closed in layers and a dressing applied.

Spinal Fusion

Spinal fusion is one of the commonly performed surgeries on the lumbar spine for degenerative disorders (Bono & Lee, 2004). Fusion usually accompanies a decompression discectomy. Spinal fusion accounts for almost 50% of all back surgery in the United States (Spinal Fusion Under the Microscope, 2007). Spinal fusion is indicated for herniated disc, degenerative disc, degenerative disc disease, degenerative spondylolisthesis, spinal stenosis, and revision of previously failed back surgery (Brady & Jackson, 2005). The spine is realigned anatomically and then fused to prevent vertebral movement (Harvey, 2005). Fusion requires bone grafts; either autograft, from self, or allograft, from a cadaver. Autografts historically have been take n from the iliac crest. Most patients complain more about the pain from the graft site than from the spinal incision. A wedge-shaped bone graft is inserted between vertebrae. After the bone graft is in place, screws, plates, and/or rods are used to stabilize the vertebrae. A spinal fusion will limit the mobility in the area and the patient may feel a permanent stiffness.

A spinal fusion can be accomplished from an anterior approach or a posterior approach.

The advantages of anterior lumbar surgery include: back muscles and nerves are not disturbed so recovery time is shorter; the fusion area is in the anterior spine, which leads to better fusion results (Brady & Jackson, 2005).

Nursing Implications
ANESTHESIA

Lumbar laminectomy with fusion is performed under general anesthesia. The major anesthetic concern is that the necessary positioning does not compromise the respiratory process. Airway and breathing are compromised by the prone position (Phillips, 2007). Blood loss from the procedure is usually minimal.

POSITION

The conventional position, when undergoing a lumbar laminectomy with fusion, is prone. The torso is supported on chest rolls or a Wilson frame. Some surgeons prefer to position the patient in knee-chest position or the lateral position for a unilateral laminectomy. The Wilson frame is an arch-shaped frame that supports the patient's torso on two longitudinal pads extending from the clavicle to the pelvis. The frame serves the same purpose as chest rolls (ie, to permit adequate expansion of the chest and abdominal excursion). The angle of the arch can be adjusted with a crank to provide optimal visualization of the surgical site. When placing the frame on the bed, the nurse should ensure that it is positioned so that the crank is extended over the side of the bed and is freely movable. The frame should be in the lowest position before the patient is transferred to it. The frame should be covered with cloth to protect the patient from direct contact with it. Each side of the frame must be covered separately to avoid a sling effect, which can compromise respiration and abdominal excursion.

In the absence of a frame, chest rolls are used. These may be commercially available rolls of foam or silicone gel material, or sheets or bath blankets may be rolled to an appropriate size and secured with tape. Gel rolls offer superior protection over standard rolled linen; however, the gel rolls have a tendency to slide out from under the patient and precautions should be taken to secure them. Any roll should extend from the level of the clavicle to the pelvis and be firm enough to elevate the patient's chest off the bed. The surgeon may wish to use another roll transversely under the pelvis, in addition to the chest supports. This helps to decrease pressure on the vena cava.

The nurse should also prepare the bed with a doughnut headrest for the head, padding for the knees, and pillows or a gel roll to go under the lower legs. Two padded armboards are also needed. Pneumatic compression devices should be applied to the leg. This promotes venous return during the surgery. The patient is anesthetized on the transport stretcher. A Foley catheter is usually not necessary because this is a fairly short procedure. The eyes are protected with eye pads taped in place.

The patient care team turns the patient onto the surgical table. The anesthesia provider controls the head and the airway. At least one team member stands at each side and one at the feet. More help may be necessary for a large patient. At a signal from the anesthesia provider, the patient is turned slowly and smoothly. The anesthesia provider is responsible to support the head and neck along with the endotracheal tube during the transfer to the surgical table. The transfer stretcher/bed is removed. The patient's arms are pronated on padded armboards, with the elbows flexed and the lower arms parallel to the body. Care must be taken not to overextend the shoulder. Pillows or a gel roll is placed under the lower legs and are adjusted to prevent plantar flexion of the feet, and the toes should be free from pressure. Pedal pulses should be palpated to ensure that knee flexion is not compromising arterial circulation. Gel-filled doughnuts are placed under the knees to relieve pressure points on the patella. The head is turned to one side with a doughnut headrest, preventing pressure on the ear. There must be no pressure on the eyes. The breasts and the male genital are checked to confirm that these areas are not compressed. A thermal blanket may be placed over the legs. A safety strap is secured over the upper thighs.

Establishing and Maintaining the Sterile Field

Before preparing the skin, the nurse may apply a plastic drape with an adhesive edge over the buttocks to isolate that area from the surgical site. Preparation includes the lumbar area and extends to the lower scapulae, to the gluteal fold, and laterally on the torso to the supporting devices. After the patient is prepared, the scrub person hands the surgeon a folded towel to blot the area to be incised. A marking pen or scalpel is used to mark the incisional line while landmarks are still visible. The incisional line may be cross-hatched for ease of approximation at closure. A plastic incise drape may be used, followed by four towels to square off the incision area. These are secured with towel clips or staples. A fenestrated sheet or square draping is used next. The sheet is attached to intravenous poles at the head of the patient for access by the anesthetist. The Mayo stand is placed over the patient's legs.

Equipment and Supplies

Supplies needed for the procedure include laminectomy instruments, a marking pen, a self-retaining spinal retractor, curettes, Cobb elevators, a plastic incise drape, patties, Gelfoam, and bipolar and monopolar electrosurgery generators. Some surgeons use a Taylor retractor with a rolled gauze bandage attached to the handle for retraction. The end of the bandage is dropped off the field and weighted with hanging weights used for traction. Power equipment is usually not needed for a laminectomy. If the laminectomy is to be accompanied by spinal fusion, additional bone instruments, straight and curved osteotomes, and gouges are needed.

During the procedure, the surgeon uses a variety of rongeurs and punches. Each time that material is removed, the surgeon holds out the instrument to be cleaned. The scrub person should be ready with a damp sponge to remove any debris from the instrument as the surgeon holds it. The nurse must also be aware that some of this material is a specimen that needs to be removed from the sponge and placed in the appropriate container.

SPECIMENS AND CULTURES

Specimens generated in this procedure are disc material and ligamentum flavum. Cultures normally are not taken.

LABORATORY AND DIAGNOSTIC STUDIES

Diagnostic tests to prove disc herniation are myelogram, computed tomography, and magnetic resonance imaging.

Procedure

During the procedure, radiographs should be anticipated for disc localization. A spinal needle is inserted into the disc space, and a lateral radiograph is taken. The x-ray cassette is either suspended on a Mayo stand with adhesive tape and positioned at the side of the patient outside the sterile field or placed in a sterile cassette cover and propped along the patient's side within the sterile field. The radiograph confirms that the surgeon is dissecting at the correct level.

INCISION AND EXPOSURE

After the patient is prepared and draped, the incision is made vertically in the midline. Finger pressure on gauze sponges provides hemostasis while coagulation of vessels is performed. Cutting current is used with the electrosurgical pencil to incise fascia and muscle. The muscles are dissected from the lamina and spinous processes are packed back by pushing opened gauze sponges around the bony structures with Cobb elevators. When hemostasis is achieved, the sponges are removed and a self-retaining retractor is placed.

DETAILS

Rongeurs are used to remove lamina, the ligamentum flavus is incised with a No. 15 blade on a No. 7 knife handle, and a window is created. Surgical patty strips are placed into this incision for protection and hemostasis. The nerve root and dura are retracted. Hemostasis of epidural vessels is performed with bipolar coagulation. Disc rongeurs are used to remove disc material. The area is irrigated and hemostasis in ensured. All sponges are removed and accounted for.

CLOSURE

The wound is closed in layers, and a pressure dressing is applied. Care must be taken in the transfer of the patient to their bed. Adequate help is needed in the transfer from the prone position to the patient's bed.

Postprocedure Care

After the procedure the patient remains in bed for only a short time. Many patients ambulate during the first 24 hours after surgery, and early ambulation is a factor in reducing the length of hospital stay. The majority of patients are discharged within a week of the surgery.

Potential Complications

Complications that may occur include pain, numbness, impaired muscle function, incontinence, impotence, urinary retention, and CSF leak.

Vertebralplasty/Kyphoplasty

There are over 700,000 osteoporotic vertebral compression fractures each year in the United States. Vertebral compression fractures produce modest to severe pain and loss of vertebral height. Vertebral compression fractures occur when the load placed on the spine exceeds the ability of the bone within the vertebral body to support it. The combination of bone loss and vertebral disc degeneration in older adults weakens the spinal column. (Hanna & Letizia, 2007). Conservative treatment includes bed rest and pain management; healing takes place in six to twelve weeks. Conservative management is not successful in 15–20% of the patients because of the inability to tolerate the pain and prolonged bedrest (Shen & Kim, 2006).

Vertebralplasty and Kyphoplasty are both treatments for vertebral compression fracture. Both involve the percutaneous injection of bone cement into the fracture site. Kyphoplasty involves an additional step; a deflated balloon is placed into the fracture site and inflated. The cavity created is filled with bone cement. This additional step restores vertebral height. The discussion that follows will be for Kyphoplasty; however, setting up for a vertebralplasty will be almost identical.

Vertebralplasty is a percutaneous injection of bone cement in the area of a vertebral compression fracture. The cement hardens and stabilizes the fracture. The procedure does not restore normal vertebral height. The procedure can be done as a same-day surgery procedure.

Kyphoplasty is also a treatment for vertebral compression fractures. A percutaneous balloon is inserted into the fracture area. The balloon is inflated creating a cavity. The cavity is filled with bone cement. Stabilization of the fracture along with vertebral height is restored. Kyphoplasty is a minimally invasive procedure for the treatment of vertebral compression fractures. The procedure can reduce back pain, improve back function and quality of life, and restore vertebral body height. No more than three vertebral fractures can be reduced at the same time because of the potential from microembolization of cement and bone marrow (Hanna & Letizia, 2007).

The patient under general anesthesia is placed in the prone position with appropriate positioning devices and gel padding. Using fluoroscope imaging through a 5 mm incision a working cannula is placed through the pedicle and a deflated balloon is guided into the fractured vertebral body. The balloon is inflated, with contrast medium reducing the fracture and elevating the superior endplate. A bilateral approach is utilized using two balloons. Fluoroscopic images are obtained and when the fracture has been reduced the balloons are deflated and removed. This process created a void that serves as a repository for the bone cement. Bone cement is injected under constant and low pressure. Approximately 3.5 to 8.5 mL of cement is injected into the vertebral body. The procedure takes less than one hour per fracture. Pain is significantly decreased and activities of daily living are reported to improve after the procedure (Hanna & Letizia, 2007).

Anterior Cervical Decompression and Fusion
Conservative Treatment

Conservative treatment consists of rest, avoidance of flexion of the area, use of a cervical collar, analgesics, nonsteroidal anti-inflammatory medication, and physical therapy. For those who do not respond, surgery may be indicated.

Indications

Anterior cervical discectomy and fusion is used to treat degenerative cervical disc disease that is not relieved by conservative therapy. The intervertebral disc accounts for 25% of the height of the cervical vertebral column. As disc disease progresses, it loses water content and narrows the disc space. Many people also develop osteophytes and they can compress or irritate the cervical nerve root. Herniated discs protrude into fissures which develop in the annulus. If this occurs, it can cause pain and numbness. The degenerative process can also cause spinal stenosis (narrowing of the spinal canal) which compresses the spinal cord or vessels supplying the spinal cord resulting in cervical myelopathy (Cherry, 2002). Symptoms include numbness, weakness, and clumsiness of the arms and weakness of the legs.

Anterior cervical discectomy and fusion has proven to be successful in the treatment of symptoms caused by cervical degenerative disease. The procedure has a high success rate and a low rate of complications (Cherry, 2002).

Nursing Implications

The anterior approach offers the advantage of a direct approach of the disc space without removal of lamina. The disc is removed and the space is occupied with a bone graft, a cage made of carbon fiber, titanium, plastic composite, or an artificial disc. The bone graft can be an allograft or an autograft.

ANESTHESIA

The anesthesia provider will need to assess any limitations the patient has in jaw and neck movement in anticipation of intubating the patient. Fiberoptic intubation may be required.

POSITION

The patient is transferred to the surgical table and after induction of anesthesia the patient is positioned. The head is placed in a doughnut made of foam or gel. A rolled sheet may be placed under the shoulders to hyperextend the neck. Arms are placed at the patient's side with the palmer surface of the hands against their body. The arms are then secured with a draw sheet. The shoulders are then pulled down toward the feet and secured with wide three-inch tape. This aids in fluoroscopic visualization of the surgical site.

ESTABLISHING AND MAINTAINING THE STERILE FIELD

Prepping and draping are completed, time out is done, and an incision is made. Dissection is initiated with hemostasis controlled with the use of monopolar and bipolar electrosurgery. Dissection will continue until exposure of the disc space is completed. The disc level will be confirmed with an x-ray. Disc will be removed with a pituitary rongeur, curettes, and Kerrison rongeurs. A distraction device will be utilized that creates visualization of the disc space, removal of the disc, and preparation of the implant device. The sterile draped microscope will be moved into position for better visualization of the intervertebral space. Remaining disc will be removed and the space will be explored. Hemostasis will be controlled with Thrombin-soaked Gelfoam sponges, bone wax, and saline-moistened patties. A high-speed drill will be used to prepare the space for the implant (Cherry, 2002).

EQUIPMENT AND SUPPLIES

A warming blanket is placed over the patient to aid in maintaining the patient's normal body temperature. The x-ray equipment is moved into place and images are obtained to verify the correct surgical level and ensure a quality image can be obtained. Monopolar and bipolar electrosurgery is essential. Standard cervical instrumentation will be required along with a microscope, vertebral body distraction system, plating system, drill, self-retaining retractors, C-arm type fluoroscopy unit, lead aprons, fiberoptic intubation setup, and an implant for the removed disc.

Implants

Traditionally a bone graft has been used; either from the patient's iliac crest or from cadaver bone. The iliac crest donor site (autograft) is a source of postprocedure pain and discomfort for most patients. The cadaver bone (allograft) comes in many shapes and sizes and it can be trimmed if needed.

Synthetic material may be used in place of a bone graft. Cages can be made of carbon fiber, titanium, and composite plastic, polyetheretherketone (PEEK). The synthetic material offers immediate biochemical support and elimination of local side effects at the donor site. The cages have an open space in the middle for packing with demineralized bone or synthetic bone grafts. These bone grafts have demonstrated effective fusion without complications (Kahraman, Daneyemez, Kayali, Beduk, & Akay, 2006). On newer implants plating is optional. The advantages of using cages are a smaller incision, less operative pain, shorter operative pain, and shorter hospital stays.

PEEK
Polyetheretherketone

After the appropriate implant has been selected it is put into position, usually with a bone impactor, fluoroscopic images will be taken to verify correct placement and alignment. The vertebral body distracter is removed and any bleeding will be controlled. The correct size plate will be selected and holes drilled into the vertebral body for the screws. Most screws are self-tapping. The plate is secured in place with the screws. The plate provides additional stability at the surgical site by preventing extrusion of the implant during the early healing stages of the fusion (Cherry, 2002). Final x-rays are taken to confirm the position of the hardware and the implant.

Closure

The wound is irrigated with an antibiotic solution or normal saline. The wound is closed in layers and counts are completed and reported to the surgeon. Dressings are applied and a cervical collar may be applied. The type and size should be determined long before closing so it is available at the end of the procedure. The neurosurgeon may evaluate the patient for movement and strength in all of their extremities and evaluate them for neurological deficits before they are moved to PACU.

Postoperative Care

The patient should be monitored for neurological deficits and for airway constriction from postprocedure edema.

Potential Complications

Complications can include hoarseness, which is usually temporary; however, it can be permanent; dysphasia, which is temporary; wound infection; injury to the spinal cord or nerve roots; dura tears; non-unions; graft extrusion; and screws that loosen (Cherry, 2002).

Posterior Discectomy

The posterior cervical approach is used for laminectomy for decompression, tumor removal, cordectomy, discectomy, and fusion. If a posterior discectomy is performed, only the extruded disc fragments are removed. The annulus is not entered (Hickey, 2002).

Equipment and Supplies

Three-pin headrest with traction pulley and weights, fluoroscopic x-ray equipment, a high-speed drill such as the Midas Rex, standard cervical laminectomy instruments including retractors and monopolar and bipolar electrosurgery are commonly used equipment. A warming blanket should be utilized to maintain the patient's normal temperature. Compression pneumatic stocking pump and sleeves should also be used. If a postprocedure cervical collar is going to be used, the type and size should be procured.

Drugs and Solutions

Antibiotics, both IV and for irrigation, topical Thrombin, and Gelfoam.

The patient is brought into the OR and anesthesia induction will be on the transfer stretcher. If the patient has limited movement in the neck, fiberoptic intubation may be required. While the patient is still in the supine position, leads for neurologic monitoring will be put in place. Positioning devices will need to be verified and be available before induction on anesthesia. A 3-pin headrest may be used with or without traction. The patient is transferred to the prone position with careful attention to the alignment of the head and neck. Appropriate positioning aids will be added; foam blocks under the head/face, gel rolls under the torso, gel doughnuts under the knees, and rolls under the ankles to relieve pressure off the feet. For male patients the genitalia will be checked so they are pressure-free and for females the breasts will need to be checked to determine they have not been compromised. A final check is made to pad all bony prominences. The arms will be placed at the sides and secured with a draw sheet and a safety strap is applied.

X-rays are obtained and the correct level is identified and the incision site is marked. The skin is prepped and the area is draped. A midline incision is made and soft tissue dissection is completed. The correct disc level is identified with an x-ray. Hemostasis is accomplished with both monopolar and bipolar electrosurgery, moistened patties, and Thrombin-soaked Gelfoam. A laminectomy is performed using a high-speed drill, rongeurs, and Kerrisons. Disc material is removed with pituitary rongeurs and curettes. If a fusion is going to be performed, an allograft or autograft will be needed and instrumentation for plating. (Ferrara, 2007) The wound is irrigated with antibiotic saline. Counts are completed as the wound is closed. Sutures or staples can be used for skin. Dressings are applied and the cervical collar is applied. The patient is transferred to the supine position onto the patient's bed.

Artificial Disc

Artificial disc replacement is now available and is an alternative to discectomy and fusion. Artificial intervertebral disc replacement involves removing a disc through an anterior approach and replacing it with synthetic one. What makes this modality appealing is it replaces the traditional anterior discectomy and fusion. Artificial disc replacement relieves pain while preserving range of motion, something a fusion cannot do (Artificial Intervertebral Disc Replacement for Symptomatic Cervical Disc Disease: What's the State of Evidence?, 2008). Artificial disc replacement preserves spinal motion but also recreates the natural function of the disc. In traditional fusions, they may fail and the bone does not heal or fuse. Immobilization of the fused spinal segment can cause increased stress at adjacent levels; some studies indicate it occurs in 36% of all fusions (Bajnoczy, 2005). The benefits of artificial discs include: it restores the natural kinetic motion of the spine, maintains disc height, and provides stability without causing adjacent segment disease. The artificial discs contain two metallic endplates with a free-floating polyethylene core. Some of the endplates have an osteoconductive coating to stimulate bone growth and aid in permanent fixation. The challenge has been developing a long-term device that will not wear out, loosen, or be expelled (Bajnoczy, 2005). Time and multiple studies will answer those questions.

Resorbable Anterior Cervical Plates

Resorbable anterior cervical plates are available as a replacement for traditional titanium cervical plates. Theoretical advantages include better postprocedure images and since the titanium plate is only needed until the fusion takes place, a resorbable plate may offer some advantages. Recent studies indicate the use of a resorbable plate may result in a loss of some of the advantages of using titanium plating (Bindal, Ghosh, & Foldi, 2007). New to the market, time and further research will indicate the advantages of these plates.

CONCLUSION

The challenges in neurosurgical nursing will be in keeping up with technology. Advances in technology will improve surgical outcomes. Remaining on the cutting edge of technology is paramount in providing the best treatment options for neurosurgical patients.

REFERENCES

1. Artificial intervertebral disc replacement for symptomatic cervical disc disease: What's the state of evidence? (2008, January). Supplement to *OR Manager*, 24, (1).

2. Bajnoczy, S. (2005). Artificial disc replacement-evolutionary treatment for degenerative disc disease. *AORN*, 82, 191–206.

3. Bearden, B.G., Conrad, B.P., Horodyski, M., & Rechtine, G.R. (2007). Motion in the unstable cervical spine: comparison of manual turning and use of the Jackson table in prone positioning. *Journal of Neurosurgery Spine*, 7, 161–164.

4. Bindal, R.K., Ghosh, S., & Foldi B. (2007). Resorbable anterior cervical plates for single-level degenerative disease. *Operative Neurosurgery* 61; 305–308.

5. Bono, C.M. & Lee, C.K. (2004). Critical analysis of tends in fusion for degenerative disc disease over the past 20 years: Influence of technique on fusion rate and clinical outcome. *Spine*, 29, 455–463.

6. Bowen, B. (2007). Orthopedics. In J.C. Rothrock, *Alexander's Care of the Patient in Surgery* (pp. 704–798). St. Louis, MO: Mosby.

7. Brady, S. & Jackson, S. (2005). Anterior lumbar interbody fusion-advances in spinal fusion technology. *AORN*, 82, 817–823.

8. Cherry, C. (2002), Anterior cervical discectomy and fusion for cervical disease. *AORN*, 76, 996–1008.

9. Devlin, V.J. & Schwartz, D.M. (2007). Intraoperative neurophysiologic monitoring during spinal surgery. *Journal of American Academy of Orthopedic Surgeons*, 15, 549–560.

10. Drummond, J.C. & Patel, P.M. (2000). Neurosurgical Anesthesia. In R.D. Miller, *Anesthesia* (pp. 1855–1899). Philadelphia, PA: Churchill Livingstone.

11. Epstein, N.E. (2005), Intermittent pneumatic compression stocking prophylaxis against deep vein thrombosis in anterior cervical spinal surgery: a prospective efficacy study in 200 patients and literature review. *Spine*, 30, 2538–2543.

12. Ferrara, D.L. (2007). Neurosurgery. In J.C. Rothrock, *Alexander's Care of the Patient in Surgery* (pp. 799–862). St. Louis, MO: Mosby.

13. Gobbi, D.G., Comeau, R.M., & Peters, T.M. (2000). Ultrasound/MRI overlay with image warping for neurosurgery. In *Lecture Notes in Computer Science* (pp. 106–114). Retrieved January 10, 2008, from http://www.bic.mni.mcgill.ca/research/groups/igns/US/us_home.html.

14. Hanna, J. & Letizia, M. (2007). A treatment for Osteoporotic vertebral compression fractures. *Orthopedic Nursing*, 126, 342–346.

15. Harvey, C.V. (2005). Spinal surgery patient care. *Orthopedic Nursing*, 24(6), 426–440.

16. Hickey, J.V. (2002). *The Clinical Practice of Neurological and Neurosurgical Nursing*. Philadelphia, PA: J.B. Lippincott.

17. Kahraman, S., Daneyemez, M., Kayali, H., Beduk, A., & Akay, M. (2006). Polyetheretherketone (Peek) cages for cervical interbody replacement: clinical experience. *Turkish Neurosurgery*, 16, 120–123.

18. Manna, E.M., Ibraheim, O.A., Samarkandi, A.H., Alotaibi, W.M., & Elwatidy, S.M. (2005). The effect of prone position on respiratory mechanics during spinal surgery. *Middle East Journal of Anesthesiology*, 18: 623–630.

19. Palese, A. & Infami, S. (2006). The experiences of nurses who participate in awake craniotomy procedures, *AORN Journal*, 84: 811–826.

20. Phillips, N. (2007). *Berry & Kohn's Operating Room Technique* (11th ed.). St. Louis, MO: Mosby.

21. Price, P. (2007). Diagnostic Procedures. In J.C. Rothrock, *Alexander's Care of the Patient in Surgery* (pp. 277–290). St. Louis, MO: Mosby.

22. Price, P. & Price, B.D. (2001). In Caruthers, B.L. & Price, P. *Surgical Technology for the Surgical Technologist* (pp. 824–880). Clifton Park, NY: Delmar Thomson Learning.

23. Rigamonti, A., Gemma, M., Rocca, A., Messina, M., & Beretta, L. (2005) Prone versus knee-chest position for microdiscectomy: a prospective randomized study of intra-abdominal pressure intraoperative bleeding. *Spine*, 30, 1918–1923.

24. Robinson, J.B., Sun, C.C., Bodurka-Bevers, D., Im, D.D., & Rosenshein, N.B. (2000). Cavitational ultrasonic surgical aspiration for treatment of vaginal intraepithelial neoplasia. *Gynecologic Oncology*, 78, 235–241.

25. Sala, F., Beltramello, A., & Gerosa, M. (2007). Neuroprotective role of neurophysiological monitoring during endovascular procedures in the brain and spinal cord. *Neurophysiology Clinical*, 37, 415–421.

26. Sala, F., Manganotti, P., Tramontano, V., Bricolo, A., & Gerosa, M. (2007). Monitoring of motor pathways during brain stem surgery: what we have achieved and what we still missing? *Neurophysiology Clinical*, 37, 399–406.

27. Shen, M. & Kim, Y. (2006). Vertebroplasty and Kyphoplasty: Treatment techniques for managing osteoporotic vertebral compression fractures. *Bulletin of NYU Hospital for Joint Disease*, 64(4), 106–113.

28. Spinal fusion under the microscope. (2007, March). *OR Manager*, 23, 5 & 7.

29. Tanner, J., Moncaster, K., & Woodings, D. (2007). Preoperative hair removal: a systematic review. *Journal of Perioperative Practice*, 17, 118–121, 124–132.

30. Wagner, M. & Stenger, K. (2005).Unruptured intercranial aneurysms: using evidence and outcomes to guide patient teaching. *Critical Care Nursing Quarterly*, 28, 341–354.

31. Weinzieri, M.R., Reinacher, P., Gilsbach, J.M., & Rohde, V. (2007). Combined motor and somatosensory evoked potentials for intraoperative monitoring: intra- and postoperative data in a series of 69 operations. *Neurosurgery*, 30, 109–116.

32. Wright, I. (2007). Cerebra aneurysm—treatment and perioperative nursing care. *AORN*, 85, 1172–1182.

CHAPTER 27

Urological Surgery

Jason Bitner

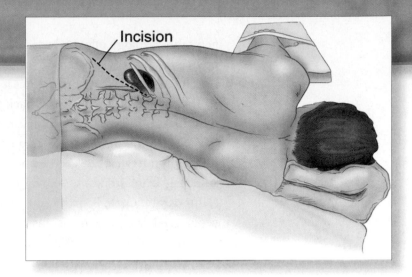

Incision

INTRODUCTION

This chapter describes urological procedures as they pertain to the nursing and the operative and invasive procedure team. Content includes anatomy of the genitourinary system for the male and female, a discussion of the management and care of the patient undergoing a urological operative procedure, and the role of the nursing staff, descriptions of various procedures and urological instruments, and potential complications.

A team approach is essential in carrying out urological surgery. The nursing team plays a major role in the care of the patient before, during, and after a urological operative or invasive procedure. Key components of this role include assessment and planning for each patient. Safe positioning often presents a challenge, particularly for elderly and compromised patients having procedures in the lateral and lithotomy positions. See Chapter 8 for in-depth information concerning patient positioning. As with all operative and invasive procedures, the nurse advocates for the patient during the procedure. The nurse provides and directs patient care and ensures that nursing care team members correctly prepare and operate the sophisticated equipment associated with urological surgery such as lasers, ureteroscopes, and lithotripsy instruments. After the procedure, the nurse evaluates the patient's response to the nursing care given and provides education that assists the patient in the rehabilitation process.

Urological surgery investigates and manages diseases of the urological system in both males and females to include diseases and malformations of the adrenal glands, kidneys, ureters, bladder, male genitalia (penis, urethra, prostate gland, and scrotum), and female

Chapter Contents

genitalia. Urology offers a broad spectrum of treatment modalities, which include open procedures, endoscopic procedures, laser therapy, lithotripsy, and robotics, which have made open procedures less invasive.

The practice of urology goes back to antiquity. Illustrated and written documents describe procedures such as circumcision and lithotomy. Circumcision is present in Egyptian hieroglyphs depicting circumcision. Ancient specialists practiced lithotomy. Hippocrates, however, admonished, "I will not use the knife, even upon those suffering from stones, but I will leave this to those who are trained in this craft" (Hippocratic Oath, Fourth Century B.C.E.). Since that time, urological surgery has progressed from circumcisions and lithotomies to a specialty that encompasses a wide range of diseases and procedures to include operative intervention for trauma to the genitourinary system and cancer therapy. Surgery provides solutions for many congenital abnormalities that affect the urinary tract. The past 20 years have also brought about dramatic changes in the approach to stone disease with the evolution of equipment such as the extracorporeal shock wave lithotriptor and sophisticated endoscopic and laser equipment. In addition, the urologist manages and treats complications involving the bladder and the ureters that may result from standard surgical procedures on adjacent organs (eg, colon or uterus).

ANATOMY

Abdominal Wall

An operative procedure on the urinary tract requires incisions through the abdominal wall musculature. The abdominal wall, which extends from the rib cage to the bony pelvis, consists of anterior, anterolateral, and posterolateral walls.

Two paired, segmented muscles, surrounded by fascial layers, form the anterior abdominal wall (**Fig. 27.1**). Known as the rectus abdominis muscles, they extend from the pubic crest to fifth, sixth, and seventh ribs, where they insert. A fibrous envelope called the rectus sheath surrounds these muscles. This sheath represents

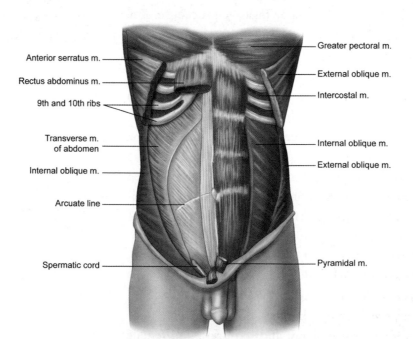

Anterior serratus m.
Rectus abdominus m.
9th and 10th ribs
Transverse m. of abdomen
Internal oblique m.
Arcuate line
Spermatic cord

Greater pectoral m.
External oblique m.
Intercostal m.
Internal oblique m.
External oblique m.
Pyramidal m.

Figure 27.1

Layers of the anterior abdominal wall.

the continuation of the fascial layers from the anterolateral abdominal wall. In the midline, a dense fibrous tissue known as the *linea alba* separates the rectus muscles. Inferiorly, between the umbilicus and the pubic bone on which it inserts, can be found a small triangular muscle, the pyramidal muscle.

Strong muscles make up the flank. The anterolateral abdominal wall consists of the external oblique, internal oblique, and transversus abdominis muscles (see **Fig. 27.1**). The fibers of each muscle course in a different direction to provide strength and support to an area of the body with a great deal of mass and little skeletal support, except for the spine. At the inferior aspect of the anterolateral abdominal wall in the inguinal area exists a communication between the abdominal cavity and the inguinal canal, the internal ring. This represents an area of potential weakness through which hernias may develop. In addition, the spermatic cord in the male and the round ligament in the female course through the internal ring of the inguinal canal. Three muscle groups comprise the posterolateral abdominal wall: deep, superficial, and intermediate. The superficial group consists of the external oblique muscle and latissimus dorsi muscle. The serratus posterior inferior, internal oblique, and sacrospinal muscles comprise the intermediate group. In the deep group are the transversus abdominis, quadratus lumborum, and psoas muscles (**Fig. 27.2**).

After the retroperitoneum has been entered through an incision in the abdominal wall, access to the kidneys, ureters, and adrenal gland is possible by reflecting the peritoneal contents with or without entering the peritoneum.

Each kidney weighs 150 g in the average adult man and 135 g in the woman (**Fig 27.3**). The kidney has a convex lateral border. Near the center of the medial aspect of each kidney is a shallow depression, the renal hilum, through which pass

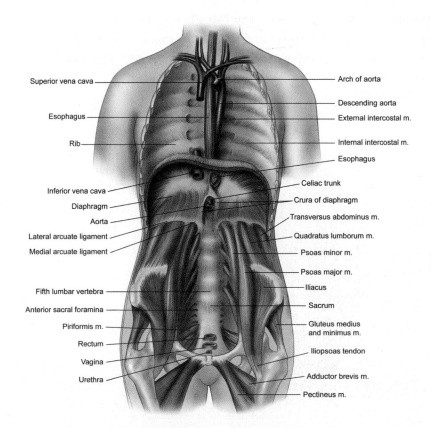

Figure 27.2

Cross-section showing the deep muscles of the abdominal wall (transversus abdominis, quadratus lumborum, and psoas muscles).

Superior vena cava
Esophagus
Rib
Inferior vena cava
Diaphragm
Aorta
Lateral arcuate ligament
Medial arcuate ligament
Fifth lumbar vertebra
Anterior sacral foramina
Piriformis m.
Rectum
Vagina
Urethra

Arch of aorta
Descending aorta
External intercostal m.
Internal intercostal m.
Esophagus
Celiac trunk
Crura of diaphragm
Transversus abdominus m.
Quadratus lumborum m.
Psoas minor m.
Psoas major m.
Iliacus
Sacrum
Gluteus medius and minimus m.
Iliopsoas tendon
Adductor brevis m.
Pectineus m.

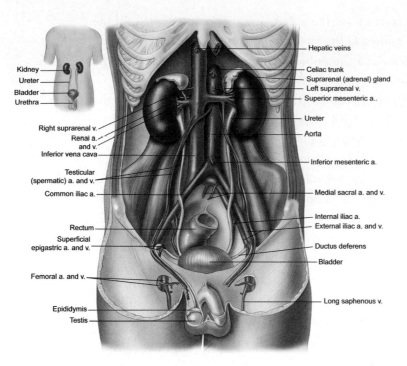

Figure 27.3

Posterior abdominal wall showing the relationship of the urinary system, genital system, and great vessels.

the renal artery, vein, nerves, and lymphatics, and the renal pelvis. The central part of the kidney, the renal sinus, is occupied by the major urine collecting system, the renal pelvis, which branches out into two or three major calyces. These, in turn, branch out into minor calyces. Between the minor calyces are the renal papillae, which are projections of medullary renal tissue. There is a wide variation in the anatomy of the pelvis and the calyces.

A fibroelastic capsule covers the kidney and extends over the organ into the renal sinus to merge with the ends of the calyces. A number of small capsular vessels penetrate the capsule. The renal tissue is divided into medulla and cortex (**Fig. 27.4**). When the kidney is incised and bivalved, one can observe that the medulla is composed of

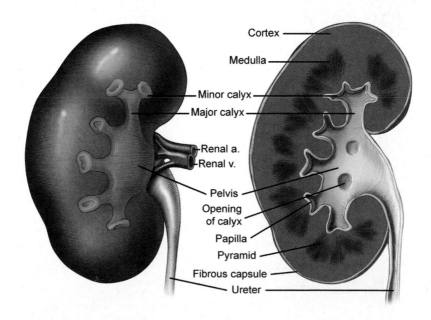

Figure 27.4

Entire and sagittal view showing the relation of calyces to the kidney as a whole.

striated groups of tissue called the renal pyramids. The tops of the pyramids actually form the renal papilla. The striations of the renal pyramids represent the linear arrangement of the renal tubules. The cortex has a more granular appearance. Refer to a standard textbook of nephrology for information concerning microanatomy of the kidney.

In 70% of individuals, there are single left and right renal arteries. Both arise from the aorta, the right renal artery being higher than the left. Before entering the hilum of the kidney, the renal artery usually divides into anterior and posterior divisions. Again, some variation in the anatomy may be found, with some patients having two or more arteries supplying one kidney. Within the kidney, the arteries further branch into interlobar, or arcuate and interlobar, arteries. A single vein drains the kidney into the inferior vena cava. The renal vein is situated anterior to the artery. On the left side, there are two veins draining into the renal vein, one from the adrenal and one from the gonad.

Surrounding the kidney and adrenal gland is a thick layer of fat known as perinephric fat, which in turn is covered by a layer of connective tissue, known as Gerota's fascia. More fatty tissue is found outside Gerota's fascia, further helping to cushion the kidney.

Several major organs are in close proximity to the kidneys. The right lobe of the liver, the descending duodenum, and the hepatic flexure of the colon are adjacent to the right kidney; and on the left, the stomach, the spleen, the splenic flexure of the colon, the pancreas, and the small intestine are close to the kidney.

Adrenal Gland

An adrenal gland lies on top of each kidney (see **Fig. 27.3**). As mentioned earlier, perinephric fat covers the adrenal glands and they appear as thin, bright yellow structures. The right adrenal is triangular, whereas the left one is elongated. Blood supply to the adrenal glands consists of three small arteries. An artery coming from the renal artery supplies the lower portion of the adrenal gland. A branch from the aorta supplies the middle portion, and the upper portion gets a branch from the phrenic artery. The suprarenal veins drain the adrenal glands. The right vein drains into the inferior vena cava and the left vein drains into the left renal vein or the left inferior phrenic vein.

Ureters

Urine produced by the kidney collects into the calyces, which coalesce to form major calyces. These in turn drain into the renal pelvis. The pelvis opens into the ureteropelvic junction. The ureter courses down to the bladder in the retroperitoneum and enters the bladder on its posterior aspect at the ureterovesical junction (**Fig. 27.3**). Much like the small intestine, the ureter is a hollow, muscular tube that uses peristalsis to propel urine toward the bladder. Along its course, the ureter is in close relationship with several organs of importance; on the right, the duodenum, and the body of the pancreas, the ascending colon, and the iliac vessels; and on the left, the tail of the pancreas, the descending colon, and the iliac vessels. In the pelvis, the ureter is in close proximity to the vas deferens and the seminal vesicles in the male and the ovaries, the uterus, and the vagina in the female.

Bladder

The bladder is a hollow, muscular organ that rests anteriorly in the pelvis and is contained in a layer of retroperitoneal tissue (fat and connective tissue). Its role is storing urine and its shape changes as it fills (**Fig. 27.5**). The detrusor muscle forms the bulk of the bladder. Anatomically, the bladder can be described as having two lateral walls, a posterior wall, and a dome. At the base of the bladder, a triangular area can be seen, the trigone. The angles of the triangle are formed by each of the ureteral orifices and the bladder neck. The dome of the bladder is in contact with the peritoneum.

The blood supply to the bladder arises from branches of the internal iliac artery, the superior and inferior vesical arteries, and a number of smaller vessels. Venous drainage occurs through several venous plexuses, which drain into the internal iliac vein. These vessels are found in the lateral and posterior ligaments of the bladder, which are located deep in the pelvis.

Urethra

The urethra extends from the bladder neck to the urinary meatus. In the female, the urethra is short (34 cm) and runs through the layers of the perineum anterior to the vagina. Muscular sphincter mechanisms that ensure urinary continence surround the proximal part of the urethra. The male urethra is substantially longer and can be divided into two segments as it extends from the bladder neck to the tip of the penis (**Fig. 27.5**). The posterior, or membranous urethra, traverses the urogenital diaphragm and is surrounded proximally to the bladder by the prostate gland and by the muscle fibers of the urethral sphincter. The anterior urethra, which extends from the urogenital diaphragm to the urethral meatus, has three parts: bulbar, penile, and glandular. The erectile tissues of the penis surround the anterior urethra. Several structures can be identified within the urethra: the striated sphincter, the verumontanum with the openings of the ejaculatory ducts, and the lobes of the prostate gland.

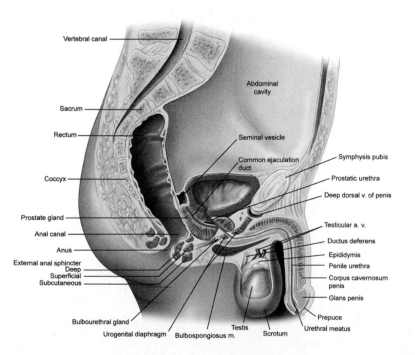

Figure 27.5

Midsagittal section of the male pelvis and external genitalia.

Pelvic Floor Musculature

Several muscles that essentially create a semicircular structure within the pelvic bones form the base of the pelvis or pelvic floor. These muscles include the Ievatorani, which has two main portions, a pubovisceral portion, and a diaphragmatic portion; the coccygeus; the obturator internus; and the piriformis. Laterally, the iliacus muscle covers the greater pelvis.

The Perineal Musculature

The perineum is usually divided into two triangles joined at the base: the urogenital triangle and the anal triangle. Musculature of the urogenital triangle consists of three superficial pairs of muscles: the median bulbocavernosus, the right and left ischiocavernosus, and the superficial transverse perinei.

The deep perineal musculature of the urogenital triangle includes two parts: the deep transverse perineal muscle and the urethral sphincter muscle. The anal triangle consists of a superficial fascia and dense fatty tissue that fills the space surrounding the rectum and the levator and obturator internus muscles.

Male Genital System

The male genital system includes the prostate gland, the seminal vesicles, the vas deferens, the epididymis, and the testes (**Fig. 27.5**). The penis and scrotum are discussed separately. The prostate gland lies at the base of the bladder and can be examined only by digital rectal examination. It is roughly the size of a walnut, and it encircles the urethra. The prostate gland has been thought to be composed of several lobes, which are not readily apparent on cxamination. In the older man, the prostate enlarges by growth of adenomatous tissue (nonmalignant) in the lateral and anterior lobes. The prostate is covered by a dense capsule, and it is fixed to the pelvic floor by investments of parietal fascia and by the endopelvic fascia. The blood supply to the prostate comes from a branch of the inferior vesical artery. The dorsal vein of the penis drains into the plexus of veins (the plexus of Santorini) on the anterior aspect of the prostate. Venous drainage of the prostate occurs via hypogastric veins.

To understand better the anatomy of the male genital system, one can follow the passage of the sperm from the testis to the urethra. After spermatozoa are formed in the testis, they are moved to the epididymis, which is a structure lying alongside and on top of the testis. The epididymis is formed by the convolution of the epididymal duct, which stores sperm. The next structure encountered is the vas deferens, which courses from the scrotum to the prostate through the inguinal canal and the pelvis, posteriorly and then medially. The vas deferens passes between the ureters and the posterior aspect of the bladder. The seminal vesicles are paired structures sitting at the back of the bladder that communicate with the vas deferens. The vas ends at the ejaculatory duct, which opens into the urethra on either side of the verumontanum.

Penis

The penis is composed of erectile tissue organized in three distinct cylindrical bodies: two corpora cavernosa and one corpus spongiosum through which courses the urethra. Each corpus is enclosed in a thick fascia, the tunica albuginea corporis spongiosi. Surrounding this fascia is a fibrous envelope known as Buck's fascia. The corpora end in the glans penis, which is covered by the prepuce. The meatus of the urethra is found at the tip of the glans.

Scrotum

The scrotum contains both testes in separate pouches. The scrotal skin covers the dartos muscles, which in turn cover three thin fascial layers derived from the abdominal wall. The testis measures 4.5 cm in length, 3 cm in width, and 2 cm in thickness and is covered by the tunica albuginea testis. The mass of the testis is made up of coiled seminiferous tubules, where spermatozoa are made. Blood supply to the testis is provided by spermatic vessels that arise from the aorta on the right and the renal artery on the left and course down in the retroperitoneum parallel to the ureters and through the inguinal canal in the spermatic cord to the testes.

INSERTION OF PENILE PROSTHESIS

The first implantation of a prosthesis for male erectile dysfunction was performed in 1936 when Borgoras implanted a rib in the penis to provide rigidity (Culley, 2002). Penile prostheses are divided into two categories: rigid and semi-rigid devices and inflatable prostheses. The rigid and semi-rigid devices are made of two malleable rods. Each rod is composed of silicone elastomer with a metal or alloy core. When the devices are placed within the penis, a permanent degree of rigidity is provided to allow vaginal penetration and sexual intercourse. Self-contained penile prostheses consist of a pump, a cylinder, and a reservoir, all in a single unit. The pump is squeezed just below the head of the penis to fill the cylinder and achieve erection. Inflatable penile prostheses consist of two hollow silcone cylinders, an abdominal reservoir, and a scrotal pump. The pump is squeezed to fill the cylinders and achieve erection. **Figure 27.6** shows the different types of penile prostheses.

The inflatable penile prosthesis consists of several parts: a reservoir, which is placed in the abdomen extra-peritoneally, a pump placed in the scrotum, connecting tubing, and paired cylinders placed within the corporal bodies. A hydraulic mechanism allows the filling of the paired cylinders, which impart tumescence and rigidity to the penis. The patient activates the device to achieve an erection and then deactivates it to achieve a flaccid state.

Indications

Indications for the insertion of a penile prosthesis include organic impotence not amenable to medical treatment and psychogenic impotence in which conventional therapy has failed. Patients who wish to undergo placement of a penile prosthesis must undergo an extensive medical and psychiatric evaluation. They should be

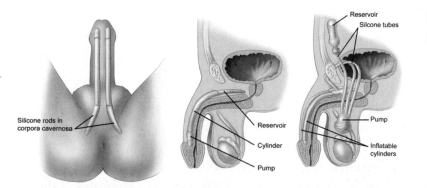

Figure 27.6

Penile prostheses.

informed that normal erectile tissue is destroyed at the time of the procedure to place the corporal rods or cylinder and that they will never be able to attain a normal erection. However, it should be stressed that, in most cases, a prosthesis does not affect sensation, ejaculation, or orgasm.

Related Procedures

A related procedure includes the insertion of the artificial genitourinary sphincter. The device is placed around the urethra in selected cases of urinary incontinence. Components of the sphincter include a reservoir, pump, connecting tubing, and a cuff that is placed around the urethra. The patient operates the pump, which is placed in the male scrotum or in the labia majora of the female, to open or close the cuff.

Nursing Implications
Anesthesia

Insertion of a penile prosthesis can be performed under general or regional anesthesia. If the patient is awake during the procedure, the circulating nurse must make sure that conversation is kept to a minimum and is relevant to the procedure at hand. Transfusions are not generally required.

Position

Positioning of the patient depends on the operative approach. If a suprapubic incision is planned, place the patient in the supine position. If a perineal approach is planned, place the patient in the low lithotomy position.

Establishing and Maintaining the Sterile Field

As for the insertion of any prosthetic device, perform an extensive skin preparation. The area is prepped with a suitable antiseptic solution following standard operative preparation guidelines. Antibiotics may also be given before the procedure. A plastic adhesive drape should be provided to the scrub person for the draping procedure. If the patient is awake, the circulating nurse should make sure that a screen is setup with an unsterile drape so that the patient does not watch the preparation and the procedure.

In creating a sterile field, the scrub person uses a plastic adhesive drape to isolate the rectal area from the field when the patient is in the low lithotomy position. Other draping requirements for the supine and low lithotomy positions are routine. All components may be submerged in an antibiotic solution.

Equipment and Supplies

Table 27.1 lists the equipment and supplies for insertion of a penile prosthesis. The circulating nurse should also have available all components of the type of the prosthesis selected for the patient. As a general precaution, have available two of each component in case of inadvertent contamination or problems. Before the procedure begins, the scrub person prepares the manufacturer's recommended solutions. During the tissue dissection, the scrub person carries out normal role requirements. As the corpora are dilated, the scrub person should announce the size of the dilator

Table 27.1	Equipment and Supplies for Penile Prosthesis Insertion

Adhesive drape, plastic

Basin set

Drain, 7 mm Jackson-Pratt

Drape packs appropriate for patient position

Electrosurgery pencil

Foley catheter, 14 Fr Foley with a 5 mL balloon

General urology set

Mayo stand covers

Needle counter

Patient return electrode

Pushers, Kitner dissectors

Scalpel blades Nos. 10 and 15

Skin marker

Soft tissue dissection set

Sponges, 4 × 8 radiopaque

Sponges, small laparotomy, radiopaque

Suture (select chromic and synthetic suture based on surgeon preference; usually sutures include 0, 2-0, and 3-0 synthetic braided and monofilament suture ties and on Swedgeon cutting needles)

Syringe, Toomey

Syringe, 20 mL

Syringe, 60 mL

Syringe, Asepto

Yankauer suction with tubing

as it is handed to the surgeon. The dilators should be kept in order so that the scrub person can easily move forward or backward in the sequence. In addition, the scrub person should also be familiar with the loading of the Furlow instrument so that the cylinder can be loaded and ready for insertion by the surgeon.

Physiological Monitoring

During the procedure, the circulating nurse records all blood loss and irrigation. Urine is not routinely emptied from the bladder during this procedure.

Specimens and Cultures

There are no routine specimens and/or cultures for this procedure. If the patient is having a prosthesis removed for infection, the circulating nurse sends several cultures for microbiological examination.

Drugs and Solutions

Drugs and solutions necessary for the penile prosthesis procedure include sterile water for irrigation; sterile saline for irrigation; contrast media, and neomycin and polymyxin B (Neosporin G.U. irrigant).

Physician Orders and Laboratory and Diagnostic Studies

Patients with erectile dysfunction may have either psychological problems or systemic diseases known to affect erectile capability. These include vascular disease (eg, arteriosclerosis), neurological disease (eg, multiple sclerosis), and endocrine or metabolic diseases (eg, diabetes mellitus). These patients, therefore, may need an evaluation before the procedure that includes a chest radiograph, a complete set of laboratory data, and an electrocardiogram (ECG). Other diagnostic studies may include penile ultrasonography, probe Doppler analysis of the penile vasculature, nocturnal penile tumescence studies, and, as required, angiographic evaluation of the penile vasculature. These studies help to document erectile dysfunction and provide the indications for operative management.

ECG
Electrocardiogram

Procedure

Several operative approaches can be used to insert penile prostheses. **Table 27.2** lists the possible incisions for penile prosthesis insertion. In the early years of penile prosthetic procedures, the devices were introduced through a dorsal midline penile incision with the patient in the supine position. More recently, a perineal approach has been advocated with the patient in the low lithotomy position. Parenteral antibiotics are administered before the procedure.

Incision and Exposure

The incision is brought sharply down to the corpora cavernosa, which are easily recognized by the white tunica albuginea. The tunica is then opened longitudinally for 34 cm. The intracorporal space containing the erectile tissue is then dilated with Hegar dilators proximal to the ischial tuberosity and distal to the end of the corpora cavernosa at the glans. The space is then copiously irrigated with antibiotic solution, and a prosthesis of the appropriate size is inserted after careful measurement of the corporal space. The procedure is repeated for the opposite side.

Details

Components of the inflatable penile prosthesis can be placed either through an incision extending from the base of the penis over the pubis or through a small scrotal or penoscrotal incision with the patient in the supine position and a urethral catheter inserted. An inflatable prosthesis necessitates placement of the reservoir

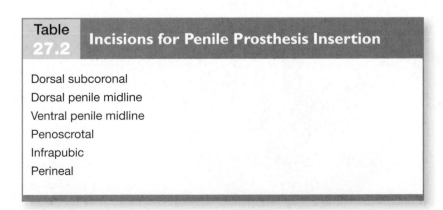

Table 27.2	Incisions for Penile Prosthesis Insertion
Dorsal subcoronal	
Dorsal penile midline	
Ventral penile midline	
Penoscrotal	
Infrapubic	
Perineal	

in the paravesical space, medial to the epigastric vessels. The pump is placed in a subdartos scrotal pouch on the right for the right-handed patient or on the left for left-handed patients. Pump, reservoir, and penile cylinders are connected by tubing, which has been cut at an appropriate length and placed in such a way that it neither kinks nor is under tension. Before closure, the operative field is irrigated with copious amounts of antibiotic solution. **Figure 27.7** shows the insertion of a rigid penile prosthesis using a perineal incision.

Closure

Closure is done with absorbable suture material in several layers.

Postprocedure Care

Nursing care is relatively simple. Patients may have the urethral catheter removed on the first postprocedure day. Ice should be applied to the groin to prevent excessive swelling. Parenteral antibiotics should be administered for at least 24 hours, and patients should be discharged on a regimen of oral antibiotics for at least 7 days. The patients should be instructed to watch for any signs of local infection.

Potential Complications

The risk of infection is the primary complication. If the prosthesis becomes infected, it must be removed and antibiotics administered. Late complications include severe pain from an inappropriately sized prosthesis, skin or urethral erosion, urinary retention, skin necrosis from increased local pressure, and mechanical failure in the case of an inflatable prosthesis. Over time, longterm complications may occur. Most problems are due to cylinder leak, tubing kinks, and aneurysmal dilation of the

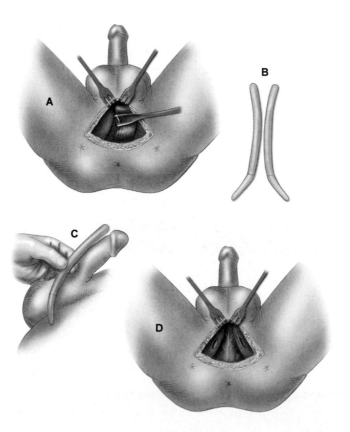

Figure 27.7

Insertion of a rigid penile prosthesis using a perineal incision.

corpora. Rarely, erosion of the reservoir into the bladder and large bowel has also been reported. Because of such complications, there should be extended and careful followup for patients with penile prostheses and artificial genitourinary sphincters.

CIRCUMCISION

Circumcision is the operative removal of the foreskin, or prepuce.

Indications

The practice of circumcision is ancient. It can be a religious rite for newborns and young boys but is not an operative necessity, except in certain rare specific instances when the foreskin cannot be retracted easily (phimosis), when the foreskin cannot be brought back over the glans (paraphimosis), or when infection causes posthitis or balanoposthitis. Circumcision of the newborn has been the focus of controversy. It is one of the most commonly performed operative procedures in the United States. Scientific studies show some medical benefits of circumcision. However, these benefits are not sufficient for the American Academy of Pediatrics to recommend that all infant boys be circumcised. **Table 27.3** lists the pros and cons of circumcision as defined by the American Academy of Pediatrics. Circumcision in the adult is performed for phimosis, paraphimosis, and balanoposthitis.

Nursing Implications
Anesthesia

In most adult patients, circumcision is performed under local anesthesia with a penile or caudal block and moderate sedation/analgesia. Children will receive general anesthesia.

Position

Patients are placed in the supine position.

Establishing and Maintaining the Sterile Field

In adults and children, the penis is prepared with a povidone iodine solution. Hair removal is not performed before the procedure. The penis is draped into the sterile field.

Because most circumcisions are performed under local anesthesia with moderate sedation/analgesia, care should be taken not to cover the face of the conscious patient while establishing the sterile field. The scrub person should have the local anesthesia ready for injection by the surgeon when the surgeon asks for it, to avoid anxiety on the patient's part while waiting for the anticipated injection. No special supplies are required.

Equipment and Supplies

Table 27.4 lists the equipment and supplies for circumcision.

Physiological Monitoring

Physiological monitoring of the patient includes all of the guidelines for the care of patients receiving local anesthesia with moderate sedation/analgesia. Urinary catheterization is not routinely performed.

Table 27.3	Pros and Cons of Circumcision

Pros

- [ ] A slightly lower risk of urinary tract infections (UTIs)
  - A circumcised infant boy has about a 1 in 1,000 chance of developing a UTI in the first year of life.
  - An uncircumcised infant boy has about a 1 in 100 chance of developing a UTI in the first year of life.
- [ ] A lower risk of getting cancer of the penis
  - This type of cancer is very rare in all males.
- [ ] A slightly lower risk of getting sexually transmitted diseases, including HIV, the virus that causes AIDS
- [ ] Prevention of foreskin infections
- [ ] Prevention of phimosis, a condition in uncircumcised males that makes foreskin retraction impossible
- [ ] Easier genital hygiene
- [ ] Social reasons
  - Many parents choose to have it done because "all the other men in the family" had it done or because they do not want their sons to feel "different."
- [ ] Religious or cultural reasons
  - Some groups such as followers of the Jewish and Islamic faiths practice circumcision for religious and cultural reasons.

Consequences

- [ ] Fear of the risks
  - Complications are rare and usually minor but may include bleeding, infection, cutting the foreskin too short or too long, and improper healing.
- [ ] Belief that the foreskin is needed
  - Some people feel the foreskin is needed to protect the tip of the penis.
  - The tip of the penis may become irritated and cause the opening of the penis to become too small.
  - Can cause urination problems that may need to be surgically corrected.
- [ ] Belief it can affect sex
  - Some feel that circumcision makes the tip of the penis less sensitive, causing a decrease in sexual pleasure later in life.
- [ ] Belief that proper hygiene can lower health risks
  - Boys can be taught proper hygiene that can lower their chances of getting infections, cancer of the penis, and sexually transmitted diseases.

Adapted from American Academy of Pediatrics (2008). Reasons parents may choose circumcision. Retrieved 31 August 2008 from AAP Website: http://www.aap.org/publiced/BR_Circumcision.htm.

Specimens and Cultures

Cultures are not usually required, and the operative specimen is the foreskin, or prepuce. Process the specimen according to hospital policy.

Drugs and Solutions

Provide sterile saline for irrigation, neomycin and polymyxin B (Neosporin G.U. irrigant), and a local anesthetic (according to the surgeon's request).

Table 27.4	Equipment and Supplies for Circumcision

Basin set

Circumcision drape pack

Electrosurgery pencil

Drape pack

Gauze, petrolatum

Marking pen

Needle, 25 $^{5}/_{8}$-gauge

Patient return electrode

Plastic tray or minor dissecting set

Scalpel blades No. 15

Sponges, 4 × 8 radiopaque

Suction tubing

Suture (select chromic and synthetic suture based on surgeon preference; usually 3-0 and 5-0 chromic ties and 5-0 chromic on Swedgeon needle)

Syringe, 10-mL

Procedure

In the adult, the procedure is performed on an outpatient basis. Most newborn circumcisions are performed by the obstetrician or pediatrician with a device such as the Plasti bell, Gomco clamp, or Mogen clamp. When a clamp device is used for the circumcisions, contact of the electrosurgical active electrode with the clamp, such as the Gomco clamp, will greatly increase current flow and can result in unintended, catastrophic injury (Covidien, 2007).

Incision and Exposure

In the adult, two incisions are made: one on the outer skin and one approximately 3 mm from the corona of the glans.

Details

Small vessels are electrocoagulated and ligated. The subcutaneous tissue is then removed with scissors. **Figure 27.8** shows the sleeve resection technique of circumcision.

Closure

Both skin edges are reapproximated with either running or interrupted 5-0 chromic catgut. This stitch can be subcuticular. A light dressing may be applied.

Postprocedure Care

The suture line may be covered with petrolatum gauze to prevent adherence to underwear or bedclothes. Instruct patients not to rub or wash the penis vigorously for at least a week. The patient should apply petrolatum jelly for 23 days to protect the suture line.

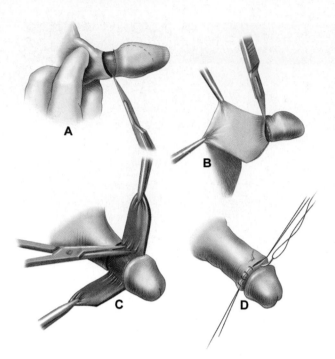

Figure 27.8

Sleeve resection technique of circumcision. (A) The coronal unction on the skin is outlined and incised circumferentially, following the V shape of the frenulum on the ventral surface. (B) The foreskin is retracted, the adhesions are thoroughly broken, and a circumferential incision is made in the mucosal skin just proximal to the coronal sulcus. (C) The sleeve of the skin between the two incisions is excised. (D) The skin edges are reapproximated, yielding a good cosmetic result.

Potential Complications

Immediate complications of circumcision include hemorrhage, removal of insufficient or excessive foreskin, infection, urinary retention (from too tight a bandage), and meatitis. Longterm complications include meatal stenosis, skin breakdown, and urethrocutaneous fistula.

TESTIS PROCEDURES

Orchiectomy

Orchiectomy, or orchidectomy, is the term used to refer to the operative removal of testes.

Indications

There are several reasons to remove testes. In the pediatric population, testes may be removed if, at the time of the procedure, they are found to be atrophic or nonviable (eg, prolonged ischemia from torsion). A testis may also be removed if it harbors a tumor with a malignant potential. Growth of adenocarcinoma of the prostate has been found to be hormonally dependent. By removing the testes, the source of male hormones, one can palliate the progression of advanced prostate cancer.

Orchiectomy can be either unilateral or bilateral and either simple or radical. Bilateral orchiectomy is reserved for patients with prostate cancer who require endocrine control of their malignancy. Indications for unilateral orchiectomy are testicular maldevelopment when the testis is not believed to be worth salvaging because of small size, testicular trauma when the testis is thought to be nonviable because of the extent of the damage, prolonged testicular torsion with irreversible ischemic changes, severe infection with the presence of testicular abscess, and testicular malignancy. In radical orchiectomy for testicular malignancy, the cord and surrounding fat are removed as far up as the internal ring. This requires an inguinal approach. The incision is the same as for inguinal herniorrhaphy. Simple orchiectomy refers to the removal of the testis, the cord structures being divided at any level. The epididymis is usually removed with the testis. Simple orchiectomy can he performed through either an inguinal or a scrotal approach.

Vasectomy

Vasectomy is an operative form of contraception. Ligation and division of the vas deferens is performed through a small incision in the upper scrotum. This outpatient procedure can be done with local anesthesia with or without moderate sedation/analgesia or general anesthesia.

Indications

Any man wishing to be provided with a reliable method of birth control is a candidate for vasectomy.

Hydrocelectomy

Hydroceles are collections of fluid around the testis. The fluid is usually contained between the tunica albuginca and the tunica vaginalis (**Fig. 27.9**). There are two categories of hydroceles: congenital and acquired. Congenital hydroceles are seen in the male pediatric population. A persistent communication between the peritoneum and the scrotum allows fluid to accumulate around the testis. In most male infants, this communication closes by age 2, but in 6%, it persists, usually in association with an inguinal hernia (Lee, DuBois, & Shekherdimian, 2006). In the adult, acquired hydrocele frequently develops because of a local inflammatory process such as infection of the testis or epididymis. Tumor and trauma are also known to cause the development of a hydrocele. A spermatocele is a similar accumulation of fluid located not around the testis but above the testis.

Indications

Surgery performed for congenital hydrocele is different from acquired hydrocele. The purpose of hydrocele procedures in the pediatric population is to alleviate the communication between the peritoneum and the scrotum and to fix the inguinal hernia. In the adult population, the procedure is elective and its goal is to remove the pocket of accumulated fluid. The approaches are therefore quite different and are described separately. Indications for adults include pain secondary to the size of the hydrocele, unacceptable scrotal appearance, and the patient's request for removal of the hydrocele.

In the child, a history of waxing and waning scrotal swelling localized to one or both sides is typical. The swelling is usually asymptomatic, but some redness of the scrotal skin may appear. The swelling may become considerable and alarming to the parents. The adult patient has a persistent, non-painful swelling around the testis, which may be come quite cumbersome because of its size. A history of trauma or of epididymitis may be elicited.

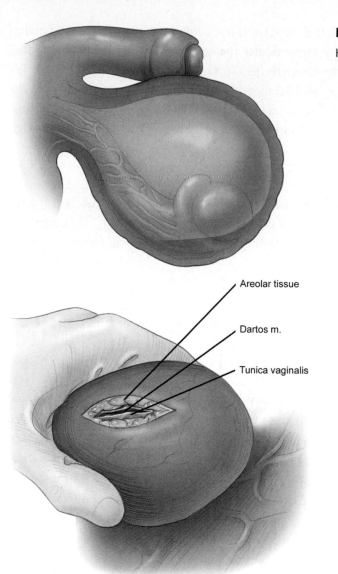

Figure 27.9
Hydrocele.

Areolar tissue

Dartos m.

Tunica vaginalis

On physical examination, the testis itself may be hard to palpate because of the surrounding fluid. If a light is placed against the testis, the testis will trans-illuminate. In the child, the cord is thickened, a feature referred to as the silk glove sign.

Related Procedures

Similar and related procedures include orchiopexy (testicular fixation), testicular biopsy, and insertion of testicular prosthesis. Orchiopexy is performed through an inguinal incision in cases of maldescent or through a scrotal incision for cases of torsion. Testicular torsion is a urological emergency, and the procedure should be performed for suspected testicular torsion with minimal delay. Fixation of the testis can be done by either placing the testis in a dartos pouch made under the scrotal skin in cases of maldescent or by fixing the testis in place with three or four tacking stitches in the scrotal cavity. Indications for testicular biopsy include evaluation for male infertility.

Nursing Implications

Anesthesia

Procedures on the testis and scrotum may be performed with the use of local, regional, or general anesthesia. Routine nursing care of these patients is practiced. Blood loss is usually insignificant. Most patients are extremely apprehensive before the procedure. Helping to reassure and comfort the patient before and during anesthesia may be necessary.

Position

Patients are placed in the supine position. No special positioning equipment is required. If the patient is awake, the nurse should make sure that he is in a comfortable position before draping.

Establishing and Maintaining the Sterile Field

The patient's abdomen, from the umbilicus to the upper thigh, including the scrotal area, is then prepped with the preferred solution. If the patient is awake, a drape should be placed as a barrier to prevent him from watching the preparation, and/or procedure. In the establishment of the sterile field, the penis is usually not included in the operative field.

Equipment and Supplies

The scrub person must be prepared for an inguinal or scrotal approach. In addition to the soft tissue dissection set, a Weitlaner self-retaining retractor should be available. During the procedure, the spermatic cord is isolated and secured by sliding a Penrose drain around it. The small Penrose drain may also be used at the end of the procedure for drainage of the wound.

Table 27.5 lists equipment and supplies for hydrocelectomy.

Physiological Monitoring

With pediatric patients, all sponges should be weighed. In addition, the circulating nurse records blood loss and irrigation. The bladder is not usually emptied during these procedures.

Specimens and Cultures

Cultures are not routinely performed during these procedures, unless an infection is present or suspected. **Table 27.6** lists the possible specimens related to testis procedures. Besides the specimens listed in **Table 27.6**, send any abnormal tissue found to pathology.

Drugs and Solutions

Provide sterile saline for irrigation, neomycin and polymyxin B (Neosporin G.U. irrigant), and a local anesthetic (if necessary). Fill the ice bag for use during transport of the patient to the postanesthesia care unit.

Physician Orders and Laboratory and Diagnostic Studies

A precise diagnosis can be obtained with ultrasonography. Routine laboratory studies are obtained before the procedure.

Table 27.5	Equipment and Supplies for Hydrocelectomy

Drape pack
Elastic bandage for possible pressure dressing
Electrosurgery pencil
Fluff dressing
Ice bag (fill before the patient goes to the postanesthesia care unit)
Minor dissection set
Needle counter
Package of Kling wraps for possible pressure dressing
Patient return electrode
Pushers (Kitner dissectors)
Scalpel blades Nos. 10, 11, and 15
Scrotal support (small, medium, and large)
Self-retaining (Weitlaner) retractor
Skin marker
Small Penrose drain
Sponges, 4 × 8 radiopaque
Sponges, small laparotomy, radiopaque
Suction tubing
Suture (select chromic and synthetic suture based on surgeon preference; usually sutures include 0, 2-0, 3-0, 4-0 chromic, silk, and synthetic braided sutures)
Syringe, 10-mL with 25 g $^{5}/_{8}$ needle
Syringe, Asepto

Table 27.6	Possible Specimens Related to Testis Procedures

Procedure	Specimen(s)
Simple orchiectomy	Testis, epididymis, and spermatic cord
Radical orchiectomy	Testis, epididymis, spermatic cord, and surrounding fat
Bilateral orchiectomy	Both testes
Testicular biopsy	Biopsy specimen of the testis
Hydrocelectomy	Redundant sac from the hydrocele
Vasectomy	Segment of vas deferens

Procedure for Orchiectomy

Orchiectomy may be performed with the use of general, spinal, or local anesthesia, and most patients are admitted for a same-day procedure. Preprocedure preparation and antibiotics are unnecessary. Diagnostic studies are limited to routine studies, except that serum markers are obtained if testicular cancer is present. These include alpha-fetoprotein and human chorionic gonadotropin beta subunit. These markers are elevated in certain specific types of germ cell tumors of the testis and have an important role in monitoring the management of these patients.

Inguinal Approach

INCISION AND EXPOSURE

Both inguinal and scrotal approaches are described. The inguinal approach is performed by making an incision parallel to the inguinal ligament, two fingerbreadths above and extending just above the pubic tubercle to the mid-inguinal point. The incision is brought down through subcutaneous tissue and fat to the fascia of the external oblique muscle. The fatty covering of the fascia is cleared away to expose the external inguinal ring. The fascia is then opened from the external ring up to the internal ring. The spermatic cord is then exposed lying in the inguinal canal. It is then dissected carefully and freed up. Care is paid to two small sensory nerves that course in close proximity to the cord, the iliohypogastric and ilioinguinal nerves.

DETAILS

The testis can then be brought into the field by traction. The lower pole of the testis is attached to the scrotum by remnants of the gubernaculuni. These are tied and divided with absorbable sutures. The cord can then be clamped, ligated, and divided with absorbable sutures at the level of the internal ring, and the testis is removed. **Figure 27.10** shows a left orchiectomy following trauma.

CLOSURE

After inspection for hemostasis, the fascia of the external oblique is closed with absorbable suture material. Care should be given to inspection of the scrotal cavity

Post-accident Condition

A. A left hemiscrotal transverse incision is made exposing the testicle.

Swelling of the scrotum

Anterior view

Testicle

Enlarged anterior view

Figure 27.10

Left orchiectomy.

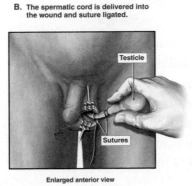

B. The spermatic cord is delivered into the wound and suture ligated.

Testicle

Sutures

Enlarged anterior view

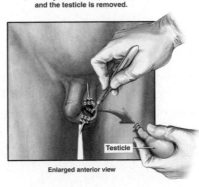

C. The spermatic cord is severed and the testicle is removed.

Testicle

Enlarged anterior view

where hematomas may form. If an incipient hematoma is noted, drainage of the scrotum may be accomplished with a small Penrose drain. The skin should be closed with an absorbable suture (4-0 polyglactin 910), with a subcuticular stitch for cosmetic purposes.

Scrotal Approach

INCISION AND EXPOSURE

Simple orchiectomy may be performed through a scrotal incision. The skin of the scrotum is put under stretch, and a longitudinal incision is made through the layers of the scrotum. The last layer is the tunica vaginalis. After this layer is opened, the glistening white covering of the testis is observed and a small amount of fluid can be found.

DETAILS

The cord structures are identified above the upper pole of the testis. Clamping, ligation, and division of the cord are done.

CLOSURE

The scrotum is closed in two layers with absorbable suture after careful inspection for hemostasis. Again, drainage of the scrotum can be accomplished by the use of a small Penrose drain. The skin is closed with 4-0 polyglactin with an interrupted stitch.

Procedure for Vasectomy

Incision and Exposure

The patient usually receives local anesthesia (1%–2% lidocaine). An incision is made either on each side of the scrotum or along the median raphe. The vas deferens must be palpated before the incision is made, separated from the surrounding tissue, and then firmly held in place.

Details

After the skin incision is made, the vas is dissected free over 12 cm and then divided. A 1-cm segment is removed, and both ends are occluded with small metal clips. Needle point electrosurgery can be used to fulgurate the vasal lumen to prevent recanalization. Closure is carried out in two layers. The skin can be closed with a subcutaneous stitch. **Figure 27.11** shows a close-up cutaway view of the vas deferens after a vasectomy has been performed. Individual sperm are shown trapped behind the barrier created by the sutures that were placed in the procedure.

Postprocedure Care for Orchiectomy and Vasectomy

Place a compression dressing around the scrotum. Tell the patient to wear a scrotal support for 7–10 days. Ice should be applied to the groin area for 24–36 hours.

Tell the patient that he should consider himself fertile until the results of one or two semen analyses are obtained 6–8 weeks after the procedure. Other forms of contraception must be used until then. The procedure is reversible, but fertility can be expected in only 30%–40% of cases by reanastomosis of the vas (vasovasostomy).

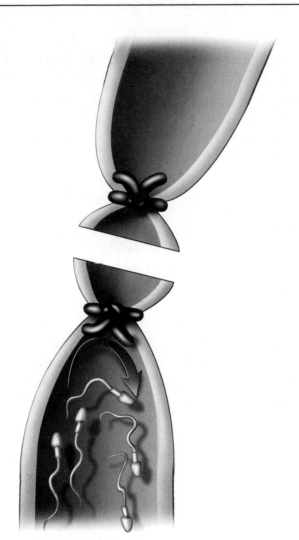

Figure 27.11
Vasectomy.

Procedure for Hydrocelectomy

The procedure is usually done on an outpatient basis.

Incision and Exposure

Pediatric hydrocele is treated similarly to pediatric hernias. Preparation and incision are made over the inguinal area. Dissection is aimed at mobilizing the cord and the hydrocele. The principles of pediatric hydrocelectomy are to interrupt the communication between the peritoneum and the scrotum by ligating and dividing the processus vaginalis. Several techniques are used to treat adult hydrocele operatively. A transverse mid-scrotal incision is used.

Details

The testis and hydrocele can be delivered into the field. The hydrocele can then be opened, and the redundant sac may be removed, leaving a 5 to 10 mm rim of tissue. Hemostasis is carried out, and the edge of sac is oversewn with 4-0 absorbable suture in a continuous locked fashion. The cut edges of the hydrocele sac can also be brought behind the testis and oversewn to each other. Other techniques have been developed to allow drainage of the fluid. These include "window" procedures and repositioning of the hydrocele sac around the testis.

27

Closure

Closure of the scrotal incision is done in two layers with absorbable suture. The deep layer is closed with a running stitch, and the skin layer should be closed in interrupted fashion. Placement of a Penrose drain is recommended for cases in which hematoma may develop. Wound infection and scrotal abscess occur rarely. Hydroceles may recur, and reoperation may be indicated. Hydrocele recurrence is due to inadequate dissection of the hydrocele sac, allowing reaccumulation of fluid within it.

Postprocedure Care for Hydrocelectomy

Care should include the application of an ice pack to the scrotum for at least 1.2 hours to minimize swelling and pain. Instruct the patient to wear an athletic support and limit activities. Patients are sent home with a prescription for pain medication and are seen 1 week after the procedure.

Potential Complications

Complications include hematomas and infection. These complications can be prevented by achieving proper hemostasis and by observing careful sterile techniques. Longterm complications occur rarely. A small number of patients describe chronic local pain that may be due to nerve injury to the ilioinguinal or iliohypogastric nerves.

HYPOSPADIAS REPAIR

Hypospadias is a congenital anomaly of the penis in which the opening of the urethra is found on the ventral surface of the penis (**Fig. 27.12**). This abnormality is believed to result from incomplete embryological development of the distal urethra. Ventral curvature of the penis is frequently found in patients with the more severe forms of hypospadias and is due to fibrous tissue bands found on the ventral aspect of the penis. It is called chordee. Undescended testes and inguinal hernias may be found in association with hypospadias.

Epispadias is a congenital abnormality of the penis in which the meatus is located on the dorsum of the penis. This condition is rare. Some patients with more

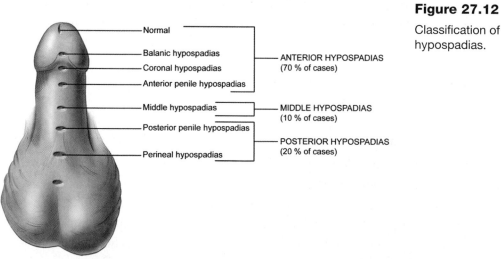

Figure 27.12

Classification of hypospadias.

severe forms of hypospadias may have ambiguous genitalia and require further evaluation to rule out an intersex condition. Anatomically, the penis of the patient with hypospadias demonstrates an anomalous meatus; dorsal hooded foreskin, which is deficient on the ventral aspect of the penis; and frequently some degree of curvature.

The patient has usually been diagnosed at birth. Associated abnormalities (undescended testis and inguinal hernia) should be noted. Parents should provide additional information regarding the child's health and immunization status. A significant amount of parental anxiety is usually readily apparent, and the nursing staff plays a major role in alleviating both parental and infant anxiety by providing reassurance, by teaching, and by answering questions.

Indications

The main goal of hypospadias repair is to reconstruct a straight penis with a meatus placed as close as possible to the tip of the glans, allowing for straight voiding and good cosmesis. There are five major maneuvers involved in this operative repair:

1. Meatoplasty and glanuloplasty, which repositions the meatus and fashions the glans
2. Removal of the ventral curvature (chordee)
3. Urethroplasty (reconstruction of the urethra), if needed, when a deficiency in urethral length coexists
4. Cosmetic skin rearrangement over the shaft of the penis
5. Scrotoplasty (reconstruction of the scrotum), as needed

Determining the type of operative technique to use depends on the location and the degree of chordee.

Until 1980, hypospadias repair was postponed until the child was older than 3 years because of the larger size of the penis, making the procedure technically easier. However, since genital awareness occurs at about 18 months of age, surgery in the older child has been linked to psychological morbidity, such as abnormal behavior, guilt, and gender identity confusion. Currently, most surgeons attempt repair between the ages of four to 18 months, with improved emotional and psychologic results (Gatti and Kirsch, 2007).

Indications for the procedure, therefore, are any anomaly in the position of the urethral meatus in a male infant who has been diagnosed as having hypospadias.

Related Procedures

Related procedures are circumcision and meatoplasty. The latter procedure involves creating a larger urethral opening.

Nursing Implications
Anesthesia

The patient will receive general anesthesia for hypospadias repair. Children may be anxious when coming to the operative and invasive procedure suite. Allow the child to remain with a parent as long as possible. Take steps to allay the child's fear and anxiety.

Position

Place the patient in the supine position with the legs in a frog-leg position. Pad the legs so that they do not suspend over the bed. Carefully apply the safety strap above the operative area. Warm the room before the child is transferred to the operating bed. Apply warming devices as necessary to prevent heat loss from the child's body during the procedure.

Establishing and Maintaining the Sterile Field

Prep the skin from umbilicus to midthigh to include the entire genitalia. During the preparation, fully retract the foreskin and accumulated smegma. Place the electrosurgical patient return electrode according to the manufacturer's written instructions. See Chapter 37 for information concerning application of an infant patient return electrode.

Create the sterile field around the genital area of the child. If scrubbed, remember the frog-legged position of the patient's legs. The operative team must exercise care and avoid leaning on the bent legs or chest during the procedure.

Placing the draped Mayo over the feet of the patient will provide a convenient work surface for the scrub person. The scrub person should have a sterile catheter and collection device available for emptying of the child's bladder during the procedure and prepare injectable solutions, such as the saline used for artificial erection. The scrub person should exercise care while handling the smaller suture used for hypospadias repair. Use of a magnetic pad below the operative area, between the scrub person and the surgeon helps in catching stray needles.

Equipment and Supplies

Equipment and supplies for the hypospadias repair may vary according to the type of procedure. **Table 27.7** lists the basic equipment and supplies for hypospadias repair.

Physiological Monitoring

Before the incision, the surgeon drains urine from the bladder. Document this urine output as well as other urine output during the procedure. Measure blood loss in the sponges and the suction container.

Specimens and Cultures

The surgeon may send the urine initially emptied from the bladder for culture. Specimens may include redundant foreskin from the repair. Send this tissue to pathology as a routine specimen.

Drugs and Solutions

Medications and solutions include lidocaine 1% with 1:100,000 epinephrine, sterile saline solution for injection, neomycin and polymyxin B (Neosporin G.U. irrigant), and sterile saline for irrigation.

Table 27.7	Equipment and Supplies for Hypospadias Repair

Basin set

Bougies, small set

Diapers (assortment of sizes)

Drape pack

Dressing, small, Xeroform

Dressing, Tegaderm

Electrosurgery pencil

Feeding tube, 8 Fr tube (16-inch)

Hypospadias set

Infusion set, Butterfly

Needle counter

Needle, 18-gauge

Needle, 30-gauge

Patient return electrode

Rubber tourniquet, small, or rubber bands

Set of microsurgery instruments (Castroviejo needle holders, 0.5 forceps, and fine mosquito forceps)

Skin marker

Sponges, 4 × 8 radiopaque

Suction tubing

Suprapubic catheter

Suture (select chromic and synthetic suture based on surgeon preference; usually sutures range in size from 5-0 to 8-0 and Swedgeon micro needles)

Scalpel blades Nos. 10 and 15

Syringe 10-mL

Syringe, 5-mL

Urethral stent (6 Fr Silastic tubing)

Physician Orders and Laboratory and Diagnostic Studies

The patient remains NPO according to anesthesia department policy. The physician usually does not order laboratory and diagnostic studies unless clinical symptoms merit further evaluation.

Procedure

At the time of the procedure, the surgeon performs an artificial erection test by injecting sterile saline into the corpora of the penis, which has had a tourniquet placed at its base to evaluate the degree of penile curvature (chordee).

Meatal Advancement and Glanuloplasty

For patients with minimal chordee and a meatus located anteriorly, meatal advancement and glanuloplasty alleviates urinary stream deflection, abnormal appearing foreskin, and an unaesthetic meatus. The procedure is done on an outpatient basis, and the patient goes home without a urinary catheter.

INCISION AND EXPOSURE

The surgeon places a holding stitch of 5-0 nonabsorbable polypropylene suture through the glans, performs a circumcision incision below the corona, and frees up the shaft from its overlying skin.

DETAILS

A dorsal meatotomy on the ventral aspect of the glans is done, and the meatus is advanced to the tip of the penis by placing absorbable 6-0 sutures transversely. The wings of the glans are then brought back in the midline, and the glans is reshaped conically with 5-0 polyglactin 910 sutures.

CLOSURE

The redundant foreskin is removed, and the penile skin is reapproximated to the coronal margin with 6-0 or 7-0 chromic suture. A petrolatum gauze dressing is applied.

Perimeatus-Based Flap (Mathieu Procedure)

If the meatus is not adequate for a meatal advancement and glanuloplasty because it is too far from the tip of the glans or abnormal and there is minimal chordee, a meatus-based flap is used.

INCISION AND EXPOSURE

The surgeon makes parallel lines along the glanular groove and then a subcoronal incision.

DETAILS

A skin flap is raised from the skin overlying the urethra and brought over for suturing on the edges of the glanular groove (5-0 or 6-0 polyglactin 910). Alternatively, the urethral plate may be incised in the midline, thus widening it and allowing it to be reconstructed by bringing it together over an 8 Fr tube (Snodgrass).

CLOSURE

The wings of the glans are brought over to the midline, and the skin is then reapproximated with 5-0 or 6-0 chromic suture. A small (6-8 Fr) Silastic catheter may be sewn into place and left for 7–10 days. Either foam dressing or a single layer of mesh nonadherent dressing may be applied and left in place for 3–5 days.

Onlay Island Flap

When the meatus is placed too proximally (middle or posterior hypospadias) or if the ventral skin is not suitable for a meatus-based flap, the preputial skin may be used to form the missing wall of the urethra.

INCISION AND EXPOSURE

The penile shaft is dissected from its skin covering. The skin flap is then taken from the inner surface of the foreskin, having been measured to provide adequate length and width.

DETAILS

Care is taken to preserve the vascular blood supply to the skin flap, which is then transposed to the ventral surface of the penis and sutured onto the urethral plate with 6-0 or 7-0 polyglactin or polydioxanone suture. A 6 Fr urethral stent may be placed for 5–7 days to allow for urinary drainage. Alternatively, urinary drainage may be accomplished by using a 10 Fr suprapubic tube secured and left in place for 10 days. **Figure 27.13** shows an Onlay Island Flap procedure.

CLOSURE

The excess preputial skin is removed, and the skin is reapproximated with 6-0 chromic suture. A nonadherent mesh dressing or foam dressing is applied.

Tube Grafts

For extensive reconstruction of the urethra, a tube graft may be fashioned from preputial skin. Free grafts may also be used. Skin from the inner upper arm or lateral margins of the superior edge of the iliac crest is harvested, defatted, and fashioned into a tube with 6-0 polyglactin running suture. They should be non-hair bearing. The bladder mucosa and the buccal mucosa may serve as a substitute for a large deficiency in the urethra.

Postprocedure Care

The patient is awakened and returned to the postanesthesia care unit. After he is sufficiently recovered, he is taken to his parents and is encouraged to drink liberally. He should void at least once before discharge.

The parents are instructed to care for the dressing and catheter. The child is sponge-bathed until the dressing is removed. When the dressing falls off, usually within 24 hours, or two days after surgery, whichever occurs first, the child may have a tepid water tub bath without soap. Instruct the parents to soak the operative area rather than scrubbing or washing. The catheter may remain in place during the bath. The operative area is gently patted dry with a clean towel (UCSF Children's Hospital, 2007).

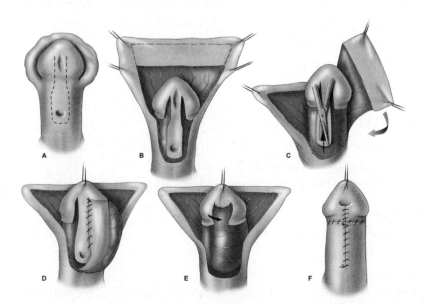

Figure 27.13

Onlay island flap. (A) spared ventral strip of urethral plate; (B) Longitudinal strip outlined on the inner aspect of the foreskin; (C) This strip is being rotated ventrally on its own separate vascular pedicle; (D and E) The foreskin strip is sutured to the ventral strip to form the neourethra; (F) Penile skin is reapproximated.

Fluid intake should be encouraged to ensure continual flushing of the urinary tract to prevent infection. Parents should monitor urine output. If the child wears diapers, the catheter will drain in the diaper. When changing the diaper after bowel movements the parents should clean the meatus and the catheter. For the older patient, the catheter is attached to a ureteral drainage bag. Patients with an indwelling catheter should be sent home on a regimen of oral antibiotics.

Most likely, patients who have undergone a meatal advancement and glanuloplasty will go home the same day. The patients are seen 7–10 days after the procedure for removal of the urethral catheter. Petrolatum may be applied to the incision. Gentle cleansing with warm water and hydrogen peroxide can be performed. The child should be monitored for fever, chills, flank pain, and foul smelling or cloudy urine, which indicate a urinary tract infection, and/or an unusual swelling or redness as well as purulence around the incision, indicating a wound infection.

Potential Complications

Blood loss is usually minimal, but in the young infant it should be monitored closely, because the penis is a well vascularized organ and may bleed significantly, leading to anemia and postprocedure hematoma. Hematoma formation may seriously compromise a delicate repair. Wound infection is rare and can be prevented with hygiene. Longterm complications include urethral strictures and urethrocutaneous fistula. These complications require further operative repair.

KIDNEY PROCEDURES

Operative procedures on the kidney are performed for infection, cancer, trauma, and rarely for stone disease.

Indications

Patients with infections of the kidney exhibit signs and symptoms related to infection. Flank pain, fever, chills, and pyuria may be present. The patient may report the presence of hematuria. Stone disease manifests with flank pain and hematuria; however, in this instance, the flank pain maybe different. It usually is severe, intermittent (colicky), and deep-seated. Signs and symptoms of infection may coexist with the presence of renal stones. Patients who harbor a renal tumor may be completely asymptomatic, except for painless hematuria. However, other symptoms include weight loss, fever, hypertension, hypercalcemia, night sweats, malaise, and varicocele, due to obstruction of the testicular vein (Sachdeva et al, 2008). Patients may have experienced blunt or penetrating injuries, which require a full evaluation, including a computed tomographic (CT) scan, intravenous urogram (IVU), and arteriogram to plan therapeutic management.

Operative procedures of the kidney can be divided into six general categories:

CT
Computed
Tomographic

- Simple nephrectomy for nonfunctional renal units resulting from obstructive uropathy, severe infection, injuries to the kidney, and congenitally nonfunctional kidneys
- Radical nephrectomy for renal cancer
- Partial nephrectomy for injuries limited to one pole of the kidney, for segmental parenchymal disease, or for tumors confined to a solitary kidney

- Nephroureterectomy for transitional cell carcinoma of the renal pelvis
- Open operative procedures on the kidney, such as anatropic lithotomy in which the kidney is opened up to remove stones, which has become extremely rare with the advent of endoscopic operative technique and extracorporeal shock wave lithotripsy
- Procedures on the renal pelvis or proximal ureter to relieve a ureteropelvic junction obstruction, which may be caused by a congenital narrowing of the most proximal portion of the ureter or by crossing vessels that press on the ureter, particularly in children

Operative Approaches to the Kidney

The flank approach avoids entering the peritoneal cavity. The incision may be transseptal, intercostal, or subcostal (**Fig. 27.14**).

The abdominal approach uses either a midline or a paramedian incision. Anterior subcostal or chevron incisions are used infrequently (**Fig. 27.15**).

The posterior lumbotomy approach uses an incision made in the back with the patient in the prone or lateral position (**Fig. 27.16**).

The thoracoabdominal approach is through the chest. The pleura may or may not be opened. A transcostal or intercostal incision may be used.

Another method is the hand-assisted laparoscopic approach for kidney procedures, which allows insertion of a hand to assist with dissection and manipulation of tissue surrounding the kidney. See Chapter 24 for a description of hand-assisted laparoscopic nephrectomy.

The operative team for urological procedures should be familiar with each approach because each requires specific patient positioning and instruments.

Related Operative Procedures

Related procedures include those on the adrenal gland, which entails a similar flank approach to the retroperitoneum.

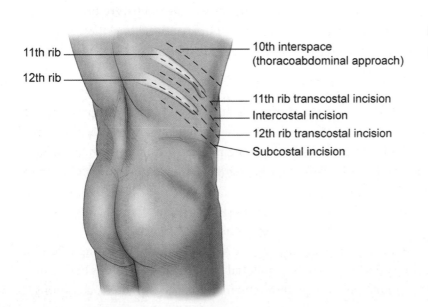

Figure 27.14

Flank incisions.

11th rib

12th rib

10th interspace (thoracoabdominal approach)

11th rib transcostal incision

Intercostal incision

12th rib transcostal incision

Subcostal incision

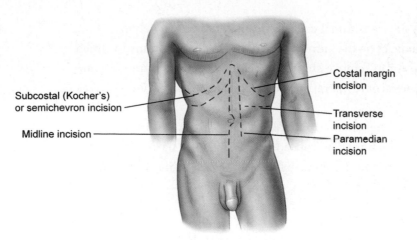

Figure 27.15

Abdominal approaches to the kidney.

Subcostal (Kocher's) or semichevron incision

Midline incision

Costal margin incision

Transverse incision

Paramedian incision

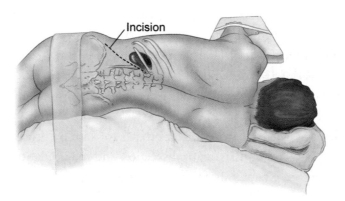

Incision

Figure 27.16

Posterior lumbotomy incision.

Nursing Implications

Anesthesia

Operative procedures for the kidney are performed under general anesthesia. This may be supplemented with an intercostal nerve block, consisting of bupivacaine with epinephrine, or with an epidural regional block, which may provide good postprocedure pain control. Blood is usually typed and crossmatched before the procedure in case a transfusion is needed. The circulating nurse and the anesthesia provider should follow hospital policy regarding blood administration.

Position

When the patient is placed in the lateral position, special consideration is given to the ventilation of both lungs. Breath sounds are checked carefully after the patient is positioned, and adjustments are made in the patient's position or the placement of the endotracheal tube as needed. See Chapter 8 for information about placing the patient in the lateral and prone positions.

Because the patient is placed in the lateral position, the nurse must consider other factors when positioning. Insert the Foley catheter before turning the patient but wait to secure the drainage tubing and bag until the positioning is completed. This will facilitate urinary drainage. Apply sequential compression stockings before turning the patient. Do not apply the patient return electrode until after positioning. If the patient return electrode is applied before positioning, it may become dislodged while the patient is being moved.

Establishing and Maintaining the Sterile Field

Patient preparation varies according to the position of the patient. If the patient is in the supine position, the area from the nipple line to the midthigh is prepared with a povidone-iodine solution. Draping is carried out in the routine fashion for this position. When the patient is placed in the lateral position, the entire back, flank, and abdomen on the operative side are prepared with a prepping solution. See Chapter 9 for a description of prepping and draping the patient for the supine and lateral positions.

The scrub person positions the Mayo stand over the patient's legs. During the procedure, the scrub person must adjust the height of the Mayo stand if the bed is raised or lowered.

Equipment and Supplies

Table 27.8 lists the equipment and supplies needs for kidney procedures. Depending on the exact procedure to be done, not all of the equipment may be necessary.

When scrubbed, have extra long instruments and an extended electrosurgical tip ready for use in deep cavities. Roll and fold 4×8 inch radiopaque sponges and place on ring forceps for blunt dissection. Place a sterile magnetic pad over the patient's hips to help control the loss of instruments and needles, especially if the patient is in the flank position.

Sterile ice may be used during partial nephrectomy. When used, the sterile ice is placed in a sterile intestinal bag and then placed around the kidney to decrease blood flow before the incision into the kidney.

Physiological Monitoring

Rapid blood loss can occur during kidney procedures. Keep a current record of sponge and suction container blood loss as well as the volume of irrigation fluids used. Assist the anesthesia provider with monitoring urine output.

Specimens and Cultures

Cultures are performed when infection is present or suspected. Specimens in kidney procedures can include all of the following:

> Kidney (right or left)
>
> Kidney and ureter
>
> Perinephric fat
>
> Kidney, adrenal gland, perinephric fat, and Gerota's fascia en bloc
>
> Upper or lower pole of the kidney
>
> Stones

Handle specimens according to hospital policy (eg, fresh, fixed, and frozen section).

Drugs and Solutions

Table 27.9 lists drugs and solutions for kidney procedures.

Table 27.8	Equipment and Supplies for Kidney Procedures

Active electrode tip cleaner

Chest tubes (according to surgeon preference)

Drain No. 10 Jackson-Pratt

Drain, Penrose drain

Drape pack

Electrosurgery pencil

Extended active electrode tip

Foley catheter and drainage bag (size according to the surgeon's request)

Hemoclips, large and medium

Hernia tape

Intestinal bag, plastic

Laparotomy set

Long instrument pack

Magnetic pad

Mayo stand cover

Needle counter

Needle, 25 gauge 1½

Nephrectomy set

Patient return electrode

Pushers, Kitner dissectors

Red rubber catheter Nos. 8 Fr or 10 Fr

Scalpel blades Nos. 10, 11, and 15

Skin marker

Skin staples

Sponges, 4 × 8 radiopaque

Sponges, large and small laparotomy, radiopaque

Sterile ice

Suction tubing

Suture (select chromic and synthetic suture based on surgeon preference; usually sutures include 1, 0, 2-0, 3-0, 4-0, 5-0 chromic and silk ties and on Swedgeon needles.

Syringe, 10-mL

Syringe, 50-mL

Syringe, Asepto

Ureteral catheters (according to surgeon preference)

Vascular set

Vessel loops

Physician Orders and Laboratory and Diagnostic Studies

Preprocedure evaluation of the patient undergoing procedures on the kidney should include functional studies of the kidney (either IVU or radioisotopic renal scan) to ensure adequate function in the contralateral kidney and an anatomical study (IVU, retrograde pyelogram, ultrasound, CT scan, magnetic resonance imaging [MRI1 scan, and/or arteriogram]).

Table 27.9	Drugs and Solutions for Kidney Procedures

Sterile saline for irrigation

Sterile water for irrigation

Neomycin and polymyxin B (Neosporin G.U. irrigant)

Hemostatic agents (according to the surgeon's choice), such as microfibrillar collagen hemostat, oxidized regenerated cellulose, and absorbable gelatin sponge

Mesh, for partial nephrectomy

Local anesthetic agent, usually bupivacaine hydrochloride with epinephrine, for local intercostal injection during closure

A patient being prepared for elective procedures may be placed on a modified bowel preparation regimen (clear liquids, enemas, and administration of magnesium citrate on the day before the procedure). Preprocedure teaching, breathing exercises, and incentive spirometry should be initiated. One dose of a parenteral broad-spectrum antibiotic should be given immediately before the procedure. Routine laboratory studies to include blood urea nitrogen, creatinine, and electrolyte determinations, complete blood cell (CBC) count, platelets, prothrombin time, partial thromboplastin time, chest radiograph, and ECG are obtained and checked. Blood should be available in the blood bank (12 U of packed red blood cells). Patients with suspected pulmonary disease should undergo pulmonary function studies and blood gas analysis to help plan the operative approach.

CBC
Complete Blood Cell

Patients found to have a urinary tract infection should be treated with the appropriate intravenous antibiotic therapy before the procedure. Certain severe infections may warrant immediate operative therapy, and in such cases, broad-spectrum intravenous antibiotic therapy should be initiated with minimal delay.

Teaching before the procedure includes a full explanation of the procedure. The patient should be reassured and told that he or she can live a normal life after a nephrectomy, provided there is good function in the remaining kidney. This kidney actually increases its function to compensate for the loss of the other kidney.

Procedures

Some basic principles must be adhered to for operative procedures on the kidney. The incision and approach must be planned according to the anatomy of the patient and to the nature of his or her disease. Preprocedure evaluation (IVU, CT scan, arteriogram, ultrasound, and MRI), which helps define the anatomy and the extent of the disease, should be available for review. Given the position of the kidney in the retroperitoneum, exposure should be adequate to provide access and control of the renal vascular pedicle.

Simple Nephrectomy

Simple nephrectomy is performed for pyonephrosis, chronic pyelonephritis with extensive destruction of the kidney, renal abscess not amenable to percutaneous drainage, congenitally malformed and nonfunctional kidney (eg, polycystic kidney disease), and severe renal damage from trauma.

INCISION AND EXPOSURE

Depending on the position of the kidney, either a subcostal 11th or 12th rib or anterior 12th rib incision is made. The layers of the abdominal wall are sharply traversed, with care being taken to achieve hemostasis and to note the location of nerves, especially the 12th thoracic intercostal nerve (which lies between the transversus abdominis muscle and the internal oblique muscle). The retroperitoneum is entered and the peritoneum is reflected medially. If the peritoneum is inadvertently opened, it can be closed with 3-0 chromic suture. Gerota's fascia is then identified. A self-retaining (Balfour or Finochietto) retractor may be placed to improve exposure.

DETAILS

Gerota's fascia is incised, and the perinephric fat is bluntly dissected from the capsule of the kidney. The kidney is then mobilized by freeing it from its fatty surroundings. The lower pole is first mobilized. The ureter is identified, clamped, and divided with metallic clips. The kidney can be retracted, and the hilum is identified. Accessory vessels to the kidney should be kept in mind, and, when found they should be clamped, ligated, and divided. The main artery and vein are then identified, dissected, and mobilized. First the artery and then the vein is doubly clamped; ligated with heavy, free ties; and divided. A set of vascular instruments should be available if difficulties are encountered in controlling bleeding from either the vein or the artery. The kidney is then removed from the field. In case of severe infection, monofilament suture or absorbable suture should be used. **Figure 27.17** shows an example of a nephrectomy.

CLOSURE

After removal of the kidney, the renal fossa is carefully inspected for signs of bleeding and hemostasis should be established. The incision is then closed, and the renal fossa can be drained by a Penrose drain. Closure in three layers is standard, with running polyglactin 910 sutures for the deep layers and interrupted suture for the external oblique layer. Skin is reapproximated with skin clips.

Posterior Lumbotomy

A posterior lumbotomy approach may be used. It may lessen pain and respiratory compromise after the procedure and allows a rapid approach to the renal artery. However, dissection of the kidney is harder. This approach is excellent for an open renal biopsy. Simple nephrectomy for injury may be performed through a transabdominal approach at the time of exploratory laparotomy. It offers the advantage of easy access and control of the renal vessels. The same principles of dissection, mobilization, and control of the renal vasculature apply.

Nephroureterectomy

Nephroureterectomy is used to remove transitional cell carcinoma involving the renal collecting system. The kidney and entire ureter with a cuff of bladder are

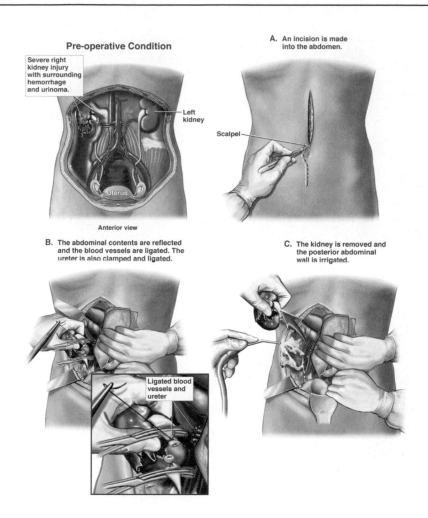

Pre-operative Condition

Severe right kidney injury with surrounding hemorrhage and urinoma.

Left kidney

Uterus

Anterior view

A. An incision is made into the abdomen.

Scalpel

Figure 27.17

Nephrectomy.

B. The abdominal contents are reflected and the blood vessels are ligated. The ureter is also clamped and ligated.

C. The kidney is removed and the posterior abdominal wall is irrigated.

Ligated blood vessels and ureter

removed en bloc. The approach for nephroureterectomy is also similar to that for a simple nephrectomy; however, a second incision or a larger incision is usually needed to obtain access to the distal ureter and its insertion into the bladder (**Fig. 27.18**). A modified Gibson incision is usually used in these cases. A cuff of bladder is removed, and the procedure on the bladder follows the same principles as those used for open prostatectomy.

Radical Nephrectomy

The indication for radical nephrectomy is renal cell carcinoma. The goal of the operation is to remove en bloc the kidney, the adrenal gland, all the perinephric fat, and Gerota's fascia (**Fig. 27.19**).

INCISION AND EXPOSURE

Several approaches can be used: thoracoabdominal, flank, or transabdominal. The thoracoabdominal and transcostal approaches are described. The thoracoabdominal approach provides excellent access to renal vessels, the aorta, the inferior vena cava, and the kidney. The pleura may or may not be entered, depending on which rib or intercostal space is entered. The choice of level of incision depends again on the position of the kidney. The patient is positioned in similar fashion as for a flank incision with more of a posterior tilt (the patient's body is at a 45-degree angle to the bed and the pelvis is at 15–20 degrees). A transcostal incision is made right over the 9th or 10th

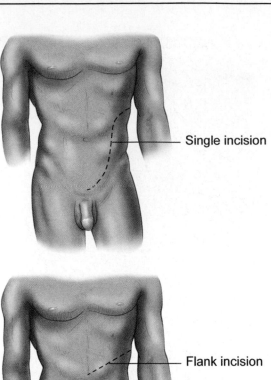

Figure 27.18

Incisions for
nephroureterectomy.

Single incision

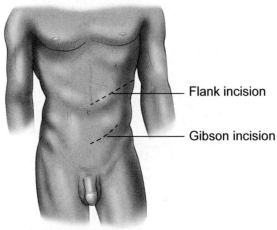

Flank incision

Gibson incision

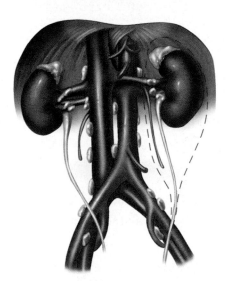

Figure 27.19

Boundaries of a left radical
nephrectomy (the dotted line
represents both the surgical
margin and Gerota's fascia).

rib, is brought down to the rib, and extended anteriorly to the lateral border of the rectus abdominis muscle. Rib resection is then carried out. This technique provides wider exposure.

DETAILS

By means of a periosteal (Alexander) elevator, the rib is dissected up on its anterior surface. A Doyen periosteal elevator is passed behind the rib, which is then freed up from the periosteum. The rib is transected as far back as possible with a rib cutter. Attention is then turned to dissecting the lower fibers of the diaphragm. The pleura is likewise dissected. The retroperitoneum is entered, and the peritoneum is incised and opened. A self-retaining (Finochietto) retractor is placed on the right side.

The liver overlies the kidney and should be retracted upward by a wide Deaver retractor. The liver should be packed with a moistened laparotomy pad before the retractor is placed. The colon is then mobilized and reflected medially by incising the avascular white line; The duodenum is likewise mobilized and reflected medially, giving access to the renal hilum, which is then carefully dissected. The renal vein and, posterior to it, the renal artery are mobilized, dissected out, ligated, and divided. Extreme care should be taken not to injure any adjacent structures.

The dissection is then carried out toward the liver along the vena cava, into which the adrenal vein drains. The vein, after being identified and mobilized, is ligated and divided. The lower pole of the kidney and the surrounding perinephric fat can then be freed up, and the ureter is identified. After the ureter is identified, it can be dissected toward the bladder and then doubly ligated with hemoclips and divided. The upper pole is then mobilized. Adrenal vessels should be clipped and divided. Blunt and sharp dissection are used, and hemoclips are applied to ensure hemostasis. After the upper pole is freed, the kidney is removed from the field and sent to the pathology department. The renal fossa is inspected for bleeding and hemostasis is ensured. The wound is irrigated.

CLOSURE

The pleura is closed, and, if necessary, a chest tube is placed. The flank incision is closed in three layers as described earlier with 1 or 1-0 polyglactin suture material. Drains are not used.

Left Radical Nephrectomy

A left radical nephrectomy is different insofar as the anatomy of the renal vein is concerned: the adrenal vein and the gonadal vein drain into it. The descending colon is dissected and reflected medially from Gerota's fascia. The great vessels are identified, and the left renal vein is dissected in front of the aorta. Both the gonadal vein and the adrenal vein are identified, dissected out, ligated, and divided. The renal artery is then localized and freed from its surrounding tissue. The artery and then the vein are further mobilized, ligated, and divided with heavy silk suture (2-0 silk). The vein is divided close to the aorta. The rest of the dissection and mobilization of the kidney follows as for the right side. Attention should be given to the left gastroepiploic artery and short gastric vessels, which may be ligated during mobilization of the upper pole of the kidney. Careful handling of the spleen and descending colon should be ensured.

Partial Nephrectomy

INCISION AND EXPOSURE

The approach to a partial nephrectomy is similar to that for the simple nephrectomy.

DETAILS

After the kidney is mobilized and freed up from its fatty surroundings, the tumor or injury should be identified in either the upper or the lower pole. If the lesion is clearly confined to either pole, partial nephrectomy can be carried out. The renal hilum is dissected out, and the vessels mobilized to provide good control of renal vasculature. A moistened umbilical tape is then placed around the kidney proximal to the hilum and cinched down to occlude intrarenal circulation (alternatively, a Rumel clamp may be used).

The renal capsule is incised, and the renal parenchyma is incised with the handle of a scalpel. The cut edge of the kidney is inspected for vessels, and these are sutured with 4-0 chromic suture placed in a figure-of-eight. The umbilical tape or clamp may be released to identify vessels that have not been sutured. The collecting system is closed with a running 5-0 or 4-0 chromic suture.

CLOSURE

The edges of the renal capsule are then brought back together with the interrupted mattress sutures of 2-0 chromic catgut. Care should be taken not to tear the friable parenchyma. Perinephric fat may be brought back over the closed capsule to provide extra tamponade. The kidney is then placed back into the gutter, and the incision is closed. One or two Penrose drains should be placed around the kidney and should be removed 25 days after the procedure.

Nephroureterectomy
INCISION AND EXPOSURE

A flank incision extended to the lower abdomen or a second incision (Gibson incision or transplantation incision) should be used. The approach to the kidney is similar to that for a simple nephrectomy. The exposure to the distal ureter and bladder is the same as for renal transplantation. Closure is the same as for nephrectomy or renal transplantation. Drains are not used.

Postprocedure Care

Postprocedure orders include intravenous administration of antibiotics for a short course, strict monitoring of vital signs and urine output, and breathing exercises with incentive spirometry. If patients experience nausea and vomiting, a nasogastric tube should be placed. The Foley catheter is left in place for 24 hours and then removed. Pain medication should be administered liberally. A chest radiograph is helpful to document or rule out pneumothorax caused by entry into the pleura. If the pneumothorax is significant (greater than 15%–20%), a chest tube should be inserted. The sequential compression stockings and device should be left in place for 2–3 days. The patient may be out of bed on the operative day and should ambulate. Intravenous fluids are administered until the patient is able to resume normal oral fluid intake. Sutures or skin clips may be removed on the day of discharge.

Potential Complications

Complications during the procedure were described earlier. There can be significant bleeding and injury to adjacent organs during renal procedures (**Table 27.10**). Both can be avoided by controlling the renal vasculature and by using careful

Table 27.10	Potential Complications of Nephrectomy	
Operative	**Postprocedure**	
Hemorrhage or shock	Wound	
Pleural or pulmonary complications	Dehiscence	
Cardiovascular complications	Infection	
Visceral injury	Hernia	
	Gastrointestinal	
	Ileus	
	Fistula	
	Pulmonary	
	Pneumothorax	
	Pneumonia	
	Atelectasis	
	Cardiovascular	
	Myocardial infraction	
	Congestive failure	
	Thrombophlebitis	
	Cerebrovascular accident	
	Shock secondary to blood loss, septicemia	
	Renal function impairment	

technique. Postprocedure complications include infections, prolonged ileus, pneumonia, wound dehiscence, and herniation. Some patients may experience varying degrees of intercostal neuralgia, which usually resolves during several months. Mortality is reported as less than 1%. Increased mortality rates are noted in patients with renal failure, azotemia, or infections.

PROSTATE PROCEDURES

Surgery on the prostate is performed for benign prostatic hyperplasia and cancer. A prostatectomy is performed for benign prostatic hyperplasia when the gland is configured in such a way that it is not amenable to transurethral resection.

Open Prostatectomy

The typical patient with symptoms of bladder outlet obstruction is older than 50 years of age. The physical examination is usually unrevealing, except in the rare cases when the patient has urinary retention and has an easily palpable bladder on examination of the abdomen. The rectal examination may help in assessing prostatic size as well as in ruling out a prostatic nodule or induration indicative of a possible malignancy.

Operative options are considered for benign prostatic hyperplasia when symptoms of bladder outlet obstruction become significant to the patient. These include urinary frequency, urgency, decreased stream, straining to void, dribbling, nocturia, and, urinary retention. Even though most men experience some degree of benign prostatic hyperplasia, only a small percentage of all men require an operation to relieve symptoms of bladder outlet obstruction because of the new availability of reasonable alternative medical and surgical treatment options (Leslie, 2006). When done, the goal of the procedure is to alleviate the symptoms and prevent further consequences of chronic outlet obstruction, such as progressive renal failure, recurrent urinary tract infections because of urine stasis, and development of bladder stones. Surgery on the prostate for benign disease can be either open or closed. Open surgery refers to procedures done through an incision that extends down to the prostatic tissue. Closed surgery refers to transurethral resection carried out through a cystoscope.

Indications

Indications for open prostatectomy are limited to significant bladder outlet obstruction, urodynamic evaluation consistent with bladder obstruction (high bladder pressure and low urinary flow), a large prostate not amenable to transurethral resection, and the presence of large bladder stones. At cystoscopy, the prostate may appear to extend into the bladder, obscuring the ureteral orifices.

Related Procedures

Related procedures include radical prostatectomy for prostatic cancer. In other related procedures to remove bladder stones and to re-implant the ureters, a similar transvesical approach is used. Several approaches to the prostate are possible: suprapubic, transvesical, retropubic, and perineal. Only the suprapubic approach will be described.

Nursing Implications

ANESTHESIA

Open prostatectomy is usually performed under general anesthesia. Occasionally, continuous epidural anesthesia is used alone or as an adjunct to the general anesthesia. Blood is typed and crossmatched for all patients for possible transfusion in the operating room. The circulating nurse assists in blood administration according to hospital policy.

POSITION

The patient undergoing suprapubic or radical retropubic prostatectomy is placed in the supine position. A small roll or sandbag is placed under the patient's sacrum. The bed is placed in a slight Trendelenburg position. Pneumatic compression stockings should be placed by the circulating nurse during patient positioning. If the surgeon also requires the table to be flexed to accentuate the patient's position, the patient's pelvic area should be over the break in the bed. In addition, if indicated, a 28 or 30 Fr red rubber catheter maybe placed in the rectum at this time and hooked to straight drainage. The electrosurgical patient return electrode should be placed at this point, avoiding the area to be prepared.

ESTABLISHING AND MAINTAINING THE STERILE FIELD

In establishing a sterile field, if the surgeon elects to remove the patient's body hair at the operative site, the patient is clipped from umbilicus to midthigh. A preparation using the prescribed solution covering the same area is performed. A sterile towel is placed under the penis after the preparation.

During the prostatectomy, the scrub person should keep the following in mind:

A Foley catheter is inserted, with sterile technique, at the start of the procedure.

Urine is drained at intervals from the clamped catheter and must be measured.

A bladder irrigation kit should be available for instillation of fluid into the bladder.

The prostate specimen is removed.

During the reanastomosis of the urethra and bladder, free needles as well as Swedgeon sutures may be used.

Extra long instruments and an electrosurgery extension tip may be needed.

EQUIPMENT AND SUPPLIES

Table 27.11 lists equipment and supplies for open prostatectomy.

Table 27.11	Equipment and Supplies for Open Prostatectomy

Active electrode tip cleaner

Basin set

Bookwalter retractor

Deaver retractor, extra deep

Drain, Penrose or Jackson-Pratt (according to surgeon preference)

Drainage bag, straight with urine meter

Drape pack

Electrosurgery pencil

Extended active electrode tip

Foley catheter irrigation set

Foley catheter, silastic, 30-mL balloon (according to surgeon preference)

Hemoclips, large and medium

Laparotomy set

Long instrument pack

Magnetic pad

Malecot catheter, silastic (for suprapubic tube according to surgeon preference)

Needle counter

Patient return electrode

Prostatectomy set

Pushers, Kitner dissectors

Red rubber catheter, 28 Fr or 30 Fr (rectal tube)

Scalpel blades Nos. 10, 11, and 15

Skin marker

Skin staples

Spleen roll

Sponges, 4 × 8 radiopaque

Sponges, large and small laparotomy, radiopaque

Suction tubing

Suture (select chromic and synthetic suture based on surgeon preference; usually sutures include, 0, 2-0, 3-0, 4-0, 5-0 chromic and synthetic ties on Swedgeon needles)

Toomey syringe

Ureteral catheter

Vessel loops

Physiological Monitoring

During the procedure, the circulating nurse maintains accurate blood loss records, including sponge and suction container blood loss and irrigation. Urine drained onto the field via the sterile catheter must also be measured and recorded.

Specimens and Cultures

Cultures are not routinely performed during prostatectomy unless an infection is suspected. Specimens include prostate gland with surrounding tissue and pelvic lymph nodes for frozen section examination (for radical prostatectomy only).

Drugs and Solutions

Drugs and solutions delivered by the circulating nurse include normal saline for irrigation (warm), neomycin and polymyxin B (Neosporin G.U. irrigant), and lubricant (KY jelly).

Physician Orders and Laboratory and Diagnostic Studies

Before the procedure, the patient undergoes routine laboratory assessment (CBC, platelet count, electrolyte panel, blood urea nitrogen, and creatinine measurements), ECG, chest radiograph, and an evaluation of the upper urinary tract by either ultrasound or IVU. At least 4 units of blood or expanders should be available in the blood bank before the procedure. Many patients donate their own blood before the procedure for possible autologous transfusion during the procedure.

The patient may administer a Fleets enema at home the night before the procedure, as well as a perineal, genitalia, and lower abdomen povidone-iodine preparation. Parenteral antibiotics may be administered before the procedure.

Procedure

The patient is placed in the supine position. The lower abdomen, genitalia, and perineum are prepared with the prescribed solution. The penis is included in the field.

Incision and Exposure

A suprapubic incision is made in the midline to the fascia, which is sharply incised, taking care not to enter the bladder prematurely (**Fig. 27.20**). The peritoneum is identified and reflected toward the patient's head, and the bladder is dissected from its lateral attachments by blunt dissection.

The bladder is filled with 200–300 mL of saline and then opened. A self-retaining (Balfour) retractor is then placed, and the dome of the bladder is packed with several moist sponges, The ureteral orifices are identified, and if they are hard to identify, ureteral stents (5 Fr) are placed. Using electrosurgery, a circumferential incision is made below the bladder neck.

Details

Blunt dissection is then carried out to shell out the prostatic adenoma. After the adenoma is removed, there may be brisk bleeding. The prostatic fossa is packed with a warm laparotomy pad or spleen roll, which is left in place for at least 5 minutes. The fossa is then reinspected and 1-0 chromic suture may be placed at the 5 and 7 o'clock

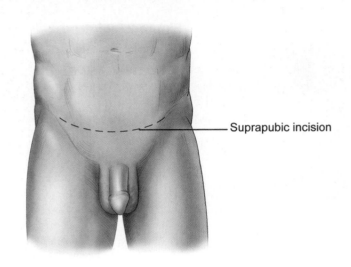

Figure 27.20
Suprapubic incision.

— Suprapubic incision

positions. A Foley catheter is placed and the balloon is inflated with 60–100 mL of fluid. Traction on the Foley catheter helps tamponade bleeding from the prostatic fossa.

CLOSURE

The bladder is then closed in two layers with either chromic or Vicryl absorbable suture material. A suprapubic catheter may be placed. Drainage of the perivesical space may be accomplished by either Jackson-Pratt drains or Penrose drains. The fascia is then closed with nonabsorbable suture. Subcutaneous and skin closure are performed in the standard fashion.

Postprocedure Care

After the procedure, the patient should be given parenteral antibiotics and kept well hydrated. The urine output should be monitored carefully. The Foley catheter and suprapubic tube should be checked periodically to ensure patency and irrigated gently to dislodge any clots. Drainage from the wound should be monitored. CBC and electrolytes should be checked for at least 2 days after the procedure. The drains can be removed on day 3 or 4 if the drainage is scant. The suprapubic tube may be removed 4 days after the procedure. A cystogram may help to ascertain if the bladder is closed and leak free before removing the Foley catheter, which is done 1 or 2 days later.

Potential Complications

Bleeding may be significant during the procedure, and all patients should be warned that they might need a transfusion. Retrograde ejaculation is an anticipated occurrence after prostatectomy.

Stricture disease and bladder contracture may occur later, causing recurrent voiding symptoms. Other complications include incontinence, impotence, potential injuries to intra-abdominal organs, and persistent bladder leak which may require prolonged bladder drainage.

Robotic Prostatectomy

Recent developments in computer, mechanical, and laparoscopic technology have allowed the development of a robotic surgical system. The system enables the surgeon to operate the robot without actually being in the sterile field. Robotic instruments

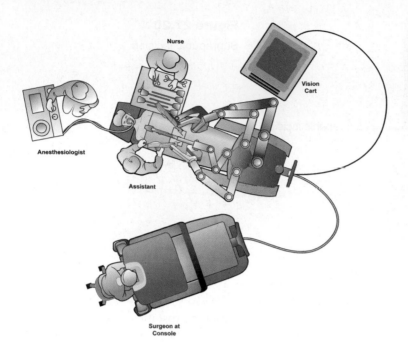

Figure 27.21

Robotic prostatectomy.

Source: Photo/Illustration courtesy of Intuitive Surgical, Inc., 2008.

also offer greater articulation than traditional laparoscopic instruments, thus allowing increased and more precise internal mobility (**Fig. 27.21**). The surgeon is also able to view the operation in three dimensions instead of two in traditional laparoscopy. Robotic prostatectomy allows for a less invasive approach than open prostatectomy. Compared to an open approach, robotic prostatectomy offers potential advantages such as shortened hospital stays, less pain, decreased risk of infection, and the possibility of a faster return to normal activity of daily living.

Nursing Implications

GENERAL GUIDELINES

Set up and test the robotic equipment before it is used on the patient. The nurse must make sure the camera is aligned, the light is functional, and the robotic arms and cartridges are in working order.

ANESTHESIA

General anesthesia is used and an epidural catheter may be placed for pain control. The anesthesia provider places a nasogastric tube prior to the incision.

POSITION

A safety strap is placed across the chest. The patient begins in a supine position and then progresses to steep Trendelenburg (>20–30 degrees). The patient's legs are separated via a split leg table or Allen stirrups. Tuck arms to the sides using sleds for stability and protection. Pad bony prominences and pressure points.

ESTABLISHING AND MAINTAINING A STERILE FIELD

Establishing and maintaining a sterile field presents many challenges for the nurse. First, the nurse must drape the robotic arms and maintain arm sterility from room traffic. In addition, the light cord and camera must remain covered with sterile drapes throughout the procedure. If the surgeon opts to remove hair, electric clippers may be used.

The abdomen, penis, scrotum, perineum, and thighs are prepped with the solution of choice. The patient is draped to expose these areas. An 18 F 5cc Foley catheter is inserted.

EQUIPMENT AND SUPPLIES

In addition to the items listed in **Table 27.12**, all of the previous supplies for an open prostatectomy should be available for the procedure in case there is a conversion to open prostatectomy.

PHYSIOLOGICAL MONITORING

Physiological monitoring is similar to that of a prostatectomy, except that the nurse and surgical team should be aware of abdominal pressure, and aware of complications of steep Trendelenburg position.

SPECIMENS AND CULTURES

Cultures are not routinely performed during prostatectomy unless an infection is suspected. Specimens include prostate gland with surrounding tissue and may include the pelvic lymph nodes for frozen section examination.

DRUGS AND SOLUTIONS

Drugs and solutions delivered by the circulating nurse include the following: 0.25% Marcaine, 0.9 % normal saline irrigation, sterile water, and indigo carmine.

PHYSICIAN ORDERS AND LABORATORY AND DIAGNOSTIC STUDIES

The orders and testing are similar to the orders for prostate cancer.

Procedure

INCISION AND EXPOSURE

The surgeon places trocars and cannulae using conventional laparoscopic techniques in the positions illustrated in **Figure 27.22**. Next, the surgeon insufflates the abdomen and retracts and repositions the colon and small bowel away from the operative area before moving the robotic cart in place.

DETAILS

The circulating nurse, guided by the surgeon, rolls the patient cart into place between the patient's legs, locks the wheels to prevent rolling, and makes sure that the operating arms are high enough to clear the patient's legs (**Fig. 27.23**). The camera is then docked to the patient cart, followed by the appropriate instruments on the robot arms. The instrument arms are manipulated to place them in a position where they may move freely as well as have access to the trocars.

The surgeon begins the robotic portion of the procedure by freeing the bladder from its anterior and lateral attachments. The surgeon then opens the endopelvic fascia and mobilizes the prostate from the urogenital diaphragm by dissecting up to the dorsal venous complex. After ligating the dorsal venous complex, a plane is established for apical prostate dissection.

Table 27.12	Equipment and Supplies for Robotic Laparoscopic Prostatectomy

Allis forceps, 6" narrow × 2	Patient return electrode
Band-Aids, large	Retractor, Harrington, small
Basin set	Retractor, vein
Bean bag positioner	Robotic light cord
Bioclusive	Robotic parts set
da Vinci robot cart, console, and tower	Robotic scope and camera
Disposable camera drape	Robotic trocars and caps
Disposable instrument arm drapes	S retractors
Dover strap	Scalpel blades, No. 10, 15, and 20
Drain, Blake with trocar,19 Fr round Blake	Scope warmer
Drain, Jackson-Pratt, 100-mL reservoir	Sponges, 4 × 8 radiopaque
Dressing, abdominal	Steri-strips
Dressing, Dermabond	Suction, Poole
Electrosurgery generator	Suture (select suture based on surgeon preference; usually includes chromic, silk, and absorbable and nonabsorbable synthetic suture, free ties and Swedgeon with appropriate needles)
Electrosurgery Pencil	
Endoscopic clip applies	
Endoscopic fan retractor	
Endoscopic gastrointestinal anastomosis staplers	Syringe, Asepto
Endoscopic paddle retractor, 12-mm	Syringe, Toomey
Endoscopic pouch specimen retriever	Syringes, 10-, 30-, and 60-mL
Fanfold drape, large	Telfa
Fluffs, sterile	U-bar set
Foley catheter, 20 Fr with 5- or 30-mL balloon)	Umbilical tapes
Gauze dressing, petrolatum	Ureteral catheters available
Gore suture passer	Urine drainage bag
Laparoscopic grasper	Vessel loops
Leggings, sterile	Video monitor, second
Ligaclip applier, large	
Micro scissors and tips	

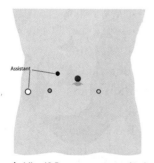
da Vinci® Prostatectomy (3-Arm)

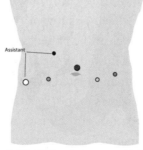
da Vinci® Prostatectomy (4-Arm)

Figure 27.22

Port placement for robotic prostatectomy.

Source: Photo/Illustration courtesy of Intuitive Surgical, Inc., 2008.

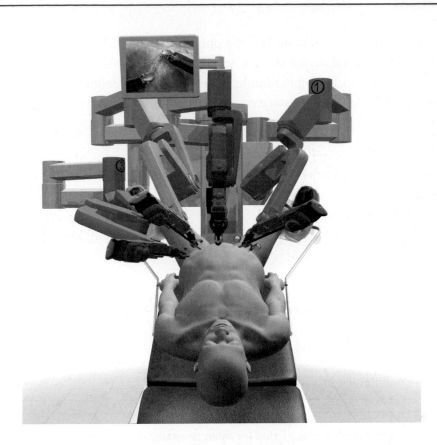

Figure 27.23

Placement of the patient card for robotic prostatectomy.

Source: Photo/Illustration courtesy of Intuitive Surgical, Inc., 2008.

The bladder neck junction is then identified and transected, followed by transection of the vas deferens and seminal vesicles. Since the neurovascular bundle is very close to the seminal vesicle, electrosurgery should be used sparingly, if at all. The surgeon dissects the prostate posteriorly via an opening created in Denonvilliers fascia and then performs an apical dissection of the prostate, followed by transection of the urethra and then urethrovascular reanastomosis. When the specimen is freed, it is retrieved with an endo-pouch through one of the 12 mm trocar sites.

The laparoscopic incisions are closed in the normal fashion by the surgeon.

Postprocedure Care

After recovery in the postanesthesia care unit, the patient is transferred to a surgical or urological unit for 24–72 hours. Ambulation begins as soon as practical on the operative day. Spirometry and deep breathing exercises should be performed. Intake and output should be carefully measured, and urine should be frequently assessed for hematuria. Pain control medications and antibiotics should be administered according to surgeon preference.

Radical Retropubic Prostatectomy (Nerve Sparing)

This procedure involves removal of the entire prostate gland, including the prostatic urethra, the seminal vesicles, and vas deferens, with subsequent reconstruction of the bladder neck and proximal urethra.

Indications

Radical retropubic prostatectomy is believed to be the most effective form of treatment for patients younger than age 70 years with prostatic cancer limited to the

PSA
Prostate Specific
Antigen

prostatic capsule. On physical examination, the only notable feature is a palpable nodule or induration on rectal examination, usually picked up on routine examination. Patients may also have ultrasound findings as well as elevated results of a prostate specific antigen (PSA) test. The history is unremarkable.

Nursing Implications
ANESTHESIA
Radical retropubic prostatectomy is performed under general anesthesia and continuous epidural anesthesia as an adjunct. The continuous epidural catheter may later be used for postprocedure pain control. Blood is typed and crossmatched for all patients. The circulating nurse assists in blood administration according to hospital policy.

POSITION
The patient is placed in the same position as for an open prostatectomy.

ESTABLISHING AND MAINTAINING THE STERILE FIELD
The patient is prepared and draped as described for an open prostatectomy. The sterile field is also maintained in a similar fashion.

EQUIPMENT AND SUPPLIES
Use the same equipment and supplies listed for open prostatectomy in **Table 24.11**.

PHYSIOLOGICAL MONITORING
Physiological monitoring is similar to that done during the open prostatectomy. In this procedure, rapid and significant blood loss can occur when the surgeons are working on the dorsal venous complex. Both the scrub person and the circulating nurse should prepare for this potential event.

SPECIMENS AND CULTURES
During lymph node dissection, right and left obturator lymph node specimens are sent to the laboratory for frozen section examination and diagnosis. The lymph node dissection may be performed laparoscopically. The radical prostatectomy specimen consists of the entire prostate gland, including the prostatic urethra, the seminal vesicles, and the vas deferens.

DRUGS AND SOLUTIONS
Drugs and solutions delivered by the circulating nurse include normal saline for irrigation (warm), neomycin and polymyxin B (Neosporin G.U, irrigant), lubricant (KY jelly), and indigo carmine (administered by the anesthesia provider to observe urine flow).

PHYSICIAN ORDERS AND LABORATORY AND DIAGNOSTIC STUDIES
Before the procedure, the patient should undergo PSA determination, cystoscopy and needle biopsy of the prostate, bone scan, chest radiography, IVU, and CT and/or MRI to rule out any spread of the tumor. As for the suprapubic prostatectomy, blood loss may be significant and the patient should have at least 4 units of banked blood available.

Procedure

INCISION AND EXPOSURE

The bladder is approached in a manner similar to that described earlier. Before radical prostatectomy, a bilateral staging pelvic lymphadenectomy is carried out. This may be done laparoscopically. The lymph node packets lying in an area limited anteriorly by the external iliac vein, inferiorly by the pelvic side wall, and posteriorly by the obturator nerve up to the bifurcation of the great vessels are then removed on the right and then on the left. The lymph nodes are sent for frozen section examination. If the lymph nodes do not contain tumor, attention is then turned to the prostatectomy.

DETAILS

With the Bookwalter self-retaining retractor in place, the bladder is retracted toward the abdomen. A Foley catheter has been inserted into the bladder. The anterior surface of the prostate is revealed and the endopelvic fascia identified and incised. The dorsal venous complex and puboprostatic ligaments are then ligated and divided. The urethra is palpated and dissected from the rectum with a right-angled clamp. The urethra is cut, revealing the Foley catheter, which is also cut and its bladder end grasped. This then allows the prostate to be lifted up, and further dissection of the posterior aspect of the prostate is carried out to reveal the lateral pedicles. These pedicles contain the neurovascular bundles, which should be preserved to decrease the risk of impotence. The lateral pedicles are then divided with hemoclips. Further posterior dissection is necessary to remove the seminal vesicles and divide the vas deferens; the specimen is then removed. **Figure 27.24** shows a retropubic prostatectomy for prostate cancer.

CLOSURE

The bladder is brought down to the urethra, and a Foley catheter (24 Fr 30-mL balloon) is placed in the bladder. The bladder is anastomosed to the urethra with interrupted sutures. Drains are placed on either side of the bladder (either Penrose or closed suction devices), and closure is accomplished in a manner similar to that used for suprapubic prostatectomy. After the procedure, the Foley catheter is left in place for 3 weeks to allow the urethrovesical anastomosis to heal.

Postprocedure Care

Patients may be admitted to the intensive care unit the first night after the procedure for close monitoring.

Nursing care focuses on measures to prevent thromboembolic sequelae, such as the use of knee-high antiembolism stockings, and pneumatic or sequential compression stockings. Respiratory care via incentive spirometry is provided every 4 hours while the patient is awake. In addition, patients ambulate the day after the procedure.

Postprocedure pain control is accomplished by a number of alternatives, such as an epidural catheter that can be injected by an anesthesia provider or the patient-controlled pump. Also used are intramuscular and oral pain medications, as well as patient controlled intravenous pain medication.

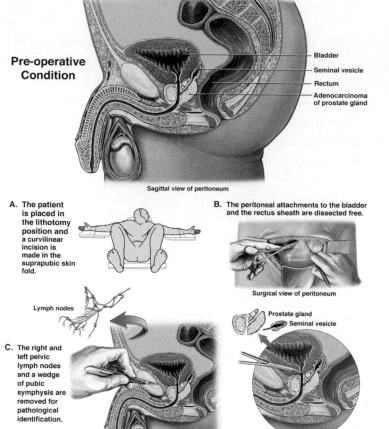

Figure 27.24

Prostate cancer with radical retropubic prostatectomy.

Pre-operative Condition

Bladder
Seminal vesicle
Rectum
Adenocarcinoma of prostate gland

Sagittal view of peritoneum

A. The patient is placed in the lithotomy position and a curvilinear incision is made in the suprapubic skin fold.

B. The peritoneal attachments to the bladder and the rectus sheath are dissected free.

Bladder

Surgical view of peritoneum

Lymph nodes

C. The right and left pelvic lymph nodes and a wedge of pubic symphysis are removed for pathological identification.

Prostate gland
Seminal vesicle

D. The urethra is transected with scissors and the prostate gland is and seminal vesicles are removed.

The Foley catheter functions as a stent, bridging the urethral bladder neck anastomosis. The nurse must monitor the patency and functioning of the Foley catheter at all times.

The nurse is also responsible for strict intake and output measurements and for maintaining the Foley catheter in straight drainage. Minimal manipulation of the Foley is necessary to avoid aggravation of the anastomosis. Irrigation, if done at all, is usually done by the physician.

Additional orders are as follows:

> Vital signs per postoperative protocol Jackson-Pratt drain that is connected to bulb suction, which is reconstituted every shift
>
> Nothing by mouth until the patient expels flatus
>
> Nothing per rectum
>
> Intravenous 5% dextrose in half-normal saline solution with 10 mEq/L of potassium chloride at 125–150 mL/hour

Medications:

> Pain relief medications
>
> Antibiotics per surgeon guidelines
>
> Antacids

Laboratory studies:

> CBC and platelet count
>
> Electrolytes, blood urea nitrogen, and creatinine determinations after the procedure

Potential Complications

Complications during the procedure include hemorrhage and injury to nerve structures and to the rectum, which may be entered inadvertently. Rectal injury can be closed in two layers, provided the patient has received a bowel preparation after the procedure.

Thrombophlebitis and pulmonary emboli are early postprocedure complications and can be minimized by the use of sequential compression devices and early ambulation. Disruption of the urethrovesical anastomosis may occur, leading most often to permanent incontinence and urine leak. This can be prevented by keeping the Foley catheter in place for an adequate length of time. Late postprocedure complications include urinary bladder incontinence and impotence. The incidence of these complications is based on age, height, weight, and preexisting conditions.

RADICAL CYSTECTOMY AND DIVERSION

Cystectomy refers to the removal of the bladder, which is usually performed for invasive bladder cancer. Certain rare conditions, however, may also lead to removal of the bladder: intractable bleeding from hemorrhagic cystitis, pyocystis (chronically infected bladder), severe painful symptoms from interstitial cystitis, and severe cases of neurogenic bladder. Simple cystectomy refers to removal of the bladder only. Radical cystectomy is recommended for cancer therapy and includes removal of the bladder and iliac and obturator lymph node packets. In the male, the peritoneum covering the bladder, the ureteral stumps, the seminal vesicles, the prostate, and a small part of the membranous urethra are also removed (**Fig. 27.25**). In the female, the uterus, the anterior vaginal wall, the ovaries, the fallopian tubes, and the entire urethra are excised (**Fig. 27.26**). In addition, a procedure to divert the stream of urine is performed. Since the 1950s, the standard of care has been the Bricker ileal loop diversion. Other techniques of diversion include colon conduit, ureterosigmoid diversion, and cutaneous ureterostomy.

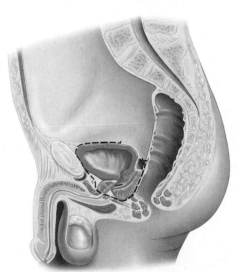

Figure 27.25

Simple cystectomy in the male means removal of the bladder with a portion of the overlying pelvic peritoneum, the ureteral stumps, the prostate, the seminal vesicles, and a portion of the membranous urethra.

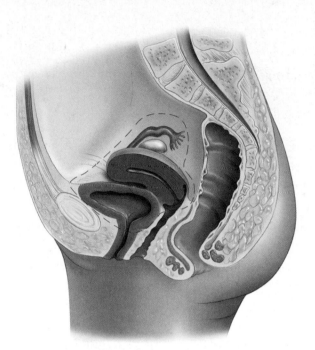

Figure 27.26

In the female patient, the uterus, ovaries, fallopian tubes, and a portion of the vaginal vault and urethra are included in the surgical specimen.

Indications

Bladder cancer is usually found in patients older than age 50 and only rarely in younger patients. Gross or microscopic hematuria is present in 85% of cases. Patients may also note bladder irritability with increased frequency of urination, dysuria, and urgency. The diagnosis is made at cystoscopy when biopsy and transurethral resection of the lesion is carried out. The physical examination is usually unrevealing.

A general indication for radical cystectomy is transitional cell carcinoma of the bladder, which is invasive into the detrusor muscle. Diagnosis is confirmed by microscopic examination of bladder biopsy material obtained during cystoscopy. If the tumor extends into the urethra, urethrectomy should also be done.

Related Procedures

Partial cystectomy may be performed in selected patients, thus preserving voiding function. Several other operative procedures, including an open bladder procedure for stone disease, prostatectomy, and ureteral reimplantation, employ a similar approach to the bladder.

Nursing Implications
Anesthesia

Patients undergoing a radical cystectomy and diversion procedure are given a general anesthetic. Continuous epidural infusion may be used to supplement the general anesthetic as well as to help control pain after the procedure. Blood is typed and crossmatched for possible transfusion. If an autologous blood supply has been arranged, these units should be administered first. The circulating nurse should follow hospital policy while assisting the anesthesia provider with blood transfusion. The circulating nurse should locate and have available a blood warmer and a pressure bag for transfusion.

Position

Place the patient in the supine position with a small roll under the sacrum. For urethrectomy, place the patient in the relaxed lithotomy position. If using the low lithotomy position, support the patient's feet with Allen stirrups. In addition, the nurse should follow routine precautions when placing the patient in the lithotomy position. A 28–30 Fr red rubber catheter is inserted to act as a rectal tube. Apply thigh-high antiembolism or pneumatic compression stockings to the patient before the preparation begins.

Establishing and Maintaining the Sterile Field

The patient is prepared from the nipple line to the midthigh with the prescribed solution, including the penis in men and the perineum and vagina in women.

Establishing and maintaining the sterile field is challenging for the scrub person. Leg drapes must be used if the patient is in the low lithotomy position. When the patient is in the lithotomy position, the Mayo stand can usually be brought between the legs and placed over one leg. Care must be taken to avoid leaning on the patient's legs by the members of the operative team. Some surgeons need to work between the open legs during the procedure. Because the surgeons usually sit down, care must be taken to avoid contamination of other areas owing to changes in the height of the sterile field. If the Bookwalter self-retaining retractor is used, the pieces should be kept together on one small table so that the retractor can be moved from side to side of the operative field during placement of the retractor pieces.

The scrub person should have enough extra cartridges for the reusable disposable stapling device as requested by the surgeon.

Equipment and Supplies

Table 27.13 lists equipment and supplies for a radical cystectomy.

Physiological Monitoring

Blood loss during the radical cystectomy and diversion can be sudden and severe. The circulating nurse must measure and record sponge and suction container blood loss, irrigation, and urine output. The circulating nurse should also assist the anesthesia provider in the estimation of blood and urine volume on the drapes.

Specimens and Cultures

Cultures are not usually indicated in this procedure, unless an infection is suspected. Specimens include the following:

Right and left distal ureter for frozen section

Right and left iliac, and obturator lymph node packets for routine processing

For males: bladder, peritoneum covering the bladder, ureteral stumps, seminal vesicles, prostate, and small amount of the membranous urethra

For females: bladder, uterus, anterior vaginal wall, ovaries, fallopian tubes, and entire urethra

Drugs and Solutions

Drugs and solutions include sterile lubricant, sterile normal saline for irrigation, and neomycin and polymyxin B (Neosporin G.U. irrigant).

Table 27.13	Equipment and Supplies for Radical Cystectomy

Active electrode tip cleaner

Allis clamps, small

Basin set

Bookwalter retractor

Deaver retractor, extra deep

Drape pack

Drapes, leg (for lithotomy position)

Electrosurgery pencil

Extended active electrode tip

Foley catheter irrigation set

Foley catheter, 24 Fr silastic with 30-mL balloon (according to surgeon preference)

Gastric and bowel pack

Gastrostomy tube per surgeon request

Hemoclips, large and medium

J diversion stents × 2

Jackson-Pratt drain (according to surgeon preference)

Laparotomy set

Long instrument pack

Magnetic pad

Malleable bladder blades for Balfour retractor (if used)

Needle counter

Package vessel loops

Patient return electrode

Pushers, Kitner dissectors

Red rubber catheter (rectal tube), 28 or 30 Fr

Scalpel blades Nos. 10, 11, and 15

Silastic Malecot catheter (or suprapubic tube according to surgeon preference)

Skin marker

Skin staples

Spleen roll

Sponges, 4 × 8 radiopaque

Sponges, large and small laparotomy, radiopaque

Stapling devices with appropriate reloading units

Suction tubing

Suture (select chromic and synthetic suture based on surgeon preference; usually sutures include 0, 2-0, 3-0, 4-0, 5-0 chromic, and synthetic braided and monofilament suture ties and on Swedgeon needles, and retention sutures)

Syringe, Asepto

Syringes, 3- and 50-mL

Toomey syringe

Towel drape (Steri-drape)

Ureteral catheter

Urine drainage bag with meter, straight

Urostomy pouch

Vascular set

Vessel loops

Webster cannula

Physician Orders

Patients are admitted the day of the procedure unless their other medical history warrants an overnight stay the day before. Physician orders include:

> Clear liquid diet before the procedure; nothing-by-mouth status after midnight the night before the procedure
>
> Intravenous 5% dextrose in half-normal saline with 10 mEq/L of potassium chloride at 100 mL/hour
>
> Incentive spirometry teaching
>
> Enterostomal therapy consultation
>
> Bowel prep as prescribed
>
> Oral and parenteral antibiotics before the procedure

Laboratory and Diagnostic Studies

Before undergoing cystectomy and diversion, the patient undergoes routine laboratory evaluation (as described for prostatectomy), chest radiography, ECG, bone scan, IVU, and CT.

Procedure

Incision and Exposure

A midline abdominal incision is made from the upper abdomen to the pelvis, around the umbilicus, and at least 45 cm away from the medial aspect of the stomal site. The peritoneal cavity is entered, and abdominal and pelvic exploration is carried out. The self-retaining retractor is placed (Balfour or Bookwalter), and the intestines may be packed superiorly with moist towels.

Details

The peritoneum overlying the ureters on either side is opened, and the ureters are dissected out, doubly ligated with clips, and divided. The proximal ends of the ureters may be sent for frozen section examination to ensure that they are free of tumor. The ureters are left clamped to allow them to dilate. This facilitates the anastomosis between the bowel and the ureter. A tunnel is then made in the mesentery of the sigmoid colon so that the left ureter can be brought over to the right side.

Pelvic lymph node dissection is carried out on both sides; both obturator and iliac packets are taken. At the end of the dissection, the lateral pelvic walls and vessels should be free of any lymphatic tissue.

The bladder is dissected from the pelvic wall. In the female, dissection of the female genital organs is carried out. The ovarian and uterine vessels are ligated and divided. With a povidone-iodine soaked sponge in the vagina, the vaginal cuff is removed and oversewn with a 10 chromic running suture. The lateral pedicles containing blood supply and lymphatic drainage to the bladder are then identified.

Division of the lateral pedicles of the bladder is then performed posteriorly. Anteriorly, in the male, a maneuver similar to that for the radical suprapubic prostatectomy is used to divide the endopelvic fascia, the dorsal venous complex, and the urethra. In the female, the entire urethra is grasped at the bladder neck, dissected to the vulva, and removed with the bladder. Care is then taken to dissect the posterior aspect of the bladder, avoiding any injury to the rectosigmoid.

A loop of ileum is selected and measured to be approximately 15 cm in length, and the mesenteric vascular pedicle is prepared. The ileum is divided either between two clamps or with a gastrointestinal anastomosis stapler (GIA). The conduit is placed in an infra-mesenteric position, and the ileum is re-anastomosed. The mesenteric defect is closed. The ureters are then anastomosed to the ileal loop. The ureters may be attached to the proximal end of the loop or directed into the loop by making small circular openings in the distal part of the loop. Ureteroileal anastomosis is then performed with interrupted sutures of 4-0 chromic catgut. Before completing the anastomosis, ureteral stents (single J 6 Fr) are placed up to the kidney and brought through the stoma. After completion of the ureteroileal anastomosis, a circular incision in the abdominal wall is made at the site of the stoma. Subcutaneous fatty tissue is removed, and a cruciate incision is made in the fascia. The ileal loop is then brought through the anterior abdominal wall and a stoma is fashioned.

The pelvis is then carefully reinspected and hemostasis is established. Urine output from the ureteral stents should be carefully monitored, and the stents can be irrigated to ensure patency. The abdominal contents are reinspected and replaced in an anatomical position. **Figure 27.27** sows the major steps for establishing an ileal conduit following radical cystectomy. **Figure 27.28** shows the Bricker method of ureteral placement for ileal loop cutaneous diversion.

Closure

The ileal loop is placed in such a way that neither loop nor ureter is kinked. Drains are then placed in the pelvis and close to the ureteroileal anastomosis. The anterior abdominal wall is closed in a standard fashion. Skin staples are used to reapproximate the skin. Some surgeons recommend placement of a gastrostomy tube before closure.

Postprocedure Care

After the procedure, the patient may be taken to the intensive care unit for a 24-hour observation period. During that time, careful monitoring of urine output and vigorous fluid replacement may be necessary to keep up with third spacing (loss of fluid from the intravascular space into the soft tissues and the abdominal cavity). Early ambulation and vigorous pulmonary toilet should prevent postoperative pulmonary complications. Postprocedure orders include the following:

- Obtain vital signs per postoperative routine.
- Strictly monitor intake and output.
- Continue ECG and arterial catheter monitoring.
- Connect the nasogastric tube to low intermittent suction.
- Connect the gastrostomy tube to gravity drainage.
- Connect the Hemovac to suction.
- Perform chest physiotherapy and incentive spirometry every 2 hours while the patient is awake.
- Maintain intermittent compression devices at all times.
- Administer postprocedure pain medications.
- Administer antibiotics intravenously for 24–48 hours.
- Give antacids.

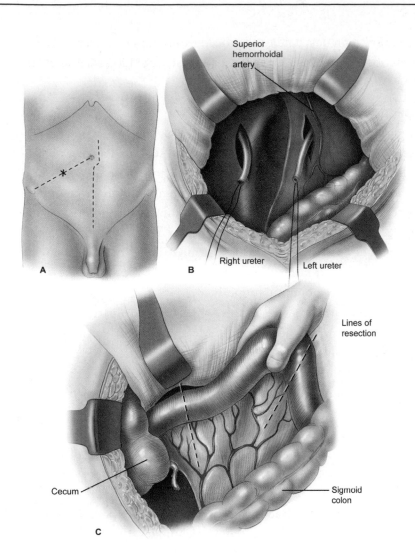

Figure 27.27

Major steps of an operation for ileal conduit, urinary diversion. (A) Location of the ileal stoma; (B) Ureters freed; the left ureter is brought under the base of the mesosigmoid; (C) Location of the ileal segment.

27

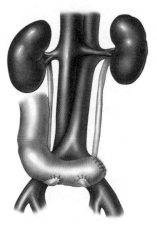

Figure 27.28

Bricker method of ureteral placement for ileal loop cutaneous diversion.

Skin staples are removed on day 7 after the procedure. The ureteral stents are left in place for the prescribed time. The patient is usually discharged 5–7 days after the procedure.

Potential Complications

Immediate complications of a radical procedure on the bladder are those encountered with any extensive procedure that also involves bowel surgery. Patients require large amounts of fluid to keep up with losses and third spacing. Blood loss may also be significant. After the procedure, every measure to prevent pulmonary complications and deep venous thrombosis and/or pulmonary embolism should be taken. Early ureteroileal anastomosis disruption may occur and require reoperation. Small bowel obstruction may develop from adhesions formed in the peritoneal cavity. Parastomal hernia results from a fascial defect at the level of the stoma. Revision may be required if the loop does not drain properly.

Late complications include ureteroileal stenosis, which leads to obstruction of the flow of urine from the kidney to the ileal conduit. Metabolic disturbance may also develop in the form of metabolic acidosis.

Most complications from the procedure are related to the ileal loop diversion. Close patient followup and monitoring is therefore mandatory.

ENDOSCOPY

Direct observation of the entire urinary tract is possible with the use of refined endoscopic techniques. Cystoscopes allow visualization of the bladder while ureteroscopes allow visualization the upper urinary tract. Biopsy and resection of suspicious lesions, as well as stone extraction and resection of the prostate, can be performed endoscopically. The various endoscopic techniques, their applications, and the equipment used to carry them out are described.

Cystoscopy

Cystoscopic evaluation provides insight into the patient's urological condition. It is primarily a diagnostic tool.

Indications

Patients with hematuria (gross or microscopic), voiding dysfunction, recurrent infection, stone disease, and fistulas should undergo cystoscopy. The procedure may be done under local anesthesia on an outpatient basis.

Related Procedures

Related procedures include urethroscopy and ureteroscopy.

Nursing Implications

Cystoscopic equipment, like all other endoscopic equipment, is composed of a light source, sterile irrigation fluid (water or saline for cystoscopy), a working sheath, an obturator, and a set of optical lenses (0, 30, 70, and 120 degrees). The lenses are made up of a fiberoptic bundle that conveys light from the light source to the tip of the cystoscope. The light bundles are angulated at the tip of the cystoscope to direct light into the field of vision. A variety of fiberoptic cystoscopes and video attachments are available.

Bridges and deflector mechanisms permit the introduction and passage of ureteral stents. Through these components, electrosurgical devices (Bugbee electrode), electro hydraulic lithotrite electrodes, and laser fibers may be introduced. Cold cup biopsy forceps may also be passed through the sheath to biopsy urethral or bladder lesions. Flexible cystoscopes are available for patients unable to be placed in the lithotomy position or cannot tolerate rigid cystoscopy.

Urine may be sent at the time of cystoscopy for culture, and bladder washings may be obtained for cytological examination. Associated diagnostic studies, such as JVU or renal ultrasonography, should be available for review.

Procedure

During the procedure, the cystoscope is carefully advanced under direct vision. Examination of the urethra, the prostate in the male, and the bladder is carried out. Suspicious lesions should be sampled with the cold cup biopsy forceps. Areas of bleeding may be fulgurated with the Bugbee electrode. Imaging of the ureters and upper collecting system may be performed by retrograde injection of contrast material with bulb-tipped catheters. Ureteral catheters may also be placed at the time of cystoscopy. **Figure 27.29** shows a cystoscopy.

Postprocedure Care

After the procedure, the patient should be instructed to increase his or her fluid intake for 24–48 hours and warned of possible symptoms such as urgency, frequency, and burning on urination. Gross hematuria can be expected. The patient should be given a prescription for oral antibiotics to be taken for 3–5 days. If the patient is unable to void or experiences fevers and chills, he or she should report immediately to the physician.

Transurethral Resection of the Prostate

Resection for benign prostatic hypertrophy may be accomplished endoscopically if the prostate gland is of moderate size and if it does not extend into the bladder, obscuring the ureteral orifices. Resectoscopes are similar to cystoscopes but include

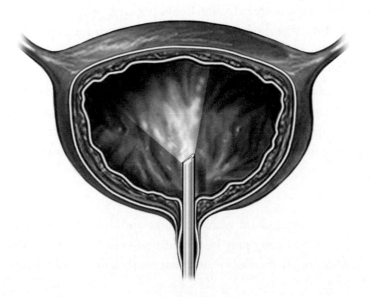

Figure 27.29

Cystoscopy of the bladder.

additional components. There are different types of resectoscopes: McCarthy, Nesbit, Iglesias, Baumrucker, and continuous-flow resectoscopes. Elements of the resectoscopes are the obturator, sheath, working element, cutting loops, laser fibers, and lens. Isotonic nonhemolytic and nonelectrolyte irrigation fluid (1.5% glycine solution) provides a clear view during the procedure.

Indications

Indications for transurethral resection of the prostate are similar to those for suprapubic prostatectomy.

Related Procedures

Related procedures include transurethral resection of bladder tumors, endoscopic extraction of bladder tumors, and endoscopic resection of urethral strictures and posterior urethral valves.

Nursing Implications

An isotonic solution such as glycine, sorbitol, or mannitol should be used for irrigation during the procedure. If a hypotonic fluid, such as water, is absorbed into the large venous sinuses that are exposed or unroofed during transurethral prostate surgery, intravascular hemolysis can occur. Normal saline, even though an isotonic solution, should not be used because the electrolyte composition of the solution dissipates the electrosurgery current, preventing adequate cutting and coagulation of tissue. However, caution must still be exercised because absorption of large amounts of glycine, sorbitol, and mannitol can cause hyponatremia, confusion, and visual disturbances (Leslie, 2006). **Table 27.14** lists irrigating solutions for various urological endoscopic procedures, as well as positioning and prepping guidelines.

During the procedure, keep the irrigating fluid at the lowest height possible to maintain an adequate flow. Placing the irrigation fluid at a height of 60 cm should provide sufficient pressure for the procedure. Raising the height to 70 cm, however, can have a negative effect on fluid absorption (Leslie, 2006). The use of a high-flow, low-pressure fluid warmer specifically designed for the delivery of TURP irrigation fluid can help in controlling pressures.

Patients having a transurethral resection of the prostate are at increased risk for hypothermia because of room-temperature irrigation fluids, particularly if continuous-flow irrigation is used. In addition, absorption of large amounts of body fluid can affect normothermia. Other causes include long resection times, increased prostate size, small body size, and low body weight. Ambient temperature in the operating room is another important factor. Reduce the patient's risk for alteration in normothermia by warming irrigating fluid to body temperature and applying warming devices such as warming blankets and other appropriate thermal devices. No significant increase in blood loss has been found with the use of irrigating fluid warmed to body temperature (Leslie, 2006).

Procedure

The surgeon should check the equipment with the nurse and may elect to dilate the urethra by using sounds. Cystoscopy may be performed before resection. The resectoscope sheath and obturator are then lubricated generously and passed into the

Table 27.14	Position, Preparation, and Irrigation Solutions for Patients Undergoing Endoscopic Procedures		
Procedure	**Position**	**Area Prepared**	**Irrigation Solution**
Cystoscopy	Lithotomy	Perineum, genitalia, and lower abdomen	Water or saline
Transurethral resection of the prostate	Lithotomy	Perineum, genitalia, and lower abdomen	Glycine, sorbitol, mannitol
Transurethral resection of the bladder	Lithotomy	Perineum, genitalia, and lower abdomen	Water of saline
Ureteroscopy	Lithotomy	Perineum, genitalia, and lower abdomen	Water or saline
Percutaneous nephrolithotomy	Prone[†]	Nephrostomy[††]	Saline

[†] Pillows under chest, hips, and legs
[††] Tube site and surrounding area

urethra and then to the bladder. The working element with lens and cutting loop is then inserted. Light cord, irrigation tubing, and electrosurgical cord are connected. Current setting for cutting and coagulation should be set and the patient return electrode applied by the circulating nurse. The surgeon controls the delivery of current via a foot pedal. Resection of the prostate is then carried out. Landmarks for resection are the ureteral orifices and the verumontanum. Careful monitoring of bladder filling by irrigation fluid should be performed to prevent overdistension and possible bladder rupture. A continuous flow resectoscope allows drainage to help prevent overdistension. The enlarged lobes of the prostate are removed piecemeal, leaving the capsule intact. Bleeding vessels are coagulated with cutting loops. Blood clots and prostatic chips are then removed by manual irrigation of the bladder with either an Ellik evacuator or a Toomey syringe placed on the resectoscope sheath. The prostatic chips are sent to the pathology department for microscopic examination.

After evacuation of the bladder, the prostatic fossa is carefully reinspected for bleeding points and residual chips. These should be removed. The resectoscope sheath is then removed, and a Foley catheter is inserted (two- or three-way, 22 or 24 Fr, with 30m-L balloon). Traction on the Foley catheter helps tamponade persistent venous ooze from the prostatic fossa. Isotonic saline solution for continuous bladder irrigation may be started, and the Foley catheter is attached to a 2000-mL drainage system. If continuous bladder irrigation is used, careful monitoring of the system is mandatory. **Figure 27.30** shows a transurethral resection of the prostate.

Postprocedure Care

Postprocedure observation includes monitoring of urine output, mental status, and abdominal girth. Routine laboratory evaluation should be obtained for at least 2 days (CBC, electrolyte, blood urea nitrogen, and creatinine determinations). The bladder irrigation may be discontinued when the urine is clear or light rose colored, and the Foley catheter is removed on the day of discharge.

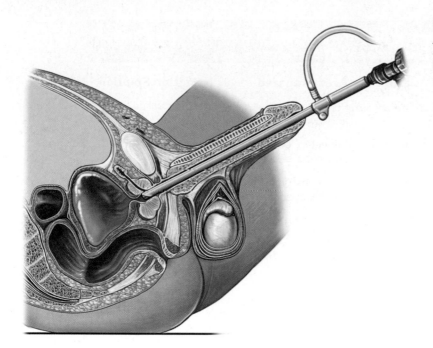

Figure 27.30

Transurethral resection of the prostate.

Photoselective Vaporization of the Prostate

Photoselective vaporization of the prostate (PVP) is a minimally invasive technique for treating benign prostatic hypertrophy. PVP uses an 80-watt potassium-titanyl-phosphate (KTP) to treat benign prostatic hypertrophy. The technology uses a 532 nm wavelength that is highly absorbed by oxyhemoglobin and minimally absorbed by water. As the laser beam is applied vaporization occurs within tissue where vapor bubbles form and burst the collagen matrix. The generated heat produces a coagulation zone, which achieves hemostasis (Sancha et al, 2007).

Indications

The indications for PVP are similar to those of a transurethral resection of the prostate.

Related Procedures

Related procedures include transurethral resection of the prostate, and resection of urethral strictures.

Nursing Implications

Studies show that anticoagulation therapy is not a contraindication to photoselective vaporization of the prostate provided the patient's overall medical condition is stable. However, antiplatelet and anticoagulation (warfarin) medications such as aspirin and warfarin should be discontinued before the procedure, if possible. If a high-risk patient requires the procedure, heparin or an equivalent high-molecular-weight anticoagulant should replace warfarin. The patient should receive appropriate prophylactic antibiotics before the procedure. Maintain the patient's normothermia by applying appropriate interventions, if necessary. Apply full-length sequential compression stockings according to facility protocols for policies for deep vein thrombosis prophylaxis (Sancha et al, 2007).

ANESTHESIA

The patient will have general or spinal anesthesia this procedure. For patients who cannot tolerate the preferred method of anesthesia, such as those with significant cardiac risk, periprostatic block with moderate sedation/analgesia is an option if the patient has a relatively small prostate (Sancha et al, 2007).

POSITION

The surgeon will sit or stand when performing the procedure. If the surgeon chooses to sit, provide a chair with a back and armrests. Place the patient in a modified lithotomy position with the legs in stirrups (Sancha et al, 2007).

EQUIPMENT AND SUPPLIES

Table 27.15 lists equipment and supplies for photoselective vaporization of the prostate.

PHYSICIAN ORDERS AND LABORATORY AND DIAGNOSTIC STUDIES

Before treatment, patients should have laboratory performed relative to their health status. Additional testing may include digital rectal exam, PSA test, urinalysis, uroflow test, as well as a prostate needle biopsy.

Table 27.15	Equipment and Supplies for Photoselective Vaporization of the Prostate

- 80-W potassium-titanyl-phosphate (KTP) laser
- Laser fiber
  - 600 µm core diameter and is equipped with 1800 µm quartz cap
  - Side-firing
- Continuous flow laser cystoscope which accepts the laser fiber
- 30° telescope (it is also possible to use a 12° scope) with a 7 Fr inner laser bridge and an external sheath with a beak visual obturator
- Self-sealing nipple to avoid water leakage around laser fiber
- Video system with camera cover to prevent water penetration
- Filtering laser mechanism for camera protection
- Pump, continuous flow, gravity, or suction (optional)
- Irrigation system, saline, room temperature
- Urethral dilators or Otis urethrotome plus lubricant (standby)
- Catheter (standby)
  - Latex or silicone
  - Catheters, Fr 16–20, large bore catheters (usually necessary for this procedure)
  - 2- or 3-way (irrigation is usually not necessary)
- Laser goggles
- Suprapubic trocar (optional)
- Resectoscope and electrosurgery generator (standby)
- Chair with arm rest (optional)

Adapted from Sancha, F. G.; Bachmann, A; Choi, B. B.; Tabatabaei, Muir, G. H. Photoselective Vaporization of the Prostate (GreenLight PV): Lessons Learnt After 3500 Procedures. *Prostate Cancer and Prostatic Dis.* 2007, 10(4):316–322.

Procedure

The surgeon must use a video system for the procedure. Set up the camera equipment with a special 532 nm lens filter, which protects the camera. Insert the lens filter between the camera and the telescope. Keep the filter dry before and during the procedure to avoid image distortion. The surgeon will use a laparoscopy sheath to protect both the camera and the filter during the procedure. Before starting the procedure, check the white balance. All members of the operative team should wear laser goggles specifically filtering the 532 nm wavelength. When wearing these goggles the operative team should note any color distortion that may occur, such as the blue triangle on the laser tip indicating direction. This triangle may appear in a different color. Adhere to facility laser safety protocols. The entire operating team should understand about color distortion, which presents safety challenges, particularly when using color-coded medications and instruments (Sancha et al, 2007).

The procedure is done with a 30° lens. This lens, however, does not visualize the beak at the tip of the external sheath of the laser cystoscope. In order to minimize local damage and possible bleeding when introducing the laser cystoscope, an optical obturator should be used. This obturator along with gentle introduction of the cystoscope through the urethra, particularly with a large median lobe prostate, will help limit damage (Sancha et al, 2007).

After irrigation is started, the anatomy of the urethral sphincter and prostate is viewed, and the position of the ureters and the bladder neck noted. Next, the optical obturator is removed and replaced with the laser carrier and then the laser fiber is introduced and placed at a distance from the telescope lens to avoid damage to the latter or to the beak of the cystoscope (Sancha et al, 2007).

Set the power at 80 W for laser vaporization. The laser is activated perpendicularly in lateral side-to-side slow, sweeping movements as compared to back and forward actions of a TURP resectoscope loop. The formation of bubbles when the laser is activated indicates effective vaporization. A long continuous period of vaporization achieves optimal debulking. During vaporization, tissue may adhere to the tip of the fiber. When this happens, the tip should be cleaned by turning off the laser, removing the fiber, and cleaning the tip with gauze. Another technique involves turning off the laser, and then with the laser fiber still in the cystoscope, removing the tissue at the end of the tip by rubbing in an upward motion towards the tip of the fiber against previously lasered tissue (Sancha et al, 2007).

Postprocedure Care

The patient is discharged home after recovery from the procedure. An antibiotic is usually prescribed for 3–5 days and patients return to normal activity of daily living within 3 days.

For elective patients who have received general anesthesia, postprocedure catheterization depends on surgeon preference. If needed, the catheter will remain from a few hours up to overnight. However, some patients require longer catheterization because of urinary retention, a large prostate, old age, anticoagulant therapy, or failure to void secondary to bladder neck or prostatic urethra swelling or inflammation (Sancha et al, 2007).

Complications

Usually, the patient does not experience clinically significant bleeding during PVP (Sancha et al, 2007). Other complications that may occur include, but are not limited to, urinary retention, bladder spasms, and dysuria.

Prostate Seed Implant

Prostate seed implant (PSI) is a procedure that is performed for the treatment of some patients with prostate cancer. The procedure uses radioisotope (iodine 125 or Palladium 103) to deliver radiation (brachytherapy) directly to the prostate. The placement of radioactive seeds into the prostate is a treatment option best performed on patients with a low to moderate grade (well or moderately differentiated) adenocarcinoma of the prostate, who have a low to minimally elevated serum PSA, and a low risk of extension of the tumor outside of the prostate.

PSI
Prostate Seed Implant

Related Procedures

Related procedures include cystoscopy and prostatectomy.

Nursing Implications

The patient is given general or spinal anesthesia. The nurse should take precautions in using the high lithotomy position as discussed in Chapter 8. The nurse must also adhere to radiation safety and radiology safety guidelines.

PHYSICIAN ORDERS AND LABORATORY AND DIAGNOSTIC STUDIES

The orders and testing are similar to the previously mentioned orders for prostate cancer.

Table 27.16 Equipment and Supplies for Prostate Seed Implant
Basin
Cystoscopy drape pack
Cystoscopy set
Cystoscopy tubing
Dover catheter strap
Grid map template
Kelly clamp, straight, 5½-inch
Kidney stone filter
Medications (Bacitracin ointment and Conray contrast dye 60%)
Prostate seeds and needles
Silastic catheter, 16 or 18 Fr
Sterile lubricant
Sterile ruler
Sterile water for irrigation
Syringe, Asepto
Ultrasound machine with rectal probe
Urine drainage bag

EQUIPMENT AND SUPPLIES

Table 27.16 lists equipment and supplies for prostate seed implant.

Procedure

At a time before the procedure, an ultrasound probe is inserted into the rectum and the size of the prostate gland, its exact location in addition to the location of the rectum, seminal vesicles, and bladder are assessed. The actual volume of the prostate gland is then calculated. The radiation dose is then reviewed by the radiation oncologist and dosimetrist or physicist, and adjustment to the location of the seeds is then made and documented and mapped on a grid to be placed operatively via a template.

Place sequential compression stockings on the patient. Place the patient in the high lithotomy position with Allen stirrups. If necessary, clip the perineum. The penis and perineum are prepped and the scrotum is taped to allow perineal exposure. A urethral catheter is inserted, contrast dye is placed into the bladder, and the catheter is clamped. The patient is then draped with a fenestrated drape to allow exposure.

A sterile ultrasound probe is inserted into the rectum to visualize the prostate. A grid for seed mapping is superimposed on the image. A corresponding grid is secured to the foot of the bed to guide seed placement. Seeds are implanted in the prostate using a perineal approach via needles through the corresponding holes in the grid. After implantation is completed, the bladder is drained via the Foley through a stone filter to assure no seeds were inserted into the bladder. The Foley is then attached to a drainage bag and secured with a Dover strap. A cystoscopy is often performed to ensure that the bladder is intact. The remaining needles should be disposed of according to the facility's radioactive waste policy.

Postprocedure Care

Postprocedure care and orders are similar to those of cystoscopy. The patient is often discharged home on the day of surgery, and radiation safety precautions are reinforced.

Transurethral Resection of Bladder Tumor

Transitional cell carcinoma of the urinary tract covers a broad spectrum, from superficial lesions to aggressive, invasive tumors. It is also ubiquitous but most frequently found in the bladder. It is also known to recur and therefore necessitates careful followup.

At the time of evaluation for bladder tumor, panendoscopy of the urethra and bladder is carried out. Random biopsy specimens of the bladder and bladder washings for cytological examination are obtained. Radiological imaging of the entire urinary tract should be performed before the procedure. Tumors that are found to invade into the muscle layer of the bladder are treated with radical cystectomy. At the time of transurethral resection, bladder tumor, adjacent mucosa, and a portion of the bladder wall are removed to evaluate the extent of invasion by the tumor.

Procedure

The setup, instruments, and procedure are similar to those for transurethral resection of the prostate. A retrograde pyelogram may be performed at the same time. Sterile water or normal saline may be used for irrigation fluid. Electrosurgery is used to ensure hemostasis after resection of the tumor. A large Foley catheter (22 or 24 Fr) is left in place after the procedure for 24–48 hours.

Superficial bladder tumors may be treated with the Neodymium Yttrium Aluminum Garnet (Nd YAG) laser. The laser beam is transmitted through a flexible glass fiber passed through the cystoscope sheath. Bladder tumors are coagulated by pulses of laser beam. There is minimal bleeding associated with the procedure, and the operating time is short. No catheter drainage of the bladder is necessary, and the procedure can be done on an outpatient basis.

Postprocedure Care

Postprocedure care in patients having undergone transurethral resection of bladder tumor is similar to that after transurethral resection of the prostate. Bladder irrigation is not used.

Ureteroscopy

Ureteroscopy is another transurethral endoscopic evaluation of the upper urinary tract. The procedure is done with a long, narrow, rigid, or flexible endoscope that enables access to the upper urinary tract: ureter, pelvis, and calyces. Because it entails the use of biopsy forceps, baskets, and laser attachment, ureteroscopy is both a diagnostic tool and a therapeutic instrument.

Indications

Table 27.17 lists indications for ureteroscopy.

Related Procedures

Related procedures include any endoscopic procedure.

Physician Orders and Laboratory and Diagnostic Studies

Typical admissions orders include routine laboratory evaluation as described earlier. Intravenous antibiotics are recommended before and after the procedure because of pyelorenal backflow of urine and irrigation fluid during the procedure.

After the procedure, urine output monitoring is important. Most patients have ureteral stents left in place and require careful urine output measurement. Irrigation of the stent may be necessary to alleviate obstruction by either clot or stone fragments. Most patients experience pain similar to that of renal colic and bladder spasm and will require analgesics for 24–48 hours after the procedure.

Stent removal may be performed as early as 48 hours after the procedure. Further radiological studies may be carried out before removal of the ureteral stents.

Procedure

Ureteroscopy necessitates cystoscopic examination. The ureteral orifice is identified, and a cone-tipped retrograde ureterogram with preinjection and postinjection films is taken to identify the course of the ureter. A disposable ureteral access catheter may be used to maintain access. A floppy tipped guide wire is then passed up the ureter to the pelvis under fluoroscopic guidance. The lower ureter is then dilated by either bougies (up to 16 Fr) or balloon dilator. The ureteroscope is then passed into the bladder, through the ureteral orifice, and carefully advanced up the ureter to the pelvis along the guide wire.

Table 27.17	Indications for Ureteroscopy

Evaluation and Treatment of Urothelial Tumors

Direct visualization

Biopsy

Selective cytological evaluation

Electrocoagulation

Resection

Laser photocoagulation

Followup

Evaluation and Treatment of Ureteral Obstruction

Examination and localization of stones and ureteral strictures

Guide wire placement

Ureteral dilation

Stone disintegration and/or retrieval

Internal ureterotomy

Stent placement

Evaluation and Treatment of Upper Urinary Tract Bleeding

Localization of bleeding sites

Diagnosis

Treatment

Foreign Body Retrieval

Displaced or fragmented ureteral stents

Extraction of broken instrument parts

Identification, biopsy, and treatment of papillary tumors may then be carried out. Stones, the most common indication for ureteroscopy, can be extracted with a basket or three-pronged grabber or disintegrated with ultrasonic equipment or an electrohydraulic lithotripter.

After diagnosis and treatment has been achieved, a retrograde study of the ureter and pelvis should be done to check the integrity of the upper urinary tract. A ureteral stent is then left in place after removal of the ureteroscope. Foley catheter drainage of the bladder is carried out for 24–48 hours.

Postprocedure Care

Postprocedure care for ureteroscopy is similar to that for percutaneous endoscopy.

Percutaneous Endoscopy of the Renal Pelvis (Percutaneous Nephroscopy)

Percutaneous puncture of the urinary collecting system has become possible with the development of fluoroscopy and nephrostomy tube drainage. The basic principle is to obtain access to the collecting system under radiographic guidance and place a tube into it, which is then used as a track. The track can be dilated to allow the passage of a nephroscope. The nephroscope permits visualization of the collecting system. Stones may be fragmented and extracted under direct vision.

Indications

The principal indication for percutaneous nephroscopy is stone removal. Nephroscopy may also be employed to diagnose and treat urothelial tumors not accessible by ureteroscopy.

The large majority of patients have staghorn calculi (large infectious stones that take up most of the collecting system). The patient may therefore have a history of urinary tract infection. Flank pain and recurrent urinary tract infection are common presenting symptoms.

The patient undergoes radiological evaluation and placement of a nephrostomy tube in the radiology suite. Radiographs must be available for review. Routine evaluation before the procedure should be carried out. Preprocedure parenteral antibiotic therapy is mandatory, and the patient should have blood available in the blood bank. Urine must be sent for culture to identify possible pathogens.

Procedure

With the patient in the prone position under epidural or general anesthesia, and under fluoroscopic guidance, a wire is advanced through the nephrostomy tube down the ureter to the bladder. The nephrostomy tube is then removed and the track is dilated with Teflon dilators (12–30 Fr). A working sheath is passed over the largest dilator and the nephroscope is inserted through the sheath. Examination of the collecting system is carried out. Stones may be extracted directly, if they are small enough to be grasped and passed through the sheath, or they are fragmented with the ultrasonic probe or a laser. A flexible nephroscope may be used to gain access to the calyces. After extraction or disintegration of the stones, the collecting system is reinspected and contrast material is injected to ensure the integrity of the system. A larger nephrostomy tube (22 Fr Malecot) is placed through the working sheath, which is then removed. The nephrostomy tube is sewn into place and a sterile dressing is applied. The patient keeps the nephrostomy tube in place for approximately 2 weeks, at which time it is removed after radiographic evaluation of the collecting system. Similarly, the nephroscope can be used to diagnose urothelial tumor of the collecting system in selected patients. Laser photocoagulation may be used to treat these cancerous lesions.

Postprocedure Care

Postprocedure orders are similar to those for ureteroscopy. Urine output should be monitored carefully and parenteral antibiotics may be administered as prescribed. Laboratory studies include CBC and electrolyte, blood urea nitrogen, and creatinine determinations.

Nursing Implications for All Endoscopy Procedures
Anesthesia

Endoscopic procedures can be performed with the use of general, regional, or local anesthesia. During general or regional anesthesia, the circulating nurse should assist the anesthesia provider in any way possible. If an anesthesia provider is not present during the local endoscopic examination, a registered nurse should monitor the patient. In these patients blood samples are not routinely typed and crossmatched for blood transfusion. The circulating nurse assists in blood administration according to hospital policy.

Position

Positioning requirements vary according to the type of procedure being performed. In each of these positions, routine precautions for positioning should be followed (Chapter 8).

When positioning the patient, the circulating nurse must consider whether the image intensifier will be used during the procedure. The patient must be positioned on the bed so that the area in question is clear of any object that would interfere with the image picture of the patient's body part. A few companies manufacture a special endoscopy table. This table offers many advantages in the positioning of patients and the use of radiological studies.

Establishing and Maintaining the Sterile Field

Clipping is not usually performed for endoscopic procedures. The preparation is usually done with a prescribed solution, encompassing the appropriate area (**Table 27.14**).

During many endoscopic procedures, a scrub person may not be required after the instruments are set up and the patient is prepared and draped. Of supreme importance during the draping is the creation of a dry environment to avoid strikethrough contamination. Sterile, adherent, impervious drapes should be used to provide a barrier when draping the patient. In addition, the operative team wears impervious gowns. Protective eyewear and waterproof shoe covers are also recommended. If the rectum is to be isolated from the operative area, an impervious transurethral resection drape should be used.

All endoscopic equipment such as telescopes, sheaths, obturators, and bridges are delicate instruments. The scrub person should use care when handling these items and instruct the operative team in this routine as necessary.

Equipment and Supplies

Equipment and supplies used during an endoscopic examination also vary according to the procedure. **Table 27.18** lists equipment and supplies for endoscopy procedures.

Physiological Monitoring

Blood loss is not usually severe during endoscopic procedures but, because of the nature of endoscopy, blood loss estimation is more difficult. Irrigation fluid is used to wash out blood and usually flows into a drain of some type. Screens can be used to catch stones, tissue, and so on, but do not filter smaller particles.

Specimens and Cultures

Routine bladder washings and/or right and left ureteral washings are sent for cytological examination and routine culture and sensitivity testing. Specimens may

Table 27.18	Equipment and Supplies for Endoscopy Procedures

Cystoscopy

Cystoscopy set

Foley catheter, silastic, size per surgeon preference

Irrigation fluid, 3000 mL

Sponges, 4 × 8 radiopaque

Transurethral resection drape pack

Transurethral resection Y tubing

Retrocath Insertion

Catheter deflecting mechanism

Drainage bag, ureteral

Ureteral catheter, according to surgeon preference

Ureteroscopy

Cystoscopy set

Drainage bag, ureteral

Foley catheter, silastic

Guide wires

Impervious plastic drapes

Irrigation fluid, 3000 mL

Sponges, 4 × 8 radiopaque

Transurethral resection drape pack

Transurethral resection Y tubing

Ultrasound probe

Ureteral catheters

Ureteroscope, angled and flexible

Ureteroscope, semirigid or flexible

Percutaneous Nephroscopy

Catheter, Malecot, 20, 24, 28, or 32 Fr, according to surgeon preference

Drainage bag, urine

Impervious drapes

Percutaneous nephrolithotomy tray

Plastic set

Scalpel blade, No. 10

Sponges, 4 × 8 radiopaque

Suction tubing

Suture, 2-0 monofilament suture on cutting needle

Syringe, 20-mL

Syringe, bulb

Transurethral resection Y tubing

Ultrasonic probe

Transurethral Resection of the Prostate and Bladder

Foley catheter, silastic with 30-mL balloon, size according to surgeon preference

Irrigation fluid, 3000 mL

Resectoscope set

Sponges, 4 × 8 radiopaque

Syringe, 20-mL

Transurethral resection drape pack

Transurethral resection flow pouch system and extension set

Transurethral resection Y tubing

include stone fragments, bladder chips, prostate chips, bladder biopsy specimen, prostate biopsy specimen, and kidney or ureter biopsy specimen.

Drugs and Solutions

Drugs and solutions are important to endoscopic examination. The continuous, uninterrupted flow of the desired irrigation solution allows surgeons good visualization of the area (**Table 27.14**). In addition, during resection of tissue or stone dissolution, the irrigation provides a timely removal of debris. Listed below are the drugs and solutions used for urological endoscopic procedures:

> Solution for bladder washings and urinary tract washings
>
> Dye for contrast visualization via radiograph
>
> Sterile water for irrigation
>
> Sterile saline solution for irrigation
>
> Glycine solution

Lubricant KY jelly

Lidocaine Urojet for local procedures

Laboratory Studies

Before a patient undergoes endoscopy of the upper urinary tract (either ureteroscopy or percutaneous nephroscopy), routine laboratory tests are required. Urinalysis and urine culture are often obtained.

Postprocedure for All Endoscopy Procedures

After an endoscopic procedure, the patient may have an indwelling ureteral catheter or stent. The stent will be placed in the renal collecting system and exit through either the skin or the bladder and urethra. Careful monitoring of urine output through various catheters and stents is required.

Postprocedure orders include the following:

- Admit patient to a regular unit or discharge home
- Ascertain that the patient's condition is stable
- Obtain vital signs per postop protocol
- Strictly monitor intake and output (output should be recorded for each drainage device)
- Call physician if there is any evidence of drainage device occlusion
- Administer antibiotics as prescribed
- Administer postprocedure pain relievers

Potential Complications

Cystoscopy and Transurethral Resection

Injuries to the urethra and to the bladder, incontinence, erectile dysfunction, retrograde ejaculation, and persistent voiding symptoms are potential complications of transurethral resection of the prostate. Some patients may experience post–transurethral resection syndrome caused by dilutional hyponatremia and experience the sudden onset of tachycardia, hypotension, tachypnea, and mental status changes. This is a life-threatening situation, and therapy is aimed at rapid correction of the electrolyte imbalance.

Ureteroscopy

Ureteral perforation and disruption, urinary extravasation, instrument breakage, bleeding, and infection can occur. The principal long-term complication of ureteroscopy is the development of ureteral strictures.

Percutaneous Nephroscopy

The most significant immediate complications are infection or sepsis and hemorrhage. Extravasation of contrast material outside the collecting system can also be seen but is usually not a problem, provided there is adequate drainage of the collecting system. Injury of adjacent structures is possible but rare. Approximately 5% of patients experience a pleural effusion, which resolves spontaneously over time.

REFERENCES

1. Alba, Linea. (2008). Abdomen. Wikipedia, the free encyclopedia. Retrieved 27 August 2008 from Wikipedia website: http://en.wikipedia.org/wiki/Linea_alba_(abdomen).

2. Covidien (2007). *Force Triad User's Manual.* Boulder, CO: Author.

3. Culley, C.C. (2002). *Urologic Prostheses: The Complete, Practical Guide to Devices, Their Implantation and Patient Follow Up.* Totowa, NJ: Humana Press Inc.

4. Dartos (2006). The Free Dictionary. Retrieved 27 August 2008 from The Free Dictionary Website: http://medical-dictionary.thefreedictionary.com/dartos.

5. Gatti, J.M. & Kirsch, A.J. (2007). Hypospadias, eMedicine. Retrieved 28 August 2008 from eMedicine Website: http://www.emedicine.com/PED/topic1136.htm.

6. Hippocratic Oath (4th Century B.C.E.). Translated by Michael North, National Library of Medicine, 2002. Retrieved 27 August 2008 from NLM Website: http://www.nlm.nih.gov/hmd/greek/greek_oath.html.

7. Lee, S.L., DuBois, J.J., & Shekherdimian, S. (2006). Hydrocele, eMedicine. Retrieved 27 August 2008 from http://www.emedicine.com/med/TOPIC2778.HTM.

8. Leslie, S.W. (2006). Transurethral resection of the prostate. eMedicine. Retrieved 28 August 2008 from eMedicine Website: http://www.emedicine.com/MED/topic3071.htm.

9. Sachdeva, K., Makhoul, I., Javeed, M., & Curti, B. (2008). Renal cell carcinoma. eMedicine. Retrieved 29 August 2008 from the eMedicine Website: http://www.emedicine.com/med/TOPIC2002.HTM.

10. Sancha, F.G., Bachmann, A., Choi, B.B., Tabatabaei, Muir, G.H. (2007). Photoselective vaporization of the prostate (GreenLight PV): Lessons learnt after 3500 procedures. *Prostate Cancer and Prostatic Dis.,* 10(4):316–322.

11. UCSF Children's Hospital (2007). Postoperative instructions for Hypospadias repair. Retrieved 29 August 2008 from UCSF Children's Hospital Website: http://www.ucsfhealth.org/childrens/medical_services/urology/hspadias/hypospadias_postop.html.

27

CHAPTER 28

Orthopedic Surgery

Rose Moss

Jay Bowers

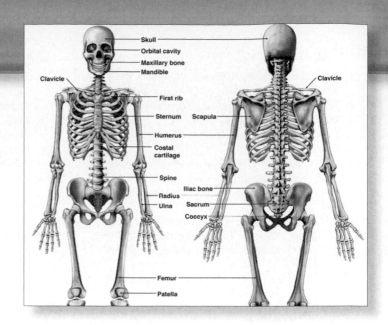

INTRODUCTION

The term orthopedic is derived from the Greek words orthos, meaning straight, and pais, meaning child, since orthopedic surgeons originally dealt with bone deformities in children (*The Free Dictionary*, 2008). Orthopedic surgeons treat deformities, diseases, and injuries of bones and joints and their related structures, which include tendons, ligaments, muscles, and nerves. The specialty focuses equally on the prevention and the correction of a deformity or disability and not just on surgical intervention.

ANATOMY

The musculoskeletal system is comprised of bones, joints between bones, muscles, tendons, ligaments, and cartilage. As a whole, it is responsible for body shape and support, protection of internal organs, and locomotion.

Bones

The skeletal system consists of 206 bones, which comprise the supportive framework of the body and its appendages (**Fig. 28.1**). Bone forms by the process of ossification through either an intramembranous or an endochondral phase. Bone from intramembranous ossification forms directly from osteoblasts without a preexisting cartilage model and is normally found in flat, irregular, and short bones and in the diaphysis of the long bones. The process begins with the secretion of an intercellular substance composed of calcium salts, by osteoblasts. This deposit of calcium salts is known as calcification. Osteoblasts, surrounded by the matrix of calcium salts, form a network of trabeculae, which become entrapped and then fuse. The trapped

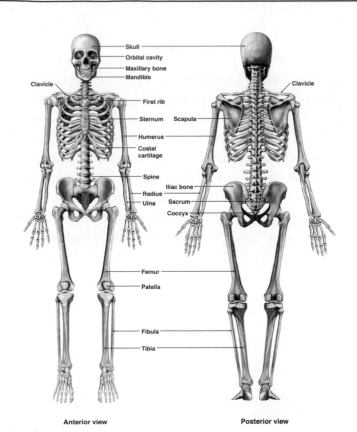

Figure 28.1

The Skeletal System.

cells are then termed osteocytes. The periosteum is formed by the fibrous membrane that surrounds the growing bone mass.

The second type of ossification is endochondral, referring to bone formation by replacement of a preexisting cartilage model. Found in the growth and development of most long bones, it is the process used in fracture healing. The first step involves the calcification of cartilage, which is subsequently removed by cells called osteoclasts. Osteoblasts then repopulate the area and secrete osteoid. Most bones develop from a combination of intramembranous and endochondral ossification. In the diaphyseal, or shaft portion of the bone, blood vessels, along with osteoblasts, arise from the newly formed periosteum and, by means of intramembranous ossification, allow bones to grow circumferentially. The epiphyseal ends of the bone use endochondral ossification. This provides longitudinal and, to a lesser degree, circumferential growth. As the ossification proceeds, the cartilaginous model grows in length at the epiphyseal ends. The area between the diaphysis and the epiphysis is called the growth plate: it remains cartilaginous until early adulthood, to allow an increase in bone length. At maturity, longitudinal growth ceases and bone replaces the growth plate.

Bones formed by endochondral and membranous ossification remodel themselves continuously, with the destruction of old bone and the formation of new bone. This remodeling and replacement vary in different parts of the body, depending on body needs and injury.

Bones are classified according to their shape: short, long, flat, and irregular. Long bones are those of the limbs (eg, femur and humerus) and are longer than they are wide. Bones of the ankle and wrist are classified as short and are about equal in length and width. Examples of flat and irregular bones are the ribs and the vertebral column.

Joints

A joint refers to the junction between the articular surfaces of two or more bones (**Fig. 28.2**). Movable joints are the fulcrums for movement. These areas are further classified according to the degree of movement at the articulation. The immovable, or fibrous, joints are those in which the joint cavity is absent and the primitive joint plate develops into a fibrous tissue. If the amount of tissue is minimal, it is known as a suture, as in the flat bones of the skull. Articulations with larger amounts of fibrous tissue are called syndesmoses. The tibiofibular joint is an example. The second type of joint is the slightly movable, or cartilaginous, type. Cartilage grows between the articular surfaces of the bones and is eventually replaced by bone, as in the epiphyseal plate, or remains throughout life, as seen between vertebral bodies. Synovial joints

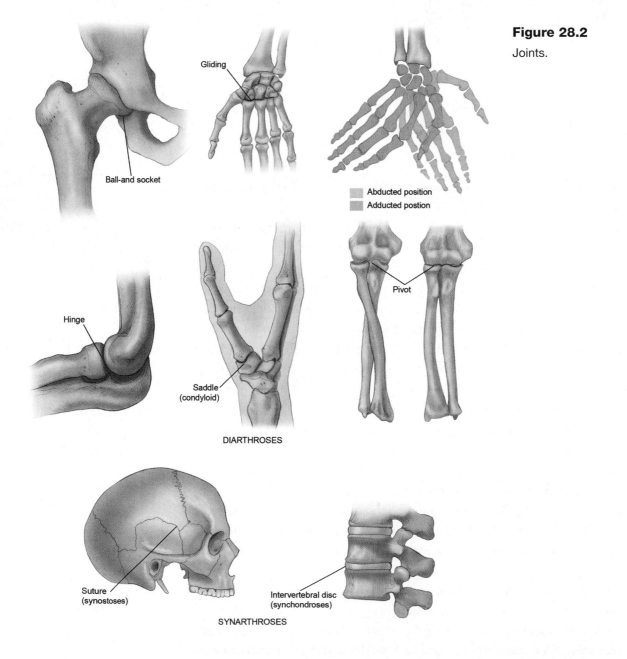

Figure 28.2

Joints.

are freely movable and are surrounded by a protective capsule of connective tissue. The synovium is a membrane that lines the joint cavity on all but the articular surfaces. Synovium secretes a fluid rich in mucins, which, owing to its viscosity and lubricating quality, reduces friction on the articulating surfaces (**Table 28.1**).

Muscles

Bones and joints cannot move by themselves, but rely on the contraction of muscles (**Fig. 28.3**). The muscular system consists of voluntary skeletal muscles, visceral muscle (also called smooth muscle), connective tissue, blood vessels, nerves, and lymphatics. Skeletal muscles provide stability to articulations and maintain the posture of the body. Skeletal muscle cells are enclosed in a membrane called the sarcolemma. Elongated cells, or muscle fibers, which contain thin and thick fibrils, constitute the body of skeletal muscle. Thin myofibrils are composed of the protein actin and the thick myofibrils of the protein myosin. These cylindrical fibrils produce a faint longitudinal striation. The elongation of the cells makes skeletal muscle efficient at producing a shortening when contracted.

Sarcomeres, which are the contractile elements in voluntary skeletal muscle, differ in arrangement from those in cardiac or smooth muscle. When a muscle contracts, thin actin filaments slide between the myosin filaments. This change, and not a shortening of the filaments, explains muscle contraction.

Table 28.1	Types of Synovial Joints	
Joint	**Description**	**Example**
Hinge	These joints act like a door hinge, allowing flexion and extension in just one plane.	Elbow (between the humerus and the ulna)
Gliding (planar)	These joints allow a wide variety of movement, but not much distance.	Carpals of the wrist
Pivot	This is where one bone rotates about another.	Elbow (between the radius and the ulna)
Saddle	Saddle joints, which resemble a saddle, permit the same movements as the condyloid joints.	Thumb (between the metacarpal and carpal)
Condyloid	Condyloid joints are where two bones fit together with an odd shape (eg, an ellipse), and one bone is concave, the other convex. Some classifications make a distinction between condyloid and ellipsoid joints.	Wrist
Ball and socket	These joints allow a wide range of movement.	Shoulder and hip joints

Wikipedia (2008). Synovial Joint, last modified on 12 July 2008. Retrieved July 30, 2008, from http://en.wikipedia.org/wiki/Synovial_joint.

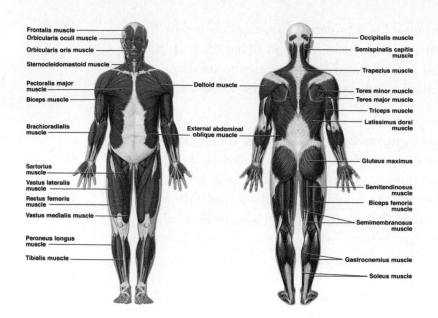

Figure 28.3

Muscles.

Skeletal muscles respond rapidly to stimuli but tire more readily than smooth muscle. The voluntary nervous system controls skeletal muscles, which respond to the will of the individual. Muscles consist of two parts: the muscle fibers, or belly, and the tendons. Tendons are the fibrous connective tissue that attaches to the skeleton. The end, which is called the head, is attached to a fixed structure and is termed the origin, which remains stationary. The end attaches to the more movable part, which is the insertion. Sometimes the origin of a muscle attaches directly to the periosteum, whereas the insertion is usually tendinous. Skeletal muscles are held together by connective tissue called the *epimysium*, dividing the muscle into bundles, or fasciculi. The tissue surrounding the fasciculi is the *perimysium*. The *endomysium* is the connective tissue that extends and surrounds each muscle fiber.

Muscle shapes vary according to their function. They may be long, short, broad, narrow, or irregular. Muscle fibers also vary in arrangement, relating directly to the strength of a muscle. Muscle function depends on a good vascular supply and sufficient innervation from the spinal or cranial nerves. **Table 28.2** lists the terms used to describe the types of skeletal muscle contraction. **Table 28.3** lists the terms used to describe the effects of muscle contractions on the joints of the body in the anatomical position.

Vertebral Column

The vertebral column protects the spinal cord and forms the flexible longitudinal axis of the skeleton (**Fig. 28.4**). It is composed of a series of bones called *vertebrae*. Between each vertebra are pads of fibrocartilage, or *intervertebral discs*. The vertebral column is also the point of attachment of many skeletal muscles of the back, and supports the head. The spinal cord passes through the vertebral canal, which is formed by the vertebrae. Impulses to and from the spinal cord, through spinal nerves, pass through openings (*intervertebral foramina*) between adjacent vertebrae.

Thirty-three vertebrae constitute the vertebral column. The vertebrae are classified according to the regions of the body they occupy: seven cervical, twelve thoracic, five lumbar, five sacral, and four coccygeal. Each vertebra is divided into two parts that together form the vertebral foramen. The body, or the anterior portion,

Table 28.2	Types of Skeletal Muscle Contraction
Isometric	Increase in tension without movement or change in muscle length, with the ends remaining fixed
Isotonic	Constant tension but changing length
Twitch	Single contraction of one muscle fiber in response to one nerve impulse, followed by relaxation
Tonic	Longer lasting contraction than twitches, produced by multiple impulses and without relaxation between; tautness without movement
Fibrillation	Quivering or spontaneous contraction of individual fibers
Convulsions	Involuntary, violent tetanic contraction of muscle groups followed by relaxation

Table 28.3	Terms Used to Describe the Effects of Muscle Contraction
Flexion	Decrease in the angle between two bones (eg, bending knee)
Extension	Increase in the angle between two bones (eg, straightening leg at the knee)
Abduction	Movement away from the midline (eg, lift arm from side)
Adduction	Movement toward the body
Rotation	Movement of a bone around an axis, either its own or that of another bone; medial or lateral rotation
Supination	Lateral rotation of the forearm; palm up
Pronation	Medial rotation of the forearm; palm down
Eversion	Outward rotation of the foot; sole outward
Inversion	Inward rotation of the foot; sole inward
Circumduction	Flexion, extension, abduction, and rotation

is the thickest part. Its surfaces are flattened and rough, which allows attachment to the intervertebral disk. Anteriorly, the body has a few small foramina, which enable the passage of nutrient vessels. Posteriorly, irregular apertures for the channel of the basivertebral veins from the body of the vertebra are present.

The vertebral arch consists of two pedicles and two laminae, from which emerge seven processes (**Fig. 28.5**). The pedicles are short, thick structures that appear from the posterolateral sides of the body. Posteriorly and medially from the pedicle ends are the broad, flat laminae that join in the midline. The spinous process is the projection posteriorly and interiorly from the point of junction of the laminae. On each side where the laminae and pedicles meet is the transverse process, which extends laterally. The spinous and transverse processes provide the attachment of muscles and ligaments.

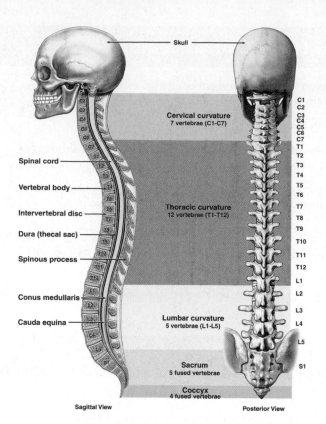

Figure 28.4

The vertebral column.

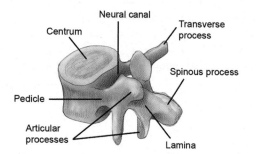

Figure 28.5

The vertebral arch.

Vertebral bodies are the weight-bearing structures of the vertebrae. As the vertebral column descends, each vertebra has to carry more weight. To accommodate, the bodies become more massive and the intervertebral discs increase in size and thickness. The vertebral canal differs only slightly in size, and the spinal cord remains approximately the same size throughout. Where the spinal cord increases slightly in diameter, the vertebral foramina also enlarge.

When viewed anteriorly or posteriorly, the vertebral column appears almost straight, except for a slight lateral curve to the right. The lateral view shows four normal curves: cervical, thoracic, lumbar, and sacral. Abnormal column curves are common. *Scoliosis* refers to an abnormal lateral curve, *kyphosis* to an excessive posterior thoracic curve, and *lordosis* to an inward lumbar curve (Medline Plus, 2008). Spinal ligaments bind together and strengthen the vertebral column, as well as limit its movement. Anterior, posterior, and lateral ligaments run the length of the vertebral column and connect the bodies of adjacent vertebrae. Restraining ligaments are present between vertebral arches, and adjacent spinous processes are connected by interspinous ligaments. Supraspinous ligaments adjoin over a group of spinous processes.

Shoulder and Upper Extremity

The point of attachment of the upper extremity to the axial skeleton is the *shoulder girdle* (**Fig. 28.6**). There is no articulation of the shoulder to the vertebral column. The anterior girdle is formed by the clavicle, which communicates anteriorly and in the midline with the sternum, and laterally with the acromion process of the scapula. The latter attachment forms the acromioclavicular joint. The scapula forms the posterior part of the shoulder girdle. Below the acromion, the glenoid forms an articulation with the humeral head. This joint, surrounded by a loose capsule, is a very shallow ball-and-socket joint that allows considerable motion. The coracoid process, which is at the lateral end of the superior border anteriorly, provides muscular attachment.

The *humerus*, which is the longest and largest bone of the upper extremity, has many distinct landmarks: greater and lesser tuberosities, anatomical neck, and the surgical neck, which is the site of most humeral fractures. The upper surface of the greater tuberosity is the area of insertion of the tendons of the rotator cuff. The subscapularis, supraspinous, infraspinous, and teres minor tendons compose the rotator cuff. The distal portion of the humerus articulates laterally with the radius and medially with the ulna at the olecranon.

The *radius* and *ulna* are the bones that form the forearm. The radius rotates around the ulna, which is medial. The proximal end, or head, articulates with the distal end of the humerus. The biceps tendon attaches to a tuberosity below the radial head. Distally, the radius divides into two articular surfaces. The distal surface communicates with the carpal bones of the wrist, and the medial side communicates with the distal end of the ulna.

Wrist and Hand

The wrist, or *carpus*, and hand consist of three parts: the carpals, or wrist bones; the metacarpals, or bones of the palm; and the phalanges, or bones of the digits (**Fig. 28.7**). The wrist is composed of two transverse rows of the eight carpal bones. Each carpal bone has several smooth articular surfaces for contact with adjacent bones and coarse surfaces for the attachment of ligaments. There are few

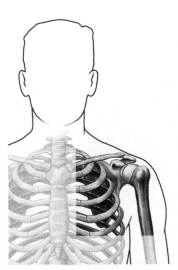
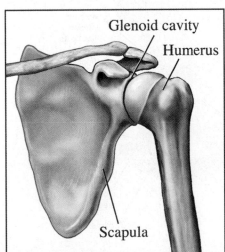

Figure 28.6

The shoulder and upper extremity.

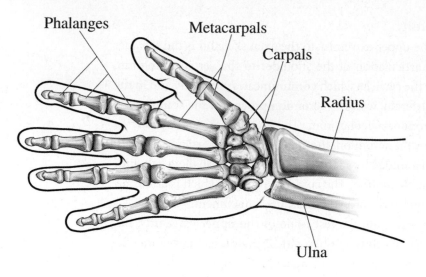

Figure 28.7

The bones of the wrist and hand.

tendinous or muscular attachments to the wrist bones. Consequently, the tendons that insert into the metacarpals and phalanges primarily cause movement of the carpal bones. There are five metacarpal bones, whose heads form the knuckles; the distal articulation is with its proper phalanx; and, proximally, they articulate with the distal carpal bones. The phalanges consist of 14 bones in each hand. There are three bones in each finger and only two in each thumb.

Pelvic Girdle and Femur

The pelvic girdle's function is to support and stabilize the lower extremities and protect underlying organs. Two hipbones, which join anteriorly at the pubic symphysis, form the pelvic girdle and, posteriorly, each attaches to the sacrum laterally (**Fig. 28.8**). Each hipbone is the fusion of three other bones: the ilium,

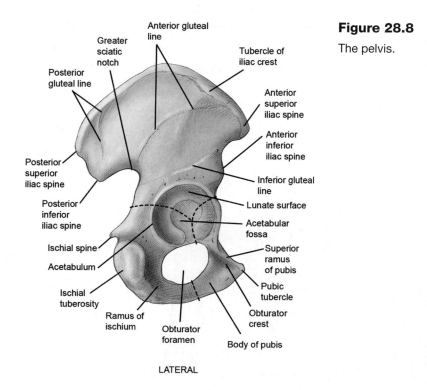

Figure 28.8

The pelvis.

the ischium, and the pubis. The sacrum, the coccyx, and both hipbones form the pelvis. The pelvis is further divided into the greater, or false, pelvis, which is the flaring posterior portion, and the lesser, or true, pelvis, which lies below the brim. The ilium is the large upper flaring portion of the hipbone. The iliac crest is the superior border of the ilium and ends anteriorly and posteriorly in the superior iliac spines. Muscles of the abdominal wall attach beneath on the inferior iliac spines. Gluteal muscles attach on the outer surface of the ilium. The ischium is the lowest and strongest part of the hipbone. At the point of the lateral fusion of the ilium, the ischium, and the pubis, is the acetabulum. This area is a socket into which the head of the femur fits.

The rounded smooth head of the femur extends superiorly and medially and articulates with the hipbone at the acetabulum. This union forms the hip joint. The hip joint is a ball-and-socket joint that is surrounded by a capsule, ligaments, and muscles. The acetabulum is deep in the anteroposterior direction and deepened by a fibrocartilaginous rim called the *glenoid labrum*. This rim provides stability of the position of the head of the femur. The capsule is a strong, thick extension from the acetabulum to the intertrochanteric line of the femur that is weakened in areas posteriorly and inferiorly. The iliofemoral ligament strengthens the hip joint anteriorly, and the pubofemoral and ischiofemoral ligaments reinforce the joint anteriorly and posteriorly. Intracapsularly, the ligamentum teres loosely attaches the femoral head to the acetabulum and channels vasculature to the head of the femur.

The *femur*, similar to the humerus, has distinguishing markings. The proximal end consists of the femoral head and neck, the upper shaft, and the greater and lesser trochanters (**Fig. 28.9**). The greater trochanter is the insertion point of the abductor and short rotator muscles. The distal femur ends in two condyles, which articulate with the tibial condyles. Anteriorly, the femoral condyles are separated by a smooth depression called the *intercondylar groove*. This groove is the articular surface for the patella. The posterior condyles project slightly, and the space between them forms a deep fossa, the intercondylar fossa. The femoral shaft bows anteriorly and directs the distal end of the femur more medially.

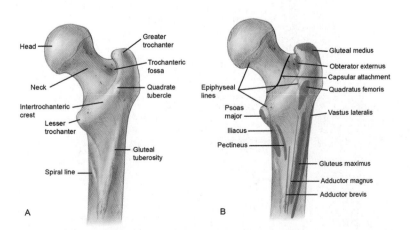

Figure 28.9

(A) Posterior aspect of the proximal right femur.
(B) Attachments and epiphyseal lines.

Knee Joint and Lower Extremity

The intercondylar fossa of the femur receives the intercondylar eminence of the tibia when in flexion. The articulating condylar surfaces of the tibia form two facets, which are deepened by cartilages into fossae to accept the distal femoral condyles. The patella, or kneecap, is a triangular bone found anteriorly in the intercondylar groove of the distal femur. The patella does not articulate with the tibia at any point, but the posterior surface communicates with the femur. It is held in position by ligaments and muscles and is united with the patellar tendon on its anterior surface.

The *knee joint* consists of all the previously mentioned articulations (**Fig. 28.10**). The bones that form the knee joint are connected by extra-articular and intra-articular structures (**Fig. 28.11**). Extra-articular attachments are the collateral ligaments, the quadriceps muscle, and the capsule. These structures provide support for the knee joint medially, laterally, and anteriorly, respectively. Anteroposterior support is provided by the anterior and posterior cruciate ligaments, which are intra-articular. The knee joint is a diarthric joint that allows flexion and extension, but also some glide as the joint approaches complete extension.

Between the articular surfaces of the femur and the tibia are two discs, or menisci. These medial and lateral semilunar cartilages provide lateral support to the weight-bearing joint. Each meniscus is attached to the capsule, with the ends attached to the upper articular surface of the tibia. The inside of the joint capsule is lined with a synovial membrane that secretes a clear viscid lubricating fluid. The synovial fluid bathes the menisci and prevents extreme wear and tear. Often, injuries to ligaments or menisci cause an inflammatory response and an increase in the production of the synovial fluid.

The *tibia*, the larger medially placed bone, articulates proximally with the fibula and the femur and distally with the talus and the fibula (**Fig. 28.12**). The smooth, concave, medial, and lateral condyles articulate with the femoral condyles. They are separated by an intercondylar eminence that projects upward. The intercondylar

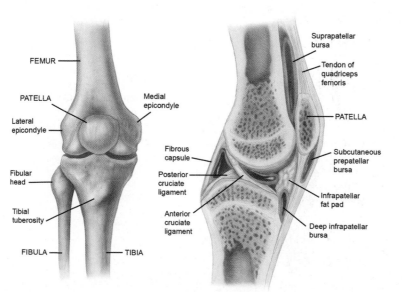

Figure 28.10

(A) Anterior view of the knee joint. (B) Sagittal section of the knee joint.

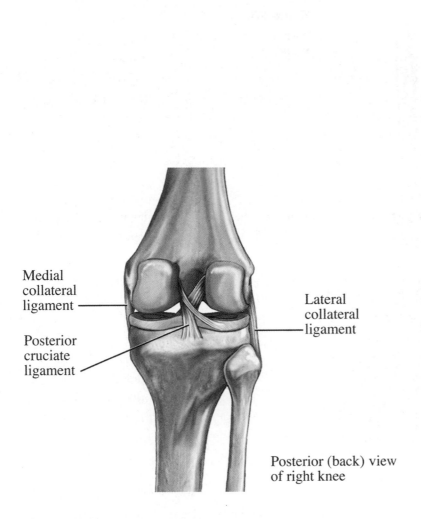

Medial
collateral
ligament

Lateral
collateral
ligament

Posterior
cruciate
ligament

Posterior (back) view
of right knee

Figure 28.11

Posterior view of knee joint.

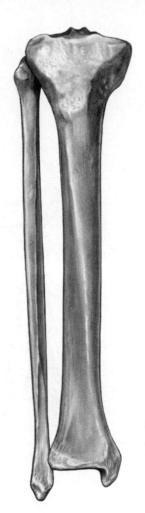

Figure 28.12

Anterior view of the bones
of the right lower leg.

28

fossa is anterior and posterior to the eminence. The *fibula* is the long, narrow bone running laterally to the tibia. Its expanded proximal head articulates with the tibia. Distally, it extends to the lateral malleolus and articulates with the talus.

Ankle Joint and Foot

The hinge joint formed by the distal end of the tibia or medial malleolus, distal end of the fibula or the lateral malleolus, and the proximal end of the talus is called the *ankle joint* (**Fig. 28.13**). The joint is surrounded by a capsule and connected by ligaments, which extend from the malleoli to the calcaneus and navicular bones.

The bones of the foot include 7 tarsal bones, 5 metatarsal bones, and 14 phalanges. The talus is an irregularly shaped bone that fits into a mortise formed by the malleoli and articulates with the calcaneus and navicular bones. The calcaneus is the heel bone and provides support to the talus. The posterior surface of the calcaneus is the attachment site of the Achilles tendon. The talus bone accepts all the body weight and transfers a large portion to the calcaneus and a portion to the anterior tarsal bones. There are five metatarsal bones, which lie anterior to the tarsals. The metatarsals articulate proximally with the cuneiforms and distally with the corresponding phalanges.

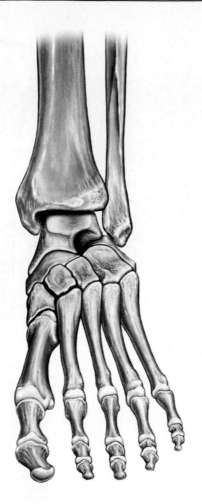

Figure 28.13

The bones of the right foot and ankle.

The foot bones are arranged lengthwise and crosswise to form supportive arches. Because of the ligaments and tendons that bind the bones together, the arches are elastic and not rigid. The arches distribute weight over the entire foot, provide rigidity and strength to the foot as a lever, provide a protective area for the vessels and nerves of the sole of the foot, and absorb shock. The arches are supported by several tendons, ligaments, and muscles.

SPECIAL INSTRUMENTS, SUPPLIES, AND EQUIPMENT

Varieties of special accessories, in addition to routine operating equipment, are required in orthopedic suites. Equipment, instruments, and supplies may vary from facility to facility.

Fracture Table

The fracture table is used for a variety of orthopedic procedures. The design allows traction to be released, maintained, or increased as necessary on the operative extremity. Rotation of the extremity during the procedure can be adjusted. Anteroposterior (AP) and lateral radiographs can be taken during the procedure without disruption of the extremity. Easy application of body cast and hip spicas is also possible with a fracture table. Additional personnel to hold the extremity are not necessary. An important aspect of the fracture table is that personnel are knowledgeable about its application and proper use of accessories.

AP
Anteroposterior

Nursing Implications

Place the patient in a supine position (**Fig. 28.14 A**), with the pelvis supported by a supplementary table top which is translucent to imaging. Wrap the operative foot in a soft bandage before placement in the operative boot attachment. The non-operative leg may be placed in a second boot or positioned in a well-leg support or padded board. Achieve traction by stabilizing the pelvis against the vertical perineal post. The patient is in the proper position when the well-padded perineal post is in contact with the perineum, but is not exerting excessive pressure on the ischial tuberosities or genitalia. Place both arms across the patient's chest, or extend one on a padded armboard for access purposes. Flex the ipsilateral arm and adduct it as far as possible on the chest to avoid contusion of the elbow or ulnar nerve by the image intensifier and to allow unobstructed access to the operative site. Place padding under the elbow and under the strap used to secure the arm in position. Check the radial pulse to confirm that the restraint to the arm is not too tight. Apply body supports if anticipating lateral tilting of the *table-top* to obtain greater exposure of the operative site. The degree of abduction of the legs depends on the physician's preference. Abduction, however, must not allow interference with positioning of the lateral x-ray machine. If a calf rest is used, position it distal to the fibular head to avoid pressure on the peroneal nerve.

When using the lateral position, secure the patient on the fracture table by a well-padded radiolucent post. Place the post ventrally in the area of the anterior superior iliac spine (**Fig. 28.14 B**). Complete stabilization by placing an additional padded post between the upper and lower thighs. Protect the genitalia from injury caused by pressure from the post. Place a pressure reduction roll caudad to the dependent axilla. Gently secure the arms on a padded double armboard. Place the uninjured leg on a padded board or in a leg holder.

Tourniquets

The surgeon may use a pneumatic tourniquet to obtain a bloodless field when operating on an extremity. A properly applied tourniquet compresses the vessels sufficiently to stop arterial blood flow and no more. If tourniquet pressure exceeds venous pressure and not arterial pressure, the extremity continues to fill with blood. This will impede the exit of blood and lead to the retention of an excessive amount of blood in the extremity. A tourniquet below arterial pressure, but above venous pressure, is worse than no tourniquet at all. Completely loosen and remove

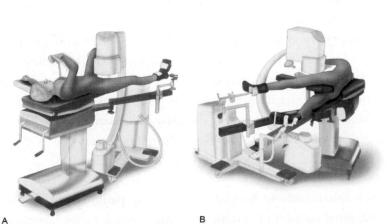

A   B

Figure 28.14

Supine (A) and lateral (B) positioning of patient on a fracture table.

Source: AMSCO Healthcare, Pittsburgh, PA.

the tourniquet at the end of the procedure to ensure venous drainage. Do not use excessive pressure because of the potential risks for irreversible ischemia and nerve damage; the minimum effective inflation pressure should be used (AORN, 2008a). Newer tourniquets use limb occlusion pressure (LOP) technology. This is based on the patient's systolic blood pressure plus a numeric value as the tourniquet pressure setting to be adequate for occlusion of blood flow but vital for tissue survival. See Chapter 11 for information concerning limb occlusion pressure.

LOP
Limb Occlusion
Pressure

Nursing Implications

Select an appropriate sized cuff. The ends must overlap 3–6 inches. Apply the cuff after padding the skin with smooth, soft padding such as Webril. Place the tourniquet as high as possible on the extremity. Do not pinch the skin folds or genitalia. The connecting hose should lead away from the patient; this will help prevent kinking and loosening, and allow for easy access. Elevate and then wrap the extremity distal to proximal with a 4- or 6-inch (10 or 15 cm) elastic (Ace) wrap or Esmarch rubber bandage to exsanguinate the limb. Prep solution must not pool under the cuff. Place an impervious drape over the tourniquet to reduce the risk of pooling and possible chemical burns.

Record tourniquet times on the nursing record. Inform the physician about tourniquet inflation times. The Association of periOperative Registered Nurses (AORN) recommends tourniquet times of 60 minutes for upper extremity for an adult or pediatric patient; 90 minutes for an adult lower extremity; and 75 minutes for a pediatric lower extremity (AORN, 2008a). With the physician's approval, release the tourniquet for 15 minutes following the above times. After the reperfusion period, with the physician approval, reinflate the tourniquet for the same amount of time. This process of tourniquet-timed application and reperfusion can be sustained until the operation is completed. See Chapter 11 for more information concerning pneumatic tourniquets.

Spinal Frames and Positioning Devices

Most orthopedic operations are performed with the patient in the supine position. To operate on a patient in the prone position, however, it is necessary to use special positioning devices that allow proper respiratory function and permit flexion at the operative site. Most physicians favor a particular set of equipment while performing spine operations. The following are some available choices: Morgan disk pads, Wilson convex frame, Relton-Hall frame (four-poster frame), Andrews spinal table (knee-chest frame), Jackson spinal table (radiolucent top and/or frame), Hastings, and chest rolls. With Morgan disk pads, the pelvis is flexed at 90 degrees to maximize exposure of the operative site. A Wilson convex frame, which can be radiolucent, provides adjustable flexion of the lumbosacral spine without flexion of the operative bed. An Andrews spinal table is used for exposure of a large number of vertebrae for spinal fusions. Chest rolls are custom made or made by rolling and taping sheets or large foam pads together; they are used when flexion is not necessary.

Nursing Implications

Set up the Jackson spinal table with chest pads and hip pads. Thigh pads may also be used for additional support in specific procedures and for specific patients.

Center the patient's iliac crests on the hip pads. Suspend the legs in a sling or place them on leg supports. Pad the sling and leg supports with gel or pillows to elevate and support the legs and to protect the toes from pressure.

The Andrews spinal table has special gel pads under the patient's chest, shoulders, and knees that reduce the possibility of pressure ulcer development. Place the patient in the prone kneeling position and support with thigh, tibial, and iliac crest supports. Place soft bolsters under both sides from just distal to the axillae to the iliac crests. Avoid exerting pressure on the axilla. This position allows the abdomen to hang free, improves respiration, and decreases operative bleeding caused by pressure on the vena cava. Use padded or covered bolsters. Place the pads under the knees and the dorsa of the feet to protect the toes from pressure.

No matter what table is used, abduct the patient's arms to slightly less than 90 degrees and place them on padded arm boards or at the patient's sides to avoid brachial plexus injury. For additional security, secure an extra safety strap around the thorax and tabletop. Exercise caution not to impede respiratory excursion.

Adjust the patient's weight to avoid pressure on the knees. Position the head on a small pillow, doughnut, or padded head support. Exercise caution to protect the airway. Frequently check the eyes during the procedure for any signs of pressure. Check the breasts and genitalia to ensure that these areas are free from compression and twisting. Before the start of the procedure, do a final check for all risk areas. During the procedure, examine potential pressure points and immediately resolve any problems that are found. Document positioning interventions and pressure point checks.

Bone Cement

Bone cement (methyl methacrylate) is often used to hold a metal or synthetic prosthesis in place. Methyl methacrylate is a respiratory, eye, and skin irritant (AORN, 2008b). Because the fumes from the cement are toxic to the respiratory system, use vacuum mixers with fume extraction whenever possible. Wear eye protection to prevent contact with eyes. Do not wear soft contact lenses during the mixing of bone cement, as the fumes may cause an adverse reaction. Don a second pair of gloves when handling methyl methacrylate to prevent the cement from permeating and irritating the skin. Always follow the manufacturer's recommendations for mixing methyl methacrylate and wear the required personal protective equipment (AORN, 2008b).

Methyl methacrylate has two components, one a liquid and the other a powder. When mixing, place the powder in the mixing unit, and add the liquid in accordance with the manufacturer's written instructions. Continuously mix the cement for the time specified. Mixing time varies with the humidity and temperature of the air.

Manually operated insertion cartridges and devices are frequently used in total joint replacements. Transfer the bone cement from the mixing unit to the cement guns while it is still pourable. If directed by the manufacturer's written instructions, place the cement in a centrifuge to increase the fatigue strength and provide a homogeneous mixture.

Nursing Implications

Prior to use, personnel should receive training about the properties, handling characteristics, mixing, and application of the bone cement (**Table 28.4**).

Table 28.4	Bone Cement Precautions

- ☐ Always add the entire liquid component to the entire powder component when mixing the cements.

- ☐ To prevent any possible contamination of the cement with glass fragments, do not break the ampoule(s) over the mixing vessel.

- ☐ Before mixing the powder and liquid, ensure that components have the same lot number, since the monomer and polymer components are individually formulated for each batch.

- ☐ The liquid component is volatile and flammable. Properly ventilate the operating theater. Do not expose the liquid component and its vapors to a naked flame.

- ☐ Avoid continuous inhalation of the liquid vapors, which may have a soporific effect. In addition, excessive exposure to the concentrated vapors may cause irritation to the respiratory tract and eyes.

- ☐ Ignition of monomer fumes caused by use of electrosurgery and electrocautery devices at surgical sites near freshly implanted bone cement has been reported.

- ☐ Avoid contact of monomer with the skin or mucous membranes. The liquid component is a powerful lipid solvent, which might cause contact dermatitis in susceptible individuals. The wearing of a second pair of surgical gloves and strict adherence to the mixing instructions will diminish the possibility of hypersensitive reactions; also, the use of a cement gun/syringe overcomes contact dermatitis. Do not allow the liquid component to come into contact with rubber.

- ☐ Exercise caution during the mixing of the two components to prevent excessive exposure to the concentrated vapors of the monomer, which may produce irritation of the respiratory tract, eyes, and possibly the liver.

- ☐ If the liquid component comes into contact with the eyes, wash with copious amounts of water. Concentrated vapors of the liquid component may have an adverse reaction with contact lenses. Inform personnel wearing contact lenses and limit their exposure. Follow guidance from contact lens manufacturers regarding exposure to irritating and noxious vapors.

- ☐ As the monomer is volatile and flammable, evaporate any waste liquid component under a well-ventilated hood or absorb by an inert material and transfer to a suitable container (which does not react with the monomer) for disposal. The polymer component and waste powder may be disposed of in a landfill.

- ☐ Use a vacuum mixing system to reduce setting time of the cement. The surgeon should read the manufacturer's instructions and be familiar with the mixing system together with the cement prior to use.

- ☐ DePuy CMW antibiotic bone cements are supplied sterile for single use only. Do not re-use. Sterility is only guaranteed if the packaging is unopened or undamaged. Resterilization of any components of the cements must not be attempted.

- ☐ There is no evidence of safety for the use of bone cement in pregnancy or lactation. The bone cement should not be used during the first trimester of pregnancy, and should only be used in life-threatening illnesses during the rest of the pregnancy period.

Adapted from Medsafe, Information for Health Professionals, Data Sheet, DePuy CMW 1 Gentamicin Bone Cement, DePuy CMW 3 Gentamicin Bone Cement, 26 August 2006, accessed 30 July 2008, http://www.medsafe. govt.nz/Profs/Datasheet/CMWGentamycinbonecement.htm.

Note the initial time of preparation. Keep the physician informed of the consistency of the remaining mixture. Have additional gloves ready for the operative team. Don these in the presence of adherent cement. Use a suction device to evacuate bone cement fumes from the mixing unit. Keep the operative site and operative field free from any loose particles of bone cement.

The acute adverse health effects of exposure to methyl methacrylate also include chest tightness, dyspnea, headache, lethargy, and the sensation of heaviness in the extremities; chronic effects include reduced lung function and cardiovascular disorders (EPA, 2007). Serious adverse events, some resulting in fatal outcomes, associated with the use of bone cement include myocardial infarction, cardiac arrest, cerebrovascular accident, and pulmonary embolism (US FDA, 2007). **Table 28.5** outlines the adverse effects of bone cement.

Power Equipment

The use of all powered instruments eliminates the need for many hand-operated tools, thereby reducing operating time. Fingertip control allows the physician to

Table 28.5	Adverse Effects of Bone Cement

The following serious and frequent adverse reactions may occur during or following the use of bone cement but are not necessarily directly related to the acrylic bone cement itself. The surgeon should be aware of these reactions and be prepared to treat such reactions if they are encountered.

☐ Serious: Myocardial infarction, cerebrovascular accident, cardiac arrest, sudden death, pulmonary embolism, and anaphylaxis.

☐ Most frequent: Transitory fall in blood pressure, elevated serum gamma-glutamyl-transpeptidase (GGTP) up to 10 days postoperation, thrombophlebitis, hemorrhage and hematoma, pain and/or loss of function, loosening or displacement of the prosthesis, superficial or deep wound infection, trochanteric bursitis, short-term cardiac conduction irregularities, heterotopic new bone formation, and trochanteric separation.

☐ Other reactions reported:
- Hypoxemia
- Heterotopic new bone
- Trochanteric separation
- Cardiac arrhythmia
- Bronchospasm
- Adverse tissue reaction
- Pyrexia due to allergy to the bone cement
- Hematuria
- Dysuria
- Bladder fistula
- Local neuropathy
- Local vascular erosion and occlusion
- Transitory worsening of pain due to heat released during polymerization
- Delayed sciatic nerve entrapment due to extrusion of the bone cement beyond the region of its intended application
- Intestinal obstruction because of adhesions and stricture of the ileum due to the heat released during cement polymerization

Adapted from Medsafe, Information for Health Professionals, Data Sheet, Depuy CMW 1 Gentamicin Bone Cement, Depuy CMW 3 Gentamicin Bone Cement, 26 August 2006, accessed 30 July 2008, http://www.medsafe.govt.nz/Profs/Datasheet/CMWGentamycinbonecement.htm.

28

control speed and power instantly. Power tools, whether air, electrical, or battery powered, can be used in a variety of ways, including drilling or cutting the bone, shaping the joint, and inserting screws.

Nursing Implications

Personnel should know how to properly use power equipment and understand the manufacturer's recommended cleaning and lubricating processes, as well as sterilizing instructions. Prior to use, ensure that routine maintenance of power equipment has been performed according to the manufacturer's recommendations.

Power equipment can generate heat, which can damage bone cells and normal tissue. Irrigation of the operative site may decrease generated heat and contain debris.

Specific Orthopedic Instruments

In addition to the basic instruments needed on all cases, **Table 28.6** lists instruments needed for orthopedic procedures.

Nursing Implications

Safe patient care during orthopedic procedures requires proper use of instruments in conjunction with routine maintenance. When handling sharp instruments exercise care to avoid injury. Use of a neutral zone will reduce risk for injury to the operative staff. Because of the weight, bulkiness, and sharp edges of many orthopedic instruments, wrap instruments separately or in groups based on function and place in the bottom of the instrument pan. Maintain and protect sharp edges during sterilization and storage with commercial tip protectors.

Arthroscopic and Video Equipment

Innovations in arthroscopic and video equipment have resulted in improved visualization and enhanced cutting capabilities during arthroscopic surgery. Instru-

Table 28.6	Special Orthopedic Instruments
Elevators	Used to strip the periosteum and to expose the bone
Retractors	Contoured to fit around a bone or a joint when placed in proper position; designed so that muscles are neither cut nor torn
Rongeurs	Used to remove soft tissue directly around the bone, cut into the bone, and remove small portions of bone; smooth or jagged edges
Osteotomes or chisels	Used for cutting the bone; chisel has a tapered side, which is required when a finer, straighter cut is desired
Bone clamps	Used to grasp a fragmented bone and hold it in place until a fixating device can be applied
Curettes	Used for scraping, shaping, and removing bone, particularly cancellous

ment design and powerful illumination enable the physician to clearly see pathological lesions that need operative correction. A fiberoptic arthroscope with sheaths allows direct visualization of a joint. The sheath protects the delicate joint tissue during the operative procedure. Sharp and blunt trocars inserted through the sheath enable the physician to access the joint. Arthroscopes come in a variety of diameters (1.7–4 mm) and lens angles (0–120 degrees) to provide different views of the joint, with the 30-degree arthroscope being the most common choice for the knee joint. Arthroscopy sheaths are larger in diameter that arthroscopes, usually by 0.5 mm; lengths are the same. Irrigation valves on the sheath allow water inflow, outflow, and suction. Each sheath also has a locking mechanism to secure it to the arthroscope.

Arthroscopic procedures require copious irrigation to remove joint fluid and debris, improve visualization, and distend the knee. The solutions used include 1000- to 5000-mL bags of normal saline or lactated Ringers solution. Elevating the irrigating system at a height of 6–8 feet above the operative field improves the pressure that maintains distention and, hence, visualization. The use of an arthroscopy irrigation pump also improves solution flow and provides positive and negative pressure, which enables the physician to assess the condition of the tissue under both pressurized and non-pressurized states.

A high-intensity light source and a light cable enable the arthroscopist to view the posterior portion of a joint. The light cable transmits light through fiberglass strands to the arthroscope. Exercise care when handling fiberoptic light cords. The irreparable fragile fiberoptic strands easily break. While many arthroscopes have a standardized connection, some arthroscopes may require a different type and size of light cable and connector. Some may require an adapter to accommodate the light cable. Controls on the light source enable the intensity of the light to be adjusted.

A video camera allows transmission of the image from the arthroscope to the video monitor. Video monitoring allows the surgical team to view the procedure and anticipate the needs of the physician. The magnified image makes viewing easier. High-definition cameras, with superb resolution, have replaced tube cameras in arthroscopic surgery. The cameras attach directly to the arthroscope.

Other equipment used in an arthroscopic procedure includes grasping forceps with and without ratchets, scissors, loose-body graspers, a shaver and abrader system, and wide-angle video arthroscopes. Diagnostic accessories such as high-flow or rotatable diagnostic cannulas, sharp trocars, conical obturators, probes, and curved and straight disposable shaver blades, complete the arthroscopic setup.

Nursing Implications

Failure of the video or irrigations systems can disrupt an arthroscopy and jeopardize patient safety. Consistent maintenance and proper storage of equipment greatly enhances the probability that the procedure will proceed without incident. Handle arthroscopes separately; a scratch on the lens may distort the viewed image. Examine all instruments and equipment before and after each use. Consult the manufacturer's written instructions regarding cleaning, sterilization, maintenance, and function. See Chapter 11 for more information concerning video equipment.

JOINT ARTHROSCOPY

Diagnostic arthroscopy allows direct visualization of the interior of a joint through the specially designed fiberoptic arthroscope. Joints explored by the arthroscope include the knee, shoulder, hip, ankle, wrist, and elbow. Since the advent of this technology, the ability to accurately diagnose and treat joint injuries has dramatically increased. Operative knee arthroscopy enables the physician to repair cruciate ligament or meniscal tears, obtain biopsy specimens, and view and remove loose bodies. With the advent of this procedure, the number of arthrotomies (ie, incision into the joint) has significantly decreased. When indicated, the operative arthroscopy has many advantages over the standard arthrotomy procedures, including a reduced length of stay, a lower risk of operative complications, and a more rapid return to normal activities (Science.jrank. org, 2008). In addition, joint arthroscopy is usually performed as an outpatient procedure.

Indications

The range of indications for both diagnostic and therapeutic arthroscopic procedures continues to expand (Katz & Gomoll, 2007; Medline Plus, 2006; Rao, Yokota, & McFarland, 2004):

- ankle arthroscopy is especially useful for soft tissue impingement syndromes, synovitis, and fractures;
- knee arthroscopy is useful for meniscal tears, injury or damage to the patella, damaged ligaments or cartilage, or synovial defects;
- hip arthroscopy is useful for management of femoral acetabular impingement, labral tears, loose bodies, and chondral lesions;
- wrist arthroscopy has provided novel approaches for ligament tears, synovitis, and fractures;
- elbow arthroscopy has been helpful in the management of synovitis and osteoarthritis due to osteophytosis; and
- shoulder arthroscopy is often indicated for several pathologies, such as rotator cuff disorders, glenohumeral instability, and biceps anchor superior lesions.

Related Procedures

Occasionally, failure to successfully complete the procedure through the arthroscope may require an arthrotomy.

Ankle Arthroscopy
Nursing Implications
ANESTHESIA

General anesthesia, spinal, or epidural anesthesia are options for ankle arthroscopy. General anesthesia is preferred, because it allows for precise control of relaxation; however, since most ankle procedures are done on an outpatient basis, short-acting agents are used (Strobel, 2001).

POSITION

Place the patient in the supine position with the operative leg placed in an arthroscopic leg holder (as for knee scopes). The leg hangs free so that the knee is flexed to approximately 90 degrees (Wheeless, 2007). A tourniquet is used; exsanguination is preferred for more complex procedures, such as arthroscopic fracture treatment and arthrodesis (Strobel, 2001).

ESTABLISHING AND MAINTAINING THE STERILE FIELD

Since ankle arthroscopy is done in a fluid medium, waterproof draping of the operative field with disposable materials is required (Strobel, 2001). After the tourniquet has been placed and/or the limb has been wrapped for exsanguination, the operative limb is prepped. The contralateral leg is draped first; then a sterile surgical glove is pulled on the operative foot to cover the toes. The foot is then passed through the aperture of the waterproof extremity sheet. This sheet is secured about 15 cm proximal to the ankle; the glove on the foot is also secured to prevent slipping.

EQUIPMENT, SUPPLIES, AND INSTRUMENTS

Ankle arthroscopy developed from the principles of knee arthroscopy; therefore, the same instruments were used initially. However, as experience developed, smaller instruments, distraction, and fluid management systems have evolved (Moyes, 2007). Therefore, the equipment and supplies for ankle arthroscopy are the same used for arthroscopy procedures (see **Table 28.7**), with the exception of smaller scopes and miniaturized instruments.

PHYSIOLOGICAL MONITORING

Nursing care of the ankle arthroscopy patient during the procedure focuses on patient support before the induction of anesthesia and protection of the patient's musculoskeletal, skin, and peripheral vascular systems. Periodically assess and monitor pressure points throughout the procedure. Examine the area beneath the tourniquet before applying and after removing the cuff, and document according to facility policy and procedure. Closely monitor tourniquet pressure settings and time and verbalize to the physician.

SPECIMENS AND CULTURES

Specimens and cultures vary according to individual pathological examination findings. Routinely, an excised portion of the damaged cartilage or bone is removed and sent for definitive studies.

DRUGS AND SOLUTIONS

Since electrosurgical instruments will be used, the joint should be distended with a nonelectrolyte solution (Strobel, 2001). Adequate distention pressure is maintained with a gravity-flow system, controlled by raising or lowering the height of the reservoir bag. However, because the joint capsule is very thin in some sites, a high distention pressure should be avoided.

PHYSICIAN ORDERS AND DIAGNOSTIC STUDIES

Before the procedure the patient's medical history will be reviewed and the patient will have a complete physical examination. In addition to the routine orders listed in

Table 28.7	Equipment, Supplies, and Instruments for Arthroscopy

Equipment	Supplies	Instruments
Abrader	18-gauge, 3½-inch spinal needle	2 Army-Navy retractors
Adjustable intravenous (IV) pole	2 20-mL Luer-Lok syringes	2 needle holders
Arthroscopic operative system	2 4 × 4 dressing sponges	2 Senn retractors
Electrosurgery generator	2 60-mL Luer-Lok syringes	2 Z-retractors
Fiberoptic light cable and source	2 6-inch elastic bandages	4 Allis clamps
Lateral knee post (arthroscopic leg holder)	2 6-inch Webril bandages	4 mosquito clamps
Shaver	25-gauge, 5/8-inch needle	6 hemostats
Tourniquet and cuff	30 mL Lidocaine 1% with 1:100,000 epinephrine	6 towel clips
Video camera and control unit	30-mL Lidocaine 1%	Adson forceps with teeth
Video monitor	4 × 8-inc radiopaque sponges	Anterior knee retractor
	4-0 Vicryl (cutting needle)	Arthroscope with sheaths
	6 3-L bags of normal saline	Arthroscopic instruments
	6-inch Esmarch bandage	Basket forceps
	Skin antiseptic agent and prepping supplies (according to the surgeon's preference)	Intra-articular shaver
		Scissor
	Assorted arthroscopic surgical blades (according to the physician's preference)	Suction punch
		Bandage scissors
	Clippers	Dandy nerve hook
	Egress cannula	Light cable
	Electrosurgery supplies	Meniscus clamp
	Impervious stockinet	Metzenbaum scissors
	Inflow tubing	No. 12 Frazier suction
	Ioban Steri-Drape	Nos. 3 and 7 knife handles
	Kling bandages	Small Weitlaner retractor
	Normal saline, 500 mL	Smillie knife
	Skin marker	Suture scissors
	Steri-Strips	Tissue forceps with teeth
	Suction tubing	

MRI
Magnetic Resonance Imaging

CT
Computerized Tomography

TENS
Muscle Stimulation Treatment

Table 28.8, scans of the affected joint (ie, magnetic resonance imaging [MRI], computerized tomography [CT], and arthrogram) are often ordered. In some cases, an exercise regimen or muscle stimulation treatment (TENS) may be recommended to strengthen muscles around the joint prior to surgery (*Encyclopedia of Surgery*, 2008).

Procedure
INCISION AND EXPOSURE

The ankle is first distended with approximately 30 cc of saline (Moyes, 2007). The anteromedial portal is established just medial to tibialis anterior at the level of the joint line carefully avoiding the saphenous nerve. The anterolateral portal is

Table 28.8	Routine Physician Orders*

- ☐ Hematology profile
- ☐ Urinalysis
- ☐ Chest radiograph
- ☐ EKG (for patients with history of cardiac disease)
- ☐ NPO for 4 hours prior to the procedure

*Orders may vary depending on physician preferences and facility protocols.

then created using transillumination, avoiding the superficial branch of the lateral popliteal nerve. A full diagnostic inspection of the anterior compartment is then completed. The posterolateral portal is created next, localizing the entry point with a spinal needle, followed by a full inspection of the posterior compartment. Using these three portals, a full systematic ankle examination can be carried out.

DETAILS

Loose fragments of bone, cartilage, or ligament can be identified and removed through the small portals in the joint capsule; occasionally, small accessory incisions may be needed to remove larger fragments of tissue found within the joint (Ray, 2008). Injured regions of the joint surface will usually display an obvious defect or a loose flap of cartilage; however, the joint surface will often appear normal, but gentle probing will expose an area of exceptional compliance compared to the surrounding cartilage. These soft areas are regions of cartilage injury and will require removal of the damaged cartilage. The physician will drill small holes through these soft zones in order to promote readhesion of the cartilage in some cases. In areas of obvious defect in the cartilage surface, the damaged cartilage is removed down to normal cartilage. Following the removal of damaged cartilage, the exposed underlying bone is drilled repeatedly to facilitate bleeding into the base of the injured area. A blood clot will form across the full dimensions of the defect; over time this blood clot is converted to cartilage. While the repaired cartilage is not of the same quality as the original cartilage, it does reestablish near normal surface-to-surface contact. In some cases, small plugs of normal cartilage and bone can be removed from one location within the ankle joint, and placed into an area of cartilage injury (Ray, 2008).

Arthroscopy has also been used to assist with the repair of fractures that involve the surfaces of the ankle joint (eg, pilon or talar fractures). In these cases, arthroscopy is used to visualize the fractured joint surface during the repair to ensure accurate realignment. Ankle arthroscopy has also been used to visualize the joint during removal of the articular cartilage prior to fusion of the ankle joint (Ray, 2008).

CLOSURE

The small portal incisions are closed with monofilament, nonabsorbable sutures or staples. The area is covered with dry, sterile, gauze dressings and wrapped with a compression dressing.

28

Postprocedure Care

After the procedure, patients may be placed in a removable cast boot or splint to keep the ankle at 90 degrees to the leg; however, gentle range of motion is recommended on a regular basis after surgery. Patients are usually non-weight bearing for 7–14 days after the procedure and then are allowed to weight bear as tolerated. If a large cartilage lesion was either drilled or excised, the patient will remain non-weight bearing for up to 4 weeks. The actual duration of non-weight bearing will depend on the extent of the injury and the type of treatment. It is common for patients to undergo physical therapy after surgery, especially if they had a prolonged period of pain and disuse before the procedure (Ray, 2008).

Potential Complications

The complications that may occur with ankle arthroscopy include infection, blood clot formation, swelling or bleeding, or damage to blood vessels or nerves; rare instrument breakage has also been reported (*Encyclopedia of Surgery*, 2008).

Knee Arthroscopy

Nursing Implications

ANESTHESIA

Patients have several anesthetic options for knee arthroscopy, including general, spinal, epidural, and peripheral nerve blocks (ie, sciatic or femoral) (Sargent & Dunfee, 2005). Regional blocks, as the sole anesthesia or in conjunction with general anesthesia, are becoming more popular and assist with decreasing postprocedure pain. Sole local infiltration may result in undue discomfort from the tourniquet or leg holder during a prolonged procedure and even prevent an adequate examination. Some physicians may use an intra-articular injection of lidocaine at the beginning of the procedure to distend the knee and minimize bleeding. Depending on the type of anesthesia, some surgeons use bupivacaine at the end of the procedure for post-procedure pain.

POSITION

Place the patient in the supine position. Align the head with the body. Extend both arms on padded armboards with the palms up. Brachial plexus injury may occur if extension of the arm is greater than 90 degrees. When requested by the physician, position the arm on the operative side at the side and tuck under the draw sheet, with the fingers and elbows close to the body. Pad the tucked arm with foam and place a folded towel to prevent skin-to-skin contact, thus eliminating the risk for an alternate-site burn from the electrosurgical current (Covidien, 2007). Secure the patient with a safety strap placed loosely across the abdomen. Exercise caution to prevent restriction of respiratory excursion. If necessary, attach additional knee holders to the operative bed for more specific positioning. Caution team members not to lean on the patient. Assess vulnerable pressure points such as the occiput, scapula, olecranon, sacrum, ischial tuberosity, and calcaneus, and apply padding as necessary. Protect the eyes from corneal abrasions or irritation with eye patches. Place the marked operative extremity in a foot-holding device, which elevates and supports the extremity during skin preparation.

Apply the tourniquet to the operative extremity, following the technique and procedures mentioned earlier (refer to the discussion of equipment). Determine and confirm the tourniquet settings with the surgeon.

ESTABLISHING AND MAINTAINING THE STERILE FIELD

If the surgeon orders hair removal, remove it from the operative site with a single-use electric or battery-operated clipper or by means of a depilatory. If the presence of hair will interfere with the procedure, hair removal should be performed the day of surgery, outside of the operating or procedure room (AORN, 2008c). Prep the limb circumferentially with an antimicrobial product, extending the length of the leg from ankle to midthigh according to manufacturer's instructions. If using an alcohol prepping solution, do not allow the solution to pool on or under body parts; allow the solution to dry before draping. Do not use electrosurgery or another ignition source in the presence of flammable substances such as alcohol or alcohol vapors.

When establishing the sterile field, use impervious drapes to establish sterile fields for arthroscopy procedures.

While the assistant holds the operative limb with a sterile towel, remove the foot from the holder. The scrub person or physician applies sterile stockinet, telescopes it down the entire leg, and secures it around the foot and ankle with a sterile bandage or wrap. Next, the scrub person uses a large drape to cover the nonoperative limb.

The scrub person then places a hinged impervious sheet under the operative leg on the sterile field formed by the first drape, and unfolds the drape to the sides and over the end of the bed. After removing the paper backing, the scrub person secures the tails around the top of the limb and the stockinet. Next, a large drape is placed over the upper part of the patient, followed by another large drape. The final large drape is placed over the impervious sheet and secured to the upper sheets around the top of the limb with towel clips. Custom drape packs may require alternative methods of draping. After application of the drapes, the physician fenestrates the stockinet and, if required, applies a plastic adhesive drape to the incisional area. Drapes should be secured to withstand any manipulation during the procedure.

Place the tourniquet controls on the operative side within easy reach of the anesthesia provider and the circulating nurse. Position the arthroscopy video equipment and the irrigating fluid system on the nonoperative side. Ensure that the operating physician can easily see the video monitor. Position the tourniquet and irrigating system out of direct view to avoid distracting the operative team or interfering with the view of the video monitor.

All members of the operative team must monitor the sterile field. Arthroscopy provides some unique challenges to the scrub person because of switching of instruments and the arthroscope from portal to portal during the procedure, frequent irrigation fluid spills throughout the case, and disruption of the sterile field because of movement of the joint from full flexion to full extension. The scrub person should anticipate this during draping.

EQUIPMENT, SUPPLIES, AND INSTRUMENTS

Equipment, supplies, and instruments for knee arthroscopy are listed in **Table 28.7**.

PHYSIOLOGICAL MONITORING

See Physiological Monitoring discussion under Ankle Arthroscopy.

SPECIMENS AND CULTURES

Specimens and cultures vary according to individual pathological examination findings. Routinely, an excised portion of a meniscus is removed and sent for definitive studies. Other diagnostic studies that may be required are anaerobic or aerobic cultures or a cell count of synovial fluid in the presence of a septic joint.

DRUGS AND SOLUTIONS

Depending on the type of anesthesia, additional local infiltration is often required. Commonly, lidocaine 1% with 1:100,000 epinephrine is used. Adjustments and calculations of the solution by the circulating nurse may be needed if it is not premixed by the supplier.

PHYSICIAN ORDERS AND DIAGNOSTIC STUDIES

Patients are admitted the day of the procedure. In addition to the routine orders listed in **Table 28.8**, the physician may order anterior-posterior (AP), and lateral radiographs. These films complete the evaluation, identify loose bodies and fractures of the patella, distal femur, and proximal tibia, and assist in diagnosing chondromalacia patella. In addition, the physician may order magnetic resonance imaging (MRI) to assist in detecting meniscal and ligamentous tears and soft tissue injury.

Procedure

INCISION AND EXPOSURE

Knee arthroscopy may be performed with or without tourniquet control. If a tourniquet is used, the operative extremity is either elevated several minutes before inflation or exsanguinated with a 6-inch (15 cm) Esmarch bandage.

Arthroscopy begins with an incision in the anterior superior lateral quadrant or medial aspect of the suprapatellar pouch. A stab incision, made with a No. 11 or 15 blade, is followed by the insertion of a cannula with a sharp or blunt trocar. If a sharp trocar is used, after the periarticular tissue and joint capsule are pierced, a blunt trocar replaces the first trocar. The blunt trocar permits entry through the synovium without any damage to the articular surfaces. An effusion, if present, may be removed at this time and sent to the laboratory. The blunt trocar is exchanged for the arthroscope. With the knee in full extension, the irrigating system is attached and opened to distend the knee.

Additional stab wound incisions are made horizontally just above the joint line, again with a No. 11 or 15 blade for three portals in the knee joint.

DETAILS

Light cables are connected to the arthroscope, and irrigation from the inflow tubing continues. The arthroscopy equipment (camera monitor, light source, arthroplasty unit and foot pedal, and printer) is brought into the visual field by the circulating nurse and arranged for optimal visualization by the surgeon.

The arthroscope is then directed into the medial compartment for examination. The medial joint surfaces, synovium, menisci, and anterior cruciate ligament are thoroughly examined. A blunt probe is inserted through the third portal. Soft tissue can be manipulated closer to the arthroscope with the use of the blunt probe, thus providing a better view of the operative field. The probe may be exchanged with the motorized intra-articular shaver if debridement of meniscal tears or lesions is documented. After the evaluation of the medial compartment, the arthroscope is replaced by the blunt probe, and inspection of the lateral compartment is performed in a similar manner. The undersurface of the patella and the suprapatellar pouch is visualized by inserting the arthroscope through the infrapatellar lateral portal. The intra-articular shaver may be inserted into the infrapatellar medial portal for debridement of lesions. Instruments may be repositioned so all aspects of the patella are visualized. The burr is used to cut through the subchondral bone to a depth of 1 mm.

During an arthroscopy, manipulation of the knee is required to bring all of the recesses into view. Thorough evaluation of the medial compartment might necessitate a valgus force on the knee with external rotation of the tibia. A varus stress is applied with internal rotation of the tibia while the lateral compartment is being evaluated. The most difficult area to examine is the posterior compartment of the knee. The posterior cruciate may be seen through a posterolateral or posteromedial portal.

Removal of a loose body is accomplished with arthroscopic grasping forceps. The visualization of a loose body sometimes presents a problem to the arthroscopist. Ballottement of the popliteal and suprapatellar compartment may facilitate the search for a loose body.

Multiple cutting tools may be utilized during a single procedure. They include knives, basket forceps, scissors, motorized burrs, and punches.

CLOSURE

The small stab incisions are closed with a suture of choice on a cutting needle, followed by application of Steri-strip bandages. The area is covered with dry, sterile, gauze dressings and wrapped with a compression dressing (6-inch [15 cm] Webril followed by 6-inch [15 cm] Ace bandages). **Figure 28.15** shows an example of knee injuries with arthroscopic repair.

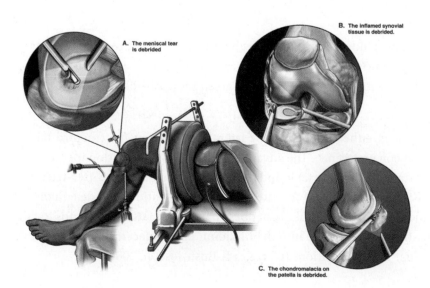

A. The meniscal tear is debrided

B. The inflamed synovial tissue is debrided.

C. The chondromalacia on the patella is debrided.

Figure 28.15

Arthroscopic knee repair.

Source: Nucleus Medical Art.

Postprocedure Care

The patient gradually increases activity as tolerated and avoids excessive use of the extremity for 48 hours. Encourage the patient to elevate the leg while sitting or lying down for seven days. During the first 72 hours, in addition to elevating the extremity, the patient should apply ice packs, 20 minutes on and 20 minutes off. If swelling increases, activity should decrease. Instruct the patient to do quadriceps-strengthening exercises (straight-leg lifts). Suggest rest and elevation for pain. If pain does not subside, the patient should take prescribed pain medication and not return to normal activity. The patient should not forcefully bend the knee until given permission by the physician or drive an automobile until pain and swelling have subsided enough to allow good mobility. The dressing remains intact for 48 hours, after which it may be removed and an adhesive bandage applied for several days. Creams or lotions should not be applied to incisions unless prescribed by the physician. The patient may shower 48 hours after the procedure. Bathing or soaking of the extremity should be avoided for 4 days. Instruct the patient to contact the physician if any of the following occur: fever greater than 101°F (38.3°C), increased pain not relieved by pain medication prescribed, and redness or swelling in the calf. A return visit is scheduled 7 days after the procedure.

Potential Complications

Knee effusion frequently develops during the first few days after the procedure. This painfully tense effusion may be relieved by aspiration of the knee joint. Infection, which is uncommon, should be considered if erythema, excessive pain with motion, and fever are present. Thrombophlebitis and pulmonary embolus, although rare, are treated with anticoagulants. Neurapraxia is a condition due to prolonged use of the tourniquet during the procedure that is managed by observation until symptoms resolve. Hemarthrosis is an occasional complication that is usually associated with cutting of vascularized tissue within the knee and that may necessitate aspiration if it does not resolve. Decreased range of motion due to hemarthrosis and subsequent adhesive capsulitis may require manipulation of the knee joint.

Hip Arthroscopy
Nursing Implications
ANESTHESIA

General, spinal, or epidural anesthesia may be used for hip arthroscopy. Epidural anesthesia is an appropriate alternative to general anesthesia, if an adequate block providing muscle relaxation can be achieved (Carreira & Bush-Joseph, 2006).

POSITION

Place the patient in either the supine or lateral position on the fracture table, depending on surgeon preference. The advantages of the supine position include the readily available standard fracture table and traction equipment and the user-friendly layout of the OR; the advantages of the lateral decubitus position include enhanced instrument maneuverability, particularly in obese patients, as fatty tissue tends to fall out of the way; and easier entrance into the hip joint. Portal placement and surgical technique is similar in both positions (Carreira & Bush-Joseph, 2006).

Using the fracture table, place the involved hip in abduction at 25° and in slight extension. Flexion is avoided to prevent pulling the sciatic nerve closer to the joint. The contralateral hip also is abducted to facilitate access of the c-arm and is placed under slight traction to stabilize the patient. A well-padded perineal post then is positioned against the pubic ramus and ischial tuberosity, providing lateralization of the proximal medial thigh. Because of the tough connective tissue capsule and the stability of the ball and socket joint itself, a distractive force must be applied to the extremity to provide proper visualization during the procedure. Using a tensiometer, a traction force of 25–50 pounds is applied, with the goal of 8–10 mm distraction. A vacuum is created within the joint, which is later ablated with instillation of joint fluid or air, thereby decreasing the required traction force. The joint capsule becomes more lax after a few minutes of traction, which thereby reduces the force needed to maintain an adequate joint space. Once adequate distraction of the joint has been achieved, the traction is released during prepping and draping to reduce total traction time, which should be limited to less than 2 hours (Carreira & Bush-Joseph, 2006).

ESTABLISHING AND MAINTAINING THE STERILE FIELD

A plastic drape with an adhesive edge is placed on the patient to protect the perineal area; the surgical skin prep is then performed by the circulating nurse. After the prep solution has dried, the sterile field is established with adhesive barrier drapes placed along the four sides of the sterile field as follows (Shugars & More, 2005):

- superiorly, just above the anterior-superior iliac spine;
- inferiorly at mid-thigh;
- medially, just lateral to the perineal post; and
- laterally, just posterior to the greater trochanter.

A clear, adhesive isolation drape with an incorporated suction pouch is then placed over the surgical field.

EQUIPMENT, SUPPLIES, AND INSTRUMENTS

Generally, standard arthroscopy equipment can be used (see **Table 28.7**) except in obese individuals (Wheeless, 2008a).

PHYSIOLOGICAL MONITORING

See Physiological Monitoring discussion under Ankle Arthroscopy.

SPECIMENS AND CULTURES

Specimens and cultures vary according to individual pathological examination findings. Routinely, an excised portion of tissue or bone is removed and sent for definitive studies. Other diagnostic studies that may be required are anaerobic or aerobic cultures or a cell count of synovial fluid in the presence of a septic joint.

DRUGS AND SOLUTIONS

The hip joint is usually irrigated with an appropriate arthroscopic irrigant as ordered by the physician during the procedure to improve visualization and flush out the debrided tissue. Upon completion of the case, the surgeon may inject local anesthetic into the joint to reduce postprocedure pain and facilitate discharge from the facility (Buly, 2008).

Physician Orders and Diagnostic Studies

In addition to the routine orders listed in **Table 28.8**, two elements of preprocedure planning are critical for hip arthroscopy (Carreira & Bush-Joseph, 2006):

- The hip ROM must be evaluated to determine the presence of contractures. If a contracture is present, the hip must be left in that position to allow for adequate distraction and visualization.

- Radiographs should be completed to identify spurs or dysplasia. Large spurs may block entrance into the joint, and hips with dysplasia have been shown to have poorer outcomes.

Procedure

Hip arthroscopy has evolved more slowly than arthroscopy of the other joints (ie, knee and shoulder) because the hip joint is much deeper and therefore more difficult to access (Buly, 2008).

Incision and Exposure

It is necessary to use traction to distract the joint under anesthesia. This distraction temporarily opens the joint space by approximately ½ inch to allow insertion of the scope and instrumentation without damage to the labrum and cartilage. Two small skin incisions are made; occasionally a third or fourth incision may be necessary, depending on the type of procedure (Buly, 2008).

Details

The landmarks for placement of the portals include the superior margin of the greater trochanter and the anterior superior iliac spine. The entrance site for the anterolateral portal is the most anterior aspect of the superior margin of the greater trochanter; the posterolateral portal site is at the most posterior aspect of the same margin (Carreira & Bush-Joseph, 2006).

The three standard portals used for hip arthroscopy are anterolateral, anterior, and posterolateral (Carreira & Bush-Joseph, 2006). The anterolateral portal site is placed first because it is the safest from the femoral and sciatic neurovascular structures. This portal penetrates the gluteus medius muscle before entering the lateral aspect of the capsule at its anterior margin; it provides the best visualization of the anterior wall and labrum. An 18-gauge 6-inch spinal needle is introduced at the landmark noted above, and is directed into the joint space under fluoroscopic guidance. The joint is then distended with approximately 40 mL of fluid and the intracapsular position of the needle is confirmed by the backflow of fluid. A superficial skin nick is made, followed by a switching wire fed through the spinal needle into the joint space; the spinal needle is then removed. A 5.0-mm arthroscopic cannula with obturator is passed over the wire into the joint space. Fluoroscopic assistance may prevent scuffing of the articular surface of the femoral head with the obturator. The switching wire is then removed and a 30° scope is used first to inspect the joint, followed by a 70° scope for further visualization, as well as placement of the remaining portals.

The anterior portal is placed next, with both fluoroscopic guidance and arthroscopic visualization to ensure proper entrance through the joint capsule. This portal penetrates the muscle belly of the sartorius and the rectus femoris before entering the anterior capsule; it provides the best visualization of lateral labrum. The skin landmark is determined as the bisector of two lines: one drawn distally from the anterosuperior iliac spine and the other drawn transversely from the superior margin of the greater trochanter. The spinal needle is introduced at this landmark and oriented toward the joint space, aiming approximately 45° posteriorly and 30° medially. Once the joint has been entered, a superficial skin nick is made to avoid damaging the lateral femoral cutaneous nerve branches. The switching wire then is used, allowing removal of the spinal needle as well as passage of the cannula with obturator over the wire.

The posterolateral portal insertion site is placed last; this portal penetrates both the gluteus medius and gluteus minimus prior to entering the lateral capsule at its posterior margin and provides the best visualization of posterior wall and labrum. The spinal needle is oriented horizontally and medially. The sciatic nerve should be well posterior and the superior gluteal nerve well superior to this insertion site (Carreira & Bush-Joseph, 2006).

After these three standard portals are established, the joint can be visualized from several perspectives to assess the pathology; it can be viewed with or without fluid distension. Most hip arthroscopy procedures require the use of multiple portals for the proper positioning of hand instruments, power shavers, and electrosurgery devices and the accomplishment of a variety of intra-articular procedures (Carreira & Bush-Joseph, 2006). **Figure 28.16** shows right hip injuries with arthroscopic repairs.

CLOSURE

A drain is usually not necessary unless the patient has an infection (Shugars & More, 2005). The small portal incisions are closed with monofilament, nonabsorbable suture or staples; sterile dressings are then applied.

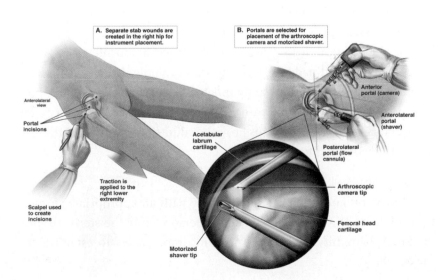

Figure 28.16

Hip arthroscopy.

Source: Nucleus Medical Art.

Postprocedure Care

In PACU, the nurse monitors the patient for cardiac and respiratory complications, inspects the dressings for excessive bleeding, manages the patient's pain, and also assesses the neurovascular status of both of the patient's lower extremities and compares this to the initial baseline assessment (Shugars & More, 2005). Patients are usually discharged with crutches, but can often return to full weight-bearing a few days after the procedure. Physical therapy may also be ordered during the postprocedure period to increase strength and range of motion. If the microfracture technique is used, it may be necessary to delay weight bearing for as long as 6 weeks after the procedure (Buly, 2008).

Potential Complications

Potential complications associated with hip arthroscopy include (Wheeless, 2008a):

- injury to the lateral femoral cutaneous nerve;
- neuropraxia of the pudendal or sciatic nerves;
- permanent injury to the sciatic nerve;
- sciatic nerve palsy (this is more likely to occur in conditions such as traumatic dislocation of the hip);
- pressure necrosis of the foot or perineum due to excessive force and duration of traction;
- chondral injury; and
- infection.

Wrist Arthroscopy

Nursing Implications

ANESTHESIA

General anesthesia is frequently used for wrist arthroscopy, however, regional anesthesia (eg, axillary block or Bier block) with sedation is also an option (Ricks, 2007). Factors to consider when deciding on the type of anesthesia include the patient's medical history, physician and patient preference, as well as the recommendation of the anesthesia provider.

POSITION

Place the patient in the supine position. After anesthesia has been induced, rotate the OR bed so that the patient's operative arm is in the center of the OR to provide complete access to the surgical field (Ricks, 2007). Place a tourniquet high on the patient's upper arm over soft padding; it is important to note that a tourniquet is always placed before the procedure, but rarely inflated because bleeding is minimal during wrist arthroscopy (Ricks, 2007). Secure the patient's arm to the extremity table with padding and a hook-and-loop strap; this provides counter traction when the arm is positioned later in a distraction tower.

ESTABLISHING AND MAINTAINING THE STERILE FIELD

Prep the operative hand and arm circumferentially with an appropriate surgical skin preparation solution. The physician and scrub person apply the sterile drapes, including a stockinet, extremity sheet, and medium drape sheets to establish the sterile field (Ricks, 2007).

EQUIPMENT, SUPPLIES, AND INSTRUMENTS

The equipment, supplies, and instrumentation commonly used for arthroscopic procedures (see **Table 28.7**) may also be used for the wrist; however, smaller-diameter arthroscopes and instrumentation are needed. Instrumentation typically used includes a 2.7-mm, 30-degree arthroscope as well as small instruments such as basket forceps (2–3 mm in diameter; 6 cm in length); an angled probe (1.5–2.0 mm in diameter; 40 mm in length); curved and straight grasping forceps, and a motorized shaver (Weisler & Poehling, 2002).

PHYSIOLOGICAL MONITORING

See Physiological Monitoring discussion under Ankle Arthroscopy.

SPECIMENS AND CULTURES

Specimens and cultures vary according to individual pathological examination findings. Routinely, an excised portion of tissue or bone is removed and sent for definitive studies. Other diagnostic studies that may be required are anaerobic or aerobic cultures or a cell count of synovial fluid in the presence of a septic joint.

DRUGS AND SOLUTIONS

The physician injects normal saline (about 5 mL–10 mL) into the wrist joint to distract the carpal bones (Ricks, 2007). The joint is usually irrigated with an appropriate arthroscopic irrigant, as ordered by the physician during the procedure, to improve visualization and flush out the debrided tissue.

PHYSICIAN ORDERS AND DIAGNOSTIC STUDIES

Before the procedure in addition to the routine orders listed in **Table 28.8**, the physician will obtain imaging studies of the hand and wrist (eg, MRI, radiographs, or arthrogram) and also perform provocative tests to locate the pain; these tests involve manipulating the hand in order to reproduce the pain (AAOS, 2007).

Procedure

INCISION AND EXPOSURE

The physician applies traction to the patient's arm with the sterile finger traps and wrist tower in order to distract the carpal bones and provide space for insertion of the surgical instrumentation (Ricks, 2007). Once the arm is secured in the traction device, the physician carefully marks the areas for portal placement, avoiding any underlying vessels, nerves, or tendons. Usually, wrist arthroscopy is performed through portals placed on the posterior side of the wrist (Ricks, 2007). After the physician injects the normal saline to distract the carpal bones, the skin incisions are made; a small hemostat is used to bluntly dissect into the joint capsule.

DETAILS

The arthroscope and instruments are then inserted through the portals. The arthroscopic cannula with a blunt trocar is inserted into the joint first; the trocar is removed and the arthroscope is inserted through the cannula (Ricks, 2007). The fluid inflow tubing is attached from the pump to the cannula; the physician also inserts an 18-gauge injectable needle into the joint capsule, which is connected to extension

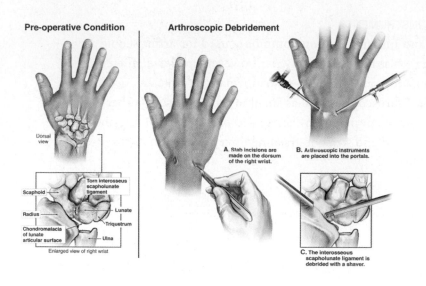

Figure 28.17

Wrist arthroscopy.

Source: Nucleus Medical Art.

tubing to act as an outflow port. Additional portals are placed as indicated by the patient's existing pathology; the physician then thoroughly inspects the joint, switching the scope to different portals as needed to obtain the best visualization. The majority of wrist abnormalities (eg, unresolved wrist pain, triangular fibrocartilage complex injuries or tears, ligament tears, fractures, foreign or loose bodies, ganglion cysts, arthritis, and carpal instability) can be diagnosed and treated with arthroscopic surgery; it may also be used to smooth bone surfaces and excise inflamed tissue (Ricks, 2007; AAOS, 2007). **Figure 28.17** shows wrist injuries with arthroscopic repairs.

CLOSURE

Upon completion of the procedure, the small skin incisions are closed with sutures; a bulky dressing is applied; sometimes a plaster splint is used to immobilize and rest the wrist (AAOS, 2007; Ricks, 2007).

Postprocedure Care

The patient is transported to the PACU by the anesthesia provider and circulating nurse. The PACU nurse monitors the patient's vital signs during recovery from anesthesia; in addition, he/she ensures that the patient's operative wrist remains elevated and applies an ice pack to decrease pain and swelling (Ricks, 2007). Discharge instructions for postprocedure care include (Ricks, 2007):

- keep the surgical wrist elevated until the postprocedure office visit, usually within four to seven days;
- keep the surgical wound dry;
- take analgesics (either prescription or over-the-counter) as ordered for postprocedure discomfort; and
- reinforce the dressing to control normal bleeding and fluid leakage.

Potential Complications

Complications during or after arthroscopic wrist surgery are rare, but may include infection, nerve injuries, excessive swelling, bleeding, scarring, or tendon tearing (AAOS, 2007).

Elbow Arthroscopy

Nursing Implications

ANESTHESIA

General anesthesia is often indicated for elbow arthroscopy because it provides complete muscle relaxation and comfort for the patient; however, intrascalene or axillary blocks can also be used. While IV regional anesthesia is also an option, the use of dual tourniquets on the upper arm compromises exposure and also causes vascular engorgement and edema, thereby interfering with optimal visualization of the joint (Meyers & Carson, 2002).

POSITION

Apply the tourniquet as high as possible on the upper arm. Place the patient in the supine position with the scapula at the edge of the OR bed and the shoulder abducted 90 degrees. Connect the hand or forearm to a "finger trap" or other type of wrist support; the arm is then connected to an overhead suspension device so that the elbow is flexed to 90 degrees. A single sterile towel, covered by a transparent plastic drape, may be used to cover the forearm wrist support (Meyers & Carson, 2002). The patient may also be placed in the prone position, with a sandbag placed under the antecubital fossa (Wheeless, 2008b).

ESTABLISHING AND MAINTAINING THE STERILE FIELD

Place a rolled towel under the shoulder and axillary region. The arm is elevated and supported; a circumferential scrub is performed with an appropriate antimicrobial agent. Typically, the entire arm including the axilla and hand are prepped. Following the skin preparation, the elbow is extended with the upper arm abducted; a surgical drape is then wrapped around the elbow and secured on the posterior side of the upper arm (Strobel, 2001).

EQUIPMENT, SUPPLIES, AND INSTRUMENTS

The equipment, supplies, and instrumentation commonly used for the arthroscopy (see **Table 28.7**) may also be used for the elbow, however, smaller-diameter arthroscopes and instrumentation may be needed.

PHYSIOLOGICAL MONITORING

See Physiological Monitoring discussion under Ankle Arthroscopy.

SPECIMENS AND CULTURES

Specimens and cultures vary according to individual pathological examination findings. Send excised tissue, bone (fragments, radial head), and loose bodies to pathology for examination.

DRUGS AND SOLUTIONS

The joint is usually irrigated with an appropriate arthroscopic irrigant as ordered by the physician during the procedure to improve visualization and flush out the debrided tissue. The physician may also inject a local anesthetic into the joint for postoperative pain control.

PHYSICIAN ORDERS AND DIAGNOSTIC STUDIES

Before the procedure in addition to the routine orders listed in **Table 28.8**, the physician will obtain an MRI and radiographs of the joint to assess the soft tissues (cartilage, tendons, and ligaments) surrounding the bones as well as the bones themselves, which may have irregularities such as spurs; placement of the portals may also be guided by these findings (Altchek, 2003).

Procedure

INCISION AND EXPOSURE

Arthroscopic surgery on the elbow is challenging because of the anatomy of the joint; the bones are in close proximity and the nerves and blood vessels are located very close to the joint (Shoulderdoc, 2008). With a standard supine approach, anterolateral, anteromedial, and posterolateral portals are used.

DETAILS

The anterolateral portal is often established first and can be used for instrumentation as well as visualization of the lateral aspect of the radial head (Wheeless, 2008b). With the elbow flexed 90 degrees, the portal is located 3 cm distal and 1–2 cm anterior to the lateral epicondyle, which brings the portal just anterior and proximal to the radial-capitellar articulation with the portal driven toward the center of the trochlea. The elbow is kept flexed during trochar insertion since extension brings the radial nerve 3 to 7 mm closer to the joint. Some physicians prefer to establish the anteromedial portal first. The elbow should be flexed 90 degrees as the portal is established; placed 2 cm anterior and 2 cm distal to the medial epicondyle under direct vision, since the *median nerve* lies 1 to 2 cm anterior and lateral to this portal. The posterolateral portal is located through the center of the *anconeus triangle;* when the anterior aspect of the joint is being visualized, the posterolateral portal can be used as an outflow portal. The posterolateral portal can also be used to visualize the posterior elbow structures including the olecranon fossa; the use of a 70-degree arthroscope facilitates visualization of the radiocapitellar joint; this portal allows debridement of the capitellum, in the case of osteochondritis dissecans (Wheeless, 2008b). **Figure 28.18** depicts elbow arthroscopy for repair of ulnar nerve injury.

CLOSURE

The small portal incisions are closed with monofilament, nonabsorbable sutures, or staples. The area is covered with dry, sterile, gauze dressings and wrapped with a compression dressing.

Postprocedure Care

The elbow is kept elevated when not in use for the first postprocedure day to reduce swelling. The patient is instructed to use the elbow as tolerated. If the procedure was performed for improving range of motion or for the treatment of arthritis, an indwelling catheter may be inserted for brachial plexus block anesthetic if the neurologic exam is normal in the PACU; the patient is also started on a full range of motion on a continuous passive motion (CPM) device the same day. All circumferential

CPM
Continuous Passive Motion

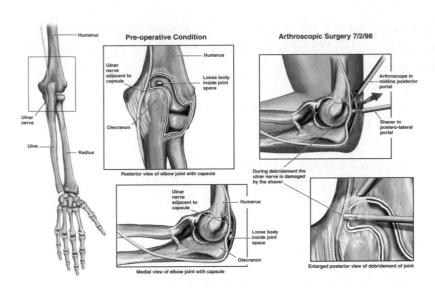

Figure 28.18

Elbow arthroscopy.

Source: Nucleus Medical Art.

dressings must be removed to avoid skin damage during CPM; only an elastic sleeve should be used to hold the absorbent dressing in place (O'Driscoll, 2002).

Potential Complications

The potential complications associated with elbow arthroscopy are similar to those with any arthroscopic procedure, including infection, problems associated with tourniquet use, instrument breakage, and neurovascular complications (Meyers & Carson, 2002).

Shoulder Arthroscopy

Nursing Implications

ANESTHESIA

General or regional anesthesia are both options for shoulder arthroscopy (Strobel, 2001). General anesthesia is often preferred because of the potential circulatory compromise with the beach chair position, and it provides both the most effective muscle relaxation and the option for controlled hypotension if the field of vision is obscured by excessive intraoperative bleeding. The intrascalene plexus block is preferred for postprocedure pain relief.

POSITION

The two most common positions used for shoulder arthroscopy are the lateral decubitus and beach chair (Strobel, 2001). The position selected depends on the physician's experience and the planned procedure.

Lateral Decubitus   In this position, the patient is placed in the lateral position with his/her back even with the edge of the OR bed. The torso is supported by side rests placed anteriorly at the level of the thoracic outlet and posteriorly at the level of the pelvis or with a vacuum beanbag positioning device. Bony prominences are carefully padded. This position requires a special shoulder traction system that allows adjustments in abduction, anteversion, and distraction; a forearm wrap connects the arm securely to the overhead traction device without the risk of compression injury to the soft tissues. The arm is positioned in approximately 45 degrees of abduction, and 15 degrees of anteversion with 4–8 kg of traction to prevent brachial plexus injury.

Beach Chair In this position, one important consideration is that the full circumference of the shoulder must be accessible during the procedure. An extended head rest, which supports the head and positions the shoulder past the edge of the OR bed so that it is accessible both anteriorly and posteriorly, is used (**Fig. 28.25**).

ESTABLISHING AND MAINTAINING THE STERILE FIELD

Establishing the sterile field is dependent upon the patient position (Strobel, 2001).

Lateral Decubitus Cover the patient with a drape prior to skin preparation to protect the skin from the prep solution. Prep the arm with the appropriate antimicrobial solution, wrap it with a sterile drape, and then secure it in the traction device. Drape the shoulder area with two sterile aperture drapes, one placed from the axillary side, one placed from the cranial side.

Beach Chair In this position, place a towel under the patient's shoulder to protect the skin from the skin prep solution; the arm is abducted at the shoulder during the skin preparation. Place sterile drapes covering the patient to the chest. A waterproof adhesive aperture drape is then placed over the shoulder from the cranial side; a smaller adhesive drape is placed from the axillary side. Wrap the arm with a waterproof towel drape secured with adhesive tape. Pull the cranial drape over the patient's head to form a screen for the anesthesia provider, who is seated next to the contralateral shoulder.

EQUIPMENT, SUPPLIES, AND INSTRUMENTS

Standard arthroscopic equipment, instruments, and supplies are used for shoulder arthroscopy (see **Table 28.7**); however, a large-bore sheath (ie, 6 mm) should be used to deliver adequate fluid pressure for distention (Strobel, 2001).

PHYSIOLOGICAL MONITORING

See Physiological Monitoring discussion under Ankle Arthroscopy.

SPECIMENS AND CULTURES

Specimens and cultures vary according to individual pathological examination findings. Routinely, an excised portion of tissue or bone is removed and sent for definitive studies. Other diagnostic studies that may be required are anaerobic or aerobic cultures or a cell count of synovial fluid in the presence of a septic joint.

DRUGS AND SOLUTIONS

Because electrosurgery instruments and shavers will be used, the joint is distended with a nonelectrolyte solution (Strobel, 2001). A local anesthetic with epinephrine is also injected into the joint to reduce bleeding.

PHYSICIAN ORDERS AND DIAGNOSTIC STUDIES

Before the procedure in addition to the routine orders listed in **Table 28.8**, the physician will obtain an MRI and radiographs of the joint to assess the soft tissues (cartilage, tendons, and ligaments) surrounding the bones as well as the bones themselves.

Procedure

INCISION AND EXPOSURE

Three portals are made in the shoulder joint: posterior, anterior superior, and anterior inferior. Prior to creating the portals, the physician must palpate the bony structures around the shoulder (Strobel, 2001). The primary landmarks are the clavicle, acromioclavicular (AC) joint, acromion, coracoid process, and scapular spine. The posterior portal is used as the primary portal for insertion of the arthroscope. It is placed approximately 2–3 cm inferior and 1–2 cm medial to the posterolateral corner of the acromion. The two anterior portals are used for instrumentation and inflow.

AC
Acromioclavicular

DETAILS

The shoulder joint is expanded with the appropriate irrigation solution. The physician will examine the entire joint to assess the cartilage, tendons, and ligaments of the shoulder. The physician will perform repairs with various instruments (eg, blunt hook to retract tissues, a shaver to excise damaged tissues, or a burr to remove bone) inserted through the additional portals. The physician will also examine the subacromial space to evaluate the area above the rotator cuff, excise inflamed or damaged tissue, remove a bone spur, or repair a rotator cuff tear. Upon completion of the procedure, the fluid is drained from the shoulder. **Figure 28.19** depicts arthroscopic shoulder surgery.

CLOSURE

The small portal incisions are closed with monofilament, nonabsorbable sutures, staples or Steri-strips, if preferred by the physician. The area is covered with dry, sterile, gauze dressings and wrapped with a compression dressing. The shoulder is often placed in a sling, a sling and swath, or a brace.

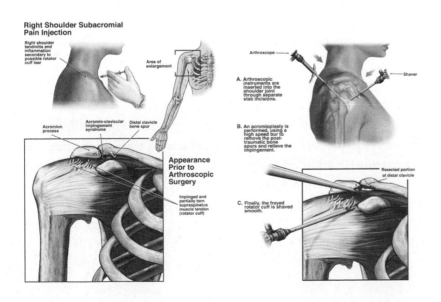

Figure 28.19

Shoulder arthroscopy.

Source: Nucleus Medical Art.

Postprocedure Care

After the procedure the PACU nurse will monitor the patient's vital signs, manage his/her pain, and assess the operative wound. The amount of movement allowed and the time until the patient can resume moderate exercise is dependent upon the type of procedure. Recovery is often augmented with physical therapy exercises targeting specific muscle groups to help the shoulder strengthen and recover in a manner that supports the procedural repairs.

Potential Complications

The potential complications associated with shoulder arthroscopy include (Medline Plus, 2007):

- bleeding;
- infection;
- nerve damage;
- stiffness of the shoulder joint;
- failure of the procedure to relieve the symptoms;
- failure of the repair to heal; and
- weakness of the shoulder.

BUNIONECTOMY

A bunion is a deformity characterized by lateral angulation of the metatarsophalangeal joint of the great toe, with enlargement and the development of a bursa, termed a hallux valgus. There is medial rotation of the great toe on its long axis, and the extensor tendon of the long toe is displaced laterally. Hallux valgus is more frequently seen in females, and there appears to be a familial tendency. Poorly fitting shoes, degenerative arthritic changes, flat feet, and a wedging of bone causing a medial angulation of the first metatarsal, are known contributory causes. The pain of hallux valgus may be due to traumatic arthritis, pressure on the digital nerves, and compression and inflammation of the overlying bursa. Atrophy of the articular cartilage may occur and become extensive.

Indications

Operative intervention is for the relief of symptoms, mostly being pain, and not for cosmetic reasons.

Related Procedures

There are numerous procedures to correct a hallux valgus deformity. Other deformities, such as hammertoes or corns, may also be associated with the bunion and may necessitate correction. In addition to the excision of the exostosis, various procedures may also use partial resection of the first metatarsal head (Mayo procedure), partial resection of the first proximal phalanx (Keller procedure), tendon transfer to lateral portion of the first metatarsal (McBride procedure), or osteotomy of the first metatarsal (Mitchell procedure).

Nursing Implications

Anesthesia

General anesthesia or an ankle block with monitored anesthesia care is generally used.

Position

Position the patient supine, close to the end of the operative bed or stretcher. Place the operative extremity on a wedge to facilitate access.

Establishing and Maintaining the Sterile Field

After applying the tourniquet just above the ankle or on the thigh, prep the area in the routine orthopedic fashion with an antimicrobial solution. The prep area includes the entire leg below the tourniquet including the ankle, foot, and between the toes. Drape the operative extremity in the same fashion as for an arthroscopic procedure of the knee. The stockinet and drapes, however, are taken to just above the knee.

Place the tourniquet controls on the nonoperative side within easy access of the anesthesia provider and circulating nurse. Prevent kinking of the tourniquet hose.

Equipment and Supplies

Table 28.9 lists equipment, supplies, and instruments for bunionectomy.

Drugs and Solutions

The physician may order antibiotic irrigation solution.

Physiological Monitoring

The same principles of nursing care during the procedure apply to all operative patients. Closely monitor pressure points and tourniquet pressure and times. Document care according to facility policy and procedure. After deflation of the tourniquet, calculate blood loss based on suction collection and sponge saturation. Check and document neurovascular status after any extremity procedure.

Specimens and Cultures

Send the resected portion of the metatarsal head or proximal phalanx to pathology.

Physician Orders and Diagnostic Studies

The patient is admitted the day of surgery. For laboratory studies, refer to the discussion of arthroscopy of the knee. The physician may order weight-bearing AP, and lateral radiographs of bilateral feet. These radiographs document a valgus deformity of the great toe at the metatarsophalangeal joint (the base of the proximal phalanx is subluxed laterally), the presence of a medial exostosis on the first metatarsal head, and a varus deformity of the first metatarsal.

Procedure

Incision and Exposure

An incision is made with a No. 15 blade over the dorsomedial aspect of the metatarsal head, giving access to the exostosis. Retraction is minimal, owing to the prominent metatarsal head. Additional exposure may be achieved with Senn retractors

Table 28.9	Equipment, Supplies, and Instruments for Bunionectomy	
Equipment	**Supplies**	**Instruments**
Basin set	1500 mL of normal saline	¼-inch osteotome (hand)
Electrosurgery generator	2 2-0 Vicryl on a cutting needle	½-inch osteotome (hand)
Nitrogen power source	2 No. 1 Vicryl on a cutting needle	2 Adson forceps with teeth
Power microsagittal saw and blade	2 povidone-iodine scrub brushes	2 needle holders
Prep leg holder	4 0.065 Kirschner wires	2 No. 3 knife handles
Tourniquet and cuff	4 × 4-inch dressing sponges	2 ribbon retractors
	4 × 8-inch radiopaque sponges	2 Senn retractors
	4-0 Prolene on a cutting needle	2 sponge-holding forceps
	4-inch Webril	2 tissue forceps with teeth
	4-inch Webril	4 Allis clamps
	6 No. 15 blades	4 Kocher clamps
	6-inch Esmarch bandage	4 mosquito clamps
	Alcohol (according to the surgeon's preferences)	6 towel clips
	Drape pack	Assorted drill bits and drill
	Electrosurgery supplies	Bandage scissors
	Hinged impervious sheet	Bunion retractors
	Impervious stockinet	Freer periosteal elevator
	Ioban Steri-Drape	Hand drill and key
	Irrigation syringe	Heiss retractor
	Kling bandage	Key periosteal elevator
	Skin antiseptic agent and prepping supplies (according to the surgeon's preference)	Mallet
	Skin marker	Metzenbaum scissors
	Steri-Strips	Microsagittal power saw and blade
	Suction tubing	No. 12 Frazier suction
		Pin cutter
		Power wire driver
		Small bone rongeur (double action)
		Small curet
		Suture scissors

placed dorsomedially and dorsolaterally to the exostosis. The bursa is excised and retracted with the Senn retractors.

The incision is curved over the metatarsophalangeal joint dorsally. Caution is taken to avoid the extensor hallucis longus tendon. It is then curved back along the medial aspect of the shaft of the first metatarsal, continuing 2–3 cm from the metatarsophalangeal joint.

The deep fascia is incised with a No. 15 blade, keeping in line with the incision, and then followed down to the dorsomedial aspect of the metatarsophalangeal joint.

The dorsal digital branch of the medial cutaneous nerve, along with the skin flap, is retracted laterally with a small right-angled retractor. The joint capsule is incised, leaving the proximal end attached to the proximal phalanx.

Details (*Keller Procedure*)

The periosteum of the proximal phalanx and first metatarsal is incised with a No. 15 blade. The covering is removed from the bone by a Key periosteal elevator. Again, caution is taken to preserve the flexor hallucis longus on the plantar surface of the proximal phalanx. Small bunion retractors are inserted on each side of the midphalanx. These retractors function as bone levers.

The proximal half of the proximal phalanx is then cleanly resected across the middle of the shaft with a 1/4-inch hand osteotome and a small sharp-pointed bone cutter. The cut surface of the distal fragment is examined for projecting bone spurs. Any remaining, uncut bone is removed with a small bone rongeur. Small Metzenbaum scissors dissect any bursa from the underlying bone on the medial side. The exostosis is removed with the 1/4-inch hand osteotome. Fixation is achieved with the insertion of a 0.065 Kirschner wire through the proximal phalanx and the first metatarsal with a power drill or wire driver.

Closure

The tourniquet is deflated, and hemostasis is achieved with electrosurgery or hemostats. The wound is copiously irrigated with an antibiotic solution. The capsule is revised with a continuous 2-0 absorbable suture to promote stability of the soft tissues and great toe. The skin is closed with an interrupted 4-0 nylon suture. The incision is covered with dry, sterile gauze dressings, with attention to the area between the great and second toes. A bandage of 4-inch (10 cm) Webril followed by a posterior plaster splint is applied. The toe is splinted in 5 degrees of flexion and slight varus position.

Figure 28.20 shows an example of bunion deformity of the right foot with surgical repairs.

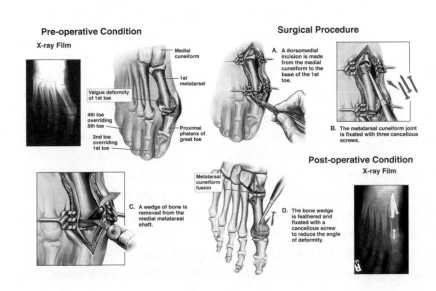

Pre-operative Condition
X-ray Film

Medial cuneiform
1st metatarsal
Valgus deformity of 1st toe
4th toe overriding 5th toe
2nd toe overriding 1st toe
Proximal phalanx of great toe

Surgical Procedure

A. A dorsomedial incision is made from the medial cuneiform to the base of the 1st toe.

B. The metatarsal cuneiform joint is fixated with three cancellous screws.

C. A wedge of bone is removed from the medial metatarsal shaft.

Metatarsal cuneiform fusion

D. The bone wedge is feathered and fixated with a cancellous screw to reduce the angle of deformity.

Post-operative Condition
X-ray Film

Figure 28.20

Bunion deformity of the right foot with surgical repairs.

Source: Nucleus Medical Art.

Postprocedure Care

Although the procedure is performed on an outpatient basis, the patient and family must understand the importance of postprocedure care. Instruct the patient concerning bed rest or resting with the leg elevated higher than heart, for 48 hours. During the first 24 hours, the patient should apply ice packs (20 minutes on and 20 minutes off). After the initial 48 hours, if tolerated, the patient is allowed up with crutches; however, the patient still elevates the operative extremity when seated, lying down, or if increased pain or swelling occurs; elevation continues until the symptoms subside. Antibiotic coverage is provided for 24 hours. Pain medication is prescribed. Before discharge, the patient receives crutch walking and boot cast walking training.

Discharge occurs in three to ten hours, depending on the ability to ambulate, or overnight if there is bleeding or complications. The patient sees the physician in ten days for suture removal. Encourage the patient to maintain nutritional status and fluid volume. No bathing is allowed until the sutures are removed. The patient may take a shower if able to keep the foot dry. A bunion shoe is used for 6 weeks. High-heeled shoes are not allowed without physician approval. Instruct the patient about the signs of infection: redness, warmth, point tenderness, swelling, and drainage. The patient should report signs of infection or paresthesias or numbness of the great toe to the physician. Encourage the patient to perform straight-leg raises and active ankle range-of-motion exercises. If inserted, Kirschner wire removal is done in 4–6 weeks.

Potential Complications

The deformity may redevelop or occur at any point after the procedure. Hallux varus deformity occurs because of overcorrection of the valgus deformity and may create a new deformity that requires correction. Necrosis of the wound edges may occur because the skin on the medial aspect of the metatarsophalangeal joint is thinner and may not heal as well. In addition, the bursa may have been inflamed, which can complicate the procedure. Numbness or paresthesias are due to transection of the medial dorsal cutaneous nerve during incision and may persist for up to a year. Severed nerves or the development of neuromas may require further treatment. Excessive capsular tightening during reconstruction, fibrous tissue formation, or scarring of the extensor hallucis longus may limit motion of the metatarsophalangeal joint. Nonunion or avascular necrosis of the osteotomy may occur. Infection is also possible.

EXCISION OF A GANGLION

A ganglion is a cystic swelling overlying a joint or a tendon sheath. One large cyst usually develops and is either unilocular or multilocular. Multiple small accessory cysts usually lie adjacent to the large cyst. The ganglion consists of a dense fibrous capsule surrounding a thick, sticky, clear odorless fluid. The cystic fluid has the consistency of soft jelly. The cyst is bound to joint and/or tendon by dense tissue.

Two theories explain why ganglia develop. In one theory, the dense collagenous tissue of the wrist degenerates and leads to the formation of multiple small cysts containing mucin. Small cysts over time may coalesce into one large cyst. The other theory postulates a deficit in the joint capsule or tendon sheath, permitting a protrusion of synovial tissue. The communicating channel between the protruding tissue and the joint becomes obliterated, and a cyst remains as a pedicle or adhesion. Additional cysts may be formed if the defect in the capsule or sheath persists.

A ganglion occurs most frequently about the wrist but may appear adjacent to the wrist. The usual location, at the wrist, is the dorsum between the long extensor of the thumb and the extensor to the index finger. It may be traced down to the articulation between the lunate and the scaphoid. When the ganglion is over the volar aspect of the wrist, it appears between the brachioradialis and the flexor carpi radialis tendons. In the palm of the hand, ganglia develop from the deep pulley of the finger flexors over the metacarpal heads.

Indications

Ganglion excision is indicated for persistent discomfort that does not respond to medical treatment and when the ganglion interferes with range of motion.

Related Procedures

Nonoperative and operative treatments are available for ganglion cysts. Frequently, however, nonoperative methods are unsuccessful and operative excision is required. Nonoperative procedures include the following: aspirating the cyst fluid with a 21-gauge needle and injecting the remaining tissue with a corticosteroid or a sclerosing agent; rupturing the cyst by means of an external force; and using roentgenographic therapy (a 1.5-erythema dose repeated in 1 month).

Nursing Implications
Anesthesia

The procedure can be performed under local anesthesia, a regional block, or general anesthesia.

Position

Place the patient in the supine position. Extend the operative arm on a hand table. Do not extend the arm greater than 90 degrees. Place the nonoperative arm on a padded armboard with the palm up. Secure the patient by placing a safety strap 2 inches (5 cm) above the knees. Check to ensure that the patient's legs remained uncrossed. Align the head in anatomical alignment with the body. During preparation of the operative field, gently turn the head away from the operative side. Protect vulnerable pressure points such as the occiput, scapula, olecranon, sacrum, ischial tuberosity, and calcaneus with additional padding, especially if the patient is under general anesthesia.

Raise the operative arm on an arm support or bolster positioned under the upper arm. Apply the appropriate-sized tourniquet high on the upper arm.

Establishing and Maintaining the Sterile Field

With the arm elevated, prep the hand, including all fingers, to just above the elbow. Place sterile stockinet over the hand; the arm is held suspended and the arm support removed. Telescope the stockinet to above the elbow. Cover the hand table with a large sterile drape. Use a fenestrated drape as a single-layer drape that covers the patient's body.

Equipment, Supplies, and Instruments

Table 28.10 lists equipment and supplies for excision of ganglion.

Table 28.10	Equipment and Supplies for Excision of Ganglion	
Equipment		**Supplies**
Basin set	1500 mL of normal saline	Alcohol (according to the surgeon's preferences)
Electrosurgery generator	2 3-0 silk on a cutting needle	Bipolar cord and forceps
Hand table	2 3-0 Vicryl on a cutting needle	Drape pack
Tourniquet and cuff	2 4 × 4-inch dressing sponges	Electrosurgery supplies
	2 4-0 nylon on a cutting needle	Impervious hinge sheet
	2 povidone-iodine scrub brushes	Impervious stockinet
	4 No. 15 blades	Irrigating syringe
	4 × 8-inch radiopaque sponges	Kling bandage
	4-inch Esmarch bandage	Skin antiseptic agent and prepping supplies (according to the surgeon's preference)
	4-inch Webril	Skin marker
	5-0 chromic on a cutting needle	Prep tray
		Suction tubing

Physiological Monitoring

See the discussion of bunionectomy.

Specimens and Cultures

Send the ganglion sheath to the pathology laboratory for definitive testing. A synovectomy might be performed and synovial tissue sent to the pathology for rheumatology studies.

Drugs and Solutions

The physician may order an antibiotic irrigation. Follow healthcare facility guidelines for dosages and preparation protocols.

Physician Orders and Diagnostic Studies

In addition to routine orders listed in **Table 28.8**, the physician may order bilateral AP, and lateral radiographs of the wrist and hand, which may reveal calcification in the tendon or sheath.

Procedure

Incision and Exposure (*Dorsal Approach*)

The physician exsanguinates the operative extremity with an elastic bandage, and then inflates the tourniquet. With the forearm pronated, a longitudinal incision is made on the dorsal aspect of the wrist with a No. 15 blade. The incision extends across the wrist joint midway between the radial and ulnar styloids, beginning 3 cm proximal and 5 cm distal to the wrist joint. The skin is retracted on both sides with the aid of skin hooks. A 3-0 silk suture on a cutting needle can also be placed on each side as a traction stitch. The subcutaneous fat is incised, in line with the skin incision, with small Metzenbaum scissors. The extensor retinaculum is exposed. The retinaculum over the extensor carpi radialis longus and brevis is incised with a No. 15 blade. This is the compartment on the radial side of the Lister tubercle. The sharp dissection is carried out in the same fashion on the ulnar edge of the cut retinaculum. The extensor retinaculum should be preserved. The tendons are mobilized and lifted from their beds in an ulnar and radial direction. The underlying radius and joint capsule are exposed. The incision is taken down to the retinaculum before the ulnar and radial flaps are elevated to protect the radial nerve in the subcutaneous fat.

Details

The joint capsule is incised longitudinally with a No. 15 blade. The dissection continues subcapsularly on the radial and ulnar sides of the radius, thus exposing the entire distal end of the radius and carpal bones. As long as the dissection (at the level of wrist) remains subperiosteal, the radial artery remains protected. The tendons on both sides of the Lister tubercle are carefully inspected for any ganglion or satellite lesions. The cysts are released from tendon attachment with small Metzenbaum scissors. The cysts are then carefully dissected from their base. A large cuff of joint capsule tissue is also removed to prevent recurrence. The tendons at the level of the Lister tubercle are retracted with small right-angled retractors, and the wrist joint and capsule are thoroughly inspected for any smaller cysts. Any defects in the joint capsule or tendon sheaths are repaired with a running 5-0 chromic suture on a cutting needle.

Closure

After copiously irrigating the wound with antibiotic irrigation, the physician closes the joint capsule with a continuous 5-0 chromic suture on a cutting needle. The subcutaneous tissue is then irrigated and closed with a 3-0 Vicryl interrupted suture on a cutting needle. The skin is closed with an interrupted 4-0 nylon suture on a cutting needle.

The incision is covered with a dry, sterile gauze dressing. A bandage of 3- or 4-inch (7.5–10 cm) Webril followed by a neutral volar splint is then applied. The tourniquet is deflated after compression is achieved by the Webril. The patient's arm is positioned in a sling for additional support and comfort.

Figure 28.21 shows an example of a ganglion cyst removal.

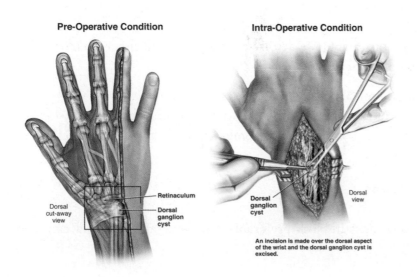

Figure 28.21

Ganglion Cyst Removal.

Source: Nucleus Medical Art.

Postprocedure Care

Usually the patient goes home the same day of surgery. Instructions include rest at home with the extremity higher than the heart for 72 hours and longer if increased pain or swelling occurs. During the first 24 hours, the patient should apply ice packs (20 minutes on and 20 minutes off). Antibiotics may be administered for 24 hours after surgery. Instruct the patient to bathe the extremity only after sutures have been removed. Pain medication is ordered and instructions given to the patient and family. Tell the patient to report signs of infection (redness, warmth, point tenderness, swelling, and drainage) and paresthesias to the physician. A followup appointment is scheduled in 10 days. Splint removal occurs in 3 weeks. After cast removal, the patient begins active range-of-motion exercises.

Potential Complications

Excessive capsular tightening during reconstruction, fibrous tissue formation, and scarring of extensor tendons may cause limitation of motion. Scarring of the radial nerve may cause neuromas. A remaining defect in the capsule or the tendon sheath or a remaining cyst may cause recurrence of the ganglia. An underlying systemic inflammatory condition may lead to infection.

CARPAL TUNNEL RELEASE

Carpal tunnel syndrome refers to the compression of the median nerve as it passes through the carpal canal, also known as the carpal tunnel. Carpal tunnel release involves transecting the transverse carpal ligament to allow for more space in the canal, thereby decompressing the median nerve. Causes of carpal tunnel syndrome include repetitive hand motions, traumatic injuries, or various systemic processes such as pregnancy, obesity, diabetes mellitus, amyloidosis, or thyroid disease.

Indications

Indications for carpal tunnel release include persistent pain or paresthesia that does not respond to non-operative treatment and significant median nerve dysfunction that can be documented clinically or electro-diagnostically.

Related Procedures

Treatment for carpal tunnel syndrome includes operative and nonoperative methods. Operatively, carpal tunnel release can be performed either open or endoscopically. Nonoperative treatment includes the following:

- the use of nonsteroidal anti-inflammatory medications;
- the use of volar wrist splints keeping the wrist in neutral flexion; and
- injecting the carpal canal with a combination of a local anesthetic and corticosteroid.

Nursing Implications
Anesthesia

Local or regional anesthesia is preferable, but general anesthesia can also be used.

Position

Patient positioning is as described for excision of a ganglion. The same safety measures are also followed.

Establishing and Maintaining the Sterile Field

Position, prepare, and drape the arm as described for excision of a ganglion.

Equipment, Supplies, and Instruments

Table 28.11 lists equipment and supplies for carpal tunnel release.

Physiological Monitoring

See the discussion of excision of a ganglion.

Specimens and Cultures

Sometimes the surgeon does a tenosynovectemy and sends the tenosynovial tissue to the pathology department.

Drugs and Solutions

The surgeon irrigates the incision with normal saline or antibiotic irrigation before wound closure.

Physician Orders and Diagnostic Studies

In addition to routine orders listed in **Table 28.8**, the physician may order AP and lateral radiographs of the hand and wrist. Sometimes the physician orders a special radiograph called a carpal tunnel view, which may reveal an osseous pathological process.

Procedure (Open Technique)
Incision and Exposure

The operative extremity is exsanguinated with an elastic bandage, and the tourniquet is inflated accordingly. With the forearm supinated, a longitudinal

Table 28.11 Equipment and Supplies for Carpal Tunnel Release		
Equipment		**Supplies**
Basin set	4 × 8-inch radiopaque sponges	Electrosurgery supplies
Electric battery tourniquet and cuff	2 4-0 nylon sutures	Extremity sheet
	3 No. 15 blades	Impervious split sheet
Electrosurgery generator	3-0 silk suture	Non-adherent dressing
Extra sitting stools	4 × 4-inch dressing sponge	Skin antiseptic agent and prepping supplies (according to the surgeon's preference)
Hand table	4-inch impervious stockinet	
Low instrument table	4-inch Esmarch bandage	PSS 500 mL
Low side table	4-inch Kling bandage	Single gown
	4-inch Webril	Prep tray
	60-mL syringe	Suction tubing
	Drape packs	Towel pack

incision is made on the volar aspect of the hand with a No. 15 blade. The incision is made parallel and ulnar to the thenar musculature. It is gently curved and can be extended proximally to cross the wrist crease if necessary. The incision is carried only through the skin. The skin is retracted on both sides with the aid of skin hooks. The subcutaneous tissue is dissected bluntly with tenotomy scissors, being careful to identify and preserve any palmar cutaneous nerve branches. A Heiss retractor is used to aid in exposure, and the palmar fascia is divided with small Metzenbaum scissors or a No. 15 blade. The transverse carpal ligament is completely exposed.

Details

The median nerve is identified proximally as it enters the carpal canal, and the vascular arch is identified just distal to the transverse carpal ligament. The transverse carpal ligament is transected along the ulnar side to avoid the recurrent motor branch of the median nerve. The ligament is divided with small Metzenbaum scissors or a Beaver blade, being very careful to avoid damaging the underlying median nerve. The nerve and flexor tenosynovium are inspected, and a tenosynovectomy is performed if indicated. The release is completed by dividing the distal portion of antebrachial fascia with Metzenbaum scissors, again being careful to protect the median nerve.

Closure

The wound is copiously irrigated with normal saline or antibiotic irrigation, and the tourniquet is deflated. Meticulous hemostasis is achieved with bipolar electrosurgery. The transverse carpal ligament is left open. The wound is again copiously irrigated with normal saline. The skin is closed with an interrupted 4-0 nylon suture on a cutting needle.

The incision is covered with dry, sterile gauze dressings. Bandage of 3- or 4-inch (7.5–10 cm) Webril. A neutral volar splint is then applied. The patient's arm is positioned in a sling for additional support and comfort.

Figure 28.22 shows an example of carpal tunnel syndrome and surgical release.

Postprocedure Care

The extremity is kept elevated for 72 hours or if increased pain or swelling occurs. During the first 24 hours, the patient should apply ice packs (20 minutes on and 20 minutes off). Tell the patient to report signs of infection such as redness, warmth, point tenderness, swelling, and drainage, and any paresthesias, to the physician. Bathing resumes after suture removal. A followup appointment is made in 10 days. Splint removal is done in 3 weeks. The patient begins active range-of-motion exercises after the cast removal.

Potential Complications

Infection may occur. Fibrous tissue formation and immobilization in a splint may cause limitation of motion. Neurovascular injury to the median nerve or its branches, the ulnar nerve, or the vascular arch is possible. Incomplete release or development of adhesions may lead to recurrence.

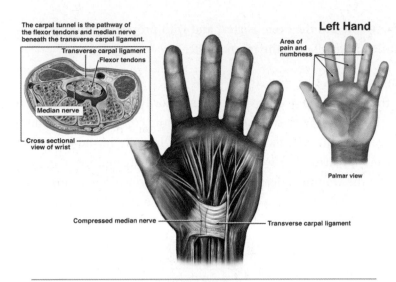

The carpal tunnel is the pathway of the flexor tendons and median nerve beneath the transverse carpal ligament.

Transverse carpal ligament
Flexor tendons
Median nerve
Cross sectional view of wrist

Left Hand

Area of pain and numbness

Palmar view

Compressed median nerve — — Transverse carpal ligament

Figure 28.22

Carpal tunnel syndrome and surgical release.

Source: Nucleus Medical Art.

Surgical Release

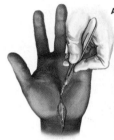

A. An incision is made in the palm and wrist to expose the carpal tunnel.

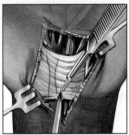

B. The transverse carpal ligament is incised.

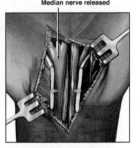

Median nerve released

C. The median nerve is freed from compression.

OPEN REDUCTION AND INTERNAL FIXATION OF THE FRACTURED ULNA

Ulnar shaft fractures require perfect apposition and alignment for the restoration of normal function. Consequently, the physician often repairs the fracture by fixation with plates. The fracture is described in relation to its location in the bone (metaphyseal, diaphyseal, or epiphyseal) and with regard to its rotation, angulation, and displacement. These fractures generally occur as the result of a fall on an outstretched arm, but there is usually a component of direct force as well. Fractures of the ulna alone are rare, but fractures of both the ulna and the radius can occur at any age.

There are often angulation and shortening, causing a deformity because of problems that are special to the forearm. Muscle groups that pull at oblique angles between the radius and the ulna tend to misalign the fracture ends and cause the deformity. The type of deformity depends on the level of the fracture. If closed fractures are left displaced, they lead to not only a deformity but also a limitation of rotation of the forearm. There is also the risk of ischemic damage to the forearm muscles, leading to severe loss of function of the hand.

Indications

Open reduction is a method in which the fracture site is opened and the fragments are united into correct anatomical position. Intramedullary nails and compression plates are most commonly used for internal fixation. The latter are most suitable for fractures of the ulna. Applied to the bone cortex, and with proper techniques, substantial compression can be applied to the fracture site.

Related Procedures

Many transverse fractures of the forearm heal satisfactorily by closed reduction and application of a plaster cast. With fractures that are more complex, open reduction is necessary. In general, internal fixation is not used initially in the treatment of open fractures of the forearm. The wound is usually first treated by irrigation and debridement. After the wound is healed, a procedure may be done to insert an appropriate internal fixation device (eg, a compression plate and an intramedullary rod) or an external fixation device may be applied.

Nursing Implications

Anesthesia

General anesthesia is preferable, but a regional anesthetic may be used.

Position

Position the patient as described for an excision of a ganglion. The same safety measures are also followed.

Establishing and Maintaining the Sterile Field

See the discussion of the excision of a ganglion.

Equipment, Supplies, and Instruments

In addition to the equipment, supplies, and instruments for an open reduction and internal fixation of the ulna listed in **Table 28.12**, this case will require some items used for a Silastic wrist joint implant (**Table 28.13**).

Physiological Monitoring

Neurovascular status in the affected arm should be assessed every 15 minutes. The potential for a neurovascular deficit related to soft tissue swelling and trauma to the bone should be of great concern. In addition to tourniquet times and pressures, blood loss should be measured, documented, and reported to the surgeon and the anesthesia provider.

Specimens and Cultures

Send any resected or fragmented bone not used as an allograft to the pathology laboratory for conclusive testing.

Drugs and Solutions

For an open wound, the physician will frequently use a pulsatile lavage system to irrigate the wound with the routine antibiotic irrigation. The physician removes any debris, bone fragments, and/or fracture hematoma particles before the reduction of bone ends and again before closure.

Physician Orders and Diagnostic Studies

In addition to the routine tests listed in **Table 28.8**, the physician may order neurovascular checks every 2 hours, IV fluids, elevation and immobilization of the

Table 28.12	Equipment, Supplies, and Instruments for Open Reduction and Internal Fixation of the Ulna	
Equipment	**Supplies**	**Instruments**
Electrosurgery generator Nitrogen power source X-ray machine and cassettes	2 2-0 Vicryl sutures 3000-mL bags of normal saline 4-inch roll of casting material Arm sling Electrosurgery supplies Pulsatile lavage system X-ray cassette cover or image intensifier cover Skin antiseptic agent and prepping supplies (according to the surgeon's preference)	*The following are used in addition to instruments for a Silastic wrist joint implant (Table 28.13)* ½-inch osteotome 2 four-prong rakes (sharp) 2 medium Weitlaner retractors 6 Kelly clamps Appropriate drills, and taps for use with the fixation device Assorted bone clamps (Lowman, Lambotte) Bone cutter (double action) Cobb periosteal elevator Fixation device (eg, compression plates and screws) Plate benders Power drill

extremity, application of ice packs as needed, analgesics taken as needed, venous thromboembolism (VTE) prophylaxis, and consults for physical therapy and occupational therapy. AP and lateral radiographs of both bones of the forearm, including the wrist and elbow joints, are also ordered.

VTE
Venous Thromboembolism

Procedure

Incision and Exposure

Place the patient supine on the bed with the operative extremity on an armboard. Exsanguination of the limb is achieved either by elevation or by application of an Esmarch bandage.

The forearm is fully pronated to expose the subcutaneous border of the ulna. A linear, longitudinal incision with a No. 15 blade is made over the fracture site. The length of the incision depends on the amount of bone that is to be exposed. Deep fascia is incised along the same line as the skin incision distally. Exposure is achieved with the use of Army-Navy retractors. Dissection is carried down to the subcutaneous border of the ulna. The periosteum is incised longitudinally over the ulna with a Cobb periosteal elevator, and the incision is continued around the bone to reveal the flexor and extensor aspects.

The ulnar nerve and the ulnar artery are preserved if the flexor carpi ulnaris is stripped from the ulna subperiosteally. If the dissection strays into the substance of the muscle, the nerve may be damaged.

Table 28.13	Equipment, Supplies, and Instruments for Silastic Wrist Implant Joint		
Equipment	**Supplies**	**Instruments**	
Nitrogen power source	1500 mL normal saline	¼-inch osteotome (hand)	
Power micro drill	2 3-0 silk sutures on a cutting needle	½-inch osteotome (hand)	
Pulsatile lavage		2 Army-Navy retractors	
Silastic trial sizers and implants	2 3-0 Vicryl sutures on a cutting needle	2 bunion retractors	
Small microsagittal saw and blade	Skin antiseptic agent and prepping supplies (according to the surgeon's preference)	2 ribbon retractors	
		Bone curets (assorted)	
Tourniquet and cuff	4 × 4-inch dressing sponges	Key periosteal elevator	
Hand table	4 × 8-inch radiopaque sponges	Mallet	
Electrosurgery generator		Senn retractors	
Basin set	4-0 nylon suture on a cutting needle		
	4-inch Esmarch bandage		
	Prep tray		
	4-inch Webril bandage		
	6 No. 15 blades		
	Bipolar electrosurgery cord and forceps		
	Drape packs		
	Impervious hinged sheet		
	Impervious stockinet		
	Irrigating syringe		
	Kling bandage		
	Medium pineapple burr		
	Skin marker		
	Suction tubing		

The fracture site is irrigated with an antibiotic solution, and both ends are carefully cleaned with a small curette.

Details

Apposition and alignment of the fracture must be perfect if normal function is to be restored. The reduction is achieved and maintained with the aid of a Lowman or a Lambotte bone clamp. A plate is chosen and contoured with the plate benders. The length of the plate should ensure that a minimum hold of six good cortices is possible on either side of the fracture line. One side of the plate is drilled through the hole nearest the fracture site. It is drilled in a neutral position through both cortices. A drill guide for the plate is used to ensure accurate direction of the drill bit. The hole is measured to the opposite cortex with a depth gauge. While the scrub person is retrieving the appropriate screw, if not using self-tapping screws, the hole is tapped to accept the screw. The screw is then inserted.

For the first hole on the opposite side of the fracture line, the load guide is used. This offsets the drill hole to move the bone by 1 mm in a compressive action. The arrow on the drill guide must be pointing toward the fracture site. The same procedure follows as just described. When the desired compression is achieved, the neutral guide is used in the remaining holes. Any bone loss at the fracture site should be filled with autogenous cancellous bone graft to strengthen the fixation. The wound is again copiously irrigated with an antibiotic solution.

Closure

The physician closes the fascia with an interrupted 2-0 Vicryl suture on a cutting needle and the skin closure with an interrupted 4-0 nylon suture. After applying sterile gauze dressings and then a 4-inch (10 cm) Webril bandage, a posterior plaster splint is applied.

Figure 28.23 shows an example of an ulnar fracture with fixation.

Postprocedure Care

Radiographs are taken in the postanesthesia care unit. Allow the patient out of bed as tolerated. Diet is also as tolerated. If the patient had general anesthesia, incentive spirometry is done every 2 hours during waking hours. Antibiotic coverage is prescribed for 24 hours with administration of analgesics as needed. VTE prophylaxis is continued. Occupational therapy is consulted. Blood studies include a CBC with differential count and a blood chemistry panel-7 test on the morning after the procedure and in 2 days. Sutures are removed in 2 weeks. A cast is applied with the elbow at 90 degrees in 2 weeks and left on for 10 weeks.

Potential Complications

Complications may include infection, neurovascular compromise due to pressure on nerves and vessels or the pressure of a splint or cast, and decreased mobility from the immobility imposed by a splint or cast.

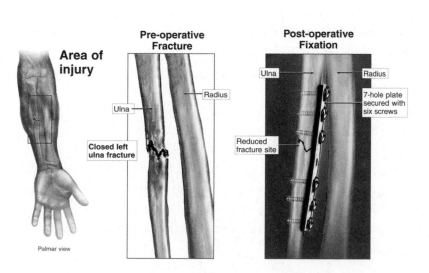

Figure 28.23

Ulnar fracture with fixation.

Source: Nucleus Medical Art.

PROSTHETIC REPLACEMENT OF THE FRACTURED HUMERAL HEAD

Fractures of the proximal humerus are common, especially in the elderly. In fact, they are the most common humeral fracture. The reason for the increase in incidence in the elderly is osteoporosis. The most common mechanism of proximal humeral fractures is a fall on outstretched hands. Severe trauma docs not necessarily play a significant role; the distance may be from standing height or less. In younger individuals, the resulting fracture is often more serious and severe trauma may be the cause. The position of the arm and hand during the initial injury is a major factor. Excessive rotations of the arm in the abducted position or a direct blow to the side of the shoulder are also mechanisms of injury. Metastatic disease may significantly weaken the bone; and with minimal activity or trauma, a pathological fracture can occur.

In any arthroplastic procedure, the objectives are to relieve pain, to improve mobility, to maintain stability, and to improve function. Some proximal fractures may be treated conservatively; some displaced fractures or fracture dislocations may necessitate more invasive therapy. Malunion and nonunion of fractures may shatter the balance of forces across the shoulder girdle and thus lead to an impingement.

An understanding of the classification system for fractures of the proximal humerus is necessary to initiate proper management. The Near classification, which is commonly used, identifies the four major fragments of the proximal humerus and their relationship to each other (**Fig. 28.24**).

Indications

Humeral head prosthesis may be indicated for a fracture of the anatomical neck if internal fixation is not feasible. For other selected cases of osteoporotic three-part fractures, head-splitting fractures, and four-part fracture-dislocations, prosthesis is generally indicated.

Related Procedures

Numerous techniques and devices have been proposed to treat proximal humeral fractures. The choice depends on several factors: the type of fracture, the quality of the bone and soft tissue, and the age and reliability of the patient. Alternative methods of fixation include intramedullary nails, plates and screws, staples, wire, and suture material.

Nursing Implications
Anesthesia

Many patients scheduled for shoulder procedures have numerous medical conditions. Rheumatoid arthritis frequently damages other joints; these patients need support and protection during anesthesia to avoid pain or further damage. General or regional anesthesia is considered. A number of regional anesthetic techniques may be used for shoulder procedures.

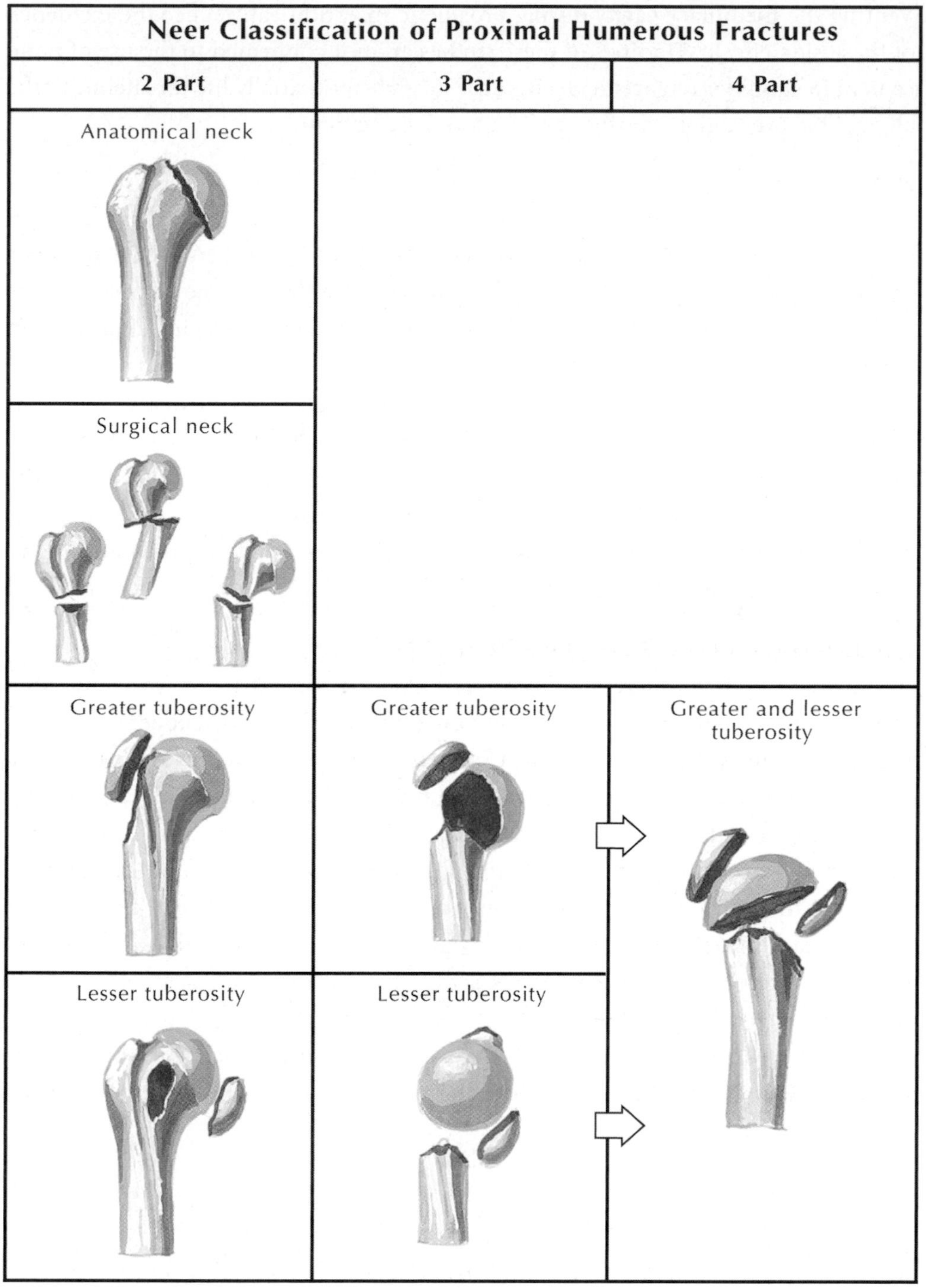

Neer Classification of Proximal Humerous Fractures		
2 Part	**3 Part**	**4 Part**
Anatomical neck		
Surgical neck		
Greater tuberosity	Greater tuberosity	Greater and lesser tuberosity
Lesser tuberosity	Lesser tuberosity	

Figure 28.24

Neer Classification of the Proximal Humerus Fractures.

Source: Netter Images.

Shoulder replacement is facilitated by the use of polymethyl methacrylate cement. A number of problems have been reported immediately after the insertion of the cement including hypotension and cardiac arrest. It is thought that the liquid monomer produces a reduction in peripheral vascular resistance, which causes the cardiopulmonary changes.

Fat and bone marrow emboli to the lungs may result from high intermedullary pressures. Oxygen desaturation has also been documented after cement application.

Venting the medullary cavity during prosthetic insertion can reduce the incidence of these side effects. Findings of these studies are not confirmed to the use of bone cement in shoulder replacements. Because it can be potentially life threatening, take all possible precautions during application of the cement.

Position

Place the patient supine, in a beach chair position (**Fig. 28.25**). Align the lateral aspect of the head with the lateral aspect of the bed. Raise the affected shoulder forward by placing a padded sandbag beneath the scapula. Flex the table 45 degrees at the waist and 30 degrees at the knees. Secure the patient by placing a safety strap across the patient's knees to prevent sliding. Place the patient's head in a padded doughnut-shaped headrest. Use additional straps across the patient's head and chest to ensure that the patient remains safely immobilized. Prevent pressure on the patient's face/eyes and malalignment of the cervical spine. Place a pillow under the patient's knees to reduce back strain during the procedure. Protect the nonoperative arm by securing it at the patient's side. Use adequate foam padding and folded hand towels to prevent skin-to-skin contact.

Establishing and Maintaining the Sterile Field

If preferred by the surgeon, remove hair from the operative site in the holding room before patient arrives in operating room. Do not shave; use clippers. The areas included are the upper arm from the elbow to the midsternum, including the axilla and the midback. With the patient's arm suspended in a finger-trap positioning device, prep the affected extremity from the wrist to the superior aspect of the shoulder area and to the base of the neck. Include the posterior portion of the shoulder, including the lateral aspect of the scapula, and the anterior and lateral chest wall to the nipple line. Prep the axilla last due to higher bacterial counts in that area. Prevent pooling of prep solution beneath the patient. Use a plastic adherent drape to protect the patient's face and hairline.

The scrub person or assistant holds the arm with a sterile towel while the circulating nurse removes the finger traps. Next, the physician or assistant places impervious

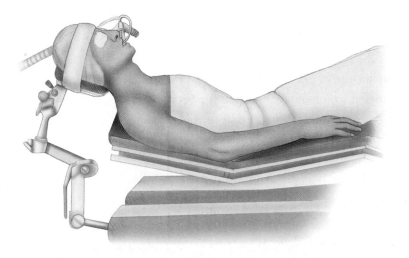

Figure 28.25

Beach chair position.

stockinet over the hand and telescopes it to above the elbow. The sterile area is squared off with sterile towels held in place with towel clips. A drape sheet is placed under the operative extremity and unfolded over the patient's torso and lower body. A second drape sheet is taken cephalad and fastened to create a barrier between the anesthesia provider and the operative team. A hinged impervious sheet is placed beneath the operative arm and secured around the area of the skin preparation. An additional layer of drapes is placed as described above and fastened with towel clips. The skin is covered with an adhesive drape, with careful attention to the axilla. The stockinet may be secured with a Kling or Coban bandage.

The bed is positioned as for procedures performed on the upper extremity. The Mayo stand is positioned across the patient's feet and the instrument table beside the scrub person. An additional sterile, padded Mayo stand may be positioned under the operative extremity for added support.

Equipment, Supplies, and Instruments

Table 28.14 lists the equipment, supplies, and instruments used for a prosthetic replacement of the fractured humeral head.

Physiological Monitoring

In addition to the measures in the discussion of anesthesia, carefully calculate blood loss throughout the procedure. View sponges for blood amount and measure contents of suction devices. The physician will document the estimated blood loss in the postprocedural note.

Specimens and Cultures

Send the humeral head to the pathology department for a definitive diagnosis.

Drugs and Solutions

The physician may order antibiotic irrigation. Follow healthcare facility guidelines for dosages and preparation protocols.

Physician Orders and Diagnostic Studies

In addition to the routine tests listed in **Table 28.8**, the physician may order a coagulation profile, occupational and physical therapy consults, immobilization of the extremity, VTE prophylaxis, analgesics as needed, bed rest, and vital signs every 4 hours. Shoulder radiographs, to include AP, axillary lateral, and Grashey[1] views are usually ordered.

Procedure

Incision and Exposure

Beginning over the distal clavicle, an anterior skin incision is made with a No. 10 blade approximately 1.5 cm medial to the acromioclavicular joint. The incision is extended distally and slightly laterally to the coracoid process, ending 1.5 cm medial to the deltoid insertion. The skin edges are freed from the underlying deep fascia and held apart by small rake retractors.

The deep fascia is incised with a No. 15 blade in line with the skin incision, and the cut edges are retracted to identify the deltopectoral groove. The pectoralis major and deltoid muscles are separated with small Metzenbaum scissors.

Table 28.14	Equipment, Supplies, and Instruments for Prosthetic Replacement of the Fractured Humeral Head		

Equipment	Supplies	Instruments
Basin set	1500 mL normal saline	2 Crile forceps
Electrosurgery generator	2 cement mixing bowels	2 dull Hohmann retractors
Pulsatile lavage	2 impervious May stand covers	2 medium Weitlaner retractors
	2 packages of small laparotomy sponges	Bone hook
	3 1-0 Vicryl suture	Cement gun
	3 2-0 Vicryl suture	Cement restrictor and inserter
	4 × 4-inch dressing sponges	Cobb periosteal elevator
	4 × 4-inch radiopaque sponges	Fukuda retractor
	4-0 Vicryl suture	Large double-action rongeur
	500 mL normal saline	Pulsatile lavage tips
	6 No. 10 blades	Required in addition to equipment for Silastic wrist implant are trial prosthesis and reamers
	Adhesive drape	Right-angle tip for cement gun
	Arm sling	Suction drain
	Drape packs	
	Electrosurgery supplies	
	Impervious hinged sheet	
	Impervious stockinet	
	Irrigating syringe	
	Kling bandage	
	Skin antiseptic agent and prepping supplies (according to the surgeon's preference)	
	Prep tray	
	Skin marker	

The cephalic vein is identified and retracted medially along with the pectoralis major muscle. The medial portion of the deltoid muscle is separated from the clavicle over a distance of 2–3 cm. This is performed by Metzenbaum scissors after the muscle has been separated from the underlying tissues. A small rim of muscle should be left attached to the bone to aid reconstruction at the end of the operation.

The pectoralis major and the deltoid are separated widely with a blunt Weitlaner retractor to reveal the coracoid process and coracobrachialis and biceps muscles. The coracoid process is stripped of soft tissue with a Cobb elevator, and the distal portion is separated with a ¼-inch straight osteotome. The fascia surrounding the biceps muscle is divided with Metzenbaum scissors. The muscle origin is marked distally to the coracoid and the muscles reflected distally with the attached fragment. Caution is taken to protect the musculocutaneous nerves, which enter the deep surface of the conjoined muscles.

The inferior and superior borders of the subscapularis muscle are defined by the stretch of the muscle on lateral rotation of the humerus. The borders are freed from the surrounding tissue with Metzenbaum scissors, and the lateral tendinous portion is divided. A small right-angled retractor is placed over the tendon. All branches of the cephalic vein are cauterized from the deltoid muscle. The subscapularis muscle belly is retracted with holding sutures of No. 1 Vicryl suture inserted proximally. The subscapularis is divided proximal to its insertion into the humerus. Another retraction stitch may be placed to retract the distal portion of the muscle laterally.

The anterior aspect of the shoulder capsule is exposed and incised vertically with a No. 15 blade. Retraction of the flaps of the capsule with small Kelly-Richardson retractors exposes the head of the humerus and the anterior rim of the glenoid fossa.

Details

The Kelly-Richardson retractors are removed, and a Cobb elevator is placed in the shoulder joint. The humerus is extended and placed in external rotation. The shoulder joint is dislocated, and the humeral head is slid anteriorly. The humeral head is cleared of all osteophytes for better visualization of the shoulder joint. With the elbow flexed at 90 degrees, the forearm is aimed at the operating physician's midline and the humerus is externally rotated 30 to 35 degrees.

With a ½ inch straight osteotome, the physician marks the osteotomy cut downward and medially from the superolateral point of the humeral head. The cut is continued distally and medially 45 degrees to the axis of the humerus with a microsagittal saw. The head is removed with an osteotome and a large towel clip if necessary. All remaining osteophytes around the circumference of the proximal humerus are trimmed.

The humeral reamer is placed 0.5 cm posterior to the bicipital groove and 1 cm medial to the lateral edge of the cut osteotomy surface. The appropriate trial humeral component is seated until the base of the prosthesis touches the osteotomized humeral surface. The rotation of the trial component can be adjusted, and trial reduction is performed.

The trial component is removed, and the intramedullary canal is irrigated with a pulsatile lavage of antibiotic irrigation. An intramedullary cement restrictor is inserted and the canal is thoroughly dried. The humerus is levered slightly laterally with a Cobb elevator and exposure of the proximal humerus achieved with Kelly-Richardson retractors. Polymethyl methacrylate is injected into the humeral canal with a cement gun, and the humeral component of the correct size is impacted into position. Excess cement is removed with a Cobb elevator or curette from around the prosthesis. When the cement has set, any apparent or potentially loosened fragments of cement are removed. The wound is irrigated again, and the humeral component is reduced to the glenoid.

Closure

The physician or assistant closes the horizontal and vertical limbs of the subscapularis incision with an interrupted No. 1 Vicryl suture on a cutting needle. After placing a suction drain in the distal aspect of the subdeltoid space, the deltopectoral interval and subcutaneous tissues are closed with an interrupted 2-0 Vicryl suture on a cutting needle. The skin is closed with a subcuticular 4-0 Vicryl suture. A dry, sterile gauze dressing is applied to the incision followed by a shoulder immobilizer.

Figure 28.26 shows an example of left humerus fracture and prosthetic replacement.

Postprocedure Care

The patient does coughing and deep breathing exercises every 2 hours while awake. Antibiotic coverage is provided. During the first 72 hours, ice packs are applied, 20 minutes on and 20 minutes off. Analgesics are administered as needed. Blood studies include a CBC, prothrombin time, and partial thromboplastin time the morning after surgery and in 5 days. Radiographs are taken in the recovery room. Neurovascular checks are done every 2 hours for 24 hours. The patient is allowed out of bed as tolerated. Diet is as tolerated. VTE prophylaxis is continued. A shoulder immobilizer is used for 1 week, then at night for 4 weeks. Active exercises of the hand are instituted in 24 hours, with passive motion of the shoulder and pendulum exercises in 36 hours. Isometric exercises are done in 1week. The patient is discharged in 2–3 days.

Potential Complications

Infection may occur. Because of operative technique or improper bone stock loosening may occur. Improper component size, overcorrection of muscular reconstruction, or instability of the shoulder joint may result in some loss of motion or strength.

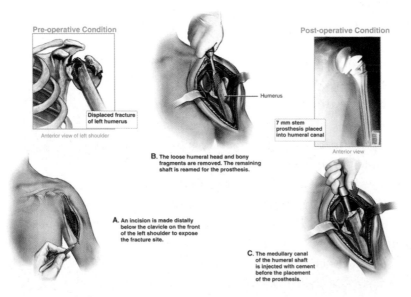

Figure 28.26

Left humerus fracture and prosthetic replacement.

Source: Nucleus Medical Art.

OPEN REDUCTION AND INTERNAL FIXATION OF THE HIP

Fracture of the hip refers to a fracture of the proximal one third of the femur that extends up to 5 cm below the lesser trochanter. Most commonly, the fracture occurs through the neck or the intertrochanteric region of the femur, but it is also seen in the subtrochanteric region. Hip fractures are classified as either intracapsular or extracapsular. Intracapsular fractures occur within the hip joint capsule and are capital (fractures of the femoral head), subcapital (fractures just below the head of the femur), and transcervical (fractures of the neck of the femur). Extracapsular fractures are outside the joint capsule through the femur's greater or lesser trochanter, in the intertrochanteric area, or in the subtrochanteric location.

Indications

Treatment of hip fracture consists of realigning the fragments by either closed or open methods, followed by the operative insertion of an internal fixation device.

Related Procedures

The choice of procedure in the treatment of a hip fracture depends primarily on the type of fracture and secondarily on the patient's general physical condition, and the length of the time since the fracture was sustained. Ultimately the decision is based on the surgeon's preference and judgment. The following is a list of possible operative interventions for the various intracapsular and extracapsular fractures.

- *Capital and subcapital*: The principles of treatment for capital and subcapital fractures are prosthetic head replacement for severely comminuted fractures or those that are severely displaced for a prolonged period. Closed reduction and pinning are appropriate for fractures relatively nondisplaced or impacted and can be reduced adequately.
- *Transcervical*: This type of fracture is treated the same as for capital and subcapital.
- *Intertrochanteric*: Intertrochanteric fractures heal readily in traction (8–12) weeks). However, this prolonged bed rest increases the patient's risk of complications. Thus, the preferred method of treatment is open reduction and internal fixation with a sliding screw and slide plate.

Nursing Implications

Anesthesia

The operation is performed most frequently under general anesthesia because the patient's position on the fracture table for a prolonged period can be uncomfortable. However, some anesthesia providers use epidural or spinal anesthesia for patients with compromised pulmonary or cardiac function. If the fracture is produced by severe trauma, there may be extensive bleeding into the soft tissue. Because of the relative abundance of the blood supply in the cancellous segment of the femur, an intertrochanteric fracture is a severe injury. Due to the high incidence of complications including blood loss, shock, fat embolism, pulmonary embolism, and pneumonia, vital signs, oxygen saturation, ECGs, pulmonary status, and urine output are carefully monitored during and after the procedure.

Position

Position the patient on the fracture table as previously described. The affected limb is held in slight medial rotation so that the patella is directed about 15 degrees inward. The unaffected limb is abducted almost fully and locked in this position by clamping the appropriate swivel surface of the table. The injured limb is abducted about 30 degrees and locked in this position. Pad and tape the arm on the operative side across the patient's chest to allow easy movement of the x-ray machine and C-arm.

Move the mobile x-ray image intensifier into position between the abducted lower extremities. Place the tube close up against the inner side of the sound knee and direct it horizontally toward the neck of the femur on the injured side.

Establishing and Maintaining the Sterile Field

Position the operative lights to ensure adequate lighting on the operative limb. Position the fracture table in the room so the operative team and equipment can be located on the operative side.

Prep the area from above the iliac crest to the knee as described earlier. The leg need not be prepped circumferentially but as medially and posteriorly as possible.

Apply the clear plastic Steri-Drape by removing the paper backing from the adhesive portion. Next, center the adhesive portion over the incisional area and apply. While fan folding, open the drape, and fold the upper portion over the shower curtain pole that is attached to the fracture table by C-clamps.

Equipment, Supplies, and Instruments

Table 28.15 lists the equipment, supplies, and instruments required for open reduction and internal fixation of a hip.

Physiological Monitoring

See the discussion of anesthesia.

Specimens and Cultures

A bone sample may be sent to the pathology laboratory, if there is suspicion of a pathological fracture without any evidence of traumatic injury.

Drugs and Solutions

The routine antibiotic irrigation is used.

Physician Orders and Diagnostic Studies

In addition to routine tests listed in **Table 28.8**, the physician orders vital signs every 4 hours, physical therapy, and occupational therapy consultation, administration of analgesics as needed, prophylactic antibiotics, and Foley catheter connected to gravity drainage, VTE prophylaxis, typing and crossmatching of blood, and AP and lateral hip radiographs.

Table 28.15	Equipment, Supplies, and Instruments for Open Reduction and Internal Fixation of Hip	
Equipment	**Supplies**	**Instruments**
Basin set	100 mL normal saline	2 Adson forceps
Electrosurgery generator	3 2-0 Vicryl sutures	2 Beckman retractors
Nitrogen power source	3 No. 1 Vicryl sutures	2 Bennett retractors
	3 No. 10 blades	2 Cobb periosteal elevators
	3 packages of large laparotomy sponges	2 Ferris Smith forceps
	4 × 4-inch dressing sponges	2 Lowman bone clamps
	Clear plastic drape	2 sponge sticks
	Electrosurgery supplies	2 Weitlaner retractors
	Irrigating syringe	3 needle holders
	Marking pen	4 Kocher clamps
	Medium Hemovac	6 curved hemostats
	Needle counter	6 Kelly clamps
	Skin antiseptic agent and prepping supplies (according to the surgeon's preference)	Appropriate hip compression system, drill bits, and implants
	Skin staples	Assorted curettes
	Suction tubing	Bandage scissors
		Bone hook
		Double-action bone cutter
		Mallet
		Mayo scissors
		No. 10 knife handle
		Power drill
		Small and large rongeurs
		Suture scissors
		Yankauer suction tip

Procedure

Incision and Exposure

The incision is made on the lateral aspect of the hip, extending from the greater trochanter distally, with a No. 10 blade. The length of the incision depends on the length of the implant. Weitlaner retractors are placed under the subcutaneous fat. The fascia lata is split in the direction of the incision distally with Mayo scissors. Proximally, the slit is extended upward into the tensor fascia lata muscle, again with Mayo scissors. Beckman retractors can now replace the Weitlaner retractors. The deeper muscle layer, the vastus lateralis, is retracted anteriorly with a Bennett retractor. Any remaining muscle fibers overlying the lateral aspect of the femur are divided by a vertical cut straight onto the bone with Mayo scissors. The periosteum is stripped over a length of 7–10 cm from the base of the greater trochanter downward with a Cobb elevator.

Details (*Intertrochanteric Fractures*)

With traction applied to the operative extremity, a guide pin is inserted under image intensification using a power drill. The level of insertion varies with the angle of the plate used. The lesser trochanter helps to verify the point of entry. The guide pin enters just opposite the tip of the lesser trochanter for a 135-degree angle plate and 2 cm lower for a 150-degree angle plate. The guide wire position is checked using AP and lateral views. Ideal pin position is slightly inferior to the center of the femoral head on the view and slightly posterior on the lateral view. The depth of the guide pin should be within a distance of 1 cm of the articular surface of the femoral head. This length should be confirmed with a direct measuring gauge. An additional stabilization pin may be inserted at the time, if necessary, parallel to the guide pin. The length of the guide pin is measured, and the reamer is prepared accordingly. The lag screw is determined by the direct measuring gauge. This measurement permits 5 mm of compression.

The reamer is then adjusted and slid over the guide wire and driven on through the femoral neck into the head. Penetration of the reamer should be checked radiographically. The appropriate plate and lag screw are assembled into the insertion wrench. The entire assembly is then placed over the guide wire and introduced into the channel. The lag screw is driven past the fracture site and its depth is checked periodically radiographically and with a depth gauge in both planes. The insertion wrench is removed, and the plate is impacted over the lag screw. The plate is attached to the femur with a Lowman bone clamp, and the guide wire is removed. Some traction can be released, and manual impaction of the fracture fragments can be performed if necessary. The screws of the side plate are inserted by means of the same technique discussed for open reduction and internal fixation of the fractured ulna. The compression screw is engaged into the end of the lag screw and tightened judiciously. It is important not to overtighten the screw, lest the threads of the lag screw pull through the bone.

Closure

Closure of the vastus lateralis muscle and the fascia lata is done in layers with No. 1 Vicryl suture on a cutting needle. A wound suction device is placed between these layers. Subcutaneous fat is closed with 2-0 Vicryl suture on a cutting needle. Skin is approximated with staples. A dry, sterile gauze dressing is applied to the incision.

Figure 28.27 shows an example of an open reduction and internal fixation of a left hip fracture.

Postprocedure Care

Check vital signs every 4 hours, and neurovascular status every 2 hours. Administer analgesics as needed. Continue antibiotics and VTE prophylaxis. Allow the patient out of bed, as tolerated, the next day. Radiographs are taken in the recovery room and on the morning after the procedure. Hematology and chemistry studies are completed after the procedure and the next morning. Incentive spirometry is done every 2 hours. Depending if the patient goes to rehab, discharge occurs in 5–14 days, with a cane or walker.

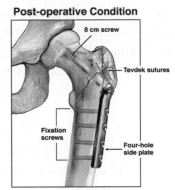

Figure 28.27

Open reduction and internal fixation of left hip fracture.

Source: Nucleus Medical Art.

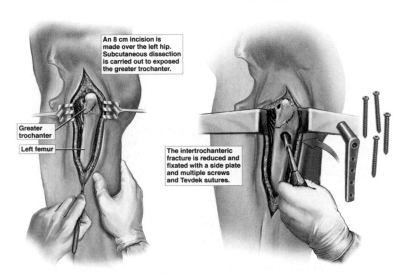

Potential Complications

Complications include fat embolism, breakage of fixation device due to additional injury or poor bone quality, and pin penetration into the acetabulum due to improper technique or poor bone. Infection may also occur.

OPEN REDUCTION AND INTERNAL FIXATION OF THE FEMUR WITH AN INTRAMEDULLARY ROD

The femur is the largest bone in the body. The fractures seen in this location are due to high-velocity and high-energy accidents. Consequently, these fractures frequently are associated with other fractures and/or other internal injuries.

Indications

The femur heals slowly. If a patient were treated with traction alone, it would take as long as 4–6 months for healing. Therefore, methods of treatment have been devised in an attempt to gain earlier ambulation during the healing period.

Classification of the degree of comminution of the fracture and its location is most important. Femoral fractures can be classified as open or closed. Those that are open need immediate operative debridement, stabilization, and secondary closure. The fracture can also be classified as simple, comminuted, or segmental. The anatomical locations of femoral shaft fractures are divided into subtrochanteric, midshaft, and distal shaft. Each area lends itself to specific types of treatment.

Open intramedullary nailing of the femur involves inserting a nail after reduction and operative exposure of the fracture. Intramedullary fixation is the treatment of choice for closed uncomminuted and severely comminuted fractures through the midshaft. Subtrochanteric fractures can also be treated with interlocking intramedullary fixation devices.

Related Procedures

Closed intramedullary nailing is a method used to nail shaft fractures without exposing the fracture site. The fracture site may be manipulated to enable the nail to cross the fracture, but the fracture site is not seen.

Nursing Implications
Anesthesia

The same principles apply as for open reduction and internal fixation of the hip.

Position

Place the patient on the fracture table in the supine or in the lateral decubitus position. The foot of the affected extremity is placed in the traction boot with 15 degrees of internal rotation. The fractured side is placed in 15 to 30 degrees of hip flexion with the unaffected side in neutral position.

Establishing and Maintaining the Sterile Field

Routine orthopedic preparation is completed.

Sterile drapes are placed distally and proximally to the prepped area. A large adhesive povidone-iodine drape is placed over the prepared area covering the thigh circumferentially.

Equipment, Supplies, and Instruments

Table 28.16 lists the equipment, supplies, and instruments used an open reduction and internal fixation of the femur with an intramedullary rod.

Physiological Monitoring

The same principles apply as for open reduction and internal fixation of the hip.

Specimens and Cultures

See the discussion of open reduction and internal fixation of the hip.

Drugs and Solutions

The routine antibiotic irrigation is used.

Physician Orders and Diagnostic Studies

Table 28.8 lists routine orders. Other orders include NPO for 4 hours prior to the surgery if not trauma or emergent, bed rest with immobilization, physical therapy and occupational therapy consultation, VTE prophylaxis, typing and crossmatching of 4 units of blood, administration of analgesics as needed, AP and lateral radiographs, vital signs every 4 hours, neurovascular checks every 2 hours, and antibiotic coverage. See the discussion for open reduction and internal fixation of the hip.

Table 28.16	Equipment, Supplies, and Instruments for Open Reduction and Internal Fixation of the Femur with an Intramedullary Rod	
Equipment	**Supplies**	**Instruments**
Basin set	1000 mL normal saline	Appropriate intramedullary fixture devices and instruments: reamers, drills, drill guides, impactors, guide wires
Electrosurgery generator	15 large laparotomy sponges	Assorted osteotomes
	4 2-0 Vicryl sutures	Curved awl
	4 No. 10 blades	Flexible intramedullary reamers
	4 No. 2 Vicryl sutures	Heavy pliers
	4 × 4-inch dressing sponges	Tissue protector
	5 small laparotomy sponges	
	50–mL syringe	
	Adhesive loban drape	
	Electrosurgery supplies	
	Irrigating syringe	
	Marking pen	
	Medium Hemovac	
	Needle counter	
	Skin antiseptic agent and prepping supplies (according to the surgeon's preference)	
	Suction	
	Table drapes	

Procedure

Incision and Exposure

With a No. 10 blade, a longitudinal incision is made on the posterolateral aspect of the thigh. The distal part of the incision is on the lateral femoral epicondyle and continues proximally along the posterior portion of the femoral shaft. The exact length of the incision depends on the degree of comminution of the fracture. Weitlaner retractors are positioned to retract the subcutaneous fat layer. The deep fascia is incised with a No. 10 blade in line with its fibers and the skin incision. The femoral and sciatic nerves are in the internerve plane between the vastus lateralis and the hamstring muscles. Caution is taken to identify and maintain these structures.

The vastus lateralis is followed posteriorly to the lateral intermuscular septum (which covers the hamstring muscle). The muscle is reflected anteriorly with a Beckman retractor, and dissection between muscle and septum is performed with Mayo scissors. Ligation or coagulation of the branches of the perforating arteries is accomplished to gain hemostasis. The dissection is continued until the femur is exposed. The periosteum is incised longitudinally and stripped off the muscles covering the femur with a Cobb periosteal elevator.

Details

After the fracture site is exposed, the bone ends are cleared so that reduction is accurate. The proximal fragment is reduced to the distal fragment with an internal fracture alignment device. When perfect reduction has been secured by manipulation and application of traction, the fracture is held together with a Lowman bone-holding forceps.

An oblique incision 2 cm distal to the proximal tip of the greater trochanter is made with a No. 10 blade and continued proximally and medially for 8–10 cm. Weitlaner retractors are positioned, and the fascia of the gluteus maximus is incised with a No. 10 blade in line with the skin incision. The gluteus maximus is divided in line with its fibers with Mayo scissors. Weitlaner retractors are removed and replaced with Beckman retractors for deeper exposure.

The trochanteric fossa is palpated, and a curved awl is introduced manually in line with the femoral shaft. This step is verified with AP and lateral radiographs. The entry portal can be further enlarged with the awl. A tapered T-handle reamer is inserted, and the metaphyseal canal is enlarged.

A ball-tipped guide wire is introduced to the level of the fracture. The ball tip is to facilitate retrieval of a reamer head should it break off. The position of the wire is checked with the intensifier because the wire may take a false course. A skin protector is placed over the proximal skin edges during reaming and insertion of the nail.

Flexible reamers of graded sizes are passed over the guide wire in order of increasing diameter. Reaming should begin with the smallest diameter, and only moderate pressure should be applied on the power tool. The process is repeated until the canal has been enlarged to the desired size. AP and lateral views are periodically checked during the reaming process. Manufacturer's recommendations to over ream ensures inserting a nail in an adequately reamed femoral canal. The proper nail size must be investigated. Inserting a nail too large can cause severe bone splitting and comminution. Systems vary as to nail diameter and stated size. Most manufacturers recommend reaming of 1 to 1.5 mm greater than the desired diameter for midshaft fractures. A flexible, cannulated exchange tube is passed over the ball-tipped guide wire to maintain reduction when the wire is removed. A nail guide wire is then inserted and the medullary tube removed.

The correct length of the nail is determined from the known length of the guide wire within the bone. A nail length gauge can determine the correct nail size. The nail should be allowed to penetrate to within 2–3 cm of the lower articular surface of the femur but not as far for fractures above midshaft. The type and size of the nail is also dependent on patient characteristics and fracture classification.

The scrub person attaches the appropriate nail on the nail insertion device. The nail is placed so that its curvature matches that of the femur: horizontally when the patient is in the lateral decubitus position. With the use of the correct handle to control rotation, the physician inserts the nail. The nail guide wire is removed after the nail has entered the distal fragment by several centimeters. Repeated observations with the image intensifier show if distraction is occurring and will allow preventive measures to be taken. The nail should be felt to drive on with each blow. With the length of the nail calculated correctly, when hammered into its optimal position the head of the nail should have disappeared within the bone just at the point of entry.

Stable fractures of the isthmus may be treated by means of the conventional unlocked method. Fractures proximal to the isthmus necessitate a proximal locking screw, whereas fractures that are more distal should be locked with one or two distal screws. All unstable fractures should be locked distally and proximally, thereby maintaining length and preventing rotation.

Closure

See the discussion of open reduction and internal fixation of the hip.

Figure 28.28 shows an example of an open reduction and internal fixation of the femur with an intramedullary rod.

Postprocedure Care

Obtain vital signs every 4 hours, with neurovascular checks every 2 hours. Administer analgesics as needed. Continue antibiotic coverage and VTE prophylaxis. Radiographs are taken in the recovery room and on the morning after the procedure. Diet is as tolerated. If the fracture site is stable, ambulation is done as soon as possible. Chemistry and hematology panels are done the morning after the procedure and for 2 days. Incentive spirometry is performed. Immediately following the procedure, the patient begins quadriceps setting and plantarflexion and dorsiflexion exercises. Discharge occurs in 4–10 days.

Potential Complications

Infection may occur. Nonunion can be caused by a nail that is too small, a fracture too proximal or distal in the shaft, or a nail that cannot completely fill the canal and control rotation. Fat embolism is always a potential complication when there is a fracture of a long bone and is especially associated with intramedullary nail insertion. Peroneal nerve injury may be due to externally applied pressure from splints or traction devices. Loss of fixation and migration of the nail are due to failure to accomplish fixation.

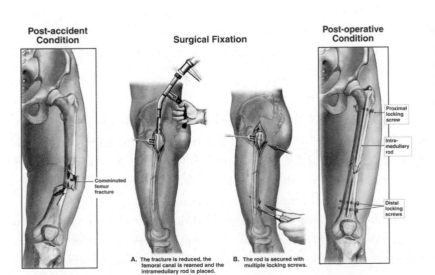

Post-accident Condition

Surgical Fixation

Post-operative Condition

Comminuted femur fracture

Proximal locking screw

Intra-medullary rod

Distal locking screws

A. The fracture is reduced, the femoral canal is reamed and the intramedullary rod is placed.

B. The rod is secured with multiple locking screws.

Figure 28.28

Open reduction and internal fixation of the femur with an intramedullary rod.

Source: Nucleus Medical Art.

TOTAL JOINT ARTHROPLASTY

Arthroplasty is the operative reformation of a joint, in which both joint surfaces are replaced with artificial materials.

Total Hip Arthroplasty

In a total hip arthroplasty, both of the articulating surfaces of the hip joint are replaced. The hip is replaced by an acetabular component made of high-density polyethylene and a femoral component made of metal. Implant placement may be with or without bone cement; however, the implant material must have a precise finish and placement.

Indications

The primary goals of a total hip arthroplasty are to relieve pain and to increase mobility and stability of the joint. The indications for total hip arthroplasty are severe primary rheumatoid arthritis, osteoarthritis, inactive inflammatory arthritis, ankylosing spondylitis, congenital dysplasia, traumatic arthritis, osteonecrosis, and failed femoral osteotomy.

Related Procedures

Three common types of hip arthroplasty are the hemiarthroplasty, the total hip arthroplasty, and the total hip surface replacement arthroplasty. In a cup arthroplasty, the acetabulum and the head of the femur are reamed down to an untraumatized surface and an appropriately sized metal cup is fitted over the head of the femur; this procedure has been replaced by the other two. The total hip surface replacement arthroplasty consists of reaming out the acetabulum and implanting an acetabular cup while the femoral head is only reamed down to accept a metal femoral cap.

Nursing Implications

ANESTHESIA

The procedure is performed under general or spinal anesthesia. Some orthopedic surgeons insist on transient hypotensive anesthesia during the procedure. The anesthesia provider may be willing to do this by pharmacological means.

Blood loss during the entire procedure must be well controlled, and, if possible, circulating blood volume should be maintained throughout the operation. The same anesthetic and nursing interventions apply as for the replacement of the proximal humerus during the cementing stage.

POSITION

The anesthetized patient is rolled onto his or her side with the operative hip up. The pelvic and lumbar area is firmly stabilized anteriorly and posteriorly with padded positioners attached to the bed. Care is taken not to restrict normal respiratory excursion. The anterior positioner should be tightened to allow the insertion of a hand between the positioner and the patient's abdomen.

The patient's arms are positioned on a well-padded double armboard and secured with straps or tape, or a lateral arm holder. A soft chest roll is positioned under the upper thorax. Safety measures as discussed earlier are followed for all pressure-point areas.

ESTABLISHING AND MAINTAINING THE STERILE FIELD

With the patient secured safely in the lateral position, the operative extremity is placed in a preparation holder and abducted. An unsterile hinged sheet is placed between the patient's legs and covering the perineum. The hinges are taken over the gluteal fold posteriorly and to the groin anteriorly. The surgical site is prepared from below the rib cage, including the buttocks posteriorly, to midcalf circumferentially. The gluteal fold and the groin are prepped last because they are considered wet prep areas containing more contamination.

With the patient in the lateral position and the affected extremity abducted in the leg holder, the limb is held by an assistant with a sterile towel while the circulating nurse removes the holder from the ankle.

A sterile drape sheet is placed over the foot of the bed while an impervious stockinet is telescoped over the foot to above the knee. The towels holding the extremity are then discarded. A sterile drape sheet is placed over the down extremity to the groin. A sterile impervious hinged sheet is placed directly over the previously placed hinged sheet. Another drape is placed over the hinged sheet and fastened with towel clips. A sterile drape sheet is placed over the patient's upper torso to the level of the waist (prepared area).

A second sheet follows in a similar fashion. Side sheets are placed and fastened beneath the affected extremity, in the groin area, and around the prepared area and clipped together at the top. Sterile adhesive drapes are taken around the thigh and knee circumferentially. A second adhesive drape is taken over the incision site and under the groin. Special attention is taken to seal the groin area carefully during the draping procedure. The stockinet may be fastened with a sterile Kling or Coban bandage.

EQUIPMENT, SUPPLIES, AND INSTRUMENTS

Table 28.17 lists the equipment, supplies, and instruments used for a total hip arthroplasty.

PHYSIOLOGICAL MONITORING

See the discussion of anesthesia.

SPECIMENS AND CULTURES

Routinely, a portion of the joint capsule and the femoral head are sent to the pathology department for definitive studies. Specimens might be sent to the rheumatology department for investigational purposes. Cultures are taken if indicated.

DRUGS AND SOLUTIONS

See the discussion of prosthetic replacement of the proximal humerus.

PHYSICIAN ORDERS AND DIAGNOSTIC STUDIES

Orders and studies include NPO status for 4 hours prior to surgery; activity as tolerated; diet as tolerated; AP and lateral radiographs (bilaterally); antibiotic prophylaxis; VTE prophylaxis; typing and crossmatching of 4 units of blood; transport to the operative and invasive procedure suite in a bed with an overhead frame and trapeze; EKG; chest radiograph; urinalysis; hematology profile; and physical

Table 28.17	Equipment, Supplies, and Instruments for Total Hip Arthroplast

Equipment	Supplies	Instruments
Electrical power source for saw (if applicable)	2 suction tubing	Charnley hip retractor
Electrosurgery generator	15 large laparotomy sponges	2 Beckman retractors
Nitrogen power source	15 small laparotomy sponges	2 Weitlaner retractors
Pulsatile lavage	Electrosurgery supplies	2 Ferris retractors
	Bulb syringe	2 Ferris Smith forceps
	6 No. 10 blades	2 Adson forceps
	60-mL syringe	2 No. 3 knife handles with teeth
	Suction drain	2 No. 3 long knife handles
	Skin marker	10 Kelly clamps
	4 No. 1 Vicryl sutures	10 curved hemostats
	4 2-0 Vicryl sutures	8 towel clips
	Alcohol	4 Allis clamps
	Cement gun cartridges	4 Mayo-Hegar needle holders
	Lavage irrigation tips	Yankauer suction tip
	Long-straight shower head	9-inch long smooth forceps
	Impervious stockinet	Suture scissors
	2 adhesive drapes	Canal finders
	Kling bandage	Mallet
	Impervious hinger sheet	Assorted curets
	3000 mL normal saline	Assorted straight and curved osteotomes
	Methyl methacrylate	Long double-action rongeur
	Cement mixing bowls	Long Metzenbaum scissors
	Skin staples	Assorted curved curets
	4 × 4-inch dressing sponges	Small double-action rongeur
	Skin antiseptic agent and prepping supplies (according to the surgeon's preference)	Cobb elevator
	Mayo stand cover	Impervious hinged sheet
	Disposable Yankauer suction tips	4 sponge sticks
		Bone hook
		Ligamentum teres knife
		Power saw: reciprocating or oscillating
		Saw blade
		Long Frazier suction tip
		Bandage scissors
		Acetabular positioner
		Femoral impactor
		Acetabular trials
		Femoral trials
		Femoral broaches
		Acetabular reamers
		Appropriate screws and drill bits
		Power neck elevator
		6-mm drill bit
		8-mm drill bit
		Box osteotome

therapy and occupational therapy consultation. Autologous blood may be donated by the patient 10–14 days prior to the procedure.

Procedure

INCISION AND EXPOSURE

The proximal, anterior, and posterior margins of the greater trochanter are identified by palpation. The skin incision is made with a No. 10 blade just below the most prominent part of the greater trochanter, toward the greater sciatic notch. Subcutaneous fat is incised with another No. 10 blade and retracted with Weitlaner retractors. The incision is extended posteriorly to expose the gluteus maximus fascia. The fascia lata, just below the most prominent portion, is incised with a No. 10 blade. Beckman retractors or Charnley retractor may now replace the Weitlaner retractors for optimum exposure. Hemostasis is maintained with electrosurgery.

The gluteus maximus muscle is bluntly divided with Mayo scissors along the line of its fibers. The bursal tissue over the greater trochanter is excised with the Mayo scissors. The posterior aspect of the hip is exposed, and the gluteus maximus tendon is released.

DETAILS

The thigh is internally rotated, and a Hohmann retractor is placed under the border of the gluteus medius and over the gluteus minimus. The Hohmann retractor is retracted anterosuperiorly, and the piriform and the insertions of the short external rotator muscles are identified. The external rotators are cut with the electrosurgery unit. The Hohmann retractor is repositioned at the lesser trochanter and the inferior aspect of the hip capsule. Internal rotation of the hip followed by the release of the piriform tendon at its femoral insertion improves exposure of the joint.

A No. 1 Vicryl suture is placed on the ends of the cut external rotators for later identification and reattachment. The detached rim of the external rotators is peeled off the hip capsule toward the posterior rim of the acetabulum.

A longitudinal incision is made in the superior hip capsule as far anteriorly as possible from the acetabular rim to the greater trochanter with a No. 10 blade on a long handle. The capsule along the rim of the acetabulum is further incised.

The hip is flexed and adducted with a bone hook placed around the femoral neck. The femoral head is lifted out of the acetabulum during longitudinal traction and internal hip rotation. If intact, the ligamentum teres is cut with a teres knife or a No. 10 blade. After dislocation, the tibia is placed in a vertical position with the foot pointed upward and the hip in flexion, adduction, and internal rotation. The femur is pushed posteriorly and upward by the first assistant.

The femoral neck elevator is placed under the neck to expose the area completely. The neck is resected 1.5–2 cm above the beginning of the lesser trochanter with a reciprocating or oscillating saw. The cut stops at the greater trochanter. Next, it is resected vertically to meet the horizontal cut. The femur is internally rotated and the neck is elevated with a bone hook. The capsulectomy is completed all around with a No. 10 blade on a long handle to provide an excellent view of the acetabulum. Soft tissue or osteophytes should be cleaned from the acetabular fovea.

28

A Hohmann retractor is placed under the remaining neck with the tip up over the anterior margin of the acetabulum into the pelvis. The acetabulum is reamed in a concentric manner with a power reamer starting with the smallest size. Manufacturer's recommendations vary with regard to final reamer size and specific components (cemented and noncemented).

The reamer should be directed medially, and overreaming should be avoided. Anchor holes are created in the acetabulum to enhance cement fixation. They are made with a long 6- or 8-mm drill bit and are undercut with a curved curette. When proper size and position of the cup have been established, the acetabulum is irrigated with a pulsatile antibiotic lavage. Reamed bone debris and blood are removed to open the interstices of cancellous bone. Bleeding should be controlled with electrosurgery.

The proper acetabular component (cemented or porous) is delivered to the sterile field by the circulating nurse. The appropriate positioner and impactor are readied, along with drill guides and drill bits for a noncemented component.

The polymethyl methacrylate is prepared as discussed earlier and injected into the acetabulum with a cement gun. The bone cement may be manually impacted, or an acetabular cement compressor may be used. When the cement can be handled, the selected acetabular component is pushed into the cement of the acetabulum. The excessive cement is trimmed with a curette from the rim of the acetabulum. When the position is satisfactory, the positioner is removed and replaced by an impactor until there is complete cure of the cement. The area is then again copiously irrigated to remove any loosened cement.

For a porous-coated acetabular component, the implant is inserted and impacted at the desired inclination. If screws are required, screw holes are drilled through the holes in the component to avoid penetration of the inner cortex of the pelvis or the sciatic notch. A drill guide is used when drilling, and the length is measured with the appropriate depth gauge. The selected screw is inserted and fully seated within the screw hole. The permanent polyethylene liner is then impacted into the acetabular shell.

The initial preparation of the femur is started with a hollow box chisel, starting in the middle of the longitudinal axis of the femoral neck, and directed parallel with the femoral neck. The canal is entered with a tapered reamer or a flexible reamer. The femoral canal is further prepared with a series of broaches, which correspond to the size of the final implant. In general, the smallest broach is used first and the size of the broach increased until cortical bone is reached. If the prosthesis has a collar, an oscillating saw is used to adjust the collar against the medial aspect of the femoral neck cortex. A trial femoral head and neck are then placed on the final broach and a trial reduction is performed.

When the surgeon is satisfied with the preparation, the trials are removed and the canal prepared in the same manner as the acetabulum. A cement restrictor is inserted into the femoral canal prior to insertion of the femoral component. The selected femoral prosthesis is delivered onto the field and cement preparation begins again. The bone cement is injected into the canal via a long nozzle on the cement gun, starting distally at the cement plug. The prosthesis is then inserted and impacted. Cement is trimmed from around the stem collar, and gentle pressure is maintained until the cement is completely hardened.

The selected femoral head implant is placed onto the femoral component and impacted. The hip is reduced and placed through a range-of-motion test. The wound is copiously irrigated with the pulsatile lavage. Any loose pieces of cement or potentially loose pieces are removed.

CLOSURE

The previously placed sutures are identified and reattached to the greater trochanter. A suction drain is placed in the hip joint. The fascia lata is closed with interrupted No. 1 Vicryl suture, and a second suction drain is placed. The gluteus maximus is also closed with an interrupted No. 1 Vicryl suture.

The subcutaneous fat is closed with interrupted 2-0 Vicryl sutures. Skin is approximated with skin staples. The incision is covered with dry, sterile gauze dressings. A hip abduction brace is applied immediately after the procedure.

Figure 28.29 shows an example of arthritis of the left hip with total hip replacement.

Postprocedure Care

The patient is placed at bed rest overnight with an abduction brace. He or she is allowed out of bed with physical therapy the morning after the procedure. Fifty percent weight bearing is prescribed for 6 weeks with crutches. Radiographs are taken in 6 weeks. Abductor strengthening exercises are taught. Vital signs are taken every 4 hours, with neurovascular checks every 2 hours. A radiograph is obtained in the recovery room and the morning after the procedure. An elevated toilet seat and hip chair are advised. Blood studies include a CBC, prothrombin time, and partial thromboplastin time the morning after the procedure and in 5 days. VTE prophylaxis is continued and analgesics administered as needed. Antibiotic coverage is prescribed. Urinalysis, culture, and sensitivity testing are done in 5 days. The patient is discharged in 3–5 days.

Potential Complications

Infection may occur. Hip dislocation is due to excessive flexion and internal rotation. Prosthesis loosening is due to infection, fracture, dislocation, and migration of implants. Thrombophlebitis is possibly due to preprocedure screening radionuclide scans.

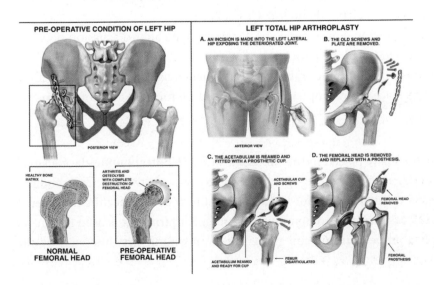

Figure 28.29

Arthritis of the left hip with total hip replacement.

Source: Nucleus Medical Art.

Total Knee Arthroplasty

In total knee arthroplasty (TKA), the distal femur is replaced with the metal component of the prosthesis; the plastic component is placed on the proximal tibia in order to produce a smooth articulating surface. In most cases, the undersurface of the patella is also replaced with a plastic component so that it articulates with the femoral surface.

Indications

The primary indication for TKA is to relieve pain, which is significant and disabling, caused by severe arthritis (Palmer & Cross, 2004). If dysfunction of the knee is causing significant reduction in the patient's quality of life, this should be taken into account. Correction of significant deformity is an important indication but is rarely used as the primary indication for surgery (Palmer & Cross, 2004).

Related Procedures

Several operative procedures should be considered in patients with degenerative disease of the knee (Palmer & Cross, 2004):

Arthroscopic debridement may be indicated in mild degenerative joint disease with mechanical symptoms and recurrent persistent effusions.

Proximal tibial valgus osteotomy should be considered only for patients with medial tibiofemoral compartment disease, stable collateral ligaments, and a correctable varus deformity of the knee joint.

A distal femoral varus osteotomy can be considered for patients with lateral tibiofemoral compartment disease, stable collateral ligaments, and a valgus deformity of the knee joint.

Nursing Implications
ANESTHESIA

Most patients who undergo TKA are elderly with comorbid diseases. Patients must have good cardiopulmonary function to withstand anesthesia, as well as a blood loss of 1000–1500 mL over the perioperative period. Routine preprocedure electrocardiography should be performed on elderly patients; in addition, patients with ischemic heart disease, congestive heart failure, and chronic obstructive airway disease should be seen by a medical specialist (Palmer & Cross, 2004).

The decision for regional or general anesthesia is made after discussion between the anesthesia provider and the patient; the decision is affected in part by the medical condition of the patient. Epidural anesthesia is beneficial because the indwelling catheter is left in place 48–72 hours after the procedure for pain control (Palmer & Cross, 2004).

POSITION

The patient is usually placed in the supine position (Hohler, 2008). Place a small blanket roll under the hip on the operative side to prevent the hip from abducting. The physician may prefer a foot-holder apparatus; if used, place the non-sterile device to the OR bed prior to prepping and draping. A tourniquet is used to control bleeding; apply a properly fitting cuff at the site of maximum circumference on the thigh of the operative limb; use soft, wrinkle-free, nonlinting padding underneath the tourniquet; ensure that the cuff is not twisted. Protect the patient's skin underneath the cuff by placing an adhesive drape around the distal circumference of the cuff (Hohler, 2008).

ESTABLISHING AND MAINTAINING THE STERILE FIELD

Prepare the operative limb using a broad-spectrum germicidal agent; begin the skin preparation at the knee and move up to the tourniquet; using another prep sponge, prep down to the ankle, unless otherwise specified by the physician (Hohler, 2008). After the patient's skin is prepped, the physician and scrub person place the sterile drapes. Drape the nonoperative leg first; drape the operative leg using a surgical glove or other drape to cover the foot and toes, then pass the foot through the aperture of an extremity sheet. Secure this sheet proximal to the ankle as well as the foot to prevent slipping. After the patient is draped, the physician may exsanguinate the operative limb by applying an elastic wrap prior to inflation of the tourniquet (Hohler, 2008).

EQUIPMENT, SUPPLIES, AND INSTRUMENTS

Table 28.18 lists the equipment, supplies, and instruments used for a total knee arthroplasty.

PHYSIOLOGICAL MONITORING

Monitor and document pressure points and tourniquet pressure and times. With the deflation of any tourniquet, blood loss is calculated on the basis of suction collection and viewing of sponges.

SPECIMENS AND CULTURES

Routinely, the excised portions of the femur and tibia are sent to the pathology department for definitive studies. Specimens might be sent to the rheumatology department for investigational purposes. Cultures are taken if indicated.

DRUGS AND SOLUTIONS

The physician may order antibiotic irrigation. Follow healthcare facility guidelines for dosages and preparation protocols. During closure, the physician may choose to prepare the femur, tibia, and sometimes the patella by applying platelet-rich plasma (PRP) to the bony surfaces and tissues to enhance the healing process (Hohler, 2008).

PRP
Platelet-Rich Plasma

PHYSICIAN ORDERS AND DIAGNOSTIC STUDIES

Preprocedure laboratory evaluation should include the following (Palmer & Cross, 2004):

- Complete blood count, sedimentation rate, prothrombin time, and activated partial thromboplastin time (PT/PTT)—routine preprocedure evaluation of coagulation studies is not necessary except in patients with a history of bleeding, alcoholism, or previous liver disease.
- Urinalysis to rule out occult urinary tract infection

Table 28.18	Equipment, Supplies, and Instruments for Total Knee Arthroplasty		

Equipment	Supplies	Instruments
Electrical power source for saw and drill	2 suction tubing	2 Richardson retractors
Electrosurgery generator	15 small laparotomy sponges	2 Hohmann retractors
Nitrogen power source	Electrosurgery supplies	2 Weitlaner retractors
Pulsatile lavage	Bulb syringe	2 Adson forceps
Pneumatic tourniquet	No. 10 knife blades	2 No. 3 knife handles with teeth
	60-mL syringe	8 Kocher clamps
	Suction drain	10 Kelly clamps
	Skin marker	10 curved hemostats
	4 No. 1 Vicryl sutures	8 towel clips
	4 2-0 Vicryl sutures	4 Allis clamps
	Alcohol	4 Mayo-Hegar needle holders
	Cement gun cartridges	Yankauer suction tip
	Lavage irrigation tips	Smooth forceps
	Straight shower head	Suture scissors
	Impervious stockinet	Canal finders
	2 adhesive drapes	Mallet
	Kling bandage	Assorted curets
	Impervious hinger sheet	Assorted straight and curved osteotomes
	3000 mL normal saline	Double-action rongeur
	Methyl methacrylate	Metzenbaum scissors
	Cement mixing bowls	Assorted curved curets
	Skin staples	Small double-action rongeur
	4 × 4-inch dressing sponges	Cobb elevator
	Skin antiseptic agent and prepping supplies (according to the surgeon's preference)	4 sponge sticks
	Mayo stand cover	Bone hook
	Tourniquet cuffs and appropriate padding supplies	Power osteotomy saw
		Saw blades
		Frazier suction tip
		Bandage scissors
		Depth gauge
		Appropriate screws and drill bits
		AP cutting alignment guide
		Distal cutting alignment guide
		Cutting block
		Spacer block
		Power drill
		Drill bits
		Burrs
		Box osteotome
		Trials and implants as ordered by the physician

- Radiographs for the assessment of the patient with knee arthritis:
  - Standing AP view
  - Lateral view
  - Patellofemoral view
  - Long leg radiographs to assess malalignment
  - Standing radiographs with the knee in extension or in 45 degrees of flexion
- Routine use of a chest roentgenography is not usually performed as a screening tool; it is indicated in patients with cardiopulmonary disease or in patients with clinical signs identified upon preadmission testing.
- Electrocardiography is performed in elderly patients and in patients with a history of cardiac problems.

Procedure

INCISION AND EXPOSURE

The knee joint is usually approached anteriorly through a medial parapatellar approach, although some surgeons may use a lateral or subvastus approach (Palmer & Cross, 2004). An incision is made directly over the front of the knee. After dissecting through the skin, the tendon of the quadriceps muscle is identified over the front of the knee; an incision is made through this muscle along the medial side of the patella. The knee is then opened and the procedure is performed.

DETAILS

Cuts are made into the distal femur perpendicular to the mechanical axis, usually using an intramedullary alignment system; this is then checked against the center of the hip. Further cuts are made to the anterior and posterior femur, as well as "chamfer" cuts. The proximal tibia is cut perpendicular to the mechanical axis of the tibia using either intramedullary or extramedullary alignment rods. Restoration of mechanical alignment is vital to allow optimum load sharing and prevent eccentric loading through the prosthesis. A sufficient amount of bone is removed so that the prosthesis recreates the level of the joint line; this permits accurate balance of the ligaments around the knee and prevents alteration in patellar height, which can have a detrimental effect on patellofemoral mechanics. Because of preprocedure deformity, some ligaments around the knee are contracted. These ligaments are carefully released in a step-wise fashion to balance the soft tissues around the knee and provide optimum knee kinematics, Patellofemoral tracking is assessed with trial components and balanced if necessary with a lateral release or medial reefing procedure. If the patellofemoral joint is significantly diseased, it can be resurfaced with a polyethylene button. The physician must recreate the original width of the patella (Palmer & Cross, 2004).

Once the final prosthetic components have been selected, they are cemented into place with polymethyl methacrylate cement. If an uncemented system is being used, press-fit and bony ingrowth provides the short-term and long-term fixation of the prosthesis. The tourniquet is deflated before the wound is closed to allow accurate hemostasis (Palmer & Cross, 2004). **Figure 28.30** depicts a total knee arthroscopy procedure.

CLOSURE

Upon completion of the procedure, the knee joint is usually drained and the surgical incision is closed with monofilament, nonabsorbable suture, or staples. The

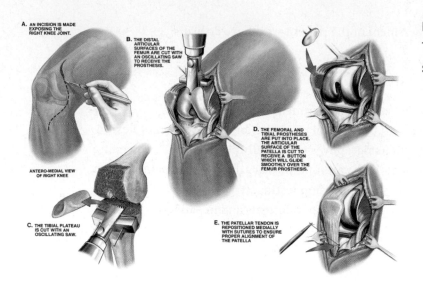

Figure 28.30

Total knee arthroplasty.

Source: Nucleus Medical Art.

operative site is dried and sterile dressings are applied while the knee is in extension. If PRP is used as noted above, a drain is usually not inserted (Hohler, 2008). The patient is usually placed in a knee splint or immobilizer. Foot pulses are checked at the end of the procedure.

Postprocedure Care

The patient is recovered in the PACU where the nurse assesses the patient and monitors vital signs, pain status, wound dressings and drain, as well as respiratory and circulatory status for approximately one hour as the patient emerges from anesthesia (Hohler, 2008). Adequate hydration and analgesia are essential during this time of high physical stress. Analgesia is provided through continuation of the intraoperative epidural, patient-controlled intravenous analgesia, or oral analgesia. At this early stage, the patient begins knee movement sometimes using a continuous passive motion (CPM) machine and exercises ; drains are usually removed within 24 hours; the patient is encouraged to walk on the second postprocedure day (Palmer & Cross, 2004). Discharge is only recommended once wound healing is satisfactory, knee flexion of 90 degrees has been achieved, the patient is considered to be safe and supported in the home environment, and no complications are present (Palmer & Cross, 2004).

Potential Complications

Potential perioperative complications include DVT, blood loss, infection, early hemorrhage, wound breakdown, and intraoperative fractures (Cross, 2008).

REPLANTATION

Replantation is commonly known as reimplantation or reattachment surgery. The goal after traumatic amputation is successful restoration of function, and circulation to the amputated part, thus providing a functional reimplanted part. Replantation of amputated parts has been performed on amputated fingers, hands, forearms, feet, ears, lips, penis, and even an amputated tongue (Wikipedia, 2008).

Nursing Implications

Anesthesia

General or regional anesthesia is generally used depending on the anticipated length of the procedure, and the body part that needs to be reattached. Regional anesthesia is preferred due to the associated trauma risk factors of the original injury (Canale & Beaty, 2007; Goldner & Urbaniak, 1983).

Position

Place the patient in the supine position. Align the head with the body. Position the arms at the patient's sides on padded arm boards, with palms up. Brachial plexus injury may occur if extension of the arm is greater than 90 degrees. If the body part to be reattached belongs to one of the upper extremities, that extremity is placed on an arm table instead of an arm board. Use a warming device to maintain normothermia. Apply a tourniquet to the operative extremity if distal space is adequate (Canale & Beaty, 2007; Goldner & Urbaniak, 1983).

Establishing and Maintaining the Sterile Field

While an assistant holds the operative extremity, prep the extremity, making sure that there is no pooling of prep solution under the tourniquet. Drape the extremity in the usual fashion with an impervious drape sheet. Place a down drape on the arm table or operative bed and then lay the extremity on the down drape. Cover the rest of the body with sterile drapes to insure a sterile field. Use an Esmarch bandage to exsanguinate the extremity (Canale & Beaty, 2007; Goldner & Urbaniak, 1983).

Physiological Monitoring

Monitor and document pressure points and tourniquet pressure and times. With the deflation of any tourniquet, blood loss is calculated on the basis of suction collection and viewing of sponges. Time is an important factor in reimplantation surgery. Time from the accident to the time of revascularization is critical for the survival of the extremity. In addition, neurovascular status is assessed and documented (Canale & Beaty, 2007; Goldner & Urbaniak, 1983).

Procedure

The amputated body part is usually taken into the operating room prior to the patient to ensure that the surgeon has ample time to prepare the body part for reimplantation. The body part should be wrapped in saline-soaked gauze and placed in iced saline. The affected extremity is then irrigated and debrided before the amputated part is reattached. Tendons and vascular structures are identified and ends are cleaned for anastomosis. Loupes or a microscope may be needed depending on the size of the vessels, nerves, and tendons and the surgeon's preference. The bones involved should be stabilized with Kirschner wires. Tendon repair is completed. The digital veins are repaired, followed by repair of the digital artery. If the ischemic time has been prolonged, digital vessel repair may precede repair of tendons and nerves. **Figure 28.31** shows an example of replantation of an avulsed thumb (Canale & Beaty, 2007; Goldner & Urbaniak, 1983).

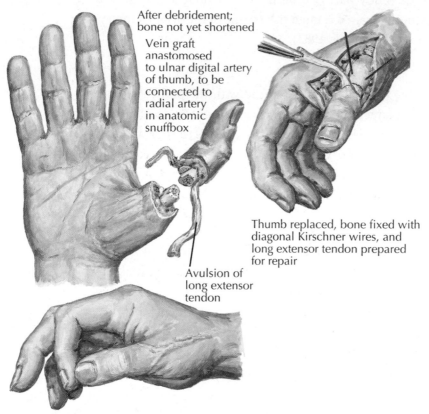

After debridement; bone not yet shortened

Vein graft anastomosed to ulnar digital artery of thumb, to be connected to radial artery in anatomic snuffbox

Thumb replaced, bone fixed with diagonal Kirschner wires, and long extensor tendon prepared for repair

Avulsion of long extensor tendon

Good functional result. Thumb readily opposes to index finger despite shortening

Figure 28.31

Replantation of an avulsed thumb and midpalm.

Source: Netter Images.

Replantation of Midpalm

Amputation through metacarpals with thumb, index and middle fingers on severed part, and ring finger longitudinally amputated. Debridement complete, but bones not yet shortened

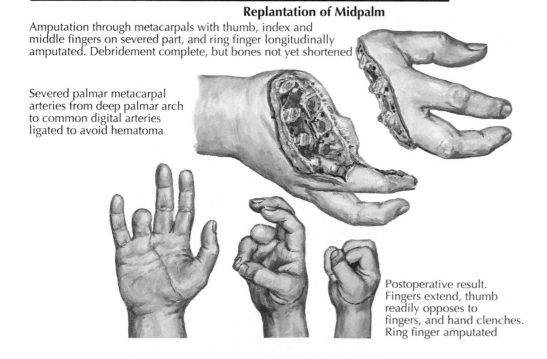

Severed palmar metacarpal arteries from deep palmar arch to common digital arteries ligated to avoid hematoma

Postoperative result. Fingers extend, thumb readily opposes to fingers, and hand clenches. Ring finger amputated

Closure

The skin is approximated and the incision is covered with dry, sterile bulky dressing and/or splint is applied (Canale & Beaty, 2007; Goldner & Urbaniak, 1983).

Postprocedure Care

Skin color, turgor, and temperature are carefully monitored. Any change in temperature below 30 degrees is considered a sign of circulatory compromise. Dressing changes are not usually done until the 10th post-op day unless there are changes in any of the above. The extremity should be elevated to help prevent venous pooling (Canale & Beaty, 2007; Goldner & Urbaniak, 1983).

Potential Complications

The major complication of replantation is the survival rate, however, infections are also common. The average survival rate of replants is 80%. Necrotic tissue should be evaluated and irrigated and debrided as needed (Canale & Beaty, 2007; Goldner & Urbaniak, 1983).

ENDNOTE

1. With a successful exposure, the Grashey view demonstrates the glenohumeral joint space, superoinferior head subluxation, joint congruity, joint degeneration, and other articular abnormalities. The radiological technician obtains this view by positioning the posterior surface of the scapula flat onto the radiography film, resulting in a view that is 45° oblique to traditional shoulder anterior-posterior radiography (Afsari, A., and Mehlman 2004).

REFERENCES

1. Afsari, A., & Mehlman, C.T. (2004). Anterior glenohumeral instability. Retrieved July 29, 2008 from http://www.emedicine.com/orthoped/topic464.htm.
2. Altchek, D.W. (2003). Elbow arthroscopy. Retrieved August 13, 2008 from http://womensportsmedicine.org/conditions_14230.asp.
3. American Academy of Orthopaedic Surgeons. (AAOS). (2007). Wrist arthroscopy. Retrieved August 18, 2008 from http://orthoinfo.aaos.org/topic.cfm?topic=A00001.
4. AORN (2008a). Recommended practices for the use of the pneumatic tourniquet in the perioperative practice setting. *Perioperative Standards and Recommended Practices.* Denver, CO: AORN, Inc: pp. 483–495.
5. AORN (2008b). Recommended practices for a safe environment of care. *Perioperative Standards and Recommended Practices.* Denver, CO: AORN, Inc: pp. 351–373.
6. AORN (2008c). Recommended practices for preoperative patient skin antisepsis. *Perioperative Standards and Recommended Practices.* Denver, CO: AORN, Inc: pp. 537–555.
7. Buly, R.L. (2008). Arthroscopy of the hip. Retrieved August 7, 2008 from http://www.hss.edu/conditions_14162.asp.
8. Canale, S.T., & Beaty, J.H. (2007). *Campbell's Operative Arthroscopy,* 11th ed. Philadelphia, PA: Mosby Elsevier.
9. Carreira, D. & Bush-Joseph, C.A. (2006). Hip arthroscopy. Retrieved August 12, 2008 from http://www.orthosupersite.com/view.asp?rID=17203.
10. Covidien. (2007). *Force Triad™ electrosurgical generator users guide.* Boulder, CO: Covidien.
11. Cross, M.J. (2008). Complications of total knee arthroplasty. Retrieved August 11, 2008 from http://www.emedicine.com/orthoped/TOPIC384.HTM.
12. Encyclopedia of Surgery. (2008). Arthroscopic surgery. Retrieved August 12, 2008 from http://www.surgeryencyclopedia.com/A-Ce/Arthroscopic-Surgery.html.
13. Environmental Protection Agency (EPA). (2007). Methyl methacrylate. Retrieved July 30, 2008 from http://www.epa.gov/ttn/atw/hlthef/methylme.html.
14. Goldner, R.D., & Urbaniak, J.R. (1983). Replantation in the upper extremity. *Orthopedic Surgery. Update Series*; 2; Princeton, NJ: Continuing Education Professional Education Center, Inc.: pp. 1–8.

28

15. Hohler, S.E. (2008). Total knee arthroplasty: past successes and current improvements. *AORN Journal*; 87(1): pp. 143–158.

16. Katz, J.N., & Gomoll, A.H. (2007). Advances in arthroscopic surgery: indications and outcomes. *Current Opinions in Rheumatology*; 19(2): pp. 106–110.

17. Medline Plus. (2006). Knee arthroscopy—series: indications. Retrieved July 30, 2008 from http://www.nlm.nih.gov/medlineplus/ency/presentations/100117_2.htm.

18. Medline Plus. (2008). Medical encyclopedia: lordosis. Retrieved July 30, 2008 from http://www.nlm.nih.gov/medlineplus/ency/article/003278.htm.

19. Medline Plus. (2007). Shoulder arthroscopy. Retrieved August 14, 2008 from http://www.nlm.nih.gov/medlineplus/ency/article/007206.htm.

20. Meyers, J.F. & Carson, W.G. (2002). Elbow arthroscopy: supine technique. Retrieved August 13, 2008 from http://books.google.com/books?id=1Uq3bmM6qwcC&pg=PA665&lpg=PA665&dq=elbow+arthroscopy+medical+description+procedure&source=web&ots=zRpGkdSewv&sig=PIHSXZQYmfxZP7Uv-qGhL9d1g_M&hl=en&sa=X&oi=book_result&resnum=7&ct=result#PPA665,M1.

21. Moyes, S. (2007). Ankle arthroscopy. Retrieved August 12, 2008 from http://www.ankle-arthroscopy.co.uk/surgeon/.

22. O'Driscoll, S.W. (2002). Elbow arthroscopy. Retrieved August 13, 2008 from http://www.maitrise-orthop.com/corpusmaitri/orthopaedic/115_odriscoll/odriscollus.shtml.

23. Palmer, S.H., & Cross, M.J. (2004). Total knee arthroplasty. Retrieved August 7, 2008 from http://www.emedicine.com/orthoped/TOPIC347.htm.

24. Rao, A.G., Yokota, A., & McFarland, E.G. (2004). Shoulder arthroscopy: principles and practice. *Physical Medicine & Rehabilitation Clinics of North America*; 15(3); pp: 627–642.

25. Ray, R. (2008). Arthroscopy of the ankle and subtalar joints. Retrieved August 12, 2008 from http://www.podiatrynetwork.com/document.cfm?id=55.

26. Ricks, E. (2007). Wrist arthroscopy. *AORN Journal*; 86(2): pp. 181–188.

27. Sargent, C.A., & Dunfee, M.T. (2005). Knee block anesthesia for arthroscopic procedures. *AORN Journal*; 82(1): pp. 20–36.

28. Science.jrank.org. (2008). Arthroscopic surgery—benefits of arthroscopic surgery, development of the procedure, the operation, types of arthroscopic surgery. Retrieved August 20, 2008 from http://science.jrank.org/pages/528/Arthroscopic-Surgery.html.

29. Shoulderdoc. (2008). Elbow arthroscopy. Retrieved August 13, 2008 from http://www.shoulderdoc.co.uk/article.asp?article=5.

30. Shugars, R.A., & More, R.C. (2005). Arthroscopic hip surgery. *AORN Journal*; 82(6): pp. 976–998.

31. Strobel, M. (2001). Manual of arthroscopic surgery. Retrieved August 12, 2008 from http://books.google.com/books?id=iRbbX0rr6dIC&dq=anesthesia+options+ankle+arthroscopy&source=gbs_summary_s&cad=0.

32. *The Free Dictionary*. (2008). Orthopedic surgery. Retrieved July 30, 2008 from http://medical-dictionary.thefreedictionary.com/Orthopedic+surgery.

33. US Food & Drug Administration (FDA). (2007). Class II special controls guidance document: polymethylmethacrylate (PMMA) bone cement; guidance for industry and FDA. Retrieved July 30, 2008 from http://www.fda.gov/cdrh/ode/guidance/668.html.

34. Wheeless, C.R. (2007). Ankle arthroscopy. Retrieved August 12, 2008 from http://www.wheelessonline.com/ortho/ankle_arthroscopy.

35. Wheeless, C.R. (2008a). Hip joint arthroscopy. Retrieved August 12, 2008 from http://www.wheelessonline.com/ortho/hip_joint_arthroscopy.

36. Wheeless, C.R. (2008b). Elbow arthroscopy. Retrieved August 13, 2008 from http://www.wheelessonline.com/ortho/elbow_arthroscopy.

37. Wiesler, E.R., & Poehling, G.G. (2002). Arthroscopy of the wrist: operating room set up and technique. *Operative Arthroscopy*, 3rd ed. Retrieved August 18, 2008 from http://books.google.com/books?id=1Uq3bmM6qwcC&pg=RA1-PA729&lpg=RA1-PA729&dq=wrist+arthroscopy+operative+procedure&source=web&ots=zRpHegXhtz&sig=oijysHcQyxQ3ranjgYMBpMbwnYo&hl=en&sa=X&oi=book_result&resnum=2&ct=result#PRA1-PA729,M1.

38. Wikipedia. (2008). Replantation. Retrieved August 21, 2008 from http://en.wikipedia.org/wiki/Replantation.

CHAPTER 29

Gynecological and Obstetrical Surgery

Joyce A. Cox
Mary A. Rogers

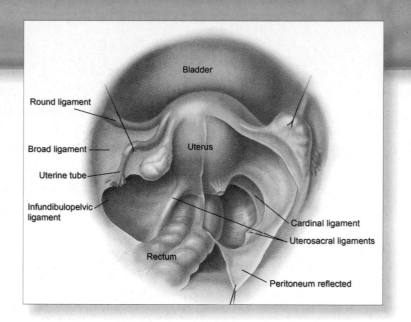

INTRODUCTION

Gynecological surgery refers to all operative and invasive procedures that involve the female reproductive organs and related structures (bladder, vasculature, rectum, musculature, and lymphatics), particularly those situated in the pelvis and perineum. From an operative perspective, the reproductive structures include the uterus, the cervix, the ovaries, the fallopian tubes, the vulva, and the vagina. With the advancement of technology, many gynecological procedures are now performed using minimally invasive techniques. The addition of robotics has allowed many complex minimally invasive procedures to be performed with added precision.

Obstetrical surgery refers to operative procedures on the gravid uterus. Obstetrical procedures include cerclages and cesarean sections.

Fetal surgery is operative intervention by reaching inside the uterus to help a fetus that has a correctable problem. The UCSF Fetal Treatment Center comments that "… it is surprisingly new because our ability to detect fetal problems has advanced so rapidly over the last few decades. While many diseases can now be accurately diagnosed before birth by genetic and imaging techniques, only a few require intervention before birth." Animal research began in the 1960s and the first human fetal interventions were performed in the early 1980s (The Regents of the University of California, 2008).

This chapter includes the most frequent gynecological and obstetrical operative procedures, as well as an overview of fetal operative procedures (DeCherney & Nathan, 2003).

Chapter Contents

ANATOMY
External Genitalia

The external genitalia consist of the mons pubis (veneris), the clitoris, the labia majora and minora, the hymen, Bartholin's glands, and the orifice of the vagina (**Fig. 29.1**). Collectively, the external genitalia are referred to as the vulva. The mons pubis is an area of fatty tissue and coarse skin that lies over the symphysis pubis. After puberty, this area is covered with hair. The clitoris is an erectile structure; it is located beneath the anterior commissure formed by the labia majora and is partially hidden by the anterior ends of the labia minora. It is analogous to the corpora cavernosa in the male. The labia majora are long folds of skin filled with subcutaneous fat that run downward and backward from the mons pubis. The labia majora are embryologically homologous to the scrotum of the male. The labia minora are two delicate folds of fat-free, hairless skin. They lie between the labia majora, and their lateral surfaces are in contact with the smooth surfaces of the labia majora. They enclose the vestibule of the vagina, into which the vaginal and urethral orifices enter. The hymen is a thin mucous membrane that partially covers the entrance of the vagina in young females. The membrane remains intact until coitus but its presence is not reliable as a test of virginity. Analogous to Cowper's glands in the male, Bartholin's glands lie on either side of the vagina and behind the hymen. They secrete mucus or lubricant at the time of coitus.

Internal Genitalia

The internal genitalia include the vagina, the uterus and its ligaments, the ovaries, and the fallopian tubes (**Figs. 29.2** and **29.3**).

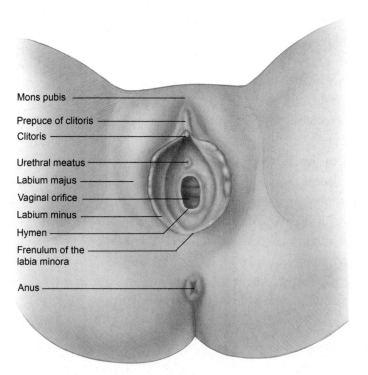

Figure 29.1

External genitalia.

Mons pubis

Prepuce of clitoris

Clitoris

Urethral meatus

Labium majus

Vaginal orifice

Labium minus

Hymen

Frenulum of the labia minora

Anus

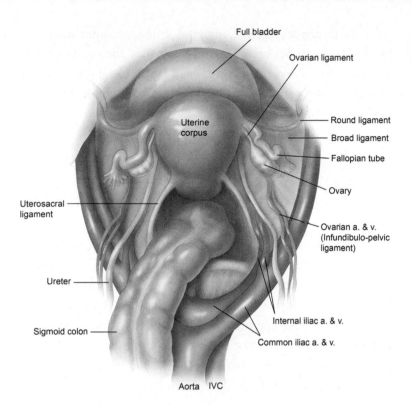

Figure 29.2

View of the organs in the female pelvis.

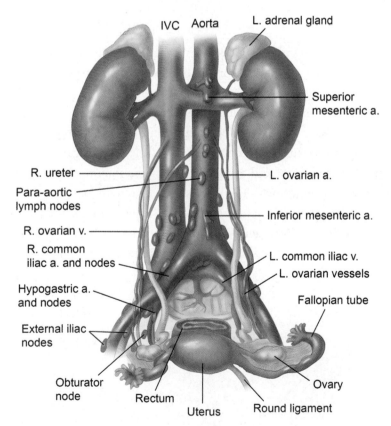

Figure 29.3

Lymphatic drainage of the female internal genital organs.

Vagina

The vagina is a muscular membranous tube that forms the passageway between the uterus and the vulva. It lies posterior to the urinary bladder and anterior to the rectum. The vagina has four walls: two lateral, one anterior, and one posterior. Its anterior wall is in contact with the cervix, the base of the bladder, the terminal parts of the ureters and the urethra. Its posterior wall is connected to the rectum.

The vagina consists of three layers: an internal mucosal lining, an outer muscular coat, and an erectile layer of tissue in-between. During pregnancy, the muscular coat increases, and the mucosal lining allows for dilation of the birth canal during labor and birth. The vagina receives the penis and semen during intercourse and is the passageway for the menstrual flow and for the fetus during birth.

Uterus

The uterus is a hollow, thick-walled, pear-shaped muscular organ that is approximately 7–8 cm long and 4–5 cm wide. It is composed of three layers: (1) the perimetrium, or outer layer; (2) the myometrium, or middle layer, which consists of smooth muscle; and (3) the endometrium, or inner layer, which lines the hollow shell. During pregnancy, the uterus becomes extremely large. It returns to almost its original size by approximately 3 months after delivery; this shrinkage can be hastened by breastfeeding. After menopause, the uterus always becomes smaller. The uterus consists of three areas: (1) the body, or corpus: (2) the isthmus; and (3) the cervix, which is the lower portion located at the upper end of the vagina. Under normal conditions, the uterus is ante-flexed, or bent forward, between the cervix and the body, but many women have retroflexed, or posterior uteri (**Fig. 29.4**). The major function of the uterus is to contain and nourish the fetus from the time of fertilization and to expel the fetus at the time of birth.

Uterine Ligaments

The uterus is suspended by eight ligaments: two broad, two round, two uterosacral, and two cardinal (**Fig. 29.5**). The broad ligaments help form a barrier extending across the pelvic cavity. These double folds of peritoneum hold the uterus in a normal position. Enclosed in the free edge of each broad ligament is a fallopian tube. The round ligaments are two rounded bands continuous with the wall of the uterus. Each round ligament runs between the layers of the broad ligament and across the pelvis to the inguinal canal and attaches to the labia majora. These ligaments help suspend the uterus anteriorly. The uterosacral ligaments pass from the sides of the cervix toward the sacrum deep in the pelvis to the peritoneum and superior to the levator ani muscle. The uterosacral ligaments are responsible for holding the uterus in its normal position in the pelvis. The cardinal (Mackenrodt's) ligaments

Figure 29.4

Normal and abnormal uterine positions.

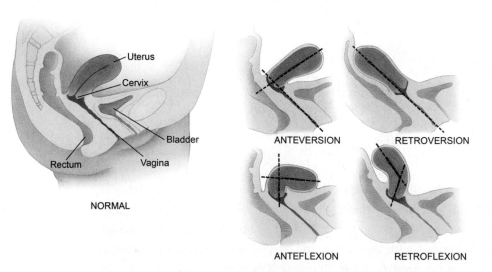

Uterus

Cervix

Bladder

Rectum

Vagina

NORMAL

ANTEVERSION

RETROVERSION

ANTEFLEXION

RETROFLEXION

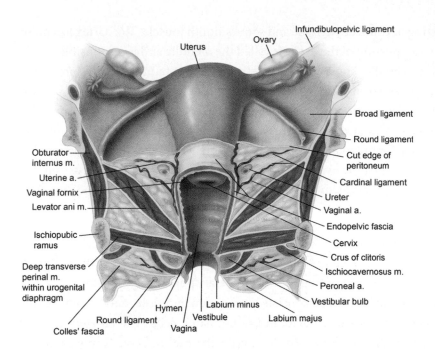

Figure 29.5

Coronal section of the pelvis at the level of the uterine isthmus and ischial spines, showing the ligaments supporting the uterus.

help prevent prolapse of the uterus and consist of fibrous sheets that extend from the level of the isthmus to the lateral pelvic fascia (**Fig. 29.6**).

In addition to the eight ligaments, the uterus has peritoneal folds. They are posterior (rectouterine) and anterior (vesicouterine); the posterior, which is behind the uterus, forms a deep fold in the peritoneum, and the anterior fold is between the bladder and the uterus.

Ovaries

The ovaries are analogous to the testes in the male. Normally two in number, the almond-shaped glands lie on either side of the uterus. Each ovary is attached to the uterus by the ovarian ligament and to the lateral pelvic walls by the infundibulopelvic ligament, which contains vessels and nerves. The ovary has an outer portion, called the

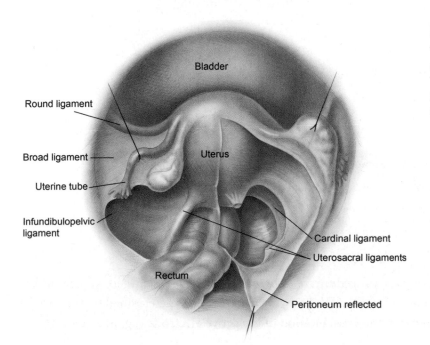

Figure 29.6

The uterus and ligaments as viewed from above. The peritoneum has been reflected back to show the cardinal ligament.

cortex, consisting of connective tissue and some smooth muscle. The cortex has many follicles. The inner portion of the ovary is called the medulla and is responsible for the vascularity of the gland. It consists of connective tissue containing nerves, blood, and lymphatic vessels. The ovary is responsible for the production of eggs (ova), and the two female hormones: estrogen and progesterone. These hormones are responsible for the maintenance and development of secondary sexual characteristics, the preparation of the uterus for pregnancy, and the development of the mammary glands. The ovary has two ligaments: the ovarian ligament, which attaches to the uterus, and the infundibulopelvic ligament, which contains the ovarian artery. The blood supply of the ovary comes from the ovarian and uterine arteries.

Fallopian Tubes

The fallopian tubes are a pair of ducts that are about 7–12 cm long. They connect the uterus to the ovaries and provide a means to transport the eggs from the ovaries to the uterus. Each fallopian tube consists of an inner, a middle, and an outer layer. The inner mucosa consists of ciliated and non-ciliated cells. The ciliated cells aid in the movement of the ovum toward the uterus, the middle layer is muscular and consists of an inner circular layer and an outer layer of smooth muscle. The serosa, or outer layer of the fallopian tube, is made up of connective tissue.

The fallopian tube is divided into four parts: (1) the infundibulum, or fimbrial end, which is funnel-shaped and opens into the abdomen; (2) the ampulla, which is the longest part of the fallopian tube, receives the oocyte from the fimbria, and is the site where fertilization usually takes place; (3) the isthmus, which joins the horn of the uterus; (4) and uterine portion, which is the short segment that transverses the wall of the uterus. The fallopian tubes lie in the free edges of the broad ligament of the uterus called the mesosalpinx.

SPECIAL SURGICAL INSTRUMENTS AND EQUIPMENT

Gynecological instrument sets may include the following:

> Basic GYN Abdominal Set
>
> GYN Endoscopy Set
>
> Vaginal Procedure Set
>
> Major Set
>
> Minor Set
>
> D&C Set
>
> Laparoscopy Set
>
> Hysteroscopy Set
>
> Endoscopic supplies
>
> Cesarean Section Set

Electrosurgical Unit

Many gynecological procedures require the use of an electrosurgery generator that has monopolar and bipolar capabilities. Power selection is determined on the basis of the type of generator, the configuration of the active electrode (eg, needle tip versus ball electrode), the tissue involved, and the desired tissue effect (cutting, desiccation, or fulguration). See Chapters 11 and 17 for additional information on electrosurgery.

Laser

Carbon dioxide, neodymium yttrium-aluminum-garnet (Nd: YAG) and potassium titanyl phosphate (KTP) lasers are used with select gynecological procedures. They can be used for treating vulvar and cervical lesions, endometriosis, leiomyomas, and for accomplishing tubal reconstruction.

KTP
Potassium Titanyl Phosphate

ROBOTICS

Robotic surgery enables the surgeon to perform more complex operative procedures using a minimally invasive approach. Robotic operative procedures can mean less pain and scarring, less blood loss, reduced risk of complications, shorter hospital stays and quicker recovery. Use of robotics in minimally invasive procedures (MIP) provides a three-dimensional view increasing depth perception during the procedure. Because the primary surgeon sits at a console while operating, his/her operating ergonomics and comfort are greatly improved. The surgeon's ergonomics are further enhanced by creating a computer interface between the surgeon's hands and the instrument tips. This gives more natural movement of the surgeon's hands into the desired movement of the robotic instrument. As outlined by Francis and Winfield, care of the robotic surgical patient differs only slightly from non-robotic care. The overall content of pre-procedure care does not need to be altered for patients undergoing robotic intervention. Francis and Winfield (2006, p. 103) comment that "... intraoperative nursing functions are affected the most by medical robotic technology. Nursing personnel must know how to properly connect, calibrate, and setup the equipment pieces for the surgical robotic system. They must also be familiar with the robotic instrumentation needs for each type of procedure, including how to properly load, handle, and clean these specialized instruments. The nursing personnel should also understand the robotic system well enough to know how to troubleshoot problems for the primary/non-sterile operative surgeon at the robotic surgical system and the surgeon at the patient's side. The patient-side surgeon assists the primary/non-sterile operative surgeon by exchanging sterile instruments, retracting patient tissues, and manipulating non-robotic sterile instruments used to assist the procedure." (page 103 see insert) The ability of the nursing personnel to interpret and react to messages displayed on the robotic television monitor is critically important to the flow and success of the procedure. If it is necessary to abort the robotic procedure, nursing personnel must be familiar with removing the robotic system and setting up for a non-robotic procedure. Postprocedure care is similar to non-robotic procedures (Francis & Winfield, 2006).

MIP
Minimally Invasive Procedure

POSITIONING

Positioning for gynecological/obstetrical procedures should provide optimum exposure for the procedure and access to IV lines and monitoring devices. AORN *Perioperative Standards and Recommended Practices* (2008) emphasizes that "attention must be given to patient comfort and safety, as well as circulatory, respiratory, musculoskeletal, and neurologic structure. The procedure, surgeon preference, and patient condition determine equipment used for positioning" (AORN, 2008 p. 497).

Supine

In supine (dorsal recumbent) position, the patient lies flat on her back. The head generally rests on a small pillow. Arms may be positioned on padded arm boards or tucked at the sides. If the arms are placed on arm boards, soft wrist restraints may be applied. If the arms are tucked at the sides, the fingers should be straight with palms toward the body and 2 inches of insulation such as a bath towel or folded sheet should be applied between the patient's arms and hands to prevent skin-to-skin contact. A safety strap is placed two inches above the knees.

Trendelenburg

In Trendelenburg, the patient lies flat on her back with the table tilted so that the upper torso is lowered and the feet are raised. The patient's knees must lie over the break in the bed to ensure safe, anatomic positioning.

Lithotomy

Beginning with the patient in supine position, the legs are raised simultaneously and abducted to expose the perineal area. The legs may be placed in high stirrups or low stirrups. Both right and left stirrups need to be at the same height. Legs should be raised and knees flexed, in a slow, smooth motion. After the legs are secured in the stirrups, the lower end of the OR bed is lowered. The buttocks are moved to be even with the end of the bed. The arms are supported on arm boards or tucked at the patient's sides. Extreme diligence must be used to assure hands and fingers are out of the way when the end of the bed is raised. Severe hip flexion as well as abduction of the hip joint must be avoided. When the legs are removed from the stirrups, they must be lowered simultaneously. The legs should be lowered slowly to allow for gradual hemodynamic changes. Distal lower extremity pulses should be evaluated before, during, and after this position. Proper patient positioning is the responsibility of all members of the surgical team to protect the patient from injury.

SKIN PREPARATION

The purpose of skin preparation is to reduce the incidence of postprocedure operative site infection. An adequate skin prep removes soil and microorganisms from the skin with the least amount of tissue trauma while arresting rapid regrowth of microorganisms. The operative site should be examined prior to the skin prep. Any hair removal from the operative site should be done according to physician preference and/or policies and procedures in the practice facility. Using sterile technique, the skin prep should start at the cleanest area and move to less clean areas. The incisional area is ordinarily prepped first moving outward. A soap solution of the surgeon's choice should be used to perform the primary scrub. Surgeon's preference may warrant painting the operative area with a topical antimicrobial solution. Care should be taken to avoid pooling of the solution under the patient's body. Gynecological surgery includes vaginal vault preparation with normal saline or solution of surgeon's choice. This is done prior to the incisional prep.

DILATATION AND CURETTAGE

Dilatation and curettage (D&C) is a procedure in which the cervical os is enlarged using graduated-sized dilators. A sharp curette is then used to scrape the endometrium.

D&C
Dilatation and Curettage

Indications

Dilatation and Curettage (D&C) is useful in providing a definitive diagnosis for abnormal uterine bleeding. It is the most common minor gynecological procedure performed. D&C is performed when the pain associated with menstruation suggests an abnormality of the uterus; when bleeding is abnormal, irregular, heavy, or postmenopausal; and after an incomplete abortion.

Related Procedures

Related procedures are hysteroscopy, dilatation and evacuation (D&E), and uterine polypectomy.

D&E
Dilatation and Evacuation

Nursing Implications

Anesthesia

D&C can be performed with a regional block and sedation or general anesthesia. General anesthesia in the patient allows the surgeon to perform a better pelvic examination.

Position

The procedure is performed with the patient in the lithotomy position with high stirrups. Refer to the section on positioning.

Establishing and Maintaining the Sterile Field

A skin prep of surgeon's choice is used to prepare the operative site, which should include the perineum and the vagina. A double-folded sheet is placed under the buttocks, with leg drapes applied next. Last, an open sheet is placed over the abdomen. The surgeon sits for this procedure. The instrument table is placed closest to the surgeon's dominant arm.

Equipment and Supplies

Instruments from a D&C set are used and should be placed on the table from left to right in the order that the surgeon will use them.

Physiological Monitoring

No special monitoring is needed for this procedure.

Specimens and Cultures

D&C usually yields two specimens: endocervical and endometrial curettage specimens. Both specimens are routinely sent to the pathology laboratory.

Drugs and Solutions

If the procedure is performed with a general anesthetic, no other drugs are needed. However, if it is performed with sedation, a local or regional block anesthetic is required.

Physician Orders

This procedure is usually performed as an outpatient procedure. The patient should have NPO orders.

Laboratory and Diagnostic Studies

Preprocedure testing depends on the age and medical condition of the patient and the type of anesthesia. The patient's preprocedure testing may include CBC, ECG, urinalysis, and electrolyte values.

Procedure

Incision and Exposure

No incision is needed for this procedure. A Sims retractor or a weighted speculum is placed in the vagina for exposure.

Details

A straight catheter is used to empty the bladder and then removed. The lip of the anterior cervix is grasped with a tenaculum. A sound is carefully inserted into the endometrial cavity to determine the depth and direction of the uterus. A curette is used to scrape the cervical canal. Dilators are used to dilate the cervical os to at least 8 mm. A polyp forceps is used to explore the cavity for polyps. A sharp curette is advanced into the fundus and moved back and forth until all of the endometrium is sampled. A nonadherent dressing is placed over the retractor to collect the curettage specimens. The tenaculum is removed, and the site is checked for a cervical tear or any bleeding. If a tear or bleeding is discovered, pressure is applied, and electrosurgery or a ligature is used to achieve hemostasis. The speculum is then removed.

Closure

No closure is needed.

Postprocedure Care

The patient is taken to the PACU. Perineal pads are checked for heavy bleeding and clotting and cramping are also noted. The patient is discharged the same day. The patient is instructed to take her temperature twice per day for 1 week and report to the surgeon if it is more than 100°F (37.8°C). Acetaminophen or ibuprofen should be used for mild pain. Activity may be increased gradually during the first 24 hours.

Potential Complications

Potential complications are bleeding, infection, and uterine perforation (Guido & Stovall, 2006).

SUCTION CURETTAGE

Suction curettage, also referred to as Dilatation and Evacuation (D&E), is the vaginal evacuation of the products of conception with a suctioning device (Tulandi, May 11, 2007).

Indications

Suction curettage is performed to remove any remaining tissue that was not expelled during an incomplete abortion.

Related Procedure

D&C is a related procedure.

Nursing Implications

Anesthesia

Suction curettage can be performed under cervical block with or without sedation or performed under general anesthesia.

Position

Suction curettage is done with the patient in the dorsal lithotomy position with high stirrups.

Establishing and Maintaining the Sterile Field

The perineum and the vagina must be prepped with a scrub solution of physician's choice. A double-folded sheet is placed under the buttocks, with leg drapes applied next. Lastly, an open sheet is placed over the abdomen. The surgeon sits for this procedure. The instrument table is placed closest to the surgeon's dominant arm. The suction machine is placed on the same side as the instrument table. The suction tubing is passed over the patient's leg and attached to the suctioning machine.

Equipment and Supplies

    D&C tray

    Paracervical block tray (if regional anesthesia is preferred)

    Suction machine with tubing and various-sized curettes

The scrub person should test the suction apparatus when it is attached to the suction machine, making sure that proper suction levels are attained. The circulating nurse turns the machine on when the surgeon is ready for suctioning.

Physiological Monitoring

The circulating nurse should monitor blood loss and inform the anesthesia provider if blood loss is excessive.

Specimens and Cultures

The specimen (products of conception) is routinely sent to the pathology laboratory.

Drugs and Solutions

Oxytocin may be added to the IV solution to enhance uterine contractions.

Physician Orders

This procedure is usually performed as an outpatient status. The patient should have NPO orders.

Laboratory and Diagnostic Studies

Preprocedure testing depends on the age and medical condition of the patient and the type of anesthesia. The patient's preprocedure testing may include ECG, urinalysis, and electrolyte values. CBC should be obtained. If the patient is Rh-negative, she should receive immune globulin after the procedure.

Procedure

Incision and Exposure

No incision is made for this procedure. Exposure is obtained by a weighted speculum.

Details

The bladder is emptied with a straight catheter, which is then removed. After the cervix is exposed, it is grasped with a double-toothed tenaculum or ringed forceps. A uterine sound may be passed through the cervix to check the length and direction of the cavity, but is usually not used because of the softness of the uterus. Dilators, preferably Pratt dilators, are used to dilate the cervix to at least 6 mm to allow for the No. 6 curette. The amount of dilatation depends on the length of gestation. Suction tubing is applied to the curette, and the suction machine is turned on. The curette is rotated in a 360-degree arc and withdrawn slowly. It is reintroduced several times to ensure that all products of conception are retrieved. A sharp curette is used to check for completeness of the procedure. The specimen is collected in the gauze sack in the suction apparatus. When the procedure is completed, normal saline or sterile water is run through the tubing. This ensures that all tissue is collected in the gauze sac. The surgeon examines the tissue for anatomical parts, and then it is placed in a specimen container.

Closure

No closure is required for this procedure.

Postprocedure Care

The patient is taken to the PACU for a short time. Perineal pads are checked for heavy bleeding and clotting and cramping. The patient is discharged the same day and is instructed to take her temperature twice per day for 1 week and report to the surgeon if it is more than 100°F (37.8°C). Acetaminophen or ibuprofen should be used for mild pain. Activity may be increased gradually during the first 24 hours. The patient is given ergonovine maleate 0.2 mg (200/mg) orally every 4 hours for six doses; this aids the uterus in contracting to prevent excessive bleeding. Some vaginal discharge can be expected for a few days after the procedure.

Potential Complications

Infection, hemorrhage, and perforation of the uterus are possible complications.

HYSTEROSCOPY

Hysteroscopy is the insertion of a fiberoptic hysteroscope into the uterus which aids in the visualization of the entire uterine cavity (Guido & Stovall, 2007).

Indications

Hysteroscopy is performed for diagnostic and therapeutic purposes, including infertility, suspected abnormal tissue, adhesions, uterine polyps, and submucosal myomas.

Nursing Implications

Anesthesia

General anesthesia is choice for this procedure.

Position

The procedure is performed with the patient in the lithotomy position with high stirrups. Refer to the section on positioning.

Establishing and Maintaining the Sterile Field

A scrub solution of surgeon's choice is used for the preparation, which includes the perineum and the vagina. The patient is draped with a half sheet under the buttocks, then leg drapes, and finally with an open sheet across the abdomen. The instrument table should be on the surgeon's dominant side. The hysteroscopy insufflator should be on the patient's side, close to the instrument table, positioned so that the surgeon may see the pressure monitor for carbon dioxide flow rate. The surgeon sits for the procedure.

Equipment and Supplies

    D&C tray

    Hysteroscope

    Light cord

    Light source

    Hysteroscopy insufflator

    Straight catheter

    Sponges

Physiological Monitoring

If glycine is used to aid visualization, the amounts should be carefully monitored.

Specimens and Cultures

If the procedure is done in conjunction with a D&C, curettage specimens are possible. Depending on the patient's history, a polyp or a submucosal myoma may be obtained. All specimens are routinely sent to the pathology laboratory.

Drugs and Solutions

Carbon dioxide is used for insufflation; glycine is the medium used by most surgeons when resection is necessary.

Physician Orders

This procedure is usually performed as an outpatient procedure. The patient should have NPO orders.

Laboratory and Diagnostic Studies

Preprocedure testing depends on the age and medical condition of the patient and the type of anesthesia. The patient's preprocedure testing may include CBC, ECG, urinalysis, and electrolyte values.

29

Procedure

Incision and Exposure

No incision is made for this procedure. Exposure is obtained by a weighted speculum.

Details

Before the hysteroscope is inserted, the system should be checked. The circulating nurse checks the gas pressure, turns on the machine, closes the insufflator's switch, adjusts the intrauterine pressure and carbon dioxide flow rate to zero, turns on the flow rate, and adjusts the flow rate with the insufflator to deliver 25–30 mL/minute. After the system is checked, the bladder is emptied with a straight catheter, which is then removed. The cervix is grasped with a tenaculum. The cervix is dilated to accommodate the entrance of the hysteroscope into the cervical os. The hysteroscope is passed through the cervical os and the carbon dioxide valve on the hysteroscope is opened, and the hysteroscope is advanced. The endocervical and endometrial cavities are explored, as well as the fallopian tubes. D&C may be performed (Pascholpoulos et al, 2006).

Closure

No closure is required for this procedure.

Postprocedure Care

The patient is taken to the PACU for a short time. Perineal pads are checked for heavy bleeding and clotting and cramping is also noted. The patient is discharged the same day. The patient is instructed to take her temperature twice per day for 1 week and report to the surgeon if it is more than 100°F (37.8°C). Acetaminophen or ibuprofen should be used for mild pain. Activity may be increased gradually during the first 24 hours.

Potential Complications

Complications are rarely seen in hysteroscopy.

LAPAROSCOPY

Laparoscopy is the visualization, examination, and/or observation of the peritoneal cavity by way of optics. The procedure may be diagnostic, therapeutic, or both (Stovall, 2007).

Indications

The indications for gynecological laparoscopy are numerous. It is used for, but not limited to, diagnosis and treatment of endometriosis, assessment of infertility, diagnosis and treatment of ectopic pregnancy, assessment of the capability for tubal restoration, checking for recurrence of ovarian cancer, and checking for suspected uterine perforation during D&C or D&E (Schenken, 2007).

Nursing Implications

Anesthesia

The procedure is performed under general endotracheal anesthesia.

Position

The patient is placed in the modified lithotomy position. The patient's legs are angled to accommodate the surgeon when working in the abdomen; a 15-degree Trendelenburg position is used to displace the intestines from the abdomen to the diaphragm. The arms are extended on boards; they are not abducted more than 90 degrees. They also may be placed alongside of the patient, with care not to injure the patient's hands and fingers.

Establishing and Maintaining the Sterile Field

The electrosurgical patient return electrode is placed on the patient according to the manufacturer's instructions. See Chapter 11 for additional information. Skin scrub of surgeon's choice is used to prepare the operative site (refer to section on skin preparation). The patient is draped as follows: a half sheet is placed under the buttocks; leg drapes are applied; a laparotomy sheet is placed over the abdomen; the arms are covered with opened plain sheets if the laparotomy sheet does not include arm covers. Abdominal instruments and vaginal apparatus are kept separate. A small square table can accommodate the vaginal instruments, and a large table is used for the abdominal instruments. The surgeon is positioned to the patient's right, with the abdominal instrument table closest to the surgeon's dominant arm. The nonsterile monitor, insufflator, and light source are on the patient's left in perfect view of the surgeon. The sterile assistant is positioned at the foot of the bed, managing the vaginal instruments. If another assistant is available, he or she is positioned on the patient's left. The circulating nurse is available to connect and manage the accessories being used in the procedure (eg, camera). The scrub person should check that all equipment is functioning properly and that optics equipment are clear and provide good visualization.

Equipment and Supplies

Laparoscopy set

GYN endoscopy set

Physiological Monitoring

A Foley catheter is inserted into the patient's bladder and usually discontinued at the end of the procedure.

Specimens and Cultures

A D&C may be performed with the procedure; therefore, curettage specimens are possible. All specimens are routinely sent to the pathology laboratory.

Drugs and Solutions

Normal saline (0.9% sodium chloride) with indigo carmine is used to check for tubal patency. Normal saline or lactated Ringer's solution may also be used to irrigate the pelvis.

Physician Orders

Patient instructions may include NPO instructions, administering a Fleet enema, and skin preparation including clipping hair and showering.

Laboratory and Diagnostic Studies

Preprocedure testing depends on the age and medical condition of the patient and the type of anesthesia. The patient's preprocedure testing may include CBC, ECG, urinalysis, and electrolyte values.

Procedure

Incision and Exposure

No incision is made for the vaginal part of the procedure. Exposure of the cervix is obtained with a Sims retractor. The abdominal incision is made with a No. 11 blade, through the umbilicus.

Details

After the patient is placed in the lithotomy position, the hips are extended to allow access to the abdomen. A Foley catheter is inserted into the bladder and attached to a urinary drainage bag. Next, a Sims retractor is used to expose the cervix, and a tenaculum is used to grasp the cervix. If D&C is scheduled, it is performed at this time. A Jarcho or Sparkman cannula is inserted into the cervix and attached to the tenaculum to allow manipulation of the uterus.

Attention is now focused on the abdomen. Towel clips or manual grasping are used to elevate the sub-umbilical area of the abdominal wall. A small incision is made with the No. 11 blade. The abdomen is elevated to allow easy advancement of the Verres needle. After the needle is in place, the carbon dioxide tubing is attached. One liter of carbon dioxide is allowed into the peritoneum, after which tympanic sound of percussion is tested at the suprapubic region, to indicate free diffusion of the gas in the peritoneal cavity. When abdominal pressure is 14 mm Hg, there is usually adequate distention.

The Verres needle is removed at this time. The incision is extended to allow for the 10- or 12-mm trocar and sleeve. After the sleeve is in the cavity, the trocar is removed. The laparoscope is inserted into the sleeve and the gas reconnected. The uterus is manipulated by holding the vaginal apparatus already in the vagina.

If a second puncture is needed, the lower abdominal wall is illuminated with the laparoscope to select an avascular site for the incision. A small incision is made. A 3- or 5-mm trocar and sleeve are used. The surgeon may look through the laparoscope and use the second incision for operative instruments. A third or fourth port is sometimes used for extensive laparoscopic procedures.

Indigo carmine may be injected through the Jarcho or Sparkman cannula to check for tubal patency. Via the laparoscope, the dye may be seen flowing through the fallopian tubes and any obstruction noted.

Closure

The laparoscope is removed from the sleeve. Carbon dioxide is forced out of the abdomen. The sleeve is removed. If a second puncture apparatus was used, it is removed in the same manner. All incisions are closed with the surgeon's choice of suture. Antibiotic ointment and adhesive bandages are used for dressings. The vaginal apparatus is gently removed, and the cervix is checked for any bleeding. Pressure is used to stop any bleeding that may occur.

Postprocedure Care

The patient is taken to the PACU for a short time. Any bleeding is checked and noted. The patient is instructed to take her temperature two times per day for 1 week and report to the physician if it is more than 100°F (37.8°C). Acetaminophen should be used for mild pain. Activity may be gradually increased. Referred pain may be experienced in the shoulder. The patient is discharged the same day.

Potential Complications

Infection and hemorrhage are potential complications.

LAPAROSCOPICALLY ASSISTED VAGINAL HYSTERECTOMY

Laparoscopically assisted vaginal hysterectomy (LAVH) is the removal of the uterus and cervix (hysterectomy) and possibly the tubes and ovaries via the vagina after the laparoscope is used to resect the ovaries, lyse adhesions, and/or resect endometriosis (Reich, 2007).

LAVH
Laparoscopically Assisted Vaginal Hysterectomy

Indications

LAVH is indicated when there is a need for hysterectomy in the presence of pelvic floor relaxation with or without pathological processes such as pelvic and abdominal adhesions, endometriosis, fibroids, and/or adnexal disease. The avoidance of an abdominal incision is one of the major advantages (Falcone & Covey-Levy, 2007).

Nursing Implications

Anesthesia

The procedure is performed with general or spinal anesthesia. In some cases, the patient should be typed and screened so blood can he readily available if necessary.

Position

The patient is placed in the modified lithotomy position with the hips extended. During the procedure, the bed should be tilted in deep Trendelenburg position. Refer to the section on positioning.

Establishing and Maintaining the Sterile Field

A skin prep of surgeon's choice is used to prepare the operative site, which should include the perineum and vagina. A Foley catheter is inserted and hooked to straight drainage. The electrosurgical patient return electrode is placed on the patient according to the manufacturer's instructions. Drapes are applied as follows: A half sheet is placed under the buttocks. Leg drapes are then applied followed by a laparotomy sheet with an opening over both the abdomen and perineum. The instruments for the vaginal and abdominal portions of the procedure should be placed on separate tables. The surgeon is positioned on the patient's left side with the instrument table and scrub person close to the patient's leg. Before beginning the procedure, the scrub person should make sure that all equipment is functioning properly. There should be two monitors, one for the surgeon and one for the assistant. If another assistant is available, he or she should be positioned at the foot of the table.

Equipment and Supplies

> Laparoscopy set
>
> Hysteroscopy set
>
> Vaginal set
>
> Magnetic pad
>
> All other basic and laparoscopic supplies per surgeon's preference
>
> Endoscopic supplies
>
> Irrigation system and probe
>
> Camera cover
>
> CO_2
>
> Verres needle or blunt trocar
>
> CO_2 insufflator
>
> Satellite monitor
>
> Insufflator
>
> 0 degree laparoscope

Physiological Monitoring

Physiological monitoring is carried out by the anesthesia provider.

Specimens and Cultures

Specimens include the uterus and cervix. In some instances, the fallopian tubes and ovaries may be included. All specimens are routinely sent to the pathology laboratory unless otherwise ordered.

Drugs and Solutions

No drugs other than anesthetic are needed for this procedure. Normal saline is used to irrigate the pelvis.

Physician Orders

The patient is instructed to have nothing to eat after 8 p.m. and no liquids after midnight the night before the procedure. A Fleet enema may be ordered.

Laboratory and Diagnostic Studies

Preprocedure testing depends on the age and medical condition of the patient. The patient's preprocedure testing may include CBC, ECG, urinalysis, and electrolyte values. Blood typing and screening is recommended.

Procedure

Incision and Exposure

After the patient is placed in the lithotomy position, the hips are extended to allow access to the abdomen. The cervix is exposed with a heavy weighted speculum and a Deaver or right-angle retractor. A cannula is inserted into the cervix and attached to a tenaculum. Attention is then focused on the abdomen. Towel clips or manual grasping are used to elevate the umbilicus. An incision is made into the umbilicus with a No. 11 blade.

Details

The Verres needle is then inserted through the umbilicus into the abdominal cavity. The carbon dioxide tubing is attached. Enough carbon dioxide is allowed to enter the abdominal cavity to maintain approximately 14–15 mm Hg of intra-abdominal pressure. A 12-mm trocar is then inserted into the abdomen through the umbilicus. Two to three other incisions are made. One incision is made suprapubically in the midline, into which a 5 to 12 mm trocar is inserted, and incisions are also made in the left and right lower quadrants, lateral to the deep epigastric vessels. Adhesions, if present, are lysed to allow for exposure of the pelvic organs. The ureters must be identified to avoid injury. The retroperitoneal space is entered lateral to the infundibulopelvic (IP) ligament by holding traction on the ovary. After isolation at the IP ligament, the gastrointestinal anastomosis (GIA) stapler is used to cut the IP ligament. Electrosurgery of the IP ligament, followed by excision, may be performed instead of stapling. The tissue between the ovary and the round ligament is coagulated and divided by sharp dissection. The vesicouterine peritoneum is divided to allow for separation of the bladder from the uterus. At this point, the rest of the procedure is carried out vaginally. After the procedure, the laparoscope is used to check for hemostasis. The pelvis is lavaged with copious amounts of normal saline. Before removing the laparoscope, the carbon dioxide is allowed to escape. The laparoscope is used to visualize the ports and the operative site to check for hemostasis. The laparoscope is then removed.

IP
Infundibulopelvic

GIA
Gastrointestinal Anastomosis

Closure

The larger ports are closed by suturing the fascia as well as the skin with 3-0 and 4-0 polyglactin, respectively.

Postprocedure Care

The patient is taken to the PACU for observation and is admitted for 1–2 days. Refer to the discussions of vaginal hysterectomy.

Potential Complications

Potential complications include hemorrhage, bladder injury, bowel injury, ureteral injury, and infection.

TOTAL ABDOMINAL HYSTERECTOMY WITH BILATERAL SALPINGO-OOPHORECTOMY

Total abdominal hysterectomy with bilateral salpingo-oophorectomy entails the removal of the uterus, the cervix, the fallopian tubes, and the ovaries through an abdominal incision (Falcone & Cogan-Levy, 2007).

Indications

Abdominal hysterectomy with bilateral salpingo-oophorectomy is performed for endometriosis, uterine fibroids, pre-malignant or malignant conditions, obstetrical emergencies, and severe pelvic inflammatory disease.

Related Procedures

Related procedures are simple abdominal hysterectomy, vaginal hysterectomy, and radical hysterectomy.

Nursing Implications
Anesthesia

The procedure is performed with general endotracheal or spinal anesthesia. Two units of blood may be ordered for the patient.

Position

The patient is placed in the supine position. Refer to the discussion on positioning.

Establishing and Maintaining the Sterile Field

To minimize contamination as the cervix is pulled up into the pelvis after the uterus is freed, the vagina must be prepared internally. The preparation can be accomplished with the patient in either of two positions: the lithotomy position or the frog-leg position. The preparation should concentrate on the vagina itself. To accomplish this, sponge sticks (ring forceps) are used. After the preparation has been completed, a Foley catheter is inserted into the bladder and connected to a urinary drainage bag. The electrosurgical patient return electrode is placed on the patient according to the manufacturer's instructions. The patient is draped according to basic laparotomy technique. The Mayo stand is placed over the patient's feet. The large instrument table is placed to the scrub person's dominant side, with square tables placed behind the scrub person. The electrosurgical unit is placed at the right side of the patient's head.

Equipment and Supplies

> Abdominal hysterectomy set
>
> 60-mL syringe (if pelvic washing is to be obtained)
>
> All other basic laparotomy instruments
>
> Suture of choice

Physiological Monitoring

The circulating nurse must catheterize the patient before the surgical preparation is accomplished. A Foley catheter is inserted into the bladder and attached to a urinary bag. The circulating nurse monitors and records blood loss and irrigating fluids during the procedure. In many instances, the surgeon prefers wet sponges after the abdomen is opened. Usually, 2 U of blood are available for the procedure.

Specimens and Cultures

The uterus, the cervix, the ovaries, and the fallopian tubes are sent to the pathology laboratory. If after gross examination the surgeon believes that the ovarian specimen looks abnormal, a frozen section examination may be requested.

Drugs and Solutions

If washings are to be obtained, a 1000-mL bag of combined electrolyte solution with 5000 U of heparin is available on the scrub table.

Physician Orders

Admission and preprocedure orders may include a Fleet enema the night before the procedure, cross-matching and typing for 2 U of blood, NPO orders, and skin preparation which may include a vaginal douche and a shower.

Laboratory and Diagnostic Studies

Preprocedure testing depends on the age and medical condition of the patient. The patient's preprocedure testing may include CBC, ECG, urinalysis, and electrolyte values. If the hemoglobin level is less than 10 g/dL, the surgeon may order a blood transfusion before the procedure.

Procedure

Incision and Exposure

A midline or Pfannenstiel incision is used. An O'Connor-O'Sullivan retractor is preferred. The bowel is packed off with warm wet sponges. Before the retractor is introduced, the abdomen is explored. Bleeding is controlled with 2-0 chromic or 3-0 polyglactin ties and suture ligatures, along with the electrosurgery.

Details

The round ligaments are identified and grasped with a Heaney or Kelly clamp close to the uterine cornu. The ligaments are ligated with heavy suture and cut. After both round ligaments are cut, the anterior leaf of the broad ligament is exposed and incised with Metzenbaum scissors. The anterior leaf is pushed forward and incised, making a hole in the broad ligament. The ureters are identified so that no injury can occur. Next, the ovarian ligament and tube are clamped through the hole that was made previously. The ligament is divided and ligated. The bladder is mobilized inferiorly with scissors and forceps, away from the cervix. The uterine vessels are doubly clamped, ligated, and cut. The cardinal ligaments are then clamped, cut, and ligated. The uterosacral ligaments are clamped, cut, and tied. The bladder base is freed from the anterior vaginal wall. Curved Heaney clamps are then placed across the vaginal angles and the uterus is removed by incising the vagina below the cervix with a knife or scissors. The vagina is closed with interrupted figure-of-eight stitches with No. 0 or No. 1 polyglactin sutures (**Figs. 29.7 A–E**).

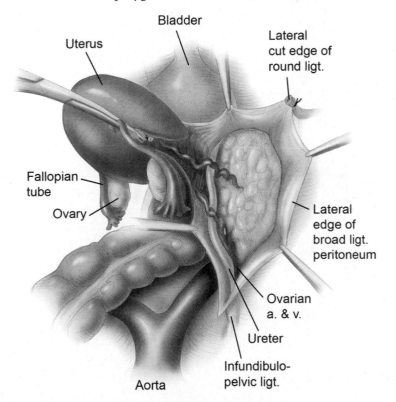

Figure 29.7A

Technique for abdominal hysterectomy. The round ligament has been clamped, cut, and tied, and the broad ligament opened.

Bladder

Uterus

Lateral cut edge of round ligt.

Fallopian tube

Ovary

Lateral edge of broad ligt. peritoneum

Ovarian a. & v.

Ureter

Infundibulo-pelvic ligt.

Aorta

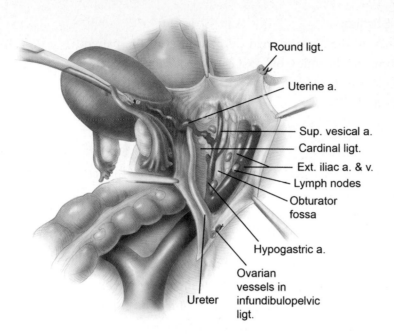

Round ligt.

Uterine a.

Sup. vesical a.

Cardinal ligt.

Ext. iliac a. & v.

Lymph nodes

Obturator fossa

Hypogastric a.

Ovarian vessels in infundibulopelvic ligt.

Ureter

Figure 29.7B

Technique for abdominal hysterectomy. The retroperitoneal space has been opened, revealing the ureter and pelvic vessels.

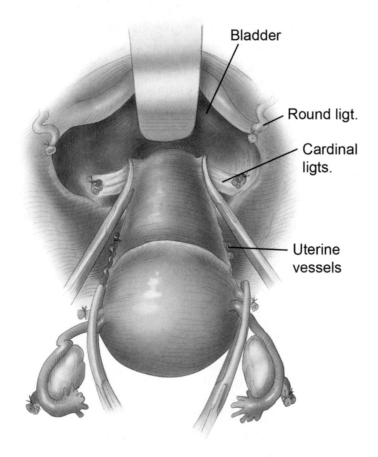

Bladder

Round ligt.

Cardinal ligts.

Uterine vessels

Figure 29.7C

Technique for abdominal hysterectomy.
The infundibulopelvic ligaments and uterine arteries have been secured, the bladder dissected off the cervix, and the cardinal ligaments clamped.

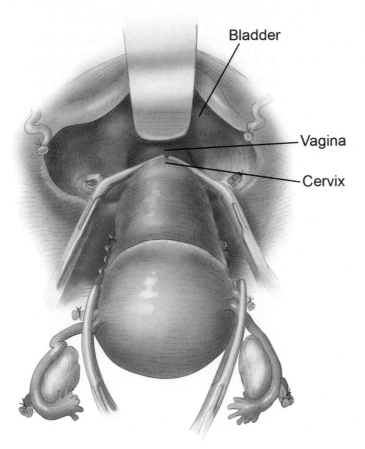

Bladder

Vagina

Cervix

Figure 29.7D

Technique for abdominal hysterectomy. Clamps have been placed across the upper vagina.

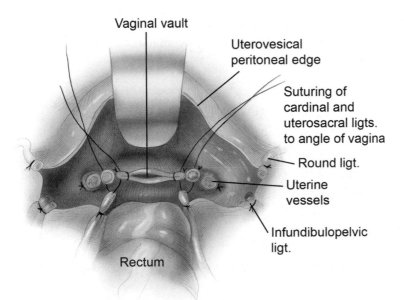

Vaginal vault

Uterovesical peritoneal edge

Suturing of cardinal and uterosacral ligts. to angle of vagina

Round ligt.

Uterine vessels

Infundibulopelvic ligt.

Rectum

Figure 29.7E

Technique for abdominal hysterectomy. The uterus has been removed, and the vaginal vault is being closed.

29

Closure

The abdomen is checked for any bleeding. All packing sponges are removed and counted. Retractors are removed. The abdomen is again irrigated with saline or lactated Ringer's solution. The peritoneum is closed with a 1-0 polyglactin suture, followed by a 1-0 polyglactin suture for the fascia layer. A 3-0 polyglactin suture is used for the subcutaneous fat. A 4-0 polyglactin suture on a cutting needle is used for sewing the skin or skin staples are applied.

Postprocedure Care

The patient is taken to the PACU, with typical orders as follows:

PCA
Patient-Controlled
Analgesia

> Measurement of vital signs
>
> Restriction to bed rest
>
> Patient-controlled analgesia (PCA) for administration of pain medications, which is discontinued when medication is tolerated by mouth
>
> NPO status; diet advanced as tolerated
>
> Antibiotics per surgeon's request
>
> Intake and output measurement (with removal of Foley catheter the morning after the procedure, if the urine is clear)
>
> Deep breathing exercises

The patient is usually discharged 2 days after the procedure.

Potential Complications

Potential complications include hemorrhage, bladder injury, bowel injury, ureteral injury, and infection.

VAGINAL HYSTERECTOMY

Vaginal hysterectomy is the removal of the uterus, the cervix, and, if necessary, the fallopian tubes and the ovaries by way of the vagina rather than through an abdominal incision (Falcone & Cogan-Levy, 2007).

Indications

Vaginal hysterectomy is indicated for benign disease or carcinoma in situ of the cervix. The vaginal approach is considered when the woman has at least a third-degree uterine prolapse and the uterus can easily be pulled into the vaginal vault. It should not be performed if the patient has extensive endometriosis, large uterine fibroids, invasive carcinoma, other suspected disease, or previous uterine suspension.

Nursing Implications
Anesthesia

General anesthesia is preferred, but spinal anesthesia with sedation is also an option.

Position

Lithotomy position with high stirrups allows best exposure for the vaginal hysterectomy procedure.

Establishing and Maintaining the Sterile Field

Preparation of the operative site should include the perineum and the vagina. A folded sheet is placed as far under the buttocks as possible. An adherent disposable drape is then applied to isolate the anus. Next, leg drapes are applied, with a large drape sheet over the abdomen. The surgeon usually sits during this procedure. The scrub person should be positioned closest to the surgeon's dominant arm. The small square table is positioned to the right of the large table; this table holds all of the retractors for the procedure. The electrosurgical patient return electrode is placed on the patient according to the manufacturer's instructions. The circulating nurse assists the scrub person with the positioning of tables. A double-folded plain sheet should be placed in the surgeon's lap. A sterile tray and magnetic pad may also be added to enable the surgeon to have frequently used instruments available at all times.

Equipment and Supplies

> Vaginal procedure tray
>
> Magnetic pad (optional)
>
> Tray with Mayo cover
>
> Foley catheter
>
> Other basic supplies
>
> A sterile tray in a Mayo cover allows the surgeon to keep some instruments (scissors, hemostats) close at hand. A magnetic pad is used to prevent instruments that may be left on the field from falling to the floor.

Physiological Monitoring

The circulating nurse is responsible for accurately measuring and recording all blood loss and local anesthetic used.

Specimens and Cultures

The uterus and the cervix are routinely sent to the pathology laboratory. Fallopian tubes and ovaries may be included, if salpingo-oophorectomy is performed.

Drugs and Solutions

One percent lidocaine with 1:200,000 epinephrine is sometimes injected into the cervix with a 10-mL syringe with either a tonsil needle or a 22-gauge needle attached. This aids in reducing bleeding.

Physician Orders

Patient instructions may include cross-matching and typing for 2 units of blood, NPO instructions, administering a Fleet enema, and skin preparation including vaginal vault douche, clipping hair, and showering.

Laboratory and Diagnostic Studies

A CBC, ECG, urinalysis, chest radiograph, and electrolyte determination must be obtained. If the hemoglobin level is less than 10 g/dL, the surgeon may order a blood transfusion before the procedure.

29

Procedure

Incision and Exposure

A weighted speculum or Sweeney retractor is placed posteriorly, with small Deaver or Heaney retractors used anteriorly and laterally.

Details

The patient undergoes straight catheterization with a Foley catheter at the start of the procedure. Retractors are positioned in the vagina. The cervix is grasped with a Jacob tenaculum to pull the uterus down into the vagina. At this point, if the surgeon believes it is necessary, the cervix is injected with 1% lidocaine with 1:200,000 epinephrine. Heavy scissors and forceps are then used to cut around the cervix and peritoneum. Metzenbaum scissors are used to enter the peritoneum. The bladder is freed from the uterus in front and from the rectum in back. The uterosacral ligaments are clamped with Heaney clamps, ligated with heavy suture, and then cut. Heaney clamps are next applied to the cardinal ligaments. After this is accomplished, the peritoneal cavity is entered and the uterine arteries are clamped, ligated, and cut. Again, heavy suture ligatures are used. The fundus of the uterus is delivered from the abdomen. The round ligaments are clamped with Heaney clamps, ligated, and cut. The peritoneum is closed with a pursestring suture of 2-0 chromic. The uterus is freed and removed from the vagina. To prevent prolapse, the cardinal ligaments are sutured to the superior angle of the vagina, with the uterosacral ligaments tied to prevent enterocele.

Closure

The vaginal cuff is closed with interrupted 2-0 catgut or 3-0 polyglactin suture. A Foley catheter is placed in the bladder at the end of the procedure. Occasionally, the vagina is packed with vaginal packing and antibiotic cream.

Postprocedure Care

PACU
Postanesthesia Care Unit

The patient is taken to the postanesthesia care unit (PACU) for a short time. Orders may include measurement of vital signs, restriction to bed rest, NPO status and then diet as tolerated, Foley catheter in place, intake and output monitored and recorded, IV administration, administration of pain medication as needed, administration of sedatives as needed, antibiotic regimen for 3 days, and CBC on the first postprocedure day.

Potential Complications

Infection and hemorrhage are potential complications. There may be increased vaginal bleeding in comparison with that after the abdominal procedure. Amount of blood loss should be recorded.

SKINNING VULVECTOMY

Skinning vulvectomy is a surgical procedure removing the vulvar skin and replacing it with a split–thickness graft (Helm, 2003).

Indications

Skinning vulvectomy is indicated to treat extensive vulvar intraepithelial neoplasia. It is primarily performed when other procedures are inadequate (Elkas and Berek, 2007).

Related Procedures

Related procedures are simple vulvectomy and radical vulvectomy.

Nursing Implications

Anesthesia

General, epidural, or spinal anesthesia can be administered.

Position

The patient is placed in the dorsal lithotomy position using low stirrups. A Foley catheter to straight drain is then inserted.

Establishing and Maintaining the Sterile Field

The perineum, vagina, and donor site must be prepped with a scrub solution of the physician's choice. A double-folded sheet is placed under the buttocks with leg drapes applied next. The surgeon sits for this procedure.

Equipment and Supplies

In addition to the instruments for vaginal hysterectomy, a skin graft tray and mesher should be available.

Physiological Monitoring

The circulating nurse monitors and records blood loss during the procedure. A Foley catheter is inserted at the end of the procedure and left in place until the graft has taken.

Specimens and Cultures

The perivulvar tissue is sent to the pathology laboratory.

Drugs and Solutions

No drugs (other than anesthetic) or solutions are needed for this procedure.

Physician Orders

Before the procedure, a bowel prep may be ordered in case there is damage to the rectum or anus. The patient must have NPO orders the evening before the procedure. Sedatives may be prescribed. Preprocedure antibiotics and medications are usually ordered.

Laboratory and Diagnostic Studies

Preprocedure testing depends on the age and medical condition of the patient. The testing may include CBC, ECG, urinalysis, and electrolyte values.

Procedure

Incision and Exposure

The skin margins are outlined with a marking pen before the incision is made. The incision is made down and through the dermis.

Details

With tension on the sides of the proposed incision, a No. 10 knife blade is used for the incision. An Allis clamp or elevated forceps are used to grasp the skin as it is dissected from the subcutaneous tissues, while keeping close to the underside of the dermis. If the clitoris and clitoral hood is involved with vulvar intraepithelial neoplasia, it can be preserved and treated with laser ablation later (**Figs. 29.8 A–C**). Hemostasis is obtained by applying pressure to the operative area. All remaining bleeding sites are coagulated with the electrosurgical active electrode. A split-thickness skin graft is taken from the inner thigh. In case the graft does not take completely, the excess skin is refrigerated for future use.

Closure

The skin graft is sewn into place with interrupted 3-0 polyglactin or silk suture.

Postprocedure Care

After a short stay in the PACU, orders are as follows: intake and output monitored, Foley catheter remains in place, administration of pain medications, dressing checks, antibiotic therapy regimen, and bed rest. Discharge is dependent on the progress of

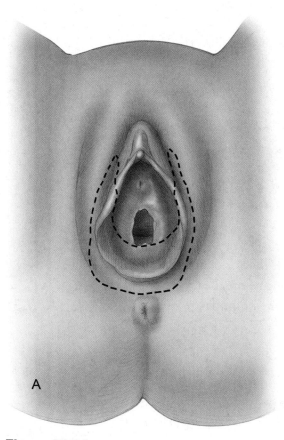

Figure 29.8A

Partial vulvectomy. The incision encompasses all involved areas with an 8–10 mm margin but spares unaffected tissue,

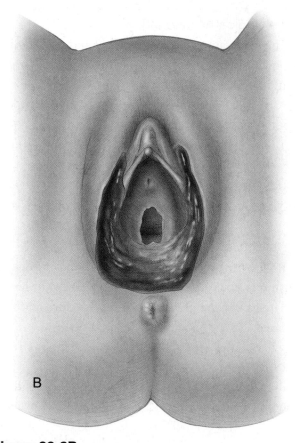

Figure 29.8B

Partial vulvectomy. Dissection is shallow down to the underlying fat.

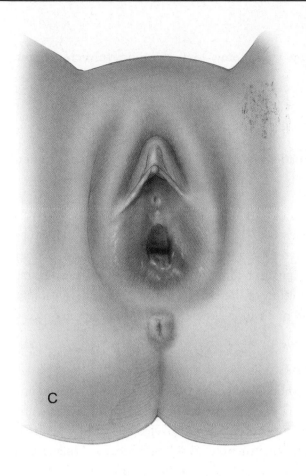

Figure 29.8C
Partial vulvectomy.
The final result shows
good cosmetic
appearance.

C

healing. Activity for the first week includes bed rest or sitting in a chair. Pulmonary embolus prophylaxis is ordered. The vulvar dressings are left in place for 4–5 days unless infection is suspected. Dressings are removed on the fifth post-op day after pain medication is given. The wound is left open if the graft has taken. Rinsing with saline or Sitz baths and drying with a hair dryer is necessary. If the graft did not successfully take, the old graft is debrided and the stored skin graft is applied. The donor site dressing is inspected daily, but left in place for 2 weeks.

Potential Complications

Infection, graft rejection, and scarring around the introitus (vaginal orifice) are potential complications.

RADICAL VULVECTOMY AND GROIN LYMPHADENECTOMY

Radical vulvectomy is the removal of the entire vulva extending down to the deep fascia of the thigh, the pubis periosteum, and the inferior fascia of the urogenital diaphragm (Helm, 2006).

Indications

Radical vulvectomy is indicated for malignant disease of the vulva. It is often performed in conjunction with a unilateral or bilateral groin node dissection.

Related Procedures

Related procedures are skinning vulvectomy, total skinning vulvectomy, and simple vulvectomy.

Nursing Implications

Anesthesia

General anesthetic is most often administered; however, epidural or spinal anesthesia can be used.

Position

Depending on the surgeon's preference, the patient may be placed in the supine position for node dissection and then placed in the lithotomy position, or she may be placed in the modified lithotomy position for both parts of the procedure. Having the perineum protrude over the bottom of the operating table enhances visibility. The sacrum is supported with a pad or cushion. Antiembolism stockings are placed on the patient's legs.

Establishing and Maintaining the Sterile Field

The area for radical vulvectomy should include the abdomen and the perineum. Skin prep solution (surgeon's choice) is used to prepare the abdomen, the perineum, and the upper thigh area. The electrosurgical patient return electrode is placed on the patient according to the manufacturer's instructions, avoiding the thighs as placement sites in case skin flaps are needed. If the modified lithotomy position is selected for the procedure, the area is draped, with both the abdomen and the perineum exposed. The rectum is draped out of the sterile field using a disposable adherent drape. If the patient is placed first in the supine position and then in the lithotomy position, extra drapes should be available. The scrub person should make sure that the tables are not contaminated when the patient is repositioned. The instrument tables are placed closest to the scrub person's dominant arm. This position should accommodate either patient positioning.

Equipment and Supplies

     Major gynecological set

     Suture of preference

     Hemoclips, large and medium

     Wound drains, large

Physiological Monitoring

A urethral catheter is inserted into the bladder and urine volume is monitored. Blood loss must be accurately measured, along with any irrigating fluids used.

Specimens and Cultures

Nodes are dissected, excised, and may be sent to the pathology laboratory for frozen section examination. If the results of the frozen section examination indicate carcinoma, the retroperitoneal nodes are then dissected. All specimens, to include the vulva, are sent to pathology.

Drugs and Solutions

No particular drugs other than anesthetic are used during this procedure. Saline or lactated Ringers solution may be used for irrigation during node dissection. Antibiotics are given per surgeon's request. In many instances, patients are pre-medicated before arriving in the operative procedure suite.

Physician Orders

Careful explanation and counseling about the effects of this procedure is necessary for all women undergoing radical vulvar surgery. A thorough bowel prep is ordered one to two days before the procedure and NPO status is necessary the night before. Antibiotics, sedatives, and other medications are ordered according to surgeon preference. Clippers are used for hair removal.

Laboratory and Diagnostic Studies

Testing usually includes a CBC with differential, prothrombin time, partial thromboplastin time, electrolyte panel, urinalysis, chest radiograph, and ECG. Other testing is ordered based on the patient's medical condition.

Procedure

Incision and Exposure

After carefully examining the patient to identify the limits of spread, a marking pen is used to identify where the skin should be incised, externally and within the vagina. Frozen sections should now be taken of the biopsies if required. A low Pfannenstiel incision is used then extended to look like a rabbit's head. **Figures 29.9 A and B**

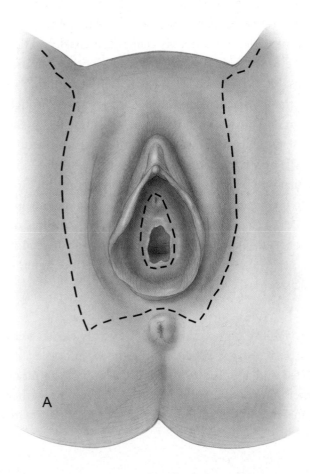

Figure 29.9A

Radical vulvectomy. Outline of the incision includes the perineum.

A

29

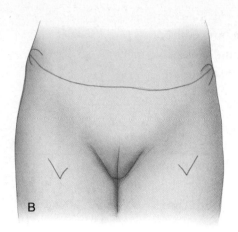

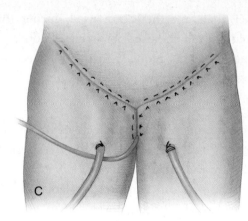

Figure 29.9B and C

Radical vulvectomy. (B) Landmarks for groin dissection incision are the iliac crests and the apices of Hunter's canal in the legs. (C) Postoperative drainage system in place.

show the outline of the incision, which includes the perineum, and landmarks for groin dissection. Handheld retractors such as Deaver retractors are used and preferred. 3-0 ties and suture ligatures are used as is electrosurgery.

Details

The skin incision is started posteriorly using a No. 10 knife blade, extends laterally on both sides and dissection is taken all the way through the subcutaneous fat to the deep fascia. The tissues are separated from the deep fascia and pubic ramus with a scalpel or scissors until the vaginal resection margin is reached. Posterolaterally, branches of the pudendal artery will require attention. Damage to the anal sphincter is avoided, while still obtaining an adequate margin around a tumor. Placing a finger in the rectum can assist in these circumstances. The femoral nerve, artery, and vein in the femoral sheath are identified. The saphenous vein is next identified, doubly clamped, incised, and tied with silk suture. Cloquet's nodes are removed and sent for frozen section examination. As mentioned, if the node results are abnormal, node dissection continues to include the deep pelvic nodes. For the lymphadenectomy, the incision goes through full thickness of the skin and 2–3 mm into the fat. The procedure is continued, and the focus is on the vulva. The inguinal flaps are passed into the lower field. The pudendal artery and vein are clamped with Crile or Mixter clamps and tied with silk suture. Allis clamps are used to retract the area that is to be removed. The remainder of the incision is made. The incision is extended to include the lateral border of the labia majora and the vestibule around the meatus, to cross the posterior fourchette, and to continue on the other side. With a No. 10 blade or Metzenbaum scissors and forceps, the dissection is made along the fascia until the perineal body is reached. The posterior vagina is elevated with an Allis clamp, and scissors are used to release the rectum.

Closure

The skin flaps are checked for viability before closure. The skin is closed with staples or interrupted vertical mattress sutures. When closing the wound, the skin above the urethral meatus is everted and apposed to the residual skin of the mons pubis. Some surgeons place marker sutures to assure the edges will come together the right way. Suction drains are inserted in the groin bilaterally, sewn in place with

2-0 polypropylene suture (**Fig. 29.9 C**). The inguinal area and then the urethra, paravaginal area, and fascia are closed with suture of surgeon's choice. Skin edges are then closed. Depending on surgeon preference, a paraffin gauze may be placed over the wound followed by a gauze dressing.

Postprocedure Care

The patient is taken to the PACU or the intensive care unit after the procedure. Routine orders are as follows:

Bed rest for 2–3 days

Sequential compression stockings

Active leg movements

Subcutaneous heparin depending on surgeon preference

Intake and output monitored

Foley catheter to straight drain

Wound inspection daily

Cleanse perineum with sterile saline after 48 hours and dry with a hair dryer

Sitz baths on day 4

Antibiotic therapy regimen

Administration of medication for pain

Low residue diet and constipating agents for 3 days if the anal sphincter or rectum were repaired

Stool softeners as ordered after 3 days

Suction drains discontinued after 3–5 days, even if still draining lymph

Discharge dependent on healing and/or wound breakdown

Potential Complications

Wound breakdown is not uncommon with radical vulvectomy. Hematomas and seromas may require evacuation. Infection, UTI, thromboembolism and osteitis pubis are potential complications. Lymphadenectomy complications include wound infection, wound breakdown and lymphedema.

PELVIC EXENTERATION

Pelvic exenteration is an extensive procedure that involves the removal of fallopian tubes, ovaries, uterus, cervix, pelvic nodes, bladder, distal ureters, rectum, and pelvic floor. Mesh is sometimes used to form a pelvic floor. This procedure is the only potentially curative option for women with central carcinoma recurrence after radiation therapy or surgery.

Indications

Pelvic exenteration is indicated in patients with carcinoma of the cervix who, after radiation therapy for stage IV disease, have a tumor that recurs and erodes into the bladder and the rectum. Pelvic exenteration is for the treatment of locally recurrent or advanced endometrial cancer. It is associated with a high operative morbidity (Hatch, 2007).

Related Procedures

Related procedures are radical hysterectomy, anterior exenteration, and posterior exenteration.

Nursing Implications

Anesthesia

In many instances, an epidural catheter is inserted before anesthesia induction and is used for pain control after the procedure. A general endotracheal anesthetic is used for the surgical procedure. Because of the length of the procedure, arterial catheters are inserted. Blood loss during the procedure can be substantial.

Position

The patient is positioned in modified dorsal lithotomy position using stirrups to support the legs. Both arms are extended on arm boards.

Establishing and Maintaining the Sterile Field

A skin prep of surgeon's choice is used to prepare the operative site, which should include the perineum and the vagina. The skin should be prepared to include the total abdomen, the upper thighs, the perineum, and the vagina. The electrosurgical patient return electrode is placed on the patient according to the manufacturer's instructions. The patient is draped with laparotomy as well as vaginal drapes. Two instrument tables are prepared for pelvic exenteration (upper, or abdominal, and lower, or perineal). Both tables are set up at the beginning of the procedure. The scrub person may be positioned to the patient's right, with the instrument table close at hand. If a Mayo stand is used, it is positioned over the patient's right leg for the abdominal part of the procedure. The electrosurgical unit is placed to the right of the patient's head.

Equipment and Supplies

    Upper table

    Major gynecology set (total abdominal hysterectomy)

    Magnetic pad

    Colostomy bags

    60-mL syringes (for washings)

    All other basic laparotomy supplies

    Skin staples

    Large wound drains

    Suture per surgeon's choice

    Lower table

    Dissecting set

    Plastic surgery set

    Surgical sponges

    Suction tubing

    Electrosurgical pencil

    Suture per surgeon's choice

    Allen stirrups with padding and holders

Physiological Monitoring

The circulating nurse is available to catheterize the patient, if requested. The catheter is removed after the ureters are severed from the bladder. Both the circulating and scrub persons should be aware of blood loss and irrigating fluids used during the procedure. Blood loss is usually substantial.

Specimens and Cultures

For each washing taken, a separate cytology specimen form must be used. Samples may be from the pelvis, right and left subdiaphragm, and right and left gutters. Specimens include the uterus, the ovaries, the fallopian tubes, the bladder, the distal ureters, the rectum, and the lymph nodes. The circulating nurse should have a sufficient number of stamped pathology laboratory forms, printed patient labels, and specimen containers for routine and frozen sections.

Drugs and Solutions

Washings are obtained during the abdominal part of the procedure. A 1000-mL bag of irrigation solution is poured from a sterile spout into a solution basin with 5000 U of heparin added. Sixty-mL syringes are filled with the solution, and Pomeroy adaptors are attached. Each washing is then placed in a sterile container. No. 16 red rubber catheters may be used to obtain gutter washings. Warm irrigation solution is available for use. Antibiotics are always given.

Physician Orders

The evening before the procedure, the patient must have a cleansing enema and shower. A regular meal is given for dinner, and NPO orders are in effect after midnight. As ordered by the anesthesia provider, a sedative is given. Sequential compression stockings are applied before the procedure.

Laboratory and Diagnostic Studies

A CBC, blood urea nitrogen measurement, creatinine clearance measurement, and liver function studies must be obtained. Chest radiography and IV pyelography are also ordered. In addition, a barium enema is often included.

Procedure

Incision and Exposure

The abdomen is entered through a low midline incision. The retractor of choice is used. All bleeding is controlled with 3-0 ties and suture ligatures, along with the electrosurgery unit.

Details

The upper abdomen is explored. The right common iliac vein and artery are identified. Washings are taken at this time. Next, the aortic lymph nodes are palpated, and any suspicious lymph nodes are removed with scissors and forceps, and sent for frozen section examination. If the nodes are reported to be normal, the procedure continues.

The peritoneal incision is extended along the external iliac vessels to the femoral canal. Again with the use of scissors and forceps, the lymphatic tissue is incised from the common iliac veins. The round ligaments (clamped with Heaney clamps) are ligated with heavy suture, cut, and tied, which opens the broad ligament. The lymphatic tissue is removed from the obturator fossa. The uterosacral ligaments are next clamped, cut, and tied at the pelvic brim.

The ureters are transected below the pelvic brim. The hypo-gastric artery and vein are clamped with Mixter clamps and tied at the bifurcation of the common iliac vessels. The lateral peritoneum of the mesentery of the rectosigmoid colon is opened. A Penrose drain is placed through an opening and used for retraction of the colon. The colon is clamped and transected with the internal stapling device). The remaining mesentery to the colon is clamped and incised down to the sacrum. The rectum is dissected from the sacrum and coccyx by blunt dissection. The stalks of rectum on both sides are clamped, incised, and tied down to the levator muscles.

The bladder is separated from the pubic symphysis. The lateral attachments of the bladder are clamped and incised on both sides. The anterior wall of the paravesical space and the posterior wall of the pararectal space are removed by dissecting the rectal stalks and bladder attachments. The urethra is exposed and transected at the level of the levator, and the vagina is transected.

The rectum is anastomosed to the descending colon. The intestinal loop urinary diversion is made from the sigmoid colon. The proximal sigmoid colon is transected with the internal stapling device. The ureters are anastomosed to the sigmoid colon. The colon is anastomosed to the rectum. A wound drain is placed in the vagina. An omental flap is made and is moved into the pelvis. The omental flap holds the intestines out of the true pelvis. Depending on the surgeon, it may not be necessary to use a perineal approach.

Closure

The abdomen is closed in the usual abdominal closure manner.

Postprocedure Care

The patient is admitted to the PACU or the surgical intensive care unit. Extensive care is required for these patients after the procedure. Typical orders include the following;

> NPO until bowel sounds return
>
> Intake and output measured
>
> Daily weights obtained
>
> Restricted to bed rest
>
> Dressing checks made
>
> Antibiotic therapy given
>
> Whole blood given as needed
>
> Potassium administered as ordered by the surgeon
>
> Heparin therapy given
>
> Drains removed when no longer productive
>
> Pain medications administered as needed

Discharge from the hospital is dependent on the patient's ability to perform self-care, normal diet, adequate physical and mental ability, minimal drug requirements, stable weight, no fever for at least 4–5 days, and understanding of possible complications.

Potential Complications

Infection and hemorrhage are the potential complications.

TUBAL LIGATION

Elective, operative, female sterilization can be accomplished abdominally, laparoscopically, or vaginally. Abdominal and laparoscopic procedures are essentially permanent. There are no absolute contraindications, but certain gynecologic disease may require sterilization by hysterectomy and bilateral oophorectomy (Stovall & Mann, 2006).

Indications

These procedures are indicated for women who desire permanent sterilization.

Related Procedures

Postpartum tubal ligations, laparoscopic tubal ligations, and mini-laparotomy sterilization are all related procedures.

Nursing Implications
Anesthesia

General anesthesia is administered for laparoscopic and mini-laparotomy tubal ligations. Spinal or epidural anesthesia may be used for postpartum tubal ligations.

Position

Depending on the surgical approach, the patient is positioned in supine or lithotomy positions.

Establishing and Maintaining the Sterile Field

A skin prep of the surgeon's choice is used to prep the abdomen. A vault prep is performed for a D&C or if a uterine manipulator is used.

Equipment and Supplies

For the laparoscopic approach, a laparoscope, camera, video system, electrosurgery unit, trocars, insufflation tubing CO_2, and other laparoscopic instrumentation is needed. Depending on surgeon preference, a uterine manipulator may be used to manipulate the uterus during laparoscopy. Skin closure suture and small dressings are needed. If a D&C is going to be performed, a D&C set is available. When performed open, instrumentation may include a major or minor instrument set along with electrosurgery unit. Suture for tying the tube and closing the skin is necessary. Abdominal dressings are needed.

Physiological Monitoring

The circulating nurse monitors blood loss, irrigating fluids, and amount of CO_2 insufflation.

Specimens and Cultures

With the abdominal approach, tissue specimens (fallopian tubes) are sent to the lab for histologic exam.

Drugs and Solutions

No particular drugs other than anesthetics are used. Irrigation for the laparoscopic approach is usually normal saline. Antibiotics are surgeon preference.

Physician Orders

Patients are instructed to be NPO the night before the proposed procedure.

Laboratory and Diagnostic Studies

CBC, urinalysis, pregnancy test, chest radiograph, and electrocardiogram may be ordered depending on patient's medical condition.

Procedure
Incision and Exposure

Mini-laparotomy approach is commonly used when the female is postpartum. At this time the uterus is enlarged and the tubes are easily visible.

Details

For the open approach, a small transverse incision is made above the pubic hairline and a Babcock is inserted to grasp and pull out the fallopian tube. The tube is tied with a heavy ligature, excised, and sent to the lab. This procedure is performed bilaterally. When performed laparoscopically, a D&C is commonly done and a uterine manipulator is inserted. An incision is made just inferior to the umbilicus and a Verres needle or non-bladed trocar is inserted into the peritoneal cavity. CO_2 is used to insufflate the abdomen. Once the abdomen is insufflated, the laparoscope is inserted and under direct visualization, a supra-pubic incision is made for the electrosurgical unit active electrode which grasps the fallopian tubes and cauterizes or occludes the tubes. The abdomen is desulfated and the incisions are closed and dressed.

Closure

The wounds are typically closed with a dissolvable skin suture.

Postprocedure Care

The patient is taken to PACU and later discharged home. If the procedure is performed laparoscopically, it is completed as an outpatient. The patient is instructed to drink plenty of fluids and is informed that she may have some referred shoulder discomfort due to some trapped CO_2 under the diaphragm.

Potential Complications

Infection, bleeding, bowel injury, and CO_2 embolus are all potential complications.

TUBOPLASTY

Tuboplasty is a widely used term that refers to several reconstructive surgical procedures performed on the fallopian tubes, which include fimbrioplasty, tubal reanastomosis, salpingostomy, and salpingolysis (Tulandi, 2007).

Indications

These procedures are performed to remove an obstruction or abnormality of the fallopian tube, thus correcting infertility and ultimately facilitating conception.

Related Procedures

Fimbrioplasty, terminal salpingostomy, salpingolysis, and tubal reanastomosis are all related procedures.

Nursing Implications

Anesthesia

The majority of tuboplasty procedures are performed with general anesthesia. The need for blood products is not anticipated during this procedure.

Position

The patient is placed in the dorsal recumbent (supine) position. After the abdomen is opened, the patient is placed in Trendelenburg position (refer to Position).

Establishing and Maintaining the Sterile Field

A skin prep of surgeon's choice is used. Side towels are used to prevent pooling of solution under the patient. The towels are removed when the prep is completed. Before draping, the electrosurgical patient return electrode is placed according to the manufacturer's instructions. The patient is draped according to basic laparotomy technique. The Mayo stand is placed over the patient's legs, with the large instrument table to the scrub person's right. The side table is placed at the patient's feet. The electrosurgical generator is placed at the right of the patient's head. If a microscope is used during the procedure, it must be draped by the scrub person, with the circulating nurse's assistance. However, most surgeons prefer to use their own optical loupes. The circulating nurse monitors and reports any breaks in aseptic technique during the procedure.

Equipment and Supplies

Basic infertility set

Bipolar cord

Small Silastic tubing

Suture boots

Microsurgical instruments

Additional supplies

Impervious split sheet

Two sterile intravenous (IV) tubing

Two sterile stopcocks

Electrosurgical patient return electrode

Electrosurgical pencil with fingertip control

Two 60-mL syringes

Sterile drape

IV
Intravenous

19-gauge needle

Assorted polyglactin sutures, size 1-0 to 7-0; ties

Swedgeon suture

For a tubal reanastomosis, diagnostic laparoscopy is most often performed before the open procedure. The surgeon visualizes the fallopian tubes to make sure that the reanastomosis can be performed. Depending on the surgeon's preference, additional equipment may include the carbon dioxide laser, laser drape, microscope, and microscope drape.

Physiological Monitoring

The circulating nurse must catheterize the patient before establishing the sterile field. A Foley catheter is inserted into the bladder and attached to a urinary drainage bag and then secured to the patient's leg with a leg band. The tubing is positioned under the patient's knee to ensure proper urinary flow. The circulating nurse is responsible for measuring and recording the amount of blood loss and irrigating fluids used during the procedure. Blood loss is usually minimal.

Specimens and Cultures

Adhesions and/or a portion of the fallopian tubes are usually the only specimens obtained from this procedure. Specimens are sent to the pathology laboratory routinely unless otherwise indicated.

Drugs and Solutions

During the procedure, several solutions are needed to moisten tissue: 1000 mL of normal saline (0.9% sodium chloride), with 5000 U of heparin or lactated Ringer's solution. The solution is hung on an intravenous (IV) pole and is transported to the sterile field by way of sterile IV tubing that has been connected to a three-way stopcock. The solution is drawn up in a 60-mL syringe. A Webster cannula is attached to the tip. Diluted indigo carmine is injected into the uterus with a 19-gauge needle to test for tubal patency (4 mL of indigo carmine in 250 mL of normal saline). In addition, a solution of 150 mL of normal saline with 25 mg of promethazine hydrochloride (Phenergan) and 4 mg of dexamethasone (Decadron) is mixed for instillation into the abdomen before the last peritoneal stitches are sewn. The solution is instilled via the IV tubing that has been used for irrigation. Lactated Ringer's solution may also be used, depending on the surgeon's preference. This solution helps to prevent pelvic adhesions. Many surgeons now use a fine film of absorbable adhesion barrier instead of the promethazine hydrochloride and dexamethasone mixture. This barrier is placed over the fallopian tubes to prevent adhesions. Antibiotics are given per the surgeon's request.

Physician Orders

The patient is instructed to administer a Fleet enema, have nothing to eat after 8:00 p.m., and have nothing to drink after midnight the night before the procedure. The patient should also take a shower. Pulsating antiembolism stockings are applied.

Laboratory and Diagnostic Studies

A complete blood cell count (CBC), electrocardiogram (ECG), urinalysis, and electrolyte measurement must be obtained. All test results should be within the normal range; otherwise, medical consultations should be obtained.

Procedure

Incision and Exposure

The incision of choice is usually a Pfannenstiel incision (**Fig. 29.10**). It is stronger than a midline incision and leaves a less noticeable scar. An O'Connor-O'Sullivan retractor is the self-retaining retractor of choice. The large intestine is packed out of the pelvis with large wet packs. For hemostasis, 3-0 ties and suture ligatures are used, along with the electrosurgery.

Details

The entire pelvis is examined by the surgeon; then attention is focused on the reproductive organs. The fallopian tubes are examined. If the obstruction is in the proximal corneal area, the distal tube is re-implanted through the cornu into the uterine cavity with 6-0 sutures. Damage to the mucosa or fimbria that results in distal tubal obstruction necessitates opening that portion of tube. A 5-0 or 6-0 suture ligature is required. If the procedure is being performed to reverse a previous sterilization procedure, the tube is reanastomosed with a 7-0 double-armed suture. Tubal adhesions are removed, and the tubes are repaired with either 4-0 or 5-0 suture.

CBC
Complete Blood Count

ECG
Electrocardiogram

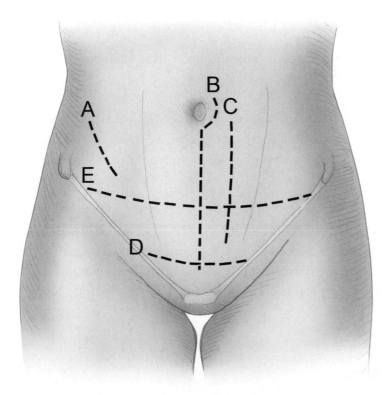

Figure 29.10

Abdominal wall incisions.
(A) McBurney, (B) Lower midline,
(C) Left lower paramedian,
(D) Pfannenstiel or Cherney,
and (E) Transverse.

29

Closure

The abdomen is checked for any bleeding. All packing sponges and retractors are removed. The abdomen is again irrigated with heparinized saline or lactated Ringer's solution. The peritoneum is closed with a 1-0 polyglactin suture, followed by a 1-0 polyglactin suture for the fascia layer. Before the last peritoneal stitches, the solution of promethazine hydrochloride and dexamethasone is instilled into the cavity, if an adhesion barrier was not used. A 3-0 polyglactin suture is next used for the subcutaneous fat. A 4-0 polyglactin suture on a cutting needle is used for sewing the skin.

Postprocedure Care

The patient is taken to the postanesthesia care unit (PACU) and remains there until vital signs are stable. Typical orders include the following:

Measurement of vital signs

Restriction to bed rest

IV administration of fluids and potassium chloride

Administration of antibiotics per the surgeon's prescription

Intake of clear liquids the first postprocedure day, then a full diet as tolerated

Administration of promethazine hydrochloride (steroid) and dexamethasone for nine doses

Intake and output measurements (with removal of the Foley catheter the morning after the procedure, provided the urine is clear)

Patient-controlled analgesia (PCA) for administration of pain medications is discontinued when medications are tolerated by mouth. The hospital stay is usually no longer than 3 days.

Potential Complications

Complications include hemorrhage, infection, and pelvic adhesions.

CERCLAGE

Cervical cerclage refers to various surgical procedures intended to mechanically increase the tensile strength of the cervix using sutures, wires, or synthetic tape. These methods reduce the occurrence of adverse perinatal events associated with cervical insufficiency (Norwitz, 2007).

Indications

Cerclage is indicated for cervical incompetency, when a woman shows an inability to carry a pregnancy to term as a result of symptomless cervical dilatation. Some causes are cervical trauma, exposure to diethylstilbestrol, prior conization of the cervix, and/or excessive muscular strain on the cervix (Varss & Norwitz, 2007).

Related Procedures

There are no related procedures to cerclage.

Nursing Implications
Anesthesia

Cerclage procedures are usually performed with general anesthesia. In some instances, epidural or spinal anesthesia may be used.

Position

The patient is placed in lithotomy position.

Establishing and Maintaining the Sterile Field

A skin prep of surgeon's choice is used to prepare the operative site, which should include the perineum and a gentle, internal vaginal prep. A double-folded sheet is placed as far under the buttocks as possible. Leg drapes are applied with an opened sheet placed low over the abdomen. The surgeon sits during the procedure and the instrument table is placed closest to the surgeon's dominant arm.

Equipment and Supplies

The cerclage tray must include several ring forceps, small narrow Deaver retractors, toothed and smooth forceps, needle holders, and No. 5 polyester fiber suture.

Physiological Monitoring

Fetal heart auscultation is done before the procedure. Blood loss is minimal.

Specimens and Cultures

This procedure yields no specimens. A urine culture is rarely taken.

Drugs and Solutions

No drugs (other than anesthetic) or solutions are used for this procedure.

Physician Orders

The patient should have nothing by mouth after midnight the evening before the procedure.

Laboratory and Diagnostic Studies

There are no tests for cervical incompetency. No laboratory testing is ordered for this procedure.

Procedure

Incision and Exposure

No incision is made for cerclage. Deaver retractors are used for exposure. A ring forceps is used to retract the cervix.

Details

The bladder is emptied with a straight in and out catheter. The cervix is retracted with a ring forceps, and a suture is placed at the junction of the vaginal mucosa and a portion of the cervical os (at the 12 o'clock position). A pursestring suture is placed in several bites around the cervix. Sutures are tied after they are all in place.

Closure

There is no closure for this procedure.

Postprocedure Care

The patient is allowed toilet privileges but otherwise should be restricted to bed rest for 24 hours. Fetal heart tones are monitored frequently. Temperature is monitored during the first 24 hours. The nurse checks for cramping and any drainage from the vagina. Indomethacin (Indocin) suppositories may be given per the physician's prescription. Patients are usually discharged the same day. After the patient is discharged from the facility, she should refrain from strenuous activity but have some form of physical exercise. The sutures are removed at 37 weeks.

Potential Complications

Potential complications include infection and premature labor.

CESAREAN SECTION

Cesarean section is an operative procedure in which the infant is delivered through an abdominal incision rather than via the vaginal route (Capeless & Damron, 2007).

Indications

The indications for performing cesarean section are varied. The most common is dystocia, a failure to progress in labor. Other indications include acute or chronic fetal distress, placenta previa, pelvic tumors, intrauterine infections, malpresentation, carcinoma of the cervix, and failed induction of labor.

Related Procedures

There are no related procedures.

Nursing Implications
Anesthesia

The cesarean section can be performed under general, spinal, or epidural anesthesia. Usually, the procedure is performed with spinal or epidural anesthesia, which poses less hazard for the patient and infant.

Position

The patient is placed in the dorsal recumbent (supine) position. To accommodate uteroplacental circulation, a 15-degree wedge should be placed under the patient's right hip.

Establishing and Maintaining the Sterile Field

A skin prep of the surgeon's choice is used to prepare the abdomen. The circulating nurse assists with the instrument tables. The large instrument table is positioned on the scrub person's dominant side. The square table with retractors is placed at the patient's feet. The patient should be draped with the usual laparotomy draping technique.

Equipment and Supplies

> Cesarean section tray (laparotomy instruments, Lister bandage scissors, episiotomy scissors) Sterile blood tube
> Bulb syringe

Suction tubing and Yankauer tip

Abdominal binder

Suture of choice

The scrub person should use haste when the infant is removed from the uterus. Suction, clamps, and umbilical scissors should be available.

Physiological Monitoring

A Foley catheter is inserted by the circulating nurse, if it has not already been done. The tubing is attached and placed under the patient's knee to allow proper drainage. The circulating nurse is responsible for measuring and recording any unusual blood loss.

Specimens and Cultures

The placenta is sent to the pathology laboratory.

Drugs and Solutions

Oxytocin is needed. An antibiotic may also be given.

Physician Orders

If the cesarean section is a scheduled procedure, the patient is NPO after midnight the evening before the procedure.

Laboratory and Diagnostic Studies

A CBC with typing and screening should be ordered. Urinalysis is also obtained.

Procedure

Incision and Exposure

Cesarean section may be performed with a midline or a Pfannenstiel incision. The uterus is usually opened with a low transverse or vertical incision (**Fig. 29.11**). To prevent damage to the fetus, only handheld retractors are used for exposure.

Details

A No. 10 blade is used to open the abdomen. After the abdomen is opened, the vesicouterine fold is identified and opened with a forceps and Metzenbaum scissors. The bladder is dissected from the lower uterine segment with blunt and sharp scissors. A knife is used to incise the uterus, with care not to injure the fetus. The uterine incision is extended with bandage scissors. The sac is opened, and the fetus is removed. The cord is doubly clamped with Kelly clamps and cut with cord scissors. The placenta is delivered manually. The surgeon then controls any bleeding; the cavity is cleansed of any blood or placental parts with a wet sponge.

Closure

Depending on the surgeon's preference, catgut or polyglactin suture may be used. The uterus is closed in one or two layers: the first layer with a continuous stitch and the next layer with an embrocating stitch. The serosa of the vesicouterine peritoneal fold is closed with a continuous stitch. Next the fascia is closed, then the subcutaneous layer, and finally the skin.

29

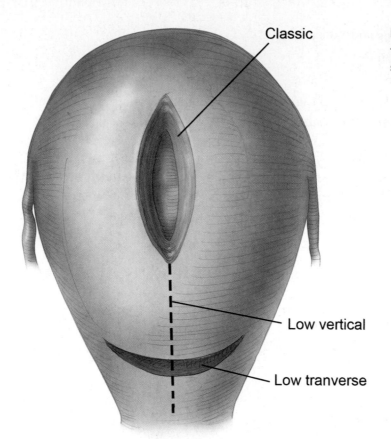

Figure 29.11

Types of cesarean section incisions.

Classic

Low vertical

Low tranverse

Postprocedure Care

The Foley catheter is maintained for 24 hours. Clear liquids are given and then a full diet as tolerated. Vital signs are monitored until the patient is stable and then every 4 hours for 24 hours. The fundus is assessed for height, tone, and location. The type and amount of lochia and the presence of clots are assessed. Dressings are checked for drainage. Intake and output are assessed for 24 hours. The Foley catheter is checked and then removed on the first postprocedure day. Bed rest is suggested. The nurse should discuss infant feeding preference with the mother, check the mother's breasts, and provide discharge instructions. The patient's length of hospital stay is usually 2–3 days.

Potential Complications

Potential complications include hemorrhage, bladder injury, bowel injury, ureteral injury, and infection.

FETAL OPERATIVE PROCEDURES

Fetal operative procedures are performed to correct a problem/deformity with the fetus before birth.

Indications

Intrauterine operative procedures have been developed for prenatal correction of obstructive uropathy, pleural effusion, twin-to-twin transfusion syndrome, amniotic band syndrome, congenital diaphragmatic hernia (CDH), congenital high airway

CDH
Congenital
Diaphragmatic Hernia

obstruction syndrome, sacrococcygeal teratoma, congenital heart disease, myelom-eningocele (spina bifida), fetal anemia, stem cell treatments, and congenital cystic adenomatoid malformations. Ideally the corrective procedure should be performed during the second trimester of pregnancy. Sacrococcygeal teratoma (SCT) is the most common tumor and is usually performed with hysterotomy on a 26-week fetus (Regents of the University of California, 2008).

SCT
Sacrococcygeal Teratoma

Related Procedures

There are no related procedures.

Nursing Implications

Anesthesia

Special anesthesia goals are the prevention of maternal hypoxia and hypotension and the maintenance of uterine blood flow. Low-dose epidural and spinal anesthetic agents are the choice. Isoflurane inhalation with 100% oxygen and muscle relaxants can be used.

Position

For an open fetal operative procedure the mother should be placed in supine position with a wedge under her right side to displace the uterine off the aorta. For fetoscopic procedures the mother is placed in lithotomy position.

Establishing and Maintaining the Sterile Field

A skin prep of the surgeon's choice is used to prepare the abdomen. The circulating nurse assists with the instrument tables. The large instrument table is positioned on the scrub person's dominant side. The square table with retractors is placed at the patient's feet. The patient should be draped with the usual laparotomy or laparoscopy draping technique.

Equipment and Supplies

Open fetal surgery:

> Cesarean section tray
>
> Stapling device to control uterine bleeding
>
> Micro instruments for fetal intervention
>
> Perfusion equipment
>
> Intrauterine monitor
>
> Fetal heart monitor

Fetoscopic approach:

> Minor instrument tray
>
> LASER instruments
>
> Electrosurgery generator
>
> Endoscopes
>
> Endoscopic monitors

29

Sonographic equipment

Ultrasonic scalpel

LASER

Perfusion equipment

Intrauterine monitor

Fetal heart monitor

Physiological Monitoring

A Foley catheter is inserted by the circulating nurse, if it has not already been done. The tubing is attached and placed under the patient's knee to allow proper drainage. The circulating nurse is responsible for measuring and recording any unusual blood loss.

The major objective during the surgery is to ensure maternal and fetal safety. Normal maternal PaO_2 must be maintained to prevent fetal hypoxia. Hypotension must be avoided by using intravenous fluids and, if necessary, ephedrine to stimulate central adrenergic stimulant action. Myometrial contractions must be monitored as well as intrauterine pressures.

Specimens and Cultures

No specimens or cultures are normally taken.

Drugs and Solutions

Ephedrine should be available to help control hypotension. Indomethacin, magnesium sulfate, and terbutaline should be on hand to stop preterm labor. Perfusion solution is available to replace amniotic fluid.

Physician Orders

Preprocedure preparation includes NPO orders for the mother and the medication Indomethacin as tocolysis to inhibit preterm labor is given during preop prep. Betamethasone, a steroid medication which accelerates the baby's lung maturity, may be given to the mother in two intramuscular doses.

Laboratory and Diagnostic Studies

Parents considering a fetal operative procedure should undergo careful evaluation and counseling by a multidisciplinary team before scheduling the procedure.

Procedure

Incision and Exposure

Open fetal surgery is performed with a midline incision. The uterus is usually opened with a vertical incision. A special stapling device is used to control uterine bleeding. Fetoscopic surgery introduces instruments through a small incision and actual manipulation is carried out in real time using endoscopic and sonographic techniques.

Details

A No. 10 blade is used to open the abdomen. After the abdomen is opened, the vesicouterine fold is identified and opened with a forceps and Metzenbaum scissors. The bladder is dissected from the lower uterine segment with blunt and sharp scissors. A knife is used to incise the uterus, with care not to injure the fetus. The uterine incision is extended with bandage scissors. The sac is opened, and the fetus is examined. Fetal manipulation is performed as planned.

Closure

Depending on the surgeon's preference, catgut or polyglactin suture may be used. The uterus is closed in one or two layers: the first layer with a continuous stitch and the next layer with an embrocating stitch. The serosa of the vesicouterine peritoneal fold is closed with a continuous stitch. Next the fascia is closed, then the subcutaneous layer, and finally the skin.

Postprocedure Care

For open fetal surgery, hospital admission for 3–7 days is necessary for monitoring and management of preterm labor. Postprocedure care includes frequent fetal heart tone checks and monitoring for uterine contractions. A tocolysis agent should be prescribed for three to five days. Subsequent delivery must be done by Cesarean section. Following fetoscopic surgery, admission is 1–5 days to monitor preterm labor.

Potential Complications

Maternal adverse effects include preterm labor and delivery, hemorrhage, and infection. Fetal adverse effects include premature closure of the ductus arteriosis and premature delivery.

REFERENCES

1. AORN (2008). *Perioperative Standards and Recommended Practices.* Denver, CO: AORN, Inc.
2. Capeless, E., & Damron, D. (2007, September 18). Cesarean delivery. http://www.uptodate.com.
3. DeCherney, A., & Nathan, L. (2003). *Current Obstetric and Gynecologic Diagnosis and Treatment* (9th ed.). The McGraw-Hill Companies, NY.
4. Elkas, J., & Berek, J. (2007, June 20). Treatment and prognosis of vulvar cancer. http://www.uptodate.com.
5. Falcone, T., & Cogan-Levy, S. (2007, March 17). Overview of hysterectomy. http://www.uptodate.com.
6. Francis, P., & Winfield, H. (2006). Medical robotics: the impact on perioperative nursing practice. *Urol. Nurs.* 2206:26(2):99–108.
7. Guido, R., & Stovall, D. (2007, May 15). Hysteroscopy. http://www.uptodate.com.
8. Guido, R., & Stovall, D. (2006, April 5). Dilatation and Curettage. http://www.uptodate.com.
9. Hatch, Ken D. (2007, June 20). Laparoscopic pelvic and paraaortic lymphadenectomy in gynecologic cancers. http://www.upttodate.com.
10. Helm, William C. (2003, January 17). Simple vulvectomy. http://www.uptodate.com.
11. Helm, William C. (2006, January 19). Radical vulvectomy. http://www.uptodate.com.
12. Norwitz, E. (2007, September 21). Transabdominal cervical cerclage. http://www.uptodate.com.
13. Owusu-Ansah, R., Gatongi, D., & Chien, P. (2006). Health technology assessment of surgical therapies for benign gynaecological disease. *Best Practice & Research Clinical Obstetrics and Gynecology* 20 (6):841–879.
14. Pascholpoulos, M., et al. (2006). Safety issues of hysteroscopic surgery. *Ann. NY Acad. Sci.* 1092: 229–234.
15. Plaxe, S., & Mundt, A. (2007, August 14). Treatment of locally recurrent or advanced endometrial cancer. http://www.uptodate.com.
16. Reich, H. (2007). Total laparoscopic hysterectomy: indications, techniques and outcomes. *Current Opinion in Obstetrics and Gynecology* 19:337–344.
17. Schenken, R. (2007, June 7). Treatment of endometriosis. http://www.uptodate.com.

29

18. Stewart, E. (2007, September 17). Overview of treatment of uterine leiomyomas. http://www.uptodate.com.

19. Stovall, T., & Mann, W. (2006, November 30). Surgical sterilization of women. http://www.uptodate.com.

20. Stovall, T., & Mann, W. (2007, January 30). Overview of gynecologic laparoscopic surgery. http://www.uptodate.com.

21. Tulandi, T. (2007, May 11). Spontaneous abortion: management. http://www.uptodate.com.

22. Tulandi, T. (2007, May 22). Laparoscopic surgery for treatment of infertility in women. http://www.uptodate.com.

23. Varss, V., & Norwitz, E. (2007, September 17). Transvaginal cervical cerclage. http://www.uptodate.com.

24. The Regents of the University of California (2008, April 3). What is fetal intervention? UCSF Fetal Treatment Center http://fetus.ucsfmedicalcenter.org/our_team/fetal_intervention.asp.

25. Women's Health Care Physicians. (2006). 2006 Compendium of selected publications. American College of Obstetricians and Gynecologists.

26. Henig, Robin Marantz. (1982, February 28). "Saving babies before birth." *New York Times*.

CHAPTER 30

Otorhinolaryn-gological Surgery

Rose Moss

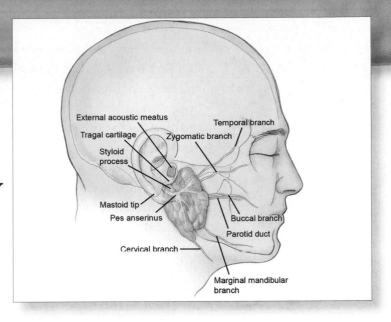

INTRODUCTION

The field of otorhinolaryngological surgery (ie, ear, nose, throat, head, and neck surgery) has diversified during the past 50 years. The numerous operative or invasive procedures involving this part of the anatomy have led to subspecialty training in certain fields. The goals of most procedures in the ear, nose, and throat and in the head and neck are the elimination of chronic infections, the extirpation of tumors, the preservation or improvement of hearing, and the manipulation of the food and air passages when obstructed or injured.

This chapter focuses on the common procedures in the ear, within the nose and paranasal sinuses, and within the soft tissues of the oropharynx and head and neck.

ANATOMY

Ears

The ears are special sense organs involved in enabling hearing as well as maintaining balance. They are divided into external, middle, and inner regions. The external ear is made up of the visible auricle and the external auditory canal. The ear and canal act as a funnel for the transmission of air vibrations that are eventually transformed into understandable sound. The external auditory canal ends at the tympanic membrane, or eardrum. The eardrum is the division between the external ear and the middle ear.

On the other side of the tympanic membrane is the middle ear cavity, or tympanic cavity. Within the middle ear cavity are the three bones that are involved in the transmission and modification of

Chapter Contents

sound energy. This energy is transported to the inner ear through the oval window. The first bone is called the malleus ("hammer"), the second is the incus ("anvil"), and the third bone is the stapes ("stirrup"). The footplate of the stapes sits within the oval window.

The inner ear is located deep within the temporal bone. It is composed of a bony portion as well as a membranous portion. The membranous portion contains a special fluid that is placed in motion when sound energy is transmitted from the tympanic membrane through the bones of hearing. Within the area called the bony labyrinth are the vestibule, the semicircular canals, and the cochlea. The vestibule and the semicircular canals are involved in balance mechanisms. The cochlea is the organ of hearing.

Nose and Paranasal Sinuses

The nose is made up of a combination of bone, cartilage, and mucous membrane (**Fig. 30.1**). The upper third of the external nose is composed of the nasal frontal, ethmoid, and maxillary bones. The lower two thirds of the nose are made up of cartilage. The internal nose contains openings on each side called the nares. The posterior openings into the nasopharynx are called choanae. The anterior skin-lined portion of the nasal cavity is called the vestibule.

The nasal septum divides the nose into two chambers lined by mucous membrane. The septum can become deviated and cause obstruction of the nasal airway. The nasal cavity communicates with the ear through the eustachian tube. The hard and soft palates divide the nasal cavity from the oral cavity. The lateral wall of the nasal cavity contains mucous membrane-lined bony projections called turbinates, or conchae (**Fig. 30.2**). Usually, there are bilateral inferior, middle, and superior turbinates. Rarely seen is a fourth turbinate called the supreme turbinate.

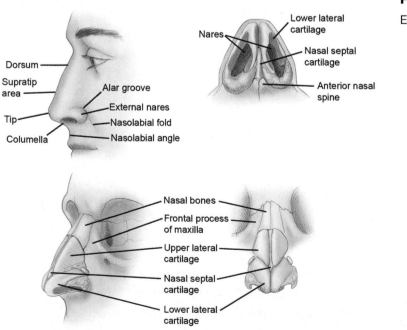

Figure 30.1

External portion of the nose.

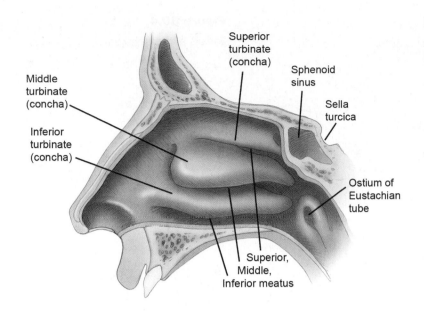

Figure 30.2

Anatomical structures of the lateral nasal wall.

The grooves between the turbinates and the lateral nasal walls are called meati. The inferior meatus contains the nasolacrimal duct opening. The lacrimal glands produce tears, which eventually flow into the nasal cavity. The middle meatus is the most important to know about. This is the one into which the maxillary, frontal, and anterior ethmoidal sinuses drain. The sphenoidal sinuses drain posteriorly and superiorly within the nasal cavity (**Fig. 30.3**).

The sinuses are air-filled pockets lined with mucous membranes. The maxillary sinuses are the largest and most accessible. The paranasal sinuses drain into the nasal cavity through openings called ostia. When these ostia become blocked, infections usually follow.

The nasal cavity has a rich vascular supply from both the external and internal carotid arteries. The proximity to the brain and the orbit makes infections within the nasal cavity and sinuses potentially dangerous.

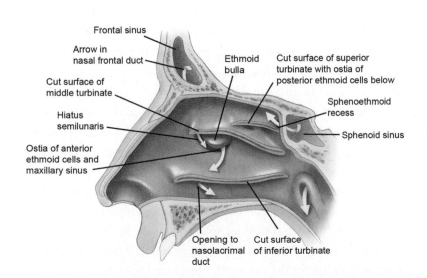

Figure 30.3

Lateral wall of the sinuses shown without turbines.

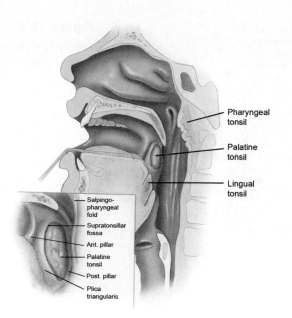

Figure 30.4

Tonsils and oropharynx.

Pharyngeal tonsil

Palatine tonsil

Lingual tonsil

Salpingo-pharyngeal fold

Supratonsillar fossa

Ant. pillar

Palatine tonsil

Post. pillar

Plica triangularis

Tonsils and Adenoids

The tonsils are found within the oropharynx, which is posterior to the oral cavity (**Fig. 30.4**). The tonsils are part of the ring of Waldeyer lymphoid tissue present in the throat. They are found between the folds of mucosa known as the anterior and posterior tonsillar pillars and are usually seen on either side of the throat when the mouth is opened and the tongue is depressed. The ease of visualization depends on the size of the tonsils.

In contrast, the adenoid tissue, which is often called a pharyngeal tonsil, is not easily visualized. The adenoid tissue is found in the nasopharynx, which is the most superior portion of the throat. Although visualization of the adenoid is occluded by the soft palate and the uvula, the adenoid pad and the nasopharynx can be seen by using a mirror. In this indirect fashion, cooperative patients can be examined.

Parotid Gland

The parotid gland is the largest of the major salivary glands. The gland is found on either side of the face in the area of the angle of the mandible (**Fig. 30.5**). The salivary glands deliver their secretory product, saliva, into the oral cavity and the oropharynx. Saliva functions as a lubricant and an acid buffer and contributes to the digestion of food. Diseases affecting the salivary glands are seen as either alterations in the production of saliva or abnormalities of the gland itself.

The parotid gland consists of two portions. There is a superficial lobe, as well as a deep lobe that is in contact with the parapharyngeal space. The parotid gland empties its contents through the parotid duct (also known as Stensen's duct). It enters the oral cavity opposite the second upper molar tooth.

The facial nerve is the most important structure associated intimately with the parotid gland. The most superficial portion of the facial nerve passes through the main substance of the parotid gland. It divides into five main branches: temporal, zygomatic, buccal, mandibular, and cervical. The mandibular branch is especially important because it lies deep under the platysma muscle in the neck.

Figure 30.5
The parotid gland.

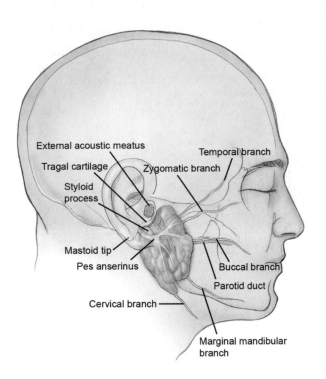

Trachea

Examination of the neck involves identification of palpable structures (**Fig. 30.6**). In infants, the most easily palpable structures are different from those in the adult. In the adult, the most prominent structure in the neck is the thyroid cartilage, or the Adam's apple. This is usually found along the midline of the neck. Immediately below this prominent cartilage is the cricoid cartilage. In adults, the cricothyroid membrane is easily palpable between the cricoid and the thyroid cartilage most of the time. The cricothyroid membrane can be entered in an emergency in most adults.

In infants up to 2 months of age, the most palpable structure is usually the hyoid bone. This horseshoe-shaped bone is found superior to the thyroid cartilage. Most infants and young children have short necks with a large amount of subcutaneous fat, which makes palpation difficult. In addition, the cartilages are much softer. Therefore, emergency access through the neck into a pediatric airway is much more difficult than in the adult.

Figure 30.6
Trachea and thyroid cartilage.

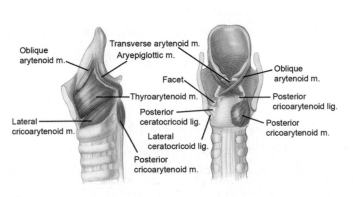

30

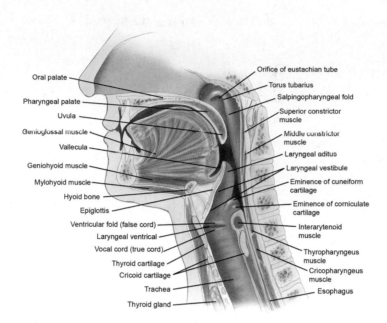

Figure 30.7

Larynx and neck.

Larynx

The larynx is found anteriorly between the lowermost portion of the pharynx superiorly and the trachea (windpipe) inferiorly (**Fig. 30.7**). It consists of three major cartilages supported by different ligaments and muscles. These cartilages are the thyroid cartilage, the cricoid cartilage directly beneath it, and the arytenoid cartilage, which articulates with the cricoid cartilage.

A function of the larynx is to modify the air being expelled from the lungs and allow this air column to be used by the tongue, cheeks, and lips to produce intelligible speech. Intelligible speech can still occur if the larynx is absent. The most important function of the larynx, however, is not speech production but protection of the respiratory passages to prevent aspiration.

Within the larynx are found the vocal cords. There are false vocal cords, which are upper folds within the larynx, and true vocal cords. The vocal cords perform the vibratory function that aids in phonation. They are innervated by the recurrent laryngeal nerve, which originates from the vagus, or 10th cranial, nerve.

SPECIAL PRECAUTIONS DURING OTOLARYNGEAL PROCEDURES

Procedures in the head and neck area present high risk for an ignition incident because of the potential for an oxygen rich environment and the use of electrosurgery and laser. Electrosurgery and laser must be used with extreme caution during head and neck procedures. See Chapters 11, 14, and 17 for more information concerning electrosurgery and laser fire hazards.

PROCEDURES OF THE EAR

The ear has been studied since ancient times. Hippocrates in 400 B.C. was the first to describe acute otitis media. In the mid-17th century, Duverney, who is often called the father of otology, published the first monograph on otology. He was the first anatomist to describe the mastoid air cells communicating with the middle ear cavity. He also established that pus coming from the ear did not originate in the brain.

Infections of the ear and mastoid were potentially deadly before the advent of antibiotics. The operations designed at the birth of otology revolved around the elimination of infection. It was not until the 19th century that operations to cure infection were successfully performed on a regular basis. In the early 1900s, the operating microscope added a new dimension to ear operations designed to cure infection and deafness. With the advent of antimicrobial agents, the necessity for operative intervention within the ear decreased dramatically. The most common surgical procedure performed in the ear today is the insertion of ventilation tubes.

Myringotomy

Definition and Indications

Myringotomy refers to a tiny incision of the tympanic membrane (eardrum) to remove thickened secretions; in most cases, a small tympanostomy tube is inserted into the tympanic membrane to aerate the middle ear for a prolonged time (MedicineNet.com, 2008a). Myringotomy is either diagnostic or therapeutic. It is usually performed on a pediatric patient who has had chronic middle ear effusions or recurrent acute otitis media. Other indications for this procedure include (MedicineNet.com, 2008a):

- Malformation of the tympanic membrane or Eustachian tube
- Downs syndrome
- Cleft palate
- Barotrauma (injury to the middle ear due to a reduction of air pressure)

Nursing Implications

Anesthesia

Most myringotomies are performed with general inhalation anesthesia. The use of intravenous (IV) catheters is usually not necessary, but the decision is made by the anesthesia provider. The procedure can be performed using local anesthesia. This type of anesthesia, however, is typically reserved for older children and adults.

IV
Intravenous

Position

The patient is placed in the supine position. After general anesthesia is induced and appropriate monitoring devices are placed, the procedure is initiated by turning the patient's head with the operative ear facing the surgeon.

Establishing and Maintaining the Sterile Field

Myringotomy is considered by some surgeons as a minor procedure. It does, however, deserve the same preparation as for any procedure. The ear is usually draped with sterile towels only. Before any sterile towels are placed, the microscope should be in position to be easily swung into the operative field. A sterile sheet may or may not be placed over the chest and body of the patient. The skin preparation is determined by the surgeon. Many surgeons use alcohol or another skin antiseptic agent. Some surgeons do not request skin preparation. If the ear is prepared, the circulating nurse

30

Table 30.1	Myringotomy Instruments
☐ Wire loop or cerumen remover	
☐ Alligator forceps	
☐ Beaver handle and myringotomy blade (No. 7100 or 7120)	
☐ 45° pick	
☐ 90° pick	
☐ Rosen pick	
☐ Nos. 3, 5, and 7 Baron suction tubes	

should include the ear, the postauricular area, and the face. The scrub person may stand next to the surgeon or across from him or her and close to the Mayo stand.

EQUIPMENT AND SUPPLIES

A dedicated myringotomy tray should be available. **Table 30.1** lists recommended instruments for a myringotomy set. The different types of ventilation tubes available can be confusing. The ventilation tube is usually chosen by the surgeon before or at the time of the procedure. Therefore, it is wise to have the ventilation tubes located where they are easily accessible to the nursing personnel. A microscope with either a 200- or a 250-mm focal length lens is most often used.

PHYSIOLOGICAL MONITORING

Myringotomies are normally quick procedures. The patient may or may not be intubated. The circulating nurse must be readily available to assist the anesthesia provider, especially during initial induction of and recovery from anesthesia.

SPECIMENS AND CULTURES

A culture may be taken to determine the type of microorganism present.

DRUGS AND SOLUTIONS[1]

Normal saline, skin antiseptic solution, and an otic antibiotic solution should be available.

PHYSICIAN ORDERS

The patient is given liquids when awake and is discharged when he or she is alert and stable, and meets all of the discharge criteria.

Procedure

EXPOSURE AND INCISION

An ear speculum is inserted in the external auditory canal while the ear is viewed under the microscope. Cerumen is usually removed with cerumen spoons. After this is completed, the ear can be irrigated with alcohol or other skin antiseptic agent. The use of a skin antiseptic is usually followed by copious irrigation with normal

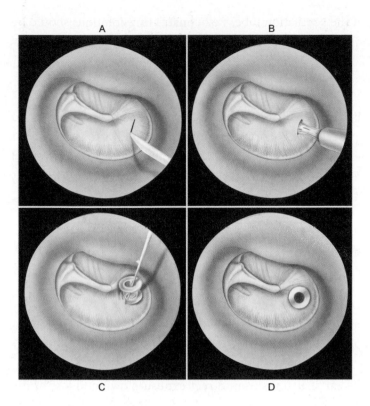

A   B

C   D

Figure 30.8
(A) Myringotomy incision,
(B) Aspiration of fluid,
(C) Insertion of ventilation tube,
and (D) Ventilation tube in place.

saline. After the tympanic membrane has been identified and described by the surgeon, a myringotomy scalpel is used to incise the tympanic membrane (**Fig. 30.8**). After the incision is made, it is imperative to have the appropriate Baron suction tips that are used to aspirate any middle ear effusion. Because some of the effusions may be tenacious, duplicate suction catheters should be available.

DETAILS

The various ventilation tubes are then inserted through the myringotomy incision using either alligator forceps or special introducers. Mounting of the ventilation tube is at the discretion of the surgeon. The scrub person should be aware of the surgeon's preference. It is important at the time of mounting of the ventilation tube that a minimal amount of contact exists between the gloves of the scrub person or the surgeon and the ventilation tube. The ventilation tube should be primarily handled with the tip of the alligator forceps or the introducer. The alligator forceps or the introducer should be handed to the surgeon so that the surgeon does not have to look away from the microscope. A 45-degree pick or a curved Rosen pick may also be used for proper positioning of the tube.

CLOSURE

After the tube is placed, an antibiotic solution may or may not be used by the surgeon. If it is used, it is introduced by placing the drops through the ear speculum or with a syringe. A cotton ball is usually placed in the ear canal after the instillation of antibiotic solutions. Occasionally, a small amount of bleeding occurs. Because blood

30

PACU
Postanesthesia Care
Unit

can occlude the lumen of the ventilation tube, vasoconstricting solutions should be available for instillation into the ear before transferring the patient to the postanesthesia care unit (PACU).

Postprocedure Care

After the procedure is completed, the patient is awakened and transported to the PACU. Because the procedure is short, the patient usually awakens quickly. If the patient is a child, the postanesthesia period can be traumatic. The child should be reunited with the parent as soon as it is feasible. There is no dressing. However, cotton may be placed in the ears.

Potential Complications

Otorrhea and bleeding may occur.

Tympanoplasty

Definition and Indications

Tympanoplasty is a broad term that has been used to refer to any procedure performed to repair perforations within the eardrum or repair defects of middle ear structures for restoring sound conduction pathways. Simple tympanoplasty can be done to protect middle ear structures from direct exposure owing to loss of the membrane cover. Tympanoplasties are classified as Types 1 through 5 (*Encyclopedia of Surgery*, 2008a):

- Type I tympanoplasty—also called myringoplasty, involves only the restoration of the perforated eardrum by grafting the area of the perforation.
- Type II tympanoplasty—this procedure is used for tympanic membrane perforations with erosion of the malleus; it involves grafting onto the incus or the remains of the malleus.
- Type III tympanoplasty—this procedure is indicated for destruction of two ossicles, with the stapes still intact and mobile; it involves placing a graft onto the stapes, and providing protection for the assembly.
- Type IV tympanoplasty—this procedure is used for ossicular destruction, which includes all or part of the stapes arch; it involves placing a graft onto or around a mobile stapes footplate.
- Type V tympanoplasty—used when the footplate of the stapes is fixed.

Nursing Implications

Anesthesia

Tympanoplasty can be performed with the use of local anesthesia, but general anesthesia is usually preferred by most surgeons. One of the techniques used is hypotensive anesthesia, which helps create a bloodless field. If nitrous oxide is used, it is discontinued before the graft is placed. Nitrous oxide diffuses into the middle ear cavity and leads to disruption of the grafting procedure.

Position

Most often, the surgeon performs this procedure while sitting. Before transferring the patient to the bed, the bed should be turned so that the patient's head rests on the foot of the bed and the feet are positioned at the head of the bed. This facilitates placement of the base of the microscope under the bed and enables the surgeon to position his or her feet under the bed. The patient is placed in the supine position, close to the edge of the bed, with the head turned and the operative ear up and stabilized. A doughnut-shaped stockinet or small headrest support device is used to stabilize the head and protect the nonoperative ear. The circulating nurse should ensure that the nonoperative ear is within the hole of the doughnut or headrest to avoid pressure on the ear.

ESTABLISHING AND MAINTAINING THE STERILE FIELD

The ear and the hair immediately around the ear may or may not be shaved. The operating microscope is placed at the head of the bed. It is draped in a sterile fashion, because it will be manipulated by the surgeon. The surgeon may examine the ear before the circulating nurse scrubs and prepares the patient. Therefore, a simple myringotomy set should be available for this purpose. After the patient's head has been positioned, the ear can be prepared with a variety of antibacterial solutions. The region to be prepared should include the ear, the postauricular area, and the face just past the midline.

The eye on the operative side is taped closed with an eye occluder. After this is done, a plastic drape with a preformed hole can be pressed onto the skin with the ear protruding through the hole. Lint-free drapes are preferred. It is imperative that gloves used by the surgeon and the scrub person be free from powder and lint. Formation of granulomas secondary to powder within the middle ear has been reported to cause irreversible hearing loss.

EQUIPMENT AND SUPPLIES

As for any otological procedure, a proper assortment of otological instruments is necessary. Most of these instruments are used in conjunction with the operating microscope. Because many of these instruments are unique for otological procedures, it is important for the scrub person to be fully familiar with the instruments. Different sets are available commercially and include a variety of fine instruments for the mobilization of tissue within a small space. Varieties of fine ossicular instruments are also essential. Appropriate suction catheters are also found within these sets. In addition to the microinstruments, a basic surgical set should also be available. This should include fine scissors, (eg, iris and Metzenbaum scissors) to harvest a graft. Bone instruments, including power drills, must be readily available if drilling becomes necessary during a simple tympanoplasty.

Table 30.2 lists a sample tympanoplasty set. Other supplies include bone wax, oxidized cellulose, absorbable hemostatic sponges, and a nerve stimulator (in rare cases the facial nerve may be encountered). The surgeon may use Silastic sheeting rather than the patient's teraporalis fascia autograft.

PHYSIOLOGICAL MONITORING

A tympanoplasty can be a short procedure or it can take several hours, depending on the surgeon's findings. If the procedure is performed using local anesthesia, constant monitoring of the patient's electrocardiogram (ECG), blood pressure, and oxygen saturation by pulse oximetry is essential. The patient is asked to lie supine with the head

ECG
Electrocardiogram

Table 30.2	Tympanoplasty Set

- ☐ Sickle knife
- ☐ Lancet knife
- ☐ Round (weapon) knife
- ☐ Flap knife
- ☐ Rosen knife
- ☐ Roller knife
- ☐ Stapes knife
- ☐ Tympanoplasty knife
- ☐ Micro-cup forceps: right, left, and straight
- ☐ Alligator forceps: fine, plain, or serrated
- ☐ Bellucci scissors
- ☐ 45° pick
- ☐ 90° pick
- ☐ Rosen pick
- ☐ Drum elevator
- ☐ Gimmick elevator
- ☐ Duckbill elevator (three sizes)
- ☐ Fisch excavators: left and right
- ☐ Microcurettes
- ☐ Iris and tenotomy scissors
- ☐ Iris forceps with and without teeth
- ☐ Tenon block

turned in one position for a period of time; therefore, the patient's comfort level is monitored constantly. Comfort measures such as padding for elbows and heels are supplied after positioning the patient on the bed. A pillow under the knees is offered to reduce pressure on the back. The patient may even be placed in a flexed (lawn chair) position for comfort, with care not to compromise adequate operating position for the surgeon.

If the patient is placed under general anesthesia, the same comfort measures are applied. The circulating nurse must be readily available to assist the anesthesia provider during induction of and emergence from anesthesia. The suction must be in close reach of the anesthesia provider.

SPECIMENS AND CULTURES

Specimens may include excess tissue used for the graft and/or remnants of the tympanic membrane. Cultures are taken as indicated by clinical findings.

DRUGS AND SOLUTIONS

Drugs and solutions that may be needed include the following:

- Lidocaine (Xylocaine) 1% with 1:100,000 epinephrine (Adrenalin)
- 1:100,000 epinephrine
- Neosporin ointment

- Colistin sulfate (Coly-Mycin) otic suspension
- Absorbable hemostatic sponges or oxidized cellulose
- Tis-U-Sol solution

PHYSICIAN ORDERS

The patient is given a regular diet. The IV catheter should be kept open until the patient is taking liquids successfully. Antiemetic and analgesic drugs are administered. The patient can ambulate depending on comfort level.

LABORATORY AND DIAGNOSTIC STUDIES

CBC, urinalysis, chest radiographs, and ECG are obtained as indicated. The surgeon may also order an audiogram with pure-tone air and bone conduction curves with adequate narrow-band masking as well as speech discrimination scores; mastoid radiographs; and computed tomography (CT) scans, which may help in determining ossicular defects and cholesteatoma size and extension.

CT
Computed
Tomography

Procedure

INCISION AND EXPOSURE

The procedure usually begins with an injection of a local anesthetic mixed with epinephrine. The injections are performed in a four-quadrant fashion within the external auditory canal. Incisions are then made within the canal skin at 6 and 12 o'clock positions. These incisions are connected with different canal microknives. This forms a flap. The flap is raised medially until the entire fibrous portion of the tympanic membrane is identified. Before beginning the procedure or at the surgeon's discretion, the graft can be taken from the temporalis muscle fascia. The incision is made within the hairline using standard surgical scalpels. The incision is carried down through the subcutaneous tissue until the fascia of the muscle can be identified (**Fig. 30.9**). A portion of the fascial layer is removed that is slightly larger than the size of the perforation to be repaired. After the graft has been harvested, it is usually given to the surgical assistant or the scrub person for preparation. The graft is prepared by compressing it between a fascia press forceps. Then it is placed on a Teflon block for drying. A dry graft allows the surgeon better pliability during the grafting stage.

30

Figure 30.9

Incision for tympanoplasty and mastiodectomy.

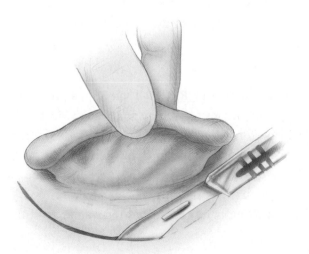

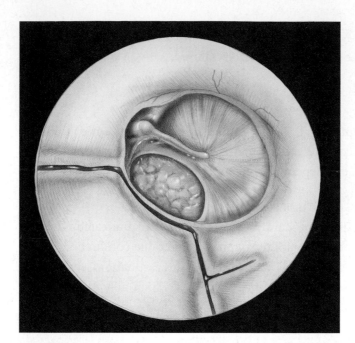

Figure 30.10

Perforation and flaps for tympanoplasty.

DETAILS

After the perforation is identified, different micropicks are used to freshen the perforation margin. This can also be done with fine curettes or cup-biting forceps. Next, the previously created tympanomeatal flap is raised superiorly (**Fig. 30.10**). Absorbable gelatin sponge is then placed within the middle ear cavity to act as a support for the graft. The graft is then taken and placed in the medial surface of the tympanic membrane. After the graft is placed in its proper position, the tympanomeatal flap is brought down to its normal position. The external auditory canal is then packed with absorbable gelatin. Antibiotic solution or ointment can also be used for this purpose.

CLOSURE

A wide variety of techniques exists for packing the external auditory canal. The scrub person should inquire as to the surgeon's preference. If a simple tympanoplasty was performed without any external incisions, the ear can be dressed in a variety of ways. Dressings are not necessary, however, if the incisions were all within the external auditory canal. A mastoid dressing is described later. The area of grafting is closed in a standard fashion using absorbable suture for the subcutaneous tissue and nonabsorbable suture for the skin.

Postprocedure Care

The patient is immediately transported to the PACU. Typical postprocedure orders include the administration of antiemetics as well as analgesics. Most tympanoplasties of the simple type can be performed on an outpatient basis. The patient is instructed to keep water away from the operative ear until further advised. If the procedure was performed through the external canal only, the dressing may be an adhesive bandage (Band-Aid). If a postauricular incision was created, however, a pressure bandage of fluffs (Kerlix) and Kling bandage is used to wrap around the head and over the operative ear.

Potential Complications

As with any wound, there is always the potential for infection within the operated area. The graft site rarely becomes infected. However, hematomas forming in this area have been reported. Additional complications include the failure of the graft to take, with a persistence of the perforation.

Mastoidectomy

Definition and Indications

A mastoidectomy is performed for eradication of infected mastoid air cells resulting from ear infections, (ie, mastoiditis or chronic otitis, or by inflammatory disease of the middle ear [cholesteatoma]); the procedure involves removal of the infected portion of the mastoid bone when medical treatment is ineffective (*Encyclopedia of Surgery*, 2008b). Mastoidectomy may or may not be done in conjunction with a tympanoplasty. In addition, a mastoidectomy may be performed along with an ossicular reconstruction.

A simple mastoidectomy involves a postauricular incision through which the air cells of the mastoid process are eradicated by drilling through the bone with burrs. The external canal and the middle ear are at times not involved (**Fig. 30.11**). A modified radical mastoidectomy involves removal of a portion of the ear canal, allowing drainage from the mastoid into the canal. The tympanic membrane and middle ear ossicles are preserved. A radical mastoidectomy is performed for severe chronic mastoiditis. In this procedure, the middle ear cavity and the mastoid antrum are combined into a large single cavity. Periodically, this cavity is inspected and cleaned on an outpatient basis. Usually, the ossicles and the tympanic membrane are entirely removed. Throughout these procedures, an additional structure that becomes important to identify and protect is the facial nerve.

Nursing Implications

ANESTHESIA

As for other ear procedures, mastoidectomy is performed using general hypotensive anesthesia. Before the procedure is started, the surgeon often injects a combination of local anesthetic with epinephrine.

POSITION

The patient's head is turned with the operative side up and stabilized. As for tympanoplasty, the bed is reversed before positioning the patient. The basic principles described earlier are also used for mastoidectomy as well as other middle ear procedures.

ESTABLISHING AND MAINTAINING THE STERILE FIELD

The sterile field is established by clipping hair behind the ear (if ordered by the surgeon) and preparing the ear and the surrounding areas with a skin antiseptic agent. The ear is covered with a plastic drape with a preformed hole. The operating microscope is also draped with a sterile plastic drape.

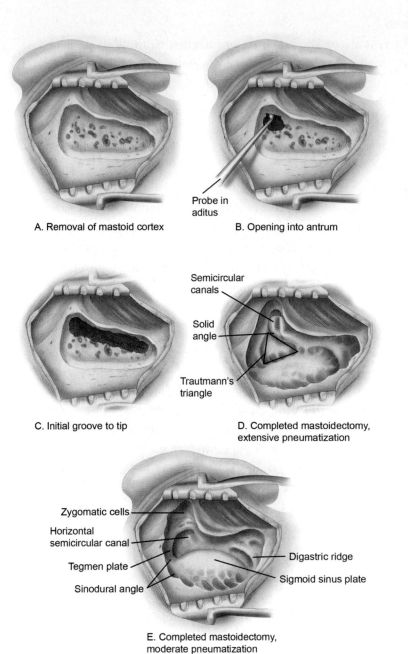

Figure 30.11

Simple mastoidectomy.

A. Removal of mastoid cortex

Probe in aditus

B. Opening into antrum

C. Initial groove to tip

Semicircular canals

Solid angle

Trautmann's triangle

D. Completed mastoidectomy, extensive pneumatization

Zygomatic cells

Horizontal semicircular canal

Tegmen plate

Sinodural angle

Digastric ridge

Sigmoid sinus plate

E. Completed mastoidectomy, moderate pneumatization

EQUIPMENT AND SUPPLIES

In addition to a tympanoplasty set, additional instruments that should be included for a mastoidectomy are outlined in **Table 30.3**. Micro ear instruments and an air-powered drill with a variety of burrs must be available. The burrs are of two types. These are designated as cutting burrs and diamond burrs. Cottonoids and cotton balls moistened with Tis-U-Sol are often used. They must always be counted. At times, solutions of diluted epinephrine are used to assist in hemostasis. Prosthetic devices for reconstruction of the ossicular chain must be readily available in a wide variety of types and sizes. Because the facial nerve is at risk during a mastoidectomy, nerve stimulators may be used to identify the facial nerve. Evoked potential audiometry can also be used to monitor the facial nerve.

Table 30.3	Mastoidectomy Instruments

- ☐ Elevators
- ☐ Incudostapedial joint knife
- ☐ Myringotomy knife
- ☐ Picks: 90° and 40° (curved, straight, and right angle)
- ☐ Knives: Guilford, tympanoplastic sickle-shaped
- ☐ Knives: Rosen, House
- ☐ Strut caliper
- ☐ Tabb knives: 45° and 90°
- ☐ Retractors: Weitlaner, Wullstein
- ☐ Rongeurs
- ☐ Suction irrigation system
- ☐ Rosen suction tube, sizes 18 to 24
- ☐ House adapter
- ☐ Absorbable gelatin sponge (Gelfoam) press
- ☐ Shea ear specula

PHYSIOLOGICAL MONITORING

During mastoidectomy, the patient is placed under general anesthesia (see the discussion of tympanoplasty).

SPECIMENS AND CULTURES

Mastoid bone fragments, granulation tissue, and/or cholesteatoma may be sent to the pathology department for study or microbiology for culture if indicated.

DRUGS AND SOLUTIONS

Drugs and solutions that should be available include the following:

- Lidocaine 1% with 1:100,000 epinephrine
- Gelfoam 100
- 1:1000 epinephrine
- Cortisporin ointment
- Cortisporin Otic suspension
- Tis-U-Sol Solution

PHYSICIAN ORDERS

The patient is given IV fluids and antibiotics. A regular diet is ordered. Antiemetic and analgesic drugs are administered. The patient is advised not to use straws with liquids and to sneeze with the mouth open.

LABORATORY AND DIAGNOSTIC STUDIES

See the discussion of tympanoplasty.

30

Procedure

INCISION AND EXPOSURE

Mastoidectomy can involve only a postauricular incision. Most often, however, the procedure is combined with a tympanoplasty. This is better known as a tympanomastoidectomy. The procedure is started by palpating the tip of the mastoid process. After external landmarks have been identified, a postauricular incision is made close to the postauricular sulcus. This incision is made with a surgical blade or electrosurgery. The microscope is usually not used for this portion of the procedure.

A dissection is carried down to the temporalis fascia superiorly and down through the periosteum just below the temporalis muscle insertion. At this time, a portion of temporalis muscle fascia is obtained if a graft will be placed later during the procedure. If the procedure is going to be combined with a tympanoplasty, external auditory canal incisions are made as described earlier.

After the tympanomeatal flap is elevated, the operation proceeds through the postauricular incision and, if necessary, through the ear canal. The postauricular incision, however, exposes the ear canal also. After the periosteum is exposed, it is elevated anteriorly with an elevator, such as a 4-mm periosteal elevator. After the external auditory canal incision is visualized through the postauricular incision, different canal instruments can be used to expose the middle ear fully through the canal. A self-retaining retractor is placed and opened widely. At this point, the air-powered drill is used with the largest available cutting burr.

DETAILS

After the dissection has proceeded beyond the superficial bony landmarks, a microscope is brought in for finer detail. Depending on the indications for the operation, the middle ear can be entered from the mastoid approach as well. It is important that the surgeon be as comfortably seated as possible. It is also important that the scrub person have a thorough knowledge of the anatomy and procedure to anticipate the use of the appropriate instruments. Ideally, the surgeon should never have to look away from the microscope for instruments. A surgeon should be able to request an instrument by name and have it handed to him or her by the scrub person.

If reconstructive procedures are indicated, the surgeon selects from a wide variety of prosthetic devices. If a tympanic membrane perforation is to be repaired, the previously harvested graft is used in a manner similar to that described earlier.

CLOSURE

The postauricular wound is copiously irrigated, and the wound is closed by approximating the previously raised periosteum. Periosteum is usually closed with absorbable sutures of the surgeon's choice. The subcutaneous tissues are then reapproximated in the postauricular area. A drain may be placed and brought out through the most inferior portion of the postauricular incision. The skin is usually closed with a nylon or polypropylene (Prolene) stitch. A subcuticular suture may be used to alleviate the necessity for suture removal later.

Again, the preference of the surgeon should be determined before the procedure is started. After the postauricular incision is closed, the ear canal is examined in the usual fashion. A variety of ear specula is used to visualize the canal. The tympanomeatal flap is replaced, and the external auditory canal is packed as previously described. After the procedure, a mastoid dressing is used. A nonadhering bandage is placed behind the ear. The postauricular incision is then supported with gauze squares. Rolls of self-adhering gauze are used to surround the head from the occiput to the forehead. Gauze may be used to place pressure on the wound to prevent a hematoma.

Postprocedure Care

The patient is transferred immediately to the PACU. After operations of the mastoid and the middle ear, it is important to assess the hearing capability of the patient as well as assess for vertigo. As soon as the patient is conscious, different tuning fork tests may be used to assess hearing. The facial nerve function is also routinely evaluated (eg, smiling, wrinkling of the nose on the operative side, and closing of the eye).

Potential Complications

Complications that may occur include hearing loss, facial nerve injury, vertigo, taste changes, bleeding and hematoma formation, and infection.

Stapedectomy

Definition and Indications

Stapedectomy is a surgical procedure in which the stapes is removed and replaced with a prosthesis; it is performed to improve the movement of sound to the inner ear (*Encyclopedia of Surgery*, 2008c). In some patients, a conductive hearing loss is identified. A common reason for this hearing loss is the formation of spongy bone within the capsule of the bony labyrinth of the inner ear. In such conditions, normal bone is replaced by vascular otosclerotic bone, which eventually involves the footplate of the stapes. The stapes thus becomes locked and unable to vibrate. This condition, commonly known as otosclerosis, is a hereditary defect. The procedure of stapedectomy with the insertion of a prosthesis has been developed to restore hearing to the ear.

The indications for stapedectomy include treatment of progressive hearing loss caused by otosclerosis, a condition in which spongy bone hardens around the base of the stapes (*Encyclopedia of Surgery*, 2008c) and also the finding of a conductive hearing loss without any evidence of other middle ear disease.

Related Procedures

Stapedotomy is a related procedure.

Nursing Implications

Anesthesia

As for other ear procedures, stapedectomy is usually performed using general anesthesia. In cooperative adults, however, local anesthesia may be used so that the patient can assist the surgeon by informing him or her of an immediate improvement in hearing.

Table 30.4	Stapedectomy Instruments
☐ Hough hoe excavators: 45° and 90°	
☐ Footplate picks: 1 mm and 2 mm	
☐ Straight pick or 30° obtuse pick	
☐ Perforator	
☐ Crimper: House and/or McGee	
☐ Strut caliper (measuring stick)	
☐ Prostheses of different sizes and shapes	
☐ House incudostapedial joint knife	
☐ Guilford-Wright joint knife	

POSITION

The patient is positioned as described for tympanoplasty.

ESTABLISHING AND MAINTAINING THE STERILE FIELD

The sterile field is established and maintained as for other ear procedures. The position of the sterile field is identical to that for other ear procedures.

EQUIPMENT AND SUPPLIES

All microinstruments for ear procedures should be available, to include fine stapes dissectors and manipulators. A variety of prosthetic devices has been described for use in this procedure. A tympanoplasty set is used with the additional instruments outlined in **Table 30.4**.

PHYSIOLOGICAL MONITORING

See the discussion of tympanoplasty.

SPECIMENS AND CULTURES

The stapes superstructure is sent for pathological study.

DRUGS AND SOLUTIONS

See the discussion of mastoidectomy.

PHYSICIAN ORDERS

See the discussion of tympanoplasty.

LABORATORY AND DIAGNOSTIC STUDIES

See the discussion of tympanoplasty.

Procedure

INCISION AND EXPOSURE

A tympanomeatal flap is raised as previously described for simple tympanoplasty. The fibrous annulus of the tympanic membrane is identified and lifted superiorly

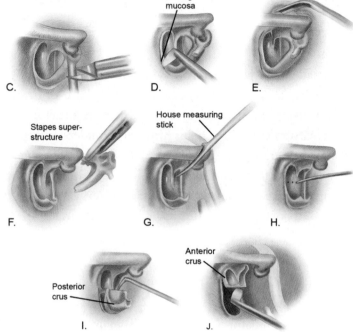

Figure 30.12
Stapedectomy procedure.

with a tympanomeatal flap (**Fig. 30.12**). Often, a small portion of bone from the edge of the bony ear canal is removed for better visualization of the joint between the incus and the stapes. The chorda tympani nerve is located in this area. Care is taken not to injure this nerve, which supplies taste to the lateral portion of the tongue on that side. Microinstruments are used to sever the connection between the incus and the stapes. The stapes bone is fractured and removed along with the remnant footplate. Some surgeons use lasers as well.

A graft is also necessary during this procedure. This graft may be vein, perichondrium, fascia, fat, or absorbable hemostatic sponges. The graft is placed over the oval window of the inner ear.

DETAILS

After the prosthesis has been selected, the previously obtained graft is placed over the oval window where the stapes footplate previously existed. A prosthesis is then inserted and connected from the incus to the graft. This restores sound conduction. If the procedure is being performed under local anesthesia, the surgeon can reposition the tympanic membrane and talk to the patient while testing for a hearing improvement. As in other microsurgical procedures, the operating microscope must be used.

CLOSURE

The tympanomeatal flap is replaced as previously described.

Postprocedure Care

Postprocedure care is the same as that for other ear procedures.

Potential Complications

Hearing loss, dizziness (vertigo), a change in taste, and injury to the facial nerve may occur.

Cochlear Implant
Definition and Indications

A cochlear implant is a small, intricate electronic device that can assist in providing a sense of sound to a person who is profoundly deaf or severely hard-of-hearing; it does not restore normal hearing, rather it can give a deaf person a useful representation of sounds in the environment, which helps him/her to understand speech (NIDCD, 2007). It works by directly stimulating any functioning auditory nerves inside the cochlea with an electric field stimulated through an electric impulse (Wikipedia, 2008a). The implant consists of two portions: an external portion that sits behind the ear and a second portion that is surgically implanted under the skin as follows (NIDCD, 2007):

- A microphone, which picks up sound from the environment;
- A speech processor, which selects and arranges sounds picked up by the microphone;
- A transmitter and receiver/stimulator, which receive signals from the speech processor and convert them into electric impulses; and
- An electrode array, which is a group of electrodes that collects the impulses from the stimulator and sends them to different regions of the auditory nerve.

Cochlear implants are indicated for children (most who receive them are between 2 and 6 years old) and adults who are deaf or severely hard-of-hearing, as well as adults who have lost all or most of their hearing later in life (NIDCD, 2007).

Nursing Implications
ANESTHESIA

The procedure is performed under general anesthesia.

POSITION

See the discussion under mastoidectomy.

ESTABLISHING AND MAINTAINING THE STERILE FIELD

See the discussion under mastoidectomy.

EQUIPMENT AND SUPPLIES

All instruments for ear procedures should be available, including a microscope and bone drill.

PHYSIOLOGICAL MONITORING

See the discussion under tympanoplasty.

SPECIMENS AND CULTURES

Bone fragments and other tissue may be sent to the pathology department for study or microbiology for culture if indicated.

DRUGS AND SOLUTIONS

See the discussion under mastoidectomy.

PHYSICIAN ORDERS

See the discussion under mastoidectomy.

LABORATORY AND DIAGNOSTIC STUDIES

In addition to the routine preoperative testing protocols, other preoperative studies include (US FDA, 2004):

- examination of external, middle, and inner ear for signs of infection or abnormality;
- various tests of hearing, such as an audiogram;
- a trial of hearing aid use to assess its potential benefit;
- exams to evaluate middle and inner ear structures, for example:
  - CT (computerized tomography) scan—to assess the shape of the cochlea. It is particularly important if the patient has a history of meningitis because it helps to ascertain if there is new bone growth in the cochlea that could interfere with the insertion of the implant; it also may indicate which ear should be implanted;
  - MRI (magnetic resonance imaging) scan;
- psychological examination to see if the patient can cope with the implant; and
- physical exam to prepare for general anesthesia.

MRI
Magnetic Resonance Imaging

A detailed evaluation by the cochlear implant team must also be conducted for those who are considered as candidates for the cochlear implant; in addition, both the preprocedure and postprocedure training are important to the overall success of the device (Levenson, 2008).

Procedure

A small incision is made in the skin just behind the ear; the surgeon drills into the mastoid bone to create a seat to hold and protect the receiver/stimulator. The surgeon then drills through the mastoid bone to the inner ear where the electrode array is inserted into the cochlea. The receiver/stimulator is secured to the skull, the incision is closed with absorbable sutures, and the head is bandaged (Wikipedia, 2008a; University of Miami School of Medicine, 2008).

Postprocedure Care

The patient may be discharged the day of surgery, or may be required to stay in the hospital for 1 to 2 days, depending on the length of the surgery. The patient may experience minimal side effects such as temporary swelling. Other side minor effects

30

include pain, changes in taste, dizziness, inflammation, and bleeding; if these do occur, they are generally temporary (Berke, 2007). Patients return to school or work within a week of surgery; activation of the implant occurs two to four weeks after implantation, allowing enough time for the incision to heal properly (University of Miami School of Medicine, 2008).

Potential Complications

The potential complications associated with this procedure include (Wikipedia, 2008a):

- skin infection;
- onset of tinnitus;
- damage to the vestibular system;
- damage to facial nerves that can cause muscle weakness, or, in severe cases, disfiguring paralysis;
- device failure, usually in cases where the incision does not heal properly; and
- destruction of any residual hearing the patient may have.

PROCEDURES OF THE NOSE AND PARANASAL SINUSES

Operations inside the nose and sinuses are primarily performed to correct obstruction or alleviate infection. Other operations have been designed to control intractable nosebleeds. Tumors within the nasal cavity and sinuses are rare. When tumors are discovered, however, extensive resection of these structures is often necessary.

Special Instruments, Supplies, and Equipment

A dedicated nasal set should always be available for procedures within the nasal cavity. This set usually includes a variety of elevators, dissectors, curved scissors, and curettes, plus nasal specula of different lengths. Dedicated sinus endoscopy sets should be readily available in operative and invasive procedure suites that provide otolaryngological services. The scrub person should be thoroughly familiar with the names of the various forceps that are often used in endoscopic sinus surgery. The use of different lasers within the nasal cavity has been undertaken.

Septoplasty (Septorhinoplasty)

Definition and Indications

Septoplasty refers to the excision of the cartilaginous or bony portions of the nasal septum that lie between the flaps of the mucous membrane and the perichondrium (**Fig. 30.13**). The goal of this procedure is to correct defects or deformities of the septum (*Encyclopedia of Surgery*, 2008d). The primary indications for septoplasty or septorhinoplasty are relief of obstruction resulting from nasal deformity. The deformity might be only within the internal nasal cavity, but it is frequently seen in conjunction with the deviation of the external nose as well. Deviation of the septum often leads to other problems besides obstruction of the nasal airflow. Severe deviations are aggravating factors in recurrent sinusitis. When there are defects of the bony framework, the bones of the nose must be reshaped. Therefore, the preprocedure evaluation of the entire external and internal nose is essential.

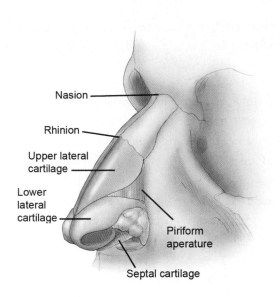

Figure 30.13
Anatomy of the nose.

Nasion

Rhinion

Upper lateral cartilage

Lower lateral cartilage

Piriform aperature

Septal cartilage

Related Procedures

Submucous resection is a related procedure.

Nursing Implications

ANESTHESIA

Septoplasty and septorhinoplasty are often performed under local anesthesia with moderate sedation. When this is done, cocaine solutions can be applied intranasally on cottonoids to provide vasoconstriction and anesthesia. Other agents often used include lidocaine in addition to oxymetazoline (Afrin). These drugs can cause adverse reactions in the patient. The initial symptoms consist of central nervous system stimulation, which is eventually followed by cardiovascular depression. Usually mild symptoms, such as mild excitation, can be seen if the patient is awake. If the patient is under general anesthesia, an increase in heart rate is frequently the only finding. If general anesthesia is going to be used for the procedure, often a throat pack is placed in the back of the throat after the patient is intubated to decrease the chance of aspiration of blood.

POSITION

The patient is placed in the supine position. A headrest should be available to stabilize the head. The same comfort measures are used as for tympanoplasty patients.

ESTABLISHING AND MAINTAINING THE STERILE FIELD

Even though the nasal membranes are contaminated, the mucus within the sinuses should be considered sterile; therefore, a sterile field is created.

EQUIPMENT AND SUPPLIES

Because illumination is provided by the endoscope, or a headlight, it must be in working order. On rare occasions, a microscope may be used. If endoscopes are used, appropriate light connectors for each type of endoscope must be available. The entire lighting mechanism must be thoroughly checked before initiation of the procedure.

The nurse should verify with the surgeon his or her preference for nasal packing and/ or splinting supplies and have these available for use at the end of the procedure.

PHYSIOLOGICAL MONITORING

The patient must be monitored at all times by vital signs measurement, ECG, and pulse oximeter. The circulating nurse must always record the amount of local anesthesia that is administered. All sponges and cottonoids must be counted. Because the cottonoids that are commonly used are small, they can present a hazard if miscounted, or not tagged. Throughout the procedure, cottonoids soaked in a vasoconstricting agent such as oxymetazoline are used. Suction must be available at all times, along with varying sizes of suction catheters.

SPECIMENS AND CULTURES

Nasal cartilage and bone and the turbinates are studied.

DRUGS AND SOLUTIONS

Drugs and solutions that should be available for this procedure include the following:

- Lidocaine 1% with 1:1000 epinephrine
- Cocaine solution or crystals
- Antibiotic ointment or cream
- Gelfoam
- Neosporin 1%
- 1:1000 epinephrine

PHYSICIAN ORDERS

The IV catheter is kept open until the patient is tolerating liquids. Analgesics are administered for pain and antiemetics for nausea. The patient is advised not to drink with straws and to sneeze with the mouth open.

LABORATORY AND DIAGNOSTIC STUDIES

PT
Prothrombin Time

PTT
Partial Thromboplastin Time

Routine CBC, urinalysis, prothrombin time (PT), and partial thromboplastin time (PTT) are ordered. Before procedures within the nose or the sinuses are started, radiographs or CT scans are often obtained to evaluate the problem fully. It is essential that these radiographs or scans are present in the operative suite.

Procedure

INCISION AND EXPOSURE

Unless endoscopes are used along with a camera and monitor, procedures inside the nose can be difficult to follow by the scrub person. The initial portion of the procedure involves the placement of local anesthetic-soaked sponges or cottonoids, as well as the injection of a local anesthetic and epinephrine solution. After this is done, an appropriate time for vasoconstriction is allowed and the nose is examined with a nasal speculum. The initial incision is made inside the nose along the tip of the nasal septum. The initial steps involve the separation of the soft tissues, which include the mucous membrane and underlying perichondrium, from the cartilaginous and bony septum. In a previously traumatized nose, this may be a difficult aspect of the operation. Different elevators, such as the Cottle elevator, are used to lift the perichondrium off the septum.

DETAILS

After the deformed portion of the septum is identified, it may be removed, straightened, or misplaced. A variety of instruments often found in nasal sets is used for this purpose. If the external nasal framework is also to be reshaped (rhinoplasty), this is accomplished using a variety of osteotomes as well as mallets.

CLOSURE

After the nose is shaped in the desired way, and the internal septal deviation is corrected, it is imperative that attempts be made to stabilize the internal and external nasal framework. This can be done in a variety of ways. Tight nasal packing has been used in the past. More commonly, however, internal nasal splints such as Doyle splints may be used to stabilize the septum. Teflon sheeting has also been used for this purpose. The internal splints are stabilized with nonabsorbable sutures. Before placement of the splints, the previously made mucosal incisions are closed using small absorbable sutures. Different ways of stabilizing the external nasal framework have been proposed. Plaster is still used and is effective. Commercially available rigid shields can protect the external nose also. At the completion of the procedure, the throat pack must be removed.

Postprocedure Care

After the procedure, the patient is transferred to the PACU. The head of the bed should be elevated to lessen edema. Analgesics are often prescribed to reduce the discomfort. At times, sedation is necessary in the postprocedure period. A nasal drip pad is often in place under the nose. Because there might be packing inside the nose, the patient is breathing primarily through the mouth. This necessitates good oral care. If the nose is packed bilaterally, humidified oxygen is often given by means of face mask. However, intake of oral fluids must not be started until the effects of the local anesthetic are gone. If oral fluids are started too early, aspiration could occur. Most septoplasties and septorhinoplasties are performed on an outpatient basis. Therefore, discharge instructions should be discussed at length with the patient.

Potential Complications

Bleeding may occur. Toxic shock has also been reported.

Functional Endoscopic Sinus Surgery

Definition and Indications

Functional endoscopic sinus surgery (FESS) refers to procedures performed on the sinus cavities with endoscopic guided resection to open sinus air cells and sinus ostia in order to restore normal drainage of the sinuses (*Encyclopedia of Surgery*, 2008e). With the advent of sinus endoscopes, the extent of visualization inside the nose as well as knowledge of its anatomy and physiology has dramatically improved.

FESS
Functional Endoscopic
Sinus Surgery

Endoscopes allow precise operations within the nasal cavity. Indications for endoscopic sinus procedures include the removal of diseased mucosa and resection of the necessary bony portions of the nasal cavity to establish natural drainage of the paranasal sinuses.

Patients have endoscopic sinus surgery only after an extensive medical and allergic evaluation. When medical treatment has failed and the patients persist with sinusitis, the surgeon often recommends operative intervention. A septoplasty may or may not be performed at the time of the endoscopic procedure. Occasionally, septoplasty becomes necessary to gain access to the nasal cavity with the endoscopes. The extent of the procedure depends on the location of the diseased mucosa and the extent of bony abnormalities within the nasal cavity and sinuses.

Related Procedures

Caldwell-Luc procedure and external ethmoidectomy are related procedures.

Nursing Implications

ANESTHESIA

Endoscopic sinus procedures can be performed using local anesthesia. However, general anesthesia is preferred because of the inability to anesthetize posterior portions of the nose. The principles previously discussed for septoplasty and septorhinoplasty must be followed.

POSITION

See the discussion of septoplasty.

ESTABLISHING AND MAINTAINING THE STERILE FIELD

See the discussion of septoplasty.

EQUIPMENT AND SUPPLIES

Of greatest importance is the availability and thorough knowledge of the appropriate equipment. Complications of the operation have occurred in the past because of lack of appropriate instrumentation. Commercially available endoscopic sinus surgery sets contain a wide variety of telescopes. The endoscopes are usually either 2.7 or 4 mm. in diameter. These have 0-, 25-, 30-, 70-, and 120-degree viewing angles (**Fig. 30.14**). Endoscopes require an external light source; therefore, precaution should be taken in case of burnout of the bulb. Also needed is a camera with a color monitor and a video recorder. A designated endoscopy cart housing all video equipment is essential.

Lasers have been advocated for use intranasally. This, however, is somewhat controversial. If the laser is used, all appropriate precautions as established by the laser safety standards of the facility must be followed.

PHYSIOLOGICAL MONITORING

See the discussion of septoplasty.

SPECIMENS AND CULTURES

Specimens of nasal cartilage and bone and of the contents of different sinuses (eg, ethmoid and maxillary) may be sent for study.

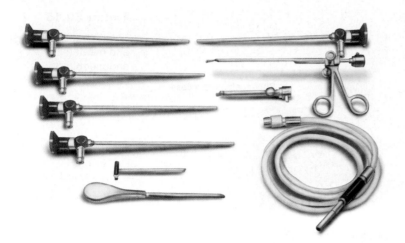

Figure 30.14
Endoscopic instruments.

DRUGS AND SOLUTIONS

See the discussion of septoplasty.

PHYSICIAN ORDERS

See the discussion of septoplasty.

LABORATORY AND DIAGNOSTIC STUDIES

Routine laboratory studies as described for septoplasty are performed. Of utmost importance is the availability of previously obtained CT scans. Because the CT scan provides the "road map" for the surgeon, the patient should not come into the procedure room unless the CT scan is readily available.

Procedure

INCISION AND EXPOSURE

The procedure is usually initiated as for a septoplasty. Local anesthetic or vasoconstricting solutions are used. These are placed intranasally on soaked cottonoids. They are placed in the area of the operation (ie, the middle meatus) (**Fig. 30.15**). The area to be operated on is injected with local anesthetic and epinephrine solutions. If a septoplasty is going to be combined with the operation, this is performed first. After the cottonoids have been left in place to allow for vasoconstriction, the operation is initiated.

Different sharp instruments, such as sickle-shaped knives and scissors, are used for the initial incisions within the middle meatus. A wide variety of straight and angled-biting forceps (usually available in the endoscopic sinus surgery sets) is used for removal of the diseased bony abnormality as well as mucosa. A wide variety of curved suction catheters is also used. The telescope is inserted intranasally and advanced into the ethmoid sinus, and if necessary the sphenoid sinus. The sinus endoscopes are used to visualize anteriorly within the nasal cavity and also into the frontal sinus.

DETAILS

Because the operation proceeds in close proximity to the eye and the brain, care is taken to identify the walls of the orbit and the base of the skull. It is important not to

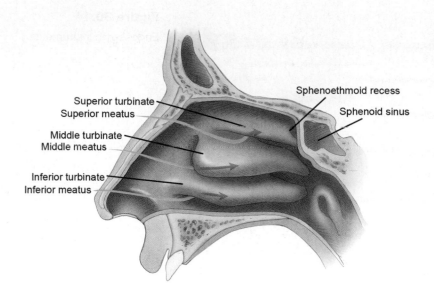

Figure 30.15

Location of turbinates and meati for endoscopic sinus surgery.

Superior turbinate
Superior meatus
Middle turbinate
Middle meatus
Inferior turbinate
Inferior meatus
Sphenoethmoid recess
Sphenoid sinus

have the eyes taped shut. If the orbit is accidentally entered, what might be perceived as nasal mucosa could be orbital contents. When pulling on these contents, movement of the eyeball is seen. This can be occluded if the eyes are taped shut.

After the diseased mucosa and bony abnormalities have been removed from within the nasal cavity, evaluation of the operative field reveals a common cavity between the anterior and posterior ethmoidal cells. However, if diseased mucosa is not encountered in the posterior portion of the ethmoidal cavity, it is not disturbed. Backward cutting antral punches are used to widen the maxillary sinus ostia.

Closure

As the procedure is concluded, hemostasis is obtained with either bipolar electrosurgery or monopolar suction electrosurgery. Because the operation is performed between the lateral nasal wall and the middle turbinate, stents are used that are later removed, to prevent the formation of scarring. Different materials have been used; commercially available Merocel sponges have been designed for this purpose. Most commonly, however, rolled absorbable gelatin film (Gelfilm) dressing is used as a stent within the operated cavity. This is removed at a later date. Usually, no drains or packing is necessary. If extensive bleeding is encountered, however, an anterior nasal pack might be left in place temporarily.

Postprocedure Care

The same nasal dressing as described for septoplasty is applied. Principles previously described are applicable in this situation as well. Of utmost importance, however, is the assessment of vision. Reports of complications stemming from swelling around the eye to blindness have been reported. It is critical that this be evaluated as early as possible. If difficulty with vision is encountered, the surgeon must be notified immediately. Further procedures might become necessary to prevent blindness. If the base of the skull has accidentally been entered, this might not be immediately known. However, profuse clear drainage from the nose may indicate cerebrospinal fluid leak. Again, the surgeon must be notified immediately.

Potential Complications

Complications may include blindness, perforation of the base of skull with subsequent central nervous system infection, injury to the lacrimal duct, and bleeding.

Caldwell-Luc Procedure

Definition and Indications

The Caldwell-Luc procedure is an intraoral procedure for entering the maxillary antrum through the canine fossa above the maxillary premolar teeth. After the maxillary antrum is opened, the sinus mucosa is stripped from the sinus wall; in addition, an intranasal antrostomy is made (*Medcyclopaedia*, 2008).

The Caldwell-Luc operation has been a standard procedure for the sinus surgeon. Additional thought and improved knowledge of the physiology of the sinuses have decreased the use of this operation. However, there are still times when tremendous amount of diseased mucosa and polyps exist within the maxillary sinus. This operation is designed to gain access to the maxillary sinus through an incision underneath the upper lip in the area of the anterior wall of the maxillary sinus. Sinus endoscopes have often been used to visualize maxillary sinus contents also. A trocar can be used to penetrate the anterior wall of the maxillary sinus. After the trocar has entered the sinus, the scope can be placed through a sheath into the sinus. This helps in assessing the extent of the maxillary sinus operation.

Related Procedures

Creation of nasal antral windows (antrostomy) is a related procedure.

Nursing Implications

ANESTHESIA

The Caldwell-Luc operation is often performed in conjunction with other intranasal procedures. Therefore, previously discussed anesthesia regimens should be followed.

POSITION

See the discussion of septoplasty.

ESTABLISHING AND MAINTAINING THE STERILE FIELD

The patient is prepared and draped as previously described for nasal procedures.

EQUIPMENT AND SUPPLIES

A general nose set is used. Also used is a Caldwell-Luc set, which includes an antral punch and Coakley antrum curettes.

PHYSIOLOGICAL MONITORING

See the discussion of septoplasty.

SPECIMENS AND CULTURES

Polyps and diseased nasal mucosa may be sent to the pathology department.

DRUGS AND SOLUTIONS

See the discussion of septoplasty.

PHYSICIAN ORDERS

See the discussion of septoplasty.

LABORATORY AND DIAGNOSTIC STUDIES

Routine CBC, urinalysis, PT, PTT, CT scan, and/or sinus radiographs are obtained.

Procedure

INCISION AND EXPOSURE

The maxillary sinus to be operated on is approached through an incision in the oral mucous membrane above the canine teeth. This mucosal flap is retracted until periosteum is incised (**Fig. 30.16**). A section of maxillary bone is cut out to gain access into the maxillary sinus.

DETAILS

Through this opening, polyps or diseased mucosa are removed. Through the nasal cavity, a flap and opening is created into the maxillary sinus through the inferior meatus. After this connection has been created, the sinus is packed with gauze impregnated with antibiotic ointment. One end of the gauze is brought out through the opening made in the nasal cavity. This packing is eventually removed through

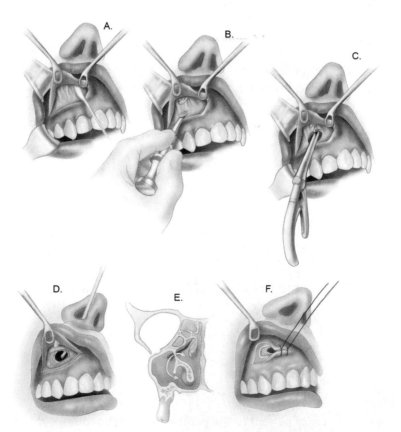

Figure 30.16

Caldwell-Luc procedure.

the nose. After the gauze is in place, care must be taken not to lose the end of the gauze that is brought out through the nasal cavity.

CLOSURE

The periosteum is reapproximated, and the mucosal incision is closed with absorbable suture.

Postprocedure Care

Postprocedure care is similar to that for other intranasal procedures previously described.

Potential Complications

Complications may include injury to the roots of the teeth in children, injury to the infraorbital nerve leading to anesthesia of the cheek, injury to the orbital contents, injury to the tooth sockets, and edema.

Closed Repair of Nasal Fracture

Definition

Closed repair of nasal fracture refers to the manipulation of a nasal fracture without incision. This procedure is often performed after trauma to the face. Intranasal manipulation can be used immediately after the injury. Occasionally, elevation of depressed bone or cartilage can be performed and the nose reshaped to its normal position.

Indications

The indications for closed reduction include unilateral or bilateral fracture of the nasal bones and fracture of the nasal septal complex that is deviated less than one half of the width of the nasal bridge; however, reduction of a nasal fracture is indicated in any patient with a significant cosmetic deformity or functional compromise (Dev, 2006). The best time for reduction may be within the first 3 hours after injury, otherwise, most believe that waiting 3–7 days is preferable in order to allow edema to resolve, and also facilitate positioning the bones correctly with more stability because inflammation and fibrosis may make the fragments less mobile. If reduction is not possible within the first 7–10 days, then the fractured segments begin forming a fibrous union (Dev, 2006).

Nursing Implications

ANESTHESIA

Most procedures to reduce the nasal cavity are most comfortably performed with the use of general anesthesia. This is especially true in children. However, local anesthesia can be used and previously described principles followed.

ESTABLISHING AND MAINTAINING THE STERILE FIELD

See the discussion of septoplasty.

EQUIPMENT AND SUPPLIES

A general nose set or designated closed nasal fracture set and a headlight are needed.

PHYSIOLOGICAL MONITORING

See the discussion of septoplasty.

SPECIMENS AND CULTURES

Typically there is no specimen.

DRUGS AND SOLUTIONS

See the discussion of septoplasty.

PHYSICIAN ORDERS

See the discussion of septoplasty.

LABORATORY AND DIAGNOSTIC STUDIES

CBC and urinalysis are performed.

Procedure

Intranasal manipulation is performed with a variety of blunt instruments. A Boies elevator is often used intranasally to elevate nasal bony depression. Different types of forceps are also available for this purpose. It is important to know that clinical evaluation of the nose is far more important than radiographic evaluation. Therefore, radiographs are not necessarily obtained. Even if the operation is performed under general anesthesia, topical anesthesia and vasoconstrictors are placed on soaked cottonoids intranasally. Previously described substances such as cocaine or oxymetazoline can be used.

After the desired reduction is obtained, it is important to stabilize the nose externally. The same principles should be used as for stabilization of the patient who has had a rhinoplasty.

Postprocedure Care

See the discussion of septoplasty.

Potential Complications

The complications of closed reduction are few. Some fractures cannot be satisfactorily reduced and that would necessitate a formal rhinoplasty at a later date. Unmanageable bleeding is rarely encountered. Nasal packing might be used temporarily to control a nosebleed after the manipulation. Additional complications have been reported if nasal packing is used, some of which are infectious, such as toxic shock syndrome.

PROCEDURES OF THE OROPHARYNX AND HEAD AND NECK

Tonsillectomy and Adenoidectomy

Definition

Tonsillectomy and adenoidectomy refer to the excision of the pharyngeal tonsils and adenoids. No operation has attracted as much attention and heated controversy.

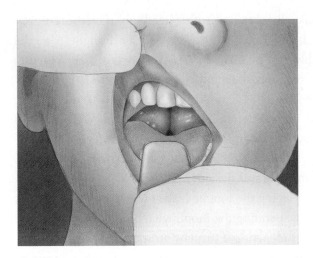

Figure 30.17

Tonsils obstructing the oropharynx.

The tonsillectomy and adenoidectomy procedure is the most common major surgery performed in children (Kavanaugh, 2008).

Indications

The indications for tonsillectomy and adenoidectomy have varied through the years. The three most common indications, however, are chronic infections, obstruction of breathing (**Fig. 30.17**), and excisional biopsy in the evaluation of tonsillar tumors. Tonsillectomy and adenoidectomy are not always performed at the same time. Different indications exist for removal of the adenoid pad only. For example, the adenoid tissue affects the middle ear. Studies revealing the effects of adenoidectomy on chronic otitis media are well known. Therefore, the decision to perform an adenoidectomy does not always include a tonsillectomy. Sometimes, a tonsillectomy alone is performed. Most adenoidal tissue involutes with age. The decision to remove it depends on the symptoms associated with an enlarged adenoid pad.

Nursing Implications

ANESTHESIA

Most tonsillectomies and adenoidectomies are performed using general anesthesia. Local anesthesia has been used successfully in adults. The discussion presented here, however, primarily refers to the patient under general anesthesia.

POSITION

The patient is usually in a supine position and is placed on the bed with his or her head at the foot. This facilitates the surgeon's comfortable access to the patient. If the patient has the procedure under local anesthesia, the semi-Fowler position may be preferable.

ESTABLISHING AND MAINTAINING THE STERILE FIELD

Tonsillectomy and adenoidectomy is not considered a sterile procedure. Hospital policy specifies whether the patient is or is not draped. The surgeon and scrub person, however, should don sterile gowns and gloves and wear appropriate head covering, eye protection, and a mask according to standard precautions guidelines. The surgeon may sit at the patient's head or stand at the side of the bed.

Lighting into the oral cavity is usually obtained with a headlight. Overhead lights, however, have been used. Lighting is superior, nevertheless, with a headlight. After the patient has been intubated, the table may be turned to suit the surgeon, The patient's head is draped to cover the eyes, which have been taped by the anesthesia provider.

If the surgeon sits at the head of the bed, a mouth gag is inserted to depress the tongue and expose the oropharynx. Most often, a Davis-Crowe or palate-type mouth gag is used for this purpose. These gags are designed to open the oral cavity while simultaneously depressing the tongue. After this is obtained, the gag is secured to a suspension apparatus. Different suspension apparatus designs are available. Most commonly, however, suspension is obtained by placing the tongue blade on a Mayo stand. This is probably the most common way of suspending the mouth gag; however, independent suspension apparatuses are superior. Independent suspension apparatuses provide free movement of the table without having the worry of the Mayo stand height or location.

Because a tonsillectomy and adenoidectomy can be a bloody procedure, appropriate suctioning with Yankauer tips is required. The incision and dissection have been described in a number of ways. A cold knife, electrosurgery, and laser have been used to perform the operation. There have been different advocates for the various techniques. No single technique is considered superior. There should be an effort, however, to decrease bleeding during the procedure. After the oropharynx is exposed, the decision is made to begin either the adenoidectomy first or the tonsillectomy. Sometimes removal of the adenoid tissue first allows more time for packing of the nasopharynx and easier hemostasis.

EQUIPMENT AND SUPPLIES

A tonsil and adenoid set is needed, as well as the surgeon-preferred mouth gag. These may range from the Jennings, to Davis-Crowe, to a palate-type mouth gag. The nurse may anticipate the use of a Davis-Crowe or McGivor mouth gag if the surgeon sits or stands at the patient's head during the procedure. The Jennings mouth gag, however, is more routinely used if the surgeon stands at the patient's side during the procedure.

The suction coagulator is necessary, and the possible use of a handswitch electrosurgery pencil should be anticipated. The foot pedal of the electrosurgery generator is necessary for the use of the suction coagulator. As for the use of all electrical equipment, the nurse should ensure that these pieces of equipment are operating correctly before the beginning of the procedure. If the laser is used, all laser precautions should be in place before the procedure.

PHYSIOLOGICAL MONITORING

The patient is monitored at all times as for previously described procedures.

SPECIMENS AND CULTURES

The right and left tonsils and adenoid tissue are sent for study.

DRUGS AND SOLUTIONS

Drugs and solutions needed for this procedure include the following:

- Normal saline
- Lidocaine 1% with 1:100,000 epinephrine

- Phenylephrine (Neo-Synephrine)
- Tannic acid
- Bismuth subgallate
- 1:1000 epinephrine
- Defogging solution (Antifog, pHisoHex)

PHYSICIAN ORDERS

The IV catheter is maintained at a keep-open rate until the patient is taking fluids without nausea and vomiting. The patient is given a soft diet. The following are administered: an analgesic of the surgeon's preference for pain (most common is acetaminophen with codeine), promethazine suppository for nausea, and dexamethasone (optional) for swelling.

LABORATORY AND DIAGNOSTIC STUDIES

Results of a CBC, urinalysis, PT, and PTT are obtained.

Procedure

INCISION AND EXPOSURE

The procedure is initiated by making a decision whether the tonsillectomy or the adenoidectomy will be performed first. The tonsillectomy is performed as follows: The tonsil is retracted with an Allis or similar tonsil clamp. Other material can be used to retract the tonsil as well. Sometimes, a 0-plain catgut suture is used on a curved urological needle. This is placed through the tonsillar tissue itself in a figure-of-eight knot. This provides good retraction without fragmenting the tonsillar tissue, which can happen with clamps. By retracting the tonsil medially, the anterior pillar is incised by whatever means the surgeon decides.

DETAILS

The incision is carried down until the capsule of the tonsil becomes visible. As previously mentioned, a knife, electrosurgery, or lasers can be used for this purpose. Using blunt and sharp dissection, the capsule of the tonsil is exposed from the tonsillar fossa. The availability of a suction coagulator helps in the hemostasis. As the dissection continues, the superior pole of the tonsil is exposed and retracted from the tonsillar fossa. As blood vessels are encountered, they may be either cauterized or tied with suture. Slipknots of 2-0 or 3-0 catgut are placed around these vessels. The tonsil dissection then continues until the most inferior portion of the tonsil is exposed. At this time, the tonsil is removed from the tonsillar fossa with a snare, or with sharp dissection using electrosurgery, laser, or scissors. After this is performed, the fossa of the tonsil is carefully inspected and any bleeding vessel is either cauterized or clamped and tied. The opposite tonsil is then removed in a similar fashion. An adenoidectomy should be performed with indirect vision using a mirror. A "blind" adenoidectomy is discouraged because the eustachian orifice can be injured.

The easiest way to expose the nasopharynx is by placing soft rubber catheters through the nasal cavity and bringing them out through the oral cavity. Before the catheters are placed through the nose, the surgeon often inspects the soft palate.

This is important to identify congenital defects of the palate that might be a contraindication to an adenoidectomy. These catheters can then be used to retract the soft palate. Using a dental mirror that has been defogged with defogging solution, the surgeon can visualize the nasopharynx. Only in this way can the eustachian tube orifices be identified and protected.

Different devices have been designed to remove the adenoid tissue. A variety of adenoid curettes are available, which are most commonly used to scrape the lymphoid tissue from the nasopharynx. Different basket punches also exist to remove any loose fragments of lymphoid tissue. The adenoidectomy is a somewhat more difficult procedure, because of the possibility of leaving fragments of lymphoid tissue in the nasopharynx. Hemostasis is usually obtained with packing as well as the suction coagulator. It must be emphasized that, when suction coagulation is used, the eustachian tube orifice must always be in full view to prevent debilitating scarring and intractable middle ear problems.

CLOSURE

Before the procedure is terminated, a final inspection is performed to evaluate for any bleeding sites. The nasopharynx can be irrigated with ice or room temperature normal saline. The stomach contents should be suctioned out before the procedure is terminated to decrease the chance of nausea and vomiting after the procedure.

Postprocedure Care

Because bleeding from the operative site is the most serious complication, this must be watched for at all times in the immediate postoperative period. Any bleeding must be reported to the surgeon immediately. When the patient is transferred to the PACU, he or she is often lying on the side. This decreases the chance of aspiration of blood or secretions. Analgesia is almost always required for the patients. The discomfort after a tonsillectomy and adenoidectomy is often underemphasized. A balance must be made between narcotic administration and depression of the central nervous system. Analgesia is attempted; however, too much sedation should he avoided to prevent aspiration.

A liquid diet is initiated only if the patient is awake enough to ask. Antiemetic medication is also often prescribed.

Potential Complications

Complications may include bleeding that can be life threatening; pain and inability to swallow, which can cause dehydration in young children; injury to the eustachian tube orifices; aspiration of blood, leading to pulmonary complications; and aspiration, leading to airway obstruction and respiratory arrest.

Parotidectomy

Definition and Indications

Parotidectomy refers to the partial or complete excision of the parotid gland. The primary purpose of parotidectomy is to remove neoplasms that occur in the parotid gland. Parotid gland neoplasms are usually benign (approximately 80%); tumors may spread from other areas of the body, entering the parotid gland via the lymphatic system (*Encyclopedia of Surgery*, 2008f). The minimal operation performed for these tumors is a superficial or lateral parotidectomy. Malignant lesions often necessitate the removal of the entire parotid gland, including the deep lobe. At times, a radical neck dissection or other more radical procedures are combined with a parotidectomy. However, for most parotid tumors, a lateral parotidectomy with preservation of the deep lobe and the facial nerve is all that is necessary.

Nursing Implications

ANESTHESIA

Operations performed on the parotid gland are always done using general anesthesia. It is critical that no neuromuscular blockade be used during the procedure. This is because identification of the facial nerve is often made not only with visualization but also by stimulation using a nerve stimulator. If blockade has been given, the nerve is not stimulated. This might lead to inadvertent severing of facial nerve branches.

POSITION

The position of the patient is supine with the affected side of the face up. A small roll underneath the shoulders, as well as a headrest, provides stabilization of the area.

ESTABLISHING AND MAINTAINING THE STERILE FIELD

This is a sterile procedure and therefore different from the previously described techniques within the oral or nasal cavities. The establishment and maintenance of the sterile field are critical and must adhere to the principles of aseptic technique. Because parotidectomy can be a lengthy procedure, padding must be provided for pressure points. After the patient is asleep and intubated and appropriate positioning has been obtained, the patient's face is prepared with antimicrobial solutions. The face is draped from the level of the forehead down to the level of the clavicle on the operative side. It is often a good practice to place a cotton ball or other type of wick into the ear canal to prevent preparation solutions from entering the ear canal.

It is important that the face be visible at all times. Stimulation of the facial nerve leads to movement of the muscles of facial expression. Therefore, the ability to see movement in the face is of utmost importance. A self-adhering plastic drape can be used to cover the entire face and neck. Some surgeons prefer not to do this and just keep the face exposed. Towels are used to create a sterile field. Lint-free sterile drapes are then used to cover the patient inferiorly and superiorily.

EQUIPMENT AND SUPPLIES

A general plastic set, a nerve stimulator, special parotid retractors, and bipolar electrosurgery unit should be available.

PHYSIOLOGICAL MONITORING

Because a parotidectomy can be a lengthy procedure, the patient's comfort and safety are important. All bony prominences are padded to decrease the risk of nerve damage and a pillow is offered for under the knees to decrease back strain. The ECG, blood pressure, and oxygen saturation are monitored by the anesthesia provider. The circulating nurse should be aware of monitoring and assist the anesthesia provider as necessary.

SPECIMENS AND CULTURES

Parotid tissue is sent to the pathology department.

DRUGS AND SOLUTIONS

No drugs or solutions are needed.

PHYSICIAN ORDERS

A regular diet is given. The IV catheter is kept open until the patient is tolerating fluids. Antiemetic and analgesic of physician's choice are administered. Facial function should be checked. The patient may be up ad lib.

LABORATORY AND DIAGNOSTIC STUDIES

CBC, urinalysis, and CT scan are obtained.

Procedure

INCISION AND EXPOSURE

The incision is made immediately in front of the ear following natural skin creases. The incision extends below the earlobe and into the neck below the angle of the jaw. The incision is carried down into the neck to provide full visualization of the facial nerve. Anterior and posterior skin flaps are developed. This incision is carried down sharply using a blade until the fascia overlying the parotid gland is seen. Monopolar electrosurgery should be used carefully because transmission of electrosurgical current to and subsequent injury of the facial nerve may occur. It is better to provide electrosurgery using a bipolar mode.

DETAILS

After the parotid fascia is identified, the next portion of the procedure involves careful dissection using curved clamps to separate the gland from the mastoid process and the cartilage of the external auditory canal. At times, there is troublesome bleeding, which can usually be controlled with bipolar electrosurgery. The tail of the parotid gland is then separated from the anterior and superior portions of the sternocleidomastoid muscle.

The most important portion of the operation is the identification of the main trunk of the facial nerve. Using a small curved or delicate Crile clamp, the parotid fascia is carefully elevated. The fascia is then transected carefully and the main trunk is identified. At times, identification is difficult. The cartilage of the external auditory canal can be used as a guide to finding the main trunk. After the main trunk is identified, the dissection proceeds anteriorly and laterally. It is critical that the dissection follow the trunk of the facial nerve. The branches of the facial nerve are identified most easily in this fashion. At times, the main trunk is not found readily. Identification of a superficial branch can be made and followed posteriorly and deeply to the main trunk. However, the safest technique is to identify the main trunk and pursue the course of the branches in a posterior-to-anterior fashion. The nerve stimulator here becomes important to trace small branches of the facial nerve. As the branches of the facial nerve become visible, the substance of the parotid gland and the lesion within it can be dissected away safely. After the freed portion of the superficial lobe is dissected from the facial nerve branches, the parotid duct is transected and ligated at the anterior wound margin.

CLOSURE

After the parotid gland and the lesion are removed from the operative field, the nerve fibers are again identified. Any areas of bleeding are either ligated with small silk ties or cauterized using bipolar cautery. The previously raised flaps are then reapproximated using 4-0 or 5-0 absorbable suture and the skin is closed using 5-0 or 6-0 nonabsorbable suture material. A small tissue drain, preferably a suction drain, may be placed in the most dependent portion of the wound.

Postprocedure Care

A firm pressure dressing (similar to the previously described mastoid dressing) is used. However, the self-adherent gauze is used in a similar fashion to a modified Barton dressing. Care must be taken to support the external ear. After the wound is dressed, the patient is transferred to the PACU. One of the most important aspects of transfer, especially if a suction drain is placed, is to prevent accidental dislodging of the suction drain.

After the patient is awake, the facial nerve can be examined by asking the patient to follow commands regarding facial expressions. Analgesics are usually ordered. The amount of discomfort is usually that of a pressure sensation from the pressure dressing. The dressing is left in place for at least 24–48 hours. After this, the dressing is changed and the wound evaluated. The suction drain is removed at the surgeon's discretion.

Potential Complications

Complications may include facial nerve injury, temporary or permanent (if a branch or main trunk is sectioned, immediate repair is indicated); bleeding with subsequent hematoma formation; recurrence of the lesion; and abnormal sweating on the side of the face.

Uvulopalatopharyngoplasty
Definition and Indications

Uvulopalatopharyngoplasty (UPPP) is a procedure used to remove excess tissue in the throat to widen the airway, in order to allow air to move through the throat more easily during breathing, thereby reducing snoring (Essig, 2008). The tissue that may be removed includes the uvula; a portion of the soft palate; excess throat tissue; tonsils and adenoids; and the pharynx. The procedure is indicated as a remedy for severe obstructive sleep apnea (OSA) believed to be caused by obstructions in the nose or pharynx.

UPPP
Uvulopalatopharyngoplasty

LA-UPPP
Laser-assisted uvulopalatopharyngo-plasty

Related Procedures

Laser-assisted uvulopalatopharyngoplasty (LA-UPPP) and tracheotomy are related procedures.

Nursing Implications

ANESTHESIA

UPPP is performed under general anesthesia.

POSITION

The patient is placed in the supine position with a small roll underneath the shoulders; a headrest is also used to provide stabilization.

ESTABLISHING AND MAINTAINING THE STERILE FIELD

Sterile drapes are placed on the patient's chest and torso to prevent soiling the clothing with secretions or blood. Eye coverage/protection/head drapes are used based on the surgeon's preference.

EQUIPMENT AND SUPPLIES

A general plastic set and bipolar cautery should be available.

PHYSIOLOGICAL MONITORING

The patient is monitored at all times as for previously described procedures.

SPECIMENS AND CULTURES

The tissues removed are sent for pathological study.

DRUGS AND SOLUTIONS

No drugs or solutions are needed.

PHYSICIAN ORDERS/LABORATORY AND DIAGNOSTIC STUDIES

The routine presurgical physical evaluation is performed. Additional preoperative diagnostic studies may include a complete polysomnogram to rule out nonobstructive causes of sleep apnea and confirmation of the site of obstruction through fiberoptic pharyngoscopy or cephalometric radiographs with tracing.

Procedure

After orotracheal intubation, a self-retaining mouth gag is placed to maintain adequate exposure. The oropharyngeal structures are carefully outlined. The lower portion of the soft palate, including the uvula, is excised. The tonsils and adenoids, if present, will also be removed at this time (see **Fig. 30.18**). Absorbable sutures are used to approximate the tissue edges.

Postprocedure Care

CPAP
Continuous Positive Airway Pressure

The patient remains in the hospital one to two nights, followed by a minimum two-week recovery period (*Encyclopedia of Surgery*, 2008g). Postoperatively, the patient may require continuous positive airway pressure (CPAP) therapy; certain analgesics

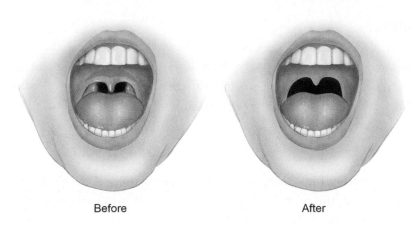

Figure 30.18
UPPP.

Before   After

are avoided since they relax the throat muscles, which can cause the throat to narrow and cause apnea episodes (Essig, 2007). The IV catheter is maintained at a keep-open rate until the patient is taking fluids without nausea and vomiting.

Potential Complications

Complications after UPPP may include (Wikipedia, 2008b):

- Sleepiness and sleep apnea related to postoperative medication;
- Swelling;
- Infection;
- Bleeding;
- A sore throat and/or difficulty swallowing;
- Drainage of secretions into the nose and a nasal quality to the voice;
- Narrowing of the airway in the nose and throat, thereby constricting breathing;
- Snoring; and
- Iatrogenically caused sleep apnea.

Tracheotomy
Definition and Indications

A tracheotomy is performed to open a direct airway through an incision in the *trachea* (Wikipedia, 2008c). Adult and pediatric tracheotomy procedures are different.

The indications for tracheotomy vary, but they are all for a maintenance of an artificial airway:

- Prolonged intubation or need to undergo ventilation
- Upper airway obstruction in which orotracheal intubation is difficult or not possible
- Pulmonary toilet and cleaning of secretions

A permanent tracheotomy is always performed when there is a laryngectomy, or removal of the voice box.

30

Nursing Implications

ANESTHESIA

Tracheotomies are often performed using local anesthesia in adults. General anesthesia, however, is preferred in the pediatric patient. A small amount of local anesthetic with vasoconstricting agents may be used to infiltrate the skin in the area of the incision.

POSITION

Several important aspects of positioning exist when performing a tracheotomy. Unless it is contraindicated, the neck is hyperextended. A roll is placed under the shoulders. In young children, the chin is pulled superiorly as much as possible. Tape may be used to help further in hyperextending a child's neck. The tape can be secured from the chin to the head of the bed. The surface landmarks of the neck are identified.

ESTABLISHING AND MAINTAINING THE STERILE FIELD

Even though the respiratory system is entered, the procedure should be considered sterile. A marking pen can be used to mark the structures that have been palpated. The skin incision can be either horizontal or vertical. The neck is prepared with a skin antiseptic agent, and sterile drapes are applied in standard fashion.

EQUIPMENT AND SUPPLIES

In a young child, appropriate pediatric instruments are required. This may include smaller curved hemostats than in an adult tracheotomy set, as well as fine tissue forceps. In addition, a wide variety of sizes and types of tracheotomy tubes are essential. A discussion of the different types of tracheotomy tubes is beyond the scope of this chapter, but sizes ranging from those small enough to fit premature infants to those suitable for the largest adult must be readily available.

PHYSIOLOGICAL MONITORING

If the procedure is performed with general anesthesia, routine care as discussed for previous procedures should be maintained. However, if the procedure is done using local anesthesia, it is vital that the circulating nurse explain the procedure and the sensations that the patient will experience before the procedure. The placement of a shoulder roll, the application of the electrosurgery patient return electrode and possible wrist restraints, and the feeling of "loss of breath" are all critical to explain to the patient. During this procedure, the nurse plays a vital role in decreasing the patient's anxiety level by being close at hand. ECG, respirations, blood pressure, and pulse oximetry are monitored throughout the procedure.

SPECIMENS AND CULTURES

No specimens are obtained.

DRUGS AND SOLUTIONS

Drugs and solutions needed for this procedure include the following:

- Lidocaine 1% with 1:100,000 epinephrine
- Lubricant jelly
- Lidocaine 4% transtracheal injection

PHYSICIAN ORDERS

The physician orders a chest radiograph, tracheostomy care as necessary, continuation of IV fluid administration, pulmonary function studies if indicated, and respiratory therapy if necessary.

LABORATORY AND DIAGNOSTIC STUDIES

CBC, urinalysis, and a chest radiograph are obtained.

Procedure

INCISION AND EXPOSURE

A vertical incision technique is described. After the skin incision has been made, it is carried deep through the platysma muscle (**Fig. 30.19A**). It is carried down until the fascia in the midline between the small strap muscles of the neck is identified. The fascia is then incised in a sharp fashion using a blade. The strap muscles are then retracted laterally. This usually exposes the thyroid gland isthmus (ie, the connection between both sides of the thyroid gland). A decision must be made at this time whether the isthmus of the thyroid gland will be transected or merely retracted (see **Fig. 30.19B**). If a decision is made to transect the thyroid gland, curved hemostats are used to dissect the gland gently from the trachea below. The gland is transected between two curved hemostats and ligated using absorbable 3-0 suture material. This facilitates visualization of the structures below.

DETAILS

The cricoid cartilage should be fully visible. As the surgeon prepares to enter the windpipe, the scrub person must have the tracheotomy tube prepared and available to be inserted. The anesthesia provider is notified that the airway will be entered. The technique of entering the airway varies in children and adults. In adults, a No. 11 blade knife can be used to cut a window of cartilage in the area of the second, third, or fourth tracheal arch (sec **Fig. 30.19C**). A flap of tracheal cartilage has also been advocated.

In young infants, however, before the airway is entered, it is important to place silk stay ties on the lateral portion of the trachea. These can be used to help bring the trachea out into the neck incision in case of accidental decannulation. Also in the pediatric population, a sharp blade that is short (a Beaver 6900 blade is ideal) can be used to incise the tracheal arches. In the pediatric population, a portion of the tracheal arch is not removed. Instead an incision is made along the third, fourth, and, at times, fifth tracheal arch.

After elevating the tracheal ring (see **Fig. 30.19D**), the surgeon places the tracheotomy tube, complete with the obturator, through the opening. The tracheotomyties

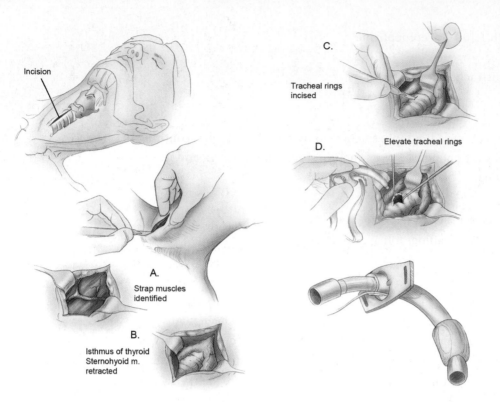

Figure 30.19
Tracheotomy procedure.

Incision

C.

Tracheal rings
incised

D.

Elevate tracheal rings

A.
Strap muscles
identified

B.
Isthmus of thyroid
Sternohyoid m.
retracted

and a syringe to inflate the cuff are attached to the tube. The obturator is removed and an inner cannula is inserted. Sterile anesthesia connectors are then used to connect a tracheotomy tube to the anesthesia machine if the tube selected is not designed with the appropriate connector.

CLOSURE

After the airway has been established, the tracheotomy tube can be secured using the tracheotomy ties usually included in tracheotomy tube sets. In addition, for extra protection, the flanges of the tracheotomy tube may be sutured to the skin of the neck.

Postprocedure Care

In the immediate postprocedure period, a chest radiograph should be obtained, especially for young infants. The possibility of pneumothorax exists in the younger patient. In addition, even small tracheotomy tubes are at times too long in the very young patient. This can cause the tracheotomy tube tip to ventilate only one side of the chest. Visualization of the tube tip on a chest radiograph helps prevent this complication. The excessive incision can be approximated using a single skin nonabsorbable suture in the young patient. However, care must be taken not to create an airtight wound. This is because air escape from a tracheotomy tube almost always occurs. If the wound is closed tightly, there can be air dissection into the subcutaneous tissues.

As the patient is transported to either the PACU or the intensive care unit, the most important portion of the transport is prevention of accidental dislodging of the tracheotomy tube. Elbow restraints should be used to prevent young children from pulling at the tracheotomy tube. If necessary, sedation is ordered by the surgeon.

Performing pediatric tracheotomies should be discouraged in settings in which pediatric intensive care units are not readily available. The nursing staff is critical in preventing accidental decannulation and subsequent tragedies. Most patients require frequent suctioning of secretions in the first 24 hours. Additional tracheotomy tubes of the size used must always accompany the patient. The previously placed tracheal stay sutures should be marked right and left. In case of accidental decannulation, these sutures may be used to elevate the trachea and aid in replacement of the tracheotomy tube. The obturator is secured to the head of the patient's bed at all times to aid in replacement of the tube.

Potential Complications

Complications may include injury to the nerves of the vocal cords; injury to large blood vessels abnormally located in the area of the incision; pneumothorax; accidental decannulation during the postoperative period, especially in children; pneumonia; infections in the area of the skin or within the trachea; formation of a tracheoesophageal fistula; tracheal stenosis; and erosion of blood vessels, leading to fatal hemorrhage.

Total Laryngectomy and Radical Neck Dissection

Definition and Indications

Total laryngectomy refers to the excision of the entire larynx with the stoma opening into the larynx being permanent; the patient breathes through the stoma and must learn to talk in a new way (MedicineNet.com, 2008b). Radical neck dissection refers to excision of a tumor, the surrounding anatomical structures, and lymph nodes on the affected side of the neck.

The primary indication for partial or total removal of the larynx and radical neck dissection is to treat cancer. Because patients undergoing laryngectomy or neck dissection are usually heavy alcohol and tobacco users, their overall medical condition must be fully evaluated. At times, preoperative or adjuvant chemotherapy is also advocated.

Related Procedures

Hemilaryngectomy or partial laryngectomy and supraglottic laryngectomy are related procedures.

Nursing Implications

ANESTHESIA

The anesthesia implications are usually identical to those described for a tracheotomy using general anesthesia. The anesthesia provider should be positioned to the side of the patient on the unaffected side of the neck. Usually, an arterial line is placed. Blood gas levels are often monitored.

POSITION

The positioning implications are usually identical to those described previously for a tracheotomy. If an accompanying neck dissection is to be performed, the head may need to be turned to the appropriate side. The comfort and safety devices described earlier for ear procedures are used.

ESTABLISHING AND MAINTAINING THE STERILE FIELD

The entire face, including the ears, the neck, and the chest to the nipple line should be prepared with a skin antiseptic agent. If necessary, the chest hair should be removed using clippers or depilatory. If a tracheostomy stoma is present, the stoma is included in the area to be prepped. The nurse must avoid getting solutions in the stoma. If the surgeon intends to obtain a graft, the thigh is prepared as well. The sterile field is created using a head and neck drape pack. Care is taken in lifting the patient's head for application of the head drape, and the anesthesia provider is informed before this is done. The patient is then draped with appropriate sterile sheets.

EQUIPMENT AND SUPPLIES

A general plastic set, a tracheostomy set, a vascular set, bipolar cautery, a headlight, a nerve stimulator, an eggcrate or gel pad for the bed, a convective warming device, a scale for weighing sponges, antiembolism stockings (these may be applied preoperatively before transfer to the operative and invasive procedure suite), a nasogastric feeding tube, a closed suction drain, bone cutters and an oscillating saw (for partial laryngectomy), a Foley catheter, and tracheostomy and/or laryngectomy tubes are assembled.

PHYSIOLOGICAL MONITORING

Most head and neck cancer cases are lengthy; therefore, a Foley catheter is usually inserted. In addition, a nasal feeding tube is usually passed through one naris down to the level of the throat. At the end of the procedure, this feeding tube is advanced into the esophagus and into the stomach. This tube is used to feed the patient in the postprocedure period.

The sponges are weighed throughout the procedure to obtain an estimate of blood loss during the procedure. The patient's temperature is also monitored with a rectal probe. An oral temperature probe is contraindicated to decrease the number of tubes in the surgical field. Blood gas and electrolyte values are monitored throughout the procedure.

SPECIMENS AND CULTURES

Contents of the radical neck dissection to include the lymphatics, the jugular vein, the 11th cranial nerve, the sternocleidomastoid muscle and the submandibular salivary gland, the ipsilateral portion of the thyroid gland, and the larynx are the surgical specimens.

DRUGS AND SOLUTIONS

Drugs and solutions required for this procedure may include those listed below:

- Lidocaine 1% with 1:100,000 epinephrine
- Oxidized regenerated cellulose (Surgicel)
- Lidocaine 4%

- Hetastarch (Hespan) for anesthesia
- Antibiotic of surgeon's preference

PHYSICIAN ORDERS

The physician orders an IV, antibiotics of choice, the use of drains to suction, nothing by mouth for 48 hours, admittance to the intensive care unit, and a chest radiograph. Vital signs are obtained every hour for 4 hours and then every 4 hours. Mouth care and tracheotomy care are given as necessary. Humidified oxygen is given per tracheotomy collar at 5 L/minute. Analgesics and antiemetics of choice are ordered. The patient is advanced to tube feeding every 4 hours and is up to a chair on the first postoperative day.

LABORATORY AND DIAGNOSTIC STUDIES

CBC, urinalysis, PT, PTT, SMA-15, electrolyte values, a chest radiograph, and CT scan are obtained.

Procedure

INCISION AND EXPOSURE

After the neck has been prepared and draped as described previously, a decision is made about the skin incision. If a laryngectomy is going to be performed without a neck dissection, the head should stay in the midline and be hyperextended. If a partial laryngectomy (ie, a vertical or supraglottic laryngectomy) is the operative procedure, appropriate horizontal incisions are planned. If the procedure is to be a total laryngectomy without neck dissection, the incision is usually a midline vertical incision or midline transverse incision.

Because the operation is most commonly performed in conjunction with a neck dissection, the incisions planned can vary at the discretion of the surgeon. The description below is for the most comprehensive of laryngectomy procedures (a total laryngectomy and radical neck dissection).

The goal of the neck dissection is to remove all lymph node-bearing tissue from the midline anteriorly to the trapezius muscle posteriorly and also from the mandible superiorly to the clavicle inferiorly. All of this tissue between the deep cervical fascia and the platysma muscle externally is removed, except for the carotid artery system and the vagus, phrenic, and hypoglossal nerves. The brachial plexus is also preserved.

The contents of the neck that are removed include the jugular vein, the spinal accessory (11th cranial) nerve, the sternocleidomastoid muscle, and the submandibular salivary gland. Sometimes, the spinal accessory nerve can be preserved.

When the operation is combined with a total laryngectomy, the larynx, the midportion of the hyoid bone, and the epiglottis are also removed. Inferiorly, the laryngectomy also includes at least one or two tracheal arches. The patient requires a permanent tracheotomy.

Various skin incisions have been described. The most common incision is an apron incision extending from the mastoid tip inferiorly to approximately two finger breadths above the clavicle across the midline and frequently to the contralateral mastoid tip. The skin flaps are then elevated, including the platysma muscle.

After the flaps have been raised, care must be exercised that the external jugular vein is not accidentally cut. The vein should instead be doubly ligated with tie and suture ligature and then transected. The inferior border of the sternocleidomastoid muscle is identified and a clamp is placed under the muscle. The muscle is then sectioned and retracted superiorly. The carotid sheath is then identified, and the internal jugular vein is isolated. Care is taken to preserve the vagus nerve also present within the carotid sheath.

DETAILS

A proximal suture ligature and a distal silk tie are placed above and below, respectively, the line of transection of the internal jugular vein. The vein is then sectioned. The muscle with internal jugular vein and associated lymph nodes and fat is raised superiorly. The radical neck dissection specimen also includes transection of the strap muscles immediately superficial to the larynx and trachea. At this time, the ipsilateral portion of the thyroid gland is transected and also taken with the specimen. The trachea is now entered, and endotracheal anesthesia is directed into the distal portion of the trachea. The upper portion of the specimen includes the tracheal arches and the entire larynx. The uppermost portion of the laryngeal complex includes the hyoid bone. The hyoid bone is transected from all the attachments to the muscles of the throat and tongue. As the dissection continues, the junction of the upper end of the esophagus with the lower end of the hypopharynx becomes visible. After this is done, the specimen, including the larynx and the upper portion of the trachea, is in connection with the radical neck specimen.

The pharyngeal defect is in the shape of a T. The remainder of the neck contents including the contents of the submandibular space, just described, is lifted superiorly. Throughout this submandibular space are large arteries and veins that necessitate suture ligatures. In addition, the duct of the submandibular gland must be ligated. After this is done, the entire specimen is attached in the posterior and superior portion. The dissection is now carried from the anterior to the posterior direction until the internal jugular vein limits the dissection. At this time, a double ligation of the internal jugular vein is performed. A suture ligature is placed as well. The vein is then transected. The remaining portion includes the tail of the parotid, which is transected along with the attachment of the sternocleidomastoid muscle. Many vessels are encountered in this area and need ligation.

CLOSURE

The entire specimen, including the larynx, is now removed from the operative field. The nasal feeding tube that was placed at the beginning of the procedure is advanced through the T-shaped pharyngeal defect until it is visible within the operative field. It is then directed into the distal esophagus and the defect is closed over it. The defect is closed in a continuous inverting fashion using an absorbable suture of the surgeon's preference. The entire neck wound is then ready for closure.

The wound is copiously irrigated with either normal saline or an antibiotic solution. A two-layer closure using absorbable suture is employed for the approximation of the platysma muscle and subcutaneous tissue. To close the skin, nonabsorbable suture or skin staples are used. The distal trachea is sutured to the skin using interrupted, nonabsorbable sutures. Two suction drains are used, taking care not to place them directly over the carotid artery (**Fig. 30.20**).

Appropriately sized laryngectomy tubes should be available. Laryngectomy tubes are similar to tracheotomy tubes, except that they are usually shorter and of wider inner diameters. The preparation of the tubes before insertion is identical to that for tracheotomy tubes.

Partial Laryngectomy

There are clinical situations when a total laryngectomy is not necessary (**Fig. 30.21**). In malignancies of the larynx for which adequate margins can be obtained, preservation of a portion of larynx is preferred. In this way, a more functional voice can

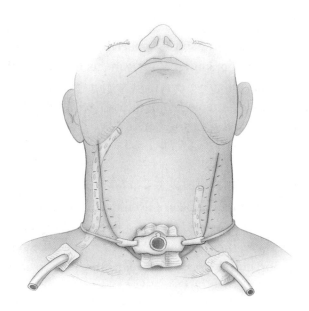

Figure 30.20

Total laryngectomy.

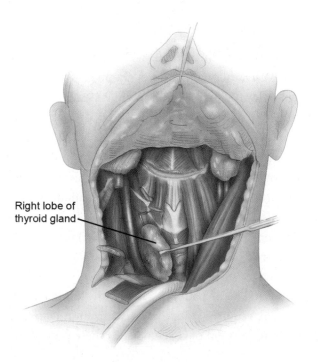

Figure 30.21

Partial laryngectomy.

Right lobe of thyroid gland

be obtained. Different procedures have been described. These include a supraglottic laryngectomy in which the epiglottis, false vocal cords, and hyoid bone are removed but the rest of the larynx is preserved. Also possible is a vertical or frontolateral hemilaryngectomy. With any conservation laryngectomies, a prophylactic tracheotomy is always performed.

Voice rehabilitation is a critical part of the short- and long-term followup of patients who have had any type of laryngectomy. Many surgeons advocate immediate insertion of a voice prosthesis after a total laryngectomy. Different types of prostheses exist. Other ways of communicating include esophageal speech, an electrolarynx, or simply a writing tablet and pencil. Before a patient undergoes a laryngectomy, extensive counseling should be given on voice rehabilitation. The nurse can make the transition to loss of the voice easier by being sensitive to the needs of this type of patient.

Postprocedure Care

After the procedure is completed, a pressure dressing is applied by some surgeons, taking care not to occlude the laryngectomy opening. Many patients undergoing a lengthy oncological procedure stay in an intensive care unit setting overnight, or longer. Analgesics and antiemetics are given. Intense humidification to the airway is given as well. Care must be taken not to dislodge the suction drains.

Potential Complications

Complications may include injury to uninvolved nerves as well as laceration of large blood vessels of the neck; injury to the lung pleura leading to a pneumothorax; necrosis of the skin and exposure of the carotid artery, leading to exsanguinating hemorrhage; fistula formation between the pharynx or esophagus and the skin after laryngectomy; recurrence of tumor; and stenosis of the remaining pharynx and esophagus.

Panendoscopy
Definition and Indications

Panendoscopy is an integral part of the care of the patients with head and neck cancers, hoarseness, dysphagia (difficulty with swallowing) and/or dyspnea (shortness of breath), and evaluation and treatment of foreign bodies or trauma. Panendoscopy is a term that refers to the endoscopic evaluation of the pharynx, larynx, upper trachea, and esophagus (Medilexicon, 2008). The endoscopic evaluations are indicated to evaluate the extent and involved anatomical structures of the primary pathology and to rule out the possibility of secondary pathological processes. Panendoscopy has most clinical application in the diagnosis and workup of head and neck cancer patients. These patients most commonly have squamous cell cancer. They classically use tobacco and alcohol, which are known co-carcinogens of the upper aerodigestive tract mucosa. Therefore, direct laryngoscopy, flexible or rigid bronchoscopy, and esophagoscopy can be performed in conjunction with biopsies of suspicious areas to rule out synchronous primary lesions, which are found in up to 5% of patients. Frequently, lesions of the larynx, base of tongue, and hypopharynx require endoscopic visualization or palpation to define the optimal treatment. In today's era of cost efficiency these procedures may be combined with the anesthetic for definitive treatment or deleted if the chest radiograph and barium swallow/esophagogram arc normal.

Related Procedures

Microdirect laryngoscopy with biopsy and bronchoscopy/esophagoscopy and foreign body retrieval are related procedures (see brief description of each procedure below).

Nursing Implications

ANESTHESIA

These endoscopic procedures are performed using general anesthesia. Previously, they were performed using topical anesthesia with or without sedation, but this is rarely done today.

POSITION

The patient is positioned supine on the table with the head at the end of the bed. The use of donut roll head supports and/or shoulder rolls varies from surgeon to surgeon but they are worth having available.

ESTABLISHING AND MAINTAINING THE STERILE FIELD

These are not sterile procedures, but sterile drapes are placed on the patient's chest/torso to prevent soiling the clothing with secretions or blood. Eye coverage/protection/head drapes are used based on the surgeon's preference.

EQUIPMENT AND SUPPLIES

The number and type of scopes should be reviewed with the surgeon before induction to ensure immediate access to the appropriate scope once the patient is asleep. The equipment and supplies for panendoscopy are outlined in **Table 30.5**.

Table 30.5	Panendoscopy Instruments

☐ Laryngoscopes (anterior commissure, Jackson, "wide mouth")
☐ Video tower
☐ Suspension arm for laryngoscope
☐ Rigid or flexible esophagoscopes
☐ Rigid or flexible bronchoscopes
☐ Light source for the above
☐ Neurosurgical 1×3-cm cottonoids
☐ Laryngoscopy suction—velvet eye
☐ Bronchoscope suction—velvet eye
☐ Tooth guard
☐ Moist Telfa pads

Optional items include
☐ Operating microscope with 350- or 400-mm lens
☐ CO_2 laser
☐ Biopsy forceps

30

PHYSIOLOGICAL MONITORING

Monitoring appropriate for general anesthesia should be done.

SPECIMENS AND CULTURES

Tissue samples should be meticulously labeled.

DRUGS AND SOLUTIONS

Saline, mineral oil, and oxymetazoline (Afrin) or another vasoconstrictor should be available.

PHYSICIAN ORDERS AND LABORATORY AND DIAGNOSTIC STUDIES

Routine preprocedure testing and evaluation by a medical doctor.

Procedure

Direct laryngoscopy is performed to evaluate the larynx, including vocal cords, epiglottis, and adjacent areas such as the base of the tongue, pyriform sinuses, lateral/posterior pharynx, and the postcricoid region. Before commencing the visualization, the teeth are evaluated for previous injury, loose/injured teeth are noted, and mucosal or mass lesions in the oral cavity are examined. The base of the tongue and pharynx are palpated for any signs of pathology. Most patients benefit from a drying agent such as glycopyrrolate. Patients who require subacute bacterial endocarditis prophylaxis should receive antibiotics; otherwise, most surgeons do not give prophylactic antibiotic coverage (so as not to mask signs of aerodigestive tract injury or perforation). A tooth guard is utilized for the dentate patient. The surgeon introduces and drives the various scopes to evaluate the larynx, pharynx, esophagus, and tracheobronchial tree. Moistening the scopes or the patient's lips with saline or mineral oil can help minimize trauma. If suction is required, the assisting nurse usually hands the device to the surgeon after the tip has been placed in the lumen of the scope. If flexible esophagoscopy is performed, many surgeons introduce the scope in the postcricoid region with direct visualization using the Jackson laryngoscope with the sleeve removed.

Flexible bronchoscopy is performed either through the endotracheal tube or by "driving" the scope beyond the cuff of the typically smaller endotracheal tube. Some surgeons extubate the patient and perform rigid bronchoscopy with or without ventilation. This is mandatory to visualize the subglottic area and proximal trachea.

The removal of the scope is the endpoint of the procedure. The laryngoscopes or bronchoscopes should not be removed from the surgical suite until the patient is awake and the airway is stable in case emergency access is needed.

Postprocedure Care

In the PACU and ensuing 24 hours, the patient is monitored for fevers, chest pain, and dysphagia, which can be associated with pneumothorax or esophageal perforation. Many surgeons obtain postprocedure chest radiographs in the PACU to evaluate for pneumothorax/pneumomediastinum and widened mediastinum.

Potential Complications

Complications may include sore throat, dental trauma, lip contusion/laceration, laryngospasm, pneumothorax, and esophageal perforation.

ENDNOTE

1. The drugs and solutions listed in this chapter are examples of the agents that the surgeon may choose to use during a procedure. The types of agents employed vary with surgeon preference.

REFERENCES

1. Berke, J. (2007). Cochlear implant surgery. Retrieved August 28, 2008 from http://deafness.about.com/od/basicsofcochlearimplants/a/cisurgery.htm.

2. Dev, V.R. (2006). Facial trauma, nasal fractures. Retrieved August 29, 2008 from http://www.emedicine.com/plastic/topic482.htm.

3. *Encyclopedia of Surgery*. (2008a). Tympanoplasty. Retrieved August 29, 2008 from http://www.surgeryencyclopedia.com/St-Wr/Tympanoplasty.html.

4. *Encyclopedia of Surgery*. (2008b). Mastoidectomy. Retrieved August 29, 2008 from http://www.surgeryencyclopedia.com/La-Pa/Mastoidectomy.html.

5. *Encyclopedia of Surgery*. (2008c). Stapedectomy. Retrieved August 29, 2008 from http://www.surgeryencyclopedia.com/Pa-St/Stapedectomy.html.

6. *Encyclopedia of Surgery*. (2008d). Septoplasty. Retrieved August 29, 2008 from http://www.surgeryencyclopedia.com/Pa-St/Septoplasty.html.

7. *Encyclopedia of Surgery*. (2008e). Endoscopic sinus surgery. Retrieved August 29, 2008 from http://www.surgeryencyclopedia.com/Ce-Fi/Endoscopic-Sinus-Surgery.html.

8. *Encyclopedia of Surgery*. (2008f). Parotidectomy. Retrieved August 29, 2008 from http://www.surgeryencyclopedia.com/La-Pa/Parotidectomy.html.

9. *Encyclopedia of Surgery*. (2008g). Snoring surgery. Retrieved August 30, 2008 from http://www.surgeryencyclopedia.com/Pa-St/Snoring-Surgery.html.

10. Essig, M.G. (2007). Uvulopalatopharyngoplasty for obstructive sleep apnea. Retrieved August 30, 2008 from http://www.aolhealth.com/procedures/uvulopalatopharyngoplasty-for-obstructive-sleep-apnea.

11. Essig, M.G. (2008). Uvulopalatopharyngoplasty for snoring. Retrieved August 28, 2008 from http://www.webmd.com/sleep-disorders/uvulopalatopharyngoplasty-for-snoring.

12. Kavanaugh, K.T. (2008). Adenotonsillectomy. Retrieved August 29, 2008 from http://www.entusa.com/tonsils_adenoid_surgery.htm.

13. Levenson, M.J. (2008). Cochlear implants. Retrieved August 28, 2008 from http://www.earsurgery.org/cochlear.html.

14. *Medcyclopaedia*. (2008). Caldwell-luc procedure. Retrieved August 28, 2008 from http://www.medcyclopaedia.com/library/topics/volume_vi_2/c/caldwell_luc_procedure.aspx.

15. MedicineNet.com. (2008a). Ear tubes (myringotomy & tympanostomy tubes). Retrieved August 28, 2008 from http://www.medicinenet.com/ear_tubes/article.htm.

16. MedicineNet.com. (2008b). Definition of total laryngectomy. Retrieved August 28, 2008 from http://www.medterms.com/script/main/art.asp?articlekey=25443.

17. *MediLexicon*. (2008). Panendoscopy. Retrieved August 28, 2008 from http://www.medilexicon.com/medicaldictionary.php?t=64705.

18. National Institute on Deafness and Other Communication Diseases. (NIDCD). (2007). Cochlear implants. Retrieved August 28, 2008 from http://www.nidcd.nih.gov/health/hearing/coch.asp.

19. US Food and Drug Administration (US FDA). (2004). Before, during, and after implant surgery. Retrieved August 28, 2008 from http://www.fda.gov/cdrh/cochlear/beforeduringaftersurgery.html.

20. University of Miami School of Medicine. (2008). Cochlear implant surgery. Retrieved August 28, 2008 from http://cochlearimplants.med.miami.edu/medical/01_Cochlear%20Implant%20Surgery.asp.

21. Wikipedia. (2008a). Cochlear implant. Retrieved August 28, 2008 from http://en.wikipedia.org/wiki/Cochlear_implants.

22. Wikipedia. (2008b). Uvulopalatopharyngoplasty. Retrieved August 28, 2008 from http://en.wikipedia.org/wiki/UPPP.

23. Wikipedia. (2008c). Tracheotomy. Retrieved August 30, 2008 from http://en.wikipedia.org/wiki/Tracheotomy.

CHAPTER 31

Ophthalmic Surgery

Brenda Ulmer

Molly McBrayer

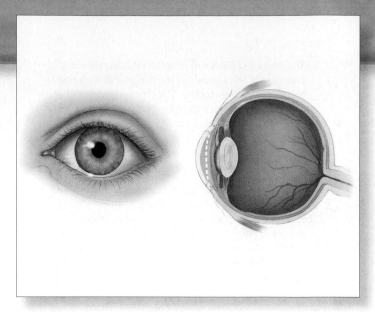

Sight is man's richest sense, his link to the world and its wealth of imagery. Vision begins with light, the abundant rain of the sun's energy falling through space to touch and warm the earth. Light projects value, tone, and shadow into nature. The eye, keen to this kaleidoscopic effect, then relates what it senses to the brain, perception's ultimate seat.

—Loel Wertenbaker (1984)

INTRODUCTION

Operative procedures involving the eye encompass ophthalmic surgery. "Ophthalmology" is a combination of the Greek words "ophthalmos," which means eye, and "logos," meaning study. Developments in the specialty of ophthalmology have advanced as have the tools available to surgeons, revolutionizing prevention, operative interventions, and cures for diseases and afflictions associated with the structures of the eye.

ANATOMY

The eyes are organs of soft tissue that are cradled inside two bony structures. Seven bones of the skull (the frontal, lacrimal, ethmoid, maxilla, zygomatic, sphenoid, and palatine) make up the sockets. A lining of fat absorbs shocks to the eyes and provides a well-lubricated area for the constant motion. When the eyes are open, the central nervous system of the body becomes exposed to outside elements. This phenomenon happens nowhere else in the human body. Because of this, any stimuli near the eye will cause the eyes to shut with lightning speed. The eyelid, also called the palpebra, is the protective covering for the eye. Its function is not only to protect and cleanse the eye but also to provide lubrication of the cornea so it does not dry out. The skin on the palpebra is the thinnest skin on the human body. There are two muscles of the eyelid—the orbicularis oculi, which closes

Chapter Contents

the lids as it contracts, and the Ievator palpebrae superioris, which opens the eye on contraction. The conjunctiva is a mucous membrane that lines the inner surface of the eyelids. It is relatively thick, except for the central portion, the cornea. The cornea is very thin, movable, and transparent.

All animals that breathe air have the ability to produce tears. The human, however, is the only one that cries. The lacrimal glands are responsible for the secretion of tears, and several ducts carry the tears from the eye to the nasal cavity for excretion. Tears contain an enzyme called lysozyme that functions as an antibacterial agent to reduce the chance of eye infections. "Crying" is when the lacrimal glands secrete excessive fluid. The result is that the nose fills with fluid as the ducts carry the excess away, while the rest spills over the edges of the eyelids. The response of "crying" is a parasympathetic nerve reaction of the central nervous system.

The six muscles that give the eye its movement are:

- Superior rectus—moves the eye upward and toward the midline
- Inferior rectus—moves the eye downward and toward the midline
- Medial rectus—moves the eye toward the midline
- Lateral rectus—moves the eye away from the midline
- Superior oblique—moves the eye downward and away from the midline
- Inferior oblique—moves the eye upward and away from the midline

The extrinsic eye muscles can be moved with great precision because the motor units contain the fewest muscle fibers. There are only 5 to 10 fibers contained in eye muscles—fewer than any other muscle in the body. The eyes are anatomically aligned, which causes them to move together. This feature of the eye involves complex motor adjustments such as the relaxation of one muscle and the contraction of its counterpart. The result of uncoordinated eye movement is termed strabismus.

The cornea is the transparent covering of the eye. It has often been referred to as "the window of the soul." It is mostly connective tissue with a thin layer of surface epithelium. The cornea is transparent because it contains few cells and no blood vessels. The cells and collagenous fibers are arranged in an unusual, regular pattern. The cornea is, however, well supplied with nerve fibers that enter at the margin and radiate toward the center. The cornea has numerous pain receptors with a low reaction threshold.

The sclera—continuous with the cornea—is the white portion of the eye. It serves as the attachment for the extrinsic muscles and protects the eye.

The middle tunic of the eye comprises the choroid coat, the ciliary body, and the iris. The choroid coat is loosely joined to the sclera and is woven with blood vessels that provide nourishment to surrounding tissues. The choroid also contains melanocytes which keep the inside of the eye dark by absorbing excess light. The ciliary body extends forward from the choroid and forms an internal ring around the front of the eye. It contains the ciliary processes and muscles. The iris is the most anterior portion of the middle or vascular tunic. It is identified as the colored portion of the eye. The iris divides the anterior chamber, which is between the cornea and the iris, and the posterior chamber, which lies between the iris and the lens. It is made of a flat bar of circular, smooth muscle fibers surrounding the pupil. By expansion and contraction, the iris controls the amount of light that enters the eye through the pupil. The pupil is the round hole in the center of the iris through which light passes. The pupil appears black because of the decreased amount of light behind it.

Aqueous humor is the watery fluid that fills the anterior chamber, or front part of the eye. The fluid provides nutrition for the surrounding parts of the eye and helps maintain the shape of the anterior chamber. The posterior chamber, which is the most distal part of the eye, has a clear, jelly-like substance which maintains its shape. This substance is called the vitreous humor.

The lens focuses light by changing the curvature of the front surface. It is a transparent, crystalline structure suspended in position by strong but delicate fibers that make up the suspensory ligament. Attached to this ligament is the ciliary body, which can change the shape of the lens to focus on objects at a variety distances.

The retina is the inner lining of the posterior chamber. It contains the layers of nerve cells that give the eye its sensitivity to light. There is a depression in the central region of the retina, called the fovea centralis that produces sharp vision.

The optic disc is in the central region of the retina and is the area where the nerve fibers from the retina leave the eye and become part of the optic nerve. A central artery and vein also pass through the retina at the level of the optic disc. The optic nerve is the bundle of nerve fibers that carry vision-related impulses from the retina to the brain. Optic nerve damage usually results in permanent loss of vision.

EQUIPMENT AND SUPPLIES

One of the most critical pieces of equipment in ophthalmic surgery is the ophthalmic microscope. It is often used with a teaching arm, also referred to as split arm. The teaching arm allows scrub personnel to view the procedure and better anticipate the needs of the surgeon. A video system with a monitor connected to the microscope that allows everyone in the room to view the procedure is a valuable aid to teaching. The ophthalmic microscopic can be equipped with a special bipolar electrosurgical unit that is attached at the base of the microscope, making it readily available for use.

The surgeon and scrubbed team members commonly sit during ophthalmic procedures, so stools must be available. The stools may be stationary, rolling, and with or without armrests, according to the surgeon's preference. Many ophthalmologists are trained with stools that roll and are designed for comfort, with curved backs and armrests, which could present a challenge in maintaining aseptic technique.

The phacoemulsification unit is an often-used piece of equipment during ophthalmic procedures. It usually has vitrectomy capabilities within the unit. Phacoemulsification units are available from several manufacturers; the specific brand is determined by the surgeon's preference.

Ophthalmic procedures are very specialized and often require specific specialty instruments. Examples of these are included in the procedure sections. There are, however, some items that are useful regardless of the type of procedure and should be on hand (**Table 31.1**). It is extremely important that the scrub person be fully familiar with all of the instruments, equipment, and supplies. Ideally, the surgeon can keep his/her vision focused on the operative site without having to look away from the microscope. The surgeon should request an instrument by name and have it placed appropriately for use, in his or her hand.

Table 31.1	Items Commonly Used in Ophthalmic Surgery

Merocel Weck Sponges

Weck Eye Spears

Weck Eye Drain

Instrument Wipe

Specialty Eye Suture

Syringes (TB, 3, 5, 10 cc)

Needles (Hypodermic and Retrobulbar)

Wetfield Cautery

Suction

4 × 4 Sponges

Balanced Salt Solution (BSS)

Methylene Blue

Eye Pads

Eye Shields

Micropore Tape

UNIVERSAL PROTOCOL

Operative site marking is imperative with ophthalmology patients. Unless bilateral procedures are being done, such as LASIK surgery, it is the surgeon's responsibility to mark the operative site. A semi-permanent marker is used with the surgeon inscribing his or her initials or YES (according to institutional policy) above the correct eye. It is unacceptable to use a sticky dot because they can easily become dislodged and reapplied to the wrong side. Additionally, a time-out is done in the operating room just before the procedure begins. All members of the team must participate in the time-out procedure.

CATARACT EXTRACTION

Definition

A cataract is a common disorder of the eye, particularly in older persons. As the cataract forms the lens or its capsule slowly loses its transparency and becomes cloudy and opaque (**Fig. 31.1**). Clear images cannot be focused on the retina. In time, the person may experience blindness.

Types of cataracts include age-related, congenital, secondary, and traumatic. Age-related cataracts develop as a result of aging. Everyone will develop cataracts if they live long enough. Each person's lens ages differently so one person may develop cataracts at 40, while an 80-year-old may show no signs of cataracts.

Congenital cataracts are usually a result of an infection. Babies may be born with cataracts or may develop them during childhood. Secondary cataracts develop as a result of diseases such as diabetes, taking medications such as steroids or diuretics, or exposure to ultraviolet light or radiation. Other factors that can increase the risk of developing cataracts include smoking, air pollution, exposure to toxins, and heavy alcohol consumption.

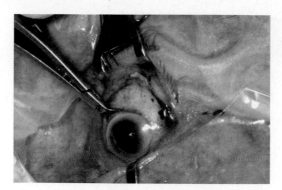

Figure 31.1
Cataract Extraction.

A cataract extraction removes the lens by a process called phacoemulsification. During phacoemulsification, the ultrasonic handpiece breaks the lens into pieces while simultaneous suction removes the fragments from the anterior chamber. An artificial lens replaces the natural lens.

Indications

Indications for cataract extraction include loss of vision and the inability to focus clearly, making activities of daily living difficult to accomplish. Corrective glasses cannot be used, because the lens is not allowing light to pass through. The only option is to remove the lens which has the cataract. Cataract extraction is the most frequently performed operative procedure in the United States, with over 1.5 million procedures done per year (Haines, 2005).

Related Procedures

There are presently no related procedures to cataract extraction.

Nursing Implications
Anesthesia

The majority of cataract extractions were once done using a peribulbar or retrobulbar block. Cataract extraction is now done with topical anesthesia, occasionally supplemented with intraocular preservative-free lidocaine. Patients generally receive monitored anesthesia care from an anesthesia provider. Propofol (Diprivan), midazolam (Versed), and fentanyl, or a combination of these, are the normal drugs of choice to provide the patient with a comfortable level of sedation during the procedure. Anesthesia for these cases is a gray area. The nurse should be aware of the type of anesthesia the patient is going to receive and whether an anesthesia provider will be present. A patient who is receiving only topical anesthesia may still need the expertise of an anesthesia provider (because of his or her health status) to ensure a safe operative course.

The peribulbar and retrobulbar blocks are prepared as follows:

- Bupivacaine (Marcaine) 0.75%, plain—15 mL
- Lidocaine (Xylocaine) 20%, plain—15 cc
- Hyaluronidase (Wydase), 150 U

The drugs are mixed in a 30-mL syringe and then divided into smaller syringes according to the surgeon's preference. All medication syringes are labeled according to AORN standards and recommended practices with medication name(s), strength, time, date, and initials of the person preparing medication and the expiration date of the medication (AORN, 2008). Different sizes of needles may be used for injection, based on the surgeon's preference. The surgeon may request a retrobulbar needle—a 23-gauge × XH-inch needle with a bevel specifically designed to be less traumatic to the blood vessels. The needle lessens the chance for a peribulbar or retrobulbar hemorrhage. Many ophthalmologists prefer to administer the peribulbar or retrobulbar block; however, it is not unusual for the anesthesiologist to administer the block.

For local or topical anesthesia, 4% topical lidocaine, tetracaine, and proparacaine (Ophthetic) are generally the drugs of choice. The drugs are liberally used during the procedure, especially during phacoemulsification. Lidocaine 1% (preservative-free only), 0.25 to 0.5 mL, may be administered when necessary, as a supplement.

•

Position

The patient lies supine on an ophthalmology stretcher or an operative bed with an ophthalmology headrest attached. There must be room at the head of the bed for the surgeon and scrub person to be seated without leg interference. The headrest is freely movable and allows the circulating nurse to position the patient's superior brow parallel to the floor. The surgeon may request that a wrist rest be attached to the bed. This aids in the surgeon's comfort and hand positioning during the procedure. A superior headrest is a half-moon shape, whereas a temporal headrest is a quarter-moon shape. Placing a pillow under the patient's knees may help alleviate back discomfort during the procedure. If the patient is to be sedated, a soft wrist restraint or securely tucked arms will prevent the patient from reaching up and contaminating the sterile field. An inexpensive but soft wrist "reminder" can be made from a Kerlix roll. A safety belt is placed over the patient's thighs to maintain safety. Older persons may be more sensitive to changes in temperature, so warm blankets should be used to assist with thermoregulation.

Establishing and Maintaining the Sterile Field

A surgical hat is placed over the patient's hair. A drop of 5% povidone-iodine (Betadine) solution is instilled in the operative eye. The circulating nurse dons sterile gloves and does a circumferential eye preparation with 5% povidone-iodine solution. After three swabs, the eye is flushed with 5 mL of 0.9% sodium chloride (NaCl). The eye is then dried with two sterile 4 × 4-inch sponges.

A nonaperture or an aperture drape is placed over the patient's eye, according to the surgeon's preference. A nonaperture drape requires that the scrub person assist the surgeon with placement. The assistant will hold the patient's eyelids open with the wooden ends of two long cotton-tipped applicators while the sticky portion of the drape is placed centrally over the patient's eye. With dull, straight Metzenbaum scissors an opening is cut to expose only the eye. The nonaperture drape fully isolates the patient's eyelashes which may be beneficial as most endophthalmitis is thought to originate from the oil gland secretion at the base of the eyelashes. This would also explain the rationale for not scrubbing the eyelashes during the sterile preparation.

The aperture drape is placed at the inner canthus of the operative eye, along the brow, and then along the cheek. One-half inch steri-strips can be used to isolate the eyelashes when using this drape. The AORN *Perioperative Standards and Recommended Practices* (AORN, 2008) do not specify whether a full-body drape must be used to maintain the sterile field. A full-body drape may be chosen, however, to help maintain patient warmth.

The surgeon sits on the patient's operative side, with the scrub person opposite, for a temporal approach. For a superior approach, the surgeon sits superior to the patient's head and the scrub person is typically to the surgeon's right. Hand dominance of the surgeon may also dictate where the scrub person sits. When a Mayo stand is used it is placed between the scrub person and the surgeon in close proximity to the operative field. In many cases, use of the Mayo stand has been discontinued because of the close proximity and the small amount of instruments. The back table should be in close enough for the scrub person to reach without contamination. The phacoemulsification unit is placed across from the scrub person so that the settings can be easily read and adjusted as needed. **Table 31.2** lists commonly used specialty instruments, equipment, and supplies.

Table 31.2	Items Commonly Used in Cataract Procedures

Lid Speculum

Alvis Forceps

Thornton Ring Fixator

Safety Blade Diamond Knife

Cystotome Needle (25 or 27 gauge)

Lens Manipulator (Connor Wand or Finzel Hook)

Phacoemulsification Unit with Accessories

Lens Folding/Lens Injector Instruments

Castroviejo Needle Holder

Slit Knife (30 or 15 degree)

Intraocular Lens

Castroviejo Needle Holder

DRUGS & SOLUTIONS:

    500 cc BSS with 0.5 cc epinephrine 1:1000 units

    Viscoelastic—Ocucoat, Healon, Viscoat, Amvisc, Duovisc

    Ofloxacin (Ocuflox), Vigamox, Zymar

    Miochol or Miostat

    Prednisolone (Pred Forte)

    Cefazolin or gentamicin

    Betamethasone

    Kerashield (soaked in 1 cc Maxitrol)

    Collagen Shield

    Pilocarpine 2% Solution

    Sterile 0.9% NaCl

Physician Orders

All patients receive drops for dilation before the procedure. The type of drops used for dilation is surgeon preference. Dilating drops are ordered in three sets 5 minutes apart, beginning on the patient's admission or approximately 1 hour before the procedure. Major delays can be avoided with timely administration of the drops. It is difficult and dangerous to perform a cataract extraction on an eye with a pupil dilated less than 5 mm. The surgeon may request antibiotic eyedrops before the start of the procedure. IV fluids, usually dextrose 5% in lactated Ringer's, are started on all patients before the procedure. The operative eye is marked according to the Universal Protocol for any case with laterality, as previously described. The marker must not come off during the operative prep and the mark must be visible during the time-out procedure prior to the start of the procedure.

Laboratory and Diagnostic Studies

The majority of patients undergoing cataract extraction are elderly with few to multiple comorbidities. Preprocedure studies are dictated by the patient's health history and facility policies. Patients older than the age of 40 are required to have an electrocardiogram, and chest radiographs are required for patients with known or suspected pulmonary problems.

Patients taking blood-thinning medications are instructed to discontinue use before the procedure. This should be confirmed with the patient. If the patient is a diabetic, whether insulin- or diet-controlled, a finger blood sugar check is done on admission for the procedure. Diabetic and cardiac patients have chemistry profiles for analysis of blood sugar, potassium, and electrolytes. A dipstick urinalysis may be done for those patients on cardiac and antihypertensive drugs.

Procedure

A lid speculum is placed to retract the eyelids. An Alvis fixation forceps or Thornton ring fixator is used to stabilize the eye. A diamond knife is used to create a groove at the limbus. A 15-degree slit knife is used to create a paracentesis on both sides of the groove. Viscoelastic is injected into the anterior chamber. A capsulorhexis is performed using a cystotome. A keratome is used to enter the anterior chamber, creating a three-step tunnel incision. A syringe filled with Balanced Salt Solution (BSS), using a 27-gauge flat-tip cannula, is used for hydrodissection. The nucleus rotator, or other lens manipulator, is used to free the lens in the capsular bag. Once the bag is free, phacoemulsification is used to divide the lens in half. Once divided, the lens is turned with a lens manipulator and divided into quarters. The lens is then removed by using the phacoemulsification unit. The irrigation/aspiration (I/A) setup aspirates the remaining cortex. The posterior capsule is polished with a silicone-tipped cannula on the I/A handpiece. A foldable intraocular lens is prepared by the scrub person for insertion. Viscoelastic is injected into the capsular bag to maintain its shape while inserting the lens. The new intraocular lens is inserted and positioned with a lens manipulator. The I/A hand-piece is used to aspirate the remaining viscoelastic. The wound is checked to ensure that proper sealing will occur. A suture may be needed if the wound is unable to seal itself properly. Injections and drops are administered and a Kerashield may be placed. An eye pad is taped in place with transparent Micropore

BSS
Balanced Salt
Solution

I/A
Irrigation/
Aspiration

31

tape, and a Fox eye shield with a cloth garter is secured over the pad to protect the eye. Surgeons who prefer no dressing may use a clear plastic eye shield.

Postprocedure Care

The cataract patient is fast-tracked to the phase II area of the postanesthesia care unit (PACU). Vital signs are monitored, and family members may be allowed sit with the patient. Alert patients are may be offered fluids by mouth. Discharge instructions are reviewed with the patient and family member, with a copy of the instructions to accompany the patient home. The IV is discontinued, and the patient is assisted to his or her transportation with a staff member and family member. All patients must have a responsible adult drive them to and from the facility on the day of the procedure. A postprocedure telephone call to assess pain control, complications, and understanding of the discharge instructions is made the day after the procedure. If a problem is assessed during the telephone call, the patient is instructed to contact the surgeon. The nurse will also contact the surgeon to assure that the patient has communicated with the surgeon.

Potential Complications

Complications of cataract surgery may include endophthalmitis (infection of the eye), retrobulbar hemorrhage, retinal damage, vitreous leak (vitrectomy), rupture of posterior capsular membrane, loss of lens fragments (floaters), and loss of vision.

MUSCLE PROCEDURES

Definition

Eye muscle procedures are done to correct strabismus. Strabismus is a malalignment of the eyes and literally means "squinting." Non-operative treatments for strabismus include patching the stronger eye to make the weaker eye muscles work, and anticholinesterase drug therapy. Effective treatment requires early recognition of the problems. An eye muscle procedure is optimal for children between four years to six years of age, but in some cases patients may be younger. The primary goals of the procedure are to preserve the patient vision, provide binocularity, and improve cosmetic appearance. **Figure 31.2** shows a muscle resection procedure.

Indications

The eyes are not in alignment due to muscle imbalance which has not responded to nonoperative treatment. It is important to correct strabismus because left uncorrected, the weaker eye will become blind from nonuse.

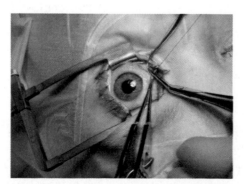

Figure 31.2
Muscle Resection.

Nursing Implications

Anesthesia

The primary patient population for eye muscle procedures are pediatrics, therefore general anesthesia is most often administered. An IV is started after anesthesia induction. An endotracheal tube may be used or the anesthesia provider may elect to use a laryngeal mask airway (LMA) to maintain the airway throughout the procedure.

LMA
Laryngeal Mask
Airway

Position

The patient is supine on an ophthalmology stretcher or an operative bed that has an ophthalmic headrest. The child's extremities are padded to provide comfort and proper positioning. Warm blankets or other heating methods, such as a forced air warmer, should be used to keep the child normothermic. A safety strap is placed over the patient's thighs during the procedure. The room temperature is maintained at 72°F (22.2°C) at minimum during the procedure.

Establishing and Maintaining the Sterile Field

After the patient is anesthetized, a surgical hat is placed over the patient's hair. A drop of 5% povidone-iodine solution is instilled into the eyes. The circulating nurse dons sterile gloves and does a circumferential eye preparation with 5% povidone-iodine solution for each eye. The eyes are prepped separately by using three swabs and then flushing with 5 mL of 0.9% NaCl. The eyes are then dried with two sterile 4 × 4-inch sponges. A bilateral aperture drape is placed over the patient's eyes and covers the full body.

The surgeon usually sits superior to the patient's head with the scrub nurse to the right of the surgeon. A Mayo stand is used, and the back table is placed to the scrub person's left and perpendicular to the bed. **Table 31.3** lists items commonly used during eye muscle procedures.

Physician Orders

All patients receiving general anesthesia are kept NPO for at least four hours prior to the procedure to reduce the complication of aspiration during anesthesia induction and airway management. No other orders are usually needed.

Laboratory and Diagnostic Studies

Pediatric patients require few preprocedure tests unless there is a known disease or illness that would warrant testing.

Procedure

The procedure is scheduled as a 2.0 recession of the left medial rectus muscle. The surgeon performs a forced duction (rotation of the eyes by the extraocular muscles). A limbal-based conjunctival peritomy is performed. The left medial rectus muscle is isolated using a small and then a large muscle hook. After isolation, the muscle is dissected from its attachments to the conjunctiva and intermuscular septum. A double-armed 6-0 polyglacin suture is passed in a double-looping fashion through

Table 31.3	Items Commonly Used in Eye Muscle Procedures

Muscle Hooks (with and without balls)

Lacrimal Duct Probe Set

Westcott Scissors

Abeli-Mason Scissors

0.12 Forceps

0.5 Forceps (with and without teeth)

Calipers

Castroviejo Needle Holders

Suture Tiers (curved and straight)

Fine Curved Hemostats

Bipolar Electrosurgical Unit (with accessories)*

DRUGS & SOLUTIONS:

    Balanced Salt Solution (BSS)

* The use of electrosurgery or electrocautery devices during procedures with the potential for an oxygen-rich environment (above 21% O_2) is extremely hazardous and can result in a patient fire. The potential for an oxygen-rich environment is present during the use of mask or nasal oxygen or with an uncuffed endotracheal tube. Refer to Chapter 14 for more information regarding fire prevention and safety during operative and invasive procedures.

the inferior and superior borders of the left medial rectus muscle near its insertion site on the globe. The muscle is carefully disinherited from the globe using the Abeli-Mason scissors. Measurements to accomplish reattachment of the muscle are taken by using the calipers and methylene blue to mark the number of millimeters needed to correct the strabismus. Reattachment to the globe is done by passing the sutures in a horizontal crossword fashion through the superficial sclera. The sutures are pulled through and tied, effecting a recession in the correct number of measured millimeters of the left medial rectus muscle. Two additional sutures of 6-0 polyglacin are placed between the muscle and superficial sclera to securely anchor the muscle to the globe and cinch it down. Closure of the wound is then accomplished by reapproximating the conjunctiva with a 7-0 chromic suture in an interrupted fashion.

Postprocedure Care

Following the procedure, the general anesthesia patient is taken to phase I of the PACU and monitored until fully awake. The parent(s) or guardians may join the patient in phase II of the PACU. Nausea and vomiting are treated with pharmacologic agents if necessary, and the patient is offered fluids by mouth to establish intake before discharge. The patient may also be required to void before discharge, depending on the policies of the facility. Discharge instructions are directed primarily toward the parent or guardian. It is stressed that special care must be taken to avoid getting the eyes wet. It is not unusual to request that two adults accompany the pediatric ophthalmic patient home so that while one adult is driving, the other adult is available to care for the child.

Potential Complications

Conjunctivitis may occur. Double vision is common for a couple weeks following a corrective procedure while the brain accommodates new visual patterns.

LASIK PROCEDURE
Definition

Laser-assisted in situ keratomileusis (LASIK) is a corneal procedure to correct farsightedness (hyperopia), nearsightedness (myopia), and astigmatism. A microkeratome or femtosecond laser is used to make a corneal "hinged flap," and the excimer laser is then used to vaporize tissue from the exposed stroma layer of the corneal bed, thus reshaping the cornea and correcting vision.

Indications

A LASIK procedure is elective because the patient has a choice about how to correct vision. Options for vision correction should be thoroughly discussed with the patient before a final decision is made. LASIK procedures have the potential to correct a wide range of refractive errors, including mild, moderate, and high myopia and astigmatisms, with few complications. Since LASIK is relatively painless and the patient has semi-clear vision immediately following the procedure, bilateral procedures are routinely done.

Nursing Implications
Anesthesia

Topical anesthesia is given using proparacaine or tetracaine eyedrops. This procedure is well tolerated by patients and has been categorized as virtually painless. For this reason, either diazepam (Valium), 5 mg orally, or lorazepam (Ativan), 2 mg sublingually, may be given 30 minutes before the start of the procedure. The patient should be instructed that when the suction is applied to the microkeratome he/she will feel a sensation of pressure but no pain. This should be reinforced during the procedure as needed.

Position

The excimer laser has an operative chair that is specially designed for the procedure and is operated by the surgeon. The patient is placed in the supine position with a beanbag head support that is inflated with a vacuum to help the patient keep his or her head in correct alignment. A warm blanket is placed over the patient, and a choice of hand positioning is offered. It is often reassuring to the patient to have the circulating nurse hold his/her hand during the procedure. Patients consistently comment on the comfort of knowing the nurse is there through the hand-holding.

Establishing and Maintaining the Sterile Field

The LASIK procedure is a clean procedure as opposed to a sterile procedure. After the administration of the topical anesthetic, povidone-iodine swabs are used to prep the operative eyes. A sterile 4 × 4-inch sponge is used to dry each eye and remove any excess povidone-iodine. Excess preparation solution will cause the microkeratome to stick when it comes in contact with the eye. A sterile 4 × 4-inch sponge is

LASIK
Laser-Assisted in situ Keratomileusis

31

Table 31.4	Items Commonly Used in LASIK Procedures

Microkeratome with Accessories
Radial Keratectomy (RK) Marker
Angled Irrigating Cannula
LASIK Flap Irrigating Cannula
Calibri Forceps
Knorr Suction Lid Speculum
Lasik Eye Drain
Powder-Free Sterile Gloves
DRUGS & SOLUTIONS:
   0.5% Tetracaine or Proparacaine Eye Drops
   Ofloxacin (Ocuflox) Solution
   Fluorometholone (FML) Solution
   Ketorolac Tromethamine (Acular) or Diclofenac (Voltaren)

placed over the nonoperative eye to allow the patient to focus on the operative side. It is common not to use any drapes or draping procedure for LASIK. Only powder-free gloves are used to avoid any inflammatory reactions.

A Mayo stand is placed to the surgeon's immediate left. The microkeratome is placed on a small preparation stand in the same general area as the Mayo stand. The microkeratome technician stands between the Mayo stand and the microkeratome. **Table 31.4** lists items that may be used during a LASIK procedure, as well as commonly used drugs and solutions.

Physician Orders

Patients may be medicated with a mild sedative on arrival to the procedure area. Five minutes before the start of the procedure, one drop each of ofloxacin, diclofenac, and proparacaine (or tetracaine) is instilled in the operative eye(s). Another drop of the proparacaine (or tetracaine) is instilled immediately before the procedure begins.

Laboratory and Diagnostic Studies

No laboratory or diagnostic studies are required for this procedure.

Procedure

The Knorr eye speculum is positioned and connected to suction. The radial keratotomy (RK) marker is impregnated with methylene blue dye and used to mark the cornea. The pneumatic suction ring is placed centrally over the pupil, and the microkeratome passed over the surface of the cornea to create the hinged flap. The suction is released, and the instrument is removed. A LASIK eye drain is moistened with BSS and placed on the eye. With the angled irrigating cannula, the corneal flap is raised nasally. The cornea is moistened with a wrung-out Merocel sponge that has been saturated with BSS. A dry Merocel sponge is then used to dry the cornea.

RK
Radial Keratotomy

The laser is then used. Each firing of the laser elicits a loud snapping noise. As the cornea is reshaped during the 20 to 80 seconds of lasing, the sound will become increasingly louder. It may be necessary to occasionally remind the patient to keep looking at the red light, adjust the patient's head position, or stop to wipe the cornea with a dry Merocel Weck sponge. After the laser portion is complete, a small drop of BSS is placed on the cornea and the irrigating LASIK speculum is used to place the cornea flap in its proper position. The surgeon is able to realign the cornea correctly using the markings made with the methylene blue dye. The surgeon will irrigate with copious amounts of BSS under the flap to make sure that debris and large amounts of air, both of which would cause non-adherence of the flap, are removed. When the flap has been positioned, the surgeon will instruct the operative staff to make note of the time. In 3 to 5 minutes the flap will start to adhere. After the noted time has elapsed, the surgeon will use a Calibri forceps to check for adherence of the flap. If it has started to adhere and appears to have a good seal, the eye speculum is removed and the patient is asked to blink gently. The surgeon uses the microscope to visualize the flap and checks to see that it has remained in position. Drops of ofloxacin, fluorometholone, and diclorfenac are instilled into the operative eye and a clear eye shield is taped into place with 1-inch Micropore tape. The same procedure is completed on the second eye.

Postprocedure Care

The patient is escorted to the phase II PACU, and vital signs are taken. The patient is offered fluids by mouth, and the discharge instructions are reviewed. Thirty minutes after the procedure the surgeon rechecks the patient's eyes with a slit lamp. The patient is then discharged home with a responsible adult.

Potential Complications

Endophthalmitis temporary or permanently blurred vision, night glare, and blindness could occur. Corneal transplantation may be necessary if problems occur with the corneal flap. Undercorrection or overcorrection of vision is possible.

PTERYGIUM EXCISION

Definition

A pterygium is a triangular growth extending from the conjunctiva and attached to the sclera. It is usually also found to be united to the cornea. **Figure 31.3** shows an example of a pterygium.

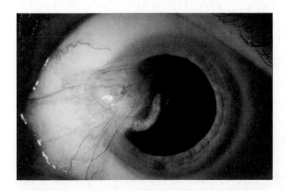

Figure 31.3

Pterygium.

Indications

A pterygium is believed to develop from chronic outside exposure, usually to the wind, dust, or ultraviolet light (sunlight). It will grow across the cornea until it invades the visual field. Pterygia do not have specific symptoms; however, they can totally encroach on the cornea and without operative treatment can eventually cause blindness. Because of a similarity in appearance, pterygia are sometimes confused with cataracts.

Related Procedures

There are no related operative procedures.

Nursing Implications

Anesthesia

A pterygium may be removed under local, regional, or general anesthesia. The decision on the type of anesthesia is made in collaboration between the surgeon and the patient. Most commonly, however, pterygium excision is done under peribulbar or retrobulbar block.

Position

The patient is placed in the supine position on an ophthalmic stretcher or on an operative bed with an ophthalmic headrest. A superior headrest is used for this procedure (please refer to Cataract Extraction, Position). The patient's arms are restrained with soft wrist restraints, and a pillow is placed under the knees to help relieve pressure on the back. A warm blanket is placed over the patient to assist in maintaining a normothermic condition.

Establishing and Maintaining the Sterile Field

A surgical hat is placed on the patient to cover the hair. A drop of 5% povidone-iodine solution is instilled in the operative eye. The circulating nurse dons sterile gloves and does a circumferential eye preparation with 5% povidone-iodine solution. After three swabs, the eye is flushed with 5 mL of 0.9% NaCl. The eye is dried with two sterile 4 × 4-inch sponges.

A nonaperture or aperture drape is utilized based on the surgeon's preference (see Cataract Extraction, Establishing and Maintaining the Sterile Field, for draping techniques). The surgeon sits superior to the patient's head, and the scrub person usually sits to the right of the surgeon. The Mayo stand is placed between the surgeon and the scrub person. Items commonly used in Pterygium excision are listed in **Table 31.5**.

Physician Orders

The type of anesthesia chosen will dictate if the patient is required to be NPO status four hours before the procedure. An IV of dextrose 5% in lactated Ringer's is started unless the patient is diabetic and then lactated Ringer's or normal saline is used.

Laboratory and Diagnostic Studies

As with cataract patients, the type of diagnostic testing done before the procedure may depend on the policies of the facility. Typical policies require that patients older

Table 31.5	Items Commonly Used in Pterygium Excision

Lid Speculum

0.12 Forceps

0.5 Forceps

Castroviejo Needle Holder

Suture Tiers (curved and straight)

Westcott Scissors

Fine Curved Hemostats

19 Gauge Irrigating Cannula

27 Gauge Irrigating Cannula

Bipolar Electrosurgery Unit with Accessories*

Fisch Drill with Diamond Burr

DRUGS & SOLUTIONS:

   Betamethasone (Celestone)

   Gentamycin

   Balanced Salt Solution (BSS)

   Beta Radiation (if Fisch Drill is NOT used)

   Maxitrol Ophthalmic Ointment

*The use of electrosurgery or electrocautery devices during procedures with the potential for an oxygen-rich environment (above 21% O_2) is extremely hazardous and can result in a patient fire. The potential for an oxygen-rich environment is present during the use of mask or nasal oxygen or with an uncuffed endotracheal tube. Refer to Chapter 14 for more information regarding fire prevention and safety during operative and invasive procedures.

than the age of 40 have an electrocardiogram, and chest radiographs are required for those patients with known or suspected pulmonary problems. Patients who are currently taking blood-thinning medications are instructed to discontinue these before the procedure. Compliance should be confirmed with the patient. Diabetic and cardiac patients will usually have a chemistry profile done before the procedure and a fingerstick sampling to test blood sugar on admission the day of the procedure.

Postprocedure Care

If the patient has had general anesthesia he or she is transferred to phase I PACU; otherwise the patient will go to phase II PACU. Vital signs are monitored and, when the patient is fully alert, he or she is encouraged to take fluids by mouth. Family members will join the patient while discharge instructions are reviewed. A copy of the instructions is given to the patient for reference at home. The patient is discharged with a responsible party. A telephone call to assess the patient's postprocedure course should be completed the day after the procedure. A postprocedure phone call is a Joint Commission recommendation as well as a patient satisfier.

Potential Complications

Corneal keratoplasty may be necessary if the cornea is damaged. Conjunctivitis, corneal ulcer, and retrobulbar hemorrhage may also occur as a result of pterygium excision.

Procedure

The lid speculum is placed in the operative eye. The Knorr eye suction speculum may be used, especially if the surgeon uses the Fisch drill. The conjunctiva is dissected away from the pterygium with the Westcott scissors and 0.12 forceps. The vascular structures of the conjunctiva are cauterized using the wet-field cautery. The pterygium is isolated on the cornea and is removed with the Fisch drill loaded with a diamond burr. The eye is well irrigated. A conjunctiva graft may be taken in close proximity to the wound, or a donor graft may be used if a primary closure cannot be accomplished. A 10-0 nylon suture is used to hold the graft in place, and 10-0 polyglactin interrupted sutures are used to secure the graft. If a donor graft is used, thrombin glue is used instead of suturing. Conjunctival injections are administered, and Maxitrol eye ointment is instilled in the operative eye. The eye is covered with two soft eye pads, and a Fox eye shield is taped over the pads with 1-inch Micropore tape for protection.

VITRECTOMY

Definition

A pars plana vitrectomy is a procedure in which the gel-like substance, vitreous humor, found in the back of the eye, is removed, providing the surgeon a clearer view of the structures in the back of the eye. **Figure 31.4** shows a vitrectomy.

Indications

A vitrectomy procedure may be done for a variety of reasons:

- to repair or prevent retinal detachment, especially when it threatens to affect the macula
- to repair tears in the retina
- to reduce vision loss caused by a vitreous hemorrhage
- to treat proliferative retinopathy that causes scar tissue formation

Related Procedures

Additional operative steps involved as part of vitrectomy may include:

- Membranectomy—removal of layers of unhealthy tissue from the retina
- Fluid-gas exchange—injection of gas into the eye such as sulfur hexafluoride (SF6) or perfluoropropane (C3F8) to hold the retina in place or temporarily seal off holes in the retina. The gases are absorbed gradually and exhaled over

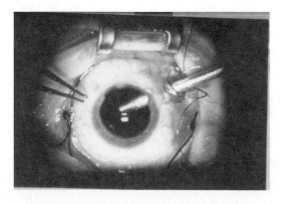

Figure 31.4

Vitrectomy.

a 3- to 8-week period, depending on the gas. Precautions after the procedure with the use of gases include no air travel, no exposure to nitrous oxide, and positioning restrictions.

- Silicone oil injection—filling of the eye with liquid silicone to hold the retina in place.
- Photocoagulation—laser treatment to seal off holes in the retina or to shrink unhealthy, damaging blood vessels which grow in some diseases such as diabetes.
- Scleral buckling—placement of a support positioned like a belt around the walls of the eyeball to maintain the retina in a proper, attached position.

Nursing Implications
Anesthesia

Most vitrectomy procedures are done with a retrobulbar block. General anesthesia may be used in some instances, or per patient request. In addition to the retrobulbar block, patients receive monitored anesthesia care with a propofol, midazolam, and fentanyl combination given by an anesthesia care provider.

The typical vitrectomy patient is geriatric. Assessment of the patient's ability to follow commands and rest comfortably while lying in the supine position is vital prior to deciding on the type of anesthesia the patient is administered.

Position

The patient is supine on an ophthalmology stretcher or on an operative bed with an ophthalmology headrest. A gel headrest is placed under the patient's head. Adequate padding for the patient's elbows and heels is essential. Soft wrist restraints are used. A pillow under the patient's knees will assist with back comfort. Normothermia is important given the age of the patient. A forced air warmer is the preferred method of temperature control.

Establishing and Maintaining the Sterile Field

After the retrobulbar block is placed, the circulating nurse dons sterile gloves. A drop of 5% povidone-iodine solution is instilled in the operative eye. A circumferential eye preparation with 5% povidone-iodine solution in completed on the operative eye. The eyes are prepped using three swabs and then flushed with 5 mL of 0.9% NaCl. The eye is then dried with two sterile 4×4-inch sponges. A nonaperture drape is placed over the patient's eyes and covers a small part of the patient's body.

The surgeon usually sits superior to the patient's head with the scrub nurse to the right of the surgeon. A Mayo stand is used, and the back table is placed to the scrub person's left and perpendicular to the bed. **Table 31.6** lists items that are commonly used during vitrectomy procedures.

Laboratory and Diagnostic Studies

Any preprocedure testing is based on the patient comorbidities. Typically, given the geriatric population, a chest x-ray and EKG, as well as a blood chemistry profile, are completed prior to the procedure. Blood sugar is tested the day of the procedure with the sample collected when the IV is started.

Table 31.6	Items Commonly Used in Vitrectomy Procedures

Iris Scissors

Speculum

Caliper

Bion with Lens

Light Pipe

Vitrector with Accessories

Soft Tip Cannula

Tamo Membrane Scraper

Laser probe

0.3 Castroviejo Forceps

Needle Holders

Tiers

DRUGS & SOLUTIONS:

   Celluvisc

   IC Green

   Kenalog 40 or Decadron

   Antibiotic (injectable or ointment)

   Atropine

   Maxitrol Ointment

Procedure

The nonaperture eye drape is cut using iris scissors. The eye speculum is placed. Using a caliper to locate the area, a 25 gauge trocar sleeve is placed for the infusion line. Once the eye is filled, the biom with lens is used to view the retina and structures in the back of the eye. Celluvisc is applied to assist with eye lubrication during the procedure. A light pipe is introduced along with the vitrector through additional sleeves. The vitrector settings are per surgeon preference. At this point in the procedure, either a membrane peel, laser probe, or perfluron is used to repair damage. If silicone oil is instilled, a 20 g MVR blade is used to make a sclerotomy site. This site is closed with 7-0 polyglacin suture.

Postprocedure Care

The patient will wear the patch and shield for 24 hours. The patient visits the physician the next day and the patch is removed. The patient should not lift or bend over for 24 hours following the procedure.

Potential Complications

Vitrectomy may cause an increase in intraocular pressure, especially in people who have glaucoma. Other risks associated with vitrectomy include bleeding into the vitreous gel, retinal detachment, corneal edema, and endophthalmitis.

CORNEAL TRANSPLANTATION

Definition

Corneal transplantation is the removal of a portion of the cornea that is injured or diseased and replacing it with a donor graft, sometimes called a button graft. The procedure is also called a keratoplasty, or a corneal graft. The procedure may be performed as a partial thickness (Lamellar keratoplasty) or full thickness (penetrating keratoplasty) graft (Rothrock, 2007). **Figure 31.5** shows a corneal transplant.

Indications

Corneal transplants are indicated for the patient who has a cornea that is scarred or cloudy and no longer permits enough light into the eye to see properly. Scar tissue may form in the eye as a result of injury, infection, abnormal eye shape, or corneal dystrophies (Ghosheh, Cremona, Ayers, et al, 2008). Conditions of the eye that are treated by cornea transplant include:

- Bullous keratopathy
- Chemical burns of the eye
- Failure/rejection of previous transplant
- Fuchs' dystrophy
- Keratoconus
- Severe corneal ulcers caused by bacterial, fungal, parasitic, or viral infections in the eye
- Severe traumatic injuries that pierce or cut the cornea
- Severe corneal edema or scarring (Cigna, 2007)

Figure 31.5

Corneal Transplant.

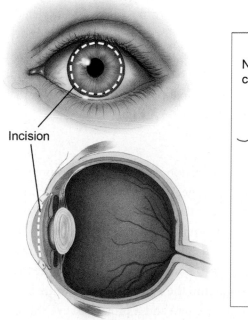

Incision

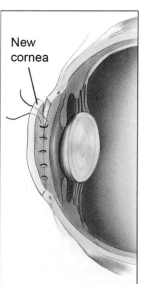

New cornea

Related Procedures

Endothelial keratoplasty which replaces diseased endothelium instead of replacing the entire cornea is a related procedure (Terry, Shamie, Chen, et al, 2008). Phototherapeutic keratectomy using the excimer laser also is a related procedure.

Nursing Implications
Anesthesia

Most corneal transplants are done with a retrobulbar block. General anesthesia may be used in some instances, or per patient request. In addition to the retrobulbar block, patients receive monitored anesthesia care with a propofol, midazolam, and fentanyl combination given by an anesthesia care provider.

Position

The patient is supine on an ophthalmology stretcher or on an operative bed with an ophthalmology headrest. A gel headrest is placed under the patient's head. Adequate padding for the patient's elbows and heels is essential. Soft wrist restraints are used. A pillow under the patient's knees will assist with back comfort. A forced air warmer is the preferred method to keep the patient warm.

Establishing and Maintaining the Sterile Field

After the retrobulbar block is placed, the circulating nurse dons sterile gloves. A drop of 5% povidone-iodine solution is instilled in the operative eye. A circumferential eye preparation with 5% povidone-iodine solution is completed on the operative eye. The eyes are prepped using three swabs and then flushed with 5 mL of 0.9% NaCl. The eye is then dried with two sterile 4 × 4-inch sponges. Sterile drapes are used according to the facility policies and surgeon's preference.

Laboratory and Diagnostic Studies

Preprocedure testing is based on the patient comorbidities. The geriatric patient may have a chest x-ray and EKG, as well as a blood chemistry profile, which is completed prior to the procedure. Blood sugar is tested the day of the procedure with the sample collected when the IV is started. Donor tissue for the transplant will be obtained for the procedure based on standards set by the Eye Bank Association of America (EBAA). The EBAA was established in 1961 and has established nationwide medical standards for the procurement and distribution of corneal tissue (EBAA, 2008).

EBAA
Eye Bank Association of America

Procedure

An eye speculum is used to hold the eye open. If a fixation ring is used, it is sutured in place. The cornea of the patient is prepared using a corneal trephine to make the initial incision. A laser or fine scissors may be used to remove the diseased tissue from the site. The donor cornea graft is prepared using a corneal trephine to cut the donor button. It is important to keep the graft moist with a solution such as Optisol GS. The donor graft is then sutured onto the patient's eye using a fine (10-0) nonabsorbable suture. Once the sutures are in place, air or Healon may be injected into the eye to keep the suture line away from the iris. Antibiotics are followed by an eye pad and a protective eye shield and are taped into place on the operative eye (Rothrock, 2007; Steen-Hall, 2008).

Postprocedure Care

The patient will wear an eye patch for about 24 hours following the procedure, but an eye shield or glasses must be worn until the eye has healed. The surgeon may prescribe antibiotics and corticosteroids for up to a year, as the healing process following corneal transplant is long. Sutures commonly remain in place for at least six months (Indiana University, 2008). The operative eye will initially feel irritated and may itch, but severe symptoms should be reported to the surgeon immediately. Vision may be blurry for several months and some surgeons may prescribe a contact lens to reduce astigmatism (*Encyclopedia of Surgery*, 2008).

Potential Complications

There are potential complications following corneal transplant. While rejection rates are low, the patient's body may reject the donor graft. One study found the average rejection time to be 35 days, so the onset of rejection is quick. The symptoms include vision decrease, eye congestion with edema, dilated vessels, and edema of the whole graft (Shi, Wang, Zhang, et al, 2008).

The complication of corneal wound malapposition may occur at the edges of the graft suture line. This may present as gapes, steps, or protrusions at the graft/host junction. One cause of this is that the graft tissue was cut too large (Kaiserman, Bahar, & Rootman, 2008).

Other complications that can occur following corneal transplant are bleeding, infection, glaucoma, and swelling of the front of the eye. Postprocedure instructions must include symptoms of the complications and when to call the surgeon.

More than 46,000 corneal transplantations are performed every year, making it one of the most frequently transplanted organs. More than 90% of all corneal transplants are successful and restore the patient's sight. Since 1961 over 549,889 corneas have been transplanted in patients ranging in age from 9 days to 103 years old. It is a safe and effective procedure that requires specialized skills and knowledge of the perioperative team (EBAA, 2008).

BLEPHAROPLASTY

Definition

Blepharoplasty can be a functional and/or a cosmetic operative procedure intended to reshape the upper and lower eyelids. Blepharoplasty is performed through incisions made along the natural skin lines of the eyelids, such as the creases of the upper lids and below the lashes of the lower lids. A lower blepharoplasty may be done from the inside surface of the lower eyelid. Initial swelling and bruising take one to two weeks to resolve. As with any plastic operative procedures, results do not stabilize for several weeks to a few months. **Figure 31.6** shows a blepharoplasty.

Indications

When excessive skin is present in the upper eyelids, the skin may hang over the eyelashes and cause visual impairment. The outer and upper parts of the visual field are most commonly affected and the condition may cause difficulty with activities such as driving or reading. During the procedure the excess tissue is removed ond/or repositioned. The surrounding muscles or tendons may be reinforced.

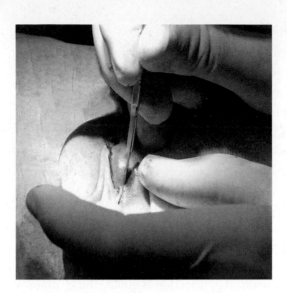

Figure 31.6
Blepharoplasty.

Related Procedures
Entropion Repair

An entropion is an inverted eyelid. The condition occurs primarily as a result of advancing age which causes weakening of certain eyelid muscles.

Nursing Implications
Anesthesia

MAC
Monitored Anesthesia
Care

The procedure is typically done with monitored anesthesia care (MAC) with a peribulbar block. Local injection or drops at the operative site of may supplement as needed.

Position

Patient is supine on the operating room table. Arms are tucked at the sides with dense foam padding to protect elbows and wrists. A gel head rest may be used, and a pillow under the knees increases comfort for the patient. A safety strap is placed across thighs as a safety precaution.

Establishing and Maintaining the Sterile Field

The surgeon will mark the incision lines before the patient is sedated or taken to the operating room. Once the peribulbar block is in place, the bilateral eyes are prepped with Technicare in a circumferential manner. Two towels with towel clips along with a split sheet are used to create a operative field. **Table 31.7** lists items that are commonly used during blepharoplasty procedures.

Physician Orders

Few orders are necessary for the patient undergoing a blepharoplasty procedure. If the patient is over 40 years, a chest x-ray may be ordered if the patient has not had a negative film within 1 year. An EKG may be requested by the anesthesia provider.

Table 31.7	Items Commonly Used in Blepharoplasty Procedures

No. 15 Blade on Safety Handle

Stevens Scissors

Tebbits Forceps

Micro Tip Active Electrode

Webster Needle Holder

Mosquitos

Baby Metzenbaum Scissors, straight

Graefe Muscle Hook

Corneal Shields

Swiss Eye Mask

DRUGS & SOLUTIONS:

   Lidocaine 1%

   Marcaine 0.5%

   Epinephrine 1:100,000

   Tetracaine Drops

   Antibiotic Irrigation for Eyes

Laboratory and Diagnostic Studies

None.

Procedure

The incisions are made with a No. 15 blade. Electrosurgery is used to control bleeding. Stevens scissors and Tebbits forceps are used to excise the excess fat and tissue. Once the excess is removed, hemostats are used to allow the assistant to expose the muscle under the eyelid. The muscle is sutured using a 5-0 nylon followed by 6-0 nylon to close the suture line. Mastisol and Steri strips are used over the suture line. Iced 4 × 4s are used over the suture lines while the other procedures are completed. The procedure is repeated for the lower eyelid and repeated on the other eye.

Postprocedure Care

Ice packs are applied to operative sites rotating 20 minutes on and 20 minutes off for the first 24 hours. The patient is instructed to apply antibiotic ointment to the suture lines twice a day for seven days.

Potential Complications

Factors which may cause complications after the procedure include preexisting dry eyes, lower lid looseness which predisposes the patient to lower lid malposition, and prominence of the eye in relation to the cheek which also can cause lower lid malposition.

REFERENCES

1. AORN (2008). *Perioperative Standards and Recommended Practices*. Denver, CO: AORN.
2. CIGNA (2007). Corneal transplant. Cigna Healthcare Coverage Position 0390. Philadelphia, PA: CIGNA Health Corporation; 1–14.
3. EBAA (2008). EBAA Medical Standards. Washington, D.C.: Eye Bank Association of America. Available at http://www.restoresight.org. Accessed August 26, 2008.
4. *Encyclopedia of Surgery* (2008). Corneal transplantation. Available at http://www.surgeryencyclopedia. com. Accessed August 26, 2008.
5. Ghosheh, F.R., Cremona, F., Ayres, B., Hammersmith, K.M., Choen, E.J., Raber, I.M., Laibson, P.R., & Rapuario, C.J. (2008). Indications for penetrating keratoplasty and associated procedures, 2001–2005. *Eye & Contact Lens*, 34(4); 211–214.
6. Haines, C. (2005). Eye health. WebMD. Accessed February 9, 2008 at http://www.webmd.com/eye-health/cataracts/health-cataracts-eyes?page 2.
7. Indiana University (2008). Corneal transplant. Available at http://www.opt.indiana.edu. Accessed August 26, 2008.
8. Kaiserman, I., Bahar, I., & Rootman, D.S. (2008). Corneal wound malapposition after penetrating keratoplasty: an optical coherence tomography study. *British Journal of Ophthalmology*, 92(8); 1103–7.
9. Rothrock, J. (2007). *Alexander's Care of the Patient in Surgery* (13th ed.), St. Louis: Mosby.
10. Shi, W., Want, T., Zhang, J., Zhoa, J., & Xie, L. (2008). Clinical features of immune rejection after corneoscleral transplantation. *American Journal of Ophthalmology*, 2008 Aug 14. (Epub ahead of print). Available at http://www.ncbi.nlm.nih.gov/pubmed. Accessed August 26, 2008.
11. Steen-Hall (2008). Corneal transplant: what is a corneal transplant? Steen-Hall Eye Institute at http://www.steen-hall.com/transplant. Accessed August 26, 2008.
12. Terry, M.A., Shamie, N., Chen, E.S., Hoar, K.L., & Friend, D.J. (2008). Endothelial keratoplasty: a simplified technique to minimize graft dislocation, iatrogenis graft failure and papillary block. *Ophthalmology*, 115(7); 1179–1186.
13. Wertenbaker, L. (1984). *The Human Body—The Eye: Window to the World*. New York: Torstar Books.

CHAPTER *32*

Trauma Care

Cecil A. King

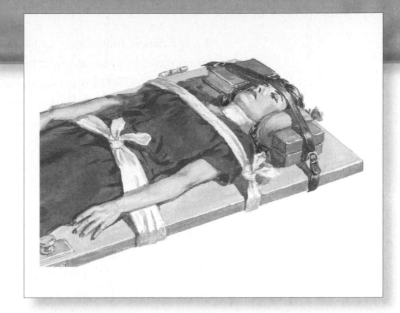

INTRODUCTION

The word trauma refers any injury, whether physical or emotional. From a medical perspective, trauma describes a serious or critical bodily injury, wound, or shock (MedicineNet, 2008). Physical injury whether unintentional (eg, sports accidents) or intentional (eg, battery) is a surgical disease. Most patients admitted to a level I trauma center require three to six operative procedures. The perioperative trauma nurse must have a strong foundation in operative and invasive procedures and be able to function as a generalist in providing expeditious care to address the complexity of the human response to traumatic injury. Trauma occurs suddenly and unexpectedly. The nurse must recognize that not only the presenting patient but also his or her family is experiencing an episode of crisis and tremendous stress in dealing with the sequelae of a traumatic incident. The trauma population presents challenges commensurate with the type and severity of injury.

Many advances in the care of the critically injured before 1960 were made by the military. Mortality rates of 8% in World War I decreased to 4.5% in World War II, to 2.5% during the Korean War, then to less than 2% by the time of the Vietnam conflict. However, it was not until 1966 that healthcare providers began to apply the military experience of trauma care to the civilian population (Beachley, 2009).

SOCIETAL IMPACT

Trauma is a major public health problem in terms of cost and years of life lost. While the concept of traumatic injury as a recognized societal affliction has remained unchanged since early civilization,

Chapter Contents

the incidence, magnitude, cause, mechanism of injury, and treatment of traumatic injury have changed significantly (Beachley, 2009). In 2004, there were 167,184 injury deaths in the US; the most common cause of injury death was motor vehicle crashes, with a total of 44, 933 deaths. Among people 65 years of age and older, falls are the most common cause of nonfatal injuries and injury death. In addition, unintentional injury accounts for over 2 million years of potential life lost before 65 years of age (Weigelt, Brasel, & Klein, 2009).

Trauma Population

Injury is the most underrecognized healthcare issue facing the US today. For people between 1 and 45 years of age, unintentional injury alone is the leading cause of death, and the fifth leading cause of death for all ages in the US. Among young people ages 15 to 24 years, three out of every four deaths were injury related in 2003. In addition, injury—unintentional, homicide and suicide combined—is the leading cause of premature death for young people and therefore is the leading cause of years of potential life lost before 75 years of age. The highest injury-related death rates are seen in the elderly; the death rates for people over 75 years of age are nearly three times those of the general population (Fowler, 2009).

Risk of injury from different causes varies by several factors: age, sex, race, income and environment. Death rates from injuries are highest among patients 75 years of age and older. The injury rate is highest for people between 15 and 34 years of age due to their participation in high-risk activities; the lowest injury rate is seen in children 5 to 14 years of age. Injury rates are highest for males between 15 to 24 years of age; the mortality risk for males is 4.6 times higher than that for females, most likely because of male involvement in hazardous activities. Native Americans have the highest death rate from unintentional injury, regardless of income; African Americans have the highest homicide rate; Caucasians and Native Americans have the highest suicide rates. The rate of unintentional injury is higher in low-income areas than in wealthy areas (Weigelt, Brasel, & Klein, 2009).

Alcohol not only contributes to trauma-producing events, it also increases the severity of injury. Alcohol abuse is a major contributing factor in motor vehicular crashes and in home, industrial, recreational, crime, suicide, and domestic violence traumatic events. There were 75,766 deaths attributable to alcohol in the US in 2001. While the involvement of alcohol in trauma has decreased by approximately 25% in the past decade, conservative estimates still implicate both alcohol and illegal drugs in 19% of the 2.2 million trauma patients who are hospitalized annually (Fowler, 2009).

Rural and urban environments have different patterns of injury: the intentional injury rate is higher in large urban areas; homicide is highest in cities. Rural areas have a higher suicide rate; in addition, the overall mortality rates from injury are higher in rural areas in comparison to urban communities. Both rural and urban environments share poisoning and falls as common unintentional injuries (Weigelt, Brasel, & Klein, 2009).

Cost

According to Whalen (2009), trauma patients average a 12-day hospital stay and it ranks second to cancer in total healthcare expenditures. The total costs of fatal and nonfatal unintentional injuries in 2003 totaled $602.7 billion, which equates to $2,100 per capita or approximately $5,700 per household. The costs to the US healthcare system for injuries that occurred in 2000 were as follows:

- $80.2 billion in medical care costs;
- $1.1 billion for fatal injuries;
- $33.7 billion for hospitalized injuries; and
- $45.4 billion for nonhospitalized injuries (70% [$31.8 billion] of these costs was attributable to injuries treated in the Emergency Department).

The economic burden must be further defined to include the cost of lost productivity; the combined economic costs for injuries that occurred in 2000 totaled $326 billion, outlined as follows:

- $142 billion for fatal injuries;
- $58.7 billion for hospitalized injuries; and
- $125.3 billion for nonhospitalized injuries.

The adverse effects of traumatic injury are more likely to occur in younger persons, relative to the negative effects of preventable diseases and smoking; the loss of productivity is likely to be the principal cost associated with injury (Whalen, 2009). **Table 32.1** lists the National Safety Council report of costs associated with the care of trauma patients.

Prevention

Prevention is the most cost-effective means of containing trauma expenditures. Traumatic death occurs in three phases. The first phase occurs at the scene of the incident. Prevention during this phase will effectively decrease mortality while containing cost. The second phase occurs within hours or days of the injury because of the sequelae of traumatic injury. Effective trauma care can somewhat decrease mortality and cost during this phase. The third and most expensive phase occurs weeks after the injury. Costs are high with this phase because of the technology required to maintain life, the expenditures associated with rehabilitation, and morbidity of those surviving their injuries. Programs that focus on prevention, coordination of care, and rehabilitation will reduce the healthcare dollars expenditure related to trauma.

Not only trauma care but also trauma prevention must be population-based and target those risk groups prone to preventable injury; a community/regional

Table 32.1	Costs Associated with the Care of Trauma Patients	
Type of Injury	**Approximate Cost in Billions**
Motor Vehicle	2003
Work	127.7
Home	99.9
Public	661

Whalen, E. (2009). Economic and administrative issues in trauma care. In McQuillan, K., Makic, M. B. E., and Whalen, E. *Trauma Nursing: From Resuscitation Through Rehabilitation,* 4th ed. St. Louis, MO: Saunders Elsevier, pp. 19–28.

population-based assessment will yield data identifying those at most risk and the type of injuries the population is most prone to (eg, rural, urban, industrial, crime, violence). The healthcare professional networking and building coalitions with multiple organizations and agencies can facilitate injury prevention programs. Mothers Against Drunk Drivers (MADD) is one such program aimed at public education, awareness, and active lobbying efforts to bring about legislative reform to decrease morbidity and mortality secondary to drunk driving.

MADD
Mothers Against Drunk Drivers

Three components necessary to consider in injury prevention include (1) to convince high-risk groups to alter their injury prone behavior, (2) to require behavior change by law (eg, seat belt laws, helmet laws), and (3) to institute passive automatic protection such as passive seat belts (Martinez, 2009). With trauma as the fifth leading cause of death and costing billions of dollars, plus the loss of productive life years, prevention remains the only means of decreasing healthcare dollars spent on trauma and the individual and public impact of this disease.

TRAUMA CENTER DESIGNATION

Whereas the trauma center is a key component of the trauma system, a trauma system encompasses all phases of care, from the field provider to rehabilitation. The actual creation of a trauma system and the trauma center designation is the function of the local emergency medical services system. Trauma systems and trauma centers focus on decreasing deaths, morbidity, and cost of trauma care. This concept is reflected in providing rapid transport, by land or air, from the scene to a center equipped to provide resuscitation and expedient treatment. Triage and transfer protocols allow the patient to reach the most appropriate facility in the least amount of time. Dr. R. Adams Cowley coined this concept and called it "the golden hour." Cowley discovered that events during the first 60 minutes after a life-threatening injury determine whether a person will live or die. Interventions instituted during the first 60 minutes after injury are more likely to reverse the cascade of shock and save life (Cowley & Dunham, 1982). Trauma centers are hospitals that demonstrate a strong commitment to providing 24-hour care to the trauma population. Such a commitment requires immediate access 24 hours a day, 365 days a year to the operative suite. The American College of Surgeons Committee on Trauma has developed specific criteria for four levels of trauma centers. Variations in geographic location, medical equipment, and needed specialists account for the different trauma level designations. The specific criteria to meet a particular level designation are published in *Resources for Optimal Care of the Injured Patient* (American College of Surgeons, 2006).

The number and level of trauma centers are determined by the specific needs of the region and reflect a population-based need. In general, level I centers must provide total care for every aspect of trauma, including prevention, education, research, and rehabilitation. Level II centers need to have extensive clinical capabilities for initial definitive treatment but not all specialties are required. Levels I and II centers are usually in urban and suburban communities. Level III centers provide services in areas not having direct access to a level I or II center (eg, rural areas). Level III centers provide rapid treatment and stabilization and must have systems in place for rapid transfer of patients to a level I or II center. Level IV centers are de facto centers because of geographic location. These centers provide advanced trauma life support before patient transfer. Some states (eg, Oregon, Washington) have developed level IV and V centers to cover large underserved rural areas (Arroyo & Crosby, 1995).

NURSING IMPLICATIONS

Two major considerations determine the impact of trauma care on the operative and invasive procedure environment: the designated level of trauma center and the patient population served.

Trauma care presents an opportunity to develop specific population-based care depending on the location and the population served. The nurse providing operative and invasive procedure trauma services must demonstrate strong core operative and invasive procedure competencies. In addition, the nurse must demonstrate competency in the various operative services required by the trauma population. As a subspecialty, trauma nursing in the operative and invasive procedure suite demands a commitment to quality care beyond the daily routine of many operative and invasive procedure suites. Consider the following factors when planning for the needs of a trauma population:

> Facility location (eg, inner city, suburban, rural)
>
> Trauma center designation (eg, level I, II, III)
>
> Types of care provided for the population served (adult and/or pediatric)
>
> Staffing requirements for trauma cases
>
> Types of injuries expected (eg, industrial, farm related, motor vehicular, gunshot wounds)
>
> Incorporation of trauma cases into the daily operative schedule
>
> Communication system used to alert personnel
>
> Distance of the operative suite from the emergency department
>
> Types of operative services provided for the population served (eg, general, orthopedic, neurosurgery)

In addition to the factors mentioned above, it is important to recognize that the needs of the pediatric patient differ greatly from those of the geriatric, adult, and pregnant trauma patient. Communication, collaboration, and coordination are key components to ensuring optimal patient outcome. Communication is paramount in ensuring that the trauma nurse obtains crucial information from various care providers to coordinate and plan for operative interventions of the trauma patient. The nurse must determine which specific operative procedures are required and in which order they will be performed.

Nursing Competencies

Safely coordinating and managing the demands of the trauma patient requires the nurse to have strong core operative and invasive procedure competencies and to function as a generalist (eg, scrub and circulate in all operative specialties). This, quality combined with critical thinking and flexibility, enhances the nurse's ability to manage the traumatically injured patient.

Experience in general, orthopedic, neurosurgical, and plastic and reconstructive procedures will only enhance the nurse's ability to address the needs of the trauma population. An educational program should evolve out of the operative services that will provide operative interventions to a specific trauma population. Community demographic and traumatic incident data can assist in predicting the types of procedures that will be provided intraoperatively to a given trauma population.

An effective orientation program should evolve around the operative services that will be provided to a specific trauma population. Identifying the trauma population that will be served and the most common types of injuries treated should form the foundation of the orientation program. A comprehensive understanding of different mechanisms of injury provides the nurse with the essential knowledge relevant to prioritizing patient care needs and the sequencing of operative procedures.

Mechanism of Injury

The broadest categories for mechanism of injury are intentional or unintentional, with intentional being the result of battery (eg, gunshot wounds) and unintentional being accidental (eg, home accidents, sport injuries). Intentional and unintentional are then considered within the two broad categories of blunt and/ or penetrating injury. As an example, was a stab wound (a penetrating injury) intentional or unintentional? Making this determination helps in understanding the pattern of injury.

Typically, mechanism of injury is discussed in relation to forces and type of energy dissipated, such as whether the injury resulted from kinetic energy (eg, motor vehicle crashes) or from thermal energy (eg, burns). Kinetic energy is further classified by blunt (eg, motor vehicle crashes) or penetrating (eg, gunshot wound) injuries. Entire texts are devoted to the various aspects of mechanism of injury. For brevity, this discussion will be limited to descriptions of injury as it relates to the more frequent pattern of injury in relation to blunt and penetrating trauma (Weigelt, Brasel, & Klein, 2009).

Blunt Trauma

Begin the assessment by determining what agent or object precipitated the injury. When identifying the mechanism of injury, be suspicious of occult injury. For example, any soft tissue injury indicates possible bony involvement until ruled out or confirmed by radiograph. Focus on predicted patterns of injury in relation to the type of force that caused the injury. Direct impact causes the greatest injury and occurs when there is direct contact of the body surface with the injuring agent; indirect forces are transmitted internally, with dissipation of energy to the internal structures (Weigelt, Brasel, & Klein, 2009). Polaroid photographs taken at the scene of the incident by field providers facilitate the assessment of potential injuries associated with the mechanism of injury.

The age and size of the patient and the agent of injury highly suggest a predictable pattern of injury. Falls, followed by motor vehicle crashes are the leading causes of traumatic brain injury. An additional problem with brain injuries is their high incidence in elderly persons who may be on anticoagulant therapy. Common causes of blunt-force injuries include motor vehicle crashes, aggravated assaults, and sports; the automobile is responsible for approximately 50% of nonpenetrating injuries (Weigelt, Brasel, & Klein, 2009).

Motor Vehicle Crashes

In motor vehicle crashes the injuries happen because of kinetic energy[1]. The speed of the vehicle (eg, velocity) increases the kinetic energy far greater than does the mass of the object (eg, patient). The combined effect of the mass and velocity in blunt trauma results in tissues being compressed. Three types of compressive forces are involved in motor vehicle crashes. The first force occurs when the vehicle collides with an object. The second force occurs when the occupant collides with an object. The third force occurs when the internal organs of the occupant collide with the resisting elements of the human body and the vehicle (Weigelt, Brasel, & Klein, 2009). **Figure 32.1** depicts the potential injury sites of an unrestrained driver.

Unrestrained front seat passengers have higher risk for craniofacial injuries because the steering wheel does not prevent the passenger from being thrown into the windshield. Extremity and pelvic injuries for front seat passengers are similar for driver and passenger. The front seat passenger, however, is more prone to a higher rate of liver injury, whereas the driver is more at risk for splenic injury. Airbags provide little protection to passengers during the lateral crash because they are designed to decrease impact during frontal crashes; however, airbags alone are not effective in reducing injury. **Figure 32.2** illustrates the more common sites of injury (eg, chest, pelvis, head, and neck) seen with the lateral impact crashes. Rear impact collisions can result in cervical spine injury due to hyperextension of the neck on impact, but spinal fractures are more common with the lateral impact collision than with the rear impact collision. Whether the driver or passenger is restrained or unrestrained does not always provide an accurate predictable pattern of injury. Compression injuries to the spleen, liver, and pancreas result from the accident victim wearing a loosely

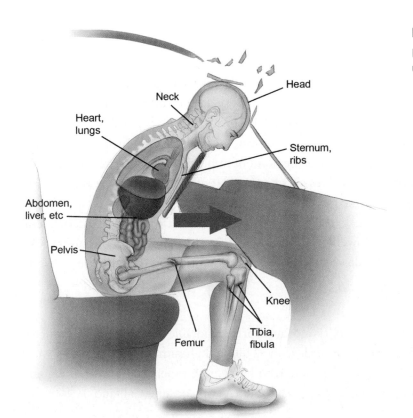

Figure 32.1

Potential injuries of an unrestrained driver.

32

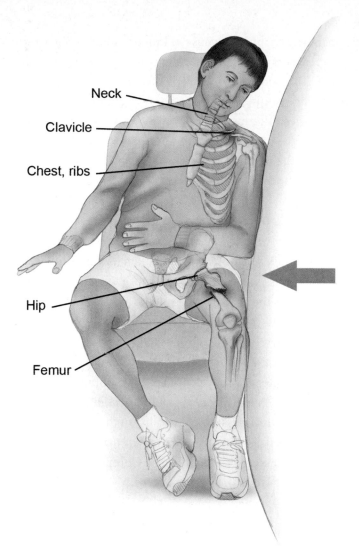

Figure 32.2

Potential injuries in a lateral-impact collision.

Neck

Clavicle

Chest, ribs

Hip

Femur

fastened lap belt too low across the pelvis. While seat belts do decrease injury morbidity and mortality, if misplaced either intentionally or unintentionally, they can actually cause an injury (Weigelt, Brasel, & Klein, 2009).

Children and adolescents have a higher rate of pedestrian-vehicle injuries than adults do. Primary injuries occur at the point of impact whether the pedestrian is an adult or child. Secondary fractures occur as a result of the pedestrian, whether adult or child, being thrown by the force.

The adult pedestrian will tend to turn away from the vehicle and thus sustain lateral impact to the upper and lower legs (**Fig. 32.3**). Lateral compression fractures of the distal femur and tibia-fibula are the more common injuries in the adult pedestrian.

Penetrating Trauma
Ballistics

The enactment of the Brady bill is indicative of the epidemic of violent trauma inflicted by firearms. Gunshot wounds cost close to $2 billion in healthcare expenditures. Most violent trauma occurs between people who know each other, that are drinking and using drugs, and have a gun nearby when the altercation occurs (Califano, 1994).

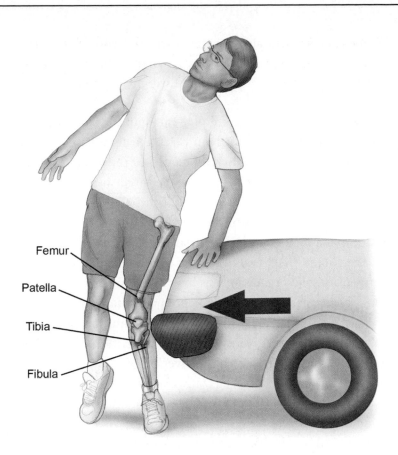

Figure 32.3

Potential injuries in the adult pedestrian struck by a vehicle.

Femur

Patella

Tibia

Fibula

Gunshot wounds are not simply cases of penetrating trauma but a combination of blunt and penetrating forces. The extent of the injury varies depending on the characteristics of the missile (eg, bullet), the type of gun, and the tissue(s) affected. The extent of injury produced by gunshot wounds will vary depending on the caliber (eg, bullet's size), velocity (eg, speed at which the bullet travels), line of flight and distance to the target, amount of energy transmitted (eg, gun power), and density of the tissues struck. Generally, the length of the gun barrel determines velocity; the longer the barrel, the higher the velocity. Low-velocity firearms propel missiles at speeds of approximately 1100 feet per second, whereas high-velocity weapons fire missiles traveling greater than 2000 feet per second (Dufresne, 1995a).

The extent of tissue injury also varies according to the missile (eg, bullet) characteristics. Deforming bullets, which are usually composed of lead, expand on impact, thus increasing the diameter of the missile. This deforming effect slows the bullet as it enters the body, transmitting more energy into the organs and tissues on impact and resulting in a larger area of injury. If small bullet fragments break off, or the energy is dispersed into dense tissue (eg, bone), fragments become secondary projectiles, resulting in massive tissue damage. Jacketed bullets, which are encased to prevent bullet deformation, result in a cylindrical wound track. Low-velocity weapons, such as a 22-caliber handgun, usually fire a deforming bullet. Most police forces prefer this weapon. The bullet and low-velocity characteristics of the weapon decrease the risk of the projectile exiting the body and harming innocent bystanders. Shotgun shells, which are fully jacketed, contain multiple small-caliber pellets. This type of shell causes massive tissue injury because the casing bursts and the pellets disperse

32

throughout the tissue. Shotgun wounds also have an increased risk of infection because of severe devitalization of tissue and contamination of the wound from shotgun wadding, clothing, skin, hair, and powder entering the wound (Weigelt, Brasel, & Klein, 2009).

Tissue cavitation is the principal mechanism of injury with gunshot wounds. Laceration and penetration of the tissue occurs as the projectile enters the body and transects the tissue. The extent of damage is directly related to the velocity of the weapon, the missile characteristics, and the density of the target tissue. The forward and lateral push of the missile through the tissue slows the missile, which causes shock waves. As the energy dissipates in the surrounding tissue, secondary shock waves occur resulting in a temporary and permanent cavitation, which further stretches tissue. Gas- or liquid-filled tissues such as the lung and bowel easily rupture, whereas higher density solid organs such as liver and bone tend to shatter (eg, fracture). Permanent cavitation is smaller than temporary cavitation and is usually the size of the caliber of the missile. Temporary cavitation is much greater with high-velocity weapons because of a much greater release of energy (**Fig. 32.4**). The more elastic the tissue the more forgiving, whereas the liver, spleen, brain, and bone have poor elasticity and suffer far greater damage (Dufresne, 1995b). More cohesive and elastic tissues experience less damage; dense tissue absorbs more kinetic energy, thereby causing greater damage (Weigelt, Brasel, & Klein, 2009).

Generally, the armament used in gunshot cases consists of rifles, shotguns, and handguns. Rifles are more powerful than shotguns and handguns, and thus inflict the most damage. Low velocity handguns usually result in limited tissue damage. The path

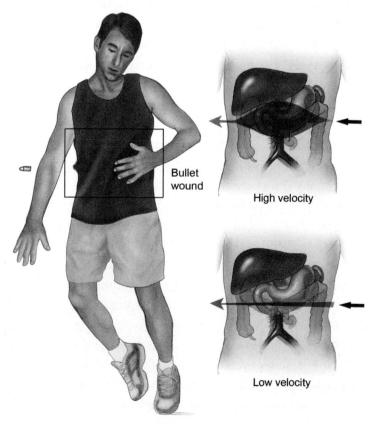

Figure 32.4

Potential injuries from a gunshot wound.

Bullet wound

High velocity

Low velocity

of the bullet causes most of the injury. In the majority of urban areas, small-caliber, low-velocity weapons cause most gunshot wounds. However, in rural areas, where hunting is common, shotgun and rifle wounds are more likely to be seen.

Stabbing and Impalement

Stab wounds and impalement injuries are low-velocity injuries. These injuries are usually obvious. However, predicting the extent of underlying injury is easier if the patient arrives with the weapon in place. If the patient arrives with the weapon removed, ask about the gender of the assailant. This information will help in predicting the extent of injury. Men tend to stab with an upward thrust, whereas women tend to stab with a downward thrust.

Injury caused by stab wounds and impaling usually depends on the point of penetration and the underlying tissues and organ(s). Unlike penetration by a deforming bullet, injury usually remains confined to the location of the stabbing or impalement. Keep in mind, however, depending on the length of the weapon, penetration of multiple body cavities can occur, resulting in significant injury.

Impalement injuries can result from a forceful impact between the object of penetration and the patient during motor vehicle crashes or falls, or from falling or thrown objects. If the patient arrives with the impaled object in place, leave it in place until an operating room is available to remove the object. The object left in place has the ability to tamponade vascular injuries and prevent exsanguination. Removing the weapon during the operative procedure allows far greater control of hemorrhage. Injuries caused by penetrating objects significantly increase the risk for bacterial contamination and usually require extensive wound debridement (Weigelt, Brasel, & Klein, 2009).

Special Populations

Pregnant women should wear the lap seat-belt low, across the bony pelvis, which could prevent ejection from the vehicle. Remember, the pregnant trauma patient presents with two patients in need of care and monitoring, not just one patient. Obstetrical consultation and collaboration is required for optimal management of the mother and fetus (eg, fetal monitoring) during the procedure to prevent fetal distress. The supine position displaces the uterus and compresses major abdominal vessels. Positioning the pregnant patient in the left lateral position can increase cardiac output and blood pressure. In the event of cardiac arrest resulting in maternal death, the decision to perform a postmortem cesarean section must be made and should be performed while cardiopulmonary resuscitation is in progress for the optimal outcome of the fetus (Smith, 2009).

Routine car restraints and air bags do not adequately prevent injury in children during motor vehicle crashes. The anatomy of infants and children makes them more vulnerable to traumatic injury; because the child's head is proportionately larger in relation to body mass than in an adult, the child's head is particularly vulnerable to injury (Moloney-Harmon, 2009). In addition, infants and toddlers are more prone to head injuries from being thrown forward during motor vehicle crashes, whereas children 4–9 years old tend to be restrained by the seat belt and therefore experience more abdominal injuries. Children struck by vehicles experience a different injury pattern than do adults who are struck by vehicles. The classic injury sustained by a child pedestrian is described as the Waddell Triad. The vehicle usually hits the child in the chest, pelvic, and shin areas, resulting in primary impact injuries to the supracondylar, patellar, and tibial areas; sternal, rib, femur, and pelvic fractures; and vessel lacerations. Next, the child is thrown backwards, usually resulting in secondary injuries to the cervical spine and skull.

Elderly drivers have higher death rates from motor vehicle crashes than younger people do. This higher mortality rate may be related to increased susceptibility to the complications secondary to trauma. The elderly also have the highest rate of trauma related to falling and being struck by a vehicle.

Nurse's Role

Successful implementation of trauma care requires systematic preplanning to ensure the availability of personnel, equipment, and supplies. Collaborative preplanning ensures an organized approach to addressing the multiple care needs of the critically injured patient. Planning should flow from the concept that *there are no emergencies.* Communication is the cornerstone of collaborative practice. The critically injured patient may require a lifesaving procedure before a definitive diagnosis. The nurse communicates as a liaison between the operative and invasive procedure suite, the emergency department, and the inpatient units. Because trauma is a surgical disease, the nurse is an important member of the trauma team. The level of interdepartmental interaction will vary among facilities. During the preprocedure phase, the nurse conducts an assessment in the emergency department or over the telephone with the emergency department nurse to determine the patient's injuries and readiness for the procedure, and to identify the proposed operative procedure(s) and any special equipment or personnel (eg, rapid infusion system).

In some facilities the nurse may assist the trauma physician outside the operative suite and invasive procedure suite with resuscitative operative procedures. The nurse's knowledge of lateral thoracotomy and tracheostomy can facilitate stabilization of the critically injured.

The nurse assumes two roles: patient advocate and plan of care coordinator. Usually, trauma patients are critically injured, intubated, in a state of altered consciousness, and thus incapable of communication or self-advocacy. No other member of the trauma team is as focal to patient safety as the nurse. A safe and rapid transport of the patient from the emergency department to the operative and invasive procedure suite requires rapid assessment and organizational capabilities to obtain needed patient information from both a number of care providers and the patient to coordinate care during the operative procedure. All trauma centers must have written policies and procedures that encompass the legal and safety rights of patients lacking decision-making capacity.

Assessment

Conducting the assessment and reporting the patient's condition in a head-to-toe, system-by-system manner will provide a holistic approach to preprocedure evaluation. **Table 32.2** lists essential information required for coordinating the care of the trauma patient during the operative procedure.

Table 32.2	Essential Information for Coordinating Care of the Trauma Patient During the Operative Procedure

- ☐ Patient's name and hospital number
- ☐ Age and sex
- ☐ Mechanism of injury
- ☐ Trauma score or Glasgow Coma Scale score
- ☐ Past medical and operative and invasive procedure history if known
- ☐ Pertinent incidents leading up to the trauma
- ☐ History of substance use (eg, alcohol, heroin)
- ☐ Preprocedure medications administered
- ☐ Blood products administered before the procedure
- ☐ Status of blood product availability
- ☐ Fluid volume replacement/resuscitation
- ☐ Airway management and method of ventilation
- ☐ Approximate time of arrival of the patient to the operative and invasive procedure suite
- ☐ Family members, family spokesperson, and location of family members waiting for information

The nursing process is a cyclical process of assessment, planning, implementation, reassessment, and evaluation of the interventions performed to determine the need for further intervention. The planning phase often occurs simultaneously with the assessment phase in the care of the trauma patient. Time is critical; therefore, focus on realistic patient outcomes based on those nursing diagnoses most applicable to the trauma population. **Table 32.3** shows the mnemonic AMPLE that can be used to focus the nurse's assessment when time is limited (Kidd, 1993).

Care Planning

Planning begins simultaneously with the initiation of assessment, often minutes before receiving the patient in the operative suite. The mechanism of injury and other relevant information obtained from the patient and other care providers will guide the assessment and planning phase of care. Do not make the error of focusing on the most obvious injury such as an open fracture. Rather, assess the patient in a holistic manner to prioritize the intraoperative interventions. For example, the patient with a closed-head injury and deteriorating level of consciousness will benefit more from an urgent craniotomy than from operative treatment of an open fracture. In addition to

Table 32.3	Rapid Assessment
A	Allergies
M	Medications/recreational drug use
P	Past medical and operative history
L	Last meal and last tetanus immunization
E	Events leading to injury

32

standard patient outcomes and nursing diagnoses as discussed in previous chapters, the trauma population all share the following nursing diagnoses.

Nursing Diagnoses and Patient Outcomes

The nursing diagnoses and patient outcomes shown in **Table 32.4** are not exhaustive in relation to the trauma patient but reflect those nursing diagnoses common to all trauma patients (Petersen, 2007). This population has an extremely high risk for fluid, electrolyte, and acid-base imbalance secondary to shock. The patient

Table 32.4	**Nursing Diagnoses and Patient Outcomes Specific to Trauma**

Outcome 1   The patient is free from evidence of impaired respiratory function.

Diagnosis	Risk Factors	Outcome Indicators
Respiratory Function, Risk for Impaired	☐ Presence of ineffective airway clearance and impaired gas exchange because of head and/or neck trauma ☐ Altered level of consciousness ☐ Aspiration ☐ Effects of anesthetic, procedure, and positioning of the patient	☐ Are blood pressure, temperature, and pulse within expected ranges? ☐ Is SaO_2 within expected range? ☐ Are conjunctiva and/or mucous membranes pink? ☐ Is the patient free from cyanosis or pallor?

Outcome 2   The patient is free from evidence of fluid volume imbalance.

Diagnosis	Risk Factors	Outcome Indicators
Fluid Volume, Risk for Imbalance	☐ Nature of injury(s) ☐ Presence of hemorrhage ☐ Shock ☐ Medications ☐ Fluid volume alteration ☐ Choice of resuscitative fluids	☐ Are temperature, pulse, and respirations within expected ranges? ☐ Are heart rate and blood pressure within expected ranges? ☐ Are peripheral pulses present and equal bilaterally? ☐ Is the skin warm to touch? ☐ Do capillaries refill less than 3 seconds? ☐ Is urine output greater than 30 mL/hr? ☐ Is specific gravity 1.010 to 1.030? ☐ Are arterial blood gases, serum electrolytes, and hemodynamic monitoring values within expected ranges?

Outcome 3   The adult patient will relate an increase in pyschological and physiological comfort.

Diagnosis	Defining Characteristics	Outcome Indicators
Fear*	☐ Feelings of dread, fright, apprehension, alarm ☐ Crying ☐ Aggression ☐ Trembling ☐ Muscle tightness	☐ Are pulse and respirations within expected ranges? ☐ Are heart rate and blood pressure within expected ranges? ☐ Does the patient differentiate between real from imagined situations?

☐ Weakness in limbs
☐ Palpitations
☐ Rapid pulse
☐ Increased blood pressure
☐ Shortness of breath
☐ Increased respiratory rate
☐ Urinary frequency/urgency
☐ Syncope
☐ Dilated pupils

☐ Does the patient describe effective and ineffective coping patterns?
☐ Does the patient identify own coping responses?

Outcome 4   The patient is free from evidence of impaired tissue integrity.

Diagnosis

Tissue Integrity, Risk for Impaired

Risk Factors

☐ Related to tissue injury
☐ Position
☐ Extending length of the procedure
☐ Open wounds
☐ Infection related to penetrating trauma
☐ Extraneous objects used during trauma care

Outcome Indicators

☐ Is the skin smooth, intact, and free of ecchymosis, cut, abrasions, shear injury, blistering, discoloration, swelling, or induration?
☐ Are incision edges approximated, free of ischemia (pallor, cyanosis, erythema)?

Outcome 5   The patient is at or returning to normothermia at the conclusion of the immediate postprocedure period.

Diagnosis

Hypothermia, Risk for

Risk Factors

☐ Cool temperature of resuscitative fluids and blood products
☐ Operative exposure
☐ Shock
☐ Environmental factors at the scene of trauma and/or the intraoperative environment

Outcome Indicators

☐ Are temperature, pulse, and respirations within expected ranges?
☐ Are heart rate and blood pressure within expected ranges?
☐ Are peripheral pulses present and equal bilaterally?
☐ Do capillaries refill less than 3 seconds?
☐ Is the skin warm to touch?
☐ Is the patient free from shivering?
☐ Is the patient free from cyanosis or pallor?

Outcome 6   The patient demonstrates and/or reports adequate pain control throughout the postprocedure period.

Diagnosis

Pain

Defining Characteristics

☐ Communication of pain descriptors
☐ Increased blood pressure, pulse, and respirations
☐ Diaphoresis
☐ Dilated pupils
☐ Guarded position
☐ Facial mask of pain
☐ Crying, moaning

Outcome Indicators

☐ Does the patient report pain control based on a recognized pain scale?
☐ Are facial expressions relaxed?
☐ Does the patient deny discomfort in non-targeted areas?
☐ Does the patient use the pain scale appropriately to describe level of discomfort?
☐ Does the patient cooperate with plan of care?

32

☐ Clenched jaws or fists

☐ Agitation

☐ Anxiety

☐ Irritability

☐ Does the patient verbalize ability to cope?

☐ Are blood pressure, pulse, and respiration within expected ranges?

☐ Does the patient report satisfaction with level of pain control?

Outcome 7   The patient is free from signs and symptoms of infection.

Diagnosis

Infection, Risk for

Risk Factors

☐ Trauma

☐ Operative procedures

☐ Contaminated wounds

☐ Existing pathophysiology at time of trauma (cancer, renal failure, hematologic disorders, diabetes mellitus, alcoholism, immunodeficiency, AIDS, hepatic disorder, respiratory disorders, immunosuppression, altered or insufficient leukocytes, and altered integumentary system)

☐ Existing compromised circulation at time of trauma (lymphedema, obesity, and peripheral vascular disease)

☐ Existing compromised host defenses at time of trauma (smoking, history of infections, and malnutrition)

Outcome Indicators

☐ Is the patient afebrile?

☐ Is the leukocyte count three to 30 days postoperative within expected range?

☐ Is the incision well approximated and free from heat, redness, induration, swelling, or foul odor?

☐ Are drians covered with sterile dressing and/or connected to continuous drainage?

Adapted from Carpentino-Moyet, L. J. (2008) *Handbook of Nursing Diagnosis* (12th ed.), Philadelphia: Lippincott Williams & Wilkins; Petersen C. (2007). *Perioperative Nursing Data Set, the Perioperative Nursing Vocabulary* (Revised 2nd ed.). Denver, CO: AORN, Inc.; AORN (2008) *Perioperative Standards and Recommended Practices*. Denver: AORN, Inc.

will arrive in the operative and invasive procedure suite with intravenous lines and invasive monitoring catheters. Consider these lines and catheters as contaminated. Most likely, the devices were placed in less than ideal conditions in the field, hospital, or emergency department environments. Replace these lines within 24 hours to decrease the risk of infection. Traumatic injuries frequently result in blood loss. A significant volume of blood may have been lost before admission to the emergency department. Whereas external blood loss from lacerations, amputations, and open fractures may be apparent, blood loss may be occult and concealed within body cavities, such as the retroperitoneal space. Injuries to the thorax may conceal a blood loss of 2 to 3 liters, and the abdominal cavity may contain as much as 6 liters. Unstable pelvic fractures result in 6 to 8 units of blood loss, whereas a femur fracture may yield 1 to 4 units of extravagated blood.

Arrange a system for rapidly infusing O-negative, non-crossmatched blood in the event of extreme blood loss. Women of childbearing years should receive Type O Rh-negative red blood cells to decrease future Rh complications and blood product incompatibility. Typing and crossmatching should be part of the initial assessment and line placement with every trauma patient.

Coordinating Operative Procedures

Because of the nature and urgency of operative intervention in the trauma population, facilities should have policies and procedures in place for obtaining informed consent in emergent situations. Frequently, the trauma patient is unresponsive or incapacitated and thus cannot sign the operative permit. The urgency of the situation may not allow the needed time to contact family to sustain or save life or limb. In addition, policies should provide guidance for patient populations such as Jehovah's Witnesses concerning their informed choice to receive or refuse blood products. A preventive ethical approach to developing policy and procedures to address these unique needs of the trauma population will prevent dilemmas in providing optimal care with respect to patient self-determination.

Staffing and Operative Suite Availability

During the final phase of planning, the nurse ensures that adequate staffing, the room, and the equipment are available to meet the needs of the trauma patient. Collaborative preplanning and communication of all personnel involved in the operative interventions of trauma patients must evolve into a systematic method of preparing the room to accommodate the multiple operative needs of the critically injured.

Communication with all members of the trauma team ensures that the necessary personnel, equipment, and room will be available to address the needs of the trauma patient. Many facilities have in place a trauma alert system, usually on beeper (eg, all members simultaneously beeped) so that all personnel are informed of their need to respond. In those facilities not having an in-house operative trauma team (eg, level III centers), notification of the operative trauma team should be initiated early in the resuscitative phase to ensure that personnel will be physically present when needed. Notification of the operative trauma team initiates the preprocedure assessment to determine the type and number of instruments, positioning needs, the type of anesthesia used, and the general setup of the room, which will depend on the procedure(s) to be performed. Staff availability can be achieved through both in-house and call teams.

There are three methods of maintaining room availability in the operative and invasive procedure suite. One is to maintain a designated trauma room. While this provides immediate room access it is costly to maintain because it is never used except for trauma cases. The second method is the next-room-out availability. This method gives priority to emergency and trauma cases over scheduled cases, while allowing the rooms to be used for scheduled cases. Whereas this method is more cost effective than having a designated trauma room, it can be upsetting to patients and their physicians when their case is delayed. A third method uses the rotational list for emergency and trauma cases. This method designates a particular room on a particular day as the room that will give priority to emergency and trauma cases. This method allows rooms to be used for scheduled cases if no trauma comes in. However, although cost effective, this has the same disadvantages in delaying elective cases as the next-room-availability method (Foss & Feistritzer, 1993).

Collaborative preplanning by the manager, trauma team leader, and anesthesia providers should focus on the room availability that will provide the facility with the more cost-effective method of room availability. Designing a schedule that designates a short room is used in some facilities based on the next-room-out method. For example, no cases longer than 2 hours are scheduled in this room with the thinking that this room will usually be the next available room within an hour.

Trauma Operative Procedures

The types of operative procedures performed will depend on the trauma population served, the mechanism of injury, and the operative services offered within the facility. Generally, emergency trauma procedures are classified as single, multi-consecutive, simultaneous, or resuscitative.

Single

A single trauma procedure should not be confused with a single procedure performed on an elective basis on a prepared patient. An example is the exploratory laparotomy performed emergently on a patient who has sustained a traumatic event that may be life-threatening. Understanding the mechanism of injury will alert the nurse to monitor for complications during the procedure.

Multiconsecutive

This patient has sustained two or more body system injuries requiring two or more operative procedures. The chief trauma physician and operative team members involved must communicate and collaborate in determining the appropriate priorities of the procedures. Each procedure is a separate operative event and is treated as such. Each procedure requires a separate set of instruments with separate sponge and instrument counts. Used instruments and equipment are removed from the room after each procedure. Constant monitoring is very important because priorities may change quickly in the critically injured patient. Examples of multi-consecutive procedures are a craniotomy followed by a tracheostomy and insertion of an intramedullary nail.

Simultaneous

During simultaneous operative procedures two separate operative teams perform two procedures at the same time. This method is used when the patient has two equally life- or limb-threatening injuries. Simultaneous procedures require careful planning of space and instrumentation. The operative fields should remain separate as much as possible to prevent cross-contamination. An example is craniotomy and simultaneous application of an external fixator.

Resuscitative

A rapid resuscitative procedure is performed on a patient who requires a simultaneous lifesaving procedure and resuscitation. This situation is extremely challenging and requires the nurse to have a basic knowledge of critical care and resuscitative procedures. Some facilities may require the nurse to have certification in advanced cardiac life support. Examples are repair of a ruptured descending thoracic aorta, gunshot wounds to the inferior vena cava, or burr holes to prevent brain stem herniation.

Use a case cart system to prepare for trauma. Case carts specific to abdominal, thoracic, neurosurgical, and orthopedic extremity injuries provide necessary instruments, supplies, and equipment for immediate use. The cart should contain instrumentation, drapes, and other supplies that can be opened rapidly to avoid unnecessary delays.

Sponge, Sharp, and Instrument Counts

Facilities not using the case cart system should develop standardized instrumentation specific to the service and type of procedures performed on the trauma patient. The specific instrument sets should allow for systematic and rapid access, while avoiding duplication.

Reducing the number and types of instruments and streamlining standardized sets improves ease and efficiency of counting procedures. Collaborative preplanning with physicians to determine the absolute essential instruments will help streamline and standardize sets. Although this may require a reorganization of sets, it should not require a greater cost outlay to purchase more instrumentation. The goal should be to avoid duplication in such a manner that each set is designed to complement the other. This approach to standardization will eliminate the need for physician preference cards. **Table 32.5** provides an example of instrumentation and supplies needed by various services to perform operative procedures on trauma patients.

Facilities that provide services to trauma patients should have preestablished policies and procedures that provide examples of when counts are to be aborted (eg, when delaying to conduct a count would jeopardize the patient's life). Assessment of the patient's condition and the urgency of the operative intervention should guide the nurse's decision as to whether or not there is adequate time to conduct the count. To ensure patient safety, the policy for aborted counts should include the appropriate documentation of the incident and followup procedures, such as abdominal radiographs after exploratory laparotomy.

OPERATIVE INTERVENTIONS

The preprocedure phase is initiated at the scene of the incident. Those patients requiring a level I or II trauma center may average 3.5 operative procedures during their hospitalization. The major procedures most commonly preformed are exploratory laparotomy, craniotomy, and open reduction with internal fixation (ORIF) of fractures. Anywhere from 50% to 75% of trauma patients experience some type of orthopedic injury (King, 1994).

ORIF
Open Reduction
Internal Fixation

Head and Neck Area

Any trauma to the head and neck area can result in cerebral, cervical spine, or craniofacial injury. Neurosurgical interventions most commonly involve a craniotomy to evacuate a hematoma or to elevate a depressed skull fracture. Insertion of a ventriculostomy catheter to monitor the intracranial pressure may be performed in the operative and invasive procedure suite or the emergency department. Craniofacial trauma results in a combination of blunt and penetrating trauma usually resulting in facial fractures requiring open reduction and internal fixation (ORIF). All patients sustaining blunt trauma or falls should be suspected of having cervical spine injury until it is ruled out by radiography. Trauma involving the head and neck area predisposes the patient to airway compromise, and a tracheostomy may be indicated emergently to maintain the patient's airway.

Table 32.5	Basic Instrumentation and Equipment for Trauma Surgery	
Service	**Instrumentation**	**Adjuncts**
General	General laparotomy set	Defibrillator/crash cart
Cardiovascular	Cardiovascular set	Internal paddles
Thoracic	Chest set	Blood warmer
		Rapid infusion system
		Autotransfusion equipment
		Cardiovascular sutures
		Vascular grafts
		Cardiopulmonary bypass
		Sternal saw
		Positioning devices
Neurosurgery	Craniotomy set	Intracranial pressure monitoring equipment
	Craniotomy	Mayfield headrest
	Cervical spine fixation set	Gardner-Wells tongs
Maxillofacial	ORIF facial/cranial implants	Padding/positioning devices
Plastics	Myocutaneous flap sets	Hypothermia blanket
Oral Surgery	Micro-instrumentation	Micro drills
	Microscope	Various drill bits
	Skin grafting equipment	Arch bars and braces
	Arch bar set	Oral surgical set
Obstetrics	General surgery set	Bladder blade
	Cord clamps	Obstetrical forceps
		Sponge sticks
		DeLee suction trap
		1 Chromic (uterine closure)
		2-0 or 3-0 Chromic or Vicryl on gastrointestinal needle for bladder flap
		Isolette
		Fetal Doppler ultrasonography

Adapted from Association of Operating Room Nurses (AORN) (1992). *Nursing Care of the Trauma Patient* (AC-ENA-051). Denver, CO: AORN.

Chest and Abdomen

Whether the injury is blunt or penetrating, the patient is frequently a candidate for pericardial window and/or exploratory laparotomy. Various facilities use different methods to assess the abdomen for injury (eg, diagnostic peritoneal lavage, computed tomography, ultrasonography). An upright chest radiograph is the easiest and most common method of assessing the chest for a widening mediastinum. Patients presenting with widening mediastinum, seen on radiograph, or penetrating chest trauma frequently require a pericardial window for definitive diagnosis and operative intervention. The left lateral thoracotomy is a resuscitative procedure and is rarely performed except on those patients presenting in full arrest. The role of the nurse during this procedure in the emergency department varies among facilities, ranging from no involvement to assisting the physician.

Patients presenting with blunt abdominal trauma frequently require an exploratory laparotomy for management of liver and splenic injury. The patient who has sustained penetrating abdominal trauma frequently will have more extensive damage, depending on the velocity of the weapon. More often than not, trauma patients ate or drank in the past 6 hours, placing them at risk for intra-abdominal contamination secondary to bowel injuries. Rapid detection, intervention (eg, bowel resection), and acute management with copious antibiotic coverage helps prevent complications such as sepsis and multisystem failure.

Genitourinary

Blunt trauma to the abdomen when the patient has a full bladder frequently results in a ruptured bladder. Penetrating trauma to the genitourinary system (eg, urethra, vagina) is usually a result of gunshot wound or laceration from bone fragments in lateral compression fractures of the pelvis. This is considered an open fracture and requires urgent operative intervention to debride the wound and stabilize the pelvis.

Orthopedic

Severe, unstable pelvic fractures can result in 40% of the circulating blood volume pooling in the pelvis. Urgent application of a pelvic external fixator will stabilize the bone fragments, providing hemostasis. Some facilities maintain a self-contained pelvic external fixator tray with battery-operated drills in the emergency department to address this urgent need.

Open fractures require emergent operative intervention to maintain viability of the affected extremity. During the procedure these fractures are usually managed with pulsatile pressure lavage with 0.9% normal saline and debridement of devitalized tissue. Traumatic fractures are treated one of three ways: intramedullary nailing, ORIF, and/or external fixation. Controversy surrounds the question of whether to do a primary closure on open fractures. Orthopedic traumatic injuries will always require reduction and fixation to maintain viability and function of the extremity and structures involved.

This discussion of operative procedures is not exhaustive, nor all-inclusive, of the various life- and limb-saving and sustaining procedures required to promote the trauma patient's involvement in the rehabilitative process. The trauma patient frequently requires sequential reconstructive and cosmetic operative procedures after acute operative stabilization.

Assessment and Intervention During the Procedure

During the procedure the nurse monitors the patient for any signs of further compromise of physiologic parameters. Continuously reassess the patient to detect and prevent further complications in the anesthetized patient. Vulnerable domains for the surgical trauma patient include positioning, fluid maintenance, and temperature regulation.

Patient Positioning

Planning the positioning of the trauma patient in the operative and invasive procedure suite begins with the assessment. Patients with pulmonary contusion tend to do poorly in the lateral position. Those patients with elevated intracranial pressure do better in the reverse Trendelenburg position and exhibit lower intracranial pressure.

Correct positioning provides optimal access to the operative area and allows the anesthesia provider access for induction and maintenance of a patent airway. When the patient has painful injuries such as open fractures, the anesthesia provider may induce and intubate on the emergency department stretcher and then move the patient to the bed. This method, however, has potential for injuring the patient if not done correctly. At minimum, four people should implement the transfer. Take care to support and correctly position the patient's entire body.

Frequently, a procedure on the trauma patient may last several hours. Road gravel and debris, if present, may further comprise skin integrity. Remove road gravel and debris from the patient's back with a portable vacuum. Assess the patient's skin integrity before the procedure and provide special positioning devices as necessary. Remember that the field provider backboard is a transfer device, not a positioning device. Remove the patient from the backboard in the emergency department. In addition, the trauma patient has the potential for cervical spine injury, therefore exercise care while transporting and positioning.

Most likely, the trauma patient will be immobile for some time after the procedure. Therefore, apply antithrombolytic stockings to facilitate venous return and prevent deep vein thrombosis. However, do not place stockings on patients presenting with lower leg injury. When simultaneous operative procedures are planned, careful planning of positioning is needed to accommodate both operative teams.

Fractured extremities may be splinted and elevated. In addition, tibial traction pins may be in place to maintain fracture reduction. Prevent further complications secondary to positioning by maintaining traction during the procedure. This may require collaboration with the orthopedic surgeon, nurse, or technician. Monitor fractures prone to compartment pressure syndrome in the anesthetized patient. When the pneumatic antishock garment has been applied in the prehospital setting, it is difficult to assess the lower extremities. The nurse should obtain a report of the skin condition from the emergency medical service providers. The pneumatic antishock garment may need to remain inflated intraoperatively to maintain the patient's blood pressure. Do not remove it until allowed by the trauma physician.

Fluid Maintenance

Trauma patients, especially those in shock, present with a fluid volume deficit requiring significant volume replacement. Plan to use autotransfusion, a rapid-infusion system, and blood products. Check the availability of blood products. Do not use autotransfusion in the presence of gastric or stool spillage into the abdominal cavity. When infusing blood products and fluids, use blood and fluid warmers, which will help maintain the patient's core body temperature.

Work closely with the anesthesia provider to estimate the blood loss and to anticipate the volume replacement needs of the trauma patient. Depending on the situation, measure the fluid volume in the suction canister in relation to irrigation used on the operative field. Also, account for the fluid volume in the autotransfusion reservoir that can be reinfused to the patient. Other methods of accounting for blood loss include the weighing of sponges, and estimating blood loss on the drapes and on the floor. The most accurate means of determining blood loss is a serial hematocrit and hemoglobin assay; not all facilities, however, have the means of performing these diagnostic studies.

Temperature Regulation

Maintaining optimal body temperature in the trauma patient presents the same challenge as maintaining fluid volume. Trauma patients are especially prone to hypothermia secondary to the use of resuscitative fluids and blood products. In addition, environmental factors at the scene of the incident, such as motor vehicle crashes in subzero weather, increase the potential for hypothermia. In response to these variables, increase the room temperature, apply a warming blanket to help restore and maintain normothermia, and warm irrigation fluids to decrease the risk of lowering the body temperature when irrigating wounds and body cavities.

Never overlook the potential for malignant hyperthermia in the trauma population. These patients present unexpectedly and usually cannot disclose a family history of anesthesia complications. Suspect malignant hypothermia in any trauma patient presenting with an unexplained increasing temperature.

Anesthesia Considerations

During induction of anesthesia, remain alert for possible cardiovascular and respiratory complications in the trauma patient. Premorbid medical conditions such as hypotension and medications may or may not be known. Patients with increased intracranial pressure are especially prone to hypertension during induction. In addition, the trauma population frequently has consumed alcohol and/or recreational drugs such as cocaine. The patient with a history of recreational drug use may require much larger doses of anesthetic agents than other patients. Patients who recently ingested cocaine are prone to serious tachycardia. Unlike patients prepared and scheduled for elective procedures, consider all trauma patients to have a full stomach. Peristalsis decreases or stops at the time of the traumatic incident. These patients are more prone to aspiration of gastric contents during the induction phase of anesthesia than is a fasting scheduled patient.

Rapid sequence induction is the preferred method when inducing trauma patients. This method decreases the risk of aspiration. During induction, assist the anesthesia provider by applying cricoid pressure to occlude the esophagus. Trauma patients presenting with hypovolemia because of severe blood loss are more prone to severe hypotensive crisis during the induction phase. Continuous monitoring of the patient by the anesthesia provider and nurse is vital to detecting and averting complications. Trauma rooms should have a crash cart with defibrillator and internal cardiac defibrillation paddles. Emergency medications may be stored in other appropriate areas of the operative and invasive procedure suite.

MEDICAL LEGAL AND ETHICAL ISSUES
Medical Legal Issues

The nurse plays a significant role in the preservation of the chain of evidence. Facility policy and procedure for the preservation of evidence should be developed in consultation and collaboration with local law enforcement officials. All types of gunshot wounds are subject to legal investigation. Protecting and preserving the evidence and its admissibility in a court of law should be a priority for any clothing or foreign objects removed in the operative and invasive procedure suite.

In general, do not cut off the patient's clothing by way of the hole created by stabbing or gunshot wounds. Remove each piece of clothing separately, place the items in plain brown paper bags, and label the bags with the patient's identifying information. Avoid placing wet and bloodstained clothing in plastic containers. Closed containers promote mold and bacterial growth, which can distort the evidence. To protect potential evidence, assess clothing and the skin for any sign of injury. If possible, take photographs of the wound. When taking photographs, place a scale, such as a ruler, in the scene being photographed. In addition, write a detailed description of the injury in the nursing notes. Do not label wounds as entrance or exit wounds. Preserve foreign matter on the skin according to guidelines developed in conjunction with the local police jurisdiction. When possible, preserve the initial appearance of the wound by not removing debris or cleansing the wound until evidence has been obtained or documented. Do not allow distortion of the wound such as inserting a chest tube through a wound or incising through it. Bullets and bullet fragments have microscopic striations that can be matched to the gun barrel that fired them. Therefore, to preserve the quality of evidence, do not use toothed or metallic instruments to handle evidence. These types of instruments can alter or change the appearance of the bullet. Place each bullet or foreign body in plain gauze and transfer into specimen cups labeled with the patient's identifying information. Maintain the chain of evidence by keeping the removed objects under surveillance until released to a local law enforcement official. Include a complete description of the appearance, retrieval, handling, and disposition of evidence in the nursing notes. Preserving the chain of evidence without altering the findings is a very important part of providing care to trauma patients who are victims of battery. Thorough and complete documentation can avert the nurse being called into court at a later date. Most law enforcement organizations provide the information (eg, phone number) needed to contact them to retrieve the evidence (Dufresne, 1995b).

Ethical Issues

The ethical issues encountered in trauma care vary. Whereas some patients present as victims, others may present as the perpetrator of violence. According to the AORN "Expectations for Perioperative Nursing," the nurse provides services with respect for human dignity and the uniqueness of the client, "unrestricted by considerations of social or economic status, personal attributes, or the nature of health problems" (AORN, 2008, p. 634).

Because of the nature and uniqueness of the demands of providing care to trauma patients, it helps to have in place a debriefing protocol as well as a nursing ethics committee to address the multiple needs of the nursing staff. Death in the operative and invasive procedure suite is a common occurrence for the nurse providing trauma care. Use of a preventive ethics approach in the development of policies and procedures can avert the multiple dilemmas that may occur in providing care to the trauma population. Facilities' policies and procedures must avert the dilemma of obtaining informed consent emergently when the trauma patient is compromised or unconscious. Also, policies that guide recognizing living wills, advanced directives, power of attorney, and the special self-determination of Jehovah's Witnesses must be in place and must incorporate the state and federal laws concerning these issues. The trauma staff must be knowledgeable of specific facility policies to effectively act as the patient's moral agent (eg, patient advocate) within the agency of permanence. As an employee of the facility, the nurse is obligated to uphold and comply with the facility's policies. This can conflict with the individual personal and religious values as a moral agent for the patient.

The allocation of resources is another dilemma when providing care to the trauma patient population. Trauma care is a very expensive use of critical care technology. Technology has advanced healthcare to a state in which almost any human can be sustained on life support. The critically injured may require massive volumes of blood products to sustain life, depleting blood bank supplies of a scarce commodity. The question of when is "enough" remains unanswered. All too frequently trauma patients are underinsured or uninsured, with the cost of care being covered in some cases by state or federal agencies and taken as a loss in other cases. The cost of providing trauma care has forced many trauma centers to close because providing trauma care is not cost effective and rarely is a return on the investment gained. Yet, as healthcare professionals are we not obligated to provide care to all who need our services?

CONCLUSION

The goals of trauma care are to prevent early death and provide definitive intervention to preserve life and function. The nurse as a trauma team member is responsible for coordinating the operative experience with these goals in mind. Failure to maintain an adequate airway and ventilation or fluid, electrolyte, and acid-base balances can have disastrous results after the procedure. Improper positioning can result in nerve and muscle damage that may be irreversible. The nurse participating in the continuum of trauma care maintains the role of patient advocate during the operative experience. A skillfully choreographed operative experience helps to reduce the risk of complications during the operative procedure and enhance the recovery process.

ENDNOTE

1. Energy which results from an object (eg, the patient) being in motion (speed).

REFERENCES

1. American College of Surgeons (ACS) Committee on Trauma. (2006). *Resources for Optimal Care of the Injured Patient*. Chicago, IL: American College of Surgeons.
2. Arroyo, J.S., & Crosby, L.A. (1995). Basic rescue and resuscitation. *Clinical Orthopaedics and Related Research;* 318, pp. 11–16.
3. AORN (2008). AORN explications for perioperative nursing. *Perioperative Standards and Recommended Practices*. Denver, CO: AORN, Inc., pp. 633–660.
4. Beachley, M. (2009). Evolution of the trauma cycle. In McQuillian, K.A., Makic, M.B.F., & Whalen, E. (Eds.) *Trauma Nursing: From Resuscitation Through Rehabilitation*, 4th ed. St. Louis, MO: Saunders Elsevier, pp. 2–18.
5. Califano, J.A. (1994). *Radical Surgery: What's Next for America's Health Care*. New York, NY: Random House, Inc., pp. 66–69.
6. Cowley, R.A., & Dunham, C.M. (1982). *Shock Trauma/Critical Care Manual*. Baltimore, MD: University Park Press, pp. 35–42.
7. Dufresne, G.W. (1995a). Wound ballistics: Recognizing wound potential. Part I: Characteristics of missiles and weapons. *International Journal of Trauma Nursing*, 1(1), pp. 4–10.

8. Dufresne, G.W. (I995b). Wound ballistics: Recognizing wound potential. Part II: Gunshot wounds—tissue response and nursing care. *International Journal of Trauma Nursing*, 1(2), pp. 37–40.

9. Foss, J., & Feistritzer, N. (1993). Perioperative care of the trauma patient. *Trauma Nursing: The Art and Science*; St. Louis, MO: C.V. Mosby, pp. 657–675.

10. Fowler, C.J. (2009). Injury prevention. In McQuillian, K.A., Makic, M.B.F., & Whalen, E. (Eds), *Trauma Nursing: From Resuscitation Through Rehabilitation*, 4th ed. St. Louis, MO: Saunders Elsevier, pp. 67–90.

11. Kidd, P.S. (1993). Assessment of the trauma patient. *Trauma Nursing: The Art and Science*; St. Louis, MO: C.V. Mosby, pp. 115–142.

12. King, C.A. (1994). Coordination and collaboration of violent trauma care. *Seminars in Perioperative Nursing*, 3(4), pp. 175–184.

13. Martinez, R.J. (2009). Psychosocial impact of trauma. In McQuillian, K.A., Makic, M.B.F., & Whalen, E. (Eds), *Trauma Nursing: From Resuscitation Through Rehabilitation*, 4th ed. St. Louis, MO: Saunders Elsevier, pp. 422–446.

14. MedicineNet. (2008). Definition of trauma. Retrieved July 31, 2008 from http://www.medterms.com/script/main/art.asp?articlekey=8171.

15. Moloney-Harmon, P.A. (2009). Pediatric trauma. In McQuillian, K.A., Makic, M.B.F., & Whalen, E. (Eds), *Trauma Nursing: From Resuscitation Through Rehabilitation*, 4th ed. St. Louis, MO: Saunders Elsevier, pp. 810–834.

16. Petersen, C. (2007). *Perioperative Nursing Data Set*, revised 2nd ed. Denver, CO; AORN. In McQuillian, K.A., Makic, M.B.F., & Whalen, E. (Eds), Inc.: pp. 17–116.

17. Smith, L.G. (2009). The pregnant trauma patient. In McQuillian, K.A., Makic, M.B.F., & Whalen, E. (Eds), *Trauma Nursing: From Resuscitation Through Rehabilitation*, 4th ed. St. Louis, MO: Saunders Elsevier: pp. 780–809.

18. Weigelt, J., Brasel, K.J., and Klein, J. (2009). Mechanisms of injury. In McQuillian, K.A., Makic, M.B.F., & Whalen, E. (Eds), *Trauma Nursing: From Resuscitation Through Rehabilitation*, 4th ed. St. Louis, MO: Saunders Elsevier, pp. 178–199.

19. Whalen, E. (2009). Economic and administrative issues in trauma care. In McQuillian, K.A., Makic, M.B.F., & Whalen, E. (Eds.), *Trauma Nursing: From Resuscitation Through Rehabilitation*, 4th ed. St. Louis, MO: Saunders Elsevier, pp. 19–28.

CHAPTER 33

Cardiac Catheterization and Electrophysiology

Russell Todd

Mark Phippen

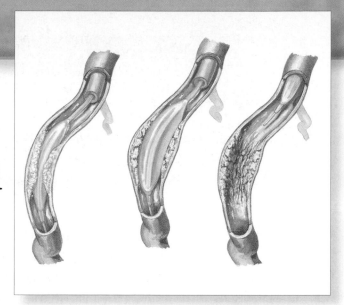

INTRODUCTION

Worldwide, 16.7 million people die of cardiovascular diseases each year. In 2001, cardiovascular disease (CVD) contributed to virtually one-third of worldwide deaths. By 2010, CVD will lead as the cause of death in developing countries. By 2020, CVD will cause nearly 25 million deaths worldwide. Globally, approximately 32 million myocardial infarctions and cardiovascular accidents occur each year, resulting in approximately 12.5 million deaths per year. Clearly, cardiovascular disease has no geographic, gender, socioeconomic, or political boundaries (American Heart Association, 2004). This chapter provides an overview of cardiac catheterization and electrophysiology.[1]

Cardiac Catheterization

Many of the deaths from myocardial infarction occur because of blocked coronary arteries secondary to atherosclerosis. Traditionally, the preferred treatment option was Coronary Artery Bypass Graft (CABG) surgery. Now technological advances, such as drug eluting stents (DES) and intravascular catheters, have created less invasive options for patients and growth for hospitals and specialists in cardiology. In 1990, surgeons and cardiologists[2] performed approximately an equal number of coronary artery bypass graft (CABG) and percutaneous coronary interventions (PCI). Today the number of operative interventions has decreased and the number of percutaneous coronary interventions has increased (**Table 33.1**).

Chapter Contents

CVD
Cardiovascular Disease

CABG
Coronary Artery Bypass Graft

DES
Drug Eluting Stents

PCI
Percutaneous Coronary Interventions

Table 33.1	2005 US Cardiac Procedures		
	Number of Procedures	**% Men**	**% Women**
Angioplasty[†]	1,271,000	874,000	397,000
Cardiac Revascularization (CABG)	469,000	325,000	145,000

[†] 1,265,000 angioplasties were percutaneous coronary interventions. American Heart Association, 2008.

Electrophysiology

Coronary atherosclerosis or other disease processes can damage heart muscle, leading to impaired cardiac electrical activity, which can result in sudden death. For these at-risk patients, electrophysiology provides a potentially lifesaving alternative. Electrophysiology tests map the exact location of the aberrant intracardiac electrical signals and provide treatment options for the patient when the standard ECG, Holter monitor, event recorder, stress test, echocardiogram, or angiogram ordered by the cardiologist cannot provide enough information to evaluate the arrhythmia. During an electrophysiology test, a physician electrophysiologist, with advanced training in the diagnosis and treatment of arrhythmias, determines the exact location of an arrhythmia, and often corrects it during the same procedure. Intervention offers a permanent cure and, in many cases, eliminates the need for heart medications (*Encyclopedia of Surgery*, 2007).

CARDIAC CATHETERIZATION

From the inception of this technology it has changed from a basic diagnostic procedure used to visualize the coronary anatomy into a dynamic care modality providing palliative care for patients with atherosclerotic coronary lesions. As technology progressed, the most dramatic changes happened in the last thirty years. In the 1970s the images were being captured on 35 mm cine radiographic film, and today imaging technology has leaped forward with digital imaging video loops and data being stored on a computer server. In the past, physicians could only view these images with special 35 mm film projectors. Now caregivers can view the images at a computer desktop display. In addition, physicians can remotely view images throughout an organization or at their office. Along with imaging, catheter technology leapfrogged with the development of angioplasty balloons and stent development. Advances in pharmacology and the development of drugs have improved outcomes and patient survival. Cardiac catheterization as a minimally invasive procedure will continue to forge a new frontier in cardiac care.

The Cardiac Catheterization Team

At the forefront of changing cardiac practice are minimally invasive interventions performed by cardiologists. The cardiac catheterization team consists of cardiologists, cardiovascular technology professionals[3], radiology technologists, and registered nurses[4]. These multidisciplinary teams provide care to patients with an emphasis on patient safety and quality outcomes. Registered nurses have led the way in helping create an environment that supports best practice, which has allowed for collaboration of all these professionals. In many instances nurses were the only professionals available to fill the gap until specialized professionals could be trained. Anesthesia professionals provide care for patients who require monitored anesthesia care, such as pediatric patients. Cardiothoracic surgeons collaborate with the cardiac catheterization team to provide care for patients requiring operative interventions.

The cardiac catheterization team should have a clear understanding of recommended practice standards for cardiac catheterization promulgated by the American Heart Association, American College of Cardiology, Society for Cardiac Angiography Intervention, and the Society for Cardiac Invasive Professionals. Skill, judgment, and knowledge of new and innovative technologies are critical for success in the modern cardiac catheterization laboratory.

History of Cardiac Catheterization

The history of cardiac catheterization has a long, innovative history beginning in 1733 with Stephen Hale. Using animal subjects and then progressing to human studies, physicians invented catheterization devices and developed techniques that have resulted in the cardiac catheterization seen today. Werner Forssman is usually credited with performing the first cardiac catheterization of a living person—himself. He was awarded the Nobel Prize, with Andre Cournand and Dickinson Richards, in 1956 (Biam, 2006).

The last 35 years have seen extensive developments which have changed cardiac catheterization from a diagnostic test to an interventional care modality, allowing the cardiologist the ability to offer minimally invasive alternatives to patients versus surgical alternatives. **Table 33.2** highlights the progress of cardiac catheterization during the past 200 years. Significant contributions by Judkins, Sones, and Gruntzig have changed the way medical care is provided by physicians. These technological developments have forged a new patient care dynamic for clinicians.

Indications

Physicians use cardiac catheterization to confirm the presence of a clinically suspected condition, define anatomic and physiologic severity, and determine the presence or absence of associated conditions. The most common indication for cardiac catheterization today is the patient with acute coronary ischemic syndrome. The goal is to identify the culprit lesions and restore vessel patency via PCI (Biam, 2006). There has been great emphasis in recent years focusing on the ST segment MI (STEMI) and Non ST segment MI (Non-STEMI) patients. National patient safety goals and Medicare guidelines have forced providers to target goals for restoring blood flow to ischemic myocardium in less than 90 minutes. Measurement of this goal starts from the time the patient enters through the Emergency Room doors to the time of the first inflation of the PTCA balloon. This benchmark data has become standard practice for facilities offering percutaneous coronary interventions (PCI). Cardiac catheterization teams will be pushing the envelope to achieve shorter and shorter door to balloon times with the goal of improving patient outcomes. Faster times to reperfusion and better systems of care are associated with reductions in morbidity and mortality rates (Bates, 2008). Further listings of clinical indications can be located at the American College of Cardiology and American Heart Association published Guidelines at each organization's website.

STEMI
ST Segment MI

Non-STEMI
Non ST Segment MI

Table 33.2	History of Cardiac Catheterization	
1733	Stephen Hale	Using animal subjects, investigated cardiac catheterization with its underlying measurements of vascular and intracardiac pressures
1844	Claude Bernard	Using animal subjects, successfully catheterized the right and left ventricles in a retrograde manner from the jugular vein and carotid arteries
1870	Adolph Fick	Famous, but brief note on the calculation of blood flow provides the basis for today's procedures
1912	Fritz Bleichroeder, E. Unger, and W. Loeb	Published descriptions of human catheterization; among the first to insert catheters into the blood vessels without x-ray visualization
1929	Werner Forsmann	Using a cadaver, guided a urological catheter from an arm vein into the right atrium; dissected the veins of his own forearm and guided a urological catheter into his right atrium using fluoroscopic control and a mirror; with the catheter in place, walked to the x-ray room with no ill effects to have his chest x-rayed; first to document right heart catheterization in humans using radiographic techniques
1940s	Andre Cournand, Hilmer Ranges, and Dickinson Rickards	Began using right heart catheterization on a regular basis in the undertaking of a comprehensive investigation of cardiac function in both normal and diseased patients
1947	H. A. Zimmerman	Developed a completely intravascular technique for human left heart catheterization; with associates, performed a simultaneous catheterization of both right and left heart; credited with the development of combined cardiac catheterization
1953	Sven-Ivar Seldinger	Developed a percutaneous femoral approach with guide wires
1958	Mason Sones	Performed first selective coronary arteriography
1964	Charles Dotter and Mel Judkins	Conceived and reported Percutaneous Transluminal Coronary Angioplasty (PTCA)
1974	Andreas Gruentzig	Invented the first experimental PTCA balloon
1970	Jeremy Swan and William Ganz	Made it possible to do cardiac catheterizations outside a conventional cardiac catheterization laboratory; credited with the balloon flotation catheter, which is widely used today in modern healthcare
1979	Andreas Gruentzig	Successfully used balloon angioplasty catheters with transluminal angioplasty techniques

Adapted from Cohn, L. H. (2008). *Cardiac Surgery in the Adult,* 3rd ed. McGraw Hill Professional, Dubuque, IA; Virtual Cardiac Cath Lab (1996), The History of Cardiac Catheterization, http://user.gru.net/clawrence/vccl/intro/hist2.htm. Accessed 13 August 2008.

Contraindications and Complications

Contraindications directly correlate to the overall physiologic condition of the patient. With the exception of patient refusal, cardiac catheterization has no absolute contraindications. **Table 33.3** lists potential risk factors that assist in determining patient suitability for cardiac catheterization.

Percutaneous cardiac interventions have a low complication rate (AHA, 2008). On occasion, however, complications do occur. **Table 33.4** lists these potential complications. In addition, while the risk is small, the literature reports risks such as

Table 33.3	Potential Risk Factors for Cardiac Catheterization

- ☐ Active gastrointestinal bleeding
- ☐ Acute stroke
- ☐ Allergy to radiographic contrast
- ☐ Electrolyte abnormalities
- ☐ Hematologic issues
- ☐ History of congestive heart failure
- ☐ Increased age
- ☐ Infection of any type
- ☐ Peripheral artery disease
- ☐ Presence of multi-vessel coronary artery disease
- ☐ Severe anemia
- ☐ Severe coagulopathy
- ☐ Severe electrolyte imbalance
- ☐ Severe uncontrolled hypertension
- ☐ Uncompensated congestive failure
- ☐ Unexplained febrile illness/or an active untreated infection
- ☐ Unsubstantiated fever
- ☐ Ventricular arrhythmias

Table 33.4	Potential Cardiac Catheterization Complications

- ☐ Air embolus
- ☐ Allergic reaction to the radiographic dye
- ☐ Aneurysm
- ☐ Arrhythmias
- ☐ Arterial occlusion
- ☐ Fistula
- ☐ Hematoma
- ☐ Hemorrhage
- ☐ Myocardial infarction
- ☐ Neuropathy
- ☐ Pseudo-aneurysm
- ☐ Retro peritoneal bleed
- ☐ Stroke
- ☐ Tamponade
- ☐ Vasovagal responses

Cohn, L. H. (2008). *Cardiac Surgery in the Adult,* 3rd ed. McGraw Hill Professional, Dubuque, IA.

33

Table 33.5	Required Monitoring Equipment for Cardiac Catheterization Procedures

- ☐ Defibrillator
- ☐ Integrated cardiac monitor with the following capabilities
  - • Hemodynamic measurement with the ability to provide full disclosure
  - • Oxygen saturation measurement
  - • Noninvasive blood pressure measurement
- ☐ Capnography monitor if the patient is intubated or ventilated
- ☐ Emergency cart with appropriate equipment, IV catheters, solutions, and medications

peripheral nerve injury, infection, pulmonary edema, and ventricular fibrillation as potential complications (Cohn, 2008).

Equipment and Supplies

Table 33.5 lists the required monitoring equipment for cardiac catheterization procedures. Disposable supplies for cardiac catheterization include a double-fenestrated patient drape, which is designed to cover the entire length of the procedural table, introducer sheaths, catheters of varying diameters, guide wires, needles of varying gauge and length, syringes, medication labels, skin marker, medicine cups, towels, towel clamps, basins, 4 × 4-inch sponges mosquito hemostat forceps, band-bags (for covering x-ray equipment and shields), surgical gowns, color-coded medication labels, No. 11 scalpel, and stopcocks. Many facilities will use prepared, custom, disposable procedural trays to facilitate setup, reduce costs, and manage inventory (AliMed, 2008; Arshad, 2006).

The cardiologist may use a Swan-Ganz flow-directed catheter to measure right heart pressures, collect blood to assess cardiac oxygen saturation, and to determine cardiac output. Right heart catheterizations with the use of flow-directed catheters that are capable of obtaining thermal dilution cardiac outputs, oximetry, and temporary pacing capabilities has evolved over the last thirty years. This treatment modality is now a vital component of the intensive care setting and provides physicians and clinicians with vital data about the patient's condition. This technology allows the nurse to provide quality, state–of-the-art care.

The cardiologist chooses a particular catheter based on vascular and cardiac anatomy, the need to opacify the coronary arteries and cardiac chambers, the degree of expected catheter manipulation during the procedure, and the chosen access site. Larger-diameter (8 French) catheters allow for greater manipulation of the catheter and facilitate visualization, but have a greater risk for trauma. Smaller-diameter catheters (4–6 French) reduce the risk of trauma. The cardiologist will use a vascular access sheath, which facilitates arterial and venous access and multiple catheter exchanges. To reduce the chance for vascular trauma, the cardiologist will advance all catheters and sheaths over a guidewire under fluoroscopy. Frequently the cardiologist uses a 150-cm, 0.035-in J-tipped guidewire for this purpose (Arshad, 2006). The equipment used by each healthcare facility will be guided by the physician's training and experience, the organization's financial contracting arrangements, and availability of the technology.

Lower Extremity Access

The access site used in the lower extremity is the common femoral artery. Access through this site requires the use of separate preformed catheters, one for the right, and one for the left coronary arteries. The cardiologist will frequently use a pigtail catheter to measure left heart pressures and perform a left ventriculogram. In order to avoid vascular complications, the cardiologist must carefully access the common femoral artery. A puncture made above the inguinal ligament or below the bifurcation of the femoral artery can increase the patient's risk for complications. Using the common femoral artery is easier than using other access sites. Another advantage is the significant safety record associated with the technique. In the past, the need for an extended time (2–6 hours) of bedrest following the procedure was the main disadvantage of using the common femoral artery for access. However, recent innovations in arterial closure devices have shortened the period of bedrest (Arshad, 2006). **Figure 33.1** shows common access sites for cardiac catheterization.

Upper Extremity Access

If the patient has significant iliac or femoral artery atherosclerosis, prior bypass grafting of these vessels, or severe obesity, the cardiologist may choose to gain arterial access from the upper extremity rather than the common femoral artery. Using

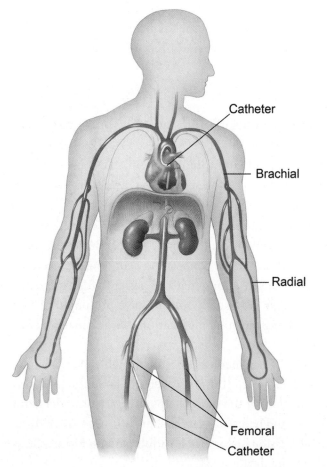

Figure 33.1

Common access sites for cardiac catheterization.

Catheter

Brachial

Radial

Femoral

Catheter

the brachial artery, the physician will insert and maneuver the catheters through the brachial artery, into the axillary and subclavian arteries, and then into the ascending aorta. Alternative access sites include the axillary artery or radial artery. Access through the axillary artery reduces the patient's risk for median nerve damage and enables the physician to compress the artery against the humerus to obtain hemostasis. Radial artery access has gained popularity with cardiologists. However, prior to accessing the radial artery, the cardiologist will perform an Allen test to verify continuity of the arterial arch in the hand; an important consideration should the radial artery occlude during or after the procedure. Radial approach reduces the patient's risk of serious vascular complications. In addition, this approach facilitates earlier ambulation. However, on occasion, the patient may experience arterial spasm when the physician uses this approach. The spasm can potentially interfere with manipulation of the catheter (Arshad, 2006).

Additional Access Sites

Although rare, atherosclerosis may affect both the upper and lower extremities, thus making it extremely difficult to access the preferred vascular access sites. In these cases, access to the descending aorta via a translumbar approach provides an alternative approach. If the patient requires catheterization of the left atrium and left ventricle, the cardiologist can use a transseptal approach. After puncturing the intra-atrial septum with a needle, the cardiologist will insert the catheter, and then advance it to the target areas. Patients with mechanical aortic valves or in need of having a true left arterial pressure taken are candidates for transseptal catheterization. For patients with aortic and mitral mechanical valves who require ventricular hemodynamic studies, the only option is a direct left ventricular puncture (Arshad, 2006).

Patient Preparation

Even though the majority of cardiac catheterizations are done on an outpatient basis, before the procedure the cardiologist obtains a complete history, does a physical examination, orders a complete blood count, blood chemistries, chest radiograph, and ECG. The cardiologist also obtains informed consent according to facility policy and procedure.

The nurse ensures that the patient receives appropriate medical education and counseling. Educational information should include what to expect during the procedure, the length of the procedure, information concerning sedation, intravenous (IV) insertion, and a description of the sensations that the patient will experience during and after the procedure. Patients are usually told to have nothing to eat or drink after 12 midnight, except for taking morning medications with a small amount of water, as directed by the physician.

During the assessment, determine what medications the patient takes. Include aspirin in this list because it affects blood clotting. Answer the patient's questions and clarify issues. Clear communication by the nurse helps the patient understand what to expect during the procedure and helps alleviate anxiety. **Figures 33.2 A, B, C, and D** show an example of an admission history for an adult patient. **Figure 33.3** shows an example of a preadmission medication list.

IV
Intravenous

Figure 33.2 A

Adult patient admission history.

Source: Inova Health System

I. Patient Information
Time of Admission: _____ Admitted from: _____
Chief Complaint/Associated Symptoms: _____

Ht. _____ Wt. _____ lb/kg ☐ Standing Scale ☐ Bed Scale ☐ Stated
Temp _____ Pulse _____ Resp _____ BP _____ Patient Identification Band on? ☐ Yes ☐ No
Emergency Contact: _____ PMD: _____

II. Allergies ☐ Latex Sensitivity ☐ No Known Allergies
If yes, Allergy Band on: ☐ Yes ☐ No Chart Labeled: ☐ Yes ☐ No Entered into Computer ☐ Yes ☐ No
Food/Drug/Substance **Type of Reaction**
_____ _____
_____ _____
_____ _____

III. Medications ☐ See attachment
Medications you are now taking, including: Non-Prescription, Aspirin, Birth Control Pills/Vitamins/Supplements/Herbal Remedies:
Drug/Dosage/Route **Last Dose**
_____ _____
_____ _____
_____ _____
_____ _____
_____ _____
_____ _____
_____ _____
_____ _____

Personal Medications: ☐ None ☐ Sent Home ☐ Inpatient Pharmacy ☐ Bedside

IV. Pain Assessment: ☐ Unable to obtain pain history due to patient condition.
Do you have any ongoing pain problems? ☐ Yes* ☐ No If yes, where _____
Do you have pain now? ☐ Yes* ☐ No If yes, where _____
*If yes to either of the above describe your pain: ☐ aching ☐ burning ☐ cramping ☐ crushing ☐ dull ☐ pounding ☐ sharp
☐ shooting ☐ sore ☐ stabbing ☐ tender ☐ tingling ☐ throbbing ☐ other_____
How often do you have pain (frequency)?_____
How long does the pain last (duration)? ☐ Continuous ☐ Intermittent ☐ With Movement
How long have you had this pain?_____
Using one of the following scales, indicate your present level of pain: now _____ at worst _____ at best _____
What level of pain is acceptable to you? _____
LEVEL OF PAIN

0   1   2   3   4   5   6   7   8   9   10
No   Hurts   Hurts   Hurts   Hurts   Hurts
Hurt   Little Bit   Little More Even More   Whole Lot   Worst

0   2   4   6   8   10

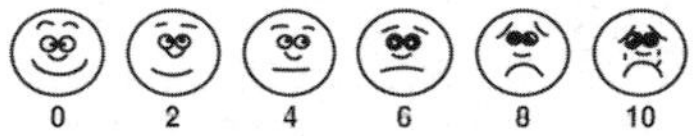

What causes or increases your pain? _____
What, if any, treatment(s) do you receive for your pain? _____
Is the treatment effective? ☐ Yes ☐ No Are the pain medications effective? ☐ Yes ☐ No
What impact does the pain have on your life and daily functioning? _____

V. Social Profile
Religious/Cultural Needs:_____ Primary Language Spoken: _____
Interpreter Needed? ☐ No ☐ Yes If Yes, specify: _____
Employed/Occupation: _____
Out of Country Recently? ☐ No ☐ Yes Where/When? _____

VI. Psychological Profile
Alcohol use: ☐ Yes ☐ No How much? _____ Last used: _____
Recreational drug use: ☐ Yes ☐ No Type & how much? _____ Last used: _____
Victim of violence/abuse: ☐ Yes* ☐ No ☐ Physical ☐ Verbal ☐ Emotional ☐ Mental
Are you thinking of taking your own life? ☐ Yes* (Contact attending MD) ☐ No
History of: ☐ Alcohol abuse ☐ Drug abuse ☐ Victim of violence abuse ☐ Suicide attempt
*If yes, referral to Social Work. ☐ Yes _____

PATIENT IDENTIFICATION

INOVA HEALTH SYSTEM
ADULT PATIENT ADMISSION HISTORY

Date: _____

Page 1 of 4

CAT # 81789 / R102904
PKGS OF 100   **MR24-00**

Anesthesia

The patient will receive a local anesthetic to prevent pain during needle access of the artery or vein. Most individuals have no sensation while the physician advances or moves the catheters during the catheterization. In addition, the cardiologist will use moderate sedation/analgesia to promote patient comfort and minimize movement during the procedure.

Anticoagulation Therapy

Most diagnostic cardiac catheterizations require minimal heparinization of the flush solutions used to maintain patency of the catheters while they are in the body with no heparin dose systemically for the patient. In some instances because of heparin

---

VII. Advance Directives Screening:
Do you have a living will or any other document which expresses your wishes or authorizes another person to make treatment decisions in the event you are unable to do so? (A two-part document in which the patient gives instructions about his or her health care and/or identifies a designated decision maker when the patient cannot speak for him or herself.)

☐ **YES** ☐ Copy of Advance Directive on chart **OR**
   ☐ If no copy *immediately* available, ask patient to provide a copy.

☐ **NO** **Would the patient like more information on Advance Directives:** ☐ Yes ☐ No
   If yes, ☐ Booklet given

☐ **PATIENT UNABLE TO RESPOND**
   ☐ Family member contacted: _____ Date: _____ Initials: _____
   ☐ Patient has Advance Directive per family ☐ Family member above will bring Advance Directive to hospital
   Comment: _____
   If no Next of Kin available, social work consult ordered in computer - Date: _____ **Initials:** _____

   Are you an organ donor? ☐ Yes ☐ No ☐ Request info ☐ Information Given

VIII. Nutritional Screening
   Check box for all that apply:
   ☐ **UNINTENTIONAL** weight loss > 10 lbs. past month
   ☐ Tube Feeding/TPN at home
   ☐ Fistula/Pressure Ulcer stage 3 or >
   ☐ Pregnant/Lactating woman (on med/surg unit)
   ☐ Nonelective surgical admit > 80 years
   ☐ Unable to take food 5 days prior to admission
   ☐ Unable to chew or swallow
   If any criteria checked, order nutrition consult in computer. Date: _____ Initials: _____

   ☐ Check box if no criteria apply; no consult required.
   Food Intolerances: _____ (Enter by CLN command)

IX. Functional Screening (not required for rehab or joint replacement patients, as therapy orders are part of routine admission orders)
   Yes ☐ NA
   ☐ The patient has *new onset* decreased ability to move in bed, get out of bed, stand up, or walk and is likely to improve with Physical Therapy intervention.
   ☐ The patient has *new onset* decreased ability to perform activities of daily living (ADL's) and is likely to improve with Occupational Therapy intervention.
   ☐ The patient has *new onset* of decreased ability to swallow, as indicated by history of aspiration pneumonia, coughing, or drooling and is likely to improve with Speech Therapy intervention.
   ☐ The patient has *new onset* of decreased ability to communicate secondary to neurological disorder, tracheostomy, and/or laryngectomy and is likely to improve with Speech Therapy intervention.
   If any criteria checked, obtain PT/OT or Speech Therapy consult order.

X. Falls Screening (check all that apply & implement Adult Fall Interventions for any box checked)

	Points		Points		Points
☐ History of Falls	(15)	☐ Urgency/Incontinence	(15)	☐ Age (older than 70 years)	(5)
☐ Confusion	(15)	☐ Dizziness/Postural Hypotension	(15)	☐ Mobility/Unable to ambulate	(5)
☐ ↑ anxiety/emotional liability	(5)	☐ Sensory deficit	(5)	independently	
☐ ↓ level of cooperation	(5)	☐ Cardiovascular or Respiratory disease	(5)	☐ Medications affecting blood pressure or	(5)
☐ Impaired judgement	(5)	affecting perfusion & oxygenation		level of consciousness	

   Score Total _____ 15 or more points = High Risk Identification.

XI. Discharge Planning Do you have someone to assist you after discharge? ☐ No ☐ Yes
   Do you have medical equipment at home/Specify: _____
   Patient/Family Living Situation: ☐ Home Independent ☐ Home/Family Care ☐ Home/Healthcare ☐ Mental Health Inst
   ☐ Retirement Community ☐ Assisted Living ☐ Skilled Nsg Fac Name of Fac. _____ ☐ Other: _____
   Social Resources: ☐ None ☐ Unknown ☐ Spouse/Partner ☐ Parent(s) ☐ Child(ren) ☐ Other Family
   ☐ Home Health ☐ Substitute Decision Maker ☐ Mental Health Service(s) ☐ Dept. of Family Services ☐ Outpatient Health Clinic
   ☐ Other: _____ Comments: _____
   What complimentary therapies do you use? ☐ none ☐ chiropractor ☐ acupuncture ☐ aromatherapy ☐ other _____

PATIENT IDENTIFICATION

INOVA HEALTH SYSTEM
ADULT PATIENT ADMISSION HISTORY

Date: _____

Page 2 of 4

CAT # 81789 / R102904
PKGS OF 100 **MR24-00**

Figure 33.2 B

Adult patient admission history.

Source: Inova Health System

HIT
Heparin Induced Thrombocytopenia

induced thrombocytopenia (HIT) syndrome, the physician may choose not to use anticoagulation, or may select an alternative anticoagulant such as Argatroban.

Cardiac catheterization in the upper extremities requires anticoagulation therapy because of the smaller arteries and the occlusive nature of the catheters. Usually the agent chosen is unfractionated heparin. Many cardiologists will also use anticoagulation therapy when accessing via the femoral artery, particularly when anticipating a long procedure with several catheter exchanges (Arshad, 2006).

Anticoagulation for the most part is now used primarily for interventional procedures. Each facility will have various protocols for anticoagulant usage. Whether the anticoagulant is unfractionated heparin or Angiomax (Bivalirudin), patient safety remains the primary concern when using these medications. Precautions should be

XII. Have you ever had, or do you have any of the following? *Check only if applicable.*

ANESTHESIA HISTORY ❑ NA	YES	If Yes, Describe
Received Anesthesia		
Anesthesia Problems		
Relatives w/anes. problems		

Previous Operations/Hospitalizations

Date		Reason

CARDIOVASCULAR ❑ NA	YES	If Yes, Describe
Chest Pain/Angina		
Congestive Heart Failure		
Phlebitis/Deep Vein Thrombosis/(Blood Clot in leg)		
Edema/Swelling		
Hypertension/High BP		
Heart Attack (MI)		
Murmur/Mitral Valve Prolapse		
Peripheral Vascular Disease		
Pacemaker/Defibrillator		

RESPIRATORY ❑ NA	YES	If Yes, Describe
Asthma, Bronchitis, COPD Emphysema, Pneumonia		
Fatigue, Night Sweats, Tuberculosis		
Sore Throat, Cough, Cold in last 2 weeks?	Duration?	
Tobacco Use	Pk/Day: # of Yrs.	
Stopped Tobacco Use:	When:	
Smoking Cessation Counseling given		
Oxygen Therapy, Recant Sputum Changes		

PATIENT IDENTIFICATION

NEUROLOGICAL ❑ NA	YES	If Yes, Describe
Alzheimer's/Dementia		
Seizures		
Mental Status Changes		
Migraines, Headaches, Head Injury		
Neuromuscular Disease		
Neurovascular Disease		
Sleep Disturbances		
Stroke/TIA		
Syncope/Fainting		

VASCULAR ACCESS ❑ NA	YES	If Yes, Describe
AV fistula, Hickman, Mediport, Groshong, PICC...		

ENDOCRINE/METABOLIC ❑ NA	YES	If Yes, Describe
Diabetes/Hypoglycemia		
Pituitary/Adrenal Disease		
Thyroid Disease		

GASTROINTESTINAL ❑ NA	YES	If Yes, Describe
Change in Bowel Routine		
Colitis/Diverticulitis		
Constipation/Diarrhea		
Gallbladder Disease		
GI Bleed		
Hemorrhoids		
Hiatal Hernia/Reflux		
Liver Disease/Hepatitis		
Nausea/Vomiting		
Ostomy		
Pancreatitis		
Ulcer Disease		

INOVA HEALTH SYSTEM
ADULT PATIENT ADMISSION HISTORY

Date: _____

Page 3 of 4

CAT # 81789 / R102904
PKGS OF 100   **MR24-00**

Figure 33.2 C

Adult patient admission history.

Source: Inova Health System

taken to have appropriate dosages, which are titrated to the patient's body surface area, and glomerular filtration rate (GFR). Often in combination with the anticoagulants, physicians will order the administration of IIb/IIIa medications Integrilin (Eptifibatide) and ReoPro (Abciximab), and oral thrombin inhibitors like Plavix (Clopidogrel bisulfate). The altering of the patient's coagulation pathway increases the patient's risk for bleeding complications.

GFR
Glomerular Filtration Rate

Cardiac Catheterization Procedure
Basic Steps of the Procedure

Cardiac catheterization procedures can take from 30 minutes to several hours, depending on the treatment modality selected, with the average length being one

XII. *(continued)* **Have you ever had, or do you have any of the following?** *Check only if applicable.*

HEMATOLOGIC/ONCOLOGIC ❑ NA	YES	If Yes, Describe
Anemia/Sickle Cell		
Blood/Clotting Disorders		
Cancer/Tumors		
HIV Infection		
Past Blood Transfusions/ Antibodies _____		
Adverse Reactions Reaction _____		

PSYCHOLOGICAL ❑ NA	YES	If Yes, Describe
Anxiety/Panic Disorder		
Have you ever had a history of psychiatric or emotional problems?		

RENAL/GENITOURINARY ❑ NA	YES	If Yes, Describe
Blood in Urine		
Incontinence		
Kidney Disease/Dialysis		
Penile Discharge/Lesion		
Prostate Disease		
Sexually Transmitted Disease		
Stones/Obstruction		

Voiding Aids: ❑ Ostomy ❑ Self Cath ❑ Indwelling Cath

INTEGUMENTARY/SKIN ❑ NA	YES	If Yes, Describe
Pressure Ulcer/Leg Ulcer/ 3rd degree burn		
Eczema/Psoriasis		

MUSCULOSKELETAL ❑ NA	YES	If Yes, Describe
Arthritis/Joint Pain		
Joint Replacement/ Any Prosthetic Devices		
Assistive Devices		
Back/Neck Pain		
Fractures		
Unable to Weight Bear		

PATIENT IDENTIFICATION

DENTAL ❑ NA	YES	If Yes, Describe
Caps, Crowns, Chipped or Loose Teeth		
Dentures/Bridgework/Retainer		
Loose Teeth		

EYES/ENT ❑ NA	YES	If Yes, Describe
Hearing Deficits/Aids		
Nose Bleeds		
Sinus Disease		
Swallowing Difficulties		
Visual Deficit/Glasses/Contacts		
Glaucoma, Cataracts, Retinal Disease		

OBSTETRIC / GYN ❑ NA	YES	If Yes, Describe
Possibility of Pregnancy		L.M.P date:
# of Pregnances _____		
# of Live Births _____		
Menopause		
Breast Changes		
Mammogram		Date:
Pap Smear		Date:
Menstrual Problems		
Vaginal Discharge		

Reason unable to complete within the first 24 hours: _____
_____

Signature: _____

Date: _____ Time: _____

Thank you for Completing this Form

Information from: ❑ patient ❑ significant other
❑ previous records ❑ transfer forms

Initiated by: _____

Completed by: _____

Reviewed by: _____ RN

Date: _____ Time Completed: _____

INOVA HEALTH SYSTEM
ADULT PATIENT ADMISSION HISTORY

Date: _____

Page 4 of 4

CAT # 81789 / R102904
PKGS OF 100   **MR24-00**

Figure 33.2 D

Adult patient admission history.

Source: Inova Health System

hour. The patient is placed in the supine position on the procedural table for most procedures. However, in some peripheral vascular procedures, the patient may be in the prone position. See Chapter 8 for more information on positioning. During patient preparation for the procedure, the clinician will establish monitoring of ECG, oxygen saturation, non-invasive blood pressure (NIBP), and hemodynamic monitoring. These vital signs will be continuously monitored throughout the procedure. The hemodynamic monitoring system allows effective documentation of all the procedural processes and integrates the clinical patient data. The access site will be prepped with an antiseptic agent at the insertion site. See Chapter 9 for information concerning establishing and maintaining a sterile field.

NIBP
Non-Invasive Blood Pressure

Anemia/Sickle Cell

MEDICATION LIST: (NOT AN ORDER SHEET) ❏ No Home Medications
INCLUDE ALL PRESCRIPTION, OTC, AND HERBAL/VITAMIN SUPPLEMENTS:

Medication Name	Concentration / Strength*	Dose	Frequency	Route	Last Given	Indication

Special
Instructions: _____

* Tablet/capsule size (ie, micrograms, mg, gm) or liquid/suspension/injection concentration (ie, mg, units / mL)

RN_____ Date _____
(admission history)

Additions by: _____ Date _____

PATIENT IDENTIFICATION

INOVA FAIRFAX HOSPITAL
PREADMISSION
MEDICATION LIST

CAT # 85924 / R092007 • PKGS OF 100

Figure 33.3

Preadmission
medication history.

Source: Inova Health
System

The cardiologist infiltrates local anesthetic agent such as Lidocaine into the access site. The patient will feel pressure but no acute pain during the needle access to the vessel. The physician uses fluoroscopy to review the anatomic structures of the patient's access site, then using palpation places a single-wall arterial needle into the vessel (**Fig. 33.4**). Once blood flow is established a short guide wire is passed through the needle, and the needle is removed over the guide wire. The cardiologist then threads a vascular sheath system over the guide wire. The sheath system has a three-way valve that prevents blood backflow. The physician then advances a long guide wire (150 cm) with the catheter using fluoroscopy antegrade over the aortic arch, and selectively engages the coronary arteries or other vessels to allow angiography of the vessel. Visualization of the vessel is enabled by radiopaque contrast media.

33

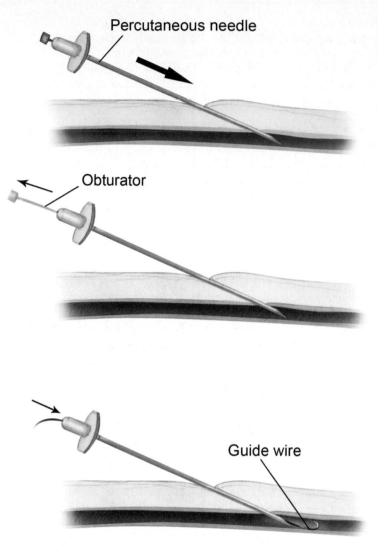

Percutaneous needle

Obturator

Guide wire

Figure 33.4

The physician places a single-wall arterial needle into the vessel.

The contrast media's atomic weight is denser than the surrounding tissue and therefore outlines the vessel wall and the course of the vessel through heart muscle. In the normal coronary arteriogram, the vessel should have a smooth appearance throughout the course of the vessel. Stenotic lesions are represented by narrowed areas in the vessel course that are different from the vessel diameter at that the part of the vessel anatomy. Catheters are designed specifically to engage vessels. The various catheter designs were developed by Judkins, Cournand, and Sones (Biam, 2006). The multiple projections of the right coronary and left coronary arteries are usually accessed using two different catheters. Various fluoroscopic angles are used to visualize the entirety of each vessel. The physician then uses this information to guide the modality of therapy.

Catheters may be advanced into the left ventricle to measure pressures and perform left ventriculography. The hemodynamic monitoring system will allow the clinician the opportunity to measure pressures in the left ventricle and across the aortic valve. The hemodynamic data provides the physician with information related to ventricular function. The physician may inject radiopaque contrast media via a specialized catheter called a "Pigtail catheter." The injection within the ventricle, which is called a ventriculogram, demonstrates the pumping function of the left ventricle. The most common data retrieved from the ventriculogram is the ejection fraction (EF). The EF is the percentage difference in ventricular volume between the end diastolic volume and end systolic volume. These various injections of contrast media will delineate structures and allow the physician to make an evaluation by digitally capturing images of the pathology using digital video technology. After all of the data is collected and reviewed, the catheters are withdrawn from the aorta using the opposite technique of placement. Due to the risk of bleeding at the access site, hemostasis is achieved by either applying manual pressure over the access site, or by deploying a closure device of some form that uses suture, arterial clip, or collagen plug to close the vessel.

EF
Ejection Fraction

Patient Care Responsibilities
During the Procedure

During the procedure, team members provide care according to their scope of practice. The goal for the patient is to provide a safe environment that allows the physician the opportunity to diagnose and treat their patients. The nurse involved in the procedure should focus primary attention to the care and monitoring of the patient. The nurse and team members document care according to facility policy. Caregivers should document the patient's physiological response to the procedure. Documentation should include vital signs, ECG, oxygen saturation levels, baseline and postprocedure peripheral pulses, and positioning, site preparation, and methods to achieve hemostasis according to facility policy and procedure.

After the Procedure

After the procedure, monitoring continues until the patient stabilizes and hemostasis at the procedure site is achieved. The patient is placed on bed rest for 4–6 hours, at a 20-degree head elevation, and with the affected leg kept straight. During this time the nurse will assess vital signs at least every half-hour for 2–3 hours, or per the facility's moderate sedation protocol. If the patient is lying on his or her side, assessment of the access site must be more frequent. Check peripheral pulses and evaluate the insertion site for bleeding and hematoma formation. Monitor hourly intake and output until the patient can tolerate oral fluids, check level of consciousness, and document all care provided.

During the recovery period, provide psychosocial and physical support. Instruct the patient concerning recommended cardiac patient diet, relaxation techniques, medications and potential side effects, and information regarding ambulation and exercise activity.

Patient Discharge

Until the early 1990s, patients having cardiac catheterization were admitted as inpatients. With the changes in healthcare reimbursement, as a cost-containment measure, facilities started performing cardiac catheterization procedures on an outpatient basis. As a result, the 23-hour length of stay for postcardiac catheterization became outdated. Patients that have only diagnostic procedures are discharged to home after a reasonable stay in the postprocedure care unit.

Patients who require an intervention routinely stay in a postprocedure care unit or designated inpatient care bed for 23 hours. These patients are routinely discharged the next day after their procedure.

Prior to discharge, each patient should receive written postprocedure and followup care instructions. These instructions should reflect the patient's individual informational needs specific to home care, response to unexpected events, and followup by the physician. The nurse should review discharge instructions with the patient and a responsible adult prior to discharge. Discharge information should include medication use and possible side effects. With respect to postprocedure side effects that would require the attention of a medical provider, the patient must clearly understand when to contact the healthcare provider for assistance.

Clearly write or provide printed discharge instructions and provide the name of the cardiologist and a contact phone number for the physician and/or cardiologist. Instructions on why and when to call may vary according to the practitioners. **Table 33.6** shows an example of what to include in the discharge instructions. Encourage the patient to ambulate. However, caution against vigorous activity for 24–48 hours. Studies demonstrate that early ambulation with selected patients undergoing diagnostic angiography through the femoral artery approach is safe and associated with acceptable bleeding complication rates (Dowling et al, 2006). The patient should limit

Table 33.6	Discharge Instructions for Cardiac Catheterization Patients

Today you have had a cardiac catheterization done by Dr. _____.

You will go home after the procedure. This list of instructions will help you understand the Do's and Don'ts after the catheterization.

Activity

☐ Do not drive for 24 hours following procedure.

☐ Do rest today and gradually increase your usual activities.

☐ If possible, avoid using stairs for the next 24 hours. If you must use the stairs, take them one at a time, leading with your unaffected leg and hold pressure on the bandaged site.

☐ Do not lift anything over 10 pounds or more for 5–7 days.

☐ Do not engage in strenuous activity for 5 days. Do not attempt anything that may cause fatigue, shortness of breath, perspiration, or chest pain.

Wound/Incision Care

☐ No tub baths, hot tubs, pools, or sitting in water for 7 days.

☐ Do not remove the occlusive dressing over the puncture site for 48 hours after your procedure.

☐ Do not apply creams, powders, lotions, or ointments to the puncture site.

☐ Do not rub, scrub, pick, scratch, or even use a washcloth over the puncture site.

☐ If the puncture site does not look like it is healing (it is red, hot to touch, has discharge) or you are running a fever over 101° F, call the physician who performed your procedure.

Diet

☐ Drink plenty of fluids, unless otherwise directed, to help wash the dye through your kidneys. You may eat as you wish.

Follow-Up Care

- ☐ You will be contacted 24 hours postprocedure by a nurse in Same-Day Surgery for followup.
- ☐ Call your cardiologist to schedule your next appointment.

Call your doctor if:

- ☐ Your arm or leg becomes numb or painful, or if there is redness or a yellow discharge.
- ☐ You have pain or numbness below the catheter insertion site (leg, toes, arm, and fingers).
- ☐ The catheter insertion site swells or bleeds. If this happens, lie down immediately on a firm surface and have someone apply pressure to the catheter insertion site for 10 minutes by pressing the heels of both hands over the lump and pushing down. If the swelling and/or bleeding does not stop, call your doctor or go to the emergency room while continuing to hold pressure on the site.

Call 911 if you have any symptoms of chest pain, shortness of breath, dizziness, fainting spells, or palpitations.

MEDICATIONS: Follow instructions on which medicines to take and which ones to stop

Medication	Dosage	Continue	How Often
_____	_____	Yes ☐ No ☐	_____
_____	_____	Yes ☐ No ☐	_____
_____	_____	Yes ☐ No ☐	_____
_____	_____	Yes ☐ No ☐	_____
_____	_____	Yes ☐ No ☐	_____
_____	_____	Yes ☐ No ☐	_____
_____	_____	Yes ☐ No ☐	_____

Emergency Phone Numbers

Physician: _____   Emergency Department: _____   Same Day Unit: _____

lifting to 10 pounds for a period of 48 hours. Patient instructions should also include the appearance of the puncture site and any response to bleeding. Encourage the patient to drink plenty of fluids in order to facilitate the elimination of dye through the kidneys. The cardiologist should confirm any changes in the patient's medication regimen and communicate the information to the patient. Instruct the patient to call the physician or go to the emergency department should chest pain, shortness of breath, dizziness, fainting, palpitations, leg numbness, or pain occur. Provide the patient with information concerning the next scheduled appointment with the cardiologist. The staff of the same-day unit should contact the patient 24 hours postprocedure for followup discussions and evaluation.

TREATMENT MODALITIES AND ADJUNCT TECHNOLOGIES

This section mentions briefly some of the various modalities and technologies now available to the cardiologist. It is not a complete listing, but only here to provide the reader with some references.

Percutaneous Cardiac Intervention

Percutaneous Balloon angioplasty's (PTCA), introduced by Dr. Gruntzig in 1977, changed the landscape of the cardiac catheterization. Once just used for diagnostic evaluation, cardiac catheterization evolved into a treatment modality offering a less invasive alternative to open heart surgery. Since the development of PTCA, there have been landmark changes in technology and pharmacology, allowing for better treatment alternatives for coronary artery disease. There will continue to be developments that will transform patient care. For example, percutaneous valvuloplasty did not exist until Cope and Ross in 1959 developed the transeptal technique (Biam, 2006). In the future, percutaneous replacement of heart valves and repair of aortic aneurysms using minimally invasive procedures will become the standard of care. The proliferation of techniques and opportunities will continue to develop, changing this exciting frontier in medicine. **Figure 33.5** shows PCTA.

Stents

Stents are named after Charles Stent (1807–1885) a dentist prominent for advancing denture making (Wikipedia, 2008). Stents were first implanted in human coronary arteries by Sigwart, Puel, and colleagues in 1986. Palmz and Schatz developed a stent

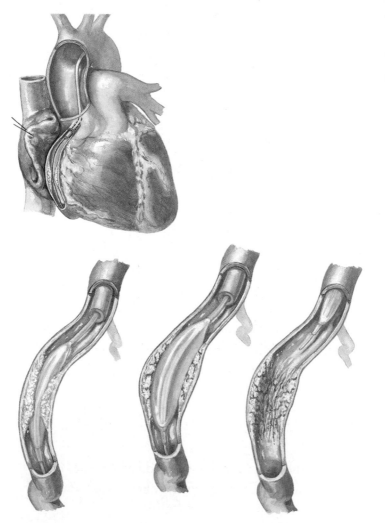

Figure 33.5

Percutaneous Transluminal Coronary Angioplasty.

Source: Netter Images

design which was first implanted by Dr. Sousa in Sao Paulo, Brazil in 1988 (Biam, 2006). Stent technology continues to evolve. Currently there are three types of stents: bare metal, drug eluting and covered stents. The future includes bio-absorbable stents. Stents are deployed over a guidewire and inflated by balloon to provide scaffolding support for an area within the vessel that is blocked by atherosclerosis. For further information related to stent design and classifications refer to *Grossmans Cardiac Catheterization, Angiography and Intervention* (2006), edited by Biam. The cardiologist's choice of a bare metal stent or drug eluting stent will depend on various factors. The cardiologist may use a drug-eluting stent to reduce the patient's risk for restenosis following angioplasty or in conjunction with angioplasty to improve the outcome. The medication used on the drug-coated stents varies with the manufacturer. Drug eluting stents have reduced the restenosis rate from the 20–30% range to the single digit range. These stents gained popularity because of the reduction in restenosis rates and reduction of interluminal endothelial hyperplasia that develops inside the stent, after the stent is deployed in the vessel. The cardiologist will take into consideration certain factors before deploying the stent. The first factor concerns stent length. Stent length must match the length of the stenosed area. The second factor concerns stent diameter versus size of the vessel in the non-stenosed section of the artery. The third factor concerns stent expansion. When deployed in the artery, the stent must expand completely to the arterial wall. Underexpansion will place the patient at risk for developing a subacute thrombosis. Usually the cardiologist sizes and assesses stent expansion during the stent deployment into the vessel and prior to removal of the coronary guide wire. The physician may require the more detailed information available through intravascular ultrasound (IVUS) imaging to ensure appropriate deployment of the stent device. As implantable devices, the FDA requires tracking via manufacturer lot number. Patients receive an owner's manual related to the stent and identification card for their records. Patient education manuals briefly outline the stenting and PTCA process and discuss the stent design. After stenting, the cardiologist places the patient on anticoagulation regimen for a year. The drugs include aspirin and drugs such as clopidogrel (Plavix) or ticlopidine (Ticlid) for a year or more. Pharmacological intervention helps prevent the thrombosis formation secondary from a reaction to the stent. Ideally, endothelial cells grow over the stent during this period and incorporate the stent into the artery, thus lowering the patient's risk for developing clots (Angioplasty.org, 2008).

IVUS
Intravascular
Ultrasound

Primary Angioplasty Versus Thrombolytic Therapy

Over the years clinical studies have indicated that patients presenting with acute myocardial infarctions experience better postinfarction outcomes if angioplasty is used to mechanically open the blocked artery, versus allowing the patient to be treated with thrombolytic therapy to open the vessel. In three trials, which enrolled 700 patients, Wijeysaundera et al (2007) reported that rescue PCI was associated with a significant relative risk reduction of 28% in the composite endpoint of all cause mortality, reinfarction, and heart failure. ACC and AHA guidelines recommend that patients presenting with active signs and symptoms of acute myocardial infarction (AMI) undergo an immediate primary angioplasty at

AMI
Acute Myocardial
Infarction

33

a PCI-capable facility (Antman et al, 2007). Usually, before the patient arrives in the Emergency Department, paramedics notify Cardiac Catheterization Laboratory staff and an Interventional Cardiologist of the patient's impending arrival. Once in the Cardiac Catheterization Laboratory, the patient undergoes a diagnostic angiogram to identify the stenosed vessel causing myocardial infarction. After identifying the vessel, the physician reopens it, which allows cardiac reperfusion. If done soon enough, primary angioplasty stops a myocardial infarction and saves heart muscle from permanent damage (CardioVascular Center at Chester County Hospital, 2008).

Intravascular Ultrasound (IVUS)

Cardiologists often use IVUS as an accessory to angiography to evaluate complex blockages in the coronary arteries (especially in the left main coronary artery) and to detect disease, which is not clearly visible during routine angiography (CardioVascular Center at Chester County Hospital, 2008).

ICE
Intracardiac
Ultrasound

Intracardiac Ultrasound (ICE)

ICE is used instead of transesophageal echocardiography. This treatment modality provides the physician with intracardiac anatomy and provides guidance in the deployment of structural heart closure devices and electrophysiology ablations.

FFR
Fractional Flow
Reserve

Fractional Flow Reserve (FFR)

FFR, which measures intracoronary pressure, is also an accessory to angiography and provides more information for the physician, especially if the patient has several areas of stenosis. Adenosine is injected into the coronary artery creating a hyperemic state. The ratio between the proximal and distal portions is called the fractional flow reserve (Kern, 2003). FFR technology allows the physician to evaluate the dynamic severity of the vascular lesion. Functional flow reserve information can guide the cardiologist in choosing whether to intervene or allow the lesion to be treated medically.

Rotational Atherectomy

The consistency of atherosclerotic plaque can be heavily calcified and, as a result, resistant to conventional PTCA and stent therapies. Rotational atherectomy used in conjunction with a stent may provide an optimum outcome to the operator. The trade product Rotoblator (Boston Scientific) uses an olive-shaped burr that has microscopic diamond particles. The burr is rotated at 200,000 rpm. The burr surface pulverizes the plaque as it is advanced along a guidewire. The particulate created is smaller than 7 microns and is absorbed through the circulation (Kern, 2003).

ELECTROPHYSIOLOGY

Clinical cardiac electrophysiology is the study of the normal and abnormal functional conduction properties of the heart (Podrid, 2001). The rhythmic pumping action of the heart occurs because of electrical impulses traveling throughout the

Table 33.7	Purpose of an Electrophysiology Study

- ☐ Diagnose the cause of bradycardia
- ☐ Diagnose the cause of tachycardia
- ☐ Provoke and diagnose arrhythmias that occur infrequently
- ☐ Expose suspected arrhythmias
- ☐ Evaluate the risk for sudden death
- ☐ Assess symptoms of unknown cause, including chest pain, shortness of breath, fatigue, and syncope
- ☐ Assess response to anti-arrhythmic therapy
- ☐ Determine the need for a pacemaker or implantable cardioverter defibrillator

Scholten, A. (2008). Electrophysiology study, *Health Information Procedures in Brief*, Ipswich, MA: EBSCO Publishing, accessed on 13 August 2008, http://healthlibrary.epnet.com/GetContent.aspx?token=b93d114e-5009-4f6a-9917-6c594254fcc7&chunkiid=35525.

walls of the atria and ventricles. These impulses originate in the sinoatrial (SA) node situated in the right atrium. Normally, the SA node spontaneously generates the impulses, which travel through specific paths throughout the atria to the atrioventricular (AV) node. The AV node relays the impulses to specialized muscle fibers throughout the ventricles. This normal conduction leads to a synchronized contraction and relaxation of the heart muscle. If these paths become damaged or blocked, or if extra pathways exist, bradycardia, tachycardia, or arrhythmias can occur and seriously affect the heart's pumping ability (*Encyclopedia of Surgery*, 2007).

Cardiac electrophysiology (EP) is a highly specialized branch of clinical cardiology (Murgatroyd, 2002). The cardiology electrophysiologist performs an electrophysiology study (EPS) to establish the cause for abnormal heart rhythms (see **Table 33.7**). The study allows the electrophysiologist to replicate an arrhythmia in the controlled environment of the Electrophysiology Laboratory and thus locate and diagnose the cause of the arrhythmia (Heart Rhythm Society, 2004; Scholten, 2008).

SA
Sinoatrial

AV
Atrioventricular

EP
Cardiac Electrophysiology

EPS
Electrophysiology Study

The EP Team

Nurses with cardiac care background have always played an integral part in providing patient care and setting up electrophysiology departments. EP procedures require a specialized team. Until recently there have been no allied health professionals trained as having an electrophysiology background. The allied health schools in the US are training personnel but the need for qualified personnel will continue to be an area of growth for the cardiac nurse and allied health professional. For further information on the EP professional please refer to the web sites in the cardiac catheterization section of this chapter.

History

The last two centuries have been monumental in the development of electrophysiology concepts and technology. In 1843 Wilhelm His published his theory in *Embryonic Cardiac Activity and Its Significance for Adult Heart Movement*.

33

Albert Kent proposed multiple muscular bridges, now known as the Mahaim fibers. Koch described the importance of anatomic landmarks relevant to the AV node. In 1916 Bachmann described interatrial-conducting fibers (Singer, 2001). Our current understanding of the cardiovascular conduction system can be traced back to Willem Einthoven's discovery of the mechanism of the electrocardiogram in 1924 (Fuster, Alexander, & O'Rourke, 2004). The developments of the last 50 years has brought to fruition the current state of cardiac electrophysiology. The landmark contributions and developments have come from cell biologists, physiologists, cardiologists, pathologists, surgeons, and electrophysiologists. From the development of the implantable pacemaker to ablative techniques for atrial fibrillation, electrophysiology continues to be a new cardiology frontier.

Indications

SCD
Sudden Cardiac Death

Each year people die of sudden cardiac death (SCD), which accounts for approximately 325,000 deaths per year in the United States. More deaths are attributable to SCD than to lung cancer, breast cancer, or AIDS. This represents an incidence of 0.1–0.2% per year in the adult population. SCD commonly is the first expression of CAD and is responsible for approximately 50% of deaths from CAD. The frequency of SCD in Western industrialized nations is similar to that in the United States. The incidence of SCD in other countries varies as a reflection of CAD prevalence in those populations (Sovari & Kocherl, 2006). Those deaths can be minimized by the use of electrophysiology studies. Patients often have symptoms prior to a syncopal event. The physician can use an electrophysiology study to guide medical and interventional therapies. A brief listing of indications for electrophysiology studies are as follows; carotid insufficiency resulting in syncopal episode or dizziness, heart block, non-sustained ventricular tachycardia, autonomic nervous system dysfunction, atrial and supraventricular tachycardias, patients with incessant ventricular tachycardia, frequent premature ventricular contractions, sudden death episodes, ventricular tachycardias, and congenital anomalies. Further listings of clinical indications can be located at the American College of Cardiology's (ACC) American Heart Association's (AHA), and Heart Rhythm Society's (HRS) published guidelines at each organization's web site.

ACC
American College
of Cardiology

AHA
American Heart
Association

HRS
Heart Rhythm
Society

Contraindications

In general, only medically stable patients without an acute medical condition that could compromise safety during the study are candidates for EPS (Guo, 2006). Contraindications to invasive EPS are listed in **Table 33.8**.

Equipment and Supplies
Disposable Trays

Disposable trays are available from many manufacturers. The general components are similar to the cardiac catheterization procedural tray but may very well have less or more components depending on the facility's needs. Cost is always a driving factor when choosing to have a custom tray designed. In addition to the disposable trays there should be adequate supplies of sterile gowns, towels, extra patient drapes, and half drapes.

Table 33.8	Contraindications to EPS

- ☐ Acute exacerbations of heart failure
- ☐ Acute metabolic or electrolyte disturbances
- ☐ Acute myocardial infarction within the past 48 hours
- ☐ Compromised hemodynamics of any cause
- ☐ Critical aortic stenosis
- ☐ Recent thromboembolic events
- ☐ Severe and extensive coronary artery disease, including left main artery disease
- ☐ Severe hypertrophic obstructive cardiomyopathy
- ☐ Severe respiratory distress
- ☐ Systemic infection
- ☐ Unstable angina

Adapted from eMedicine (2006). Program Electrical Stimulation—Contraindications. Retrieved from eMedicine Web site on 24 November 2008, http://www.emedicine.com/med/topic3578.htm.

Reusable Instrument Sets—For Implanting Devices

Most facilities have a standard basic instrument set that is used by surgeons for implantation of pacemakers and ICDs. These basic sets usually include hemostats, right-angle clamps, mosquito clamps, Mayo scissors, iris scissors, Weitlaner retractor, rakes and blunt retractors, tissue forceps, and needle drivers. The facility's operating room is a good source for these instrument trays.

Pacing and Mapping Ablation Catheters

Catheters are classified by the number of electrodes, spacing of the electrodes, curve design of the catheter, and whether the catheter is fixed or deflectable. Catheters with numerous electrodes are more rigid. Except for coronary sinus catheters, these catheters do not have a central lumen. Quadripolar catheters have four electrodes, hexapolar have six electrodes, octapolar catheters have eight electrodes, and decapolar catheters have 10 electrodes. Spacing of the electrodes on the catheter can be 10 mm, 5 mm, and 2 mm and other variations of electrode spacing depend on the catheter's intended use. Catheter electrodes are made of platinum. Some facilities will have a recycling process in place from an outside vendor for catheters that do not have lumens. The FDA guidelines state these catheters are for single use; however, cost savings initiatives have forced healthcare facilities to review options that defray costs. Rather than pursuing resterilization options for the pacing wires, the lab management might consider collecting the electrode tips of the catheters, then finding a vendor who will recover the platinum and reimburse the institution for the platinum saved.

Vascular Access

Vascular access is achieved in a fashion similar to that used in cardiac catheterization; however, the physician will be gaining access to veins versus arteries in most instances. The clinician will need to become familiar with transeptal approach for atrial fibrillation and left sided arrhythmia mapping and ablations. The most common access sites are the right and left femoral veins, and left subclavian vein or

33

right internal jugular vein for coronary sinus catheter placements. Access sites for implanted devices are usually designated by the patient's needs. The risks and complications are the same as in the cardiac catheterization section with the addition of potential pneumothorax injuries caused by subclavian access.

Patient Preparation

Preparation for the procedure is similar to the patient having a cardiac catheterization. Patients undergoing diagnostic procedures will usually just receive moderate sedation during the procedure. However, patients having implanted devices and ablation therapies will probably benefit from anesthesia support and care during the planned procedure. Nursing care responsibilities are the same as with cardiac catheterization procedures, except that the informed consent and stay after the procedure may be very different from cardiac catheterization patients. Refer to the preprocedure assessment forms (**Figs. 33.2 A–D**) in the cardiac catheterization section that refer to patient assessment and history.

Anesthesia

For basic electrophysiology studies, the patient will receive moderate sedation/analgesia. Depending on the facility, nursing personnel will give the sedation and monitor the patient's vital statistics. For implanted devices and ablation procedures, the patient will most likely receive general anesthesia.

Anticoagulation

For diagnostic procedures, most often heparinization of the flush solutions is all that is necessary. Ablative procedures and transseptal procedures of the heart require anticoagulation. Dosing of anticoagulants is physician-dependent and protocols for monitoring anticoagulation levels are facility-specific.

Electrophysiology Procedure
Basic Steps of Procedure

Patients undergoing an electrophysiology study, which is similar to cardiac catheterization, have the procedure under local anesthesia and moderate sedation/analgesia. The procedure takes 1–3 hours. Place the patient on the procedure table in the supine position. Establish monitoring with optimally filtered 12-lead ECG, oxygen saturation, and NIBP. The hemodynamic monitoring system should have the ability to provide full disclosure, and be adaptable to recording multiple intracardiac electrograms simultaneously, in addition to the surface ECG. Attach remote defibrillation pads to the patient and connect the pads to the defibrillator (Murgatroyd, 2002). Secure the hands and arms and legs with restraints for patient safety. Prep the access sites and establish the sterile field according to facility protocols.

After the administration of sedation and the local anesthetic, for a basic electrophysiology study the physician uses two venous vascular access sites, usually in the right femoral vein. Two quadripolar catheters are advanced under fluoroscopy to the high right atrium and Bundle of His. The high right atrium-pacing catheter is repositioned to the right ventricle and right ventricular outflow tract to record

EKG Intervals (Estimated Normal)

Figure 33.6

PR Interval   120-200 ms
QRS Interval   60-100ms
QT Interval   Less than half preceding interval

Basic electrophysiology
measurements.

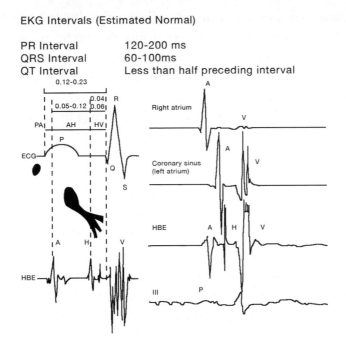

electrograms during various components of the induction protocol. During the diagnostic portion of the electrophysiology study pacing is established using a pulse generator (Bloom Stimulator) that allows for decremental adjustments to energy settings while pacing. Baseline measurement on intracardiac electrograms recorded from the catheters at the various locations within the heart are compared to surface ECG lead information and baseline data collected and documented. See **Figure 33.6** for baseline electrogram measurements.

Then, the electrophysiologist, using standard protocol, attempts to induce the patient's arrhythmia with various pacing settings that affect the refractory periods. Eventually the arrhythmia is either reproduced or not. The physician may use medications such as Isuprel or Adenosine to help with the diagnosis. Once the source of the arrhythmia or pathway is mapped, the physician can then guide his or her decision to use ablation, implant a pacemaker or defibrillator, or direct the patient to medical therapy to control the arrhythmia. In most instances the physician will pursue ablation because the reoccurrence of the arrhythmia is low and the risks to the patient are minimal.

Treatment Modalities

Ablation

The cardiac electrophysiologist inserts four vascular access sheaths for an ablative procedure; two sheaths are placed in the right femoral vein, and two sheaths are placed in the left femoral vein. Three catheters are advanced through these sheaths under fluoroscopy to positions in the heart, high right atrium, right ventricular apex, and the Bundle of His located right above the tricuspid valve. The fourth vascular access is used for the ablation catheter. Vascular access is established in the left subclavian vein and a decapolar catheter advanced into the coronary sinus. The high right atrium, right ventricle, and Bundle of His catheters are usually quadripolar. Using mapping technology, the arrhythmia is reproduced and the pathway defined. Mapping technology now provides the electrophysiologist with the integration of cardiac CT and ultrasound information, which is more accurate three-dimensional electroanatomic representation of myocardial cell depolarization. Earliest activation is represented by the color red. These maps help the electrophysiologist locate and ablate the appropriate pathway that is the source of the arrhythmia. See Chapters 11 and 17 for more information covering safe use of electrosurgical generators.

Implanted Devices

Various pacemakers and implantable defibrillators are available to the physician. Physicians usually choose which device will be implanted for their patient. However, some economic relationships might exist for the organization, and then the choice of the device will be guided by that contract relationship. Today's devices include all the newest technology. Whether single chamber, dual chamber, or biventricular in design, the patient can be assured that the organization is using the best device for them. Congestive heart failure is being more aggressively treated with use of biventricular ICDs and pacemakers. The medical industry is continuously developing better leads, and better algorithms to improve patient care and outcomes. Implanted devices are tracked by registry and reported to the FDA for tracking.

Patient Care Following Electrophysiology Studies, Device Implant, or Radiofrequency Ablation

Postprocedure care following electrophysiology studies and radiofrequency ablation, and implanted devices is similar to the care following cardiac catheterization See **Table 33.6** for discharge instructions. Patients having EP studies are sent home the same day following safe recovery from moderate sedation, and once hemostasis is achieved. Patients having radiofrequency ablation or implant will often remain in the hospital overnight for observation in a monitored cardiac care unit (*Encyclopedia of Surgery*, 2007).

CONCLUSION

Cardiac catheterization and electrophysiology can be performed safely and efficiently in an outpatient setting. The approach to interventional cardiology patients is consistent with the approach to surgical patients. Patients require on going education pre-, intra-, and postprocedure.

It is an exciting time in the field of interventional cardiology and cardiac electrophysiology. Technological advances have improved patient outcomes. Nurses must prepare for the future by learning endovascular skills that cross over into minimally invasive procedures. Remember that endovascular procedures require the blending of x-ray imaging technology with the operative suite. Imaging equipment is burdensome and often sterility issues will be compromised. Blending both areas will be a challenge but the rewards will be great. The revolution and evolution will continue to move toward the less invasive approach because of excellent patient outcomes.

ENDNOTES

1. For in-depth information, the practitioner and student should consult cardiac catheterization and electrophysiology textbooks, research, and standards and recommended practices published by professional associations.
2. The term cardiologist in this chapter refers to the interventional cardiologist.
3. Cardiovascular technology professionals are Registered Cardiovascular Invasive Specialists (RCIS) or Registered Cardiovascular Electrophysiology Specialists (RCES). These practitioners receive intense training in programs accredited by the Commission on Accreditation Allied Health Education Programs (CAAHEP), which is a branch of committee of the American Medical Association.
4. Registered nurses with advanced cardiac life support (ACLS), cardiac monitoring, and moderate sedation/analgesia skills provide nursing care to patients before, during, and after the procedures.

REFERENCES

1. AHA (2008). *Heart Disease and Stroke Statistics—2008 Update.* Downloaded 1 August 2008, from http://www.americanheart.org/downloadable/heart/1200082005246HS_Stats%202008.final.pdf. American Heart Association.
2. AliMed (2008). Medline Cardiac Catheterization Procedure Tray. Accessed 14 August 2008, http://www.alimed.com/ProductDetail.asp?style=921417&fprd=Medline+%20Cardiac+Catheterization+Procedure+Tray&oid1=&oid2=American Heart.
3. American Heart Association. (2004). Statistical Fact Sheet—Populations, *International Cardiovascular Disease Statistics.* Accessed 13 August 2008, ttp://www.americanheart.org/downloadable/ heart/1077185395308 FS06I NT4(ebook).pdf.
4. Angioplasty.org (2008). Drug-eluting stent overview, http://www.ptca.org/des.html.
5. Antman, E.M., et al. (2007). Focused update of the ACC/AHA 2004 Guidelines for the Management of Patients with ST-Elevation Myocardial Infarction; a report of the American College of Cardiology/American Heart Association Task Force on Practice Guidelines, *J Am College, Cardiology,* 2008: 51: 210–247.
6. Arshad, S. (2006). *Cardiac Catheterization (Left Heart),* eMedicine. Retrieved 13 August 2008 from eMedicine Web site: http://www.emedicine.com/MED/topic2958.htm.
7. Bates, E.R. (2008). ACC/AHA Guidelines Managing patients with ST-elevation myocardial infarction, *Cardiac Interventions Today,* March 2008, Vol. 2, No. 2, pp. 27–31.
8. Biam, D.S. (2006). *Grossman's Cardiac Catheterization, Angiography and Intervention,* 7th ed., Lippincott Williams & Wilkens, ISBN: 0-7817-5567-0, p. 5.
9. Cohn, L.H. (2008). *Cardiac Surgery in the Adult,* 3rd ed. McGraw Hill Professional.
10. Dowling, K., Todd, D., Siskin, G., & Stainken, B., et al. (2006). Early ambulation after diagnostic angiography using 4-F catheters and sheaths: a feasibility study. *Journal of Endovascular Therapy,* 9(5): 618–621.
11. *Encyclopedia of Surgery.* (2007). Electrophysiology study of the heart. Retrieved 16 September 2008 from Encyclopedia of Surgery Web site: http://www.surgeryencyclopedia.com/Ce-Fi/Electrophysiology-Study-of-the-Heart.html.
12. Fuster, I., Alexander, R., & O'Rourke, R. (2004). *Hurst's The Heart,* 11th ed. McGraw Hill, ISBN: 0-07-142264-1, p. 3–14.
13. Guo, H.M. (2006). Programmed Electrical Stimulation, eMedicine Accessed 8 September 2008, from eMedicine Web site: http://www.emedicine.com/med/fulltopic/topic3578.htm.
14. Heart Rhythm Society. (2004). EP study, accessed on 13 August 2008, www.HRSpatients.org.
15. Hoffmann, U., Ferencik, M., Cury, R.C., and Pena, A.J. (2006). Coronary CT angiography. *Journal of Nuclear Medicine,* 47(5): 797–806.
16. Kern, M.J. (2003). *The Cardiac Catheterization Handbook,* 4th ed. St. Louis, MO: Mosby, Elsevier Publishing, ISBN: 978-0-323-02247-7, pp. 511–519.
17. Murgatroyd, F.D. (2002). *Handbook of Cardiac Electrophysiology: A Practical Guide to Invasive EP Studies and Catheter Ablation,* Remedica, ISBN: 1-901346-37-4.
18. Podrid, P.J., (2001). *Cardiac Arrhythmia Mechanisms, Diagnosis, and Management,* 2nd ed., Lippincott Williams & Wilkens, ISBN:0-7817-2486-4, p. 3.
19. Scholten, A. (2008). Electrophysiology study, *Health Information Procedures in Brief,* EBSCO Publishing, accessed on 13 August 2008, http://healthlibrary.epnet.com/GetContent.aspx?token=b93d114e-5009-4f6a-9917-6c594254fcc7&chunkiid=35525.
20. Singer, I. (2001). *Interventional Electrophysiology,* 2nd ed., Lippincott Williams & Wilkins, ISBN: 0-7817-2333-7, pp. 3–45.
21. Sovari, A.A., & Kocheril, A.G. (2006). Sudden cardiac death, eMedicine, accessed 8 September 2008 from eMedicine Web site: http://www.emedicine.com/med/topic276.htm.

22. The CardioVascular Center at Chester County Hospital, Cardiac Catheterization, accessed 12 August 2008, http://www.cchosp.com/cchheart.asp?p=399.

23. Wijeysundera, H.C., et al. (2007). Rescue angioplasty or repeat fibrinolysis after failed fibrinolytic therapy for ST-segment myocardial infarction: meta-analysis of randomized trials, *J. Am. College Cardiology*, 49: 422–430.

24. Wikipedia. (2008). Charles Stent. Retrieved 16 September 2008 from Wikipedia Web site: http://en.wikipedia.org/wiki/Charles_Stent.

CHAPTER 34

Gastrointestinal Procedures

Sophia Mikos-Schild

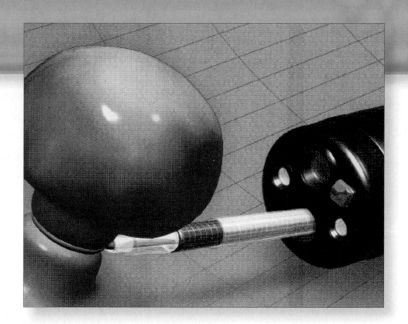

INTRODUCTION

In the 1970s and 1980s, gastrointestinal (GI) procedures were performed in the operating room suite or in a special dedicated operating room. GI procedures were seldom performed in a location other than the operating room (OR). Today, a few institutions still perform these procedures under those circumstances; however, many have a special GI laboratory with dedicated surgical personnel whose location may be away from the OR, or they may have OR staff cross-trained to float to the GI lab. In addition, these procedures may be performed at the bedside by GI nursing personnel. Other institutions may have special dedicated areas in an ambulatory setting. What used to be a trend is more commonplace with gastroenterologists opening GI laboratories in an ambulatory setting in outpatient centers or in their offices.

Gastrointestinal procedures are performed on the GI tract, which includes the upper GI region, the lower GI region, and the associated organs. Most of the procedures are performed for diagnostic or therapeutic reasons. Patients may have much anxiety regarding outcomes or may be experiencing pain caused by the pathological process. For this reason, nurses must be attuned to the needs of the clientele. Patient assessment, support, and education are important components of this process.

The GI laboratory personnel work in a fast-paced, highly technical area in which patients are monitored before, during, and after a procedure. State-of-the-art equipment is used by nursing personnel to care for patients who may have potentially life-threatening complications. It is therefore not uncommon for nurses to be advanced cardiac life support (ACLS)-certified, have become a certified gastroenterology

Chapter Contents

GI
Gastrointestinal

OR
Operating Room

ACLS
Advanced Cardiac Life Support

CGRN
Certified
Gastroenterology
Registered Nurse

CBGNA
Certification Board
of Gastroenterology
Nurses and Associates

SGNA
Society of
Gastroenterology
Nurses and Associates

OSHA
Occupational
Safety and Hazard
Administration

LPNs
Licensed Practical
Nurses

LVNs
Licensed Vocational
Nurses

GTS
GI Technical Specialist

registered nurse (CGRN) by the Certification Board of Gastroenterology Nurses and Associates (CBGNA), and to possess a high level of communication skills. In addition, the GI nurse may be working with varied personnel such as a gastroenterologist, an anesthesiologist, a nurse anesthetist, a physician assistant, a licensed vocational nurse, a GI technician, an instrument room technician, a nurse practitioner, and a patient care partner. In working in this environment, the nurse must possess a high level of specialized training.

GASTROINTESTINAL NURSING

The GI nurse is a highly trained member of the team and cares for patients with gastrointestinal problems and their families. The Society of Gastroenterology Nurses and Associates (SGNA) is an organization for GI nurses and associates whose membership included more than 8,000 members by the end of 2007. The roles they perform range from equipment management and cleaning to performing screening procedures or case management. The society defines the nursing care and standards that apply to GI nurses and has issued formal opinions on topics related to practice (**Tables 34.1** and **34.2**). The specialty requires (1) knowledge of nursing process, anatomy and physiology, moderate sedation/analgesia, pathophysiology, pharmacology, infection control, and Occupation Safety and Hazard Administration (OSHA) guidelines, and (2) the ability to use advanced technological methods for diagnostic and therapeutic endoscopy and emergency situations. The nurse must be knowledgeable in assessment, planning, intervention, and evaluation in order to provide effective care. The effective care is the result of the training required, which usually consists of on-the-job training with a mentor and physician endoscopist.

National certification in GI registered nursing (CGRN) is offered by the Certification Board of Gastroenterology Nurses and Associates (CBGNA). It requires clinical experience and successful completion of a written test that is based on a core curriculum for GI nurses. Recertification is available through the organization. A certificate is also available for licensed practical nurses (LPNs) and licensed vocational nurses (LVNs). SGNA Associates can earn recognition as a GI Technical Specialist (GTS). A certificate is an indication of competency, not of advanced practice. Advanced practice nurses such as nurse practitioners may work in a GI center. Management positions usually require advanced experience and education.

A team approach is vital to working effectively in this environment. The team works toward facilitation of an uneventful procedure. The physician, nurse, and ancillary personnel work closely for the good of the patient. The nurse acts as a patient advocate and uses assessment skills before, during, and after a procedure. Assessment skills, knowledge of procedures, and recognition of early signs of complications before, during, and after a procedure are hallmarks of the GI nurse.

In addition, the nurse needs to understand the patient's level of health and have the specialty knowledge to recognize the onset of complications and of how to manage potential patient complications. It is because of this knowledge that the nurse can take appropriate action that may prevent complications. To prevent complications during and after a procedure, the nurse must be vigilant and able to communicate with the physician and other members of the team.

Table 34.1	SGNA Position Statements

ASGE/SGNA Joint Position Statement

2004	Role of GI Registered Nurses in the Management of Patients Undergoing Sedated Procedures

SGNA Position Statements

2007	Statement on the Use of Sedation and Analgesia in the Gastrointestinal Endoscopy Setting
2006	Performance of Gastrointestinal Manometry Studies and Provocative Testing
2006	The Role of the Nurse/Associate in the Placement of Percutaneous Endoscopic Gastrostomy (PEG) Tube
2006	Statement on Minimal Registered Nurse Staffing for Patient Care in the Gastrointestinal Endoscopy Unit
2006	Statement on Reprocessing of Endoscopic Accessories and Valves
2006	Reuse of Single-Use Critical Medical Devices
2005	Role Delineation of the Advanced Practice Nurse in Gastroenterology/Hepatology and Endoscopy
2005	Role Delineation of Assistive Personnel
2005	Role Delineation of the Licensed Practical/Vocational Nurse in Gastroenterology and/or Endoscopy
2005	Role Delineation of the Registered Nurse in a Staff Position in Gastroenterology and/or Endoscopy
2004	Manipulation of Endoscopes During Endoscopic Procedures
2004	Statement on Reprocessing of Water Bottles Used During Endoscopy
2004	Role of GIRN in Management of Patient Undergoing Sedation Procedures
2001	Safe Operation of Radiographic Equipment During GI Endoscopic Procedures
1999	Performance of Flexible Sigmoidoscopy by Registered Nurses for the Purpose of Colorectal Screening

SGNA Society of Gastroenterology Nurses and Associates, Inc., Position Statements, http://www.SGNA.org, accessed 23 March 2008.

Table 34.2	SGNA Standards and Guidelines

2003	Performance of Flexible Sigmoidoscopy by Registered Nurses for the Purpose of Colorectal Cancer Screening
2007	Guidelines for the Use of High-Level Disinfectants and Sterilants for Reprocessing of Flexible Gastrointestinal Endoscopes
2005	Standards of Infection Control in Reprocessing of Flexible Gastrointestinal Endoscopes
2007	Guidelines for Preventing Allergic Reactions to Natural Rubber Latex in the Workplace
2003	Guidelines for Documentation in the Gastrointestinal Endoscopy Setting
2005	Standards of Clinical Nursing Practice and Role Delineation Statements
1996	Understanding and Influencing the Legislative Process

SGNA Society of Gastroenterology Nurses and Associates, Inc., Position Statements, http://www.SGNA.org, accessed 23 March 2008.

Communication skills are an important component both of the care of the GI patient and of the effective working relationship with the physicians and members of the team. The communication skills are needed for performance of tasks that include teaching, interpersonal relationships, establishing rapport, and communicating with members of the team.

Nurses working with team members are involved in the preparation and operation of specialty equipment such as gastroscopes, colonoscopes, lasers, electrosurgery, audiovisual equipment, and various monitoring devices. This equipment is highly sophisticated, and the nurse must be multitask-oriented while performing direct patient care in a fast-paced, changing environment.

This chapter introduces nurses to the specialized environment of the GT laboratory and its components. The focus is on discussion of anatomy and physiology and on common procedures performed in the laboratory. As the procedures are discussed, the role of the GI nurse before, during, and after a procedure is examined. Finally, the potential complications and nursing interventions are discussed briefly.

ANATOMY OF THE GI SYSTEM

The primary function of the GI, or digestive, system is to provide nutrients to the cells. The process entails ingestion (taking in of food), digestion (breakdown of food), absorption (transfer of food and nutrients into circulation), and elimination (excreting the waste products of digestion).

The GI system (**Fig. 34.1**) includes the GI tract and its associated organs. The organs include the mouth, esophagus, stomach, small intestine, and large intestine. The associated organs are the gallbladder, pancreas, and liver.

Besides pathological factors, emotions such as anxiety and stress may have an effect on the well-being of patients. These factors may contribute to stress-related symptoms such as epigastric and abdominal pain, diarrhea, or anorexia. These symptoms are associated with both organic and psychological problems and may exist concurrently or independently. Other factors such as tobacco smoking, ingestion of caffeine and alcohol products, diet, and fatigue may play a role in aggravation of disease such as ulcers or colitis.

The GI tract consists of a tube 30 feet (9.15 m) long that extends from the mouth to the anus. Its four layers consist of mucosa, submucosa, muscle, and serosa. The esophagus does not have a serosal layer but instead consists of a fibrous tissue as an outer coat. Its muscular coat has a circular layer and a longitudinal layer, which form the inner and outer layers, respectively.

The enteric nervous system coordinates the motor and secretory activities. The parasympathetic and sympathetic branches of the autonomic nervous system have excitatory and inhibitory functions. Pain is transmitted through the sensory fibers of the sympathetic system, and peristalsis is increased by the parasympathetic system.

The GI system also contains hormones and enzymes, which aid in digestion; mucus, which provides lubrication and protection; and electrolytes and fluids. Each part of the GI system works in conjunction with the other parts to assist in ingestion and propulsion of food, digestion, absorption, and elimination.

Figure 34.1

Major structures of the gastrointestinal tract.

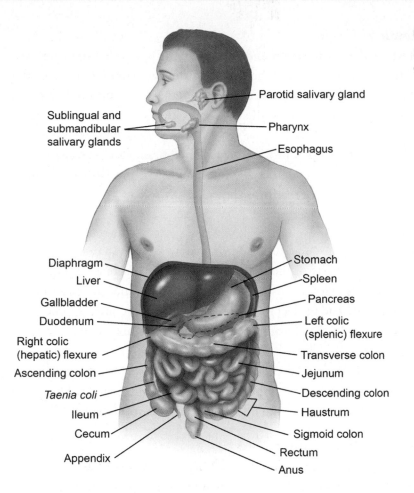

Parotid salivary gland

Sublingual and submandibular salivary glands

Pharynx

Esophagus

Diaphragm

Liver

Gallbladder

Duodenum

Right colic (hepatic) flexure

Ascending colon

Taenia coli

Ileum

Cecum

Appendix

Stomach

Spleen

Pancreas

Left colic (splenic) flexure

Transverse colon

Jejunum

Descending colon

Haustrum

Sigmoid colon

Rectum

Anus

The Mouth

The mouth includes the lips and the oral cavity, which perform speech and mastication (chewing). The tongue and palate assist in moving the food to the back of the throat and allowing the taste receptors to determine the presence of tastes such as sweetness, sourness, or bitterness. As the food is propelled back, salivary glands assist in the digestion process.

The Pharynx

The pharynx consists of the nasopharynx, laryngeal pharynx, and oropharynx. The oropharynx is the route by which the food continues from the mouth to the esophagus. It contains receptors that are stimulated by liquids or food during swallowing.

The Esophagus

The esophagus is a muscular tube that moves food from the pharynx to the stomach. It begins behind the trachea and extends to the stomach. Some of the muscles help move the food to the stomach with peristaltic action. Other muscles prevent the reflux of gastric acids from the stomach.

The Stomach

The stomach stores food, mixes it with gastric secretions, and propels it into the small intestine, where digestion takes place. It absorbs water, alcohol, electrolytes, and some drugs. The varied layers of the stomach secrete gastric juices that not only aid in digestion but also protect the body from harmful organisms.

The Small Intestine

The small intestine aids in digestion and absorption. It is a coiled tube approximately 23 feet (7 m) long and 1.0–1.1 inches (2.5–2.75 cm) in diameter; the diameter decreases to 1.0 inch (2.5 cm) at the lower end. The duodenum, jejunum, and ileum are separated from the large intestine by the ileocecal valve, which prevents reflux of its contents.

The villi (finger-like projections in the mucous membrane) secrete mucus and digestive enzymes. Working in conjunction with microvilli, the villi break down nutrients that can be readily absorbed by the body.

The Large Intestine

The large intestine is a muscular tube approximately 6 feet (183 cm) long and 2 inches (5 cm) wide. It consists of the cecum, appendix, colon, rectum, and anus. It absorbs water and electrolytes, forms feces and retains them until defecation, and secretes mucus to lubricate and protect the mucosa. The muscles contract, producing a kneading action and peristalsis. The peristalsis is caused by reflexes that act to assist in defecation.

Defecation is controlled by a relaxation of the external anal sphincter and facilitated by the Valsalva maneuver. The control is voluntary and involves fibers that produce contraction of the rectum as the urge to defecate begins to be felt.

Liver, Pancreas, and Biliary Tract

The liver is the largest organ in the body, weighing 3 pounds (1.36 kg), and has a right and left lobe. It is essential in the storage, manufacturing, transformation, and excretion of a number of substances involved in metabolism. The size of the organ and its ability to metabolize hormones and medications decrease after the age of 50, but liver function test results usually remain the same. Its lobules remove toxins and bacteria from the blood by the Kupffer cells, which line the capillaries. The cells secrete bile and are located around a central vein of the liver. The portal vein and hepatic artery carry blood to and from the liver; the blood supply is from the stomach, intestines, spleen, and pancreas. The nerve supply is obtained from the vagus and celiac plexus.

The pancreas is a long, slender gland found behind the stomach and in front of the first and second lumbar vertebrae. It consists of a head, a body, and a tail, and it has lobes and lobules. The pancreatic duct extends along the gland and enters the duodenum through the common bile duct. In its exocrine function, the pancreas contributes to digestion through the exocrine cells, which secrete pancreatic enzymes. In its endocrine function, its beta cells secrete insulin, and other cells secrete glucagon.

The biliary tract includes the pear-shaped gallbladder and the duct system. The gallbladder concentrates and stores up to 45 mL of bile. The bile is produced by the hepatic cells, is secreted into the lobules, and then drains into the right and left hepatic ducts. The ducts converge with the cystic duct (from the gallbladder) to form the common bile duct. This duct enters the duodenum at the ampulla of Vater and is closed by the sphincter of Oddi. The sphincter of Oddi opens when stimulated by food in the GI tract.

SPECIAL INSTRUMENTS, SUPPLIES, AND EQUIPMENT

GI instruments are designed to perform functions of grasping, cauterizing, visualizing, obtaining biopsy samples, and crushing. Each serves a special function during the various procedures to which patients are subjected. Knowledge in their use, care in handling, and maintenance is necessary for the nurse to achieve positive patient outcomes.

The nurse must know how to operate, care for, and maintain equipment such as a flexible fiberoptic endoscope, light sources, electrosurgical generators, lasers, monitors, pulse oximeters, and probes. Maintaining competency is also a requirement for GI nurses. The role of the educator is vital in meeting these needs. He or she can assist staff in keeping current and competent.

Care and maintenance of equipment are always as per manufacturer recommendations and are most important for keeping down repair costs, prolonging the usefulness of the instruments, and preventing accidents. Education and maintenance of competencies regarding endoscopic cleaning and high-level disinfection can be provided by the educator and through SGNA and the Association of periOperative Registered Nurses (AORN) publications.

AORN
Association of periOperative Registered Nurses

Fiberoptic Endoscope

This lighted instrument is used to directly visualize the esophagus, stomach, duodenum, colon, pancreas, and biliary tree. It consists of channels through which cytology brushes, biopsy forceps, and irrigating solutions may be passed. The adjustable dial allows the endoscope to contour into and around curvatures to permit visualization of all surfaces in the organs of the GI tract. **Figures 34.2**, **34.3**, and **34.4** show examples of endoscopes.

The light source (**Fig. 34.5**), video system, and video processor (**Fig. 34.6**), which illuminate the body cavity and enable observation of images on a monitor, are integral parts of the system. Special cameras may be attached for visualization and picture taking for documentation. Videoendoscopy is commonly performed in the GI laboratory. Television cameras are commonly mounted in an individual procedure room or available on a video cart that can be easily moved from one room to another (**Fig. 34.7**).

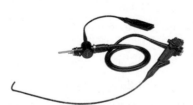

Figure 34.2

Esophagoscope (Olympus PEF-V).

Source: Courtesy of Olympus.

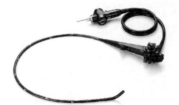

Figure 34.3

Gastrointestinal videoscope (Olympus GIF-H180).

Source: Courtesy of Olympus.

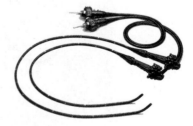

Figure 34.4

Colonoscope (Olympus CF-Q180).

Source: Courtesy of Olympus.

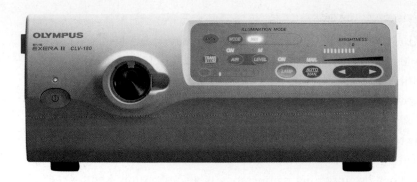

Figure 34.5

Xenon light source (Olympus CLV-180).

Source: Courtesy of Olympus.

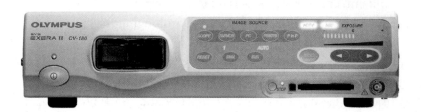

Figure 34.6

HDTV Video Processor (Olympus CV-180).

Source: Courtesy of Olympus.

Figure 34.7

Gastroenterology work station (Olympus WM-NP1 & WM-DP1).

Source: Courtesy of Olympus.

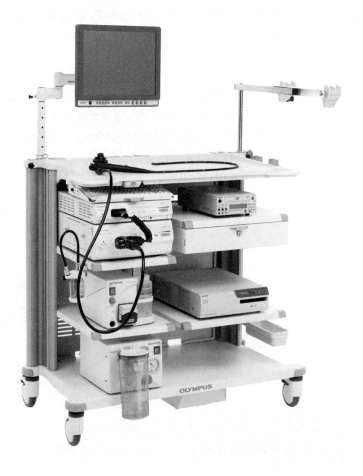

Endoscopy is commonly performed for diagnostic and therapeutic purposes. Fluoroscopy and radiography are often used in conjunction with endoscopy. Polyps, varices, bleeding sites, stones, neoplasms, and papillomas are treated. A possible, but not highly probable, complication is perforation of the structure being visualized. Patients, families, and significant others should be advised as to the signs and symptoms of perforation and other complications.

Electrosurgical Unit

Gastroenterologists routinely use electrosurgery (**Fig. 34.8** and **Fig. 34.9**) for coagulation of bleeding vessels and excision of polyps. The device is used on internal organs and vessels. Although bleeding points may also be coagulated by a laser beam or an argon coagulator, electrosurgery is used more commonly because of its accessibility and ease of use.

Familiarity with the available waveforms of cut, blend, and coagulation, the active electrode, and the correct placement of the patient return electrode is essential for safe patient care. The patient return electrode should be placed on a well-vascularized muscle mass (Ulmer, 2007). Frequently this site will be the upper thigh or the flank (Morris, 2006). Proper placement of the patient return electrode, the use of electrosurgery on a patient with a pacemaker, safety factors, and legal aspects, including documentation of skin preparation and condition, are important components of patient care. The electrosurgical unit can be safe and effective if institutional policies and procedures, as well as the manufacturer's recommendations, are followed. See Chapters 11 and 17 for more information about electrosurgery.

Laser

Laser is an acronym for "light amplification by stimulated emission of radiation." Photons, the basic units of radiation that constitute light, strike atoms, causing them to become excited and forcing the electrons of the atoms to a higher energy level. As

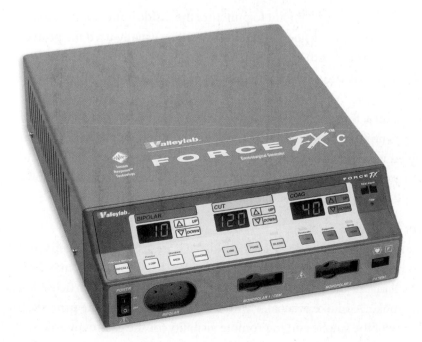

Figure 34.8

Force FX™C Electrosurgical Generator with Instant Response™.

Source: Copyright © Covidien. All rights reserved. Reprinted with the permission of the Energy-Based Devices and Surgical Devices divisions of Covidien.

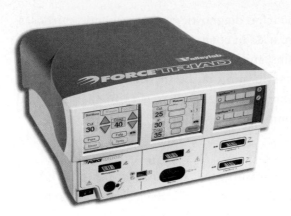

Figure 34.9

Force Triad™ Energy Platform with TissueFect Sensing Technology.

Source: Copyright © Covidien. All rights reserved. Reprinted with the permission of the Energy-Based Devices and Surgical Devices divisions of Covidien.

the electrons in an atom return to their normal lower level, they emit more photons, which further excite the other already excited atoms. As this excitation continues, a chain reaction of stimulated photons at high energy levels continues to produce energy. The captured energy powers the laser as it is amplified and metamorphosed into wavelengths of laser light. The wavelengths are either continuous or pulsed (short and of repeated duration), and the type of wavelength used determines where they will be used.

The carbon dioxide (CO_2) and argon lasers were developed in the mid-1960s. The CO_2 laser cannot be used through the flexible endoscope because the beam cannot be conducted through quartz fibers. The argon laser is used when shallower penetration and red pigmentation are needed. These two lasers are not as popular for GI procedures as the neodymium:yttrium-aluminum-garnet (Nd:YAG) laser.

The Nd:YAG laser beam scatters on impact and is not readily absorbed, as is the argon beam. The Nd:YAG beam penetrates deeper and can coagulate and more extensively destroy large tumors, excise lesions, or ablate masses. Esophageal obstruction is also treated with the laser to debulk, vaporize, or excise a tumor. Additional laser uses include coagulation of bleeding sites, malformations, polyps, fistulas, and lower bowel stenosis.

When the laser is used, care is taken not to puncture the inside lumen of the biopsy port with the sharp tip of the laser fiber. A catheter sheath is usually used for protection from the sharp tip. The sheath is pulled back enough to expose the fiber before laser activation. The tubing must be far enough from the end of the fiber to keep from being burned.

During the procedure, the laser tip is monitored to prevent damage to the end of the endoscope. Preventing damage to the tip is but one component of safety precautions to be followed with the use of the laser. Other safety precautions are used to protect the patient and personnel (**Table 34.3**). In accordance with laser precautions, the beam is focused through the endoscope and held in a self-retaining device.

Electrosurgical and Laser Plume

When electrosurgery and lasers such as the Nd:YAG are used, carcinogens and viruses may become airborne as byproducts of the smoke. The byproducts may produce a distinct smell as a result of the water, intact cells, and carbonized particles that are present in the smoke. A smoke evacuator with a filter is used during the procedure to prevent inhalation of the smoke and to promote visibility for the gastroenterologist

Table 34.3	**Laser Precautions**	
Personnel/Patient Safety	**Environmental Safety**	
1. Eye protection	1. Nonreflective surfaces	
2. Skin protection	2. Warning signs	
3. Use of noncombustible agents	3. "Standby" mode when not in use	
4. Laser plume	4. Manufacturer's written instructions	
5. Education about lasers	5. Availability of sterile water/saline and carbon dioxide fire extinguisher	
6. Protection of area from thermal injury		

Medications

Infiltration with a local anesthetic such as lidocaine (Xylocaine) or bupivacaine (Marcaine) is performed by the gastroenterologist during the local procedure. Because there is no anesthesia provider, the nurse needs to be familiar with the drugs administered during the procedure. Knowledge regarding the available concentrations, duration of action when used with or without epinephrine, maximum doses, signs and symptoms of problems (eg, allergic reactions, toxic overdose, and reaction to epinephrine) and their treatment is important to the GI nurse who is monitoring the patient. For example, according to the National Institutes of Health (NIH), a blood disorder called methemoglobinemia (MHB) can be acquired by exposure to anesthetics such as Xylocaine, benzene, some antibiotics and nitrites (Dix, 2008) In addition to medication for moderate sedation/analgesia, premedication and reversal agents may also be ordered. Knowledge of those medications is a prerequisite for competent nursing care.

An intravenous (IV) port is used to administer medication during the procedure and for access during life-threatening situations. Medications are carefully titrated, and their effects are closely monitored. The GI nurse has knowledge of monitoring equipment. The knowledge includes function, connections, and interpretation of the data. The monitoring devices include an electrocardiogram (ECG) and a pulse oximeter; the parameters to be monitored include heart rate.

NIH
National Institutes of Health

MHB
Methemoglobinemia

IV
Intravenous

ECG
Electrocardiogram

Pulse Oximeter

The pulse oximeter is used to continuously and noninvasively monitor a patient's arterial blood oxygen saturation (SaO_2) rate before, during, and after a procedure. A sensor emits light into arterialized tissue and measures the amount of light reflected by that tissue (Lesser, 2007). It is an effective and easy method for the GI nurse to detect potential problems that may not be readily evident during visual assessment. In addition, it provides an accurate means of alerting the nurse to hypoxemia before signs and symptoms occur.

During the procedure, the nurse applies a pulse oximeter on the index, middle, or ring finger, using the adhesive or finger clip sensor. Other sensors may be used on the nose, earlobe, toe, or foot (infants or neonates), as well as on the forehead, depending

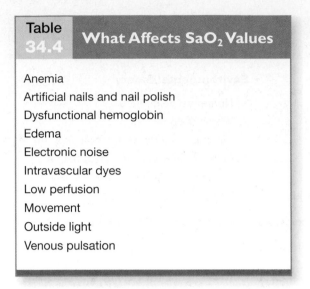

Table 34.4	What Affects SaO$_2$ Values
Anemia	
Artificial nails and nail polish	
Dysfunctional hemoglobin	
Edema	
Electronic noise	
Intravascular dyes	
Low perfusion	
Movement	
Outside light	
Venous pulsation	

on patient's size, perfusion, or movement. Which type should be used, how it works, how to apply it, and what affects SaO$_2$ values (**Table 34.4**) are just some of the clinical considerations vital to appropriate application and accurate readings.

Other Instruments and Supplies

To treat the GI patient, many accessories are available today and many more are being developed. Some are reusable and others are disposable. Products available from various manufacturers include biopsy and retrieval forceps, snares, baskets, ligators, dilators, and cytology brushes. Brief descriptions of their uses follow.

Biopsy and retrieval forceps are used to obtain mucosal samples and to retrieve foreign bodies through the endoscopic. The heads of the instrument come in varied shapes and can be autoclaved. Disposable biopsy forceps can be used in conjunction with monopolar electrosurgery to obtain mucosal biopsy samples and remove polyps.

Snares and polypectomy devices are used to remove polyps and come packaged as reusable or disposable. Their various sizes and shapes allow for quick and simple connection and use with electrosurgery. **Figure 34.10** shows an example of a polyp snare.

Wire baskets are used for endoscopic removal of foreign bodies and polyps. They may contain up to eight monofilament wires and may be used with balloon dilators to remove stones.

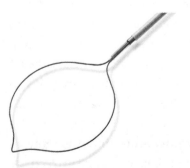

Figure 34.10

Polyp snare (Olympus PolyLoop).

Source: Courtesy of Olympus.

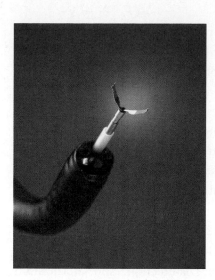

Figure 34.11

Endoscopic clipping device (Olympus QuickClip2 Long).

Source: Courtesy of Olympus.

34

Balloon dilators are commonly used to dilate strictures of the esophagus, pylorus, or colon. They are accompanied by kits with inflation devices or contain multiple-size polyvinyl chloride reusable dilators.

Cytology brushes are sterile disposable brushes used to collect brushings of cells from the lower and upper portions of the GI tract. Once the brushing of the area is completed, the device is removed from the endoscope, and the bristles are cut from the sheath and placed into a specimen container. After the procedure, the specimen container is sent to the pathology department.

Another instrument used for endoscopic procedures is an endoscopic clip placement device (**Fig. 34.11**). This device is used for endoscopic marking, hemostasis for mucosal/submucosal defects less than 3 cm, bleeding ulcers, arteries less than 2 mm in diameter, polyps less than 1.5 cm in diameter, and diverticula in the colon. The device can also be used as a supplementary method closure of GI tract luminal perforations (Olympus, 2008).

ENDOSCOPIC PROCEDURES

These procedures allow for direct visualization of the contents and walls of the esophagus, stomach, and colon. The endoscopic procedure assists in diagnosis and treatment of disease. Lasers (such as the Nd:YAG), stone retrieval baskets (snare wires), dilators, and electrosurgery may be used to treat esophageal varices, strictures, ulcers, GI bleeding, stones, and malignancies.

In general, endoscopic procedures are performed with local anesthesia, with moderate sedation/analgesia monitoring, or with general anesthesia. An IV catheter, a patient return electrode (when monopolar electrosurgery is used), laser safety glasses (when laser is used), and monitoring devices are routinely in place during the procedure. In the GI laboratory, most endoscopic procedures (eg, gastroscopy, colonoscopy, and percutaneous endoscopic gastrostomy [PEG]) are performed with local anesthesia and moderate sedation/analgesia. Endoscopic retrograde pancreatography (ERCP) is usually performed with general anesthesia and in the radiology department by GI nurses. Some procedures may be performed at the patient's

PEG
Percutaneous
Endoscopic
Gastrostomy

ERCP
Endoscopic
Retrograde
Pancreatography

bedside, as in the critical care areas. The GI nurse's role is critical because patients are medicated and sedated, which necessitates not only the maintenance of a patient's position and assistance to the physician but also physiological monitoring, psychological support, and maintenance of the airway.

Flexible fiberoptic endoscopes are used for these procedures. These endoscopes require special handling to prevent damage and cross-contamination between patients. Due to the varied infections that can be transmitted, colonization or death can result (AORN, 2008 A). For practical purposes, high-level disinfection with a cold sterilant is done between uses on different patients. This standard is defined by unit policies and should provide for the same level of care for all patients. Polices for cleaning, processing, disinfecting, and sterilizing of endoscopes should follow endoscope manufacturer written instructions, the AORN "Recommended Practices for Cleaning and Processing Endoscopes," "High-Level Disinfection," and "Sterilization in the Perioperative Setting" (see AORN, 2008a), and the Association for Professionals in Infection Control and Epidemiology (APIC) *Guidelines for Infection Prevention and Control in Flexible Endoscopy*.

APIC
Association for Professionals in Infection Control and Epidemiology

Upper Endoscopy

An example of upper endoscopy is esophagoscopy, performed to visualize the esophagus. Other endoscopic procedures are performed to visualize the mucosal lining of the stomach and the duodenum. A flexible fiberoptic endoscope is used for direct visualization. A video camera may be used to view stomach motility. Because upper endoscopy is not a sterile procedure, a high level of disinfection is important so as not to transmit disease to a patient.

Indications

Indications for upper endoscopy are listed in **Table 34.5**. Because of the potential for perforation, the nurse needs to be alert after the procedure for signs and symptoms of complications. Patient and family instructions should also be given.

Table 34.5	Common Indications for Upper Endoscopy
Abnormal Upper GI X-ray Studies	
Bleeding	
Foreign Body	
Inflammation	
Mallory-Weiss tears	
Reflux	
Strictures	
Tumors	
Ulcers	
Varicees	
Viral hepatitis	

Related Procedures

Procedures similar to upper endoscopy are gastroscopy and esophagogastroduodenoscopy (EGD).

Nursing Implications

ANESTHESIA

Anesthesia and analgesia are vital for esophagoscopy and related procedures. Patient comfort and ease of procedure are factors considered when both are provided. A topical anesthetic agent such as lidocaine (Xylocaine) or benzocaine (Hurricaine) spray is used to spray the throat, which temporarily inhibits the gag reflex. In addition, it facilitates introduction and passage of the endoscope through the esophagus. The gag reflex should be functional before the patient's discharge. The ability to drink fluids is used as a determinant of that function.

Moderate sedation/analgesia is the choice of physicians when the procedure is performed. IV sedative medications such as fentanyl (Sublimaze), midazolam (Versed), and meperidine HCL (Demerol) are often the drugs of choice to be administered to achieve sedation. The amount to be administered depends on multiple factors such as the patient's age and tolerance level. Meperidine, used for analgesia, is often combined with midazolam. Their use must be carefully monitored to prevent complications such as respiratory arrest.

POSITION

The patient is placed in a sitting position as the endoscope is introduced with a bite block in place to protect the patient's teeth. As it is advanced, the patient is placed on the left side to facilitate drainage of secretions, prevent aspiration, and facilitate passage of the endoscope.

ESTABLISHING AND MAINTAINING THE STERILE FIELD

Upper endoscopy is a clean procedure; a high level of disinfection is needed for the endoscope. A sterile field is not maintained because the oral cavity is not sterile and the endoscope is passed through it.

EQUIPMENT AND SUPPLIES

The equipment used for the procedure is listed in **Table 34.6**.

PHYSIOLOGICAL MONITORING

Basic monitoring measures for all patients include ECG, blood pressure, and pulse oximetry. Depending on the American Society of Anesthesiologists (ASA) classification of patients (see **Table 7.2**), the physiological changes may be rapid, even for patients who undergo "quick look" procedures. An unexpected drop in vital sign values may occur, and so the nurse must be vigilant in monitoring blood pressure, pulse, SaO_2, heart rate, and respiration. Monitoring equipment that produces a written strip can record unusual occurrences and aid in documentation of patient care.

SPECIMENS AND CULTURES

When specimens, washings, and cultures are collected, they remain with the nurse until after the procedure is completed. Specimens are labeled, placed in formalin or

EGD
Esophagogastroduodenoscopy

34

ASA
American Society of Anesthesiologists

Table 34.6	Upper Endoscopy Equipment and Supplies

Argon-enhanced electrosurgery supplies
Aspiration tube
Biopsy forceps
Cytology brush and solutions for washings
Electrosurgical unit
Fiberoptic endoscope and video camera (if used)
Irrigation Supplies
Light source with air infusion capability
Lubricating jelly
Protective bite block
Suction setup

saline, and sent to the pathology department. Multiple biopsy samples, washings, and cultures may be taken. Each must be carefully labeled with the patient's identification information, the date, and the site of the procedure.

DRUGS AND SOLUTIONS

Topical throat spray (Hurricaine), meperidine and midazolam, and normal saline are used.

PHYSICIAN ORDERS

The typical admission orders include a medical examination with emphasis on the GI system. A history is obtained; a physical examination is performed; and risks, complications, and alternatives are discussed by the physician. Prior endoscopy results (if any), including radiographic studies, should be available.

NPO
Nothing by Mouth

Before the procedure, the GI nurse explains the procedure to the patient and makes sure that patient has taken nothing by mouth (NPO) at least 8 hours before admission. The patient's baseline vital signs are measured before the throat is sprayed and before IV medication is administered. An IV catheter or heparin lock and monitoring equipment are standard for providing access and obtaining baseline vital signs. Vital sign monitoring is continuous during and after the procedure. Institutional policy and procedures regarding monitoring should adhere to SGNA and Association of periOperative Registered Nurses (AORN) standards for moderate sedation/analgesia. These standards recommend that during moderate sedation/analgesia, the RN should document the physiological data from continuous monitoring at 5- to 15-minute intervals and upon significant events (AORN, "Recommended Practices for Managing the Patient Receiving Moderate Sedation/Analgesia," 2008 B).

A procedure consent form must be signed before any preprocedure medication is given. Then medication such as meperidine or diazepam may be given. A local anesthetic may be sprayed on the patient's throat for upper endoscopic procedures before the endoscope is inserted. At this time, the patient is on a gurney or in a bed, the rails are up, and monitoring equipment such as the pulse oximeter, ECG, and blood pressure cuff are in working order. Depending on the physician's preference, antibiotics may also be given.

LABORATORY AND DIAGNOSTIC STUDIES

Recommended laboratory tests include, but are not limited to, a chest radiograph, ECG, complete blood count (CBC), blood chemistry and electrolyte studies, coagulation studies (prothrombin time [PT] and partial thromboplastin time IPTTI), and urinalysis. Typing and screening are not typically done.

Procedure

As the medication takes effect, a protective bite block is placed in the patient's mouth before insertion of the flexible endoscope which is covered with a water-soluble jelly. The patient is placed on the left side. As the procedure begins, the patient is instructed to breathe slowly as the endoscope is introduced into the patient's mouth. Care is taken as the endoscope is introduced slowly. The esophagus is inspected. A biopsy may be performed or laser treatment may be carried out, depending on the pathological process. Attention is paid to positioning in order to minimize discomfort and prevent injury to nerves. The patient may be sedated heavily, and the nurse may be maintaining the oral airway.

Postprocedure Care

Vital signs are checked after the procedure, as is the return of the gag reflex. Because short-acting IV drugs are given, the patient may remain in the GI laboratory for a relatively short duration; depending on the extent of the procedure, the patient may then be discharged. Recently, regulatory agencies are recommending that postprocedure patients be monitored for 1 to 1.5 hours after the administration of sedation and observation for hemorrhage, abdominal distention, and pain (SGNA, *Standards for Clinical Practice*, 2008). Patients can go home within 2 hours (Ogilvie, 2008). Typical charting after the procedure includes the use of the nursing process for an assessment, plan, outcome, and interventions (**Table 34.7**).

Discharge to family or significant others is done after the patient has been seen by a physician and discharge orders are written. Discharge criteria and disposition include those listed in **Table 34.8**. The followup appointment is made, and the physician's emergency number and instructions are given to the patient and family. Instructions should include the following (Huber, 2007):

- Do not drive or operate any electrical equipment or appliances.
- Do not sign any legal papers or make any decisions, because your judgment and perception may be impaired for 24 hours.
- Do not drink alcoholic beverages or smoke cigarettes when alone.
- Rest for several hours before resuming routine activities.
- Resume your regular diet and medications slowly as tolerated.
- Drink warm liquids and take throat lozenges or acetaminophen (Tylenol), no aspirin, for relief of sore throat.
- Call the doctor if you have shortness of breath or a constant cough.
- Call the doctor if you have chills or fever within 24 hours after the procedure.
- Call the doctor if you have persistent vomiting (with or without blood), diarrhea, black stools, fever, severe chest pain, severe abdominal pain, or distention.

CBC
Complete Blood Count

PT
Prothrombin Time

PTTI
Partial Thromboplastin Time

Table 34.7	Postprocedure Documentation

Assessment

Level of Consciousness

☐ Awake, responsive
☐ Drowsy, arouses to verbal stimuli
☐ Unresponsive
☐ No gag reflex

General Condition

☐ Stable
☐ Unstable

Vital Signs

☐ Stable
☐ Unstable

Check

☐ Tubes
☐ Drains
☐ Catheters
☐ Dressing
☐ Abdomen
☐ Bleeding
☐ IV site
☐ Level of pain
☐ Burns, bruises, cuts

Plan

Observe for

☐ Shortness of breath
☐ Chest discomfort
☐ Nausea
☐ Pain
☐ Vomiting
☐ Hemorrhage
☐ Bleeding
☐ Condition of IV site

Palpate for

☐ Abdominal distention

Monitor

☐ Vital signs per policy
☐ Draining type, amount, and color from tubes
☐ Draining type, amount, and color from catheter
☐ Draining type, amount, and color from drain
☐ Presence of gag reflex

Outcome

☐ Absence of injuries noted
☐ Discomfort tolerable
☐ Absence of abdominal distention
☐ Absence of redness or swelling at IV site
☐ Meets discharge criteria
☐ Absence of excessive bleeding
☐ Absence of seizure activity
☐ All vital signs meet discharge criteria

Nursing Observations with Intervention and Evaluation

(Note time, problem, and intervention along with RN signature in the following area)

_____
_____
_____
_____
_____

(Facility Name)	(Addressograph or Patient Sticker)

Potential Complications

Perforation is not common with the use of the flexible endoscope, but nurses must carefully monitor the patient accordingly during and after the procedure. Infection, pulmonary aspiration, bleeding, cardiac arrest, and death may also occur. Other complications include oxygen desaturation, self-limited bleeding, and local reactions to medication.

Table 34.8	Discharge Criteria and Disposition*

☐ Alert and oriented
☐ Vital signs stable
☐ Minimal nausea, vomiting, dizziness
☐ Able to ambulate
☐ Absence of respiratory distress
☐ IV discontinued _____ Site checked _____
☐ Postsedation recovery score _____
☐ Received prescriptions/emergency phone number
☐ Responsible adult present to escort patient home
☐ Physical assessment by physician before discharge orders
☐ Patient or responsible adult given discharge instructions and verbalizes understanding

Disposition:

☐ Home   ☐ Room   ☐ Other _____

Mode of Transport:

☐ Ambulance
☐ Wheelchair
☐ Stretcher
☐ Other _____

Accompanied by:

☐ Spouse
☐ Relative
☐ Friend
☐ Other _____
☐ Physician signed discharge orders
☐ Nurse completed documentation according to unit policies

Nurse's notes (Note time, problem, intervention, and RN signature)

_____

_____

_____

_____

_____

* Based on AORN and SGNA criteria.

Flexible Fiberoptic Colonoscopy/Sigmoidoscopy

During this procedure, the physician directly visualizes the rectum and entire large intestine with a colonoscope. Sigmoidoscopy is the visualization of the sigmoid colon and rectum. "It is thought that about 60% of all colorectal cancers are within reach of the sigmoidoscope," which as a result is a common procedure (Zuber, 2001, p. 1375). As the sigmoidoscope is advanced, the patient's position is changed to promote its advancement to the cecum. Polyps of the colon can be easily removed without the patient's

Table 34.9	Indications for Colonoscopy/Sigmoidoscopy
Bleeding	
Colorectal cancer screen	
Inflammatory bowel disease	
Neoplasm	
Polyps	
Strictures	

undergoing a laparotomy. Oftentimes these procedures are used to diagnose inflammation of the bowel, bleeding, or tumors and to dilate strictures.

Indications

Indications for colonoscopy/sigmoidoscopy are listed in **Table 34.9**. Because of the potential danger of perforation or hemorrhage during the procedure, the patient is observed for any complications.

Related Procedure

Proctosigmoidoscopy (rigid) is the only procedure related to flexible procedures in that it also visualizes the rectum and sigmoid colon.

Nursing Implications

ANESTHESIA

Moderate sedation/analgesia is common practice during these procedures. See prior discussion of moderate sedation/analgesia and use of sedatives and analgesics. Studies in ambulatory surgery settings suggest that the use of Propofol and S-Ketamine with monitored anesthesia care may have a less nausea and vomiting, fewer complications, and an uneventful home discharge (Hobaika, 2007).

POSITION

As the procedure begins, the patient is positioned on the left side to facilitate drainage of secretion and promote visualization. Care is taken to provide comfort and retain body heat. It is important to provide pillows to maintain support, as well as warm blankets to aid in thermal regulation. Verbal reassurance and emotional support of the patient are offered during the procedure.

ESTABLISHING AND MAINTAINING THE STERILE FIELD

Sigmoidoscopy and colonoscopy are not sterile procedures because the colonoscope is inserted into the rectum. A high level of disinfection is required. See previous discussion.

EQUIPMENT AND SUPPLIES

The instruments used for the procedure are listed in **Table 34.10**.

Table 34.10	Equipment and Supplies for Colonoscopy/Sigmoidoscopy

Colonoscope or flexible sigmoidoscope
Video camera (if needed)
Light source
Air insufflation capability
Biopsy forceps or hot biopsy forceps
Snares
Suction
Electrosurgical unit (if needed)
Cytology brushes
Baskets
Dilators
Ligators
Specimen cup
Saline
Guide wires
Dilating balloons

PHYSIOLOGICAL MONITORING

As in upper endoscopy procedures, moderate sedation/analgesia with monitoring devices is used. See the discussion in the section on upper endoscopy.

SPECIMENS AND CULTURES

As in other GI procedures, when specimens are collected, they remain with the nurse until after the procedure is completed. The specimens are labeled, placed in formalin, and sent to the pathology department. Multiple biopsy samples may be taken. Each must be carefully labeled with patient's identification information, the date, and the site of the procedure. Cultures are not routinely obtained.

DRUGS AND SOLUTIONS

Normal saline and lubricating jelly (water-soluble) are needed for these procedures.

PHYSICIAN ORDERS

The patient is instructed to follow a clear-liquid diet 2 days before the procedure and maintain NPO status for 8 hours before admission. Laxatives are administered for 1–3 days before the procedure and enemas the night before. The preparation of the bowels is accomplished with a cleanser such as polyethylene glycol (GoLYTELY) or citrate of magnesium, which must be ingested. The enema is self-administered at home or given by the nurse before the procedure. New on the horizon is the use of OsmoPrep Tablets to clean the colon before colonoscopy in adults 18 and older.

Adequate hydration is a must before, during, and after the use of OsmoPrep Tablets. Additionally, other prep includes polyethylene glycol (PEG) solution, sodium phosphate (NaP) solution, NaP tablets, and over-the-counter NaP solutions (Allen, 2007).

Laboratory and Diagnostic Studies

Laboratory work and studies are the same as those of upper endoscopy. See the discussion in the section on upper endoscopy.

Procedure

Baseline vital signs are measured, the patient is instructed about the procedure, and the patient's consent is obtained before IV sedatives and analgesics are administered. A well-lubricated, flexible colonoscope is slowly introduced and passed into the anal canal and advanced until it reaches the cecum for colonoscopy. During sigmoidoscopy, only the left side of the colon is examined, although research has found that there has been a shift of distribution of cancer toward the right side during the last few decades (Lubowski & Newstead, 2006; Kumar, 2007). A biopsy may be performed, or electrosurgery may be used to control bleeding. Other pathological processes such as polyps may necessitate the use of snare wires. The goal of positioning is to minimize discomfort and prevent injury to nerves. If the moderate sedation/analgesia is heavy, the nurse may need to maintain an airway or provide oxygen while monitoring vital signs and assisting the physician. The nurse needs to observe for abdominal distention secondary to air insufflation.

Postprocedure Care

Vital signs are checked after the procedure. The patient needs to be monitored because of the sedative effects of short-acting IV drugs. The patient may remain in the GI recovery area until ready to be discharged. The nurse observes for signs of perforation and rectal bleeding. Side effects of the drugs, such as nausea and vomiting, may be observed. Gas retention may cause cramping and discomfort for a few hours after the procedure; a sore rectum is common. The patient and significant other or family need to be advised as to preoperative and postoperative instructions. Instructions to the patient and family include the following:

- Do not drive or operate any electrical equipment or appliances.
- Do not sign any legal papers or make any decisions, because your judgment and perception may be impaired for 24 hours.
- Do not drink alcoholic beverages or smoke cigarettes when alone.
- Rest for several hours before resuming routine activities.
- Drink warm liquids and eat soft foods to help the cramps pass.
- Call the doctor if there is a large amount of bleeding; a small amount is expected if you have had a polyp removed or a biopsy performed.
- Take acetaminophen (Tylenol), not aspirin, for a sore rectum.
- Call the doctor if you have shortness of breath or a constant cough.
- Call the doctor if you have chills or fever within 24 hours after the procedure.
- Call the doctor if you have persistent vomiting (with or without blood), diarrhea, black stools, fever and chills, chest pain, or severe abdominal pain or distention (Lee, 2005; Levin, 2006).

Potential Complications

Potential complications include perforation, hemorrhage, hypotension, respiratory depression or arrest, cardiac dysrhythmia or arrest, and infection.

Percutaneous Endoscopic Gastrostomy

This procedure is commonly called a PEG procedure. A fiberoptic gastroscope is used to place a gastrostomy tube through the esophagus into the stomach and is then pulled through a stab wound made in the abdominal cavity wall. A bumper and a retention disk keep the gastrostomy tube in place.

Sterile technique is used for insertion of the tube, and the patient is sedated during the procedure. Either a push technique or a pull technique is used to insert a PEG tube. The pull technique is discussed in the Procedure section.

Indications

The PEG procedure is usually performed for patients who are unable to maintain nutritional status because of inability to swallow or to ingest sufficient amount of food to meet caloric requirements, for patients who have acquired immunodeficiency syndrome (AIDS), or for patients who have cancer of the head or neck.

AIDS
Acquired
Immunodeficiency
Syndrome

Related Procedure

The PEG technique with the push method is the only related procedure.

Nursing Implications

As in other GI procedures, patient education, consent, and monitoring are standard for PEG procedures. Two requirements for the procedure are an unobstructed GI tract and an esophagus large enough to pass the gastroscopes. A local anesthetic is used, but moderate sedation/analgesia may or may not be used, depending on the patient's condition. There are few risks associated with this procedure because it requires minimum sedation and time. These factors make it suitable for patients who are very ill and unable to undergo a procedure involving general anesthesia.

ANESTHESIA

The PEG tube is usually inserted with the use of local anesthesia and moderate sedation/analgesia. When moderate sedation/analgesia is used the GI nurse must monitor the patient while another nurse assists with the procedure. See previous discussion about moderate sedation/analgesia.

POSITION

The patient is placed in the supine position with a pillow under the knees. Soft restraints may be needed if it is determined that the patient will be unable to cooperate during the procedure. This type of medical immobilization must be explained to the patient and documented.

ESTABLISHING AND MAINTAINING THE STERILE FIELD

As with any abdominal incision, skin preparation is performed and sterile technique maintained. Depending on the physician's preference, if hair removal is needed clippers may be used. A surgical scrub followed by painting with antibacterial solution is then performed, with the use of aseptic technique.

The sterile field is created with towels and drapes, depending on hospital policy. Sterile supplies and instruments remain separate from the fiberoptic gastroscope. The insertion of the gastroscope is a clean procedure, inasmuch as the oral cavity is not sterile. Sterile technique is observed during the entire abdominal procedure.

EQUIPMENT AND SUPPLIES

A PEG tube kit is used. It contains the following items:

Percutaneous needle

Guide wire

Universal adapter

Pull tie

Silk suture

Flexible gastroscope

Percutaneous gastrostomy tube and bolster

Radiopaque tulip tip

Twist lock

Cold snare

Sterile knife and scissors

Suction and cautery may be needed, and that equipment should be readily available.

PHYSIOLOGICAL MONITORING

During the procedure, the GI nurse monitors the patient who has had moderate sedation/analgesia (see previous discussion of moderate sedation/analgesia).

SPECIMENS AND CULTURES

Specimens and cultures are not typically obtained.

DRUGS AND SOLUTIONS

A local anesthetic and normal saline are needed.

PHYSICIAN ORDERS, LABORATORY STUDIES, AND DIAGNOSTIC STUDIES

The patient usually maintains NPO status 6–8 hours before the procedure. The GI tract must be unobstructed and the esophagus large enough to allow for passage of the gastroscope. The laboratory work and studies are the same as those that are standard for endoscopy.

Procedure

Baseline vital signs are measured, the patient is instructed as to the procedure, and the patient's consent is obtained before IV sedatives and analgesics are administered. The patient is placed in the supine position, and the gastroscope is introduced through the oral cavity and passed through the esophagus into the stomach. The nurse may assist in introduction of the gastroscope while it is angled anteriorly to the left anterolateral wall of the stomach's fundus. The light of the gastroscope can be seen through the abdominal wall. The abdomen is insufflated with air.

The abdominal site is prepped with povidone-iodine (Betadine) scrub and paint, and the area is walled off with sterile towels. A local anesthetic is injected at the site, and a small stab wound is made with a No. 10 blade. The percutaneous needle is inserted into the stab wound and into the stomach lumen while being visualized through the gastroscope. A long silk suture is threaded into the lumen of the needle and passed into the stomach, where it is pulled with the forceps. A clamp is applied to the exterior distal end of the suture after the needle is removed.

The gastroscope is removed, and the suture can be seen extending out of the patient's mouth. The suture is attached to the tapered end of the gastrostomy tube. The gastrostomy tube is gently guided into the patient's oral cavity, through the esophagus, into the lumen of the stomach, and out through the abdominal wall. By means of direct visualization, the tube is secured with an internal bolster by reinserting the gastroscope and placing it snugly against the gastric wall. An external bolster is placed over the tube and snuggled up to the abdominal wall. The team makes sure that the bolsters are not compressing the tissue.

The distal end of the tube is cut, and a connector is applied. The stomach is slowly deflated, and the patient is notified that the procedure has been completed. The tube is marked at the skin insertion site. Usually, the patient has to spend less time than in an open procedure, and the PEG procedure itself is less costly and less risky.

Postprocedure Care

Vital signs are checked after the procedure. The patient needs to be monitored because of sedation by short-acting IV drugs. If the procedure is done in the GI laboratory, the patient may remain in the GI recovery area until ready to be discharged. Side effects of drugs, such as nausea and vomiting, may be observed. Gas retention may cause cramping and discomfort for a few hours after the procedure.

Feeding is usually begun within 24 hours or when bowel sounds are heard. The catheter is frequently connected to a pump for continuous feeding.

Instructions to the patient include the following:

- Do not drive or operate any electrical equipment or appliances.
- Do not sign any legal papers or make any decisions, because your judgment and perception may be impaired for 24 hours.
- Do not drink alcoholic beverages or smoke cigarettes when alone.
- Rest for several hours before resuming routine activities.
- Call the doctor if there is a large amount of bleeding from the wound site.
- Take acetaminophen (Tylenol), not aspirin, for incision site pain.
- Call the doctor if you have shortness of breath or a constant cough.
- Call the doctor if you have chills or fever within 24 hours after the procedure.
- Call the doctor if you have persistent vomiting (with or without blood), diarrhea, black stools, fever, severe chest pain, or severe abdominal pain or distention.

Potential Complications

Potential complications include infection, wound cellulitis, aspiration pneumonia, clogged tube, and accidental removal of the tube.

Endoscopic Retrograde Cholangiopancreatography

CBD
Common Bile Duct

Commonly known as ERCP, this is a procedure in which an endoscope is inserted through the mouth into the descending duodenum and into the common bile and pancreatic ducts (*ECRP*, 2008). It is a less invasive approach to biliary tract conditions previously treated entirely by surgical intervention. Often, the procedure is performed to retrieve a gallstone from distal common bile duct (CBD), to dilate strictures, to diagnose cysts, and to obtain biopsy specimens of tumors. It is a safe alternative to more invasive procedures such as surgical intervention. Krinsky and Topazian (1997) studied 1341 procedures and found that after ERCP, surgical procedures were recommended less, dropping from 41% before ERCP to 12% afterwards. The procedure is done in the radiology department because radiographs are taken with a radiographic dye that is injected into the ductal system, and a biopsy may be taken when indicated (Petty, 2003).

An innovation in ERCP is the use of SpyGlass technology which uses miniature probes with high resolution and high maneuverability to directly view patient's bile duct. The fiberoptic probe attaches to a camera head. The probe can move in four directions through a single-use access and delivery catheter. Bile duct stones can also be crushed using this system which provides another alternative to the two dimensional, black and white ERCP (Collins, 2007).

Indications

Indications for an ERCP are listed in **Table 34.11**. It is recommended for patients with abdominal pain, obstructive jaundice, or pancreatitis (Topazian et al., 1997).

Related Procedures

PTC
Percutaneous
Transhepatic
Cholangiography

Sphincterotomy, percutaneous transhepatic cholangiography (PTC), nasobiliary tube or stent, and papillotomy are related to the main procedure of ERCP.

Nursing Implications

Before the procedure, the GI nurse explains the procedure to the patient and makes sure that patient has maintained NPO status for at least 6–8 hours before admission. Monitoring equipment and an IV catheter or heparin lock are standard of care for IV access and obtaining baseline vital signs. Vital sign monitoring is continuous before, during, and after the procedure. Because this procedure is done

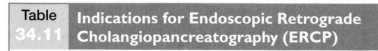

Table 34.11	Indications for Endoscopic Retrograde Cholangiopancreatography (ERCP)
Abdominal pain	
Jaundice	
Abnormal radiographic findings	
Pancreatitis (with or without gallstones)	
Strictures (malignant and nonmalignant)	
Bile duct stones	

in the radiology department, nurses must transport any needed supplies from the GI laboratory.

A procedure consent form must be signed before any preoperative medication is given. Because an IV catheter or a heparin lock is usually standard before this procedure, the nurse may be asked to administer a preoperative medication such as midazolam and meperidine or fentanyl.

At this time, the patient is on an x-ray table, and monitoring equipment such as the pulse oximeter, ECG, and blood pressure cuff are in working order. Prophylactic broad spectrum antibiotics are also usually given per physician protocol.

ANESTHESIA

Anesthesia and analgesia are critical during the procedure to minimize patient movement, which can result in perforation by the endoscope. The throat may be sprayed before the administration of sedatives. Sedatives and analgesics, such as midazolam (Versed) and meperidine (Demerol), are given during the procedure. The preoperative assessment should include the standard assessment (see the section on upper endoscopy).

As with any procedure involving moderate sedation/analgesia, the patient is monitored per institutional protocol. If the patient is under general anesthesia or deep sedation and an anesthesiologist is present, there is no need for an additional RN to monitor the patient.

POSITION

The patient is placed on an x-ray table on the left side. Attention is paid to positioning in order to minimize discomfort and prevent injury to nerves. Pillows and a safety belt are used to maintain position and to promote safety and comfort.

ESTABLISHING AND MAINTAINING THE STERILE FIELD

This is a clean procedure. Pseudomonas aeruginosa infection of the pancreatic or biliary tree from contaminated equipment has been reported (Dix, 2003). As with all procedures, care in cleaning and handling of instruments is standard protocol.

EQUIPMENT AND SUPPLIES

Equipment and supplies are listed in **Table 34.12**. These can be a standard for an ERCP cart, which can be easily transported to the radiology department before the procedure.

Table 34.12	Equipment and Supplies for Cholangiopancreatography (ERCP)

4 × 4 sponges
60-mL syringes
Water-soluble lubricant
Biopsy forceps
Varied snare wires
Balloon dilators

Physiological Monitoring

Basic monitoring equipment for all ERCP procedures includes an ECG, pulse oximeter, and blood pressure cuff. Continuous monitoring of blood pressure and continuous pulse oximetry are vital because sudden changes may occur as a result of the administration of medication for moderate sedation/analgesia. Supplemental oxygen should be available in case the SaO_2 rate falls below 90%. Monitoring is the same as for other GI procedures when performed by the RN while the patient is under moderate sedation/analgesia. When general anesthesia is used, the anesthesiologist cares for the patient.

Specimens and Cultures

If a specimen (eg, stone) is collected, it is saved in a clean, dry specimen container until after the procedure; then it is labeled and sent to the pathology laboratory for examination. Biopsy specimens and cultures are not routinely obtained.

Drugs and Solutions

The following substances are used: midazolam (Versed) and meperidine (Demerol), contrast medium, buscopan or glucagon, normal saline, and 10% lidocaine (Xylocaine) topical spray.

Physician Orders

Typical admission orders include CBC, PT/PTT, serum liver chemistry profiles, and results of previous abdominal ultrasound and other imaging studies. The patient maintains NPO status for at least 8 hours before the procedure. Typing and cross-matching are not usually needed.

Laboratory and Diagnostic Studies

Recommended tests include ECG, chest radiograph, electrolyte measurements, coagulation studies, and other radiographs that evaluate the extent of the disease. Liver function studies such as an amylase test are conducted before the procedure.

Procedure

Before the procedure, the throat is sprayed with a topical spray by the GI nurse. The patient may be sedated heavily, and an anesthesiologist or an RN may be maintaining the oral airway. A fiberoptic endoscope is inserted through the oral cavity into the descending duodenum and then into the common bile and pancreatic ducts. The ducts are cannulated, and a diluted contrast medium is injected. The physician will remove all air bubbles before injecting the medium. The catheter is advanced through the endoscope channel. This allows for direct visualization of the structures under fluoroscopy. Radiographs are taken to permanently record the results. If stones are to be extracted, a balloon or basket may be inserted to facilitate the procedure.

Postprocedure Care

Vital signs are checked, and the patient may be transferred to a recovery area in the GI laboratory or to the postanesthesia care unit (PACU). The nurse checks for a return of the gag reflex and stability of vital signs. After ERCP, patients may be

PACU
Postanesthesia Care
Unit

discharged or returned to nursing units, where they are observed for infection and perforation.

Instructions to the patient and family include the following:

- Do not drive or operate any electrical equipment or appliances.
- Do not sign any legal papers or make any decisions, because your judgment and perception may be impaired for 24 hours.
- Do not drink alcoholic beverages or smoke cigarettes when alone.
- Rest for several hours before resuming routine activities.
- Return to full activity on the day after the procedure.
- Resume your regular diet and medications slowly as tolerated.
- For mild abdominal pain and bloating, rest and drink only liquids.
- Drink warm liquids and take throat lozenges or acetaminophen (Tylenol), no aspirin, for relief of sore throat.
- Call the doctor if you have shortness of breath or a constant cough.
- Call the doctor if you have chills or fever within 24 hours after the procedure.
- Call the doctor if you have persistent vomiting (with or without blood), diarrhea, black stools, fever, severe chest pain, or severe abdominal pain or distention.

Potential Complications

Potential complications include bleeding, perforation, pancreatitis, infection (cholangitis), impacted basket, and sepsis.

Liver Biopsy

Commonly called a liver needle biopsy, a liver biopsy may be performed in the GI laboratory for diagnostic purposes. This invasive procedure is done to establish a diagnosis of hepatic disease.

Indications

The primary indication for this procedure is to obtain a specimen of hepatic tissue. Factors to consider when this intervention is chosen are (1) ability of the patient to cooperate and follow directions, (2) the patient's general medical condition, and (3) whether patient has a blood abnormality.

Related Procedures

There are no procedures related to liver biopsy.

Nursing Implications

ANESTHESIA

This procedure is usually performed with local anesthesia and moderate sedation/analgesia. The sedation should be light, to allow the patient to follow instructions regarding taking a breath, breathing, and holding a breath during the procedure.

POSITION

The patient is placed in the supine position. Because the procedure is performed while the patient is on a gurney, the patient's hands may be tied to the gurney with soft, padded restraints for medical immobilization. Standard patient teaching and documentation regarding this procedure must also be charted. Care must be taken if the patient has ascites and difficulty breathing when supine. The patient's head may need to be elevated to assist in breathing.

ESTABLISHING AND MAINTAINING THE STERILE FIELD

The skin preparation usually involves an iodophor scrub and solution or gel. The area prepped is on the right side, starting at the biopsy site, which is between the sixth and seventh or the eighth and ninth intercostal area. Sterile towels are applied and may be secured with towel clips.

EQUIPMENT AND SUPPLIES

A limited number of supplies are needed for this procedure. A local anesthetic set with needle and syringe is used to administer the local medication. It is usually done with a Silverman biopsy needle.

PHYSIOLOGICAL MONITORING

Basic monitoring devices for liver biopsy include an ECG, pulse oximeter, and blood pressure cuff. Continuous monitoring of blood pressure and continuous pulse oximetry are vital because sudden changes may occur as a result of the administration of medication for moderate sedation/analgesia. Supplemental oxygen should be available in case the SaO_2 rate falls below 90% or the patient has difficulty breathing as a result of ascites. Vital signs are monitored closely, and the patient is observed for complications such as bleeding or drug side effects during the procedure.

SPECIMENS AND CULTURES

Specimens are collected and saved until after the procedure. Each specimen is placed into a formalin container, labeled, and sent to the pathology laboratory for examination. Cultures are not routinely obtained.

DRUGS AND SOLUTIONS

Drugs and solutions required for this procedure include a local anesthetic, IV solution, and either meperidine (Demerol) and midazolam (Versed) or midazolam and meperidine. Depending on the status of the patient, meperidine may be given first for pain and then followed by midazolam for sedation. Likewise, for some patients, midazolam may be given first for sedation and then followed with meperidine for pain.

PHYSICIAN ORDERS

Typical admission orders include a medical examination with emphasis on hepatic disease. Liver function tests are used to assess the degree of functional impairment and to evaluate liver activity and reserve. Type and cross-match is usually not ordered.

LABORATORY AND DIAGNOSTIC STUDIES

Before the procedure, the coagulation status is checked (FT, clotting time, or bleeding time). An ECG, chest radiograph, and measurement of electrolyte levels are recommended.

Procedure

The patient is instructed to take several deep breaths and then to hold the breath and remain absolutely still while the needle is inserted. The Silverman biopsy needle is introduced into the liver via the transthoracic intercostal or transabdominal subcostal route. The needle is rotated to obtain a small tissue fragment. The needle is withdrawn, and the specimen is removed. As soon as the needle is removed, the patient is told to breathe normally once again. The patient is helped to the right side to compress the chest wall at the penetration site to prevent seepage of bile or blood. A compression dressing may be applied to the site.

Postprocedure Care

The vital signs are checked to detect internal bleeding. The patient should remain on the right side for about 2 hours to splint the puncture site. After this procedure, patients are usually returned to the nursing unit, where they are observed for complications. In addition, patients should remain in bed in a flat position for 10–14 hours. Slight bleeding may follow the procedure.

Instructions to the patient and family should include the following:

- Do not drive or operate any electrical equipment or appliances.
- Do not perform strenuous activity for 24–48 hours.
- Do not get dressing wet for 24 hours; remove the adhesive bandage after that time.
- Call the doctor if the biopsy site is red, swollen, or painful or is draining.
- Do not drink alcoholic beverages for 24 hours; do not smoke cigarettes.
- Resume your normal diet and current medications as tolerated.
- If you are taking anticoagulants, aspirin, or arthritis medicine, check with your doctor before resuming.
- Take acetaminophen (Tylenol) for pain unless a prescription was given.
- Call the doctor if you have an increase in bleeding from the biopsy site, severe pain, swelling, coughing up of blood, difficulty with bleeding, temperature over 100°F, or persistent shoulder pain.
- Call the doctor if you have nausea, vomiting, or any other concerns.
- Call the doctor for a followup visit and results of the biopsy as instructed.

Potential Complications

When a patient fails to cooperate with instructions to take deep breaths, hold the breath, and remain still, needle penetration of the diaphragm or liver injury can occur, and the result may be internal hemorrhage. Bile leakage into the abdominal cavity may also occur and produce peritonitis. Other complications such as shock and pneumothorax may be observed several hours after the procedure.

Pediatric Procedures

Pediatric GI procedures are unlike procedures on adults. Although children may have problems (eg, GI bleeding and indications for procedures such as abdominal pain) similar to those of adults, their care before, during, and after the procedure differs markedly. Patient education must also be tailored to meet the level of understanding of the child. Family members can reinforce that knowledge and assist in minimizing the patient's fear.

To provide good care, the GI nurse and team members must have knowledge of the growth and development of neonates, children, adolescents, and young adults. Factors such as airway management, maintenance of fluids and electrolytes, thermal regulation, nutritional needs, and the cardiovascular system differ for each population, and specialized knowledge and critical interventions are required. For this reason, many GI nurses do not have experience in treating this population unless they work in children's hospitals.

Pediatric GI procedures are usually done under general anesthesia if the patient is under 12 years old. Over 12 years old, procedures may be done using moderate sedation/analgesia if the child is able to cooperate. Sedatives must be carefully titrated to avoid potential untoward effects (American Academy of Pediatric Dentistry, 2006). Blood pressure, an ECG, and a pulse oximeter are used for monitoring. Naloxone, oxygen, suction, and pediatric resuscitation equipment must be available during and after the procedure. Pain management may be difficult in comparison with that in adults, and observations may be the key for making assessments for patients unable to verbalize.

The instruments, such as endoscopes, are specialized for this population and require the same gentle care and handling as do any fiberoptic endoscopes. When cautery is used, care in proper size of grounding pads is essential to prevent electro-surgical burns. These factors are critical because of the fragility of newborns and the susceptibility of children.

After the procedure, it is important to monitor temperature and observe for the onset of acidosis, hypotension, hypoglycemia, bradycardia, and apnea. When depression of metabolism and activity occur, the stage is set for possible cardiac arrest. The pediatric patient must be closely observed and prompt treatment initiated to prevent occurrence of postprocedure complications.

New studies point to a change in practice with use of oral bisacodyl combined with a single phosphate enema as bowel prep for children, which netted excellent results (Shaoul & Haloon, 2007). Additionally, children commonly exhibit nausea and vomiting, have sore throats, pain, and experience behavioral problems postprocedure (Mellville, 2007).

Although the care of this population is specialized, knowledge and experience of the healthcare team ensure that procedures such as PEG, polypectomy, gastroscopy, and sphincterotomy can be performed safely, cost effectively and quickly in lieu of more invasive procedures such as laparotomy.

THE FUTURE OF ENDOSCOPY

New technologies are emerging which will impact the future of endoscopic surgery in the operating room and in the endoscopy lab. The impact will be felt in a decrease in the number of endoscopic procedures performed as well as a greater number of surgical procedures due to an increase in finding of pathology. Some of the procedures include virtual colonoscopy, capsule endoscopy, and prototype robot.

CT
Computed Tomography

Virtual colonoscopy, also known as computed tomography (CT) uses a CT scanner and computer virtual realty software to view inside of the colon without using a colonoscope, sedation, or IV medication (Ahluwalia, Miser, & Bova, 2007). It can be used to screen those who have obstructive carcinoma, and elderly who cannot tolerate moderate sedation/analgesia. Although the cost is currently prohibitive, considered experimental by some insurance companies, and has some mixed results, in time it may prove to be an invaluable tool for diagnosis of cancers and colorectal polyps (Pagana, 2007).

In 2001, the FDA cleared capsule endoscopy to be used to view the entire small intestine. A patient swallows the device which is in the shape of a capsule and by peristalsis, the capsule moves through the GI tract transmitting color video images in about 8 hours. Patients continue with normal activities while wearing a set of sensors on a belt worn around the waist. When the procedure is completed, the patient returns the data recorder for processing. The capsule is excreted and there is no need for radiation ("Swallow This and Get the Picture!," 2008).

The newest technology is an autonomous earthworm-like robot that will be used for colonoscopy. The prototype robot has been tested in vitro in pig colon and can navigate freely and reliably or be stopped while it travels through the colon. It is said to squirm like an earthworm without discomfort to the patient and without causing any harm to the organs (Wang & Yan, 2007).

REFERENCES

1. Ahluwalia, J., Miser, S., & Bova, S. (2007). Virtual colonoscopy: What is its role in cancer screening? *The Journal of Family Practice, 56* (3), 186–191.

2. Allen, G. (2007). Evidence for practice. *AORN, 85* (5), 1004.

3. Alvarado, C.J., Reichelderfer, M., & the Association for Professionals in Infection Control and Epidemiology Guidelines Committees. (2000). APIC guideline for infection prevention and control in flexible endoscopy. *American Journal of Infection Control, 28,* 138–155.

4. American Academy of Pediatric Dentistry (2006). *Guideline for Monitoring and Management of Pediatric Patients During and After Sedation for Diagnostic and Therapeutic Procedures,* Reference Manual V 29 / NO 7 07 / 08. Chicago, IL.

5. AORN. (2008 a). Recommended practices for cleaning and processing endoscopes and endoscope accessories. In *Perioperative Standards and Recommended Practices,* pp. 345–350. Denver, CO: AORN, Inc.

6. AORN. (2008 b). Recommended practices for managing the patient receiving moderate sedation/analgesia. In *Perioperative Standards and Recommended Practices,* pp. 461–471. Denver, CO: AORN, Inc.

7. Collins, C. (2007, December 2007/January 2008). Utilizing new technologies in the GI suite: A case study. *EndoNurse,* 24.

8. Dix, K. (2008, December 2007/January 2008). Interference or patient safety? Benzocaine-related methemoglobinemia and restrictions at the VA. *EndoNurse,* 30–36.

9. Dix, K. (2003). *What's Lurking in Your Endoscope?* Virgo Publishing, accessed March 2008, http://www.surgicenteronline.com/articles/361feat4.html#.

10. *ERCP.* (2008). Retrieved February 12, 2008, from Boston Scientific: http://www.bostonscientific.com/procedures/ProcedureLanding.bsci.

11. Hobaika, A.B. (2007). Propofol and S-Ketamine monitored anesthesia care for colonoscopy: Implications on patients' discharge. *Internet Journal of Anesthesiology, 12* (1), 8.

12. Huber, D. (2007). Discharge instructions. *Gastroenterology Nursing, 30* (6), 451–452.

13. Krinsky, M.L. & Topazian, M.D. (1997). A novel approach to common bile duct stone extraction, *Gastrointestinal Endoscopy* 46(4):382–383.

14. Kumar, R.K. (2007). Prevalence of left-sided colorectal cancer and benefit of flexible sigmoidoscopy: A country hospital experience. *American Surgeon, 73,* 994–997.

15. Lee, E. (2005, May 17). Colonoscopy. (D. Lee, Editor) Retrieved February 12, 2008, from MedicineNet.com: http://www.medicinenet.com/colonoscopy/page4.htm.

16. Lesser, S. (2007, December 2007/January 2008). The importance of Pulse oximetry: How one technology advanced changed medicine. *EndoNurse,* 38–40.

17. Levin, T.R. (2006). Complications of colonoscopy in an intergrated health care delivery system. *Annals of Internal Medicine, 145* (12), 880–886.

18. Lubowski. D.Z., and Newstead, G. (2006). Rigid sigmoidoscopy: A potential hazard for cross-contamination. *Surgical Endoscopy, 20,* 812–814.

19. Melville, D.D. (2007). Postprocedural effects of gastrointestinal endoscopy performed as a day case procedure in children: Implications for patient and family education. *Gastroenterology Nursing, 30* (6), 426–433.

20. Morris, M. (2006). Electrosurgery in the gastroenterology suite: Principles, practice, and safety. *Gastroenterology Nursing, 29* (2), 126–131.

21. Ogilvie, A. (2008). Gastroscopy. Retrieved March 2, 2008, from netdoctor: http://www.netdoctor.co.uk/health_advice/examinations/gastroscopy. htm.

22. Olympus. (2008). QuickClip2 Long Product Description. Retrieved November 3, 2008 from http://www.olympusamerica.com/presspass/press_pass_cut/documents/QuickClip2%20Long%20brochure.pdf.

23. Olympus. (2008). Endoscope Flushing Pump EFP250. Retrieved November 3, 2008 from http://www.olympusamerica.com/presspass/press_pass_cut/documents/EndoFlush.pdf.

24. Pagana, K.D. (2007, April). Laboratory and diagnostic testing: A perioperative update. *AORN Journal*, 756–759.

25. Petty, L.R. (2003). Surgery of the liver, biliary tract, pancreas, and spleen. In J. Rothrock, *Alexander's Care of the Patient in Surgery* (12th ed., pp. 401–402). St. Louis, MO: Mosby, Inc.

26. Shaoul, R. and Haloon, L. (2007). An assessment of bisacodyl-based bowel prep for colonoscopy in children. *Journal of Gastroenterology, 42*, 26–28.

27. *Standards for clinical practice.* (2008). Retrieved February 24, 2008, from SGNA: http://www.sgna.org.

28. *Swallow this and get the picture!* (2008). Retrieved February 12, 2008, from Given Imaging: http://www.pillcam.com/ages/procedure.aspx.

29. Ulmer, B.C. (2007). Electrosurgery Self Study Guide. Boulder: Valleylab/Covidien.

30. Wang, K. and Yan, G. (2007). Micro robot prototype for colonoscopy and in vitro experiments. *Journal of Medical Engineering & Technology, 31* (1), 24–28.

31. Zuber, T. (2001). Flexible sigmoidoscopy. *American Family Physician, 63* (7), 1375–1380.

CHAPTER 35

Interventional Radiology

Brenda C. Ulmer

Melissa James Browning

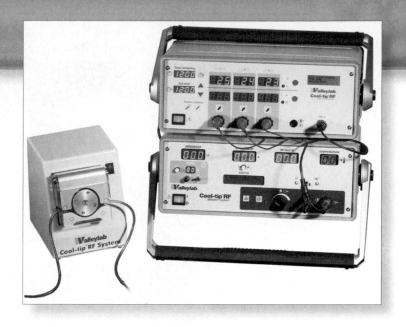

INTRODUCTION

"The apparition was so awful that Wilhelm Conrad Röntgen wondered if he had taken leave of his senses. He could hardly have been more surprised if he had looked into a mirror and no reflection stared back. It was approaching midnight on November 8, 1895. For some time scientists had been reporting bizarre apparitions when they electrified the thin gas in vacuum tubes. The English physicist William Crookes, who saw unearthly luminous clouds floating in the air, had become convinced that he was producing ectoplasm, much beloved of Victorian seances, and had turned to spiritualism as a result. In Germany Röntgen was doing similar experiments and now, alone in the night, his imagination ran wild." (Imaging Life, 2008).

The history of medical imaging began in Germany in 1895. Wilhelm Conrad Röntgen (**Fig. 35.1**) was studying the effect of cathode-ray tubes and how they emitted light. On the evening of November 8, Röntgen noticed a glowing fluorescent screen too far from the tube to be affected by the cathode rays. After many weeks Röntgen discovered that the impact of cathode rays on the glass vacuum tube had generated a new invisible ray. The rays had the power to travel across space and penetrate objects, and the images could be recorded on photographic plates. By Christmas Röntgen had written a paper on his new kind of rays, which he called "X" rays to denote their unknown quality. Wilhelm Conrad Röntgen won the Nobel Prize in 1901 for his discovery of X-rays (Imaging Life, 2008).

Chapter Contents

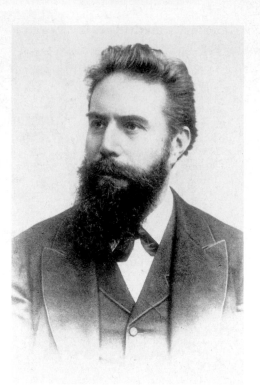

Figure 35.1
Wilhelm Conrad Röntgen (1845–1923). Munich University, Munich, Germany. Nobel Prize 1901.

The ability to visualize inside the human body without opening it revolutionized medicine. From these revolutionary beginnings the specialty of interventional radiology has emerged. The evolution of X-rays, fluoroscopy, CT, and MRI have paved the way for image-guided therapies such as radiofrequency ablation and microwave in minimally invasive cancer treatment.

INTERVENTIONAL RADIOLOGY

Imaging by radiant energy is the specialized field of medicine that encompasses radiology. Radiologists are medical doctors who have completed a four-year residency program studying the interpretation and diagnoses of radiological examinations. Following residency, extended training is available in the more specialized areas, one of which is interventional radiology. As the number of imaging technologies has expanded, so too has the field of interventional radiology. Some of the technologies used by interventional radiologists to gain access to organs and organ systems within the body include:

MRI
Magnetic Resonance Imaging

CT
Computed Tomography

- General X-rays (many types)
- Magnetic resonance imaging (MRI)
- Computed tomography (CT)
- Diagnostic ultrasound
- Fluoroscopy

The interventional radiologist uses image-guided systems along with a growing array of instruments, catheters, stents, balloons, and specialized equipment to diagnosis and treat diseases. Interventional radiology overlaps with many surgical specialties such as general surgery, cardiac surgery, and vascular surgery. For this reason, surgeons are now performing interventional radiology (IR) techniques. The advantage over traditional surgery is that IR procedures are minimally invasive, reducing the length of hospital stays and the long recovery period associated with open surgical procedures. Procedures being performed in interventional radiology suites include, but are not limited to:

- Angioplasty
- Thrombolysis
- Embolization
- Biopsy and abscess drainage
- Biliary procedures
- Genitourinary procedures
- Radiofrequency ablation
- Microwave ablation

The Interventional Radiology Team

During interventional radiology procedures a specialized team provides care. A registered nurse and radiology technologists work with the radiologist. The interventional radiologist registered nurse is a licensed professional nurse who plans and coordinates patient care in the radiology suite. Duties of the registered nurse may include:

- Provides/coordinates care by using the nursing process, including evaluation of the patient's response to care
- Responsible for patient/family education and health maintenance strategies
- Collaborates with team members to achieve patient care goals
- Demonstrates knowledge of principles of human growth and development
- Assesses data reflective of patient health status
- Interprets information to identify patient needs
- Provides professional nursing care to interventional radiology patients by:
  - Documenting patient care
  - Assisting with procedures
  - Circulating/scrubbing
  - Assisting in quality improvement process
  - Intervening in cardiac arrest/pain management
  - Managing categories of disease processes and surgical procedures
  - Serving as a resource to team members (Beth Israel Hospital, 2008)

A radiology technologist is also part of the care team. The radiology technologist has completed specialized training in the field of medical imaging. Under the direction of the physician and the registered nurse, radiology technologists produce x-ray films and imaging studies during the care of patients. The technologists assist in patient preparation and must be familiar with sophisticated imaging equipment and proper patient position to assure good images. The technologist must also know the supplies and equipment necessary to successfully treat interventional radiology patients (US Department of Labor, 2008).

The field of interventional radiology involves procedures that were once only done in operating rooms and involve most major systems within the human body. The advancements in imaging and the decreasing size of instruments and equipment have prompted the growth of minimally invasive procedures in the radiology suite as well as in the surgical suite. Abscess draining, tissue biopsies, stent placement, and vascular clot removal are a few of the procedures done in radiology suites. Among the procedures most amenable to interventional radiology are those involving cancer treatment with radiofrequency (RF) tissue ablation. The continued increase of cancer in the United States is part of the reason for growth in this field, as is the advantage of being able to treat patients with minimally invasive techniques.

RF
Radiofrequency

The number of new cases of cancer each year is staggering. In 2007, the latest year for which statistics are available, there were 1,444,920 new cases of cancer diagnosed (**Fig. 35.2**). There were 559,650 estimated deaths from cancer (**Fig. 35.3**) (American Cancer Society, 2007). Given those numbers it is not surprising that medical science and the healthcare industry continue to search for more effective methods to treat cancer. Cancer affects all parts of the body. Historically, the available treatments were surgery, chemotherapy, or radiation therapy. The advent of RF ablation techniques have given physicians and patients an additional treatment option in the fight against cancer.

SPECIALIZED INSTRUMENTS, EQUIPMENT, AND SUPPLIES

Ultrasound

In the interventional radiology suite ultrasound (sonography) is used to guide placement of the percutaneous devices used during treatment. The ultrasound unit uses sound waves to produce internal images. During ultrasound use, sound waves

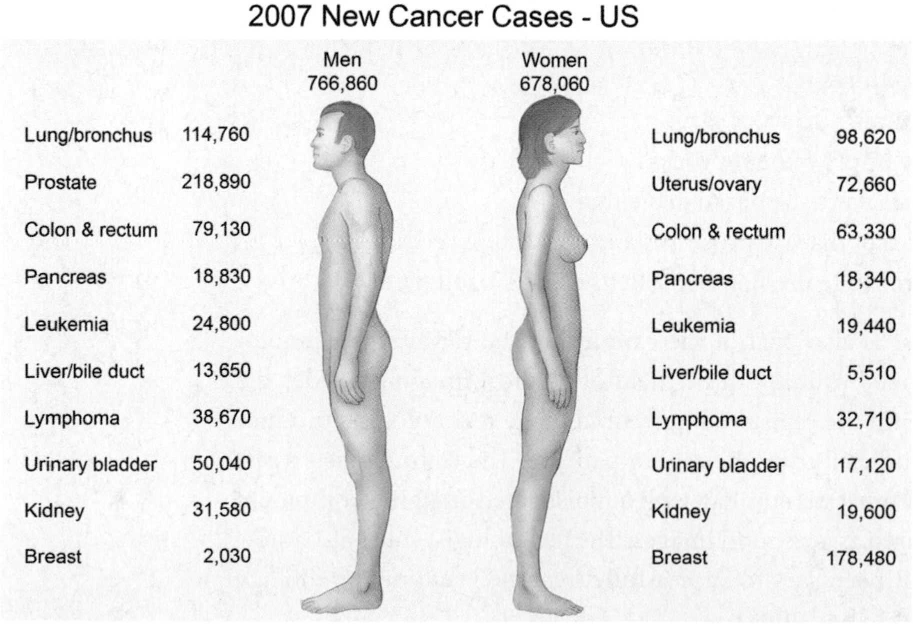

2007 New Cancer Cases - US

	Men 766,860		Women 678,060	
Lung/bronchus	114,760	Lung/bronchus	98,620
Prostate	218,890	Uterus/ovary	72,660
Colon & rectum	79,130	Colon & rectum	63,330
Pancreas	18,830	Pancreas	18,340
Leukemia	24,800	Leukemia	19,440
Liver/bile duct	13,650	Liver/bile duct	5,510
Lymphoma	38,670	Lymphoma	32,710
Urinary bladder	50,040	Urinary bladder	17,120
Kidney	31,580	Kidney	19,600
Breast	2,030	Breast	178,480

Figure 35.2

Estimated new cancer cases, 2007.

Source: Cancer Facts & Figures, 2007.

2007 Cancer Deaths—United States

Brain/Nervous System	12,740
Female Breast	40,460
Colon/Rectum	52,180
Leukemia	21,790
Liver	16,780
Lung/Bronchus	160,390
Non-Hodgkin Lymphoma	18,660
Ovary	15,280
Pancreas	33,370
Prostate	27,050
	559,650

Figure 35.3

2007 Cancer Deaths–United States.

Source: American Cancer Society, 2007.

bounce off organs and tissues like an echo to create pictures or images. The images can be viewed in "real time" on a computer monitor. Still pictures of the images can also be captured.

Radiofrequency Ablation (RFA) Devices

Radiofrequency ablation systems include a generator that produces high-frequency electrical current, and accessories that connect the patient to the equipment. The device produces high-frequency alternating current that causes ionic agitation within tissue that is converted to heat. The heat causes cellular death through coagulation necrosis (**Fig. 35.4**) (Berber, Pelley, and Siperstein, 2005).

RFA
Radiofrequency Ablation

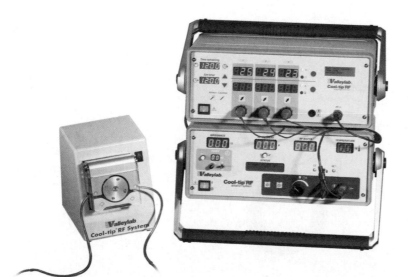

Figure 35.4

Radiofrequency ablation unit.

Source: Copyright © Covidien. All rights reserved. Reprinted with the permission of the Energy-Based Devices and Surgical Devices divisions of Covidien.

The RFA system includes electrodes that deliver the energy from the generator to the patient. The electrodes may be a single straight needle electrode, or multiple electrodes that are deployed directly into the tumor (**Fig. 35.5**).

An important component of the ablation system are the patient return electrodes, also referred to as grounding pads. The pads provide a pathway for the current to return to the RFA generator. Because of the way the current is delivered during RFA procedures it is necessary to use 2 or 4 patient return electrodes to effectively disperse the electrical current and prevent patient pad site burns. The interventional radiology team must be familiar with how the pads should be placed on the patient to assure proper function (Goldberg & Solbiati et al, 2000).

Microwave

One of the most recent treatment modalities available to the interventional radiologist is microwave ablation technology. The energy is delivered to the patient in a manner similar to radiofrequency ablation. During treatment an antenna is placed directly into the tumor. The antenna radiates an energetic field into the tissue. The microwave ablation system uses rotation of water molecules to create frictional heat, which causes higher temperatures resulting in larger ablation zones and reduced treatment times (**Fig. 35.6**). Though still in its infancy, the technology offers promise of an additional treatment method available to practitioners and patients. An important consideration with the microwave technology is that with patient return electrodes (grounding pads) are not necessary since current does not flow through the patient (Wasser and Dupuy, 2008).

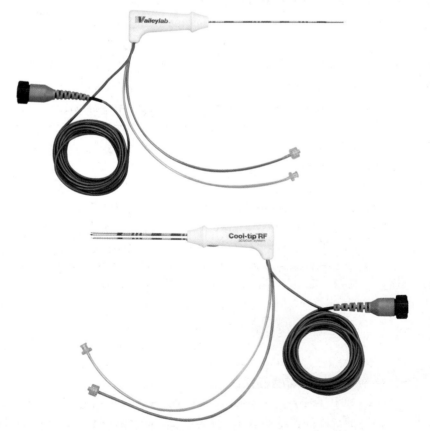

Figure 35.5

Radiofrequency ablation electrodes.

Source: Copyright © Covidien. All rights reserved. Reprinted with the permission of the Energy-Based Devices and Surgical Devices divisions of Covidien.

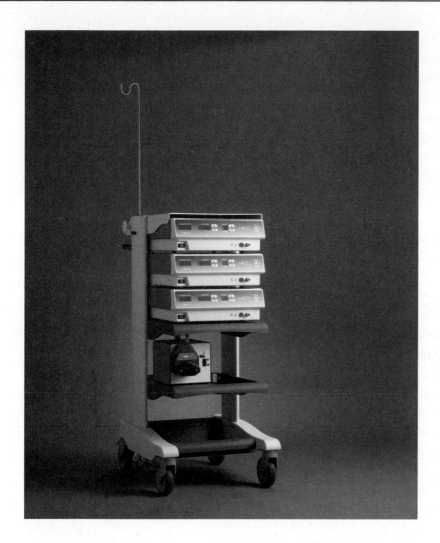

Figure 35.6

Microwave Ablation System.

35

RADIOFREQUENCY ABLATION PROCEDURES

Radiofrequency Ablation of Liver Tumors

Interventional radiology radiofrequency ablation of liver tumors is a percutaneous method that uses high temperatures to destroy cancer cells. It is a minimally invasive procedure using image-guided technology.

Indications

Ablation of liver tumors is indicated in patients with inoperable primary or metastatic tumors of the liver. Hepatocellular carcinoma (HCC) is the fifth most common cancer worldwide. It is most prevalent in Asia but the incidence is increasing in the West (Ng & Poon 2005; Ng, Lam, & Poon et al, 2003). HCC develops most frequently in patients with cirrhosis, with 60–90% of HCC tumors occurring in cirrhotic livers (Raut, Izzo, & Marra et al, 2005). Treatment options for these patients are limited. Opportunities for resection are rare due to limited normal liver parenchyma and, in addition, hepatic dysfunction caused by cirrhosis increases the risk of postoperative liver failure and death. Chemotherapy offers little to no benefit and is associated with reduced quality of life (Raut, Izzo, & Mara et al, 2005).

The liver is a common site of metastases from a number of malignancies, often from colorectal tumors via the venous drainage through the portal vein. Extra-abdominal

HCC
Hepatocellular
Carcinoma

tumors such as bronchogenic carcinoma, breast cancer, and malignant melanoma also metastasize to the liver. There is a high incidence of all of these cancer types that spread to the liver (American Cancer Society, 2007).

Related Procedures

Radiofrequency ablation of renal tumors is a similar procedure.

Nursing Implications

ANESTHESIA

Anesthesia may be local with IV sedation or general anesthesia depending on the patient and the complexity of the procedure and physician/patient preferences. Vital signs will be monitored.

POSITION

The patient is positioned in the supine position on the operating bed. Positioning devices may be used to improve access to the operative site as needed. A pillow may be placed under the patient's head and knees for comfort during the procedure.

ESTABLISHING AND MAINTAINING THE STERILE FIELD

The patient is prepped with the physician's choice of prep solution. If an alcohol-based prep solution is used, the prep should be allowed to dry to prevent flammable vapors from being trapped under the drapes. The sterile field is established with sterile towels and drapes. The sterile electrodes and other sterile supplies are delivered to the sterile field in accordance with AORN *Perioperative Standards and Recommending Practices* (AORN, 2008).

LABORATORY AND DIAGNOSTIC STUDIES

Laboratory and diagnostic studies are dictated by facility policies and health status of the patient. The studies may include:

- History and physical
- Liver imaging studies
- Chest or bone imaging studies
- Biopsy results
- Laboratory blood work (CBC, BUN/Creatinine, PT/PTT/INR)

Procedure

After the patient is positioned, prepped, and draped, local anesthesia is administered to the patient under IV conscious sedation. The radiofrequency ablation electrode is inserted into the liver under ultrasound guidance. Once the electrode is in place, the generator is activated according to manufacturer's suggested guidelines to achieve the target temperature within the lesion (**Fig. 35.7**). Activation times are dependent on the size of the tumor. Larger tumors may require multiple activations of the electrode. The development of the hyperechoic heat lesion can be observed as it forms by use of ultrasound. A margin of normal hepatic parenchyma should surround the ablated tumor to achieve adequate clean margins. After completion of the procedure, the

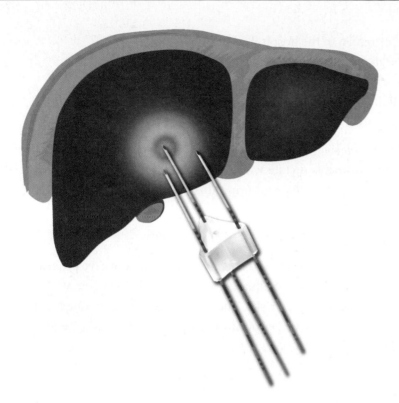

Figure 35.7

Radiofrequency ablation electrode activated within the liver.

Source: Copyright © Covidien. All rights reserved. Reprinted with the permission of the Energy-Based Devices and Surgical Devices divisions of Covidien.

35

pathway of the electrode can be cauterized as it is removed to reduce the likelihood of postprocedure bleeding (Amersi, McElrath-Garza, & Ahmad et al, 2006).

Postprocedure Care

Following radiofrequency ablation patient vital signs are monitored. Outpatients are discharged home in the company of a responsible adult after recovery from sedation when fluids can be taken by mouth and after urination. The recovery period is normally between 2–4 hours. Postprocedure pain medications are prescribed by the physician. If a patient is to be admitted for observation, then he/she is transferred to the floor (Wah, Arellano, & Gervais et al, 2005).

Some patients may develop post ablation syndrome. It is a combination of symptoms that resemble the flu. Symptoms include fever, malaise, pain, nausea, or vomiting. The symptoms can occur from 24 hours up to 10 days after ablation. Patients should be informed of the possibility of experiencing these symptoms (Wah, Arellano, & Gervais et al, 2005). Other postprocedure instructions may include:

- No strenuous exercise or heavy lifting for one week
- Do not drive or drink alcohol until complete recovery from sedation
- If taking medication, contact primary physician for instructions on resuming medications
- Soreness at the puncture site is normal
- Pain/soreness in the area of the liver is normal
- Some referred shoulder pain may occur and is normal
- Drink plenty of fluids
- Resume normal diet as tolerated

- Call physician or return to the hospital for:
  - Fever greater than 101° F
  - Inability to urinate
  - Breathing difficulty
  - Blood in urine after 3 days

Patients will normally receive followup image studies at specified periods after radiofrequency. Facility protocols dictate when the studies are done. A CT may be ordered within one month, 3 months, and 6 months (Amersi, McElrath-Garza, & Ahmad et al, 2006).

Potential Complications

Radiofrequency liver ablation is a safe and effective minimally invasive procedure with low complication rates (Livraghi, Solbiati, & Meloni et al, 2003). As with any invasive procedure, however, there are risks. The risks should be explained to the patient as part of the informed consent procedure. Risks following radiofrequency liver ablation include:

- Bleeding, hemorrhage (bleeding from liver could be delayed onset)
- Infection or abscess
- Heat injury within the abdomen
- Pad site burn
- Bile duct injuries (Amersi, McElrath-Garza, Ahmad, et al, 2006).

Radiofrequency Ablation of Renal Tumors

Interventional radiology radiofrequency ablation of renal tumors is a percutaneous method that uses high temperatures to destroy small renal tumors. It is a minimally invasive procedure using image guided technology.

Indications

In 2007 an estimated 51,190 new cases of renal carcinoma were diagnosed (**Fig. 35.2**) (American Cancer Society, 2007). The standard treatment for renal cell carcinoma has been radical nephrectomy. There are, however, patients who cannot undergo radical nephrectomy or who refuse to do so. The decreased morbidity associated with the minimally invasive ablation techniques makes the procedure an attractive alternative. Treatment of small renal cell carcinomas with radiofrequency ablation has proven to be a viable choice of therapies (Zagoria, Traver, & Werle et al, 2007).

Related Procedures

Radiofrequency ablation of liver tumors is a related procedure, as is radiofrequency ablation of adrenal masses (Mayo-Smith & Dupuy, 2004).

Nursing Implications

ANESTHESIA

Anesthesia may be local with IV sedation or general anesthesia depending on the patient and the complexity of the procedure and physician/patient preferences. Vital signs will be monitored.

35

POSITION

The patient is positioned in the supine position on the operating bed. Positioning devices may be used to improve access to the operative site as needed. A pillow may be placed under the patient's head and knees for comfort during the procedure.

ESTABLISHING AND MAINTAINING THE STERILE FIELD

The patient procedure is prepped with the physician's choice of prep solution. If an alcohol-based prep solution is used, the prep should be allowed to dry to prevent flammable vapors from being trapped under the drapes. The sterile field is established with sterile towels and drapes. The sterile electrodes and other sterile supplies are delivered to the sterile field in accordance with AORN *Perioperative Standards and Recommending Practices* (AORN, 2008).

LABORATORY AND DIAGNOSTIC STUDIES

Patients should be carefully evaluated prior to the procedure to determine the extent of the disease by diagnostic imaging techniques. Some interventional radiologists may want a definitive biopsy of the tumor(s) prior to the procedure. Other laboratory studies that may be ordered include:

- PT/PTT
- CBD
- Creatinine
- History and Physical (Hines-Peralta & Goldberg, 2004)

Procedure

After the patient is positioned, prepped, and draped, local anesthesia is administered to the patient under IV conscious sedation. The radiofrequency ablation electrode is inserted into the lesion under ultrasound or CT guidance. Once the electrode is in place, the generator is activated according to manufacturer's suggested guidelines to achieve the target temperature within the lesion. Activation times are dependent on the size of the tumor, as is the selection of the electrode. Overlapping ablations may be performed as needed (Allaf, Varkarakis, & Bhayani et al, 2005).

Postprocedure Care

Following radiofrequency ablation, patient's vital signs are monitored. Outpatients are discharged home in the company of a responsible adult after recovery from sedation when fluids can be taken by mouth and after urination. The recovery period is normally between 2–4 hours. Postprocedure pain medications are prescribed by the physician. If a patient is to be admitted for observation, then he/she is transferred to the floor.

Some patients may develop postablation syndrome. It is a combination of symptoms that resemble the flu. Symptoms include fever, malaise, pain, nausea, or vomiting. The symptoms can occur from 24 hours up to 10 days after ablation. Patients should be informed of the possibility of experiencing these symptoms (Tze, Arellano, & Gervais et al, 2005). Other postprocedure instructions may include:

- No strenuous exercise or heavy lifting for one week
- Do not drive or drink alcohol until complete recovery from sedation

- If taking medication, contact primary physician for instructions on resuming medications
- Soreness at the puncture site is normal
- Blood in the urine is normal and may be pink-tinged for up to 1 week
- Some referred shoulder pain may occur and is normal
- Drink plenty of fluids
- Resume normal diet as tolerated
- Call physician or return to the hospital for:
  - Fever greater than 101° F
  - Inability to urinate
  - Breathing difficulty
  - Red blood in urine after 3 days
  - Pain not relieved by medication
  - Pain that increases in intensity

The success of the ablation procedure should be assessed about one month after the procedure, and at intervals established by protocols following that (Hines-Peralta & Goldberg, 2004).

Complications

Radiofrequency ablation of renal tumors has been proven to be safe with a low incidence of complications. As with any invasive procedure, however, complications can occur. These should be explained to the patient as part of the preprocedure informed consent process. Complications associated with radiofrequency ablation of renal tumors include:

- Bleeding/hemorrhage
- Death
- Infection
- Thermal damage to adjacent structures
- Bile leak
- Lung collapse/pneumothorax
- Tumor seeding
- Return electrode (grounding pad) burns (Rhim, Dodd, & Chintapalli et al, 2004)

Radiofrequency Ablation of Lung Tumors

Interventional radiology radiofrequency ablation of lung tumors is a percutaneous method that uses high temperatures to destroy cancer cells. It is a minimally invasive procedure using image-guided technology.

Indications

Statistics for 2007 indicate that there were 213,380 new cases of lung cancer diagnosed (**Fig. 35.2**) (American Cancer Society, 2007). By the time lung cancer is diagnosed, 85% of the patients are inoperable. Radiofrequency ablation in selected patients may be a minimally invasive nonsurgical option for patients who have lesions of less than 3 cm in diameter (Mayo Clinic, 2008).

Related Procedures

Other radiofrequency ablation procedures are similar, but there are no other specifically related procedures to radiofrequency ablation of the lung.

Nursing Implications

ANESTHESIA

Anesthesia may be local with IV sedation or general anesthesia depending on the patient and the complexity of the procedure and physician/patient preferences. Vital signs will be monitored.

ESTABLISHING AND MAINTAINING THE STERILE FIELD

The patient procedure site is prepped with the physician's choice of prep solution. If an alcohol-based prep solution is used, the prep should be allowed to dry to prevent flammable vapors from being trapped under the drapes. The sterile field is established with sterile towels and drapes. The sterile electrodes and other sterile supplies are delivered to the sterile field in accordance with AORN *Perioperative Standards and Recommending Practices* (AORN, 2008).

LABORATORY AND DIAGNOSTIC STUDIES

Patients should be carefully evaluated prior to the procedure to determine the extent of the disease by diagnostic imaging techniques. Some interventional radiologists may want a definitive biopsy of the tumor(s) prior to the procedure. Other laboratory studies that may be ordered include:

- PT/PTT
- CBD
- Creatinine
- History and Physical
- Imaging studies

Procedure

After the patient is positioned, prepped, and draped, local anesthesia is administered to the patient under IV conscious sedation. Guide needles are inserted into the patient to create the best pathway to the lesion. The position is confirmed using ultrasound or CT followed by introduction of the radiofrequency ablation electrode. Treatment with the electrode should be in accordance with the manufacturer's recommendations of the time it will take to achieve target temperatures within the tumor. Treatment times will vary depending on the type of electrode being used and the size of the tumor. The electrode will be expanded beyond the perimeter of the tumor to create a margin of normal tissue surrounding the tumor. The radiofrequency ablation generator and the internally water-cooled electrode deliver energy automatically in pulses in response to increased impedance within the tissue. The variations in treatment times and number of ablations are patient-specific. A 2008 study by Gillams and Lees documented treatment times ranging from 3 to 53 minutes, with number of ablations ranging from 1 to 6 (Gillams & Lees, 2008).

Postprocedure Care

Following radiofrequency ablation patient vital signs are monitored. A chest x-ray may be done to rule out a pneumothorax. Outpatients are discharged home in the company of a responsible adult after recovery from sedation when fluids can be taken by mouth and after urination. The recovery period is normally between 2–4 hours. Postprocedure pain medications are prescribed by the physician. If a patient is to be admitted for observation, then he/she is transferred to the floor. Some patients may develop postablation syndrome. It is a combination of symptoms that resemble the flu. Symptoms include fever, malaise, pain, nausea, or vomiting. The symptoms can occur from 24 hours up to 10 days after ablation. Patients should be informed of the possibility of experiencing these symptoms (Tze, Arellano, & Gervais et al, 2005). Other postprocedure instructions may include:

- No strenuous exercise or heavy lifting for one week
- Do not drive or drink alcohol until complete recovery from sedation
- If taking medication, contact primary physician for instructions on resuming medications
- Soreness at the puncture site is normal
- May experience flu-like symptoms
- Drink plenty of fluids
- Resume normal diet as tolerated
- Call physician or return to the hospital for:
  - Fever greater than 101° F
  - Coughing up large amounts of red blood
  - Breathing difficulty
  - Pain not relieved by medication
  - Pain that increases in intensity

Complications

Complications associated with minimally invasive radiofrequency ablation are less than those associated with open thoracic procedures; however, as with any invasive procedure, complications may occur. Complications should be explained to the patient as part of the preprocedure consent process and include:

- Bleeding
- Pneumothorax (chest tube inserted)
- Air embolism
- Fever
- Burns to adjacent tissues
- Pneumonia
- Pleural effusion
- Nerve damage
- Return electrode (grounding pad) burn
- Death (RFA, 2008)

CONCLUSION

Radiofrequency ablation of cancerous tumors gives patients and medical practitioners an additional method to relieve symptoms and aim for a cure. Studies have indicated the minimally invasive techniques show promise for the future as the technology continues to advance. Other cancers that are currently being treated with radiofrequency ablation but to a lesser degree include bone, breast, and adrenal tumors. Patients with a diagnosis of cancer often have little hope. Adding low-risk therapies as an option to patients may help to improve the quality of life.

The author wishes to thank Melissa James Browning for her assistance.

REFERENCES

1. Allaf, M.E., Varkarakis, I.M., Bhayani, S.B., Inagaki, T.I., Kavoussi, L.R., and Solomon, S.B. (2005). Pain control requirements for percutaneous ablation of renal tumor: cryoablation versus radiofrequency ablation—initial observations. *Radiology, 237*; 366–370.

2. American Cancer Society (2007). *Cancer Facts & Figures, 2007.* Atlanta: American Cancer Society.

3. Amersi, F.F., McElrath-Garza, A., Ahmad, A., Zogakis, T., Allegra, D.P., Krasne, R., and Bilchik, A.J. (2006). Long-term survival after radiofrequency ablation of complex unresectable liver tumors. *Archives of Surgery, 141*; 581–588.

4. AORN. (2008). *Perioperative Standards and Recommending Practices.* Denver, CO: AORN Inc.

5. Berber, E., Pelley, R., and Siperstein, A.E. (2005). Predictors of survival after radiofrequency thermal ablatin of colorectal cancer metastases to the liver: a prospective study. *Journal of Clinical Oncology, 23*(7); 1358–1364.

6. Beth Israel Hospital Job Description. (2008, August 27). Registered Nurse-Interventional Radiology. Online at Monster.com. Available at http://jobview.monster.com. Accessed August 27, 2008.

7. Gillams, A.R., and Lees, W.R. (2008). Radiofrequency ablation of lung metastases: factors influencing success. *European Radiology, 18*; 672–677.

8. Goldberg, S.N., Solbiati, L., Halpern, E.F., and Gazelle, G.S. (2000). Variables affecting proper system grounding for radiofrequency ablation in an animal model. *Journal of Vascular and Interventional Radiology, 11*; 1069–1075.

9. Hines-Peralta, A., and Goldberg, S.N. (2004). Review of radiofrequency ablation for renal cell carcinoma. *Clinical Cancer Research, Vol 10*; 6328–6334.

10. Imaging Life. (2008, August 26). Imaging Life—Physics 1901. *Online Nobelprize.org.* Available at http://nobelprize.org. Accessed August 26, 2008.

11. Livraghi, T., Solbiati, L., Meloni, F., et al. (2003). Treatment of focal liver tumors with percutaneous radiofrequency ablation: complications encountered in a multi-center study. *Radiology, 226*; 441–451.

12. Mayo Clinic (August 29, 2008). Radiofrequency Ablation for lung cancer. Online a MayoClinic.org.

Available at http://www.mayoclinic.orgradiofrequency-ablation/lung.html. Accessed August 29, 2008.

13. Mayo-Smith, W.W., and Dupuy, D.E. (2004). Adrenal neoplasms: CT-guided radiofrequency ablation—preliminary results. *Radiology, 231*; 225–230.

14. Ng, L., & Poon, R. (2005). Radiofrequency ablation for malignant liver tumor. *Surgical Oncology, 14*; 41–52.

15. Ng, L., Lam, C., Poon, R., Fan, S., et al. (2003). Thermal ablative therapy for malignant liver tumors: a critical appraisal. *Journal of Gastroenterology and Hepatology, 18*; 616–629.

16. Raut, C., Izzo, F., Marra, P., Curley, S., et al. (2005). Significant long-term survival after radiofrequency ablation of unresectable hepatocellular carcinoma in patients with cirrhosis. *Annals of Surgery, 12*(8); 616–628.

17. RFA (August 29, 2008). Radiofrequency ablation of lung cancer. Online at RFAlung.com. Available at http://www.rfalung.com/treatment.html. Accessed August 29, 2008.

18. Rhim, H. Dodd, G.D., Chintapalli, K.N., Wood, B.J., Dupuy, D.E., Hvizda, J.L., Sewell, P.E., and Goldberg, N. (2004). Radiofrequency thermal ablation of abdominal tumor: lessons learned from complications. *Radiographics, 24*: 41–52.

19. US Department of Labor. (2008, August 27). *Occupational Outlook Handbook—2008–2009.* Available at http://www.bls.gov. Accessed August 27, 2008.

20. Wah, T.M., Arellano, R.S., Gervais, D.A., Saltalamacchia, C.A., Martino, J., Halpern, E.F., Maher, M., and Mueller, P.R. (2005). Image-guided percutaneous radiofrequency ablation and incidence of post-radiofrequency ablation syndrome: prospective survey. *Radiology, 237*; 1097–1102.

21. Wasser, E.J., and Dupuy, D.E. (2008). Microwave ablation in the treatment of primary lung cancer. *Semin Respir Crit Car Med, 29*(4); 384–394.

22. Zagoria, R.J., Traver, M.A., Werle, D.M., Perini, M., Hayasaka, S, and Clark, P.E. (2007). Oncologic efficacy of CT-guided percutaneous radiofrequency ablation of renal cell carcinomas. *Am J Roentgenol, 189*(2); 429–436.

CHAPTER *36*

Clinical Aspects of Operative Pain

Mary Beth Kean

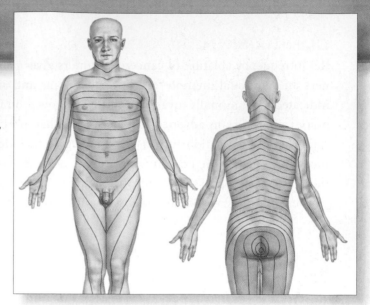

DEFINITION OF PAIN

The International Association for the Study of Pain (IASP) defines pain as "an unpleasant sensory and emotional experience associated with actual or potential tissue damage and described in terms of such damage" (Task Force on Taxonomy of the International Association for the Study of Pain, 1994). This definition reflects the complexity of the pain experience involving physiologic and interpretive/emotional components. McCaffery (1979) defines pain as "what the experiencing person says it is and exists whenever he or she says it does." This definition best reflects the subjective nature of pain and the requirement for clinicians to believe patient reports. See **Table 36.1** for a glossary of pain-related terms.

SCOPE OF THE PROBLEM

The United States Congress has designated the years between 2000 and 2010 as the Decade of Pain Control and Research. Significant efforts to improve the management of pain have yielded results in the form of published guidelines, position statements, state and federal law revisions, and, most recognizably, the Joint Commission of Healthcare Accreditation Organization's pain management standard implementation in 2001 (Gordon et al., 2002). Adherence to published guidelines combined with institutional commitment to making pain management a valued part of the culture can result in improved outcomes for postsurgical populations

Despite these efforts, patients receiving analgesics continue to experience moderate to severe pain following operative procedures

Chapter Contents

IASP
International Association for the Study of Pain

Table 36.1	Glossary of Pain Terms
Aberrant drug-related behavior	Culture-bound determination of problematic drug-related behavior ranging from unsanctioned analgesic dose escalations in times of pain flare or requesting specific medications to injecting oral formulations or forging prescriptions
Addiction	A primary, chronic, neurobiologic disease with genetic, psychosocial, and environmental factors influencing its development and manifestations; involves compulsive desire to use a drug despite continued harm
Allodynia	The presence of pain from a stimulus that is not normally painful
Analgesia	Insensibility to pain without loss of consciousness
Anesthesia	Loss of sensation and usually of consciousness without loss of vital functions artificially produced by the administration of one or more agents that block the passage of pain impulses along the nerve pathways to the brain
Central sensitization	Process by which pain is amplified and maintained centrally as in the spinal cord or brain in addition to the processes in the peripheral tissues; Thought to underlie some types of allodynia or hyperalgesia
Controlled substances	Medications regulated by law as to possession and use
Endorphins	Any of a group of endogenous peptides (as enkephalin and dynorphin) that are found especially in the brain and produce some of the same pain relief effects as the opioids
Hyperalgesia	A phenomenon whereby stimuli that are normally painful produce exaggerated pain
Multimodal analgesia	A combination regimen using two or more medications, interventional and nonpharmacologic techniques allowing for the reduced doses of medications and, therefore, reduced side effect profile
Neuropathic pain	Pain that is caused by a lesion or dysfunction of the nervous system
Neuroplasticity	The brain's ability to reorganize itself by forming new neural connections throughout life; allows neurons in the brain to compensate for injury and disease and to adjust their activities in response to new situations or to changes in their environment (MedicineNet.com, 2008)
Neurotransmitter	A substance (as norepinephrine or serotonin) that transmits a nerve impulse across a synapse
Nociceptor	A receptor for painful stimuli
Opioid induced hyperalgesia	A clinical phenomenon characterized by increasing pain in patients who are receiving increasing doses of opioids
Physical dependence	A state of adaptation that is manifested by a drug class-specific withdrawal syndrome that can be produced by abrupt cessation, rapid dose reduction, decreasing blood levels of the drug, or administration of an antagonist
Preemptive analgesia	Involves the introduction of an analgesic regimen before the onset of noxious stimuli, with the goal of preventing sensitization of the nervous system to subsequent stimuli that could amplify pain
Pseudo-addiction	A term used to describe behavior that appears like addictive "drug-seeking" behavior but is actually an effort to obtain pain relief; behaviors from pseudo-addiction are said to be distinguished from addictive behaviors when the behaviors resolve after treatment of pain

36

Somatic pain	Pain arising from somatic structures such as skin, bones, or joints and is typically well localized and worsened by palpation of the affected part
Tolerance	The loss of effect of a pharmacologic agent over a prolonged period of use, or the need to escalate the dose of the agent to maintain the same pharmacologic effect
Visceral pain	Pain arising from pathology of the visceral organs such a bowel obstruction or pancreatitis and is generally poorly localized and associated with visceral symptoms such as nausea and vomiting
Wind up	The process observed in experimental animals whereby repeated stimulation of a peripheral structure with a stimulus produces increasing central response/pain

MedicineNet.com. (2008). Retrieved 11 September 2008 from MedicineNet.com Web site: http://www.medterms.com/script/main/art.asp?articlekey=40362

at a rate of 70–80% with one-quarter experiencing pain into the late postprocedure period (Diaz & Flood, 2006). Acute postprocedure pain can be followed by persistent chronic pain in 10–50% of patients undergoing common operations such as groin hernia repair, amputation, mastectomy, and coronary artery bypass graft, and can become severe in 2–10% of these patients (Kehlet, Jenson & Woolf, 2006). Consequences of unrelieved postprocedure pain include decreased and delayed physical mobility, decreased gastric motility, increased rate of complications such as pulmonary embolism and pneumonia, increased hospital length of stay, increased hospital readmission, and decreased patient satisfaction (Diaz & Flood, 2006; Carrroll et al., 2004).

Pain has been directly associated with tremendous healthcare costs, estimated at $100 billion annually in direct healthcare expenses, lost income, and lost productivity. Chronic pain has been shown to account for greater total annual costs than other chronic conditions, including heart disease, hypertension, and diabetes (American Pain Foundation, 2008). Poorly treated chronic pain and lack of access to care has resulted in inappropriate utilization of Emergency Departments as pain patients desperately seek help (American Pain Foundation, 2008).

Advances in the science of medical imaging, genetics, and particularly pharmacogenomics promise future improvements in understanding variations in pain reports and treatment effects in patients (Smith, 2008; O'Malley, 2007). Emerging techniques in the field of robotics may result in decreased pain as procedures become less invasive.

BARRIERS TO EFFECTIVE PAIN MANAGEMENT
Professional Education

Professional education initiatives in the field of pain management have not kept pace with scientific advances, creating significant barriers resulting in inadequate pain management for patients. Barriers contributing to poor pain management originate in part from lack of dedicated standardized pain management curriculum in nursing, pharmacy, and medical schools (Ralston, 1996, Ury et al., 2002).

Knowledge deficits have not only resulted in suboptimal patient outcomes but also unfounded fears of regulatory scrutiny specifically surrounding prescribing, dispensing, and administering opioid analgesics (National Councils for State Boards of Nursing, 2007).

Inadequate professional education in pain management contributes to confusion related to drug abuse terminology as clinicians mistake symptoms of physiologic dependence and tolerance developed because of the appropriate use of opioids to treat pain as evidence of addictive disorders. Incorporating chronic pain management into practice is particularly complex and requires additional education as healthcare professionals must balance the effective and appropriate use of controlled substances for pain with risks for diversion and potential harmful contribution to substance abuse disorders (Gourlay, 2005).

Substance Abuse and Addiction

Substance abuse disorders develop because of a complex interaction of genetic predisposition, comorbid psychopathologies, environmental influence, and lack of structured access to controlled substances. Consequently, the development of substance abuse disorder is usually not a problem with the short-term use of opioids.

Pain management knowledge deficits often become most apparent when patients with known substance abuse disorders develop painful conditions or require analgesia following an operative or invasive procedure as tolerance is often not taken into consideration when analgesic doses are chosen. Inadequate analgesia combined with perceptions of lack of respect from staff can lead to cycles of antagonistic behaviors in the clinician patient relationship (Morgan, 2006). No evidence exists to suggest withholding analgesics for pain in individuals with substance abuse disorders worsens addictive disease (Alford, Compton, & Samet, 2006; Compton & Athanasos, 2003). Because of the complexity of the pain experience in these populations, effective management often requires triage to appropriate pain management and addiction disorder specialists with an approach including individualized multimodal and preemptive pharmacologic and non-pharmacologic interventions (Gourlay et al., 2005).

The American Society for Pain Management Nurses 2002 position statement identifies patients with addictive disease as having the right to be treated with respect and to receive the same quality of pain management as all other patients. Furthermore, nurses are identified as being in an ideal position to advocate and intervene for these patients across all treatment settings (American Society for Pain Management Nurses, 2002).

Cultural and Socioeconomic Considerations

Socioeconomically disadvantaged and ethnic minority populations are at particular risk for receiving inadequate analgesia (Bonham, 2001; Cintron & Morrison, 2006; Ezenwa et al., 2006). One proposed reason for ethnic disparities may relate to clinicians having difficulty identifying pain in individuals who are culturally different from themselves, resulting in unequal analgesic prescribing practices. Failure to treat pain adequately may result because the nurse could not perform a sufficient assessment due to patient-clinician language barriers (Bonham, 2001).

Evidence also suggests inadequate pain treatment can be associated with hospitals located in primarily minority communities and university medical centers when compared with hospitals located in non-minority neighborhoods (Cintron & Morrison, 2006; Morrison et al., 2000). Following discharge from the hospital clinicians should consider potential variances in opioid availability in retail pharmacies based on location in relation to ethnic and socioeconomic composition of the neighborhood where the pharmacies are located.

Clinicians should also consider evidence suggesting genetic variations account for differences in analgesic effect (Smith, 2008). Differences in response may lead to misinterpretation of behaviors when individuals with these genetic variances require increased analgesic dosing due to rapid metabolism or rotation to alternative medications for efficacy.

Subjective Report

The subjective nature of pain may create another barrier to effective management, as pain measurement is limited to primarily subjective report because there is no reliable physiologic method to measure pain's presence or intensity. Subjective pain ratings for the cognitively intact patient should be elicited routinely prior to and following analgesic administration using a validated pain scale such as a numeric rating scale (see **Fig. 18.2**).

While individuals with mild to moderate cognitive deficits can often self-report pain levels accurately, measurement becomes more complex when assessing patients who are non-verbal or have severe dementia. Recommendations for structured assessment include the use of the Hierarchy of Pain Assessment Techniques (**Table 36.2**) developed by McCaffery and Pasero (1999) and using a validated scale for pain assessment in pediatric patients or patients with dementia as discussed in the pain management in clinical practice section.

Table 36.2	Hierarchy of Pain Assessment Techniques
Self-report	Attempt to gain a self-report from the patient if possible.
Search for potential causes of pain	Assume pain is present if diagnosed with potentially painful disorders.
Observe patient behaviors	Agitation and aggression may indicate pain but may not reflect intensity.
Surrogate reporting of pain and behavior/activity changes	Adopt a multifaceted approach using observation, caregiver input, and response to treatment.
Attempt an analgesic trial	If pain is assumed to be present, start with low doses and titrate to analgesic effect as evidenced by behavioral changes or until side effects limit effect.

Adapted from Herr, K., Coyne, P., Key, T., Manworren, R., McCaffery, M., Merkel, S., et al. (2006). Pain assessment in the nonverbal patient: Position statement with clinical practice recommendations. *Pain Management Nursing, 7*(2); McCaffery, M., Grimm, M., Pasero, C., Ferrell, B., & Uman, G. (2005, December 1). On the meaning of "drug seeking." *Pain Management Nursing, 6*(4), 122–136.

RISKS FOR ADVERSE OUTCOMES FROM PAIN AND ANALGESICS

Age

The world's population is aging, with trends showing 35 million adults aged 65 and older in the US in 2006 (Federal Interagency Forum on Aging-Related Statistics, 2008). Older adults represented 38% of all inpatient admissions in 2005 and underwent 36% of the total inpatient procedures preformed. Healthcare trends indicate expected increase in hospitalized older adults, higher acuity, increased comorbidities, increased polypharmacy with drug interactions, and more hospitalized older adults with pain (Centers for Disease Control and Prevention, 2007). Although aging and pain are not synonymous, pain is a common result of conditions prevalent in the older adult population. Healthcare practitioners often have the erroneous belief that insensitivity to pain occurs with aging; the truth is vulnerability to the negative impact of pain increases with aging (Pasero, 2008).

Older adults will also often have multiple sites of chronic pain and many take analgesics on a daily basis. These patients may report operative pain as less intense than the chronic pain. In addition, the older person may not report pain as frequently as the younger person (Pasero, 2008). The protective nature of pain may be blunted in older adults, complicating diagnosis based on pain intensity and location reports such as peptic ulcers. Risk for fall with fracture also increases with age. Falls may result in painful fractures and fall risk increases the need for monitoring analgesic administration to prevent injury from side effects such as dizziness. Nurses caring for older adults must also consider vision and hearing impairments when assessing patients and providing pain management education (Rakel & Herr, 2004). When caring for older patients consider using a tool with enlarged font (Pasero, 2008). In addition, elders often have misconceptions about pain and thus require education. Misconceptions may include:

- Pain is something the patient must live with
- Expressing pain is unacceptable or is a sign of weakness
- Complaining of pain will label them as a "bad" patient
- Nurses are too busy to listen to complaints of pain
- Pain signifies serious illness or impending death
- Complaints of pain distracts clinicians from treating other diseases

Nurses providing pain management to older adult populations should consider "starting low and going slow" with analgesic titration. While some patients can tolerate regular analgesic doses, nurses may consider reducing opioid doses by 50% to start for opioid naïve elders and titrating the dose up to patient response (Buss & Melderis, 2002; Rakel & Herr, 2004).

Comorbidity Diagnoses Affecting Pharmacologic Effect

Patients with comorbidities affecting pharmacokinetics and pharmacodynamics often present with painful conditions requiring aggressive analgesia. Patients with reduced renal and hepatic clearance should receive special consideration when analgesics are administered in order to prevent analgesic effects and complications (Pasero, 2005).

Patients with decreased gastric pH and motility are at risk for alterations in drug absorption and increased gastrointestinal irritation, bleeding, and ulceration. Patients with decreased lean body mass, increased body fat, decreased total body water, and decreased albumin production may experience alterations in drug distribution. These patients have an increased risk for accumulation of lipid-soluble drugs and toxicity, faster onset of action, and longer duration of action from water-soluble drugs. Patients with decreased hepatic function resulting in altered metabolism have the potential for increased accumulation and toxicity. These patients will require longer intervals between analgesic dosing. Decreased hepatic and renal blood flow results in alterations in elimination, resulting in increased pharmacologic half-life, increased accumulation of metabolites, and potential increased toxicity (Pasero, 2008).

Obstructive Sleep Apnea

Inadequate ventilation results in the patient being unable to perform needed gas exchange, resulting in hypoventilation (respiratory depression). During hypoventilation, the patient generally has hypercapnia and respiratory acidosis. Hypoventilation can occur when patients hold their breath, have certain medical conditions, or take drugs. In addition, for patients with sleep apnea, hypoventilation may be dangerous (Answers.com, 2008). The risk of postprocedure hypoventilation increases with complex operative procedures, prolonged general anesthesia, thoracic or abdominal operative procedures, the need for postprocedure opioids, and the presence and severity of sleep apnea.

Obstructive sleep apnea is defined as a syndrome characterized by episodic, partial, or complete obstruction of the upper airway during sleep (American Society of Anesthesiologists, 2006). Risk factors suggesting the possibility of obstructive sleep apnea include BMI 35 kg/m^2, neck circumference 17 inches for men and 16 inches for women, craniofacial abnormalities affecting airway, anatomical nasal obstruction, and tonsils nearly touching or touching the midline (American Society of Anesthesiologists, 2006). Patients who have a potential diagnosis of obstructive sleep apnea have cessation of airflow during sleep, loud snoring, and/or stop breathing (apnea) for more than 10 seconds, have more than five of these episodes per hour, awake abruptly with a 'snort' as PaO$_2$ drops also called "self-resuscitation," and five to hundreds of these episodes each night. Significant others can be instrumental in reporting these symptoms, as they can be frightening to the listener. Many patients with this condition will be undiagnosed at time of the procedure, requiring increased vigilance by nurses (Windle, 2004).

PATHOPHYSIOLOGY OF PAIN
Perception and Response to Pain

Pain perception is private and subjective. No one but the person experiencing it can accurately articulate the characteristics of the pain. Although pain is perceived in the sensory cortex and is difficult to measure, it can be described as the actual awareness of painful feelings and sensations. Unfortunately, clinicians tend to have expectations of how patients should feel and respond to pain from specific operative procedures. The individual nature of pain must be appreciated and expressions of pain respected. All pain is real. When it persists in the absence of any appreciable pathology or when clinicians believe that the pain is out of proportion to physiological alteration, the validity of the pain may be questioned or doubted. It is important to recognize that when pain pathways are interrupted because of inoperative procedure, pain may persist beyond the expected duration and in ways that are difficult to detect and understand. Unlike the perception of pain, responses to pain are more a function of psychological and social variables rather than biological ones. In addition, the reaction to pain or the ability to endure it is more overt and observable by expressions or behaviors.

Nociception

Numerous types of noxious pain stimuli lead to perceptual phenomena that are processed by the sensory cortex as pain. A wide range of sensory input including tissue inflammation, tissue ischemia, and muscle spasms cause pain. A nociceptor, which is a sensory receptor that responds to painful stimuli (*The Free Dictionary*, 2008), is able to receive noxious stimuli and transmit them to the spinal cord via specific nerve fibers. Two types of first-order peripheral neurons are capable of transmitting painful stimuli: the A delta fibers, found primarily in the skin and muscle, and the C fibers, distributed throughout muscle, periosteum, and viscera. Myelinated (A-delta) fibers carry intermittent, rapid, sharp, pricking, or piercing sensations. Pain can be fairly well localized to the area or areas of tissue injury. Unmyelinated or poorly myelinated C fibers produce diffuse and dull, burning, or achy pain and are responsible for continuous, constant pain.

Pain Pathways

Second-order neurons or pain pathways of the ascending pain tracts start in the dorsal horn of the spinal cord and terminate in the thalamus. Noxious stimuli ascend to the brain via two spinothalamic pathways or tracts known as the neospinothalamic or lateral tract and the paleospinothalamic or medial tract. Sensory pain discrimination is made possible by the direct routing of painful stimuli to the sensory cortex by the neospinothalamic tract. Because the paleospinothalamic tract synapses in other parts of the brain, such as the limbic system or emotional center and the reticular formation or sleep-wake center, painful stimuli are highly influenced by affective and behavioral factors. At the level of the brain, noxious stimuli are processed in the thalamus, midbrain, and cortex. Intricate patterns of communication within the brain allow for the awareness and interpretation of pain and responses to it.

Modulation of Pain

Neuroregulators are chemical substances that modulate sensory input to the spinal cord. These substances are classified as neurotransmitters or neuromodulators. Neurotransmitters such as acetylcholine, norepinephrine, epinephrine, and dopamine exert their inhibitory and excitatory activity at postsynaptic membranes in nerve cells. Neuromodulators or endogenous opiates are protein hormones composed of large amino acid peptides named *alpha-* and *beta-endorphins* and *enkephalins*. Endorphins and enkephalins that are found in the brain seem to work as morphine-like substances, only they are more potent. Many speculate that these natural opiate-like substances produce analgesic effects that can be reversed with naloxone (Narcan), an opioid antagonist. Both endorphins, which are made in the anterior pituitary gland

and the hypothalamus, and enkephalins, much smaller peptides that are widespread throughout the brain and the dorsal horn of the spinal cord, act on highly specific opiate receptors in the central nervous system. Differences in the release and function of the endogenous opioid system may account for one of many factors that make individual responses to pain highly variable.

Physiologic Sources of Pain

Somatic Pain

Pain that arises from the nociceptors in the skin, subcutaneous tissues, bones, blood vessels, muscles, and connective tissue of the body is called somatic pain. Somatic pain is further delineated by the presence of nociceptors in the various somatic structures. Cutaneous somatic pain comes from the superficial structures of the skin and subcutaneous tissues and tends to be more localized. Deep somatic pain refers to the pain of bone, muscles, and other underlying tissues and is generally more diffuse. Patients who experience pain from the incision, muscle splitting, stretching, or cutting, and from orthopedic procedures have somatic pain (**Table 36.3**).

Visceral Pain

Activation of nociceptors in the organs and linings of the body cavities, such as the peritoneum and pleura, defines the mechanisms for visceral pain. Unlike somatic pain, visceral pain is perceived as more diffuse or poorly localized. Visceral nociceptors respond primarily to stretching, inflammation, and ischemia but do not elicit pain from the direct response of cutting. Examples of visceral pain include such conditions as peritonitis, pancreatitis, pericarditis, colitis, stretching of hollow viscera (eg, bladder spasms, intestinal gas), enlargement of organs from malignant tumors (eg, liver metastases), and in combination with somatic pain associated with the presence of tubes and drains in the chest and abdominal cavity (eg, Jackson Pratt tubes). Patients can expect visceral pain after most abdominal and thoracic operative procedures (see **Table 36.3**).

Neuropathic Pain

Neuropathic pain is a third kind of physiological pain, which occurs because of injurious insults to the peripheral nerve fibers, spinal cord, or central nervous system. Sustained injury to nerves or other parts of the nervous system is more often associated with chronic conditions and can result in central pain phenomena. Diabetes, toxic effects from chemotherapeutic agents, radiation-induced neuritis or nerve injury, and human immunodeficiency virus (HIV) infection give rise to painful peripheral neuropathies classified as neuropathic pain syndrome. Impingement or invasion of nerve fibers by cancerous growths also leads to neuropathic pain. Neuropathic pain is associated with changes in sensory modalities (allodynia, hyperalgesia, dysesthesia, and paresthesia) and sometimes motor deficits.

Acute trauma to nerve fibers, such as transection or compression of a nerve or nerves during the removal of a limb, a breast, or an organ, can lead to neuropathic pain. Phantom limb pain is perhaps one of the most common types of neuropathic pain syndromes, encountered after amputation and traumatic avulsion of

HIV
Human
Immunodeficiency Virus

Table 36.3   **Physiological Sources of Pain**

Type of Pain	Physiological Structures	Mechanism of Pain	Characteristics of Pain	Sources of Acute Postoperative Pain	Sources of Chronic Pain Syndrome
Somatic pain	Cutaneous: skin and subcutaneous tissues Deep somatic: bones, muscle, blood vessels, connective tissue	Activation of nociceptors	Well localized Constant, achy	Incisional pain, pain at insertion site of tubes and drains, wound complications, orthopedic procedures, skeletal muscle spasms	Bone metastases, osteoarthritis, rheumatoid arthritis, low back pain, peripheral vascular disease
Visceral pain	Organs, linings of body cavities	Activation of nociceptors	Poorly localized, diffuse, deep, cramping or splitting	Chest tubes, abdominal tubes and drains, bladder distention or spasms, intestinal distention	Pancreatitis, liver metastases, colitis
Neuropathic pain	Nerve fibers, spinal cord, central nervous system	Non-nociceptive injury to nervous system structures	Poorly localized or follows a nerve distribution, burning, fiery, shock-like, sharp, painful numbness	Phantom limb pain, nerve compression pain	Diabetes, human immunodeficiency virus, chemotherapy-induced neuropathies, postherpetic neuralgia, cancer-related nerve injury

36

the brachial plexus. Postmastectomy syndrome involving damage to the intercostal brachial nerve, and postthoracotomy syndrome, which occurs from injury to intercostal nerves, also represents operatively induced neuropathic pain.

Types of Pain

Acute Pain

The individual experiencing acute pain "reports the presence of severe discomfort or an uncomfortable sensation lasting from one second to less than six months" (Carpenito-Moyet, 2008, p. 69). Acute pain is an adaptive response that warns the body of impending danger. Typically, the mechanism or mechanisms for the pain are obvious, and appropriate treatment approaches are usually effective in minimizing or even eliminating the pain. Because acute pain is temporary, there is a reluctance to treat it promptly and aggressively and a failure to appreciate the long-lasting consequences and devastation that occur when severe acute pain goes unmanaged. Unfortunately, the attitude that patients must "grin and bear it" is still widely held by clinicians. Common causes for acute pain include trauma, diagnostic procedures, operative intervention, acute diseases or conditions, or exacerbations of chronic disease states. Acute pain, if untreated, may develop into chronic pain. **Table 36.4** lists the characteristics of acute pain.

Chronic Pain

Chronic pain arises from a multitude of diseases and conditions and for the most part remains poorly understood. The nature of chronic pain differs according to the types of physiological mechanisms and psychosocial circumstances surrounding the patient's life. Some chronic pain syndromes, such as those related to cancer, can progress quickly over time, whereas others, like degenerative osteoarthritis, worsen more slowly over many years. Usually chronic pain is related to some obvious pathological process, but sometimes the physiological cause of the pain cannot be identified. Prolonged noxious stimuli introduced into the nervous system can eventually lead to central nervous system dysfunction and may lead to dysfunction of parts of the nervous system. Injurious effects on parts of the nervous system can lead to neuropathic pain. **Table 36.5** lists the characteristics of chronic pain.

Table 36.4	Characteristics of Acute Pain

- ☐ Serves a biological purpose in warning the body of actual or impending tissue damage
- ☐ Is temporary
- ☐ Is generally well defined and described
- ☐ Is often associated with the physiological responses of sympathetic nervous system innervations such as elevated blood pressure and pulse, increased respirations, dilated pupils, sweating, cold and clammy skin, and restlessness or anxiety
- ☐ Often subsides with or without treatment
- ☐ Is generally more predictable than chronic pain

Table 36.5	**Characteristics of Chronic Pain**

- ☐ Rarely serves a biological purpose
- ☐ May be poorly localized and difficult to describe
- ☐ Changes over time
- ☐ Persists or recurs for an indefinite period of time (generally >2 months)
- ☐ Is rarely associated with autonomic responses
- ☐ May persist even after the physiological causes are eliminated or resolved
- ☐ May be out of proportion to direct tissue injury
- ☐ Causes more pronounced affective disorders (anxiety and depression) and behavioral responses
- ☐ Usually imposes functional, financial, and social limitations
- ☐ May be associated with peripheral and central nervous system dysfunction
- ☐ Often worsens without treatment

Table 36.6	**Classification of Chronic Pain**

Chronic Pain Related To

Cancer	Disease	Specific Conditions
Bone metastases	Rheumatoid arthritis	Migraine headaches
Enlargement or stretching of visceral or organ structures (liver metastases, pancreatic involvement, ascites)	Sickle cell anemia	Neuralgias (trigeminal, post-herpetic)
	Diabetes (neuropathy)	Fibromyalgia
	HIV (neuropathy)	Low back pain
	Peripheral vascular disease	Temporal mandibular joint (TMJ) pain
Distention of hollow viscera (intestinal or bladder distention)	Raynaud's disease	Avascular necrosis
	Inflammatory bowel disease	Postsurgical pain syndromes (postthoracotomy syndrome, postmastectomy syndrome)
Impingement on peripheral nerves or a nerve plexus (brachial plexopathy, lumbosacral plexopathy, celiacplexus involvement from pancreatic cancer)		Compression fractures from osteoporosis

The classification of chronic pain includes cancer-related pain, chronic pain related to diseases, and chronic pain related to specific conditions (**Table 36.6**). The mainstay of treatment for chronic cancer pain that is not amenable to cancer therapies is liberal use of opioid analgesics and adjuvant medications. For principles and specific interventions for cancer pain, refer to the Agency for National Comprehensive Cancer Network Clinical Practice Guidelines in Oncology (National Comprehensive Cancer Network [NCCN], 2008).

Table 36.7	Pharmacologic and Non-Pharmacologic Treatment for Pain	
Pharmacologic Treatment		**Non-Pharmacologic Treatment**
Types of Medications	*Routes of Administration*	
Opioids	Oral	Heat/cold
NSAIDS	Buccal/sublingual	TENS
Cox 2	Rectal	Cognitive behavioral therapy/biofeedback
Antidepressants	Topical/transdermal	
Antiepileptics	Nebulized	Physical therapy
Muscle relaxants	Parenteral	Massage/triggerpoint therapy
NMDA receptor antagonists	Neuraxial	Music
	Regional	Distraction

Total Pain

Total pain is a concept used to describe the interaction of physiologic pain and other sources of pain and suffering in patients, including emotional pain and other psychosocial stressors. The interaction of all types of pain gives rise to suffering as is often seen in cancer and terminally ill populations. Patients who are experiencing total pain will require multidimensional assessment and treatment to achieve effective outcomes. **Table 36.7** highlights the pharmacologic and non-pharmacologic treatment of total pain.

PHARMACOLOGIC TREATMENT

Opioid Analgesics

Opioid analgesics produce both analgesia and adverse effects by binding to receptor sites intended for endogenous opiates (endorphins and enkephalins). Opioid receptors include the mu kappa, delta, epsilon, and sigma receptors. Subclasses of opioids are grouped according to their selective activity on opioid receptors. **Table 36.8** shows dosing data for Opioid analgesics. For example, morphine-like opioids bind to mu receptors found throughout the central nervous system, typically in the periaqueductal gray matter in the brain stem, the limbic system, and the dorsal horn. The mu receptor is responsible for supraspinal analgesia, cardiovascular effects, respiratory depression, constipation, euphoria, and physical dependence. Side-effect profiles do differ for each opioid. Opioid agonists possess varying degrees of binding affinity for the mu receptor, with sufentanil possessing the highest and meperidine (Demerol) one of the lowest. Opioids influence two major hormonal systems resulting in progressive decline with chronic opioid administration in cortisol levels, increased prolactin, and decreased luteinizing hormone, follicle-stimulating hormone, testosterone, and estrogen. Chronic opioid administration may also suppress immune function (Ballantyne & Mao, 2003).

Risk Factors for Adverse Effects

Risk factors for adverse effects of opioid analgesic use include hypovolemia (dehydration, hemorrhage), vasodilation (caused by reversal of hypothermia, alteration in baroreceptor responses, histamine release), renal insufficiency, hepatic impairment,

Table 36.8	Common Opioids Used for Pain Control During the Operative or Invasive Procedure Period				
Drug	**Potency**	**Usual IV Dose**	**Peak Effect**	**Duration of Analgesia**	**Indications/Comments**
Morphine	1	2–5 mg	20 min	4–5 h	Most common choice owing to longer duration, no ceiling dose effects, titration to pain relief possible, preferred if tolerance to opioids evident, easy to convert equianalgesic doses to other parenteral or oral opioids
Fentanyl (Sublimaze)	75–125 times more potent than morphine	50–100 μg	3–5 min/IV, 20–30 min/IM	30–60 min	Effects may be prolonged in elderly, least likely to produce histamine release, useful for induction of anesthesia
Alfentanil	3–10 times less potent than fentanyl	Up to 500 μg	1.5–2 min	5–10 min	More rapidly distributed to body tissues, need for additional opioid analgesia may occur soon after emergence, used as an anesthesia adjunct, skeletal muscle rigidity may occur more rapidly than with fentanyl and sufentanil, hypotension and bradycardia when given rapidly, commonly used for short procedures but can result in light anesthesia
Sufentanil	5–7 times more potent than fentanyl	Up to 8 mcg/kg as an analgesic adjunct to anesthesia.	1.4 min	5 min	Useful for induction of anesthesia
Hydromorphone (Dilaudid)	5 times more potent than morphine	0.15–0.75 mg	0.5–1 hour	3–4 h	No active metabolites have been identified, slightly shorter acting than morphine
Meperidine (Demerol)	1/10 as potent as morphine	25–100 mg	5–7 min/IV, 30–50 min/IM	2–4 h	Has a toxic metabolite, normeperidine, that can accumulate with repeated dosing, recommended for short-term use, more likely to cause side effects associated with histamine release, may cause serious side effects with concurrent administration of MAO

Note: IV, intravenous; IM, intramuscular; MAO, monoamine oxidase

Source: RxList (2009). Sufenta, retrieved from www.rxlist.com/sufenta-drug.htm, accessed on January 20, 2009; Drug.com (2008). Hydromorphone hydrochloride, retrieved from http:// www.drugs.com/ppa/hydromorphone-hydrochloride.html, accessed on January 20, 2009.

36

older age, pulmonary diseases or conditions, and acute intoxication with alcohol or illicit drugs.

Nursing Interventions

When anticipating opioid analgesic use, identify risk factors for adverse effects from opioids. After starting therapy, monitor vital signs frequently. Have an opioid antagonist readily available. Administer small doses of an intravenous opioid at prescribed intervals until patient reports satisfactory analgesia. Assess pain level coinciding with analgesic peak using self-report pain-scale measures. Observe for accumulation of drug and associated effects. Prepare to treat opioid-induced side effects.

See **Table 36.8** for common opioids used for pain control before, during, and after the operative or invasive procedure. Opioid-induced adverse effects include nausea and vomiting, sedation, respiratory depression, hypotension, and constipation. Many of these effects can also be attributed to the impact of the procedure and the anesthetic regimen.

PCA
Patient-Controlled
Analgesia

Meperidine was commonly used for patient-controlled analgesia (PCA) and is an effective analgesic option, particularly in patients with allergies to other opioids, but has fallen out of favor due to the potential for accumulation of its neurotoxic metabolite, normeperidine. Patients at high risk for toxicity include the elderly and those with impaired renal function. Early signs of normeperidine toxicity may include myoclonus and confusion with the potential for seizures if the metabolite continues to accumulate (Pennsylvania Patient Safety Advisory, 2006). For this reason, removal of meperidine from institutional formularies or restricted use to no more than 600 mg/day for 48 hours can be used as a measure of quality of pain management services (Gordon et al., 2002).

In general, intermittent intravenous opioids are safer for patients emerging from anesthesia and those with hypothermia and coagulopathies. Fentanyl has significant advantages over morphine in the postanesthesia care unit because its rapid onset of action, shorter duration, and decreased side-effect profile make it easier to titrate to pain relief.

Nonsteroidal Anti-Inflammatory Drugs

NSAIDs
Nonsteroidal
Anti-Inflammatory
Drugs

Nonsteroidal anti-inflammatory drugs (NSAIDs) are useful adjuncts to opioid analgesics as they reduce the sensitivity of peripheral nociceptors to pain by blocking the synthesis of prostaglandins, which are hyperalgesic substances. Because these drugs can potentially cause problems with coagulation, use is generally limited to minor procedures. The side-effect profile for NSAIDs includes increased risk for bleeding, gastrointestinal toxicity, and renal impairment. Unlike moat NSAIDs, ketorolac (Toradol) is available for parenteral use. See **Table 36.7** for Dosing Data for Nonopioid.

Cox-2 Inhibitors

Cox-2 inhibitors selectively inhibit prostaglandin synthesis. Celecoxib is often used as a part of multimodal preemptive analgesia prior to elective orthopedic surgery. This medication is contraindicated in patients with renal insufficiency and sulfa allergies. Celecoxib reduces the incidence of gastrointestinal side effects and has no

effect on platelets when compared with traditional NSAIDS but carries the risk of cardiovascular side effects. Therefore Celecoxib, like all NSAIDS, is contraindicated immediately after cardiac bypass surgery.

Acetaminophen

Acetaminophen has analgesic and antipyretic effects but lacks significant anti-inflammatory properties (Diaz & Flood, 2006). It does not produce gastric irritation or affect platelet aggregation. Acetaminophen is hepatotoxic with overdose.

Antidepressants

Antidepressants exhibit analgesic properties reflecting their ability to block the reuptake of serotonin and norepinephrine in the central nervous system, increasing the activity of the endogenous pain-modulating pathways (American Pain Society, 2006). Analgesic effects of these medications are not dependant on antidepressant effects. Examples of antidepressants with known analgesic efficacy include duloxetine, and venlafaxine and Tricyclic antidepressants such as amitriptyline and nortriptyline. Caution should be used when utilizing the tricyclic antidepressants particularly in elderly populations because of their side effect profile, which includes cardiac conduction abnormalities, sedation, orthostatic hypotension, and anticholinergic effects (Fick et al., 2003).

Anti-Epileptics

Anticonvulsant medications modulate the spontaneous firing of sensory neurons associated with neuropathic pain. They can also reduce anxiety preprocedurely in orthopedic patients. These medications reduce pain with movement and can reduce the risk for developing postprocedure pain syndromes caused by neuronal plasticity. Common examples of anticonvulsants used for pain include gabapentin and pregabalin. Side effects include sedation and dizziness. These medications are increasingly being used as preemptive analgesia (Reuben et al., 2006). Preprocedure recommendations range from 300 mg to 1200 mg of gabapentin or 150 mg of pregabalin given in a single dose preprocedurely and continued for five days postprocedurely. These medications require reduced dose considerations in the presence of impaired renal function.

Muscle Relaxants

Muscle relaxants are indicated for the treatment of muscular pains and spasms from peripheral musculoskeletal conditions. The mechanism of action of skeletal muscle relaxant is largely unknown but is thought to be related to sedation for some of the medications. Common examples of muscle relaxants include baclofen, carisoprodol, cyclobenzaprine, diazepam, and methocarbamol. Baclofen can be given intrathecally for spasticity-generated pain but care must be taken to educate the patient to have an oral supply of baclofen available in the event of pump malfunction, as rapid discontinuation of baclofen in tolerant patients can result in seizure and death. Caution should be exercised when choosing agents and doses in patients with renal or hepatic insufficiency. Caution should also be exercised when administering muscle relaxants to postprocedure patients receiving opioids due to their additive sedation effect.

TENS
Transcutaneous
Electrical Nerve
Stimulation

NONPHARMACOLOGIC APPROACHES TO PAIN

Nondrug measures are useful adjuncts to analgesic therapy for both postprocedure and chronic pain and should complement, not replace, drug therapy. Physical measures such as coetaneous stimulation may provide additional relief for incisional pain or muscular skeletal pain accompanying immobility. Cutaneous stimulation techniques include transcutaneous electrical nerve stimulation (TENS), therapeutic touch, pressure, massage, vibration, and the application of heat and cold.

TENS involves the application of electrodes, attached to a battery-operated device that can deliver small electrical currents to the skin and underlying tissues. The electrodes, along with a conduction gel or substance, are placed adjacent to the incisional area or along the spine for greater distribution of pain relief. The device is adjusted to provide stimulation that is similar to the feeling of pins and needles. Heat and cold may also be beneficial for postprocedure pain relief, although direct application to the incisional area is avoided to prevent circulatory changes around the operative site. Applications of heat can relax tense muscles and reduce spasm while having a generalized calming effect. Cold packs reduce swelling and inflammation and can eliminate muscle tightness.

Except for therapeutic touch, the pain benefits of cutaneous techniques are short-lived and generally cease once the stimulation is removed. **Table 36.9** explains the indications and goals of cutaneous stimulation techniques.

PAIN MANAGEMENT IN CLINICAL PRACTICE

Pain management is practiced in many different patient care areas including preprocedure assessment and treatment units for elective operative patients, in operative and invasive procedure suites, in urgent care or emergency departments following traumatic injury, primary care facilities, and in dedicated pain management and rehabilitative facilities. Nurses providing pain management services include those practicing in physician offices, certified registered nurse anesthetists, nurses providing moderate sedation/analgesia care, postanesthesia care nurses, medical surgical nurses, and advance practice nurses providing chronic pain management care in outpatient clinics, each nursing role is essential to affect best pain management outcomes for patients.

Nursing Management of Acute Pain
Patient History

The management of acute pain for individuals undergoing elective procedures begins in outpatient operative offices and preanesthesia care units with a medical history, physical exam, and preliminary patient education regarding pain management plan of care (Barnes, 2001). Pain management plans that are initiated following traumatic injury in the emergency department or urgent care clinic do not have the benefit of time needed to coordinate an ideal plan, but thorough history and physical exam are essential. The patient history must include the history of chronic pain and chronic opioid analgesic treatment, history of substance abuse, and a patient or family history of adverse effects from anesthetics or analgesics including adjuvants, and prior history with pain management as it relates to postprocedure recovery.

Table 36.9	Cutaneous Stimulation Techniques Used to Interrupt the Pain Pathway	
Technique	**Method of Application**	**Comments**
Therapeutic touch or "laying on of hands"	The hands of the caregiver are placed on or close to the client's body	The intent to help on the part of the caregiver may contribute to the success of this technique May extend the nurse-client relationship
Pressure	A hand or other object is placed firmly over or around the painful area	Seems to relieve pain, decrease bleeding, and prevent swelling Release of pressure is associated with increased blood flow and return of pain
Massage	The hands or fingers are moved slowly or briskly over a body part A lubricant or other substance is sometimes used	Effects include muscle relaxation and sedation
Vibration	Electrical and battery-operated vibrators produce a massage effect	May decrease the intensity of the noxious (pain) stimuli
Application of heat	May be applied in a variety of ways, including short-wave diathermy, microwave diathermy, sonography, use of melted paraffin and Hubbard tank, use of hot-water bottle or heating pad, use of heat cradle and lamp, application of moist pads or towels, use of hot tub or shower, or use of gel packs	May reduce muscle spasm and decrease pain Increases the tendency for bleeding and therefore should not be used after trauma Increases edema and is not indicated if circulation is poor Use cautiously if clients have impaired sensation or cannot communicate
Application of cold	May be applied in a dry or moist way, similar to heat application Ice chips, cold towels and packs, and chilled gel packs are commonly used	May reduce muscle spasm and decrease pain Probably slows the conduction velocity of nerves Use cautiously if clients have impaired sensation or cannot communicate

When possible, include the patient's chronic pain management practitioner when developing an acute pain management plan of care for patients diagnosed with chronic pain requiring operative procedures (Hansen, 2005). Inform patients of the need to use comparatively increased amounts of analgesics for the effective treatment of pain in the postprocedure period. The patient should have a clear understanding of the need to take chronic opioid doses on the day of the procedure, if possible, to avoid withdrawal, particularly if chronic opioid doses are large. These patients may particularly benefit from regional anesthesia techniques and preemptive adjuvant administration. Chronic pain management patients requiring chronic opioid analgesia may require 2–4 times the amount of opioid analgesia required by an opioid naïve individual (Ang et al., 2004; Carol, Angst, & Clark, 2004).

Table 36.10	Pain Management for Patients Who Report a History of Substance Abuse Disorder

Establish the type of drug and amount and the time of last use.

Alert anesthesia provider and operative team of the patient's history

Observe for signs of physical withdrawal from alcohol, benzodiazepine, or opioids (agitation, delirium, elevated blood pressure, tachycardia, fever, abdominal cramping, diarrhea).

Administer opioids in sufficient amounts to prevent opioid withdrawal or administer benzodiazepine to prevent or treat benzodiazepine or alcohol withdrawal.

Expect the patient to demonstrate tolerance to opioid analgesics.

Avoid administering partial or mixed opioid antagonists and these may precipitate physical withdrawal.

Communicate the patient's history to other care providers in a respectful and professional manner.

Table 36.10 lists points the nurse should consider and communicate when participating in the formulation of pain management treatment plans for patients undergoing painful procedures who report a history of substance abuse disorder. For patients currently receiving methadone maintenance or buprenorphine for the treatment of addiction, communication with the prescribing outpatient practitioner is highly recommended (Alford et al., 2006).

Patient history should yield increased treatment consideration for individuals identified with advanced age, history, or risk factors for obstructive sleep apnea or impaired pulmonary function and history of impaired renal or hepatic function. Monitor patients with these risk factors closely during the postprocedure period for the development of adverse drug events such as opioid induced sedation and respiratory depression. Place patients suspected of having obstructive sleep apnea in a non-supine position whenever possible. In addition, patients diagnosed with obstructive sleep apnea should continue to use a continuous positive airway pressure (CPAP) device after discharge (American Society of Anesthesiologists, 2006). Communicate the need for increased monitoring in high-risk patient populations to all staff caring for the patient, particularly in the first 24 hours following procedures (Taylor & Kirton, 2005). Assessment should include level of sedation, rate, depth, and pattern of respiratory effort with traditional vital sign and oxygen saturation measurement. Oxygen saturation decreases can be a late sign of hypercarbia (carbon dioxide retention in the blood), particularly in patients receiving supplemental oxygen therapy, as it does not reflect changes in ventilation. The addition of end tidal carbon dioxide measurements may provide earlier detection of hypoventilation (Overdyke et al., 2007). Regardless of technology being used, nurses should perform routine respiratory assessments observing rate, depth, and pattern of respirations for a full sixty seconds.

CPAP
Continuous Positive
Airway Pressure

Assessment

Preprocedure physical examination should include determination of the patient's cognitive status and ability to understand and retain educational content given regarding the pain management plan of care. For individuals who are identified with

significant cognitive deficits or for patients who will be sedated after the procedure, use a non-verbal pain management scale in the postprocedure period. Cognitively impaired patients benefit from structured assessments based on the Hierarchy of Pain Assessment Techniques (**Table 36.2**) and other validated non-verbal measurement scales (McCaffery et al., 2005; Herr et al., 2006). The use of a behavioral pain scale makes assessment more effective in non-verbal populations.

Preprocedure patients who are cognitively intact should receive preprocedure education including:

* An explanation of the operative procedure
* Location of the operative incision
* Ways in which the pain will be treated
* Methods for assessing pain
* How and when to request as needed analgesia
* What to do if pain is not relieved
* Opportunities to express concerns and have these addressed

Preemptive Analgesia

Preemptive analgesia includes treatment started before and continues during an operative procedure. The proposed mechanism of action is to provide antinociceptive treatment reducing altered sensory input preventing central sensitization or wind-up and pain-related changes to the nervous system and the development of chronic pain. Preemptive analgesia often reduces opioid requirements, decreases pain, and facilitates ambulation and timely discharge. Preemptive analgesia includes epidural analgesia, local anesthetics, systemic opioids, nonsteroidal anti-inflammatories, celecoxib, gabapentin, pregabalin, and N-methyl D Aspartate blockers such as ketamine and combinations of these analgesics. Wound infiltration with bupivacaine and ropivacaine may help reduce local inflammatory response to trauma or surgery by reducing up regulation of peripheral nociceptors. Intraarticular inflammation creates opioid binding sites in animal models and opioid injected in the intra articular areas reduce inflammation (Rudolph, 2008).

Peripheral Nerve Blocks

Local anesthetics are used for peripheral nerve blocks to provide regional analgesia using the peripheral nervous system. Patients at increased risk for adverse drug events from analgesics should be evaluated for preprocedure regional anesthetic techniques, if applicable, to reduce the potential need for high doses of systemic analgesics to treat acute pain (Zaric et al., 2007).

Interscalene blocks are used for shoulder surgery, including rotator cuff and shoulder replacement. Infra- and supra-clavicular blocks are used for surgery of the hand, wrist, elbow, and distal arm. Continuous lumbar plexus and single sciatic nerve blocks are used for hip surgeries, including hip replacement and procedures for incision and drainage (**Fig. 36.1**). Continuous femoral and continuous sciatic blocks are used for knee surgeries. Continuous sciatic blocks alone are used for foot, knee, and above- and below-the-knee amputations. Continuous paravertebral blocks are used for chest wall, thoracic, breast, abdominal surgeries, and iliac crest bone graft. Single paravertebral blocks are used for inguinal hernia, prostatectomy, and hysterectomy.

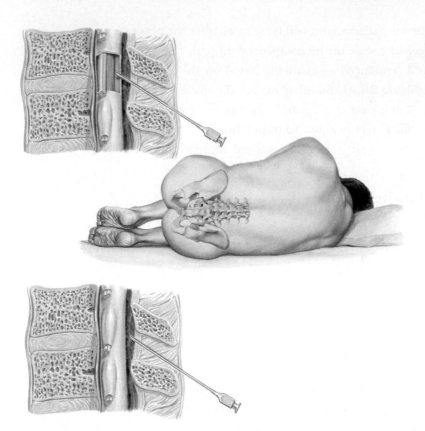

Figure 36.1

Continuous lumbar plexus and single sciatic nerve blocks.

Nursing responsibilities following peripheral nerve block include assessing the patient for pain, checking sensory and motor function, inspecting the insertion site, catheter, and dressing, and assessing for signs and symptoms of local anesthetic toxicity. When assessing sensory and motor function following femoral nerve block, look for quadriceps muscle weakness. After a sciatic nerve block and before the patient ambulates, check for foot weakness. If the continuous nerve blocks inhibit ambulation, the rate of infusion may need to be decreased and the patient may need a supportive device. Instruct the patient to ambulate only with assistance (Pizzi, 2008). Early signs and symptoms of local anesthetic toxicity include circumoral numbness, metallic taste, dizziness, blurred vision, tinnitus, and decreased hearing. Late signs and symptoms of local anesthetics include restlessness, tremors, and can progress to seizures and cardiac arrhythmias. Emergency equipment includes airway, suction, advanced cardiac life support medications and lipid emulsions that reverse the effect of local anesthetics should be readily available.

Epidural Analgesia

Epidural analgesia is the administration of a preservative-free opioid or local anesthetic, or both, into the epidural space by intermittent injection, continuous infusion, or patient-controlled methods. (**Fig. 36.2**). The subarachnoid space, which contains cerebrospinal fluid, is located just below the dura mater. Extradural fat and the epidural venous system line areas of the epidural space. An epidural catheter may be inserted in the lumbar or thoracic area. The tip should be placed in order to provide the best pain control given the type of analgesic therapy and the location of the operative incision. Lumbar epidural catheters are indicated for abdominal and lower

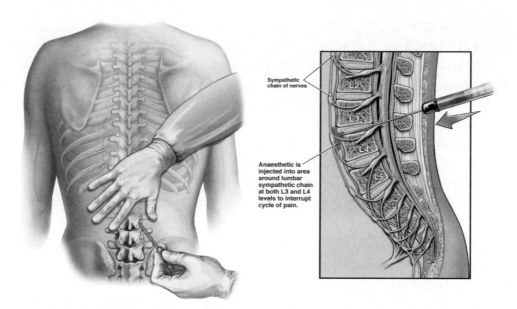

Figure 36.2

Administration of epidural analgesia.

36

extremity surgeries. Catheter placement in the thoracic region is more difficult than in the lumbar area because of narrower interspinous processes, a smaller epidural space, a steeper angle for placement, and closer proximity to the spinal cord. **Figure 36.3** shows a diagram of dermatomes, which are areas of skin associated with a pair of dorsal roots from the spine. Dermatomes can be used to identify spinal damage or neurological stenosis (Wikipedia, 2008).

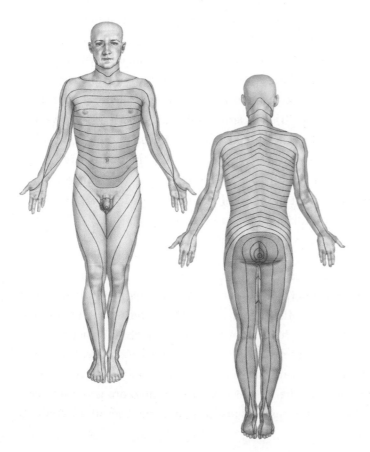

Figure 36.3

Diagram of dermatomes.

Medications

Epidural Opioids

Both opioids and local anesthetics exert analgesic effects when instilled into the epidural space, and local anesthetics in higher concentrations can produce anesthesia. Epidural opioids can act to relieve pain in a variety of ways by binding to extradural fat, being absorbed into the systemic circulation via the epidural venous system, direct delivery into the dorsal horn by the posterior radicular spinal arteries, and diffusing through the dura and entering the cerebrospinal fluid (Ferrante, 1993). Epidural opioids bind directly to opioid receptors in the spinal cord and provide far more efficient drug delivery in much lower doses than those required for systemic administration. Depending on the lipid solubility of the drug, systemic absorption of epidural opioids varies. Fentanyl, which is more lipid soluble than morphine, produces segmental analgesia so catheter location is important. In addition, it has a short duration of action (**Table 36.8**). Morphine, on the other hand, is hydrophilic and dissolves readily into the CSF toward the brain, resulting in a broad spread of analgesia across many dermatomes (Pasero, 2005). Morphine has a long duration of action making it ideal for single-bolus dose intraspinal techniques (Pasero, 2005) Epidural opioid preparations do not contain preservatives in order to avoid any caustic effects or inflammation to spinal nerves

Adverse Effects

Adverse effects of epidural opioids are respiratory depression, urinary retention, hypotension, sedation, and pruritus. The exact mechanism for epidural opioid-induced pruritus is unclear. It is probably not related to the histamine-mediated pruritus associated with systemic opioids, but to activity in the spinal cord and central-mediated processes in the brain. Whatever the cause, itching happens in about 50% of patients receiving epidural opioids and can be quite distressing. When the opioid is given by continuous epidural infusion or patient-controlled epidural analgesia (PCEA) the most effective treatment for pruritis is to decrease the infusion rate or the PCEA dose by 25–50% (Pasero, 2005). Treatment with low-dose intravenous opioid antagonists like naloxone, is effective in relieving itching without reversing analgesia but it is essential to continue to assess the patient frequently for pain control to avoid reversing analgesia. Administration of diphenhydramine (Benadryl), is effective but is thought to relieve this type of pruritus via its sedating effects and requires frequent monitoring of sedation levels.

PCEA
Patient-Controlled
Epidural Analgesia

Epidural Local Anesthetics

Epidural opioid and local anesthetic combinations offer the best form of pain control. Most epidural local anesthetics in lower concentrations produce analgesia by blocking mixed spinal nerves (both sensory and motor), thus reducing afferent sensory stimuli to the spinal cord. In higher concentrations, total anesthesia can be achieved. Ropivacaine is selective for sensory nerves and, therefore, causes less motor blockade and is associated with less cardiotoxicity than bupivacaine (Pasero, 2005). Intermittent injections of lidocaine, because it is shorter acting, are generally used to provide additional analgesia or to test the position and function of an epidural catheter.

Urinary retention is sometimes observed in the first 24 hours following an operative procedure with epidural analgesia and is most common after bolus doses of local anesthetic, which are administered during the procedure or upon emergence from anesthesia. Indwelling urinary catheters are not required with epidural analgesia; however, intermittent straight catheterization may be necessary until patients can spontaneously void.

Adverse Effects

Adverse effects of epidural local anesthetics are hypotension, urinary retention, sensory alterations, lower motor weakness, and tachyphylaxis (tolerance limiting the effectiveness of the local anesthetic).

Clonidine

Clonidine is an alpha 2 agonist thought to produce analgesia by blocking substance P interfering with the generation of an action potential. The addition of clonidine to an epidural opioid or anesthetic can prolong and intensify anesthesia and allow for decreased opioid doses. Side effects of epidural clonidine include sedation, dry mouth, bradycardia, and hypotension (Pasero, 2005).

Patient-Controlled Epidural Analgesia

Like PCA, the intent of patient-controlled epidural analgesia (PCEA) is to find the minimal amount of both a continuous rate of medication and a demand that optimally controls the patient's pain. Patients are generally given a continuous infusion of the analgesic solution and are able to self-administer a demand or bolus dose within a predetermined time (lockout) interval that is programmed into the infusion device. For dosing parameters and onset of action for both fentanyl and morphine, see **Table 36.11** Patient-Controlled Epidural Analgesia (PCEA) Guidelines.

Nursing Interventions

For administration of epidural analgesia, confer with the anesthesia provider regarding proper placement of the catheter. Ensure that the proper technology is used for continuous epidural infusion and that there are no injection site ports on the tubing so that inadvertent administration of systemic therapy into the epidural space is prevented. Check the patient's sensory level if local anesthetics have been

Table 36.11	Patient-Controlled Epidural Analgesia (PCEA) Guidelines		
Drug	**Demand Dose (mL)[†]**	**Onset of Action**	**Lockout Interval**
Fentanyl	50%–100% of continuous rate	10 min	10–20 min
Morphine	50%–100% of continuous rate	20–30 min	10–20 min

[†] PCEA demand does volumes should NOT exceed 10 mL. If the anesthesiologist's order specifies epidural demand doses greater than 10 mL, it should indicate whether any special monitoring parameters are necessary, especially if the epidural solution contains bupivacaine.

administered during the procedure or if continuous infusions of local anesthetic have been initiated. Follow nursing interventions for postprocedure care, as appropriate.

The nurse must take into consideration anticoagulant therapy administration related to the timing of insertion and removal of epidural catheters or prior to and following single-shot epidural anesthetic or analgesics to prevent epidural hematoma formation. For further information, see the guidelines published by the American Society for Regional Anesthesia. Coagulopathy and systemic infection associated with bacteremia are contraindications to neuraxial techniques.

POSTPROCEDURE NURSING INTERVENTIONS

Pain Assessment

Monitor pain levels, using an appropriate pain scale, at least every 4 hours. Assess pain levels after the administration of the PCEA demand dose (no sooner than the designated onset of action). Encourage the use of the PCEA demand dose if continuous infusion does not provide optimal pain control. If bolus doses and increased epidural analgesic doses fail to improve pain control, the anesthesiologist may check catheter placement by administering a concentrated anesthetic dose. Proper placement is verified if injection causes bilateral sensory block of the desired dermatomes (Pasero, 2005).

Respiratory Monitoring

Respiratory monitoring is appropriate only for epidural opioid administration. For these patients, monitor respiratory rate at least every two hours for the first 24 hours and, if directed to do so, after additional intermittent epidural opioid administration by the anesthesiologist or an increase in epidural opioid infusion rate. Be aware that delayed respiratory depression can occur 3–12 hours after a bolus of epidural morphine, particularly in opioid-naïve populations particularly following large bolus doses (Pasero, 2005). Do not administer additional systemic opioids without consent from the anesthesia provider managing the epidural therapy. Notify the anesthesia provider immediately and discontinue infusion as ordered should the respiratory rate fall below 10 breaths/minute after arousing the patient. Prepare to administer intravenous Naloxone (0.2 mg) or initiate a low-dose naloxone infusion as directed by the anesthesia provider.

Elimination

Check for urinary retention if indwelling catheters are not placed, and use straight catheterization as needed. Like other epidural side effects, consider decreasing the dose or analgesic and/or anesthetic. Assess bowel function, which may return earlier with epidural analgesia compared with systemic opioid therapy.

Activity

Assessment of activity is appropriate for patients receiving intermittent or continuous administration of a local anesthetic. For these patients, check sensory level. Assess motor function in bed (ability to flex hips and knees and move toes). Consult with the anesthesia provider to consider reducing infusion rate or the concentration of local anesthetic if lower motor weakness or numbness is present. Conduct a two-person assist when getting the patient out of bed for the first time if motor function in bed is intact. Take orthostatic blood pressure and pulse before getting the patient out of bed for the first time.

Level of Consciousness

Assess the level of consciousness every 2 hours for the first 24 hours and every 4 hours thereafter until therapy is discontinued, using the sedation scale shown in **Table 36.12**. Notify the anesthesia provider if the patient exhibits a sedation level of 3 (severe).

Catheter and Catheter Site

Ensure that a transparent occlusive dressing is placed over the catheter insertion site. Note any visible markings on the catheter that are indications of insertion depth and continually observe to ensure that the catheter depth does not change. Check the catheter site and dressing every shift to ensure that they are secure and that there is no evidence of bleeding or fluid leaks. Report increased pain, tenderness, and drainage at the catheter insertion site. Report new onset of lower motor weakness that may be a sign of epidural abscess or hematoma. Reinforce dressing should it become loose or wet and notify the anesthesia provider immediately. Check the catheter and tubing junction to ensure that all connections are fixed firmly. Secure the catheter and tubing to avoid tension.

Patient Teaching

Explain the purpose and expected outcomes of therapy. Reinforce proper use of the patient pendant to self-administer a PCEA demand dose. Inform the patient of the expected onset and duration of the PCEA based on the epidural analgesic or analgesics. Encourage the use of demand dose before the pain gets out of control. Caution the patient not to get out of bed for the first time without assistance and to seek assistance each time if lower motor weakness is experienced. Instruct the patient to use care when moving about to avoid tension on the catheter or tubing. Instruct the patient to notify the nurse for unacceptable relief of pain, increased drowsiness or sedation, numbness or weakness of lower extremities, difficulty urinating, pain or severe discomfort at the catheter site, headaches, and nausea or vomiting anytime during therapy or coinciding with administration of PCEA demand dose

Table 36.12	Sedation Scale
Degree of Sedation	**Description**
0 (none)	Alert
1 (mild)	Occasionally drowsy; easy to arouse
2 (moderate)	Frequently drowsy; easy to arouse
3 (severe)	Somnolent; difficult to arouse
S (sleeping)	Normal sleep; easy to arouse

Adapted from Ready, B. L., Loper, K. A., Nessly, M., & Wild, L. (1991). Postoperative epidural morphine is safe on surgical wards. *Anesthesiology,* 75, 452–456.

Interpleural Analgesia

Interpleural analgesia is accomplished through the instillation of a local anesthetic into the space between the parietal and visceral pleura. The technique is intended to selectively block intercostal sensory nerves while maintaining normal function of the internal and external motor nerves, which innervate intercostal muscles for coughing and deep breathing. The area of catheter placement depends on the type of procedure. For an open thoracotomy the catheter may be inserted before closure of the intercostal or subcostal incisions. Catheters may be placed through small incisions that are made to accommodate scopes used for video thoracoscopy. Blind insertion of the catheter for blunt chest trauma may pose greater risks for pneumothorax. Although interpleural analgesia is usually implemented after the procedure, use of the catheter before the procedure with bupivacaine has been shown to be superior to postprocedure administration in minimizing postprocedure pain and requests for additional analgesia among women having a cholecystectomy (Abdulatif et al., 1995).

Continuous infusions of local anesthetics are superior to intermittent injection in providing analgesia. Because state regulatory and institutional policies and procedures may limit the degree to which nurses can initiate and maintain interpleural infusions, nursing practices in the care of patients receiving interpleural analgesia may vary.

Patient-Controlled Analgesia

Patient-controlled analgesia is widely recognized as an effective means to provide effective pain control in the postprocedure period. Relatively small doses of morphine, fentanyl, and hydromorphone are programmed into the machine and are available to the patient initiating administration with a push of the button at a predetermined frequency.

Meperidine was commonly used for PCA and is an effective analgesic option particularly in patients with allergies to other opioids, but has fallen out of favor due to the potential for accumulation of its neurotoxic metabolite, normeperidine. Patients at high risk for toxicity include the elderly and those with impaired renal function. Early signs of normeperidine toxicity may include myoclonus and confusion with the potential for seizures if the metabolite continues to accumulate. For this reason, removal of meperidine from institutional formularies or restricted use to no more than 600 mg/day for 48 hours has become a measure of quality of pain management services. **Table 36.13** shows Patient-Controlled Analgesia (PCA) Guidelines for Opioid-Naïve Patients.

The use of continuous or basal rate infusions is controversial and is currently discouraged in opioid naïve patients or other at-risk populations such as patients diagnosed with obstructive sleep apnea in the early titration period due to the risk of opioid induced oversedation and respiratory depression. Patients and families must be given instruction about the safe use of PCA and family members must be aware of increased risk from adverse events if family members push the button for the patient, known as PCA by proxy.

Postprocedure Nursing Interventions

After the procedure, assess the patient's cognitive ability to understand and use PCA therapy. Program the device with drug, concentration, and prescribed dosing parameters. Initiate the infusion in the postanesthesia care unit. Administer a loading

Table 36.13	Patient-Controlled Analgesia (PCA) Guidelines for Opioid-Naïve Patients	
Drug	**Demand Dose**	**Lockout Interval**
Morphine	1–2 mg	6–10 min
Hydromorphone	0.2–0.4 mg	6–10 min
Fentanyl	20–50 µg	5–10 min
Sufentanil	4–6 µg	5–10 min
Meperidine[†]	10–20 mg	6–10 min
Tramadol	10–20 mg	6–10 min

[†]*Meperidine should only be used in patients intolerant to all other opioids.*
Adapted from Grass, J. A., Patient-controlled analgesia, *Anesth Analg*, 2005, 101: S44–S61.

dose, as ordered, if the patient did not receive a bolus dose of an opioid upon emergence from anesthesia. Reinforce prior teaching or introduce the principles of PCA and the operation of the device. Encourage the patient to push the patient pendant or button before the pain gets severe. Focus the patient's attention to accessing medication when needed, rather than watching the clock. Monitor vital signs according to standard postprocedure procedures. Evaluate pain levels and assess patient use before transferring the patient to the general operative unit.

Multimodal Therapy

Multimodal therapy is defined as the use of combinations of medications from more than one class of drugs, regional anesthetic techniques, and non-pharmacologic modalities to bring about additive analgesic effect and reduce side effect profile from medications. This is very different from polypharmacy where there may be multiple providers simultaneously ordering many medications often from the same class at the same time. Consideration of multimodal approaches is becoming the standard of care for the treatment of both acute and chronic pain and begins with preemptive analgesia as discussed above (Windle, 2004).

Postprocedure Period and Beyond

The nurse must continue to treat pain aggressively in the postprocedure period, using both pharmacologic and non-pharmacologic modalities to promote early ambulation and rehabilitation to prevent complications such as atelectasis from inadequate pulmonary effort and deep vein thrombosis from immobility. The nurse also ensures patients receiving opioid analgesics are adequately propylaxed for constipation. Once the patient is able to tolerate oral medications, efforts should begin to convert analgesics to the oral route with adequate strength and routine dosing with long-acting or scheduled analgesics if pain persists around the clock. Consideration must be given to calculate effective oral dosing based on effective parenteral doses. One method suggests conversion of one half of the 24-hour equianalgesic from parenteral to oral formulation to long-acting scheduled doses, and converting the remaining half to short-acting analgesics available as needed for breakthrough pain (Carol, Angst, & Clark, 2004). The nurse should also anticipate the need to taper analgesics for patients receiving around-the-clock dosing for several days. One potential taper plan is to reduce the total amount of opioids by 20% every 48 hours until the desired level is reached or the patient no longer requires opioid analgesics. Patients who have taken opioids routinely for more than a few days should be cautioned to avoid stopping the medications abruptly, to avoid the onset of withdrawal symptoms (Parran & Penderson, 2002). The nurse should also facilitate patient discharge home on adequate oral medications to promote continued recovery and reduce the potential for readmission due to uncontrolled pain.

Table 36.14 shows an example of an equianalgesic[1] chart, which provides a guideline for the administration of opioid and nonopioid pain medications. Doses and intervals between doses depend on patient response. Use the equianalgesic chart when substituting one drug for another, or when changing from one route of administration to another. The doses listed for moderate to severe pain are not necessarily starting doses. When caring for an elderly patient, initially reduce the recommended adult opioid dose for moderate to severe pain by 25% to 50%. Use a conservative starting dose of a new opioid if the patient has been receiving opioids for a long time (McCaffery & Pasero, 1999).

NURSING MANAGEMENT OF CHRONIC PAIN

Nursing management of chronic pain often requires a different approach. Patients are often treated on an outpatient basis using several different therapies including: psychology, physical therapy, occupational therapy, biofeedback, interventional techniques, as well as pharmacologic pain treatments (Arnstein, 2003). The long-term use of opioids to treat chronic pain remains controversial due to long-term hormonal effects, abuse and diversion potential, and the incompletely understood and therefore controversial considerations surrounding the development of opioid-induced hyperalgesia. However, opioids are indicated when other treatments have failed to treat pain effectively.

Chronic pain patients being considered for long-term opioid therapy benefit from risk assessment prior to therapy using a validated tool such as the Opioid Risk Tool, a pain agreement outlining rights and responsibilities for both patient and prescriber, and a structured approach to evaluation of treatment using the *Four "A" Approach*. **Table 36.15** highlights the components of the Four "A" Approach of assessing pain treatment outcomes. This approach assesses the effect of analgesia, activities of daily living, adverse drug effects, and aberrant drug-related behaviors (Passik & Kirsh, 2003; Passik & Kirsh, 2005). Patients who are identified with significant or recurrent aberrant drug-related behavior often benefit from increasing the frequency of appointments for medication refills and performing pill counts to help confirm use.

Interventional Techniques for Chronic Pain

Trigger-point injections usually involve the injection of small amounts of local anesthetic with or without steroid into myofascial trigger points or "knots" of muscle that cause significant pain and restricted range of motion to patient with myofascial pain disorders. Relief is usually immediate with variable duration of effect lasting hours to several weeks or more and can occasionally completely resolve the symptom if underlying mechanical dysfunction resolves with gentle stretching and physical therapy techniques. Trigger-point injections are typically performed in the outpatient setting.

Table 36.14	**Equianalgesic Chart**	
Approximate Equivalent Doses of Opioids for Moderate to Severe Pain		
Analgesic	**Parenteral (IM, SC, IV) Route[1,2] (mg)**	**PO Route[1] (mg)**
MUOPIOID AGONISTS		
Morphine	10	30
Codeine	130	200 NR
Fentanyl	100 µg/h parenterally and transdermally ≡ 4 mg/h morphine parenterally; 1 µg/h transdermally ≡ 2 mg/24h morphine PO	
Hydromorphone (Dilaudid)	1.5	7.5
Levorphanol (Levo-Dromoran)	2	4
Meperidine	75	300 NR
Methadone (Dolophine)	10	20
Oxycodone	—	20
Oxymorphone (Numorphan)	1	10 rectal
AGONIST-ANTAGONIST OPIODS		
Buprenorphine (Buprenex)	.04	—
Butorphanol (Stadol)	2	—
Dezocine (Dalgan)	10	
Nalbuphine (Nubain)	10	—
Pentazocine (Talwin)	60	180
Approximate Equivalent Doses of PO Non-Opioids and Opioids for Mild to Moderate Pain		
Analgesic	**Parenteral (IM, SC, IV) Route[1,2] (mg)**	**PO Route[1] (mg)**
NON-OPIOIDS		
Acetaminophen	—	650
Aspirin (ASA)	—	650
OPIOIDS		
Codeine	—	32–60
Hydrocodone	—	5
Meperidine (Demerol)	—	50
Oxycodone	—	3–5
Propoxyphene (Darvon)	—	65–100

[1]Duration of analgesia is dose dependent; the higher the dose, usually the long the duration.

[2]IV boluses may be used to produce analgesia that lasts approximately as long as IM or SC doses. However, of all routes of administration, IV produces the highest peak concentration of the drug, and the peak concentration is associated with the highest level of toxicity, eg, sedation. To decrease the peak effect and lower the level of toxicity, IV boluses may be administered more slowly, eg, 10 mg of morphine over a 15-minute period or smaller doses may be administered more often, eg, 5 mg of morphine every 1–1.5 hours.

FDA = Food and Drug Administration; NR = not recommended; ~ = roughly equal to

Adapted from McCaffery, M. & Pasero, C. (1999). *Pain: Clinical Manual*, Second Edition. Philadelphia, PA: Mosby, pp. 133, 241–243.

Table 36.15	The Four "A" Approach of Assessing Pain Treatment Outcomes
Analgesia	Assessment of analgesic effect by using a validated pain scale
Activities of daily living	Evaluation of effect of medications on activities of daily living and understanding of how good chronic pain management improves function in these domains
Adverse effects	Evaluation of adverse drug effects such as somnolence or constipation
Aberrant drug taking	Aberrant drug-related behaviors combining objective assessment and documentation of behaviors; use of random urine drug screening for both the presence of illicit drugs and drugs not prescribed by the practitioner and for absence of chronically prescribed drugs in the urine

Adapted from Passik, S., & Kirsh, K. (2003, June 1). The need to identify predictors of aberrant behavior and addiction in patients being treated with opioids for pain. *Pain Medicine*, 4(20), 186–189.

Epidural steroid injection is another example of an interventional acute and chronic pain management technique indicated for lumbar and cervical radiculopathy. These injections are usually performed on an outpatient basis.

Neuromodulation techniques for chronic pain involve electrical stimulation of the nervous system for the purpose of modulating or modifying pain. Recent technology improvements have resulted in increased frequency of use. Neuromodulation is an effective modality for the treatment of chronic neuropathic pain and can reduce the need for systemic analgesics, resulting in decreased side effect. Patient selection improves outcomes for this therapy with patients presenting with inadequate relief from systemic analgesic trial and unilateral pain of an extremity, bilateral upper or lower extremity pain, no uncontrolled diabetes, no compromised immune function, no organ transplant or chronic steroid use, no spinal stenosis at the level of electrode placement, and no aberrant opioid-related drug use behavior representing ideal candidates for therapy. Patients requiring ongoing cancer assessments with serial magnetic resonance imaging (MRI) screening, patients with history of chronic kidney stones requiring lithotripsy, morbidly obese, and those with history of infectious disease require careful consideration prior to implantation and may not be selected for therapy. Patients must have realistic expectations for pain relief. Referral for behavioral evaluation prior to operative implantation is recommended.

Nursing management for patients undergoing operative implantation include pain assessment which separates operative site ratings from underlying chronic pain condition, operative site assessment, aggressive treatment of muscle spasms, continued administration of chronic pain medications, and additional analgesics for operative pain.

Peripheral nerve blocks are often used for chronic pain syndromes and can be used for the treatment of cancer pain. Types of nerve blocks for cancer patients include: trigeminal for face, brachial plexus, interscalene, supraclavicular, infraclavicular or selective nerve blocks for upper extremity cancer pain, stellate ganglion blocks for cancer pain in the upper extremity, face and neck, intercostal for chest wall cancer pain, femoral for anterior lateral proximal lower extremity cancer pain, and sciatic for

MRI
Magnetic Resonance Imaging

posterior medial or distal lower extremity cancer pain. Celiac plexus neural blockade is indicated for intra-abdominal visceral analgesia, cancer of the stomach, pancreas, gall bladder, adrenal glands, and common bile duct cancers. Preemptive measures for celiac plexus blocks include administering fluids and clarifying pain relief. Procedure does not change disease status and the potential for loose stools. Hypogastric and ganglion impar blocks are indicated for pelvic or rectal cancer pain and do not impair urinary or fecal continence. Cervical epidural nerve blocks are indicated for pain secondary to head, face, neck, shoulder, and upper extremity malignancies and chemotherapy related peripheral neuropathies. Thoracic epidural nerve blocks are indicated for chest malignancies or for pain related to thoracotomy. Lumbar epidural blocks are indicated for pain related to abdominal pelvic and lower extremity malignancies and chemotherapy induced peripheral neuropathy.

Interventional pain management in the oncology patient can be considered for patients who fail to achieve acceptable relief of pain with systemic medications alone. Interventional techniques must also consider the patient's nutritional status, white blood count, platelet count, whether the patient will require followup MRI scans, and types of chemotherapeutic agents chosen.

Intrathecal pumps in oncology patients may decrease pain and side effects, increase activity and quality of life, allow for continuation of cancer treatment, allow weaning of oral medications, decrease hospitalizations and procedures, and decrease healthcare expenditures (Vanni, 2008). Prior to implantation of an intrathecal device, the patient undergoes a screening test to evaluate response on pain level and side effect profile. A 50% reduction in pain is often considered a positive outcome. Medications commonly administered via intrathecal route include morphine, clonidine, Ziconotide, and baclofen. Other medications are being investigated. Nursing management of implanted intrathecal pumps is similar to those outlines for implanted neurostimulators with vigilant assessment for signs and symptoms of infection. **Figure 36.4** shows the insertion of intrathecal baclofen pump.

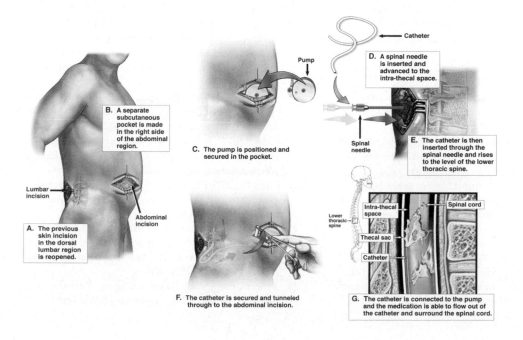

Figure 36.4

Insertion of intrathecal baclofen pump.

A. The previous skin incision in the dorsal lumbar region is reopened.

B. A separate subcutaneous pocket is made in the right side of the abdominal region.

C. The pump is positioned and secured in the pocket.

D. A spinal needle is inserted and advanced to the intra-thecal space.

E. The catheter is then inserted through the spinal needle and rises to the level of the lower thoracic spine.

F. The catheter is secured and tunneled through to the abdominal incision.

G. The catheter is connected to the pump and the medication is able to flow out of the catheter and surround the spinal cord.

Lumbar incision

Abdominal incision

Catheter

Pump

Spinal needle

Lower thoracic spine

Intra-thecal space

Spinal cord

Thecal sac

Catheter

CONCLUSION

The management of acute and chronic pain is a critical activity during the operative and invasive procedure period. Adequate pain management contributes to the patient's well-being, increases satisfaction with care, and quality of life. The nurse engaged in the care of the operative and invasive procedure patient plays a significant role in pain management by assisting the anesthesia provider in providing pain relief, administering pain medications, and caring for the patient receiving moderate sedation/analgesia.

ENDNOTE

1. The term equianalgesic means approximately the same pain relief (McCaffery & Pasero, 2007).

REFERENCES

1. Abdulatif, M., al-Ghamidi, A., Gyamfi, Y.A., et al. (1995). Can pre-emptive interpleural block reduce perioperative anesthetic and analgesic requirement? *Regional Anesthesia*, 20, 296–302.

2. Alford, D.P., Compton, P., & Samet, J.H. (2006, March, 21). Acute pain management for patients receiving maintenance methadone or buprenorphine therapy. *Annals of Internal Medicine*, 144(2), 127–134.

3. American Pain Foundation. (2008). Pain facts and figures as compared to other major conditions. Retrieved September 16, 2008, from American Pain Foundation Web site: http://www.painfoundation. org/page.asp?file_newsroom.painfacts.htm.

4. American Pain Society. (2006). Pain: current understanding of assessment, management, and treatments. Glenview, IL: American Pain Society.

5. American Society for Pain Management Nurses. (2008). Position statement: pain management in patients with addictive disease. Lenexa, KS.

6. American Society of Anesthesiologists. (2006, May). Practice guidelines for perioperative management of patients with obstructive sleep apnea. *Anesthesiology*, 104(5), 1081–1093.

7. Ang, P., Knight, H., Matadial, C., Pagan, A., Curty, R., Nieves, C., Acevedo, A. A., & Dalisay, F. P. (2004, October). Managing acute postprocedure pain: is 3 hours too long. *Journal of PeriAnesthesia, Nursing*, 19(5), 312–333.

8. Answers.com (2008). Hypoventilation. Retrieved 11 September 2008, from Answers.com Web site: http://www.answers.com/hypoventilation&r=67.

9. Arnstein, P. (2003). Comprehensive analysis and management of chronic pain. *The Nursing Clinics of North America*, 38, 403–417.

10. Ballanyne, C., & Mao, J. (2003, November 13). Opioid therapy for chronic pain. *New England Journal of Medicine*, 349(20), 1943–1953.

11. Barnes, S. (2001, April). Pain management: what do patients need to know and when do they need to know it. *Journal of PeriAnesthesia Nursing*, 16(2), 107–108.

12. Bonham, V.L. (2001). Race, ethnicity, and pain treatment: striving to understand the causes and solutions to the disparities in pain treatment. *Journal of Law, Medicine, & Ethics*, 29, 52–68.

13. Buss, H.E., & Melderis, K. (2002, February). PACU pain management Algorithm. *Journal of PeriAnesthesia Nursing*, 17(1), 11–20.

14. Carpenito-Moyet, L.J. (2008). *Handbook of Nursing Diagnosis*. Twelfth Edition. Philadelphia, PA: Lippincott Williams & Wilkins, p. 69.

15. Carroll, I.R., Angst, M.S., & Clark, J.D. (2004, November-December). Management of perioperative pain in patients chronically consuming opioids. *Regional Anesthesia and Pain Medicine*, 29(6), 576–591.

16. Cedarholm, I. (1997). Preliminary risk-benefit of ropivacaine in labour and following surgery. *Drug Safety*, 16, 391–402.

17. Centers for Disease Control and Prevention (CDC). (2007). *Advance Data from Vital and Health Statistics*, 385:1–20. Retrieved on September 16, 2008 from http://www.cdc.gov/nchs/data/ad/ad385.pdf.

18. Cintron, A., & Morrison, S. (2006, December 1). Pain and ethnicity in the United States: a systematic review. *Journal of Palliative Medicine*, 9(6), 1454–1473.

19. Clark, D. (1999). "Total pain", disciplinary power and the body in the work of Cicely Saunders, 1958–1967. *Social Science & Medicine*, 49, 727–736.

20. Compton, P., & Athanos, P. (2003). Chronic pain, substance abuse and addiction. *The Nursing Clinics of North America*, 38, 525–537.

21. Diaz, G., & Flood, P. (2006). Strategies for effective postprocedure pain management. *Minerva Anesthesiologica*, 72(3), 145–150.

22. Ezenwa, M.O., Amerger, S., Ward, S.E., & Serlin, R.C. (2006). Racial and ethnic disparities in pain management in the United States. *Journal of Nursing Scholarship*, 38(3), 225–233.

23. Federal Interagency Forum on Aging-Related Statistics. Retrieved September 16, 2008 from

http://agingstats.gov/agingstatsdotnet/Main_Site/Data/2008_Documents/Population.aspx.

24. Ferrante, F.M. (1993). Local anesthetics. In F.M. Ferrante & T.R. Vade Boncouer (Eds.). *Postoperative pain management* (p. 215). New York: Churchill Livingstone.

25. Fick, D.M., Cooper, J.W., Wade, W.E., Waller, J.L., Mclean, J.R., & Beers, M.H. (2003). Updating the Beers criteria for potentially inappropriate medication use in older adults. *Archives of Internal Medicine, 163*(22), 2716–2724.

26. Gordon, D., Pellino, T.A., Miaskowski, C., Adams, J., Paice, J.A., Laferriere, D., & Bookbinder, M. (2002, December). A 10-year review of quality improvement monitoring in pain management: recommendations for standardized outcome measures. *Pain Management Nursing, 3*(4), 116–130.

27. Grass, J.A. (2005). Patient-controlled analgesia. *Anesth Analg, 101,* S44–S61.

28. Gourlay, D., Heit, H., & Abdulaziz, A. (2005, April 1). Universal precautions in pain medicine: a rational approach to chronic pain. *Pain Medicine, 6*(20), 107–112.

29. Hansen, G. (2005, May 1). Management of chronic pain in the acute care setting. *Emergency Medicine Clinics of North America, 23*(2), 307–338.

30. Herr, K., Coyne, P., Key, T., Manworren, R., McCaffery, M., Merkel, S., et al. (2006). Pain assessment in the nonverbal patient: position statement with clinical practice recommendations. *Pain Management Nursing, 7*(2).

31. Hydromorphone hydrochloride, retrieved from http://www.drugs.com/ppa/hydromorphone-hydrochloride.html, accessed on January 20, 2009.

32. Kehlet, H., Jensen, T.S., & Woolf, C. (2006, May). Persistent postoperative pain: risk factors and prevention. *Lancet, 367,* 1618–1625.

33. McCaffery, M. (1979). Nursing Management of the Patient with Pain. (2nd ed.) Philadelphia: J.B. Lippincott.

34. McCaffery, M., Grimm, M., Pasero, C., Ferrell, B., & Uman, G. (2005, December 1). On the meaning of "drug seeking." *Pain Management Nursing, 6*(4), 122–136.

35. McCaffery, M., & Pasero, C. (1999). *Pain: Clinical Manual,* Second Edition. Philadelphia, PA: Mosby, pp. 133, 241–243.

36. McClure, J.H. (1996). Ropivacaine. *British Journal of Anesthesia, 76,* 300–307.

37. MedicineNet.com (2008). Definition of Neuroplasticity. Retrieved 11 September 2008 from MedicineNet.com Web site: http:// www.medterms.com/script/main/art.asp?articlekey=40362

38. Morgan, B. (2006, March). Knowing how to play the game: hospitalized substance abusers' strategies for obtaining pain relief. *Pain Management Nursing 7*(1), 31–41.

39. Morrison, S., Wallenstein, S., Senzel, R., & Huang, L. (2000, April 6). "We don't carry that"—failure of pharmacies in predominantly nonwhite neighborhoods to stock opioid analgesics. *New England Journal of Medicine, 342*(14), 1023–1026.

40. National Comprehensive Cancer Network. (2008, May 6). *NCCN Clinical Practice Guidelines in Oncology: Adult Cancer Pain* (Vol. 1). Fort Washington, PA: The National Comprehensive Cancer Network (NCCN).

41. National Council of State Boards of Nursing. (2007). Statement on the regulatory implications of pain management.

42. O'Malley, P. (2007). Accounting for pharmacokinetic and pharmacodynamic variability. *Clinical Nurse Specialist,* 274–276.

43. Overdyke, F.J., Carter, R., Maddox, R.R., Callura, J., Herrin, A.E., & Henriquez, C. (2007, August). Continuous oximetry/ capnometry monitoring reveals frequent desaturation and bradypnea during patient controlled analgesia. *International Anesthesia Research Society, 105*(2), 412–418.

44. Parran, L., & Penderson, C. (2002). Effects of an opioid taper algorithm in hematopoietic progenitor cell transplant recipients. *Oncology Nursing Forum, 29*(1), 41–46.

45. Pasero, C. (2003, August). Multimodal balanced analgesia in the PACU. *Journal of PeriAnesthesia Nursing, 18*(4), 265–268.

46. Pasero, C. (2005, August). Fentanyl for acute pain management. *Journal of PeriAnesthesia Nursing, 20*(4), 279–284.

47. Pasero, C. (2005). Epidural analgesic for acute pain management in adults. *American Society for Pain Management Nursing,* Lenexa, KA.

48. Pasero, C. (2008, September 4). The hospitalized older patient with pain. Presented at the American Society for Pain Management Nursing, Tucson, AZ.

49. Passik, S., & Kirsh, K. (2003, June 1). The need to identify predictors of aberrant behavior and addiction in patients being treated with opioids for pain. *Pain Medicine, 4*(20), 186–189.

50. Passik, S., & Kirsh, K. (2005, February 1). Managing pain in patients with aberrant drug-taking behaviors. *Journal of Supportive Oncology, 3*(1), 83–86.

51. Pennsylvania Patient Safety Authority. (2006, June). Demerol: Is it the best analgesic. *Patient Safety Advisory, 3*(2), 1–2.

52. Pizzi, L.J. (2008, September 5). Managing postop pain: a multimodal approach. Presented at the American Society for Pain Management Nursing, Tucson, AZ.

53. Rakel, B. & Herr, K. (2004). Assessment and treatment of postoperative pain in older adults. *Journal of PeriAnesthesia Nursing, 19*(3), 194–208.

54. Ralston, D.L. (1996). Pain management: Texas legislative and regulatory update. *Journal of Law, Medicine and Ethics, 24,* 328–337.

55. Reuben, S.S., Buvanendran, A., Kroin, J.S., & Raghunathan, K. (2006, November). The analgesic efficacy of Celecoxib, Pregabalin, and their combination for spinal fusion surgery. *Pain Medicine, 103*(5), 1271–1277.

56. Rudolph, L. (2008, September 5). Pre-emptive analgesia in the orthopedic patient: stopping the pain before it starts. Presented at the American Society for Pain Management Nursing, Tucson, AZ.

57. RxList (2009). Sufenta, retrieved from www.rxlist. com/sufenta-drug.htm, accessed on January 20, 2009. Drug.com (2008).

58. Smith, H. (2008, April 11). Variations in opioid responsiveness. *Pain Physician, 2,* 237–248.

59. Summers, S. (2000, October). Evidence- based practice part 1: pain definitions, pathophysiologic mechanisms, and theories. *Journal of Perianesthesia Nursing,* 15(5), 357–365.

60. Task Force on Taxonomy of the International Association for the Study of Pain. (1994). In H. Merskey & N. Bogduk (Eds.). *Classification of Chronic Pain: Descriptions of Chronic Pain Syndromes and Definitions of Pain Terms* (2nd ed., pp. 209–213), Seattle: IASP Press.

61. Taylor, S., Kirton, O.C., Staff, I., & Kozol, R.A. (2005). Postprocedure day one: a high risk period for respiratory events. *The American Journal of Surgery,* 190, 752–756.

62. *The Free Dictionary* (2008). Nociceptor. Retrieved 13 September 2008 from The Free Dictionary by Farlex website: http://www.thefreedictionary.com/ nociceptor.

63. Ury, W.A., Rahn, M., Tolentino, V., Pignotti, M.G., Yoon, J., McKegney, P., et al. (2002, August 1). Can a pain management and palliative care curriculum improve opioid prescribing practices of medical residents? *Journal of General Internal Medicine, 17*(8).

64. Vanni, L. (2008, September 5). Interventional pain management techniques in the oncology patient. Presented at the American Society for Pain Management Nursing, Tuscon, AZ.

65. Wikipedia. (2008). Dermatome (Anatomy). Retrieved on 12 September 2008 from Wikipedia Web site: http://en.wikipedia.org/wiki/ Dermatome_(Anatomy).

65. Windle, P. (2004, June). The challenges of pain management: Adverse effects of analgesics. *Journal of PeriAnesthesia Nursing,* 19(3), 212–216.

67. Zaric, D., Boysen, K., Christiansen, C., Christiansen, J., Stephensen, S., & Christensen, B. (2006). A comparison of epidural analgesia with combined continuous femoral—sciatic nerve blocks after total knee replace. *Anesthesia and Analgesia,* 102, 1240–1246.

Section 4
Age Specific Care

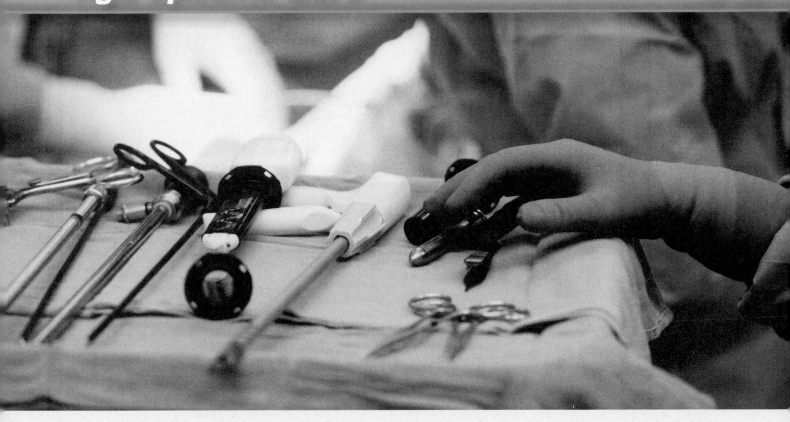

CHAPTER 37

Care of the Pediatric Patient

Kelly Kollar

Rose Moss

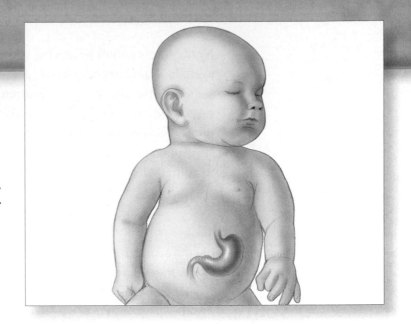

All children should be tirelessly noisy, playful, grubby-handed except at meal times, soiling and tearing such clothes as they need to wear, bringing not only the joy of childhood into the house but the dust and mud as well; in short, everything that makes the quiet and order of sickness and nursing impossible.

—George Bernard Shaw (1856–1950)

A pediatric operative or invasive procedure is not a procedure on a small adult. Not only are the procedures often exclusive to pediatric patients, but interventions throughout the procedure period also differ markedly. Pediatric patients vary from neonates to adolescents and young adults; thus, the nurse providing care during the operative and invasive procedures must possess knowledge of the stages of growth and development.

These are relatively simple statements with overwhelming implications for all staff caring for children within the operative and invasive procedure setting. The care of children is a unique and freestanding specialty. Instruments must be modified drastically for the variance in the size of pediatric patients. Appropriate-sized suture material and needles must also be available.

The impetus to develop pediatric surgery as a separate entity began with a few pioneers more than 50 years ago. The first organization for pediatric surgeons in North America was founded in 1948. Entire hospitals dedicated solely to the care of children were built. W. Potts clearly saw the need to develop pediatric surgery as a unique and separate entity when he said, "I have often wondered what sort of scar, how deep and how serious, is left on the heart of a child who is torn from his parents and suddenly tossed into a hospital environment associated in his mind with insecurity and pain" (Potts, 1956).

Chapter Contents

Now, however, most practicing clinicians in pediatric surgery believe that pain management is an integral part of care (Burrington, 1996).

In facilities that care for children, qualified pediatric nurses should be in senior positions to ensure children's needs are addressed. Often the pediatric population is poorly represented at strategic levels. The use of multidisciplinary teams including surgeons, anesthesia professionals, pediatricians, and pediatric nurses is imperative to address the specific needs of children (Smith & Dearmun, 2006).

FAMILY CENTERED CARE

Today's parents are savvy and know most organizations are adopting the philosophy of family centered care. Family centered care is complex and has broad definitions. It allows parents and families more freedom to come and go as the family sees fit. This type of care structure helps to limit anxiety and stress on families rather than having to adhere to the strict visitation guidelines of the past.

To alleviate anxiety in the pediatric population, a variety of techniques can be used. The use of other trained staff such as child life specialists, social workers, and nursing assistances, can help reduce anxiety. Age-appropriate teaching about what to expect, distraction techniques, role playing, play, and allowing comforting items to remain with the child will lower the child's anxiety level. Education of the family and child preprocedurely can take place at an anesthetic assessment visit or the day of the procedure. Efforts to educate can include traditional question answer sessions, pamphlets, or videos. Often a liaison will relay information about progress of the surgical or invasive procedure to the family. If there is not a liaison, the nurse may update the family on progress; however this should be included in preprocedure teaching so the family is not alarmed when called for the update (Wisselo, Stuart, & Muris, 2004).

Parents and children alike do not always feel like an organization is best addressing their specific needs. In the past, doctors and nurses may have come across as aloof and distant. To ensure that care is family centered, help your facility to support parents and children in their various roles. Provide access to media that parents need during their stay at the hospital. Provide children with age appropriate toys. Provide time and space for families to be together. Parents strive to comfort and support their sick child and, as care givers, nurses need to support them. Offer open communication. Consider the spiritual and emotional needs of all the members involved. Offer families choices if applicable, allow them to maintain some control, and give personalized care. A liaison or concierge can be extremely comforting to families while waiting for a surgical outcome (Miceli & Clark, 2004).

Even though family-centered care is the goal for most of today's pediatric facilities, current literature shows that it is not always optimized. Healthcare workers often find it difficult to relinquish control as parents take over some of the care of their child. Parents want to have communication about care expectations. The care providers need to communicate who is responsible for what care is given to children. Nurses are accepting of parents participating in care of their child. If work routines can be established, it can decrease the frustrations of all care providers; parents and staff (Ygge, Lindholm, & Arnetz, 2006).

CONSENTS IN THE PEDIATRIC POPULATION

For operative or invasive procedures, informed consent is required. Informed consent implies that a person legally responsible for the child having the procedure is agreeing to the procedure, after a full explanation of the procedure and alternatives to the procedure takes place. The obtaining of informed consent also includes a chance for the legal guardian to ask questions, a chance to think about all of the available options, and the right to decline the procedure (Crosbie, 2007). Typically, consent is rendered from a parent if a child is less then 18 years of age. However, if a child disagrees with the decision of the parent regarding a surgically invasive procedure, healthcare providers will strongly take their concerns into account. The aide of ethical or legal consult may advise the healthcare providers (Griffith, 2004).

There are some special considerations for obtaining consent in the pediatric population. The use of interpreter services is growing with the increasingly diverse population. Most facilities offer comprehensive interpreter services. It is not appropriate to use a child as a translator. Doing so can have legal repercussions (Lehna, 2005). The next special instance is that of an intoxicated or impaired parent who is legally responsible for giving consent for his or her child. If the procedure is nonurgent, then rescheduling until informed consent can be obtained is an option; however, if the procedure is urgent then the care providers' first duty is to the patient. If there is suspected neglect or child abuse, the care provider is mandated to report the event (Fraser & McAbee, 2004).

Another situation that needs special consideration is that of caring for a child whose family's religious beliefs are that of Jehovah's Witness. These children and families hold a belief that the consumption of blood in the form of a transfusion is forbade by God. The Jehovah's Witnesses will consent and allow for some blood components to be administered, like albumin or clotting factors, but will not allow red blood cells, white blood cells, plasma, and platelets. Sometimes the use of a cell saver may be authorized. All available options that conform to cultural and religious beliefs should be discussed prior to the procedure. The welfare of the child is the foremost concern for the healthcare provider (Wilson, 2005).

Along with obtaining consent from a parent or guardian, it is beneficial to involve the child. Involving the child gives them autonomy, self-determination, a sense of control, and a greater likelihood of cooperation in care and treatment. Children at the age of 12 are generally considered to have the ability to process information given to them for an informed consent. The role of the pediatric nurse is to act as an advocate for both the child and the family. Involving the entire family in the healthcare process can be challenging, especially if opinions differ within the family (Hallstrom & Elander, 2005).

Research in the pediatric population is heavily scrutinized to ensure that the best interest of the child is accounted for. When pediatric research is done, assent from the child 7 years or older is often obtained along with informed consent about the research from the parent or guardian. Assent ensures that the child has a voice concerning his or her own body; however, it is considered the lowest form of consent (Hallstrom & Elander, 2005). An Internal Review Board (IRB) will set up requirements for attaining assent from pediatric patients (Whittle, Shah, Wilfond, Gensler, & Wendler, 2004).

IRB
Internal Review Board

PHYSIOLOGICAL UNIQUENESS OF CHILDREN
Airway and Pulmonary Management

Children differ physiologically from adults in several areas that can affect the outcome of a procedure. Airway management is a priority because of the decreased diameter of the trachea in children. Cartilage development before muscle growth also makes the airway more prone to collapse than in the adult. If cold stress, hypoglycemia, hypovolemia, and sepsis occur, the young child is susceptible to respiratory arrest.

The lungs appear in the fourth to eighth weeks of gestation (Kovarik, 2005). The endodermal lung buds have divided into the main stem bronchi at four weeks; by six weeks, all of the subsegmental bronchi can be identified; at sixteen weeks, the number of airway generations that arise from axial pathways is similar to that found in adults; by approximately 24 weeks' gestation, the lungs are capable of extrauterine gas exchange (Kovarik, 2005). The pulmonary system is not capable of sustaining life until both the pulmonary airways and the vascular system have matured sufficiently to allow the exchange of oxygen from the air to the bloodstream across the pulmonary alveolar/vascular bed; independent life is not possible until the gestational age is 24 to 26 weeks (Coté, 2005). Alveoli increase in both size and number until the child is approximately 8 years old (Coté, 2005).

There are several anatomic differences that make respiration less efficient in infants and partially explain the high respiratory rate of infants and the rapidity with which hemoglobin desaturation can occur (Coté, 2005):

- the small diameter of the airways increased the resistance to airflow;
- the infant's airway is highly compliant and poorly supported by the surrounding structures;
- the chest wall is highly compliant, therefore the ribs provide little support for the lungs; and
- oxygen consumption is two to three times as high as it is in adults, even though dead-space ventilation is proportionally similar to that in adults.

To satisfy increased oxygen demands, alveolar ventilation in children is twice that of adults. The respiratory rate increases faster than the volume of air. This leads to decreased respiratory reserves related to functional and structural immaturity, as well as increased anesthetic requirements in relationship to size. The expired minimum alveolar concentration (MAC) of inhaled anesthetic gases required in pediatric patients changes with their age: the anesthetic requirement is lower for premature than for term neonates, and lower for term neonates than for a 3-month-old (Coté, 2005). Furthermore, the uptake of potent anesthetics is more rapid in children due to their increased respiratory rates and cardiac index, as well as a higher proportional distribution of cardiac output to vessel-rich organs (Coté, 2005).

Although textbooks state that infant lungs are not fully viable until about 24–26 weeks because of sufficient surfactant and viable lung development, infants born prior to 24 weeks' gestation can sometimes survive with the aid of lung bypass efforts such as extra-corporeal membrane oxygenation (ECMO). ECMO can be used to provide oxygen-rich blood to vital organs in the case of severe lung conditions in neonates or cardiac arrest in children (Children's Hospital, 2008). Infants are

MAC
Minimum Alveolar
Concentration

ECMO
Extra-Corporeal
Membrane Oxygenation

primarily nose breathers until the age of 3–4 months is achieved, so any obstruction can quickly lead to acute respiratory distress. The infants' smaller trachea adds a greater risk for airway obstruction (Porth, 2007). Thus infants especially those prematurely born pose a greater risk for lung compromise.

Temperature Regulation

Thermoregulation is difficult for all pediatric patients. The infant is particularly susceptible to hypothermia due to both the large ratio of body surface area to weight, as well as the limited ability to cope with cold stress (Coté, 2005). Cold stress will lead to an increase in oxygen consumption and also causes metabolic acidosis; in addition, a premature infant is even more susceptible because of very thin skin and limited fat stores (Coté, 2005). An infant may compensate for the cold by both shivering and nonshivering (cellular) thermogenesis; the minimal ability to shiver during the first 3 months of life makes cellular thermogenesis, ie, the metabolism of brown fat, the principal mechanism of heat production (Coté, 2005). Anesthetic agents can alter many of the thermoregulatory processes, especially nonshivering thermogenesis in neonates; furthermore, infants may have an increased metabolic rate for up to 12 hours after the procedure (Coté, 2005).

All areas that affect heat loss during anesthesia and surgery must be addressed for the pediatric patient. The ambient room temperature is kept at 85°F (29.4°C); all intravenous fluids should be warmed prior to infusion; the inspired gases should be humidified. Only warm irrigation fluids and skin preparation fluids are used. Pooling of fluids under the patient's body may result in chemical burns and should be avoided. Radiant heat lights are directed at the child during induction of anesthesia, skin preparation, and emergence from anesthesia. Wrapping the patient's extremities and top of the head in plastic wrap or bags helps to prevent heat loss. An underbody warming mat or forced air warming blanket device reduces loss of body temperature. Anesthetized individuals typically loose 1.6°C during the first hour of surgical or invasive procedures and longer anesthesia times cause greater temperature loss (Sessler, 2000).

A body temperature registering below 95°F (35°C) represents a cold injury that can be associated with respiratory depression, hypoglycemia, acidosis, and sepsis. The greatest risk of intraoperative hypothermia is usually manifested in the postanesthesia recovery period.

Malignant hyperthermia (MH) is an autosomal dominant disorder where the temperature rises. It involves heat produced from muscular contractions brought on by a triggering agent that can lead to hyperthermia induced death (Porth, 2007). These agents include inhaled anesthetics like: sevoflurane, desflurane, isoflurane, and halothane. There is also a strong correlation associated with MH and the use of succinylcholine, a muscle relaxant. Nondepolarizing muscle relaxants, as well as many other anesthetic drugs, are safe in this population. Screening for a family history of MH should be included in the preprocedure assessment. Risk factors for MH include over 80 genetic disorders. The initial sign that a patient may be experiencing MH would be tachycardia. The telltale sign of increased temperature is a late sign of MH, and treatment would be difficult at this stage. Treatment of MH involves cooling the patient, stopping all inhaled anesthetics, 100% oxygen, and dantrolene sodium. Dantrolene sodium is difficult to mix so additional help should be called for (Denholm, 2007). If MH has been identified

MH
Malignant
Hyperthermia

either before or after the procedure the nurse can refer the family to the Malignant Hyperthermia Association of the United States' webpage at www.mhaus.org.

Energy Stores

Infants undergoing an operative or invasive procedure may have an increased risk of hypoglycemia. Glycogen stores can be decreased in children small for gestational age and those with malnutrition and hypoxia. In addition, prolonged fasting is often associated with several adverse effects, such as an increased risk of hypotension during induction due to preprocedure hypovolemia and hypoglycemia during the procedure (Greco, 2003).

The concern of unrecognized hypoglycemia is the motivation for the routine use of glucose-containing solutions in children, particularly those who have not had food or fluids for a prolonged period or those who have diminished glycogen stores (Coté, 2005). Therefore, current anesthetic management is often modified for patients believed to be at risk for the development of hypoglycemia and also for long surgical procedures: a balanced salt solution (ie, lactated Ringer's solution) should be used for all deficits and third-space losses with 5% dextrose in 0.45% normal saline administered piggyback at infusion maintenance rates to minimize the risk of a bolus dose of glucose, thereby addressing the concern of unrecognized hypoglycemia or accidental hyperglycemia (Coté, 2005).

Various factors influence the metabolism of surgical neonates, including prematurity, operative stress, critical illness, and sepsis (Pierro, 2002). The metabolic response to operative trauma differs between neonates and adults, as follows (Pierro, 2002):

- infants have high rates of protein turnover and nitrogen retention;
- energy expenditure increases only transiently (4 to 6 hours) after major surgery in neonates;
- protein turnover and catabolism seem not to be affected by major operative procedures in neonates; and
- for neonates on parenteral nutrition, carbohydrate and fat have an equivalent effect on protein metabolism.

Hypoglycemia compounds cold stress; oxygen and fluid requirements subject the child to septic risks. Because of reduced circulating blood volume in small children, every effort must be made to prevent what may at first appear to be slight hemorrhage. Correspondingly, the administration of intravenous (IV) fluids must be monitored closely to prevent fluid overload. Increased demands for oxygen and fluid result in greater energy need which contributes to energy losses and therefore to cold stress and sepsis. Desaturation occurs much more rapidly in infants than in adults. Children and infants have less oxygen reserve then adults. Constant surveillance is needed to prevent these damaging occurrences.

The pre- and postprocedure replacement of energy stores has been greatly enhanced by the delivery of parenteral nutrition, used for children who cannot tolerate enteral feeding (Kovarik, 2005). However, the use of the GI tract for alimentation is usually the safest and most efficient approach (Kovarik, 2005). The operative insertion of various enteral feeding devices via the stomach and jejunum has also proved successful in providing nutrition for the pediatric patient's requiring supplemental nutrition.

IV
Intravenous

Fluid Balance

Maintenance of proper fluid balance in the child is a critical physiological need. Children have a larger percentage of their body weight in extracellular water than do adults; thus their needs differ from those of adults. Infants can have 70%–90% of their body weight as water. A child's increased metabolic rate also increases the need for fluids. Increased evaporative water losses come from increased surface area and a thinner epidermis. A crying child may double his or her fluid loss. Radiant heat warmers and phototherapy also increase water losses. Children who have fevers and are undergoing ventilation also require additional fluids.

To add to the difficulty of maintaining fluid balance, children have a limited renal function because the glomerular filtration rate is 25% of that of an adult. The kidneys of children are immature and have a decreased ability to concentrate urine. All these factors contribute to the need for increased administration of maintenance fluids during the procedure, but extra replacement fluids are necessary when there are major alterations in fluid shifts or balances when a child undergoes a major procedure.

Third spacing can occur in children after the procedures as a result of peritoneal irritation caused by intestinal perforation, peritonitis, or enterocolitis. During the operative procedure, capillary and lymphatic drainage can occur throughout the intestinal tract. This damage causes increased capillary permeability, which may lead to leakage of fluid, electrolytes, and proteins from the capillary space to the interstitial and intracellular spaces. The spillage of bowel contents causes a loss of gastrointestinal tone and decreased peristaltic activity. The inflammatory response causes bacteria, fecal material, and intestinal juices to pour into the peritoneal cavity, mimicking a peritoneal burn. The loss of osmotic activity from the intravascular space to the interstitial and intracellular spaces causes more fluid to leave the capillaries. Children undergoing a procedure have an increased need for fluid replacement simply because of age, which is compounded when they lose fluids from the procedure and then have a large amount of needed reserve fluid sequestered in lost spaces. Children can require 1.5 to 2 times maintenance fluids to sustain fluid volume and blood pressure after the procedure until the capillaries begin to heal and the lymphatics return to work. By 24–48 hours after the procedure, the kidneys, if they have been well hydrated, begin the process of diuresis, and fluid administration can be decreased.

Cardiovascular System

The cardiovascular system in infants and children is dependent upon the progression of structural and functional maturation; the system undergoes significant physiological changes during the first year of life (Kovarik, 2005; Coté, 2005). At birth, several events change the hemodynamic interactions so that the fetal circulation becomes adult-type circulation (Coté, 2005):

- The placenta is removed from the circulation.
- Portal blood pressure falls, which in turn causes the ductus venosus to close and blood becomes oxygenated through the lungs.
- Exposure of the ductus arteriosis to oxygenated blood causes ductal closure.

Due to the combined effects of lung expansion, exposure of blood to oxygen, and loss of low resistance through placental blood flow, pulmonary vascular resistance decreases while peripheral vascular resistance increases rapidly (Coté, 2005). The fall in pulmonary vascular resistance occurs on the first day of life and continues to decrease gradually during the next several years. An increase in the pressure on the left side of the heart, due to the rise in peripheral vascular resistance, causes the mechanical closure of the foramen ovale (Coté, 2005). Risk factors that increase the likelihood of a prolonged transitional circulation include prematurity, infection, acidosis, pulmonary disease resulting in hypercarbia or hypoxemia, acidosis, hypothermia, and congenital heart disease (Coté, 2005).

The distribution of cardiac output and functional maturity of the heart affect the response of neonates, infants, and children to medications used in anesthesia; as noted, the uptake of potent anesthetic agents is more rapid in children because of their increased cardiac index and greater proportional distribution of cardiac output to vessel-rich organs (Coté, 2005). This rapid increase in blood anesthetic levels, in addition to the functional immaturity of cardiac development, explains at least in part, why it is easy to administer an overdose to infants and toddlers (Coté, 2005).

Premature Infants

Infants born prematurely pose specific concerns for care providers. Often these infants have congenital anomalies that can challenge even the most expert clinicians. In 2006, the preterm birth rate rose slightly to 12.8%; this rate has risen 21% since 1990 (CDC, 2007a). The US fetal mortality rate in 2003 was 6.23 fetal deaths of 20 weeks of gestation or more per 1,000 live births and fetal deaths ... Over one-half (51%) of fetal deaths of 20 weeks of gestation or more occurred between 20 and 27 weeks of gestation (CDC, 2007b).

Infant death can occur for a number of reasons. The most common causes are premature birth/low birth weight, congenital anomalies, and sudden infant death syndrome. A healthy pregnancy will lower the chance for having a premature/low birth weight and the likelihood of congenital anomalies. Women who are pregnant should seek prenatal care, take folic acid and iron supplements as recommended by their physician, limit cigarette smoking and alcohol use, and maintain a healthy weight during their pregnancy (CDC, 2007c).

Congenital Anomalies

There are many types of congenital anomalies. According to the MassChips database, the distribution of birth defects in Massachusetts for 2000–2003 was as follows (MassChips, 2008):

- 34% Cardiovascular
- 26.4% Musculoskeletal
- 16.9% Chromosomal Syndromes
- 16.4% Genitourinary
- 10.5% Orofacial
- 9.7% Gastrointestinal
- 9.2% Central Nervous System Related
- 6.9% Other

The most common congenital anomalies in these categories for Massachusetts in 2000–2003 were (MassChips, 2008):

- Atrial Septal Defect (ASD)—the atrium in the heart are not properly separated
- Patent Ductus Arteriosus (PDA)—the connection between the pulmonary artery and the aorta allowing oxygen rich blood to re-circulate through the lungs
- Ventricular Septal Defect (VSD)—the ventricles in the heart are not properly separated
- Cleft Lip—with or without Cleft Palate
- Hypospadias
- Club Foot
- Polydactyly/Syndactyly
- Trisomy 21 (Down's Syndrome)

Often these anomalies can lead to one or many surgical or invasive procedures over a lifetime.

ASD
Atrial Septal Defect

PDA
Patent Ductus Arteriosus

VSD
Ventricular Septal Defect

Laboratory Studies

There are unique physiological characteristics that make children different from adults. These differences are also observed in the normal ranges for laboratory studies. **Table 37.1** presents normal findings in common preprocedure blood tests for pediatric patients.

Table 37.1	Normal Pediatric Laboratory Values for Selected Blood Tests
Blood Urea Nitrogen	
1–3 years	5–17 mg/dL
4–13 years	7–17 mg/dL
14–19 years	8–21 mg/dL
Blood Volume	
Premature infants	98 mL/kg
At 1 year	86 mL/kg (range 69–112 mL/kg)
Older children	70 mL/kg (range 51–86 mL/kg)
Carbon Dioxide, Partial Pressure (pCO$_2$)	
Newborn	27–40 mmHg
Infant	27–41 mmHg
Children	32–48 mmHg
Carbon Dioxide, Total	
Cord blood	13–29 mmol/L
<1 year	17–31 mmol/L
Adults	34–30 mmol/L
Chloride	
<1 year	96–111 mmol/L
1–17 years	102–112 mmol/L
Adults	100–108 mmol/L

Creatinine

AGE	MALES	FEMALES
1–3 days	0.2–1.0 mg/dL	0.2–1.0 mg/dL
1 year	0.2–0.6 mg/dL	0.2–0.5 mg/dL
2–3 years	0.2–0.7 mg/dL	0.3–0.6 mg/dL
4–7 years	0.2–0.8 mg/dL	0.2–0.7 mg/dL
8–10 years	0.3–0.9 mg/dL	0.3–0.8 mg/dL
11–12 years	0.3–1.0 mg/dL	0.3–0.9 mg/dL
13–17 years	0.3–1.2 mg/dL	0.3–1.1 mg/dL
18–20 years	0.5–1.3 mg/dL	0.3–1.1 mg/dL

Glucose

Premature infants	20–80 mg/dL (1.11–4.44 mmol/L)
Full-term infants	30–100 mg/dL (1.67–5.56 mmol/L)
Children & adults (fasting)	60–105 mg/dL (3.33–5.88 mmol/L)

Hematocrit

AGE	MALES (%)	FEMALES (%)
Newborns	43.4–56.1	37.4–55.9
6 months–2 years	30.9–37.0	31.2–37.2
3–6 years	31.7–37.7	32.0–37.1
7–12 years	32.7–39.3	33.0–39.6
13–18 years	34.8–43.9	34.0–40.7
>18 years	33.4–46.2	33.0–41.0

Hemoglobin

AGE	MALES (g/dL)	FEMALES (g/dL)
Newborns	14.7–18.6	12.7–18.3
6 months–2 years	10.3–12.4	10.4–12.4
3–6 years	10.5–12.7	10.7–12.7
7–12 years	11.0–13.3	10.9–13.3
13–18 years	11.5–14.8	11.2–13.6
>18 years	10.9–15.7	10.7–13.5

Oxygen Saturation

Newborns	85%–90%
Thereafter	95%–99%

Partial Thromboplastin Time

Children	42–54 seconds

Platelet Count (RBC) (Values x 10^3/mm^3)

AGE	MALES	FEMALES
Newborns	164–351	234–346
1–2 months	275–567	295–615
3–6 months	275–566	288–598
7 months–2 years	219–452	229–465
3–6 years	204–405	204–402
7–12 years	194–364	183–369
13–18 years	165–332	185–335
>18 years	143–320	171–326

Potassium

Premature infants	4.5–7.2 mmol/L
Full-term infants	3.7–5.2 mmol/L
Children	3.5–5.8 mmol/L
Adults	3.5–5.5 mmol/L

Prothrombin Time

Children	11–15 seconds

Red Blood Cell Count (Values x 10^6/mm^3)

AGE	MALES	FEMALES
Newborn—6 months	4.2–5.5	3.4–5.4
3–6 years	4.1–5.0	4.1–4.9
7–12 years	4.0–4.9	4.0–4.9
13–18 years	4.2–5.3	4.0–4.9
>18 years	3.8–5.4	3.8–4.8

Sodium

Newborns	133–146 mmol/L
Children & adults	135–148 mmol/L

Thrombin Time

Children	12–16 seconds

White Blood Cell Count (Values x 10^3/mm^3)

AGE	MALES	FEMALES
Newborns	6.8–13.3	8.0–14.3
6 months–2 years	6.2–14.5	6.4–15.0
3–6 years	5.3–11.5	5.3–11.5
7–12 years	4.5–10.5	4.7–10.3
13–18 years	4.5–10.0	4.8–10.1
>18 years	4.4–10.2	4.9–10.0

Adapted from: Soldin, S.J., Brugnara, C., & Hicks, J.M. (1999). *Pediatric Reference Ranges,* 3rd ed. Washington, DC: AACC Press; Hay, W.W., Hayward, A.L., Levin, M.J., Sondheimer, J.M. (2000). *Current Pediatric Diagnosis and Treatment,* 15th ed. New York, NY: Lange Medical Books/McGraw Hill.

PSYCHOSOCIAL IMPLICATIONS

Reactions to Hospitalization and the Operative or Invasive Procedure

Children differ from adults in their psychological responses and reactions to procedures and the environment.

It never ceases to be interesting to watch the reaction of children entering a hospital for an operation. It varies all the way from childish bravado to sheer panic. A seven-year-old boy was brought in because of a question of hernia. Examination proved there was no hernia; and as the boy left the examining room he made a gesture of wiping sweat from his brow and exclaimed, "Boy, that was a close one." A younger child clarified his position after I had explained to him that he would have to have an operation. He said, "I hate you, you stinker." Another little boy said in response to what he considered bad news, "You know what? Lions eat people, and I hope they eat you." One will not have to worry that such children will have repressions.

—Potts (1956)

The optimal approach to children facing a procedure is an overall acceptance of their behaviors. They also need information to process so that they can gain some mastery and control over their experience.

Although children's responses to hospitalization and a procedure vary, there are some fears that children commonly experience. The immediate fear is separation from loved ones and things. This includes feelings of abandonment, thoughts of punishment, and fears of rejection. The child may respond to his or her parents in various ways because of the blame he or she places on them. The child may exhibit indifference or even reject the parent. At times, the child may cling to the nurse in the presence of the parent. If the child is old enough, his or her verbalizing this anger helps to restore the parent-child relationship.

Real and fantasy fears of pain and injury include all the apprehensions regarding procedures, injections, anesthesia, and surgery. Freud (1952) noted that the child reacts more to the fantasy aroused by the procedure than to the procedure itself. It is difficult for the child to differentiate between pain from within and pain imposed from without. A child often points to his or her parents or the nurse and says, "You hurt me!" (Erickson, 1967). Fear of death has been reported to be one aspect of pain that is difficult for the child to bear (Schultz, 1971).

Honesty is essential when dealing with children and pain. They need to know when something will or will not hurt. "But woe unto him who breaks faith in promising that nothing bad is going to happen and then hurts the child" (Potts, 1956). The nature of the illness or injury affects the thoughts of the child and can produce concerns regarding body image, feelings of guilt, and fears of death.

Children in the past experienced unnecessary pain because adults feared they could not tolerate sufficient medication to alleviate the pain. Pain management in children has reached acceptance and success. Pain services have been developed in some children's hospitals to act as resources to all healthcare services and patients.

The child between the ages of 1 and 4 years seems to be most vulnerable to the effects of separation. Children aged 2–4 years show the most severe reactions. Younger children often view hospitalization as punishment for various misdeeds. Generally, before 4 years of age, separation anxiety is the greatest crisis for the child, whereas the child older than 4 years has more problems coping with the illness than the separation.

Body Image

A child younger than 2 years of age is keenly aware of body intactness and experiences fear of mutilation during medical procedures. For example, a child often is reassured if a Band-Aid is used to cover the spot of injection, thus addressing the fear of blood loss (Erickson, 1967). A child of 4 or 5 years wants to cooperate during procedures, but he or she may need some time to prepare. The child's having some say in how preparation for the procedure is accomplished helps him or her to cooperate.

The preschool child has fears of body mutilation and reacts to any violation of body integrity. These children often misinterpret the meaning of procedures. Their intense imagination often distorts explanations that they may receive. These misinterpretations often evoke anxiety and regression.

The school-age child is often outnumbered and overshadowed by younger children in the hospital setting. His or her fantasy life at this time is still vivid. Although the younger child may blame parents and other relatives for an illness, the school-age child often blames herself or himself. The child needs his or her parent when he or she is ill. Fears of death become more pronounced at this age. The responses to illness and hospitalization are usually anger and hurt. The school-age child's expression of anxiety is usually increased activity. The older child may also show regression and anxiety because of fear of genital inadequacy, muscular weakness, and loss of body control. The fear of body mutilation is more intense if the child's head or genitals are involved (Whaley & Wong, 1979).

School-age and preschool children have certain fears and reactions to procedures. They often wonder what will be done while they are under anesthesia, what will be removed, and whether or not they will die. All these fears may result in aggressive behavior if they are not resolved (Erickson, 1967).

An intact motor system helps create a good body image. A child learns about the world through muscular activity. When this activity is cut off, the child feels trapped. It is thought that immobilization may be the most difficult part of illness for the child (Erickson, 1965). The child may feel punished and threatened. The inability to move is a threat to self-preservation and promotes feelings of anxiety and aggression in the child. Immobility reactivates the dependence/independence struggle and the activity/passivity struggle. The normal reaction to restriction is preoccupation with activity.

Coping

The immobilized child gets upset from loneliness, sensory deprivation, and intolerable tension. To be inactive and prone connotes death to children, and they have to fight it. Immobility often breeds fears and fantasies (Erickson, 1965). The child may defy the restrictions or become rigid and frozen. The child cannot vent anger on those responsible for the immobility, so he or she may turn the anger inward and become depressed, withdrawn, quiet, and subdued. Some goals are to help these children feel understood and mobilize their resources to increase their control over aggression.

The child may react to hospitalization in various ways. These reactions may include regression, anger, aggression, depression, denial of illness, and withdrawal.

The child's reactions to procedures may be caused by the resentment of intrusion into his or her body or a fantasy of what is being done. These reasons may cause the child to fight to try to ward off the danger to his or her body. This fight-or-flight reaction to perceived danger is a universal response (Erickson, 1967). The child may resist the procedure in place of expressing feelings about separation and punishment. This acting-out behavior may also be exacerbated by the lack of knowledge the child may have about his or her body, lack of knowledge about what is wrong with it, and confusion over what is being done to diagnose or treat it.

Adult anger felt by the child as a result of these reactions often makes the child feel overpowered, ashamed, and angry. These feelings evoke more anxiety in the child, which in turn leads to more unacceptable behavior. The child has to learn quickly to trust the staff to establish a healthy adaptation to the hospital. If the child is unable to do this, she or he will keep feelings under rigid control or aggressively act them out.

Coping is not only important for the child, it is equally important for the parent of the child. An area of surgery that can be taxing for everyone involved is that of organ procurement. Harvesting organs is always a sensitive subject and even more so with the pediatric population. Nurses need to know their own feelings about organ procurement prior to beginning a case so they can be supportive to the family involved. Studies have shown that nurses tend to reserve their emotions concerning organ procurement until the organs are harvested and the donor body is being prepared for the morgue. Nurses tend to have difficulties with the fact that most of the time surgery saves lives; however, for organ procurement one life must end for another life to be saved (Carter-Gentry & McCurren, 2004).

Preparation for the Procedure

Preparation for the hospital needs to begin before admission to the facility. It is often necessary to prepare parents before one can prepare the child. Preparation needs to be accepted as part of the treatment. The value of good preparation often appears afterward in the speed of recuperation and freedom from neurotic symptoms. The goal is to provide the child with appropriate information so that he or she is able to master the situation or at least gain some control over the situation to cope with the impending danger that he or she may experience.

The nurse needs to understand the behavior of the family at home to really understand the child. Thereby, a family assessment has to be made, if possible, at the time of the child's admission to the facility. To assess the family, one should consider the cultural background and economic level. The development, composition, and experiences of the family should also be considered.

Information on preparatory communications should be based on how the child will feel and what he or she can do. The timing of preparation is also important. Freud (1952) stated that if the preparation is done too early, too much time is left to activate unconscious fantasies and fears. If not enough time is given, however, the ego has too little time to prepare defenses adequately

When asked to illustrate a concept or object, the child draws what he or she knows rather than what he or she sees. If a child has an erroneous idea about an object, seeing the object may correct the false idea. Showing him or her another child who has had the same procedure, however, may not help with acceptance of the same treatment.

The young child learns on the concrete level. He or she gains knowledge through the use of the senses. Meanings are associated with objects through vision and touch. The child needs to manipulate the object himself or herself. He or she has problems connecting one idea with another and connecting an idea with an object. The child cannot make generalizations or logical deductions.

Children younger than 4 years of age may not require an explanation of anatomy and physiology. One needs to stress the equipment and care used in treating these children. They do not comprehend the statement that taking medicine will make them better again. They relate more easily to concrete ideas (eg, that he or she will be able to ride a tricycle again like the little boy in a picture).

The older child wants a reason for every procedure. Equipment is not as important as specific information about what is going to happen because the child becomes more interested in what is to be done and why it is to be done. Gellert's study of the body showed that children identified contents of the body in terms of what they observed being put into or coming out of it (Gellert, 1962). Children of all ages should understand what body parts will be involved in procedures and should be reassured that no other part of the body will be operated on. Establishing trust through all the information presented to the child is as important as the preparation. The child should be asked about his or her ideas of what will happen.

Preprocedure Assessment

It is a great feat to establish trust with a pediatric patient and family within only a few minutes of meeting. A calm demeanor and confidence can ease parents' concerns; however, children take a little more to engage. Talking to the child about an interest, pets, siblings, or a toy they have brought to comfort them can make an enormous difference. Addressing the child and including them in discussions is important. Answer the child's questions as well as the family's questions.

In the preprocedure area, a past medical history is taken from the family and pediatric patient. Family centered care involves all family members in the process. The pediatric patient's current health status is determined along with allergies, vital signs, temperature, and a current weight. Accuracy in weight is important because all subsequent medications will be dosed according to weight. NPO status is also obtained in the preprocedure area. According to the American Society of Anesthesiologists (ASA), there are specific guidelines for preprocedure fasting, outlined in **Table 37.2** (ASA, 1999). Teaching about the procedure and what to expect after the procedure will take place in the preprocedure area.

ASA
American Society of Anesthesiologists

Preparing for Anesthesia Induction

Typically, infants do not display separation anxiety until between 4 and 8 months of age. This being said, most infants will easily come along with clinicians into the operative area. Parents may want to be present for induction of anesthesia. Teaching methods will need to impress upon parents that the use of parent present induction (PPI) is utilized for anxiety reduction in children. Infants will not express this anxiety, so there is no need for PPI with this age group (Taylor, 2007).

Infants are typically scheduled for the first surgery of the day to lessen the time NPO. It is vital to the preprocedure assessment to note the last time feeding occurred and whether the infant is breast or bottle fed. NPO guidelines for infants are 0–5 months, no milk or solids 4 hours before the procedure, 6–36 months, no milk or solids 6 hours before the procedure time, and greater then 36 months, no solids 8 hours before the procedure. Teaching will need to take place with the family about postprocedure feeding and use of glucose water in the recovery area (ASA, 1999).

Distraction techniques work well with infants. Use of toys and pacifiers can be beneficial during induction. Often a pacifier can remain in the infant's mouth while

PPI
Parent Present Induction

Table 37.2	Summary of Fasting Guidelines to Reduce the Risk of Pulmonary Aspiration	
Ingested Material		**Minimum Fasting Period (Hours)**
Clear liquids		2
Breast milk		4
Infant formula		6
Non-human milk		6
Light meal		6

Notes:

– These recommendations apply to healthy patients who are undergoing elective procedures.

– The fasting period noted applies to all ages.

– Clear liquids include water, fruit juices without pulp, carbonated beverages, clear tea, and black coffee.

– A light meal typically consists of toast and clear liquids.

Adapted from: American Society of Anesthesiologists. (1999). Practice guidelines for preoperative fasting and the use of pharmacologic agents to reduce the risk of pulmonary aspiration: application to healthy patients undergoing elective procedures: a report by the American Society of Anesthesiologist Task Force on Preoperative Fasting. *Anesthesiology* 90(3): pp. 896–905.

they fall asleep with mask ventilation. Also the pacifier is helpful upon extubation; it acts as an oral airway and comforts the infant.

For some age groups, a parent present induction (PPI) can be helpful in reducing the child's anxiety. Toddlers and older children benefit most from a PPI. A parent present induction should only be used for planned anesthetics when a team discussion has taken place. Use of PPI is at the discretion of the anesthesia provider. Parents should be taught about what to expect while in the operating room for the induction of their child. Children become heavy as they fall asleep. The child may move his or her arms and legs as they enter the excitement phase of anesthesia. Also their eyes may move from midline. The child may have noisy breathing and the parent should be prepared.

Preparing a parent for PPI is dependent on proper education from the healthcare team. The use of PPI has been shown to reduce both the anxiety of the child as well as the anxiety of the parent. The parent should be escorted back to the waiting by a staff member or volunteer. Children can sense when their parent is anxious and this can increase the child's anxiety. Not all children will benefit from a PPI, thus a team discussion should take place to ensure the best induction can occur (Romino, Keatley, Secrest, & Good, 2005). PPI is controversial because several studies have yielded that having a parent present for induction does not reduce the child's anxiety. Most often the mother accompanies the child for PPI and studies have shown that females' anxiety levels are higher then males. An anxious parent is less able to respond to the child's needs and may require coaching from healthcare providers to benefit their child (Kain, Mayes, Caldwell-Andrews, Saadat, McClain, & Wong, 2006).

Premedication of a child may be an option if the child or parent is not an appropriate candidate for PPI (ie, a child with a history of severe gastroesophageal reflux disease [GERD], history of MH, or a parent that is pregnant). Parents want to be present for their child's induction; however, emergencies and other situations do not allow for it. In these instances education of the parent/s is imperative. An explanation about what type of premedication is being used and its effects will greatly benefit the parent, helping to reduce their anxiety (Wisselo, Stuart, & Muris, 2004).

Some aspects of a preprocedure assessment are not as easy to determine. In today's diverse society, many individuals are experimenting with body piercing and tattooing of body parts. This is an area of concern for the nurse to ensure that there are no alternate site burns associated with the use of electrosurgery on a patient with a metal piercing. Children, adolescents, and teens need to be carefully screened for body piercing in atypical locations. Piercings are a risk for burn and altered skin integrity. Common locations for body piercings are the tongue, ears, navel, nipples, and genitalia. These areas are not always located within common site and the pediatric patient may not be forthcoming with a parent listening to the preprocedure assessment. The nurse should ask one final time before the patient goes to sleep while a parent is not with him or her if he/she has any body piercings. If the patient does have a piercing, then care should be taken to remove it and the reason should be explained to the patient (Larkin, 2004).

Methodology

Various methods have been used to prepare the child for the procedure. Play and puppet therapy can help explain procedures to the child. The child can passively observe the situation or join in with lively participation. Through this therapy, the nurse can observe the play and its effects concerning the child. Other methods that can be used to prepare the child before the actual admission are facility tours, kindergarten visits by nurses, preadmission parties, home visits by a nurse from the facility, programs presented by the school nurse concerning admission to a hospital or outpatient facility, and various pamphlets or books written by facility staff or lay people.

Before the procedure, young patients can be helped to adjust to unfamiliar surroundings by being allowed to bring a stuffed animal or other toy that can remain with them throughout their procedure experience. Allowing the patient to play with equipment (eg, a stethoscope and a blood pressure cuff) before the physical examination as well as to use the equipment on the toy at the time of the examination effectively reduces the child's anxiety.

The use of an induction room in the pediatric setting has proved invaluable. The child and a family member are escorted to a pleasant room, often decorated with cartoon characters yet fully stocked with anesthetic supplies. The room is located adjacent to the procedure suite. A family member holds the child on his or her lap, and mask anesthesia is induced. This begets a sense of security for both the child and the family member. After the child is anesthetized, the family member is directed to the waiting area while the child is transported to the procedure room. In the age range of 18 months to 4 years, the induction room works well to reduce separation anxiety.

GERD
Gastroesophageal Reflux Disease

During mask induction, children respond well to a story told in a soft tone of voice. A story featuring Oscar the Grouch from Sesame Street is especially effective: when an agent (eg, halothane) is introduced, the child can be told to imagine that the "bad" smell is from Oscar's trash can. Transparent anesthesia masks are used to decrease claustrophobia. A few drops of flavoring (eg, vanilla extract, cherry, and bubble gum) are applied to the inside of the mask to make the experience more pleasant. Again, if children are allowed to choose the flavor, they retain some sense of control.

Unlike the case for adults, children are allowed to come to the procedure suite wearing their own clothing if they are reluctant to change. They are often upset when someone removes their shoes. Particularly in the emergent situation, allowing them to retain their clothing, thus salvaging part of their sense of control, considerably reduces their anxiety. Clothing should be tagged, bagged, and returned to the parents after anesthesia induction. If children come to the procedure suite with a security item, each toy or blanket should have an identification badge.

Some methods to improve preparation for children in the future include comprehensive community involvement emphasizing parental education and children's play regarding hospitalization and procedures; special careers for people involved in teaching and preparing children for procedures; and tours of the hospital or outpatient facility on weekends and evenings to provide exposure to the environment.

Use of Cricoid Pressure

In the operating room, emergent procedures need to be treated similarly to planned procedures. Distraction techniques like the one mentioned earlier are still applicable as long as they are not hindering the emergent case. In these cases the use of cricoid pressure can reduce the risk of aspiration of stomach contents into the lungs. Proper use of cricoid pressure should result in better visualization for the provider intubating. Proper hand position for cricoid pressure is directly on the cricoid cartilage located inferior to the thyroid cartilage (Adam's apple). The force applied should be between 3–4 kg. It can be challenging to find the proper location in children for cricoid pressure, especially infants (Patten, 2006). For surgical or invasive procedures the nurse assists the anesthesia providers in intubation and intervenous placement.

ENSURING CORRECT SITE VERIFICATION BEFORE THE OPERATIVE OR INVASIVE PROCEDURE

Time Out

In recent years efforts have been introduced to reduce the amount of wrong site, wrong side, or wrong patient surgery. The existence of universal protocol including a "time out" has become a standard in practice. In 2003, The Joint Commission had several issues stated in their national patient safety goals relating to proper identification of the patient and ensuring the correct area of the body is being operated on. The Joint Commission then developed the Universal Protocol for Preventing Wrong Site, Wrong Procedure, Wrong Person Surgery™ (The Joint Commission, 2003); in 2004, The Joint Commission made these recommendations mandatory for organizational compliance.

Years before, The Joint Commission issued these mandates: in 1999, a perioperative nurse at Children's Hospital, Boston, had the foresight to see a need for site verification. In collaboration with the risk management department, this nurse developed a preprocedure checklist. The checklist verifies that the procedure was discussed with the family, patient, and surgical team. At that point the perioperative nurse caring for the child signs the checklist acknowledging that the correct site was marked by the physician who obtained informed consent. This checklist ensures that the team has agreed on the correct site/side for surgery and that site has been initialed according to the policy prior to entering the operating room. The document follows a patient into the operating room where a "time out" can be completed just prior to the time of incision. This document is a part of the medical record. **Figures 37.1** and **37.2** show examples of preprocedure checklists.

Figure 37.1

Preprocedure checklist.

Source: Children's Hospital Boston.

CHILDREN'S HOSPITAL, BOSTON, MA 02115

Additional Procedures:

Planned Procedure as written on consent: _____

Record/Documentation Verification	N/A	MD initials	Verifier initials
Operative Consent is completed and reviewed, and verified with the patient, and/or, parent/guardian.			
The operative/procedural site/side is initiated (when indicated) per policy. (Initials should be located within the area to be prepped and draped)			
Time Out was completed immediately prior to incision/invasive procedure per Policy. *(patient id, procedure, site/side, position, imaging studies, special equipment, and implants when applicable)*		**Verifier initials**	

Verifier Signature_____**Initials**_____ **Date** _____

Physician Signature_____ **Initials**_____ **Date** _____**Beeper**_____

****

Planned Procedure as written on consent: _____

Record/Documentation Verification	N/A	MD initials	Verifier initials
Operative Consent is completed and reviewed, and verified with the patient, and/or, parent/guardian.			
The operative/procedural site/side is initiated (when indicated) per policy. (Initials should be located within the area to be prepped and draped)			
Time Out was completed immediately prior to incision/invasive procedure per Policy. *(patient id, procedure, site/side, position, imaging studies, special equipment, and implants when applicable)*		**Verifier initials**	

Verifier Signature_____**Initials**_____ **Date** _____

Physician Signature_____ **Initials**_____ **Date** _____**Beeper**_____

****

Planned Procedure as written on consent: _____

Record/Documentation Verification	N/A	MD initials	Verifier initials
Operative Consent is completed and reviewed, and verified with the patient, and/or, parent/guardian.			
The operative/procedural site/side is initiated (when indicated) per policy. (Initials should be located within the area to be prepped and draped)			
Time Out was completed immediately prior to incision/invasive procedure per Policy. *(patient id, procedure, site/side, position, imaging studies, special equipment, and implants when applicable)*		**Verifier initials**	

Verifier Signature_____**Initials**_____ **Date** _____

Physician Signature_____ **Initials**_____ **Date** _____**Beeper**_____

Figure 37.2

Preprocedure checklist.

Source: Children's Hospital Boston.

Documentation in the Operative and Invasive Procedure Area

As healthcare advances, so does the technology used to record care and treatment. Many facilities are moving or have already moved to a computerized documentation system. Organizations look for a better system to increase documentation completeness, reduce costs in the long term, and methods to tract trends. All of these criteria cause healthcare organizations to look into computerized charting and documentation tools.

While the initial up-front cost of implementing a computerized documentation system may terrify hospital executives, the benefits should be considered carefully. The cost savings associated with an electronic version of documentation are well documented. Storage of paper documents alone can cost time, money, and space that all could be better utilized.

Computerized documentation holds the same potential for error as did paper documentation. Care providers using a computerized version of documentation need to instill fastidious care that documentation is complete and correct. Providers should not depend on the system to ensure complete and correct information.

The same rules apply to electronic documentation as did apply to written paper documentation. If a provider of care does not document what he or she did for the patient it is as though it never happened. This statement is true for electronic documentation, as well as written. Throughout history the nursing profession has had trouble conveying to the general public what it is that nurses do professionally. In the past, the role of a professional nurse and care provided was often attributed to medicine rather than nursing. The use of computerized documentation will better illustrate the role of the professional nurse because of the more complete documentation (Doyle, 2006).

Use of an electronic chart for documentation allows multiple users access to the same information at the same time. Unlike paper charts, when one professional had access to a paper chart, it denied other professionals access. This limited access of the past caused time constraints. Likewise, having typewritten details of care to read, rather then deciphering the handwriting of colleagues, tends to improve communication between care givers. Patient safety can be maximized with safety stops in place for medication orders, such as alerts if an allergy status is unknown, or an alert if a dose is not appropriate based on the weight of the pediatric patient (Doyle, 2006).

Electronic documentation is here to stay. It is not only environmentally friendly but organizationally friendly as well. Baccalaureate nursing programs are finally catching up with the demand and adding electronic curriculum requirements. Today's nurses need computer skills. These changes for practice will occur rapidly. The profession of nursing needs entry-level professionals who are prepared for electronic documentation.

Care needs to be impeccable to ensure patient information is safe. Passwords need to be secured and not shared. Follow your organization's rules for safe computer use by locking stations when stepping away. Viruses can attach themselves to attachments via email, so attachments should only be opened when they are from reliable sources. Delete emails containing SPAM or chain emails (Bergren, 2004).

POTENTIAL ADVERSE OUTCOMES RELATED TO A CHILD HAVING AN OPERATIVE OR INVASIVE PROCEDURE

The nurse sees many potential adverse outcomes in the young child facing a procedure. These physiological and psychological outcomes influence the role of the nurse throughout the operative and invasive period. Although nursing diagnoses vary from child to child depending on growth and development needs, there are some consistent diagnoses that affect all children.

Common nursing diagnoses, risk factors, and outcome indicators are discussed (see **Table 37.3**). Some of these are risk for infection; risk for impaired skin integrity;

Table 37.3	**Providing Care to the Pediatric Patient Does Not Compromise or Cause Injury to the Patient**

Outcome 1   The patient is free from evidence of infection.

Diagnosis	Risk Factors	Outcome Indicators
Risk for Infection	☐ Immature immune system	☐ Does the patient have a wound infection?
	☐ Lack of maternal antibodies (dependent on maternal exposures)	☐ Does the patient have a urinary tract infection?
	☐ Lack of normal flora	☐ Does the patient have an upper respiratory infection?
	☐ Lack of immunization	
	☐ Poor nutritional state	
	☐ Thin epidermis	
	☐ Small surface area	
	☐ Immature ability to handle respiratory secretions	
	☐ Inability to control bowels and bladder functions	
	☐ Surgical incision	
	☐ Anesthesia	
	☐ Invasive monitoring	
	☐ Central catheters	
	☐ Total parenteral nutrition infusion	
	☐ Ostomies	
	☐ Open wounds	
	☐ Blood sampling	
	☐ Traumatic delivery	
	☐ Trauma or accident	

Outcome 2   The patient maintains skin integrity.

Diagnosis	Risk Factors	Outcome Indicator
Risk for Impaired Skin Integrity	☐ Thin epidermis	☐ Does the patient have signs of skin breakdown?
	☐ Decrease in normal skin lubricants	
	☐ Decrease in subcutaneous fat	
	☐ Surgical incision	
	☐ Infection	
	☐ Poor nutritional state	
	☐ Drainage in contact with skin	
	☐ Open wounds	
	☐ Ostomies	
	☐ Invasive monitoring	
	☐ Application of extraneous objects, eg, electrosurgical dispersive electrode, pneumatic tourniquet, tape, casting material, adhesive drapes	
	☐ Application of chemical agents, eg, skin-prepping solutions	

Outcome 3 The patient maintains adequate fluid volume.

Diagnosis

Risk for Fluid Volume Deficit.

Risk Factors

- ☐ Large body surface area in relation to size
- ☐ Immature kidney function
- ☐ Increased fluid needs due to increase percentage of body weight in water (infant's body weight is 80 compared with adult's 50%–60% of body weight in water)
- ☐ Decreased fluid reserve
- ☐ Decreased ability to concentrate urine
- ☐ Increased volume of gastrointestinal secretions
- ☐ Surgery
- ☐ Anesthesia
- ☐ Exposed epidermis leading to increased evaporative water losses
- ☐ Poor intravenous access
- ☐ Narrow margin between adequate hydration and fluid overload
- ☐ Increased losses from the gastrointestinal tract due to nasogastric tubes and/or ostomies
- ☐ Increased fluid losses from seizures, fever, crying, time spent undergoing ventilation, suctioning, and nothing-by-mouth (NPO) status

Outcome Indicators

- ☐ Did the kidneys remain perfused and with and output of 1 mL/kg/hour?
- ☐ Was the blood pressure maintained?
- ☐ Did vital signs remain stable?
- ☐ Were the BUN and creatinine values within normal limits?
- ☐ Did the patient maintain body temperature?

Outcome 4 The patient is free from evidence of hypothermia.

Diagnosis

Risk for the development of hypothermia during the procedure period.

Risk Factors

- ☐ Ineffective temperature regulation secondary to age
- ☐ Thin epidermis
- ☐ Large body surface in relation to size
- ☐ Thin layer of subcutaneous fat
- ☐ Chemical thermogenesis in brown adipose tissue
- ☐ Exposure of epidermis to the outside environment
- ☐ Increased evaporative water loss
- ☐ Exposure of internal organs
- ☐ Exposure to cold intravenous fluids and skin preparation solutions
- ☐ Age (neonate)
- ☐ Low body weight

Outcome Indicators

- ☐ Does the patient have a core body temperature of less than 96.8°F (36°C)
- ☐ Does the conscious patient complain of feeling uncomfortably cold?
- ☐ Is the patient shivering during the procedure?
- ☐ Does the patient's skin feel cool, have pallor, or have piloerection?
- ☐ Does the patient have decreased pulse and respiration?

37

Outcome 5   The patient is free from evidence of ineffective breathing.

Diagnosis	**Risk Factors**	**Outcome Indicators**
Risk for Ineffective Breathing Patterns	☐ Age (neonate or infant)	☐ Are the patient's respirations adequate to maintain sufficient oxygen to meet cellular requirement?
	☐ Chest and abdominal procedures	
	☐ Decreased ability to handle oral secretions	☐ Is the patient's respiratory rate within normal limits, compared with baseline?
	☐ Large size of infant head compared with the adult head (attaining good "stiff" position for alignment of the airway axes is more difficult)	
	☐ Large tongue size of the infant compared with the adult tongue (laryngoscopy and visualization of the larynx are more difficult)	
	☐ Position of vocal cords in the infant (makes the airway seem anterior, resulting in difficulty when trying to visualize the larynx with laryngoscopy)	
	☐ Difference in metabolic requirements and oxygen consumption in neonates and infants (a neonate may require 6 mL/kg/minute of oxygen compared with 3 mL/kg/minute in an adult)	
	☐ Presence of fetal hemoglobin during the first 6 months of life (fetal hemoglobin has more affinity for oxygen, thus allowing more oxygen to be carried to the tissues but less to be released at the tissue level)	
	☐ Nonshivering thermogenesis to produce body heat (can be detrimental because oxygen consumption and carbon dioxide production increase)	
	☐ Alveolar minute ventilation in the neonate, which is twice that of an adult, requires an increase in ventilatory rate to meet metabolic demands for oxygen consumption	

Outcome 6   The patient is free from evidence of electrical injury.

Diagnosis	**Risk Factors**	**Outcome Indicators**
Risk for Electrical Injury (tissue burn) related to use of electrosurgery	☐ Use of electrosurgery generator not equipped with contact quality monitoring system	☐ Is the patient free from any observable signs or reported symptoms of injury related to the use of electrosurgery devices?
	☐ Use of dry adhesive return electrode	
	☐ Use of noncontact quality monitoring return patient electrode	☐ Does the patient's skin, other than the incision, remain unchanged between admission and discharge from the OR?

| Risk for Electrical Injury (ignition incident) secondary to the use of electrosurgery, laser, or other heat source | ☐ Use of high power setting
☐ Coiling of active and return electrodes
☐ Contact of active and return electrodes with metal that is attached to the patient or patient drapes
☐ Oxygen-enriched environment
☐ Use of noncuffed endotracheal tube
☐ High power settings of the electrosurgical generator
☐ Accumulation of smoke plume at the operative site | ☐ Does the patient report comfort at the dispersive electrode site after the procedure?
☐ Is the patient free from any observable signs or reported symptoms of ignition injury related to the use of electrosurgery devices, lasers, or other heat sources?
☐ Does the patient report comfort in all nontargeted areas at discharge from the OR? |

Outcome 7   The patient is free from evidence of impaired comfort [pain].

Diagnosis	**Risk Factors**	**Outcome Indicators**
Risk for Impaired Comfort (pain)	☐ Procedure ☐ Nausea and vomiting related to anesthesia ☐ Accident ☐ Trauma ☐ Diagnostic tests ☐ Lack of knowledge concerning pain management techniques	☐ Is the patient's comfort level sufficient throughout the procedure period? ☐ Does the patient verbalize comfort and control of pain?

Outcome 8   The patient is free from evidence of fear.

Diagnosis	**Risk Factors**	**Outcome Indicators**
Fear	☐ Procedure and its outcomes ☐ Lack of knowledge of expected responses to surgical or invasive procedure ☐ Anesthesia ☐ Invasive procedures ☐ Separation from parents ☐ Sensed parental fear or anxiety ☐ Lack of cognitive understanding regarding hospitalization, surgery, and invasive procedures ☐ Fantasy thoughts ☐ Active imagination	☐ Does the patient exhibit signs of control and expresses feelings (verbal and nonverbal) of security during the operative or invasive procedure period? ☐ Does the patient and family members communicate an understanding of the operative or other invasive procedure and the effects they can expect?

Adapted from: Carpentino-Moyet, L. J. (2008) *Handbook of Nursing Diagnosis* (12th ed.). Philadelphia: Lippincott Williams & Wilkins; Petersen, C. (2007). *Perioperative Nursing Data Set, the Perioperative Nursing Vocabulary.* (Revised 2nd ed.). Denver: AORN, Inc.

risk for injury (tissue burn) related to electrosurgery; risk for injury (ignition incident) secondary to the use of electrosurgery, laser, or other heat source; risk for fluid volume deficit; risk for hypothermia during the procedure; risk for ineffective breathing patterns: and alteration in comfort.

Risk for Infection

Use aseptic technique to prevent cross-contamination when working with wounds, ostomies, and central catheters, especially when they are in close proximity. Protect the thin epidermis through meticulous wound care. Keep wounds clean and protected. Prepare central catheters with povidone-iodine (Betadine) and use discriminately. Perform a preprocedure assessment of predisposing factors for infection. Perform minimal shave preparation. Follow the surgeon's preferences and aseptic technique for surgical skin preparation. Instruct caregivers on wound care after the procedure. Maintain correct wound drainage system. Maintain sterile technique by monitoring self, team members, and sterile field. Provide antibiotic irrigation as necessary. Prevent foreign bodies from entering the operative wound. Assess and document the patient's condition before the procedure to determine preexisting infection and the potential for infection. Be aware of suite air flow requirements to prevent dispersion of dust and airborne particles. Control traffic in rooms. Monitor all persons entering the procedure room for adherence to aseptic technique. Spot clean areas contaminated with fluids from the surgical field. Assist with dressing application, using aseptic technique. Provide antibiotics for irrigation and IV therapy. Note wound classification. Isolate potential contamination.

Risk for Impaired Skin Integrity

Assess and document skin integrity. Cover open wounds. Remove excess prepping solution. Prevent pooling of prepping solution. Limit pressure on the skin by using padding when positioning (pad bony prominences and support devices) (**Table 37.3**). Use nonirritating tape. Confine drainage to avoid skin contact. Place the electrosurgery patient return electrode according to the manufacturer's recommendations. Use an appropriate preparation solution (avoid pooling of the solution in contact with the skin). Limit shave preparation. Use Montgomery tapes as appropriate. Monitor the scrub team to avoid skin pressure. Carefully remove adhesive drapes. Monitor the use of the electrosurgical pencil.

Risk for Injury (Tissue Burn) Related to Electrosurgery

Return electrodes should be the appropriate size for the neonate, infant, or pediatric patient in order to prevent patient injuries (AORN, 2008). A split-plate patient return electrode intended for use with electrosurgical generators equipped with return electrode contact quality monitoring should be used for pediatric patients. Infant and neonatal return electrode pads are available today for use with contact quality monitoring systems: infant pads are used for patients weighing 2.7 kg to 13.6 kg [6 lbs to 30 lbs]; neonatal pads are used for patients weighing 0.45 kg to 2.72 kg [1 lb to 6 lbs] (Valleylab, 2007; Valleylab, 2006). However, when patient size permits, an adult-sized pad should be used to minimize the risk of patient burns (Valleylab, 2007).

Placement of the patient return electrode presents a challenge, especially for the low-weight neonate and infant. A well-vascularized, convex area in close proximity to the surgical site is preferred for application of the return electrode; avoid scar tissue, bony prominences, excessive adipose tissue, and areas where fluid may pool (Valleylab, 2007). For an infant, the preferred application site is the back or torso; for a premature infant (0.45 kg to 2.72 kg [1 lb to 6 lbs], the recommended application site is on the back, inferior to the shoulder blades and superior to the sacrum (Valleylab, 2007; Valleylab, 2006). Special clinical circumstances may require alternate application sites; if alternate sites are required, ensure maximum patient-to-return-electrode contact and minimize current levels (Valleylab, 2007). The application site should be clean and dry. See **Table 37.4** for a summary of factors that can adversely affect the pad-patient interface. During skin preparation, exercise extreme care to prevent fluid invasion of the return electrode. The condition of the patient's skin should be assessed and documented before and after electrosurgery use (AORN, 2008).

Always use electrosurgery on neonates and infants with caution. The lowest power settings that will achieve the desired surgical effect should be used (Valleylab, 2007). The maximum wattage recommendations will vary across different manufacturers. For example, when using the Neonatal REM PolyHesive™ II Patient Return Electrode (**Fig. 37.3**) on a patient weighing 0.45 kg–2.72 kg (1 to 6 lbs) with a Valleylab Force FX™C generator, the applied current should not exceed 300 milliamps (approximately 11.25 watts) nor be applied for longer than 30 seconds continually (Valleylab, 2006). Similarly, when using an Infant REM PolyHesive™ II Patient Return Electrode (**Fig. 37.4**) on patients weighing 2.7 kg–13.6 kg [6 lbs–30 lbs] the power output

Table 37.4	Factors That Contribute to Adverse Conditions at the Pad-Patient Interface

Impedance of electrosurgical return current flow when the pad is placed over areas of poor perfusion:

☐ Bony prominences

☐ Areas of scar tissue

☐ Implanted metal prosthesis

☐ Sites distal to tourniquets

Inappropriate pad placement:

☐ Over hairy surfaces

☐ Over a tattoo

☐ A pad that does not maintain uniform body contact—problems of gaping, tenting, and moisture interfere with adherence to the patient's skin

Position-related factors:

☐ A pad that is placed on the patient prior to final positioning—problems of buckling or tension may affect contact with the patient's skin

Adapted from: Association of periOperative Registered Nurses. (2008). Recommended practices for electrosurgery. In *Perioperative Standards and Recommended Practices*. Denver, CO: AORN, Inc.; pp. 315–329.

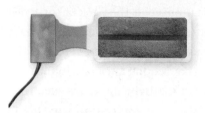

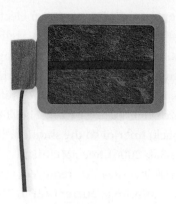

Figure 37.3

Neonatal REM PolyHesive™ II
Patient Return Electrode.

Source: Copyright © Covidien.
All rights reserved. Reprinted
with the permission of the
Energy-Based Devices and
Surgical Devices divisions of
Covidien.

Figure 37.4

Infant REM PolyHesive™ II
Patient Return Electrode.

Source: Copyright © Covidien.
All rights reserved. Reprinted
with the permission of the
Energy-Based Devices and
Surgical Devices divisions of
Covidien.

range is 0–120 watts (Valleylab, 2007). Follow the manufacturer's written instructions for determining the correct power settings for a neonatal and infant patient return electrodes.

The cut current, because it has lower voltage than the coagulation current, is preferable. Desiccation, as well as tissue cutting, can be achieved with the cut current. If the physician chooses to desiccate tissue with the coagulation current, a generator equipped with a coagulation desiccation mode, which uses lower voltage, is preferred.

During the procedure, the scrub person should keep the active electrode free of eschar buildup. A clean electrode requires less power to do the same work as a dirty one because eschar buildup has higher resistance and will impede the passage of the current (Ulmer, 2008). In addition, eschar buildup on the active electrode tip causes the entire electrosurgery unit to function less effectively and also serves as a fuel source, which can lead to a fire (AORN, 2008).

The physician should be familiar with the literature findings on electrosurgical effects on small patients; he/she may wish to consider using bipolar electrosurgery, which does not require a return electrode (Valleylab, 2007; Valleylab, 2006). The manufacturer's recommendations must be followed when using electrosurgery generators, patient return electrodes, active electrodes, and accessories.

Risk for Injury (Ignition Incident) Secondary to the Use of Electrosurgery, Laser, or Other Heat Source

Fire is always a consideration when doing a pediatric procedure because of the tendency to use uncuffed endotracheal tubes. Leakage of oxygen and nitrous oxide (heat causes the thermal breakdown of nitrous oxide, which releases oxygen) from the tube may result in an oxygen-enriched environment. Electrosurgery must not be used in the presence of an oxygen-enriched environment. See Chapter 14 for more information concerning fire prevention and safety during electrosurgery.

Risk for Fluid Volume Deficit

Assess the patient's condition before the procedure with laboratory results and determine the potential for problems (eg, dehydration and electrolyte imbalances). Communicate with anesthesia personnel and the procedure team. Beware of the decreased circulating volume of infants and children and the importance of effective retraction and suctioning to increase visualization and to reduce potential blood loss. Also be aware of effective use of suture material and the electrosurgery pencil for achieving homeostasis and identification and clamping of a bleeding vessel. Have instruments for clamping and suturing readily available for ligating vessels. Monitor electrosurgery generator power unit settings and keep the pencil tip clean for effective use. Keep a clean laparotomy pad available. Be prepared to use hemostatic agents (eg, oxidized regenerated cellulose). Measure irrigation fluids and assist in blood loss calculations. Assess and document the preprocedure fluid volume status and the potential for fluid balance problems. Maintain fluid therapy. Have available IV solutions and blood products, hemostatic agents, a large volume of laparotomy sponges and sutures for homeostasis, and supplies for pressure dressing. Monitor intake and output. Keep a running total of fluid in suction containers, and display bloody laparotomy sponges for an estimation of bloody loss. Document and report to the PACU problems with fluid volume and interventions.

Risk for Hypothermia During the Operative or Invasive Procedure Period

Perform a preprocedure assessment including laboratory data results, paying specific attention to the patient's age and the presence of anemia. All infants, but especially premature infants, have difficulty maintaining body temperature. Anemic patients are at risk for hypothermia. Keep the patient covered during transport. Increase the OR temperature to 85°F (29.4°C). Position the patient on a heating blanket protected with sheets at 100°F (37.7°C). Have warming lights available. Place plastic around the extremities and top of the head to reduce heat loss. Monitor the patient's temperature and skin color. Minimize the area of the operative site preparation to limit the area of skin exposed to circulating air. Cover as much skin area as possible during draping. For abdominal surgery, reduce heat loss by placing plastic bags around the bowel. Achieve good exposure through retraction and suctioning to allow abdominal contents to remain in the abdominal cavity when possible. Arrange for a radiant heat warmer in the PACU. Document and report to the PACU staff any problems with the patient's body temperature.

Risk for Ineffective Breathing Patterns

Assess the respiratory status and NPO status before the procedure and communicate with anesthesia personnel and the procedure team. Monitor the color of blood during the procedure. Position the patient for maximal lung expansion appropriate for the procedure. Monitor the team to prevent decreased ventilation due to pressure on the chest. Assess the color of the patient's blood. Assist anesthesia personnel during anesthesia induction and intubation. Do not use a pillow under the head during intubation. Augment head extension by placing a rolled towel under the shoulders, if necessary. Listen for changes in the pulse oximeter. Assist with physical control of the patient during early induction. Assist with suctioning for visualization and with forceps for nasal intubation. Apply cricoid pressure to prevent laryngospasm, if needed. Assist with medication administration if laryngospasm occurs. Document and report to the PAC problems with airway management. Carefully monitor oxygen therapy. Avoid cold stressors. Decrease the energy requirements of the child to decrease oxygen consumption. Arrange for respiratory support equipment for the procedure suite, PACU, or intensive care unit.

Alteration in Comfort (Pain)

Assess the patient's comfort level or level of pain. Provide support for the parents. Collaborate with anesthesia personnel to manage pain. Reposition the patient, if necessary. Provide local medication, as necessary.

Fear

Explain to the child the procedures that he or she will experience in terms of sensations. Allow the child to express concerns through the use of therapeutic play (have the child bring a favorite toy). Show children the equipment they will see (preprocedure teaching party). Plan preparation according to each child's developmental level (see earlier). Involve children in their own care. Have parents present during anesthesia induction, if appropriate. Provide information to parents and take action to reduce parental anxiety and fear. Provide periodic reports to the parents during the procedure. Provide a quiet environment.

PROCEDURES

The nurse prepares for each of the following cases in a similar manner. The differences in each procedure are discussed.

Inguinal Herniorrhaphy
Definition

Inguinal herniorrhaphy is one of the most common pediatric operations performed (Hebra, 2006). Inguinal hernia is a type of ventral hernia that occurs when an intra-abdominal structure, such as bowel or omentum, protrudes through a defect in the abdominal wall (**Fig. 37.5**); most hernias that are present at birth or that occur in childhood are indirect inguinal hernias (Hebra, 2006). The processus

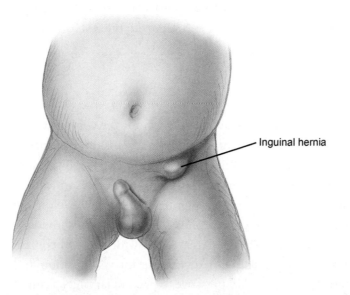

Figure 37.5

Protruding inguinal hernia.

Inguinal hernia

vaginalis is an outpouching of the peritoneum attached to the testicle that follows behind as it descends retroperitoneally into the scrotum; when obliteration of the processus vaginalis fails to occur, an inguinal hernia results (Hebra, 2006). While the exact incidence of indirect inguinal hernia in infants and children is unknown, the reported incidence ranges from 1%–5% (Hebra, 2006). Premature infants are at increased risk for inguinal hernia, with incidence rates of 2% in females and 7%–30% in males; approximately 5% of all males develop a hernia during their lifetime (Hebra, 2006).

Indications

The indications for inguinal herniorrhaphy include the following presenting factors and patient history (Hebra, 2006):

- The infant or child presents with an obvious bulge at the internal or external ring or within the scrotum. The parents will typically provide a history of a visible swelling or bulge, which commonly is intermittent, in the inguinoscrotal region in boys and inguinolabial region in girls.
- The swelling may or may not be associated with any pain or discomfort. More commonly, pain is not associated with a simple inguinal hernia in an infant. However, the parents may perceive the bulge as being painful when, in reality, it causes no discomfort to the child.
- The bulge commonly occurs after crying or straining, but often resolves at night while the child is sleeping.
- If the patient or the family provides a history of a painful bulge in the inguinal region, the presence of an incarcerated inguinal hernia must be suspected. Patients with an incarcerated hernia generally present with a tender, firm mass in the inguinal canal or scrotum. The child may be fussy, unwilling to feed, and crying inconsolably. The skin overlying the bulge may be edematous, erythematous, and discolored.

The physician will examine the child in both supine and standing positions (Hebra, 2006). The physical examination of a child with an inguinal hernia typically reveals a palpable, smooth mass that originates from the external ring lateral to the pubic tubercle; the mass may only be noticeable after coughing or performing a Valsalva maneuver, but it should be reduced easily (Hebra, 2006). On occasion, the physician may feel the loops of intestine within the hernia sac; in girls, feeling the ovary in the hernia sac is not unusual; in boys, palpation of both testicles is important to rule out an undescended or retractile testicle (Hebra, 2006).

Pediatric inguinal herniorrhaphies are usually done on an outpatient basis.

Nursing Implications

General anesthesia is administered. In young children, endotracheal anesthesia is used, whereas mask anesthesia is often used in older children. After induction, a caudal anesthetic is administered to control pain during and after the procedure. If a caudal anesthetic is not used, ilioinguinal block is performed by the surgeon during the procedure.

Procedure

The hernia is repaired by high ligation of the sac at the level of the internal ring. A transverse skin crease incision is made in the natural folds of skin in the inguinal region. The subcutaneous tissues are dissected along the spermatic cord through Scarpa fascia down to the external ring. In young patients, the internal ring lies just below the external ring, which makes it possible to achieve high ligation without incising the external oblique muscle, as is necessary for older patients. The hernia sac is visualized and, in males, the vessels and vas deferens are identified.

A clamp is placed on the sac, and the vessels and vas deferens are gently stripped from the hernia sac by grasping connective tissue, being careful never to grasp the vas deferens. In females, the hernia sac is identified with the round ligament. The fallopian tube is attached at the neck of the sac and must be avoided during ligation. Preperitoneal fat is identified, ensuring high ligation. The hernia is reduced, and an instrument such as a slotted spoon may be used. The hernia sac is placed through the narrow slot, and the bowl of the spoon prevents structures from entering the sac. The sac is ligated at the level of the internal ring with suture according to the surgeon's preference. A portion of the sac is usually removed and sent for routine pathological examination. Occasionally, the internal ring must be narrowed with a few sutures placed from the transversalis fascia to the inferior aspect of the ring. The external oblique muscle, if opened, and Scarpa fascia is closed with interrupted suture. The skin is closed, usually with a running subcuticular suture, and dressings are applied (adhesive strips or collodion a fast drying, occlusive liquid).

Postprocedure Care

Discharge from the outpatient unit takes place after the effects of general anesthesia have dissipated and the patient is able to retain oral fluids. Because of the caudal anesthesia or the ilioinguinal block, immediate postprocedure pain is not usually a problem and later pain can be controlled with acetaminophen. Young pediatric patients usually have no activity restrictions, and older pediatric patients can usually resume strenuous activities in 2–3 weeks. The skin suture for pediatric patients is usually absorbable, thereby eliminating the need for suture removal. The dressings are kept dry for approximately 1 week. Special instructions for cleaning the area should be given to parents who have infants in diapers.

Potential Complications

Possible complications include recurrence, accidental ligation of sac contents, and damage to the spermatic cord during dissection from the sac.

Repair of Hydrocele or Undescended Testis
Definition

A hydrocele (**Fig. 37.6**) is a collection of fluid within the processus vaginalis (PV), which produces a swelling in the inguinal region or scrotum (Collins, 2006). An inguinal hernia occurs when the abdominal organs protrude into the inguinal canal or scrotum; inguinal hernia and hydrocele share a similar etiology and pathophysiology and therefore may coexist (Collins, 2006). During fetal development, the testicle is located within the peritoneal cavity; as the testicle descends through the inguinal

PV
Processus Vaginalis

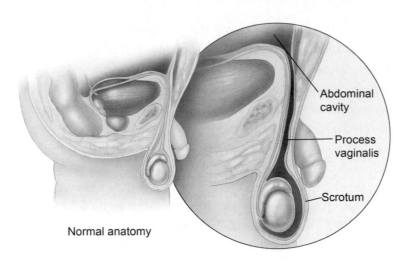

Figure 37.6

Hydrocele.

Abdominal cavity

Process vaginalis

Scrotum

Normal anatomy

canal and into the scrotum, it is accompanied by a saclike extension of peritoneum, known as the PV (Collins, 2006). After the testicle descends, the PV obliterates in the healthy infant and becomes a fibrous cord with no lumen; thus, the scrotum loses its connection with the abdomen. Without this connection, neither abdominal organs nor peritoneal fluid can make their way into the scrotum or inguinal canal. If the PV does not close, it is referred to as a patent processus vaginalis (PPV). If the PPV is small in caliber and only large enough to allow fluid to pass, the condition is referred to as a communicating hydrocele; if the PPV is larger, allowing ovary, intestine, or other abdominal contents to protrude, the condition is referred to as a hernia (Collins, 2006).

The procedure is similar, with the addition of opening the hydrocele, draining the fluid, and often removing a portion of the sac to prevent reaccumulation.

Undescended testis (cryptorchidism, **Fig. 37.7**) is the most common—genital problem encountered in pediatrics (Kolon, 2006). Even with over 100 years of research, many aspects of cryptorchidism are not well defined and remain controversial (Kolon, 2006). Overall, cryptorchidism is seen in 3% of full-term newborn boys,

PPV
Patent Processus
Vaginalis

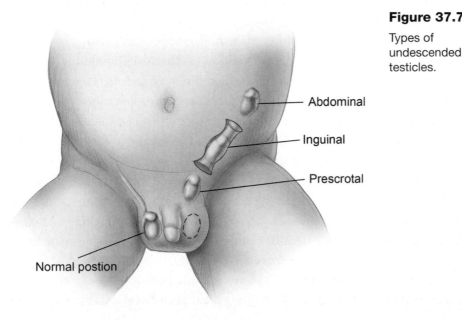

Figure 37.7

Types of undescended testicles.

Abdominal

Inguinal

Prescrotal

Normal postion

decreasing to 1% in boys aged 6 months to 1 year; the prevalence rate in premature boys is 30% (Kolon, 2006). In a healthy neonate after birth, the testicle is surrounded by a closed cavity (Collins, 2006).

The procedure is inguinal herniorrhaphy or ligation of the PPV, mobilization of the testis, and orchidopexy (fixation of the testis in the scrotum), usually by placing the testis in a pouch formed under dartos muscle.

Indications

Hydroceles should be repaired if they (Collins, 2006):

- Fail to resolve before the child reached 2 years of age
- Cause discomfort
- Enlarge or are clearly waxing and waning in volume
- Are unsightly
- Become infected

Indications for surgical correction of cryptorchidism include (Kolon, 2006):

- Possible improved fertility
- Self-examination for testis mass (cancer)
- Correction of associated hernia
- Prevention of testicular torsion
- Avoidance of injury against pubic bone
- Psychological effects of empty scrotum

There are no contraindications for intervention of undescended testis in prepubertal boys (Kolon, 2006).

Nursing Implications

The operative and invasive procedure nursing team selects equipment and supplies and organizes the room. For this procedure, an electrosurgery unit and, for infants, a warming blanket and possibly warming lights are used. Supplies consist of basic draping materials, gowns, gloves, x-ray detectable sponges, electrocautery handpiece, No. 15 scalpel blades, basins, dissecting sponges (eg, peanuts or Kittner dissecting sponges), syringes and a needle for local anesthesia if ilioinguinal block is to be done, dressings (usually adhesive strips or collodion), and, for larger patients, a Penrose drain to surround the spermatic cord. The suture packages are opened according to the surgeon's preference to include suture on taper needles for ligation of the sac and closing the external oblique muscle and fascia and usually fine absorbable suture on a cutting needle for a subcuticular skin closure.

Instruments, as always in pediatric surgery, are modified for patient size. Curved and straight mosquito clamps, dissecting scissors, smooth forceps (often vascular forceps) for manipulation of the hernia sac, forceps with teeth for opening and closing, small retractors, a Babcock or Allis clamp to place around the spermatic cord, and, if desired, a hernia spoon are prepared.

Because most inguinal hernia patients are admitted as outpatients, the nurse meets the patient and the family in the holding area. The patient and the procedure are verified, the chart is reviewed, and the surgery permit and the history and physical examination results are noted, paying special attention to whether the procedure involves left, right, or both sides. The patient and family are questioned as to allergies and NPO status. As discussed earlier, the patient and the family are evaluated, and appropriate nursing interventions are used. They are escorted to the induction room or the patient is taken to the procedure suite.

Procedure

General anesthesia is induced by mask for most children with IV induction used primarily in adolescents. Constant assessment by the circulating nurse of the patient is required during induction. Endotracheal tubes are usually inserted in young patients, whereas in older patients anesthesia is usually maintained by mask. Standard anesthesia monitors are applied: electrocardiographic monitor, blood pressure monitor, and pulse oximeter. As for all infants and young children, maintenance of normal body temperature is important. Wrapping the extremities and head prevents heat loss.

The patient is placed in a supine position, and the skin is prepared with povidone-iodine scrub and/or paint (or other solutions) from the umbilicus to the midthigh. Care is taken to prevent pooling of the povidone-iodine solution. Burns can occur when the skin is in contact with povidone-iodine and a warming blanket. Warm sterile saline is placed on the back table, along with any local anesthetic if an ilioinguinal block is to be administered.

The scrub person assists in draping and places the sterile Mayo stand over the foot of the table. The positions of the surgical team members must be monitored when the patient is an infant to prevent pressure on small extremities. As always, although hemorrhage is rare, the scrub person must be prepared with clamps, electrosurgery, or suture. During sac manipulation, forceps without teeth (preferably vascular forceps) should be used to avoid tearing the sac, which may lead to recurrence. Because of the use of small incisions in pediatric surgery, the scrub person may be required to assist in retracting. The portion of the hernia sac removed, which is often small, is sent for routine pathological examination.

Potential Complications

One complication of this procedure is recurrence. One possible cause is tearing of the sac beyond the internal ring. The first assistant must provide adequate exposure, especially considering the size of the incision. Use of only smooth forceps when handling the hernia sac is essential. Another complication is injury to the vas deferens. Adequate exposure and handling of only surrounding tissue, never the vas deferens, are critical.

Pyloromyotomy
Definition

Pyloromyotomy is the treatment of choice for congenital hypertrophic pyloric stenosis (**Fig. 37.8**). Pyloric stenosis, also called infantile hypertrophic pyloric stenosis (IHPS), is the most common cause of intestinal obstruction in infancy; the incidence of IHPS is 2–4 per 1,000 live births (Singh, 2008). IHPS occurs secondary to hypertrophy and hyperplasia of the muscular layers of the pylorus, thereby causing a functional gastric outlet obstruction (Singh, 2008).

IHPS
Infantile Hypertrophic Pyloric Stenosis

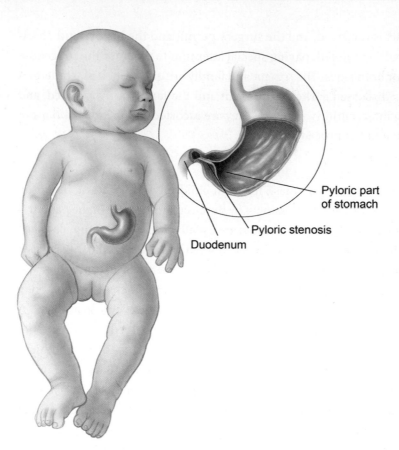

Figure 37.8
Pyloric stenosis.

Pyloric part of stomach

Pyloric stenosis

Duodenum

Indications

Patients usually present with symptoms at approximately 3 weeks of age, but may occur from 1 to 18 weeks (Singh, 2008). The presenting symptoms include (Singh, 2008):

- nonbilious vomiting or regurgitation, which may become projectile (up to 70%), after which the infant is still hungry;
- emesis, which may be intermittent or occur after each feeding; the emesis may become brown or coffee-colored due to blood secondary to gastritis or a Mallory-Weiss tear at the gastroesophageal junction;
- signs of dehydration and malnutrition such as poor weight gain, weight loss, marasmus, decreased urinary output, depressed fontanelles, dry mucous membranes, poor skin turgor, lethargy, and shock; and
- jaundice, which is corrected upon correction of the disease.

Upon physical exam, up to 60–80% of the infants with IHPS may have a firm, nontender, mobile, hard pylorus, approximately 1–2 cm in diameter, described as an "olive," present in the right upper quadrant at the lateral edge of the rectus abdominus muscle (Singh, 2008). This is best palpated after the infant has vomited, when he/she is calm, or when the gastric contents have been removed via nasogastric tube (Singh, 2008).

Although the condition is being recognized earlier with the resultant decrease in severity of symptoms, dehydration and acid-base imbalances are still a major concern.

Nursing Implications

Laboratory studies that should be drawn include electrolytes, pH, BUN (blood urea nitrogen), and creatinine levels should be drawn at the time of obtaining intravenous access (Singh, 2008). The classic electrolyte and acid-base imbalance of pyloric stenosis includes hypochloremia, hypokalemia, and metabolic alkalosis (Singh, 2008). Electrolyte abnormalities are dependent on the duration of symptoms; furthermore, dehydration may result in hypernatremia or hyponatremia, which may lead to prerenal renal failure (Singh, 2008). Appropriate IV therapy is initiated, and the procedure is usually performed within 24 hours of hospitalization.

BUN
Blood Urea Nitrogen

Procedure

General anesthesia is induced via endotracheal tube. The Ramstedt procedure consists of splitting the muscle of the hypertrophic pylorus, leaving the mucosa intact. The Ramstedt technique does not reapproximate the muscle, although this was used in the past. A right transverse incision is made through subcutaneous tissue; external oblique, internal oblique, and transversus abdominis muscles; and the peritoneum. An incision is then made through the muscle of the anterior pylorus from the junction of the pylorus and duodenum to the antrum of the stomach (2–3 cm). A blunt instrument is used to split the muscle fibers (often curved jaws of a hemostat or a pyloric spreader) with care to avoid perforation of the mucosa. Air can be placed in the stomach per nasogastric tube to check for perforations. The pylorus is returned to the abdominal cavity and, after verification of hemostasis, the incision is closed according to the surgeon's preference. Adhesive strips and possibly a small dressing are applied.

Postprocedure Care

The nasogastric tube is removed when the patient has completely recovered from anesthesia, unless there has been a perforation, in which case it is usually left in place for 24–48 hours. The patient is begun on oral feedings 6–8 hours after the procedure. The surgeon's preferences result in a variety of feeding regimens, usually beginning with sugar water and progressing to weak formula and then to full-strength formula. Because vomiting continues to be of concern, the infant's head is elevated after feeding and the child is placed on his or her right side.

Potential Complications

Complications of this procedure are rare. There is danger of peritonitis if a mucosal tear goes unrecognized and consequently unrepaired. Failure to split the muscle completely could result in unrelieved projectile vomiting.

Bowel Resection for Necrotizing Enterocolitis
Definition

Necrotizing enterocolitis (NEC) is characterized by necrosis of the mucosa of the colon and/or small intestine (**Fig. 37.9**). NEC is the most common gastrointestinal medical/surgical emergency occurring in neonates and represents a significant clinical problem: it affects approximately 10% of infants weighing less than 1500 g, with mortality rates of 50% or more, depending on the severity of the disease, compared

NEC
Necrotizing
Enterocolitis

Cross section of inflamed small intestine

Figure 37.9

Cross section of an inflamed small intestine.

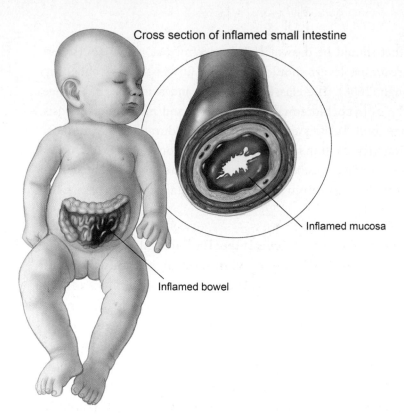

Inflamed mucosa

Inflamed bowel

with a mortality rate of 0%–20% in infants who weigh more than 2500 g (Springer, 2007). While it is more common in premature infants, it is also seen in term and near-term infants (Springer, 2007). Although the exact etiology of NEC remains unknown, research suggests that its cause is multifactorial: ischemia and/or reperfusion injury, exacerbated by the activation of proinflammatory intracellular cascades, may play a major role; in addition, cases that cluster in epidemics suggest an infectious etiology (Springer, 2007).

NEC is more prevalent in premature infants: the average age of onset is reported to be 20.2 days for babies born at less than 30 weeks' estimated gestational age (EGA), 13.8 days for babies born at 31–33 weeks' EGA, and 5.4 days for babies born after 34 weeks' gestation (Springer, 2007). Term infants develop NEC much earlier, with the average age of onset within the first week of life or, sometimes, within the first 1–2 days of life (Springer, 2007).

EGA
Estimated Gestational
Age

Indications

The clinical presentation of NEC includes nonspecific aspects of the history, such as vomiting, diarrhea, feeding intolerance, and high gastric residuals after feedings; more specific GI tract symptoms include abdominal distension and frank or occult blood in the stools (Minkes, 2008). The principle indication for surgical intervention is perforated or necrotic intestine; the most convincing predictor of intestinal necrosis indicating a need for surgery is pneumoperitoneum (Minkes, 2008). Additional indications for surgical intervention include erythema in the abdominal wall, gas in the portal vein, and positive paracentesis (Minkes, 2008). Radiography will show multiple areas of small-bowel dilation and if perforation has occurred, free air in the abdomen.

Nursing Implications

Before the procedure, the patient is kept NPO, IV therapy and antibiotic therapy is begun, and a nasogastric tube is inserted.

Procedure

The guiding principle of surgical intervention for NEC is to resect only perforated and conclusively necrotic intestine and to make every effort to preserve the ileocecal valve (Minkes, 2008). The abdomen is entered via a right transverse incision just below the umbilicus, using electrosurgery to ensure hemostasis; care must be taken at the time of entry into the peritoneal cavity to avoid injury to any dilated loops of intestines (Minkes, 2008). The abdominal cavity is then carefully inspected for evidence of necrosis and perforation, paying particular attention to the right lower quadrant, since the terminal ileum and proximal ascending colon are most commonly involved (Minkes, 2008). If a single area of bowel is resected, a proximal ostomy and distal mucus fistula are created (Minkes, 2008). Primary anastomosis is not generally recommended due to the risk of ischemia at the anastomosis, which can lead to increased incidence of leakage, stricture, fistula, or breakdown; however, intestinal resection with primary anastomosis may be safely performed in select cases in which the patient demonstrates a clearly demarcated small segment of injured bowel with normal-appearing residual intestine and is in good condition with no evidence of sepsis, coagulopathy, or physiologic compromise (Minkes, 2008). A feeding gastrostomy tube may be inserted. The abdomen is closed with interrupted suture on taper needles and subcuticular skin closure is performed.

Postprocedure Care

Intravenous fluid and antibiotic therapy are continued after the procedure. There may be a need for ventilatory assistance. The enterostomies are drained into closed containers (small ostomy bags are available). Takedown of the enterostomies is done when the infant is fully recovered.

Omphalocele and Gastroschisis Closure
Definition

An *omphalocele* is a defect in the anterior abdominal wall at the umbilicus; it consists of an avascular membranous sac with a wide base into which the liver has herniated (**Fig. 37.10**). Gastroschisis is an opening usually to the right of the umbilicus that has no sac and results in small intestine and possibly large intestine protruding from it. This bowel is abnormally thick and edematous, and the opening in the abdominal wall is small. Gastroschisis and omphalocele are among the most frequently encountered congenital anomalies in pediatric surgery; the combined incidence of these anomalies is 1 in 2,000 births (Glasser, 2007).

Indications

Infants with these defects are often identified prenatally; associated problems, such as defects in other organ systems or chromosomal abnormalities, are known before birth (Glasser, 2007). A child with gastroschisis may have malabsorption, either from an in-utero injury to the intestine or from a partial bowel obstruction (Glasser, 2007). In addition, anomalies of intestinal fixation may accompany abdominal wall

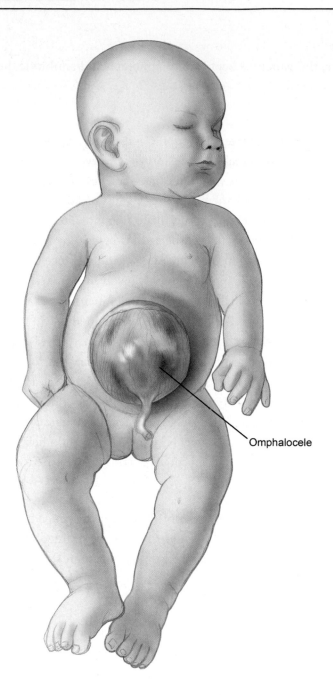

Figure 37.10
Omphalocele.

Omphalocele

defects; midgut volvulus is a potential complication, as is atypical appendicitis if the abnormally located appendix was not previously removed (Glasser, 2007). These children may also exhibit symptoms of gastroesophageal reflux, Hirschsprung disease, or both (Glasser, 2007).

Nursing Implications

Before the procedure, care must be taken to avoid pressure or traction on the sac or herniated bowel. Sterile saline-soaked dressings are applied.

Procedure

Closure of both conditions is similar. In the omphalocele, the sac may be resected and the liver returned to the abdominal cavity, and the abdominal wall is repaired.

The sac may also be left in place to prevent abdominal contents from adhering to the skin. Often, removal of the sac is necessary to stretch the abdominal wall to accommodate the abdominal contents. In gastroschisis, the defect is enlarged and the bowel is returned to the abdominal cavity and primary closure is attempted. In both cases, if the abdominal wall is too tight to allow primary closure, a "silo" of material such as Silastic sheeting may be constructed, which is sutured to the abdominal wall to cover the defect. The silo is compressed daily; forcing the abdominal contents to gradually enter the abdominal cavity until primary closure can be obtained.

Postprocedure Care

After the procedure, hyperalimentation and antibiotic therapy are used.

Potential Complications

Observation for edema of the lower extremities is necessary to detect pressure on the inferior vena cava that results when the abdominal cavity is closed under too much tension. Especially with gastroschisis (because the defect causes exposure of the bowel with no sac to protect it), infection is a concern.

Repair of Esophageal Atresia with Tracheoesophageal Fistula
Definition

Esophageal atresia (**Fig. 37.11**) describes a congenitally interrupted esophagus; one or more fistulae may be present between the malformed esophagus and the

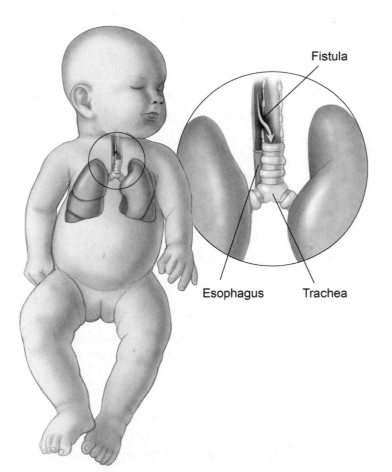

Figure 37.11

Esophageal atresia.

Fistula

Esophagus   Trachea

37

Table 37.5	Variations of Esophageal Atresia
Type	**Description**
A	Esophageal atresia without fistula, also called pure esophageal atresia (10%)
B	Esophageal atresia with proximal TEF (<1%)
C	Esophageal atresia with distal TEF (85%)
D	Esophageal atresia with proximal and distal TEFs (<1%)
E	TEF without esophageal atresia or so-called H-type fistula (4%)
F	Congenital esophageal stenosis (<1%)

Saxena, A.K. (2008). Esophageal atresia with or without tracheoesophageal fistula. Retrieved May 10, 2008 from http://www.emedicine.com/ped/TOPIC2950.HTM.

TEF
Tracheoesophageal Fistula

VACTERL
Vertebral defects, Anorectal malformations, Cardiovascular defects, Tracheoesophageal defects, Renal anomalies, and Limb deformities

trachea (Saxena, 2008). The lack of esophageal patency prevents swallowing; this problem prevents normal feeding, and may also cause infants to aspirate, literally drowning in their own saliva, which quickly overflows the upper pouch of the obstructed esophagus (Saxena, 2008). If a tracheoesophageal fistula (TEF) is present, fluid (either saliva from above or gastric secretions from below) may flow directly into the tracheobronchial tree (Saxena, 2008). The variations of esophageal atresia, and the approximate incidence in all infants born with esophageal anomalies, are described in **Table 37.5**.

Other associated anomalies include vertebral defects, anorectal malformations, cardiovascular defects, tracheoesophageal defects, renal anomalies, and limb deformities (VACTERL); these anomalies that should be readily apparent upon physical examination; if any of these anomalies are present, the presence of the others must be assessed (Saxena, 2008). The VACTERL syndrome occurs when 3 or more of the associated anomalies are present and occurs in approximately 25% of all patients with esophageal atresia (Saxena, 2008).

Indications

The patient has initial symptoms of drooling, frothy saliva, choking, and cyanosis. Gastric secretions enter the lungs through the fistula and result in recurrent chemical pneumonitis. On radiographic examination, air is seen in the intestine if there is a fistula between the trachea and the lower pouch. Attempts to pass an esophageal tube are unsuccessful.

Nursing Implications

Before the procedure, the patient may need ventilatory assistance. Antibiotics are initiated as well as IV therapy. The patient is kept NPO.

Procedure

The repair is accomplished by restoring continuity of the esophagus while ligating the fistula. The patient is placed on his or her left side with the right arm extended above the head. Thoracotomy is performed through an incision in the fourth intercostal space. Every attempt is made to avoid perforation of the thoracic cavity. By using either moist sponges or peanut gauze on the forceps, the parietal pleura is dissected away from the chest wall, proceeding posteriorly but also dissecting superiorly and inferiorly as well; a small mechanical Finochietto-type rib retractor is placed in the open thoracotomy site, and the pleural dissection proceeds to a point medial to the azygos vein (Saxena, 2008). The azygos vein is ligated and divided with fine silk. This extrapleural dissection then allows retropleural repair of the esophagus. Care is taken to avoid the vagus nerve. The upper pouch can be identified by having anesthesia personnel put pressure on a bougie inserted into the esophagus. The lower esophagus and fistula are identified, and the fistula is ligated proximal to the trachea and divided. The upper pouch is spatulated to facilitate anastomosis of the two pouches. The other varieties of this condition are repaired in similar fashion.

If the distance between the upper and lower pouches in the condition without fistula can be seen radiographically to be large, dilation with mercury-filled bougies is performed periodically according to the surgeon's preference, with the hope that eventually primary an anastomosis can be performed. If the distance is too great, colon interposition may be necessary.

A retropleural drain is usually placed. Suture on taper needles is used to close muscle layers and subcutaneous tissues, and a fine suture on a small cutting needle is used for subcuticular closure of the skin.

Postprocedure Care

After the procedure, IV fluid therapy, administration of antibiotics, and chest tube connection to drainage are necessary treatments.

Potential Complications

Complications include a possible tracheal edema due to dissection of the trachea, leakage of the anastomosis, and tracheomalacia (softening of the tissue of the trachea with resultant collapse of a segment), resulting in a need for aortopexy.

Repair of Congenital Diaphragmatic Hernia
Definition

Congenital diaphragmatic hernia (CDH) is a condition in which viscera herniate into the chest cavity, prompting the need for removal (**Fig. 37.12**); CDH occurs in 1 out of every 2,000–3,000 live births and accounts for 8% of all major congenital anomalies (Steinhorn, 2006). Emergency surgery is performed because of the severity of the symptoms. Acute respiratory distress and respiratory and metabolic acidosis make this condition life-threatening. The hernia is usually on the left side, with the contents being the small intestine, the stomach, the left lobe of the liver, the spleen, and most of the colon. The right-sided hernia usually involves the liver and some small and large bowel.

Indications

CDH is diagnosed based on prenatal ultrasonography findings in approximately half of affected infants (Steinhorn, 2006). Infants may have a prenatal history of

CDH
Tracheoesophageal Fistula

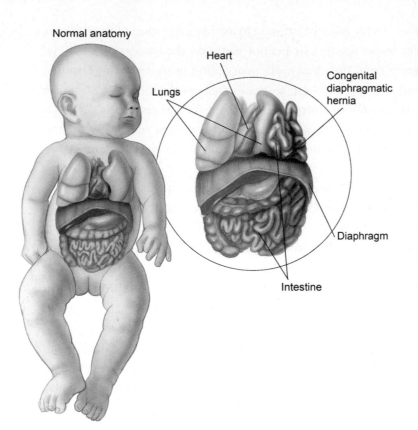

Normal anatomy

Heart

Lungs

Congenital diaphragmatic hernia

Diaphragm

Intestine

Figure 37.12

Congenital diaphragmatic hernia.

polyhydramnios and most commonly present with respiratory distress and cyanosis in the first minutes or hours of life, although a later presentation is possible; the respiratory distress can be severe, requiring aggressive resuscitative measures (Steinhorn, 2006).

Infants frequently exhibit a scaphoid abdomen, barrel-shaped chest, and signs of respiratory distress, such as retractions, cyanosis, and grunting respirations (Steinhorn, 2006). In patients with left-sided posterolateral hernia, auscultation of the lungs reveals poor air entry on the left, with a shift of cardiac sounds over the right chest; in patients with severe defects, pneumothorax signs (eg, poor air entry, poor perfusion) may also be present (Steinhorn, 2006).

Nursing Implications

Before the procedure, a nasogastric tube is placed. 100% oxygen is administered, and ventilator assistance is given if needed. An umbilical arterial catheter is inserted for drawing blood for blood gas determination. Judicious use of vasoactive agents may increase cardiac output without affecting systemic or pulmonary vascular resistance (Steinhorn, 2006).

Procedure

Anesthesia is induced with awake intubation. The repair is accomplished by replacing the contents of the hernia in the abdominal cavity and closing the defect. If the hernia is on the right side, a transthoracic approach may he used. More commonly, the hernia is on the left side and an abdominal approach is used. A left subcostal incision is made. The hernia contents are reduced, and the sac is resected if present.

The posterior and anterior margins of the diaphragm are approximated with suture of the surgeon's preference. If the posterior margin is absent, suture may be placed around the ribs. A prosthetic material such as Dacron or Silastic may be used to close the defect. Chest tubes are placed. If the abdominal cavity is too small to accommodate the contents of the hernia without placing too much pressure on abdominal organs, the skin only may be closed to increase the space. A gastrostomy tube is usually placed.

Postprocedure Care

After the operation, the patient will be on mechanical ventilation, for days or weeks, depending on the size of the hole in the diaphragm (American Pediatric Surgical Association, 2008). The baby will be started on feedings as soon as intestinal function returns, but this may take some time, in addition, babies with CDH usually have some form of GERD, which may make feeding more difficult (American Pediatric Surgical Association, 2008).

Potential Complications

Potential long-term complications include chronic lung disease and gastroesophageal reflux; in addition, these patients are assessed for developmental delays due to prolonged hospitalization and ventilation requirements (Children's Hospital of Wisconsin, 2008).

Nissen Fundoplication
Definition

Persistent GERD is one of the two most frequent disorders for which infants and children undergo abdominal surgery (Jaksic, 2008). Nearly all infants have some degree of gastroesophageal reflux (**Fig. 37.13**); if this reflux is transient it does

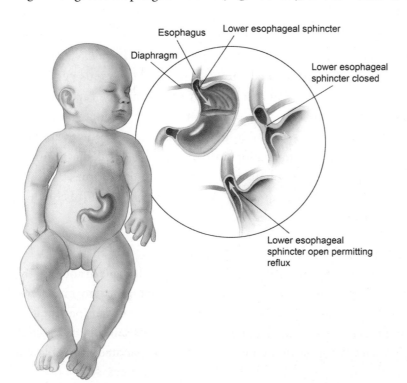

Esophagus
Lower esophageal sphincter
Diaphragm
Lower esophageal sphincter closed
Lower esophageal sphincter open permitting reflux

Figure 37.13

Gastroesophageal reflux in the infant.

not cause any morbidity; however, if the reflux is pathologic and persistent, it can cause feeding difficulties, failure to thrive, aspiration or respiratory complications, esophagitis, and esophageal stricture (Jaksic, 2008). Nissen fundoplication is performed to treat persistent GERD and is the most common operation performed today; it involves wrapping the gastric fundus 360° around the distal esophagus (Jaksic, 2008).

Indications

The primary indication for surgical intervention in children with GERD is failure of medical therapy; other indications include the complications described above, including a history of recurrent aspiration events (with or without pneumonia); apnea or near-miss sudden infant death syndrome (SIDS); reactive airway disease; refractory emesis; failure to thrive; esophagitis; esophageal stricture; Barrett esophagus; and associated anatomic anomalies (eg, large hiatal hernia) (Jaksic, 2008).

SIDS
Sudden Infant Death
Syndrome

Nursing Implications

Preprocedure planning for antireflux surgery in children is critical. Since many children have malnutrition, chronic aspiration, pneumonia, or pulmonary dysfunction, it is critical to assess and optimize the patient's nutritional and pulmonary status before surgery (Jaksic, 2008). In malnourished children, preprocedure supplemental nutrition should be considered; any ongoing pulmonary infection or pneumonia should be adequately treated (Jaksic, 2008).

Procedure

Nissen fundoplication may be done laparoscopically or open. The procedure consists of wrapping a portion of the fundus of the stomach circumferentially around the distal esophagus. Endotracheal general anesthesia is induced. The patient is placed supine, and a mercury-filled bougie or nasogastric tube is passed into the distal esophagus to ensure that the wrap is not too tight. A midline incision is made. The stomach is separated from the spleen at the proximal greater curvature. The short gastric vessels are ligated and divided with care to avoid the vagus nerve. The distal esophagus is mobilized, and a Penrose drain or umbilical tape can he placed around the esophagus, which can be used to provide traction to facilitate placement of sutures through the gastric and esophageal muscles at the site of the wrap. Prevention of movement of the fundoplication into the posterior mediastinum is accomplished by suturing the diaphragmatic hiatus to the fundoplication. A feeding gastrostomy may be formed, and closure with interrupted sutures and subcuticular closure of the skin is performed.

Postprocedure Care

While some surgeons believe a nasogastric tube should be left in place and that the gastrostomy tube should be left to drain to gravity until evidence of normal bowel function (eg, return of bowel sounds) is observed, this is not always done, particularly if a laparoscopic approach is used (Jaksic, 2008). The patient should be fed a clear liquid diet by mouth with the appropriate diet reinstated, as tolerated. If the patient is to be fed through a gastrostomy tube, the selected liquid diet should be started slowly and then progressively change to the goal diet, as tolerated; although little evidence supports the practice in children, many surgeons believe that postoperative return of bowel function is faster after laparoscopic surgery and advance the diet more quickly than after open surgery (Jaksic, 2008).

Potential Complications

After bowel function returns, the nurse must be vigilant for the signs of complications, which occur more commonly in children with neurologic impairment than in otherwise healthy children (Jaksic, 2008). Postprocedure complications may occur early or late and include (Jaksic, 2008):

Early complications:

- retching, which occurs most often in children with neurologic impairment and those who retch preoperatively;
- gas bloat—patients with this complication are usually unable to vomit;
- dysphagia;
- atelectasis;
- pneumonia;
- wound infection or dehiscence; and
- small-bowel obstruction due to adhesions.

Late complications:

- bowel obstruction; and
- wrap failure, which may include a wrap disruption, a slipped wrap, herniation of the wrap into the chest, or an excessively tight wrap. Patients with wrap failure usually present with symptoms or dysphagia or those associated with recurrent reflux.

Kasai Procedure

Definition

The Kasai procedure, or hepatic portoenterostomy, is performed for the treatment of biliary atresia (**Fig. 37.14**). Biliary atresia occurs within the first two months of life when there is a blockage of the bile duct connecting the liver to the gut; eventually this blockage will cause the accumulation of bile in the liver that leads to damage and scarring of the liver cells; if left untreated, this scarring will cause liver failure and the need for liver transplantation (The Children's Hospital, 2008). The pathology of the extrahepatic biliary system widely varies in these patients; the following classification is based on the predominant site of atresia (Schwartz, 2007):

- Type I involves obliteration of the common duct; the proximal ducts are patent;
- Type II is characterized by atresia of the hepatic duct, with cystic structures found in the porta hepatic; and
- Type III (>90% of patients) involves atresia of the right and left hepatic ducts to the level of the porta hepatis.

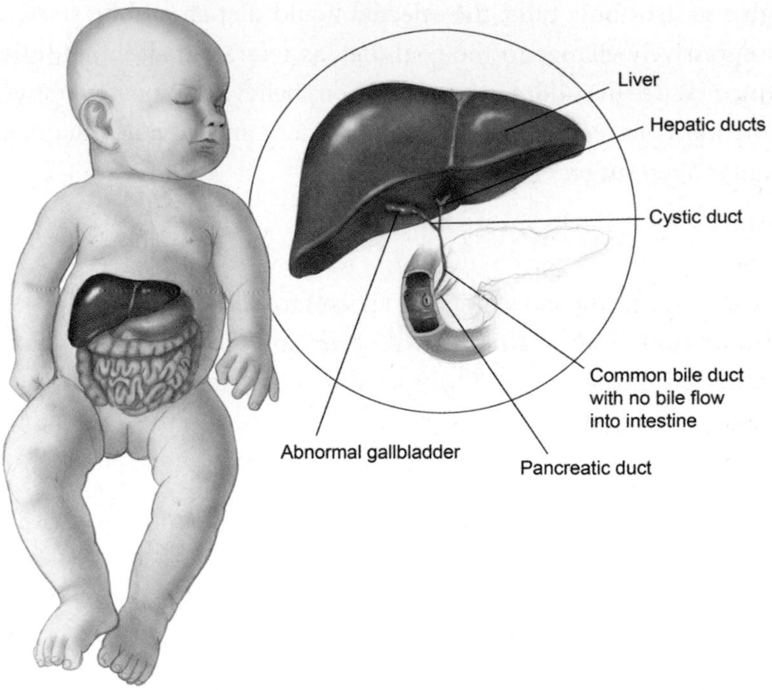

Figure 37.14
Biliary atresia.

The Kasai procedure attempts to reconstruct the bile duct with a loop of intestine; the small intestine is attached to the liver directly, allowing the bile to drain (The Children's Hospital, 2008).

Indications

In the first 2–3 weeks of life, an olive-green jaundice becomes apparent. Dark urine, light and putty like feces, hepatomegaly, abdominal distention, and failure to thrive, along with irritability and restlessness, are noted.

Nursing Implications

Since jaundice may be present with other liver disorders, other tests are performed to correctly diagnose biliary atresia, including (Cincinnati Children's, 2008):

- blood tests to detect liver function abnormalities and the etiology of the jaundice;
- radiographs to assess for an enlarged liver and spleen;
- abdominal ultrasound to detect a small gallbladder, or no gallbladder;
- liver biopsy; and
- hepatobiliary (HIDA) scan—this is a nuclear scan that determines the flow of bile.

HIDA
Hepatobiliary

Procedure

The Kasai procedure consists of resection of the nonfunctional hepatic ducts and anastomosis of the jejunum to the transected duct at the liver hilum. A right subcostal incision is made. The rectus muscle is incised to provide exposure of the right lobe of the liver. The gallbladder is mobilized, and cholangiography is performed. If patency of the biliary tree cannot be visualized, the extra hepatic ducts are removed and a Roux-en-Y procedure is performed by anastomosing a segment of jejunum to the liver hilus An end-to-side anastomosis restores intestinal continuity. The porta hepatis is often the site of drain placement. The abdomen is closed with interrupted suture, and a subcuticular skin closure is performed.

Postprocedure Care

In the immediate postprocedure period, methylprednisolone has been used as both an anti-inflammatory agent and as a nonspecific stimulant of bile salt-independent bile flow (Schwartz, 2007). In patients with chronic cholestatic conditions and bile duct patency, ursodeoxycholic acid (ie, ursodiol, UCDA) is associated with minimal toxicity and has been shown to enhance bile flow, which may improve outcomes (Schwartz, 2007). Long-term antibiotic prophylaxis may decrease the incidence of cholangitis following the procedure (Schwartz, 2007). Breastfeeding is also encouraged after the procedure when possible, because breast milk contains both lipases and bile salts that aid in lipid hydrolysis (Schwartz, 2007).

Potential Complications

Complications include intestinal obstruction and increased sebaceous gland secretion. Water-soluble vitamins are given. Drainage of bile is measured and replaced.

Cholangitis is a major complication that is confirmed by an elevated temperature, tenderness of the right upper quadrant, decreased bile drainage, and jaundice. Portal hypertension is another possible complication. If jaundice and other associated symptoms persist after surgical intervention, liver transplantation may be the treatment of choice.

REFERENCES

1. American Pediatric Surgical Association (2008). Congenital diaphragmatic hernia. Retrieved May 10, 2008 from http://www.eapsa.org/parents/resources/diaphramaticHernia.cfm.
2. American Society of Anesthesiologists. (1999). Practice guidelines for preoperative fasting and the use of pharmacologic agents to reduce the risk of pulmonary aspiration: application to healthy patients undergoing elective procedures: a report by the American Society of Anesthesiologist Task Force on Preoperative Fasting. *Anesthesiology* 90(3); pp. 896–905.
3. AORN (2008). Recommended practices for electrosurgery. In *Perioperative Standards and Recommended Practices*. Denver, CO: AORN, Inc., pp. 315–329.
4. Bergren, M. (2004). Data integrity: Beware of viruses. *The Journal of School Nursing*, 20(4); pp. 234–235.
5. Burrington, J. (1996). Pain control in children from the surgeon's viewpoint. In *Abdominal Surgery of Infancy and Childhood*, Vol. 1, W. Donnellan, J. Burrington, K. Kirnura, J. Schafer, & J. White, Eds. Luxembourg: Harwood Academic Publishers, pp. 13–18.
6. Carter-Gentry, D., & McCurren, C. (2004). Organ procurement from the perspective of the perioperative nurses. *AORN Journal*, 80(3); pp. 417–431.
7. Centers for Disease Control. (2007a). Births: preliminary data for 2006. National vital statistics report 56(7). Retrieved May 6, 2008 from http://www.cdc.gov/nchs/data/nvsr/nvsr56/nvsr56_07.pdf.
8. Centers for Disease Control. (2007b). Fetal and perinatal morality, United States, 2003. National vital statistics report 55(6). Retrieved May 6, 2008 from http://www.cdc.gov/nchs/data/nvsr/nvsr55/nvsr55_06.pdf.
9. Centers for Disease Control. (2007c). Recommendations to improve preconception health and health care—United States. MMWR; April 21, 2006; 55(RR06); 1–23. Retrieved May 8, 2008 from http://www.cdc.gov/mmwR/preview/mmwrhtml/rr5506a1.htm.
10. Children's Hospital Boston. (2008). Extracorporeal membrane oxygenation (ECMO). Retrieved February 16, 2008, from http://www.childrenshospital.org/clinicalservices/site2270/mainpageS2270PO.html.
11. Children's Hospital of Wisconsin (2008). Congenital diaphragmatic hernia. Retrieved May 10, 2008 from http://www.chw.org/display/PPF/DocID/34373/Nav/1/router.asp.
12. Cincinnati Children's. (2008). Biliary atresia. Retrieved May 10, 2008 from http://www.cincinnatichildrens.org/svc/alpha/l/liver/diseases/biliary.htm.

13. Collins, S. (2006). Hydrocele and hernia in children. Retrieved May 9, 2008 from http://www.emedicine.com/ped/TOPIC1037.htm.

14. Coté, C.J. (2005). Pediatric anesthesia. In *Miller's Anesthesia*, 6th ed, R.D. Miller, Ed. Philadelphia, PA: Elsevier, Churchill, Livingston, pp. 2367–2407.

15. Crosbie, S. (2007). Consent in practice: a case review. *Paediatric Nursing*, 19(5); pp. 34–36.

16. Denholm, B. (2007). Clinical Issues: Malignant hyperthermia; sterilization monitoring; sterilization indicators; multiple needle counts. *AORN Journal*, 85(2); pp. 403–408.

17. Doyle, M. (2006). Promoting standardized nursing language using an electronic medical record system. *AORN Journal*, 83(6); pp. 1335–1348.

18. Erickson, F. (1967). Helping the child maintain behavioral control. *Nursing Clinics of North America*, 2(4); pp. 695–703.

19. Erickson, F. (1965). When 6- to 12-year olds are ill. *Nursing Outlook*, 13, pp. 48–50.

20. Fraser, J., & McAbee, G. (2004). American Academy of Pediatrics: Clinical Report. Dealing with the parent whose judgment is impaired by alcohol or drugs: Legal and ethical considerations. *Pediatrics*, 114(3); pp. 869–873.

21. Freud, A. (1952). The role of bodily illness in the mental life of children. In *The Psychoanalytic Study of the Child*, Vol. 7, A. Freud, Ed. (Vol. 7, pp. 69–81). New York, NY: International University Press, Inc., pp. 69–81.

22. Gellert, E. (1962). Children's conceptions of the content and function of the human body. *Genetic Psychology Monographs*, 65, pp. 293–405.

23. Glasser, J.C. (2007). Omphalocele and gastroschisis. Retrieved May 10, 2008 from http://www.emedicine.com/ped/TOPIC1642.HTM.

24. Greco, C. (2003). Point-counterpoint; Point: pediatric NPO guidelines. Retrieved May 8, 2008 from http://www.pedsanesthesia.org/newsletters/2003summer/point.iphtml.

25. Griffith, R. (2004). The issue of consent and children: Who decides? *British Journal of Community Nursing*, 9(7); pp. 298–301.

26. Hallstrom, I., & Elander, G. (2005). Decision-making in paediatric care: An overview with reference to nursing care. *Nursing Ethics*, 12(3); pp. 223–238.

27. Hebra, A. (2006). Pediatric hernias. Retrieved May 9, 2008 from http://www.emedicine.com/PED/topic2559.htm.

28. Jacksic, T. (2008). Gastroesophageal reflux: surgical perspective. Retrieved May 10, 2008 from http://www.emedicine.com/ped/TOPIC2957.htm.

29. Kain, Z., Mayes, L., Caldwell-Andrews, A., Saadat, H., McClain, B., & Wang, S. (2006). Predicting which children will benefit most from parental presence during induction of anesthesia. *Paediatric Anesthesia*, 16(6); pp. 627–634.

30. Kolon, T.F. (2006). Cryptorchidism. Retrieved May 9, 2008 from http://www.emedicine.com/med/topic2707.htm.

31. Kovarik, W.D. (2005). Pediatric and neonatal intensive care unit. In *Miller's Anesthesia*, 6th ed., R.D. Miller, Ed. Philadelphia, PA: Elsevier, Churchill, Livingston, pp. 2831–2886.

32. Lehna, C. (2005). Interpreter services in pediatric nursing. *Pediatric Nursing*, 31(4); pp. 292–296.

33. Livingston, B. (2004).The ins and outs of body piercing. *AORN Journal*, 79(2); pp. 333–346.

34. MASSChips Database. (2008). Birth/death query including all congenital anomalies, Massachusetts total 1999–2003. Query ran on February 2, 2008 by: Kelly M. Kollar RN. *New England Journal of Medicine*, 272, pp. 406–414.

35. Miceli, P. & Clark, P. (2004). Your patient—My child: Seven priorities for improving pediatric care from the parent's perspective. *Journal of Nursing Care Quality*, 20(1); pp. 43–53.

36. Minkes, R.K. (2008). Necrotizing enterocolitis: Surgical perspective. Retrieved May 10, 2008 from http://www.emedicine.com/ped/TOPIC2981.HTM.

37. Patten, S.P. (2006). Educating nurses about correct application of cricoid pressure. *AORN Journal*, 84(3); pp. 449–461.

38. Pierro, A. (2002). Metabolism and nutritional support in the surgical neonate. *Journal of Pediatric Surgery*, 37(6); pp. 811–822.

39. Porth, C. (2007). *Pathophysiology: Concepts of Altered Health States*, 7th cd. Philadelphia, PA: Lippincott Williams & Wilkins, pp. 30, 211–212.

40. Potts, W. (1956). The heart of a child. *JAMA*, 161, pp. 487–490.

41. Romino, S., Keatley, V., Secrest, J., & Good, K. (2005). Parental presence during anesthesia induction in children. *AORN Journal*, 81(4); pp. 779–792.

42. Saxena, A.K. (2008). Esophageal atresia with or without tracheoesophageal fistula. Retrieved May 10, 2008 from http://www.emedicine.com/ped/TOPIC2950.HTM.

43. Schultz, N.V. (1971). How children perceive pain. *Nursing Outlook*, 19(10); pp. 670–673.

44. Schwartz, S.M. (2007). Biliary atresia. Retrieved May 10, 2008 from http://www.emedicine.com/ped/TOPIC237.HTM#section~Treatment.

45. Sessler, D. (2000). Perioperative heat balance. *Anesthesiology*, 92(2); pp. 578–596.

46. Singh, J. (2008). Pediatrics, pyloric stenosis. Retrieved May 10, 2008 from http://www.emedicine.com/emerg/TOPIC397.htm.

47. Smith, J., & Dearmun, A. (2006). Improving care for children requiring surgery and their families. *Paediatric Nursing*, 18(9); pp. 30–33.

48. Springer, S.C. (2007). Necrotizing enterocolitis. Retrieved May 10, 2008 from http://www.emedicine.com/ped/TOPIC2601.htm.

49. Steinhorn, R.H. (2006). Congenital diaphragmatic hernia. Retrieved May 10, 2008 from http://www.emedicine.com/ped/TOPIC2603.htm.

50. Taylor, E. (2007). Infant perioperative patients. *AORN Journal*, 86(5); pp. 843–848.

51. The Children's Hospital (2008). The Kasai procedure for biliary atresia. Retrieved May 10, 2008 from http://www.thechildrenshospital.org/conditions/digestive/liver/kasai.aspx.

52. The Joint Commission. (2003). Universal Protocol For Preventing Wrong Site, Wrong Procedure, Wrong Person Surgery.™ Retrieved May 8, 2008 from http://www.jointcommission.org/NR/rdonlyres/E3C600EB-043B-4E86-B04E-CA4A89AD5433/0/universal_protocol.pdf.

53. Ulmer, B.C. (2007). *Electrosurgery self-study guide.* Boulder, CO: Valleylab/Covidien.

54. Valleylab. (2007). Infant REM PolyHesive™ II Patient Return electrode. Boulder, CO: Valleylab.

55. Valleylab. (2006). Neonatal REM PolyHesive™ II. Boulder, CO: Valleylab.

56. Whaley, L., & Wong, D. (1979). *Nursing care of infants and children.* St. Louis, MO: C.V. Mosby.

57. Whittle, A., Shah, S., Wilfond, B., Gensler, G., & Wendler, D. (2004). Institutional review board practices regarding assent in pediatric research. *Pediatrics*, 113(6); pp. 1747–1752.

58. Wilson, P. (2005). Jehovah's Witness children: When religion and the law collide. *Paediatric Nursing*, 17(3); pp. 34–37.

59. Wisselo, T.L., Stuart, C., & Muris, P. (2004). Providing parents with information before anaesthesia: What do they really want to know? *Paediatric Anesthesia*, 14(4); pp. 299–307.

60. Ygge, B., Lindholm, C., & Arnetz, J. (2006). Hospital staff perceptions of parent involvement in paediatric hospital care. *Journal of Advanced Nursing*, 53(5); pp. 534–542.

37

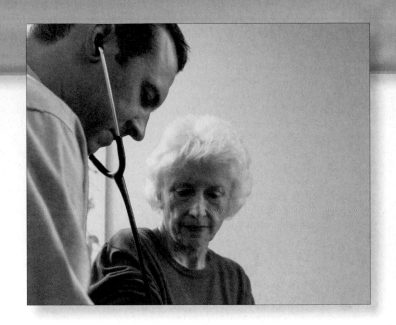

CHAPTER 38

Care of the Geriatric Patient

Charlotte Dorsey

INTRODUCTION

Healthcare financing and reimbursement, societal trends, national and state healthcare policies, and the emergence of hospitals predominately focused on acute-care services have significantly affected the delivery of healthcare to the aging population. In 2003, adults over 65 years of age comprised only 12 percent of the population, yet they accounted for one out of three hospital stays, and had a mean length of stay 1.7 days longer than the non-elderly (Russo & Elixhauser, 2006). Physiological changes and greater incidence of pathological processes associated with aging place the elderly patient at a greater risk for complications for any given operative procedure compared to the middle-aged patient.

AFFECT OF THE AGING POPULATION ON THE HEALTHCARE DELIVERY SYSTEM

Delivery methods have changed to meet the needs of the aging population. For example, in the United States, outpatient operative procedures account for more than 60% of the procedures, with speculations that the percentage will increase to nearly 75% by 2018 (eMedicine-Health, 2008). Hospitals continue to add outpatient surgery centers; more freestanding ambulatory surgery facilities continue to open. These facilities provide care relevant to the needs of the elderly.

Elderly patients benefit from outpatient operative and invasive procedures, because of convenience, lower cost, and reduced stress. However, unlike younger patients, the elderly still require thorough medical evaluations before any operative or invasive procedure to determine the most appropriate setting for the procedure. For example, while age alone does not exclude an elderly patient as a candidate for an outpatient procedure, age does affect the reaction to certain anesthetic agents and related medications. Excretion of short-acting drugs often takes a longer time. In addition, an elderly patient may also have more underlying medical conditions that could potentially make an outpatient procedure riskier (New York-Presbyterian Hospital, 2008).

LEGAL IMPLICATIONS

Informed Consent

Informed consent, while important for all patients, particularly affects the older patient because of physiological changes that may affect cognition and thus affect ability to make a reasonable decision about the proposed treatment or intervention. In order to give informed consent, patients should receive information in terms they can understand and comprehend (Guido, 2006). The person obtaining informed consent should:

1. Briefly, yet completely explain the proposed treatment and/or procedure, which would include the diagnosis and the nature or purpose of the procedure.
2. Provide the name and the qualifications of the person and assistants performing the procedure.
3. Discuss the potential for serious harm, risks, or side effects that may occur during the procedure, including death, blood loss, pain, discomfort, nausea, and vomiting.
4. Discuss the likelihood of success of the proposed treatment or procedure.
5. Explain the patient's right to refuse the treatment or procedure, which would include the prognosis if the patient refuses the proposed treatment or procedure.
6. Inform the patient that alternative care and/or support would continue should the patient refuse the proposed treatment or care.
7. Explain practical alternatives to the proposed treatment or procedure, including the risks associated with doing nothing at all.

The physician has the ultimate responsibility for obtaining informed consent (see **Fig. 38.1**). Consequently, the nurse should not explain a procedure, the possible complications, and any available alternatives for the purposes of obtaining informed consent. As necessary, however, the nurse should clarify the statements made by the physician. If the patient expresses uncertainties or has questions about the proposed treatment or procedure, the physician should provide clarification and answer questions.

Failure to obtain informed consent from the elderly patient could be construed as negligence or battery. Negligence refers to a failure to give care to a patient according to minimally acceptable standards, which includes obtaining operative or invasive procedure consent. Consent forms should contain important facts, such as major potential complications of anesthesia or the procedure. Failure to mention these facts when obtaining a patient's signature could be a breach of duties and considered negligence. Battery occurs when someone does something physical to the patient that he or she does not want done, such as wrong site operative procedures.

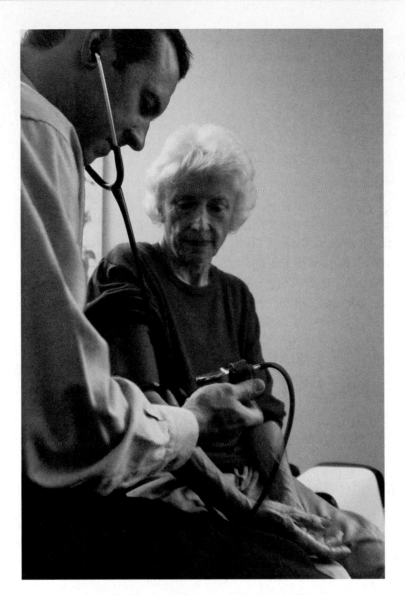

Figure 38.1

The physician has the ultimate responsibility for obtaining informed consent.

In addition to negligence and battery, other legal areas, such as giving voluntary valid consent and having competency to give consent, concern the older population. Voluntary consent means that a patient must be free to choose, and there cannot be any force, fraud, deceit, duress, constraint, or coercion to that patient. For example, a violation could occur when a patient is forced into undergoing operative intervention such as an amputation or when no alternative treatments are presented. This is not as common as coercion, in which the older adult may be manipulated into having an unwanted operative or invasive procedure.

A patient must show mental competency to sign the consent. A patient declared incompetent by a healthcare institution (de facto incompetence), may have been declared so in a court of law (de jure incompetence). In this case, an older adult's family members may provide informed consent and, in such cases, usually make compassionate and competent decisions when the patient needs an operative or invasive procedure. Priority for giving consent by family members usually begins with the spouse, followed by adult children or grandchildren, parents, adult brothers and sisters, and adult nieces and nephews (Guido, 2006).

There are four general exceptions to the informed consent requirements (Guido, 2006).

Emergencies

Emergencies require consent to prevent charges of battery; therefore, make every effort to obtain informed consent. However, in cases such as the threat of immediate death or permanent disability, obtaining informed consent is sometimes impossible because of the condition of the patient and the absence of a responsible family member or court appointed guardian. In these cases, the physician may proceed without informed consent. If this occurs, thoroughly document actions taken to obtain consent. Some facilities require written concurrence by two physicians.

Patient Waiver

The patient can waive or relinquish the right to full disclosure and still consent to the procedure.

Therapeutic Privilege

A physician or primary healthcare provider can withhold information about a patient's diagnosis or treatment when he/she feels it would be detrimental to the patient's health. Healthcare providers usually invoke therapeutic privilege if the information might hinder or complicate necessary treatment, cause severe psychological trauma, or be so upsetting that the patient cannot make a rational decision about treatment options. Before making an independent decision to withhold information, the healthcare professional should seek consultation about his or her decision. After the risk to the patient has decreased, the physician must fully disclose the previously withheld information.

Prior Patient Knowledge

When the patient knows the risk of a treatment or procedure because of experience, or when the information is known to the average patient, the healthcare professional is not required to disclose the risk.

Elder Abuse

The nurse as the patient advocate has a responsibility to recognize signs and symptoms and report elder abuse, which includes physical abuse, sexual abuse, and neglect. Physical abuse describes the inappropriate use of physical force that can result in bodily injury or physical pain. When assessing the patient, look for unexplained fractures, mysterious bruises or burns in unusual locations, sprains or dislocations, and/or unexplained head injury. Sexual abuse describes non-consensual sexual contact of any kind and ranges from unwanted touching to coerced nudity and rape. Look for genital/anal bruises or bleeding, and/or signs of sexually transmitted diseases. Assess for neglect by looking for dehydration or malnutrition, untreated bedsores, poor personal hygiene, failure to provide medical care, and unsafe or unsanitary living conditions. Determine if the suspected abuse patient has a history of healthcare hopping, meaning they rely on walk-in clinics rather than a regular physician. Psychological abuse may be more difficult to identify. Look for extreme mood changes, depression or oversedation, general fearfulness, and fear of caregivers (Mamaril, 2006).

DEFINING THE TERM ELDERLY

In the past, society considered 65 years of the age as elderly, when a person became eligible for Social Security. Over the years, however, the definition of elderly has changed. Psychologists now divide the elderly into three groups (Ebersole, Hess, Touhy, & Jett, 2005): young old, 65 to 74 years old; middle old, 75 to 84 years; and old-old, or those over 85 years of age.

According to the US Census Bureau (2007), the number of people 65 and older has steadily grown since 1990 from 28.6 million to more than 35.5 million. As life expectancy increases, so does the incidence of co-morbidity, which is the presence of one or more diseases in a patient, such as hypertension, congestive heart failure, or diabetes. These co-morbidities or chronic illnesses can affect the patient's recovery after anesthesia and operative or invasive procedures and place the patient at greater risk for postprocedure complications.

PHYSIOLOGICAL AND PSYCHOSOCIAL ASPECTS OF AGING

Physiological Changes

Cardiovascular System

Caring for an older adult patient means the nurse may have to care for a patient with cardiac problems. Cardiovascular heart disease is the leading cause of death in the United States for people over 65 years of age (National Center for Health Statistics, 2007). The most common types of heart disease include coronary artery disease (CAD) and heart failure (HF).

As people age, changes occur within the heart and the entire cardiovascular system (see **Table 38.1**). Overall heart size decreases, the left ventricular wall thickens, and the elasticity of the heart muscle and vessel walls decreases. At the same time,

CAD
Coronary Artery Disease

HF
Heart Failure

Table 38.1	Physiological Cardiovascular Changes with Aging	
Determinant	**Resting Cardiac Performance**	**Exercise Cardiac Performance**
Heart rate	Slight decrease	Slight decrease
Cardiac output	Unchanged or slightly decreased	Decreased owing to a drop in heart rate
Stroke volume	Slight increase	Slight increase
Ejection fraction	Unchanged	Increase
Afterload	Increased	Uncertain

Adapted from: McCance, K. & Huether, S. (2002). *Pathophysiology: The Biologic Basis for Disease in Adults and Children*, 4th ed. St. Louis, MO: Mosby.

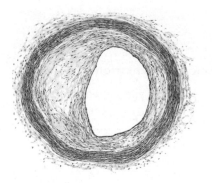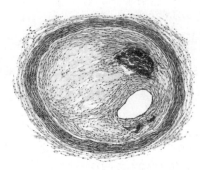

Figure 38.2

Calcification of vessels and decreased elasticity of the vessel walls.

heart valves become thicker because of lipid accumulation, collagen degeneration, and fibrosis (Meiner & Lueckenotte, 2006).

For some older patients, the cardiac conduction system may have been damaged by past ischemic attacks or from fibrotic tissue formation, affecting the nodal areas in the heart especially the sinoatrial node. In such cases, arrhythmias such as tachycardia or sinus bradycardia become more prevalent and obvious. Electrocardiogram (ECG) changes are normal for the older adult patients including increased PR, QRS, and Q-T intervals (Meiner & Lueckenotte, 2006).

Calcification of vessels and decreased elasticity of the vessel walls are very common in older adults, especially in the coronary and carotid arteries (see **Fig. 38.2**).

Cardiovascular disease (CVD) is not only the leading cause of death in the United States, but also the leading cause for hospital admissions than any other disease or condition. Common cardiac conditions in the older adult include coronary heart disease (ischemic heart disease), hypertension, congestive heart failure (CHF), arrhythmias, endocarditis, conductive disruptions, valvular conditions, and peripheral vascular disease (PVD). The most common vascular problems include chronic and acute arterial occlusions, aneurysms, phlebitis, cerebrovascular accidents (CVA), and varicosities. Operative procedures most commonly performed for disorders of the elderly cardiovascular system include revascularization procedures, and insertion of pacemakers. All general anesthetic agents may affect the aging heart because of their impact on myocardial function, preload, and heart rate.

Risk factors for cardiovascular disease fall into two categories: modifiable and non-modifiable. The non-modifiable risk factors include age, gender, race, and family history. Modifiable factors include elevated blood cholesterol levels, hypertension, diabetes mellitus, smoking, sedentary lifestyle, stress, obesity, alcohol intake, hormone intake, and excessive intake of saturated fats, carbohydrates, and salt. Adoption of healthier lifestyle has the potential to reduce or prevent the incidence of morbidity and death from CHF and stroke.

ECG
Electrocardiogram

38

CVD
Cardiovascular Disease

CHF
Congestive Heart Failure

PVD
Peripheral Vascular Disease

CVA
Cerebrovascular Accidents

Respiratory System

Normal changes in the respiratory system are related to structure and function in the elderly patient. Changes occur gradually; respiratory muscles begin to weaken, chest wall compliance begins to decrease, and elasticity in the lungs decreases (see **Table 38.2**). Skeletal defects such as shortening of the vertebral column and ossification of the costal cartilage increase stiffness or rigidity, which

Table 38.2	Physiological Respiratory Changes with Aging	

Respiratory Function	Pathophysiologic Changes	Clinical Presentation
Mechanics of breathing (decline in bellows function)	☐ Increased chest wall stiffness ☐ Loss of elastic recoil ☐ Decreased respiratory muscle strength ☐ Increased airway collapsibility	☐ Decreased vital capacity ☐ Increased reserve volume ☐ Decreased expiratory flow rates
Oxygenation (Abnormal gas exchange)	☐ Increased ventilation-perfusion mismatch ☐ Decreased cardiac output ☐ Reduced diffusing for carbon monoxide ☐ Increased alveolar-arterial oxygen gradient	☐ Arterial hypoxemia ☐ Decreased exercise tolerance
Lung defense mechanisms	☐ Decreased number of cilia ☐ Decreased effectiveness of mucociliary clearance ☐ Impaired cough mechanisms ☐ Decreased IgA production	☐ Decreased ability to clear secretions ☐ Increased susceptibility to infection (pneumonia & chronic bronchitis) ☐ Increased risk of aspiration
Upper airway obstruction	☐ Decreased upper airway muscle tone ☐ Decreased arousal ☐ Decreased ventilatory drive	☐ Increased frequency of hypopnea ☐ Increased risk of aspiration ☐ Snoring ☐ Obstructive sleep apnea
Abnormal breathing pattern	☐ Decreased responsiveness to hypoxemia ☐ Change in respiratory mechanics	☐ Increased respiratory rate ☐ Cheyne-Stokes breathing ☐ Periodic breathing

Adapted from: McCance, K. & Huether, S. (2002). *Pathophysiology: The Biologic Basis for Disease in Adults and Children*, 4th ed. St. Louis, MO: Mosby.

contributes to decreased rib mobility and reduced chest expansion. Gas exchange at the alveolar-capillary membrane becomes less effective because of fewer alveoli (Ebersole, Hess, Touhy, & Jett, 2005). These changes lead to a decrease in the vital capacity and tidal volume, as well as generalized decreased tissue oxygenation. Between the ages of 20 and 80 years, the amount of air a person can move through the lungs decreases. Because respiratory changes, like other physiological changes in the elderly, occur naturally with time, elderly patients in a state of good health adjust to the decreased oxygenation and adapt well until trauma, such as an operative procedure occurs. Trauma disrupts physiological balance and may affect the patient's breathing patterns.

In older adults, mortality and morbidity after an operative or invasive procedure often happen because of the pathophysiological changes in the aging respiratory system. Aging patients have less physiological endurance to withstand an operative or invasive procedure, as well as less energy to recover quickly. They have an increased risk of aspiration because of loss of laryngeal reflexes and an increased risk of atelectasis due to the incision, pain, and decreased postprocedure deep breathing. Consequent immobility decreases ventilation and effective airway clearance, which increase the potential for pneumonia (Meiner & Lueckenotte, 2006). The most common procedures performed in the elderly are for neoplasms of the lung (especially for patients with a long history of smoking) and endoscopic procedures. The elderly patient's ability to deliver oxygen to the tissues slightly decreases, which makes the patient more susceptible to retaining CO_2, especially after receiving medication for postprocedure pain. The most common postprocedure complications include pulmonary insufficiency, atelectasis, and pneumonia.

Musculoskeletal System

Aging patients experience changes in the muscle, bones, and joints of the musculoskeletal system. Muscle mass, tone, and strength gradually decrease over time because of a reduction in the number of muscle cells, which are replaced by fibrous connective tissue. Most likely, the weakening of motor performance in the elderly occurs because of a decline in tissue oxygenation and central nervous system functioning rather than to changes in the muscle fibers themselves. Adipose cells increase in women and decrease in men. Strength also decreases if the person does not maintain an active exercise schedule.

Bones decrease in mass for several reasons. In women, demineralization and protein matrix loss occur after menopause. Osteoporosis is twice as common in women as in men. Women have more bone resorbed than formation, leading to fragile, Swiss cheese bones. The aging body is unable to produce or use adequate calcium or phosphorus in making new bones, so bones fracture more easily and take longer to heal. Height decreases with age owing to the thinning of the vertebral disks and the general shortening of the vertebral column. Joint rigidity increases because of chronic conditions such as arthritis. This reduces the general range-of-motion ability. The legs become more resistant to passive range of motion. Tendons shrink and muscles atrophy, which further limit movement. Aging joints may deteriorate with non-inflammatory or inflammatory conditions. They may fuse or enlarge, leading to the bony joints common in the elderly.

The most common musculoskeletal procedures are for degenerative joint disease, specifically total joint replacement. These procedures often increase the quality of life for the elderly patient. Other procedures frequently performed are those for repairs of fractures and dislocations and amputations. Postprocedure complications include hemorrhage, emboli or thrombus formation, nonunion, non-healing, and infection.

Gastrointestinal System

While older adult patients have many health-related gastrointestinal complaints, these complaints are usually not life threatening. Oral and dental changes can affect the older patient's well-being, comfort, nutrition, and digestion. Teeth are lost due to periodontal disease or damage to the bone and tissue surrounding the teeth. Taste buds decline in number. Older patients also have a decreased sense of smell. These changes can make eating less pleasurable and reduce the person's appetite, leading to nutritional deficiencies. Salivary secretion decreases, causing dry mouth. Due to the dental changes and decreased saliva, food may not be chewed or lubricated sufficiently, causing problems with swallowing. Older adults may have other pathophysiological problems such as a stroke that can cause dysphagia (difficulty swallowing). The older adult can develop a decrease in esophageal peristalsis, as well as an inadequacy of the esophageal sphincter. Gastric motility and volume decrease, causing delayed gastric emptying. Delayed gastric emptying is best managed with frequent, small meals. There are also decreases in intestinal absorption, motility, and blood flow, which impairs the absorption of nutrients (McCance & Huether, 2002). Medical conditions such as diverticulosis and cholelithiasis occur more frequently in the elderly. Constipation in the older adult is most often caused by lifestyle changes such as current diet, lack of activity, and lack of fluid intake, rather than physiologic changes. During the nursing assessment, it is important to assess the patient for the symptoms of malnutrition (see **Table 38.3**). The patient should have a nutritional assessment as far in advance of the proposed procedure as possible. A good nutritional status increases the chances of an uneventful recovery and decreases potential complications. Older adults may have deficiencies in vitamins and minerals, which can delay wound healing. Anemia causes hypoxic conditions and poor

Table 38.3	Symptoms of Malnutrition
Body Area	**Signs Associated with Malnutrition**
General physical	☐ Fatigue
	☐ Dizziness
	☐ Weight loss
	☐ Decreased immune response
	☐ Irregular cravings
Hair	☐ Hair loss
	☐ Stiff, wiry hair that looks unkempt.
	☐ Light color then normal (pigmentation loss)
	☐ Hair can be pulled out with a gentle tug versus a hard pull
Skin	☐ Dull, yellow complexion
	☐ Skin color loss, including color under fingernails
	☐ Xerosis (dry, crinkled skin) looks worse visibly by moving one piece of skin parallel to the skin next to it
	☐ Tightness from excess fluids just under the skin caused by edema
Eyes	☐ Unusually bright or dull eyes
	☐ Inflamed or swollen eye lids
	☐ Softening of the cornea
	☐ Thickening of the inner surfaces of the eye lids and/or the outer layer of the eye causing a dull, lusterless or roughened surface of the eye
	☐ The blueness of the whites of the eyes may disappear

Face	☐ Wrinkles radiating out from the mouth become more pronounced when the mouth is held half open; as malnutrition increases, these lines can turn into scars
	☐ Lips can be reddened with sores
	☐ Deep cracks may be present in the corners of the mouth
	☐ The small area between the top of the upper lip and the nose can have a definite greasy, yellow scaling
Glands	☐ Swollen thyroid gland
	☐ Swollen parotid glands, enlarged as with mumps
Oral cavity	☐ Taste buds, normally covering the top of a normal tongue, can disappear
	☐ The sides and top of the mouth can appear more red in color
	☐ Sores inside the mouth
	☐ White patches of fungus growing on the tongue
	☐ Pain associated with eating because of the sores in the mouth
Teeth	☐ Decay; general corroded appearance
	☐ Paper white areas on the enamel of the tooth ranging from a few specks to the entire tooth
	☐ Brown stain, accompanied by various degrees of pitting because of decay
	☐ Gums can be red and swollen which would include all the gums, not just a spot or two between teeth
	☐ Puss oozing out of the gums from the bone below the gum line
	☐ The bones that hold the teeth in place can break down; this bone can become thin, fragile, and easily broken; as a result the teeth can easily come out
Muscles	☐ Muscle wasting
	☐ Undue degree of the folding skin on the buttocks
	☐ Jelly like feel of the remaining muscles
	☐ Lack of muscle tone; in progressed cases, the skeletal look of the body
Psychological	☐ Unresponsiveness or disinterest
	☐ Listlessness
	☐ Tiredness
	☐ Apathy
	☐ Dull spirit
	☐ Possible irritability
	☐ Poor memory

Adapted from: Malnutrition—what to look for. (2008). Retrieved July 31, 2008 from http://huntingtondisease.tripod.com/swallowing/id62.html.

tissue perfusion. Intravenous administration of electrolytes, particularly potassium, may be needed to hydrate the elderly patient before the procedure.

Some of the more common procedures of the gastrointestinal tract are colon resection for cancer or obstruction, ostomy creation, and cholecystectomy (Meiner & Lueckenotte, 2006). If enemas are ordered before the procedure, there may be incomplete emptying owing to the sluggish peristalsis of the bowel and atrophy of abdominal muscle walls. This could result in contamination of the sterile field by involuntary expulsion of feces or by leakage of feces into the abdominal cavity after the operative incision. Elderly patients are slow healers, especially after abdominal procedures, even if fecal contamination has not occurred. The risk of wound infection may be higher than in younger elderly patients because of operative contamination, poor tissue perfusion, malnutrition, or chronic diseases.

Genitourinary Tract

GFR
Glomerular Filtration Rate

BPH
Benign Prostatic Hypertrophy

Normal aging affects the genitourinary tract and renal system. Kidneys decrease in size as a person ages. In addition, blood flow and glomerular filtration rate (GFR) decreases. While the etiology of these changes remains uncertain, most likely they happen because of the aging process, or they are associated with a disease, or occur secondary to the administration of medications (Meiner & Lueckenotte, 2006). In males, glandular tissue continues to develop, which may lead to benign prostatic hypertrophy (BPH) or hyperplasia of the prostate gland. After the age of 50, the incidence of BPH increases. The urinary bladder walls become thickened, may lose muscle tone and function, and have a diminished capacity. Loss of sphincter control may also occur in elderly patients, especially women. When this happens, the accumulation of residual urine can lead to distention of the ureters, which may affect renal functioning by causing atrophy and insufficiency.

The older person is more prone to bladder and kidney infections during the operative and invasive procedure period. Aging kidneys lose some ability to filter and clear substances from the blood; tubular reabsorption increases, which may affect the patient's hydration status. The loss of renal function greatly affects the ability of older patients undergoing operative or invasive procedures to filter and clear medications and anesthetic agents from their systems. For the aging patient, protein in the urine increases, blood urea nitrogen levels rise, and the potential for electrolyte imbalance is greater.

Common genitourinary procedures are transurethral resections of the prostate, cystoscopy, and operative procedures for neoplasms throughout the genitourinary system. Postprocedure complications in the elderly include urinary tract infections, urinary retention or incontinence, hemorrhage, electrolyte imbalances, and renal failure.

Skin

The most noticeable changes of aging occur in the skin. The changes are due to both genetic (intrinsic) factors and environmental (extrinsic) factors, especially ultraviolet rays from sun exposure. The skin becomes thinner and drier. Decreased elasticity leads to wrinkles, prominence of small blood vessels, and changes in the pigmentation. The face and hands, being the most exposed skin areas, age faster than skin areas with less exposure. As the largest organ of the body, the skin serves as a barrier by preventing fluid loss and the intrusion of substances from the environment. Epidermal cells, which are flat, large, and irregular in size, reproduce slower than in young skin. For this reason, older skin appears translucent, paper-thin, smooth, and shiny. Dermis, the middle skin layer, consists of the sweat glands, blood vessels, and nerve endings, the number of which decreases with aging. These changes lead to diminished thermoregulation, decreased tactile sensation, and reduced pain perception. There is also a decrease in subcutaneous tissue and a redistribution of fat to the abdomen and thighs. Due to the decrease in subcutaneous tissue, the elderly patient's risk of developing hypothermia and physical injuries such as skin shearing, skin tears, and blunt trauma increases. For example, dragging a patient instead of lifting the patient can result in a skin burn. Aging skin is also more prone to chemical, electrical, and tape injuries because of the decreased cell reproduction and increased sensitivity. Age-related changes in the skin and vascular system, along with alterations in nutrition, elimination, and mobility, can lead to skin breakdown (Meiner & Lueckenotte, 2006).

Common operative procedures include excision of skin cancers and skin grafts and free tissue transplants for pressure sores. Healing may be delayed in the elderly, and they are more likely to have postprocedure infections.

Immune System

Age-related changes occur in virtually every body system. These changes affect an individual's ability to resist infection. Patients with underlying chronic diseases or comorbidities have a higher risk for infections. Physicians frequently prescribe multiple medications to control chronic diseases; however, these medications, such as antibiotics, anti-inflammatory agents, and steroids themselves, can impair a person's ability to resist infection.

The immune system protects the body in two ways. The first type of immunity is humoral or circulating immunity, which is initiated by immunoglobulins that are produced when exposed to antigens. Throughout the life span, a person is continually exposed to all kinds of substances and microorganisms, which are called antigens. Immunity develops as the body produces antibodies to fight against the antigens of a specific substance or microorganism. This can result from prophylactic vaccinations or from unplanned, repeated exposure to the antigen. Aging reduces a person's ability to respond to new antigens and causes increases in serum immunoglobulin concentrations In addition, immunoglobulin G (IgG) decreases with age, which leads to a higher mortality rate. IgG cells migrate from bone marrow and are part of the humoral immune system. These cells help the patient resist disease and are responsible for remembering the antigens of most bacteria, viruses, and fungi. Other immunoglobulins are IgA, IgM, IgK, and IgD. The presence of IgM is indicative of a current infection (Berman, Snyder, Kozier, & Erb, 2008).

The second type of immunity is cell-mediated or active immunity. The most well known is the T cell, which is mediated by the thymus. When exposed to an antigen, the lymphoid tissue releases activated T cells into the lymph system. The T cell is also vital in the body's resistance to infection (Berman, Snyder, Kozier, & Erb, 2008). Alteration in the cellular immune response in the aged is related to the development of neoplastic diseases, autoimmune responses, and degenerative diseases, as well as increased susceptibility to infection. Changes in the membrane of the T cell may cause functional changes in the lymphocyte response to antigens. The membrane viscosity in T cells seems to be related to the ratio of cholesterol to phospholipids in serum.

Because of these alterations in the aging immune system, the body's ability to protect itself against invasion by both endogenous (normally present within the body) and exogenous (outside the body) microorganisms decreases. The most common place for invasion of microorganisms in the healthcare facility is in the operative and/ or invasive procedure suite. The combined factors of decreased immunity, increased stress, and invasive procedures threaten the older adult with infections, which hinder recovery. Strict and conscientious adherence to the principles of aseptic technique and the monitoring and controlling of the environment are essential.

Central Nervous System

As with all the other systems in the body, aging affects the central nervous system. The changes that occur vary from person to person depending on their lifestyle, nutritional intake, genetic makeup, and tissue perfusion. Aging, however, causes some definitive changes throughout the central nervous system, some not apparent. Assess for changes to get a clear picture of the patient's mental status before the operative or invasive procedure. Baseline findings are vital to care of the elderly, so that postprocedure confusion and delirium are not attributed to senility when they are due to the anesthesia and physiological insult of the procedure (see **Table 38.4**).

Table 38.4	Common Causes of Postprocedure Confusion in Elderly Patients
Common physical causes	☐ Cerebrovascular disease
	☐ Drugs, delirium tremens
	☐ Chest infection or atelectasis
	☐ Renal infection
	☐ Abdominal sepsis (superficial or deep)
	☐ Over-full bladder or rectum
Less common physical causes	☐ Anemia (especially Vitamin B12 deficiency)
	☐ Unrecognized blood loss, other forms of anoxia
	☐ Hypothyroidism
	☐ Hepatic or renal failure
	☐ Subdural hematoma
Psychological factors	☐ Sensory distortion by bombardment or deprivation
	☐ Sleep disturbance and loss
	☐ Depression, anxiety, schizophrenia
Aggravation due to noxious stimuli	☐ Fear
	☐ Discomfort, pain
	☐ Thirst, hunger
Rare causes	☐ Hypoglycemia
	☐ Fat embolism
	☐ Hypernatremia

Adapted from: Patkin, M. (2007). Postoperative confusion: a guide to management. Retrieved August 4, 2008 from http://www.mpatkin.org/surgery_clinical/post_op_confusion.htm.

Physiologically, both the brain and the autonomic nervous system have normal deterioration with age. The aging brain loses cells, which may lead to slight shrinkage of the brain and a slight decrease in extracellular space. Degenerative changes may also occur in the autonomic nervous system. The sympathetic and parasympathetic systems become impaired owing to ganglia degeneration, and the autonomic reflex response slows. However, deep tendon reflexes remain unchanged in the healthy aging person. These changes decrease the fine motor movement ability and may affect gross motor movements. Therefore, the patient may perform psychomotor skills slowly. For example, if an ambulatory patient must learn to perform wound dressing changes before discharge from the facility, allow extra time for return demonstration. The patient may understand the concepts clearly, but may have a problem actually doing the task.

Further changes in the central nervous system may be seen in the balance of an older patient. Balance is affected because of loss of control of random movements, which originate in the brain stem and cerebellum. Vertigo or dizziness can be present because of the cerebrovascular changes. Ambulation may be further affected by a less efficient kinesthetic sense, with the older person walking with a Parkinsonian-like gait. Knowledge of these changes is particularly important for nurses working in ambulatory facilities. After the operative or invasive procedure, the normal age-related changes affecting balance and motion, combined with anesthesia and other drugs, make the patient at high risk for falls. When the patient walks, take extra care to support and protect him or her.

Other important changes are those occurring in the thermoregulatory center of the hypothalamus and in skin receptors. Postsympathetic nerve endings become less sensitive, so tolerance to heat decreases, and increases to cold. Simultaneously, the threshold for peripheral vasodilation and sweating increases. As noted, the patient can lose body heat rapidly because subcutaneous fat decreases with age. Therefore, protect older patients from hypothermia, even if they state they are not cold.

Other Sensory Changes

Vision

Aging related vision changes include both structural and functional changes. Structurally, the eyelids droop due to the loss of elasticity and skin atrophy; the drooping can interfere with vision, if it is significant. The orbicular muscle strength of the eyes decreases, which can result in ectropion or entropion. With ectropion, the lower lid rolls outward exposing the conjunctiva and can cause the eyelid not to close properly and can lead to corneal dryness and/or excessive tearing. With entropion, the lower lid turns inward, which can cause the eyelashes to scratch and irritate the cornea. The conjunctiva contains goblet cells that provide mucin that lubrication to the eye. With aging, the goblet cells produce less mucin resulting in irritation and dry eye syndrome (Ebersole, Hess, Touhy, & Jett, 2005).

Functionally, the size of the pupil decreases, affecting visual acuity, accommodation, and sensitivity to light and color. These changes are called presbyopia, or old age vision. Lenses of the eye thicken, become yellow, cloudy, and less elastic. Less light is able to pass through the thickened lens. Change in elasticity also narrows the visual field and decreases the depth perception. Night vision is decreased due to the yellowing of the lens and the changes in the size and thickening of the cornea. Fluid in the eye becomes cloudy, which reduces the amount of light

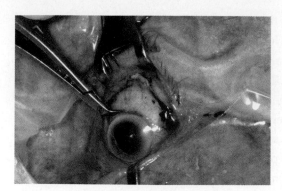

Figure 38.3
Cataract Extraction.

entering the eye. Lenses becomes yellow and transmit less violet light, which change the elderly patient's ability to distinguish colors, especially blues, greens, and violets (Meiner & Lueckenotte, 2006). For example, telling patients to take the "blue pill twice a day and the green pill at bedtime" may cause incorrect self-medication.

Disease may also affect lenses, resulting in the development of opacities, or cataracts (see **Fig. 38.3**). This is so common that cataract extraction is the most frequently performed eye surgery for the elderly. Patients admitted to healthcare facilities for procedures other than eye surgery are usually aware of their decreased vision. They may have special glasses that they feel strongly about leaving on as long as possible. Allow the patient to wear his or her glasses and make sure that they are safely secured for return to the patient after the procedure. The majority of eye procedures for the elderly are performed in ambulatory surgery centers. Several measures can be taken in these environments to promote a more comfortable atmosphere. Yellow, orange, or red colors are easier on aging eyes. Incandescent lighting, rather than fluorescent, also makes a room more comfortable for the elderly patient. Glare is irritating to older adults. For example, bright sunlight or examining lights that shine on bright floors or surfaces can be distracting. When doing admission procedures or taking histories, bright lights can be positioned behind patients rather than facing them. Window glare can be minimized with carpeting and curtains or blinds. Because eye adaptation to light takes longer with age, patients should not go from a dark to a light room, or vice versa. All rooms, such as changing rooms and bathrooms, should be illuminated the same way. Large type should be used for consent forms and other written material. Dark print facilitates reading and comprehension. Using a teaching combination of visual and audio formats and demonstrations is also helpful. By reducing the stress the elderly patient experiences because of his or her eye changes and inability to see clearly, the nurse can help make the operative or invasive procedure experience less traumatic.

Hearing

Hearing changes in both structure and function. The ear is divided into the external, middle, and inner ear. The external and middle ear are involved in hearing only. The inner ear is involved in hearing and balance. Structurally, the external ear becomes larger. The external ear loses flexibility and becomes longer and wider because of a decrease in elasticity. The auditory canal narrows, causing inward collapsing. The

ceruminal glands decrease in function, leading to thicker and dryer earwax in the canal. The wax is more difficult to remove and can be the cause of hearing impairment. In the middle ear, the eardrum thickens and appears dull, retracted, and gray. Calcifications develop between the three ear bones (malleus, incus, and stapes). The changes in the eardrum and the bone structure decrease or distort sound waves passing through the eardrum and reduce the vibrations of the bones that transmit sound (Ebersole, Hess, Touhy, & Jett, 2005). The inner ear includes both the organ of hearing, the cochlea, and the organ that is attuned to the effects of gravity and motion, the labyrinth. The balance portion of the inner ear consists of three semicircular canals and the vestibule. When normal sound vibrations change in the external and middle ear, conductive hearing loss may occur. Sensorineural hearing loss occurs when there is damage to the auditory nerve (cranial nerve VIII) in the inner ear. The third type is a mixed hearing loss, which occurs to both the conductive and sensorineural functions. There is a strong relationship between age and hearing loss in American adults; the percentages of reported hearing impairment are (NIDCD, 2008):

- 18% in adults 45–64 years of age;
- 30% in adults 65–74 years of age; and
- 47% in adults 75 years of age or older.

High-frequency hearing loss, called presbycusis, is the most common type of hearing loss and interferes with understanding speech, especially sounds such as f, g, s, sh, t, and ch (McCance & Huether, 2002). People with progressive hearing loss have difficulty screening out background noises, which interferes with hearing. Loud background sounds may drown out the quiet speech of the nurse. Elderly patients may experience difficulty interpreting and understanding fast speech. These hearing changes may adversely affect the patient's perception of the operative or invasive procedure experience. For example, if a patient is having a cataract removed under local anesthesia and there is background noise, he or she may not be able to hear instructions and may become frightened. Mechanical, sensory, and neural changes in hearing may cause fear, insecurity, or bewilderment in the elderly patient. Shouting may help an elderly patient with conductive hearing loss, but it does not help if there is neural damage. For patients with neural loss, sit near enough so that they can read lips (if they can see them). Clear enunciations, lack of mumbling, and not dropping the voice level at the end of sentences help the patient hear and understand teaching.

Touch

The sense of touch may diminish in the elderly. Diminished sensory receptors in the skin may prevent the patient from reacting to harmful stimuli, such as heat, cold, pressure, pain, and body position. This may be further affected by the decrease of circulation to the sensory receptors. Consider the safety needs of these patients and implement measures to prevent burns, pressure sores, or other skin problems due to lack of a pulling-away reaction by the patient. Patients may need to check bath water with a thermometer to prevent burns and change positions frequently to prevent pressure ulcers.

Elderly patients may have problems picking up and manipulating small articles because of the diminished sense of touch in the fingertips. They may appear clumsy when doing skills such as drawing up and self-administering insulin. Consider the patients' frustrations and creatively help them learn alternative ways to do necessary self-care skills before discharge.

Although the elderly may have lost some touch sensations, they have not lost the need for touch. Consider these psychological needs and offer to hold the patient's hand during induction of anesthesia or other stressful times during the operative or invasive procedure intervention

Taste and Smell

Taste buds are scattered throughout the mouth on the tongue, cheek, soft palate, and other parts of the mouth. A small decrease in the number of taste buds occurs around the age of 60 years. The ability to detect sweet taste seems to remain intact whereas the ability to detect sour, salty, and bitter tastes declines. Denture wearers lose some of their satisfaction in food, possibly because dentures cover the palate.

The sense of smell decreases with age and has a significant influence on food enjoyment, perhaps more significant than the decrease in taste buds. The ability to detect and identify odors begins to decrease around 30 years of age. Possible reasons for decrease in the sense of smell include nasal sinus disease, repeated viral infections, age-related changes of the central nervous system, smoking, medications, and dental changes (Ebersole, Hess, Touhy, & Jett, 2005).

Changes in taste and smell affect an elderly patient's interest in food. Elderly adults are less likely to detect the bad taste or smell of spoiled food. Reduced ability to smell also may make elderly patients unable to detect smoke, gas leaks, or other odors.

Cognitive Abilities
Memory

When older adults have a procedure done on an inpatient or outpatient basis, healthcare providers must ensure that they are as autonomous and independent as possible upon discharge, which makes teaching a priority. A working knowledge about how older adults learn will increase teaching effectiveness. In the past, learning theorists believed that the ability of older adults to learn declines after the age of 40 years and was significantly affected by age 60 years. Many healthcare workers also mistakenly view older adults as senile and incapable of learning, instead of understanding the physiological effects on cognitive ability of anesthesia, drugs, and the stress of the procedure. Furthermore, extenuating factors such as past abilities, education, disease processes, and lifestyle have been identified as affecting intelligence and learning. If older adults have retained their intelligence, they can learn, no matter what their age.

As discussed earlier, in normal aging, physiological changes in the central nervous system may affect the ability to learn. The human brain is remarkable, with a tremendous ability to learn, store, and retrieve information; this is called memory. The central nervous system regulates and performs memory tasks. Even though some older adults show a decrease in memory retrieval and reaction time, the majority of functioning remains intact and sufficient. Patients compensate for the minor

memory loss by pulling from previous learned experiences and life experiences (Ebersole, Hess, Touhy, & Jett, 2005).

The brain, as the body's largest consumer of oxygen, uses about 20% of the body's oxygen. Especially sensitive to hypoxia, after about 1 minute without oxygen, brain cells start to die. After 4 to 6 minutes, irreparable brain damage and death will occur (Memory Loss & The Brain, 2008).

In examining age-related intellectual changes in the older adult, memory has been a major focus of gerontological research. The research has divided memory into three stages (Berman, Snyder, Kozier, & Erb, 2008):

- *Sensory memory*, the fleeting perceptions of the visual, auditory, olfactory, and tactile senses are information received by the senses for an extremely brief moment;
- *Short memory*, information held in the brain for immediate use; also called recent memory; and
- *Secondary memory*, long-term memory includes all that is known such as memories of childhood friends, teachers, and events (older adults can remember things from high school, but not what they had for dinner the night before).

This research supports the opinion that older adults can learn. However, they may need to have smaller amounts of information given to them frequently before it is retained. In addition, because of retrieval problems, the patient is given written discharge instructions to take home.

Decision-Making

The decision to have an operative or invasive procedure is just one of many that older patients may have to make when they are admitted to a healthcare facility. Too often, healthcare workers, caregivers, and family members exclude the frail older adult from decisions being made about his/her own life. When an older adult is included in the discussions and decision-making process, there is greater assurance that he/she will accept and adapt to a change. Usually, older adults adjust poorly when forced into a new situation such as an operative procedure or nursing home. The healthcare team must communicate closely with both the patient and the family to make the best healthcare decisions possible. Patients with Alzheimer's disease or other forms of dementia will need the family members to take greater control in making and carrying out healthcare decisions. As discussed earlier, informed consent is the most important decision the elderly patient must make.

Learning and Teaching Implications

In the past, the educational level of older adults was lower than the educational level of younger adults, but it has been steadily increasing. Between 1970 and 2006, the percentage of older adults completing high school rose from 28% to 77.5%. About 19.5% had a bachelor's degree or more. However, the percentage of older adults who had completed high school varied considerably by race and ethnic origin (AOA, 2007). Lower levels of education can impair an older person's ability to live a healthy lifestyle, access service and benefit programs, recognize health problems and seek appropriate care, and follow recommendations for care. These factors also affect the nurse-client relationship when it comes to preprocedure and postprocedure teaching. More adults are seeking educational opportunities in later life, which promotes intellectual growth, increases self-esteem, enhances socialization, and helps the individual stay alert and involved. Erikson's seventh-stage development, Middle Adulthood (40–65 years of age) is the conflict between generativity versus stagnation. In this stage the person has a sense of achievement and productivity in career, family, and civic interests (Winters, 2008). Education provides an opportunity to avoid stagnation and isolation, keeps the brain active, and adds to the enjoyment of later life.

Adults usually function in crystallized intelligence, which is defined as knowledge, skills, and experiences accumulated over a lifetime. This type of intelligence tends to increase with age (Van Wagner, 2008). What this means is a person's life experiences enhance his or her education and ability to learn. Learning cannot proceed if the elderly patient has certain unmet needs. These needs must be considered a priority when planning education for older adults, particularly when teaching patients before or after the operative or invasive procedure. When dealing with elderly patients, consider the alignment of two need concepts: emotional reaction to having an operative or invasive procedure and Maslow's hierarchy of needs. If adults have strong anxieties, fears, or worries, memory deficits become more pronounced and it is harder for them to comprehend and retrieve information that may be vital to their welfare. After meeting the needs that may cause barriers to learning, the older adult should be emotionally capable of learning. Deal with patient pain before beginning a teaching session. If the patient is in pain he or she will have difficulty learning. External memory aids include lists, notes, and calendars, reminders from other people, and articles or items that trigger memory. Visual aids are extremely important because of the elderly patient's hearing degeneration, which adversely affects communication and understanding.

There are also strategies to counteract the physiological sensory changes that hinder communication and, therefore, decrease learning capacity. When teaching, do so in quiet surroundings; environmental distractions and background noise greatly interfere with hearing. **Table 38.5** lists one-on-one teaching strategies for elderly patients.

Many theorists consider human development as occurring throughout the entire life span. Following is a brief summary of the most well known theories, and their significance to aging. For further study, the reader is referred to psychological and development textbooks.

One of the most well known developmental theories applicable to nursing is that of Erikson, who presented a psychosocial theory of development across the age span. He believed that people go through eight stages of development during a normal life span. If the individual resolves the psychological conflicts encountered in each stage, he or she successfully progresses to the next stage. Successful mastery of each phase prepares an individual for continued development. Furthermore, a person has the ability to rework a previous psychosocial stage into a more successful outcome. According to Erikson, anticipating and accepting one's death is the final stage. Elderly adults are concerned with Stages 7 and 8. Stage 7 is *Generativity* versus *Self-Absorption* or *Stagnation* and Stage 8 is *Ego Integrity* versus *Despair*. Stage 7 occurs in

Table 38.5	**Teaching Strategies for Elderly Patients**

- ☐ Sit facing the learner so that he or she can observe lip movements and facial expressions
- ☐ Speak slowly
- ☐ Keep voice pitch low (low sounds are easier to hear than high sounds)
- ☐ Present one idea at a time; give one topic at a time
- ☐ Emphasize concrete rather than abstract ideas
- ☐ Compare new information with the person's past experiences
- ☐ Allow for a longer time for the patient to think and react
- ☐ Keep session short, because of physical fatigue
- ☐ Use audio, visual, and tactile teaching aids
- ☐ Ask for frequent feedback to move information to secondary storage
- ☐ Ask patients to set their own goals and learning needs when possible
- ☐ Remember that older adults learn what is important to them and what positively affects their lives
- ☐ Preprocedure, older adults prefer sensory information: what they will see, hear, feel, and smell

the middle adult, between 40 to 65 years of age. Middle-age adults want to establish and guide the next generation, and seeks satisfaction through productivity in career, family, and civic interests. Self-absorbed middle-age adults can become preoccupied with self. If previous conflicts are not dealt with, stagnation can occur. Stage 8 occurs in older adults or mature adults, between 65 years of age and death. Older/mature adults reflect on life accomplishments, deal with loss, and accept death with dignity, and as an unavoidable reality (Winters, 2008).

These concepts have profound implications for the nurse, because the elderly patient encounters multiple compromising situations during this period, which have the potential for robbing him or her of dignity. Ways to protect the elderly patient's dignity include calling patients by their formal name (ie, Mrs., rather than Grandma or her first name), being careful not to invade their body space without asking permission (eg, "May I listen to your stomach with this stethoscope?"), and not overly exposing the patient during preparation or transfer.

In 1953, another developmental theorist, Robert Havighurst, identified six major age periods, with the last one being later maturity which occurs in the person 60 years of age and older. He defined the aging person's necessary activities as adjusting to decreasing physical strength and health; adjusting to retirement and reduced income; adjusting to death of spouse; establishing an explicit affiliation with one's own age group; adopting and adapting social roles in a flexible way; and establishing satisfactory physical living arrangements (Wikipedia, 2008a). A period of crisis occurs at retirement. The aging person must adapt successfully to his or her new role by developing new patterns of leisure to replace what was previously society-valued work.

Usually, the nurse does not have sufficient time to assist the patient in adjusting to a particular stage of life. However, by being aware of the various life stages, the nurse may help by arranging contact of the patient with the appropriate resources to facilitate health and wellness across the developmental continuum. Some of these resources may be the family, the clinical nurse specialist, a pastoral service, a social service, and home healthcare services.

Needs Theory

Maslow defined a hierarchy of human needs as follows: physiological, safety, love/belonging, esteem, and self-actualization (Wikipedia, 2008b). During an operative or invasive procedure, the basic physiological needs of oxygen and hydration are a priority. Only after those needs are met can the other needs be addressed. Because the needs are hierarchical in Maslow's scheme, a lower need must always be met before a higher need is recognized by the person. Maslow's theory explains much about human motivation and learning. A need must be satisfied before anything else can happen. Age is not as important, according to Maslow, as the needs of an individual. However, the elderly patient may have different needs than the young because of normal physiological changes of aging.

When planning teaching for a patient related to operative and invasive procedure intervention, evaluate the needs of the patient and attend to the immediate needs first. However, obtaining information about the procedure may or may not be an overwhelming need of the elderly.

POTENTIAL ADVERSE OUTCOMES THE ELDERLY PATIENT MAY EXPERIENCE DURING THE OPERATIVE OR INVASIVE PROCEDURE PERIOD

Table 38.6 describes potential adverse outcomes that may affect the patient before, during, and after the operative or invasive procedure.

Risk for Infection

Normal, age-related changes in body systems lead to a decreased ability to protect against infection. In elderly patients, the number of organisms required to cause an infection is smaller and their response to infections is different from that of younger persons. Chronic illnesses, which are very common in older adults, can mask or mimic infections. Additionally, some medications can increase the risk of infections. Elderly patients have a decrease in specific antibody production, which causes a higher incidence and higher mortality rate from pneumonia, influenza, and infectious endocarditis.

In order to reduce the risk for infection, carefully prepare and decontaminate the skin and the operative site. Monitor the white blood cell count and differential count. Maintain optimal surgical consciousness. Use careful aseptic techniques in inserting invasive devices, especially indwelling catheters. Monitor team members' use of aseptic techniques. Document nursing care plans and their implementation. Confer with infection control personnel to obtain information about postprocedure infections.

Risk for Fluid Volume Deficit

Fluid volume deficit occurs in an elderly patient when there is a decrease in intravascular, interstitial, and/or intracellular fluid. This refers to dehydration, water loss, and electrolyte loss. Fluid volume deficit occurs due to (1) abnormal losses

Table 38.6	**Potential Adverse Outcomes the Elderly Patient May Experience During an Operative or Invasive Procedure**

Outcome 1 The patient is free from signs and symptoms of infection.

Diagnosis	Risk Factors	Outcome Indicators
Risk for Infection	☐ Immunosuppression, especially from chemotherapy	☐ Did the patient's wound heal without infection?
	☐ Presence of compromising chronic disease	☐ Did the patient experience a urinary tract infection?
	☐ Decline in respiratory system defenses	☐ Did the patient's respiratory status remain normal?
	☐ Decreased protective ability of the skin	☐ Did venous or arterial insertion sites remain free from infection?
	☐ Declining protective ability of the gastrointestinal system	☐ Was the patient afebrile following the procedure?
	☐ Aging alteration in the genitourinary system	☐ Is the leukocyte count three to 30 days following the procedure within expected range?
	☐ Operative or invasive procedure	
	☐ Anesthesia	☐ Is the incision well approximated and free from heat, redness, induration, swelling, or foul odor?
	☐ Invasive monitoring and replacement techniques	
	☐ Breaks in aseptic technique	

Outcome 2 The patient's fluid, electrolyte, and acid-base balances are consistent with or improved from baseline levels established before the operative or invasive procedure.

Diagnosis	Risk Factors	Outcome Indicators
Risk for Fluid Volume Deficit	☐ Decreased ability of the kidney to concentrate urine	☐ Did the patient experience a change in urine output?
	☐ Decreased renal functioning related to aging	☐ Does the patient have decreased venous filling?
	☐ Decreased oral fluid volume intake	☐ Does the patient have hemoconcentration?
	☐ Vomiting or diarrhea	☐ Does the patient have hypotension?
	☐ Decreased circulating blood volume	☐ Is there an increased pulse rate?
		☐ Did the patient experience an increased body temperature, pulse, and respirations?
		☐ Is the patient's urinary output greater that 30 mL/hr?
		☐ Is urinary specific gravity 1.010 to 1.030?
		☐ Are arterial blood gases, serum electrolytes, and hemodynamic monitoring values within expected ranges?

38

Outcome 3 **The patient is free from signs and symptoms of skin injury related to transfer/transport, positioning, or the use of chemicals and electrical devices.**

Diagnosis	Risk Factors	Outcome Indicators
Risk for Impaired Skin Integrity	☐ Thinning or decreased epidermis and adipose tissue	☐ Did the patient experience a disruption in skin surface?
	☐ Decreased peripheral vascular circulation	☐ Did the patient experience a destruction of skin layers?
	☐ Increased peripheral neuropathy	☐ Did the patient experience deep ulceration of body structures?
	☐ Improper transferring, moving, positioning, and padding	
	☐ Use of strong chemical antimicrobials	
	☐ Use of adhesive tape	

Outcome 4 **The patient is at or returning to normothermia at the conclusion of the immediate operative or invasive period.**

Diagnosis	Risk Factors	Outcome Indicators
Risk for Altered Body Temperature: Hypothermia	☐ Impaired thermoregulation	☐ Does the patient have a decrease in body temperature below normal range?
	☐ Diminished peripheral vascular circulation	
	☐ Administration of drugs and anesthesia	☐ Does the patient complain of being cold?
	☐ Procedure requirements (eg, renal or cardiac surgery)	☐ Does the patient's skin feel cold?
	☐ Exposure to a cold environment	☐ Does the patient show evidence of mental confusion?
	☐ Lack of adequate covering	☐ Does the patient have a decreased pulse and respiration rate?
	☐ Drug administration before the procedure	

Outcome 5 **The patient has wound/tissue perfusion consistent with or improved from baseline levels established before the operative or invasive procedure.**

Diagnosis	Risk Factors	Outcome Indicators
Risk for Altered Peripheral Tissue Perfusion	☐ Decreases in cardiac output and respiration at a cellular level	☐ Does the patient have strong peripheral pulses?
	☐ Disruption of microcirculation by mechanical pressure, positioning, and immobility	☐ Is the patient free from emboli and/or thrombus formation?

Outcome 6 **The patient demonstrates knowledge of nutritional management related to the operative or invasive procedure.**

Diagnosis	Defining Characteristics/ Related Factors	Outcome Indicators
Imbalanced Nutrition: less than body requirements	*Defining Characteristics* ☐ Emaciation	☐ Does the patient show evidence of impaired skin or tissue integrity after the procedure?

☐ Weight 10% to 20% or more below ideal body weight for height and frame

☐ Capillary fragility

☐ Inadequate food intake

☐ Pale conjunctiva/mucous membranes

☐ Tiredness

☐ Excessive hair loss

☐ Poor muscle tone

☐ Abdominal manifestation (hyperactive bowel, cramping, pain)

☐ Diarrhea or steatorrhea

Related Factors

☐ Gastrointestinal changes of aging

☐ Presence of chronic diseases

☐ Administration of drugs

☐ Use of alcohol

☐ Presence of mechanical problems

☐ Lack of ability to care for self

☐ Dysphagia or oral problems

☐ Deficient knowledge

☐ Does the patient's operative wound show signs of normal healing?

☐ Does the patient verbalize the ability to manage dietary requirements?

☐ Does the patient verbalize understanding of the importance of a balanced diet to facilitate wound healing?

☐ Does the family demonstrate willingness to obtain appropriate food and assist with meal preparation?

☐ Does the patient describe preferred foods/fluids consistent with dietary requirements that facilitate wound healing?

Outcome 7   The patient is free from injury to the musculoskeletal system.

Diagnosis	Defining Characteristics/ Related Factors	Outcome Indicators
Impaired Physical Mobility	*Defining Characteristics* ☐ Inability to move ☐ Limited range of motion ☐ Decreased muscle strength, control, or mass ☐ Impaired coordination *Related Factors* ☐ Aging musculoskeletal system ☐ Chronic disease conditions ☐ Falls ☐ Trauma to nonoperative joints ☐ Nerve damage from unrelieved pressure ☐ Presence of chronic diseases	☐ Did the patient experience an injury because of impaired physical mobility? ☐ Does the patient complain of musculoskeletal pain? ☐ After the procedure, is the patient able to demonstrate preprocedure range of motion?

Outcome 8 The patient participates in decisions affecting his or her plan of care for the operative or invasive procedure period.

Diagnosis	Defining Characteristics/ Related Factors	Outcome Indicators
Decisional Conflict	*Defining Characteristics*	☐ Did the patient verbalize understanding of treatment options?
	☐ Delayed decision-making	
	☐ Vacillation in decision-making	☐ Did the patient describe the sequence of the planned procedure?
	☐ Verbal expressions of distress or anxiety	
	☐ Physiological manifestations such as increased heart rate, respiration, blood pressure, and diaphoresis	☐ Did the patient ask questions based on information provided?
		☐ Did the patient participate in the plan of care?
	Related Factors	☐ Did the patient verbalize concerns about decisions?
	☐ Incomplete or confusing information regarding the operative or invasive procedure	☐ Did family members participate in the plan of care for the operative or invasive procedure period?
	☐ Informational overload	
	☐ Ineffective communication techniques	
	☐ Inadequate time to consider procedure implications	
	☐ Fear of procedure outcomes	

Outcome 9 The patient is free from adverse outcomes that may result from disturbed thought processes and experiences.

Diagnosis	Defining Characteristics/ Related Factors	Outcome Indicators
Disturbed Thought Processes	*Defining Characteristics*	☐ Did the patient experience an injury that can be attributed to disturbed thought processes?
	☐ Disorientation or confusion during the preprocedure period	
	☐ Failure to remember information about the procedure	☐ Did the patient experience an optimal postprocedure recovery?
	☐ Impaired attention span	
	☐ Inappropriate behavior	
	☐ Impaired perception	
	☐ Impaired judgment	
	☐ Impaired decision-making	
	☐ Egocentricity	
	Related Factors	
	☐ Sensory overload	
	☐ Disorders of memory	
	☐ Inappropriate response to commands or directions	
	☐ Inaccurate interpretation of the environment	

Outcome 10 The patient demonstrates knowledge about the operative or invasive procedure appropriate to cognitive capabilities.

Diagnosis	Defining Characteristics/ Related Factors	Outcome Indicators
Deficient Knowledge	*Defining Characteristics* ☐ Responses or questions indicate inadequate understanding, misinterpretation, and misconception of information concerning the operative or invasive period or the reason for the procedure ☐ Noncompliance with previous instructions or prescribed therapeutic regimen ☐ Inability to perform or inadequate performance of a critical self-care or rehabilitative skill ☐ Hysterical, hostile, agitated, or apathetic behaviors *Related Factors* ☐ Disturbed thought processes ☐ Uncompensated memory loss ☐ Impaired hearing, vision ☐ Inability to use teaching materials because of cultural/ language differences ☐ Fear, anxiety	☐ After receiving instruction, did the patient demonstrate that he or she understood necessary information concerning the operative or invasive procedure?

Outcome 11 An environment and informational system that the elderly patient undergoing an operative or invasive procedure can control is maintained.

Diagnosis	Defining Characteristics/ Related Factors	Outcome Indicator
Disturbed Sensory Perception	*Defining Characteristics* ☐ Inaccurate interpretation of environmental stimuli ☐ Change in amount or pattern of incoming stimuli (sensory overload) ☐ Irritability, anxiety, disorientation, sleeplessness ☐ Shows signs of decisional conflict ☐ Complaints of tiredness ☐ Complaints of muscle tension *Related Factors* ☐ Extensive information regarding the operative or invasive procedure ☐ Complexity of the operative or invasive procedure environment	☐ After intervention, did the patient exhibit any of the defining characteristics of disturbed sensory perception?

38

Outcome 12 The patient and the family copes with fear.

Diagnosis

Fear: death, mutilation, loss of body part or function, loss of independence

Defining Characteristics/ Related Factors

Defining Characteristics

- ☐ Describes the threat
- ☐ Feelings of dread, nervousness, or concern about the procedure
- ☐ Expects danger to self related to the procedure
- ☐ Restlessness, voice tremor, excessive talking
- ☐ Hand tremor and increased muscle tension
- ☐ Narrowed focus to fixed focus on the impending procedure
- ☐ Diaphoresis, increased heart and respiratory rates

Related Factors

- ☐ Deficient knowledge
- ☐ Perceived inability to control the operative or invasive procedure event
- ☐ Invasive procedures
- ☐ Anesthesia
- ☐ Surgery and its outcome

Outcome Indicators

- ☐ Was the patient able to recognize the presence of fear?
- ☐ Did the patient show evidence that he or she was handling fear in a constructive manner?

Outcome 13 The patient shows evidence of a decrease in preprocedure anxiety.

Diagnosis

Anxiety

Defining Characteristics/ Related Factors

Defining Characteristics

- ☐ Expresses apprehension, uncertainty, fear, distress, worry concerning the operative or invasive procedure or following the procedure
- ☐ Expresses helplessness concerning the impending procedure
- ☐ Overexcited, rattled, jittery behavior; restlessness
- ☐ Focus on self
- ☐ Insomnia
- ☐ Diaphoresis and increased heart rate, pulse, and respirations
- ☐ Increased tension
- ☐ Foot shuffling, hand and arm movements, trembling, hand tremor, shakiness
- ☐ Facial tension, poor eye contact, voice quivering

Outcome Indicators

- ☐ Did the patient recognize that he or she was experiencing anxiety?
- ☐ After intervention, did the physiological manifestation of anxiety continue?
- ☐ Did the patient show evidence that he or she was handling anxiety in a constructive manner?

Related Factors

☐ An impending procedure that may result in a potential, uncertain change in health, role status, or environment

Outcome 14 **The patient maintains realistic hope throughout the operative and invasive procedure period.**

Diagnosis	**Defining Characteristics/ Related Factors**	**Outcome Indicators**
Hopelessness	*Defining Characteristics*	☐ After intervention, did the patient continue to exhibits signs of hopelessness?
	☐ Passive behaviors	
	☐ Decreased talking, affect, response to stimuli, appetite	☐ Was the patient able to mobilize energy on his or her behalf?
	☐ Lack of initiative to actively participate during operative and invasive period or rehabilitation	
	☐ Exhibits behaviors that attempt to shut out others	
	☐ Increased sleep	
	Related Factors	
	☐ Nonelective or life-sustaining operative or invasive procedure	
	☐ Procedures that alter body image	
	☐ Differing opinion between the patient and the healthcare team as to the need for the procedure	
	☐ Family pressure for the procedure	
	☐ Deteriorating physiological or psychological condition	

Outcome 15 The patient effectively copes with the impending procedure.

Diagnosis	**Defining Characteristics/ Related Factors**	**Outcome Indicator**
Ineffective Coping	*Defining Characteristics*	☐ Did the patient demonstrate effective coping behavior?
	☐ Expresses inability to cope	
	☐ Does not ask for help, effectively solve problems, meet role expectation, meet basic needs	
	☐ Anxiety and fear	
	☐ Describes personal life stress	
	☐ Altered social interaction	
	☐ Destructive behavior toward self or others	
	☐ Complains of digestive, bowel, appetite disturbances	
	☐ Chronic fatigue or sleep pattern disturbance	
	☐ Attempts verbal manipulation	

38

Related Factors

☐ Patient cannot adapt to the basic
demands of the procedure

☐ Disfigurement caused by surgery

☐ Deficient knowledge

☐ Problem-solving skills deficit

Adapted from Carpentino-Moyet, L. J. (2008) *Handbook of Nursing Diagnosis* (12th ed.). Philadelphia: Lippincott Williams & Wilkins; Petersen C. (2007) *Perioperative Nursing Data Set, the Perioperative Nursing Vocabulary* (Revised 2nd ed.). Denver: AORN, Inc.

through the skin, gastrointestinal tract, or kidneys; (2) decreased intake of fluid; (3) bleeding; or (4) movement of fluid into a third space.

Monitor fluid volume replacement. Have a Foley catheter kit available. Before the procedure, assess skin turgor, edema, urine output, and oral or intravenous fluid intake. If there is significant bleeding, weigh sponges during the procedure to determine the need for fluid or blood replacement. As necessary, obtain IV fluids and blood products for replacement. Measure urine output during the procedure.

Risk for Impaired Skin Integrity

Changes in the skin begin at about 30 years of age and result in decreased protection and increased susceptibility to injury. Because of decreased cohesiveness, skin cells are replaced at a slower rate; thus, wound healing is delayed and the risk for infection is increased because the skin barrier remains broken for a longer period. Dermis and subcutaneous connective tissue become thinner, more fragile, and more prone to tear easily. Blood perfusion and the number of small blood vessels diminish. Circulation to the extremities is reduced, leading to a decrease in sensory perception.

Assess skin integrity before the procedure and document any rashes, sores, or skin disruptions. Prepare the procedure site gently and carefully. Remove hair only when necessary. When removing hair, do not shave. Apply the safety belt firmly, but avoid pressure; pad if necessary. Position the patient carefully, padding all pressure points and areas where circulation may be restricted. Use nontoxic chemicals when doing the skin preparation. Carefully decontaminate the skin to decrease postprocedure infections. Select a nonirritating, broad-spectrum antimicrobial agent for the skin preparation. If using a liquid agent, allow the skin to dry before draping. Take care not to perforate the skin with towel clamps. Have extra sterile pads available for padding if needed. Pad retraction sites with sponges or pads and maintain gentle retraction at the operative site. Wipe the procedure area with water after the procedure to remove irritating chemicals. Have paper tape or Montgomery straps available for dressing the operative incision. Use paper tape to prevent skin tape tears. Transfer the patient from the bed to the stretcher by lifting rather than dragging to prevent shearing skin tears. Use a lift sheet when possible. Evaluate all skin areas immediately after the procedure and document any changes from the preprocedure status.

Risk for Altered Body Temperature: Hypothermia

Regulation of body temperature changes throughout the life span due to changes in metabolism and within the circulatory and neurological systems. The older adult has a higher risk for alterations in core body temperature related to lower metabolic rate and a higher incidence of disease.

Assess the potential for hypothermia before the procedure. Determine the normal and present body temperature range. Assess skin color (pallor). Check the color of the hands and feet (bluish, cyanotic). Note the presence of systemic diseases, such as Raynaud disease, peripheral vascular disease, and diabetes mellitus.

Avoid unnecessary exposure of the patient to the external environment before or while preparing the skin. Cover the patient with a warm blanket or a hypothermia blanket during the procedure. If not contraindicated, use a convective warming device during the procedure to maintain the patient's temperature. Cover the patient's head with a cap or towel during the procedure. Observe vital sign monitors for evidence of hypothermic complications. If the patient's body temperature drops to 35°C (95°F) or lower, watch for shivering, ventricular fibrillation, and decreased bleeding due to vasoconstriction. Monitor for signs of hypothermia more closely if an operative procedure calls for cooling with drugs, solutions, or slush. Monitor the patient's temperature throughout the procedure. Report hypothermia potential and nursing actions implemented during the procedure to the postanesthesia care unit nurses. If hypothermia results from the operative or invasive procedure, communicate with the postanesthesia care unit nurses before the end of the procedure. This will enable postanesthesia nurses to prepare for effective warming procedures immediately after the procedure. Document and evaluate all interventions.

Risk for Altered Peripheral Tissue Perfusion

Circulating blood delivers oxygen and nutrients to tissues and removes metabolic waste products. Elderly patients may experience altered tissue perfusion secondary changes that occur in the cardiovascular system during aging.

Assess the patient's cardiac status by taking vital signs, reviewing the electrocardiogram, prothrombin time and partial thromboplastin time, and other studies as ordered. Determine if the patient has a history of clotting problems or emboli formation. Take the patient's smoking history. Assess for a history of recurrent leg ulcers. Assess the presence of chronic diseases such as diabetes mellitus, chronic obstructive pulmonary disease, malnutrition, and circulatory diseases. Before the procedure, teach the patient to flex and extend the knees and hips and to dorsiflex and extend the ankles. Have the patient demonstrate and practice these exercises. Tell the patient that he or she needs to do these exercises immediately after the procedure. If necessary, assist the patient in doing the exercises.

Position the patient carefully, ensuring that the ankles are not crossed. Avoid pressure on the feet. Before draping, check the patient for correct anatomical position, padding of pressure points, and correct alignment of joints. Apply antiembolism devices or stockings before draping the patient.

Imbalanced Nutrition: Less than Body Requirements

Obtain the patient's weight and height. Note any recent change. Assess the patient's nutrition status before the procedure. Inspect the skin for signs of nutritional deficiencies. Note signs of vitamin deficiencies: eczema; dry, rough skin; sheet hemorrhages on thighs and calves; cracking of the lips; and inflammation of the gums. Note signs of protein, zinc, or vitamin deficiencies: chronic, nonhealing skin ulcers and edema of the hands and feet. Monitor laboratory values; hemoglobin and hematocrit values may be slightly decreased.

Use and enforce aseptic technique. Note that pressure sores may develop within two hours if there is a nutritional lack of serum protein and vitamins, along with other deficiencies. Pad bony prominences well. Prepare for complications during the procedure that may arise because of undernourishment, such as bleeding problems and arrhythmias.

Impaired Physical Mobility

Elders define their health status and physical fitness in terms of their mobility. The increase in functional dependence that accompanies impaired physical mobility and its consequences can often be avoided, corrected, or minimized by shrewd nursing diagnosis and management.

Assess the patient. Inspect joints for range of motion and pain. Test the patient's muscle strength and grip strength. Observe the patient's balance when the patient is sitting and standing. Determine the patient's transferability. Assess the patient's walking ability. Test the patient's ability to flex the spine if regional anesthesia is planned. Evaluate any neurovascular deficits, such as bradykinesia and diabetic neuropathies.

When positioning for a procedure, gently transfer the patient to the bed. Monitor the patient's shoulder range of motion and do not overextend. Avoid hyperextension of the patient's elbows, knees, and neck. Assist the patient to flex the spine for regional anesthesia. Allow time for stiff vertebrae and muscles to conform to their optimal level of stretch. If obvious osteoporosis is present, logroll the patient for lateral position. When positioning for lithotomy, flex and raise both the patient's knees at the same time. Exercise extreme caution to prevent fracture of the femoral head. Ensure that the patient's fingers, hands, toes, and feet are not cramped or resting against metal before applying sterile drapes. Monitor team members to avoid their leaning or resting on the patient during the procedure. Evaluate the patient's neuromuscular status after the procedure.

Decisional Conflict

Recognize and compensate for normal aging changes that may affect the communication of preprocedure information (eg, hearing, seeing, and memory deficits). Clarify and repeat the physician's explanations as needed for comprehension and understanding. Assess the patient's decision-making ability. Consider the cultural implications of making decisions. Include appropriate family members in the decision. The patient may not be the one who makes the final decision. Provide emotional and psychological support if the patient exhibits anxiety and fear. Respect and accept the patient's final decision. Allow adequate time to ensure that all forms for consent are correctly completed.

Assessing decisional conflict is ongoing. The patient has the right to make decisions that do not follow the recommendations of healthcare providers and to change his/her mind at any time. Even with dementia or cognitive impairments, consult the patient regarding treatment decisions. If the informed consent is obtained from someone other than the patient, obtain the patient's consent as well; this may just be verbal consent. To avoid conflict and the risk of potential harm to the patient, consent for all procedures should be obtained from the older patient before beginning any treatment or procedure.

Disturbed Thought Processes

Before the procedure, assess and monitor the physiological factors that may affect the patient's thought processes. Look for hypoxia, imbalance in glucose levels, altered metabolism that could affect the central nervous system, drug interactions or adverse reactions, and central nervous system abnormalities, such as tumors and infarcts.

Note if the patient misinterprets commands or directions during the procedure. Assess the patient's ability to think and reason. Determine the patient's orientation to time, place, and event. Assess the patient's cognitive abilities and short-term memory. Verbally list a series of items and have the patient repeat them back. Normally, the patient should remember three to seven items.

Complete teaching before the procedure on one aspect of care, and ask the patient to repeat it 15 minutes later. Assign one nurse to coordinate care and to communicate with the family. Supply written reminders that may help the patient remember after the procedure (eg, place a note on the wall to practice deep breathing every hour if the patient can read and see). During the procedure, provide frequent verbal reminders (eg, ask patients not to move and to keep their hands away from their faces). Use pictures to increase recognition memory.

Document the patient's preprocedure mental status. Adjust preprocedure and discharge teaching needs to accommodate patient and family needs. Communicate decreased cognitive ability to other members of the healthcare team.

Deficient Knowledge

Knowledge deficit occurs when patients experience a lack of information or a difficulty in applying information that leads to compromises in health care. Lack of knowledge can mean that the patient does not use primary, secondary, and tertiary healthcare prevention measures. Lack of knowledge can also contribute to uninformed decision-making or to anxiety in older adults who are unprepared for healthcare experiences. Nursing interventions for older adult knowledge deficit provide the knowledge that will contribute to increased self-care and self-management skills, compliance with the therapeutic regimen, improved decision-making and decreased anxiety and fear.

Assess the patient for sensory impairments (vision, hearing) and, if present, implement appropriate interventions. Be aware of the elderly person's potential inability to hear or understand directions given to him or her during the procedure. Pay particular attention to the patient's communication needs during administration of regional or local anesthesia. Allow the patient to use communication aids as long as possible. Secure glasses or hearing aids in a safe place or give to a family member during the procedure. Sit next to the patient and speak distinctly. Face the patient so that he or she can read lips. Use large, dark print for reading matter. Draw or use illustrations for clarification. Assess the patient's knowledge level and need to know. Older patients tend to want sensory information about events that will happen during the procedure (eg, what they will hear, see, and feel), rather than procedural information. Provide teaching before the procedure. Demonstrations and patient practice of turning, coughing, deep breathing, and ambulating are vital. Tell older patients about the postprocedure environment (eg, the intensive care unit) and the presence of tubes, drains, or machines. They often worry about pain. Reassure them that the nurse will monitor them and will administer pain medication when they need it. Provide discharge instructions. For ambulatory procedures, elderly patients especially need written discharge instructions. Tell the family or caregiver about the instructions.

Disturbed Sensory Perception

Disturbed sensory perception is a state in which the person experiences a change in the amount, pattern, or interpretation of incoming stimuli (Carpenito-Moyet, 2004). Sensory overload occurs when one or more of the five senses are over stimulated and the person is unable to focus on the task. The increased quantity or quality of internal stimuli, such as pain, dyspnea, or anxiety can cause sensory overload. An increase in the quantity or quality of external stimuli, such as numerous diagnostic studies, a noisy healthcare setting, and contact with several strangers can cause sensory overload. Patients with sensory overload may complain of fatigue or sleeplessness, be restless or irritable, complain of periodic disorientation and muscle tension, have scattered attention and racing thoughts, and reduced problem-solving ability and task performance.

Recognize sensory overload by the patient's verbal or nonverbal communications. Minimize the number of people from the operative or invasive procedure team who visit the patient before the procedure. Have one contact person coordinate the total experience. Give information only at a need to-know level. Teach only vital, life sustaining self-practices, such as taking medication and performing dressing changes after the procedure. Provide anticipatory sensory information about the procedure. Develop with the patient a mutually agreed-upon method for him/her to signal a need for help. Teach the family about the impact of sensory perceptual alterations, including recommendations for care.

Fear

Fear describes the experience of physiologic or emotional disruption related to an identifiable source that is perceived as dangerous (Carpenito-Moyet, 2004). Identify the source of the fear by direct observation and questioning, and by indirect measurement of changes in physiologic state. Objective characteristics of fear include increased heart rate, blood pressure and respiratory rate, pallor, pupil dilation, increased alertness, and fight/flight behaviors. Subjective characteristics of fear include increased tension, apprehensive, and impulsiveness.

For moderate to extreme fear, notify the anesthesia provider and physician before the procedure. Recognize that overwhelming, realistic fear may interfere with other nursing and medical goals. Establish a relationship before the procedure, so that the patient believes that he or she has an ally during the procedure. Allow the patient an opportunity to share fears before the procedure. Use active listening techniques. Offer to arrange contact with other healthcare team members if the patient desires, such as a chaplain, a social services worker, or a hospice nurse.

Anxiety

Anxiety describes the state in which the individual experiences feelings of uneasiness or apprehension and activation of the autonomic nervous system in response to a vague, nonspecific threat (Carpenito-Moyet, 2004). Although a normal human response, anxiety becomes a problem when it is prolonged and interferes with a patient's daily life.

Assess the patient's anxiety level before the procedure. Consider the physiological effects of the operative or invasive procedure on the elderly patient and anticipate needs during the procedure. Consider the effects of increased immunosuppression, decreased blood flow with decreased urine output, increased vasoconstriction, and increased respiratory and heart rates. Consult the physician or anesthesia provider for preprocedure anti-anxiety medication if needed. Strengthen the patient's support systems by including the family and significant others during preprocedure teaching. Assess the patient's past coping skills (how did he or she react to stress in the past?). Use a quiet, confident demeanor with the patient. Answer or clarify questions in a positive way to instill hope. Teach relaxation and breathing techniques. Provide a therapeutic environment. Assist in maintaining a quiet and supportive atmosphere during the procedure. Ask for supplies in a quiet voice, do not talk during anesthesia induction, and maintain minimal conversation if the patient has a local anesthetic. Take precautions to protect the patient from noxious sounds if the patient has received a local anesthetic.

Hopelessness

Hopelessness describes a sustained, subjective, emotional state in which a person sees no personal choices or alternatives available for solving problems or achieving what is desired (Carpenito-Moyet, 2004). Feelings of hopelessness may be associated with numerous losses experienced during life, such as the loss of physical health; loss of family members and friends due to death; and changes in work, leisure activities, and residence. Hopelessness leads to an inability to mobilize energy to perform daily activities, decreased decision-making capabilities, giving up, and isolation.

Assess the presence of hope by seeing if the patient can discuss the future, actively question all treatments, and mobilize resources in his or her own defense. The hopeless patient may exhibit passive behavior; have decreased verbalization, affect, and response to stimuli; exhibit despondent verbal cues; and lack initiative and involvement in care. Maintain hope by telling the patient and the family that the patient will be given the best care during the operative or invasive procedure period. Reassure the patient that the physician and the patient care team are the best available. After the procedure, tell the patient what he or she will be able to do after the discharge from the facility. However, avoid being overly hopeful or cheerful. Aging patients may feel that their despair and sorrow are considered unimportant.

Ineffective Coping

Ineffective describes a state in which a person experiences an inability to manage internal or environmental stressors adequately due to inadequate resources (eg, physical, psychological, behavioral, and/or cognitive) (Carpenito-Moyet, 2004). Sickness, life-threatening disease, loss of loved ones, loss of autonomy, loss of roles, loneliness, isolation, and the reality of death are more likely to occur in the older adult. The ability to handle stressful situations and the use of coping mechanisms will vary from person to person. While some adults develop a remarkable tolerance to stress through a lifetime of coping with stress, others find that even small changes trigger excessive stress. During the assessment, differentiate the reactions to stressful situations that are part of normal life and those that represent ineffective coping.

Assess the autonomic stress response of the patient: measure pulse, respiration, and blood pressure. Observe for signs of self-neglect. Assess the patient's mental status. Support the patient. Assess coping skills and communicate with other members of the healthcare team regarding the patient's status. Identify ineffective coping with operative or invasive procedure crises. Be aware that different cultures may have different ideas and behaviors regarding the appropriateness of a particular coping response. Report potential coping problems to members of the operative or invasive procedure team. Identify the patient's stress level. Define behavior characteristics. Note verbalizations of an inability to cope. Note an inability to meet the healthcare personnel's expectations regarding surgery. Intervene if the patient exhibits destructive behavior, such as pulling out IV or indwelling catheters. Enlist the aid of the family, volunteers, or other potential network support persons so that the procedure may proceed without incident.

Provide an atmosphere of acceptance. Provide information concerning the diagnosis, treatment, and prognosis. Explore previous methods of dealing with life problems. Encourage verbalization of feelings, perceptions, and fears. Identify the patient's strengths and abilities. Provide constructive outlets for anger, hostility, and concerns. Observe the degree of family support and involve the family in the care of the patient.

CONCLUSION

Elderly patients experience physiological and psychological changes because of aging. Nurses providing operative and invasive procedure care must assess for these changes and plan appropriately to ensure a quality experience for the patient.

REFERENCES

1. Administration on Aging (AOA): US Department of Health and Human Services. (2007). A profile of older Americans: 2007. Retrieved July 11, 2008, from www.aoa.gov/prof/Statistics/profile/2007/2007profile.pdf.
2. Berman, A., Snyder, S.J., Kozier, B., and Erb, G. (2008). *Kozier & Erb's Fundamentals of Nursing: Concepts, Process, and Practice*, 8th ed. Upper Saddle River, NJ: Pearson Education, Inc.
3. Carpenito-Moyet, L.J. (2004). *Nursing Diagnosis: Application to Clinical Practice*, 10th ed. Philadelphia, PA: Lippincott Williams & Wilkins.
4. Carpentino-Moyet, L.J. (2008). Handbook of nursing diagnosis (12th ed.). Philadelphia: Lippincott Williams & Wilkins.
5. Ebersole, P., Hess, P., Touhy, T., & Jett, K. (2005). *Gerontological Nursing and Healthy Aging*, 2nd ed. St. Louis, MO: Elsevier Mosby.
6. eMedicineHealth. (2008). Outpatient surgery. Retrieved August 4, 2008 from http://www.emedicinehealth.com/outpatient_surgery/article_em.htm.
7. Guido, G. (2006). *Legal and Ethical Issues in Nursing*, 4th ed. Upper Saddle River, NJ: Prentice-Hall, Inc.

8. Malnutrition—what to look for. (2008). Retrieved July 31, 2008, from http://huntingtondisease.tripod.com/swallowing/id62.html.

9. Mamaril, M.E. (2006). Nursing considerations in the geriatric surgical patient: the perioperative continuum of care. *Nursing Clinics of North America* 41(2): 313–328.

10. McCance, K., & Huether, S. (2002). Pathophysiology: The Biological Basis for Disease in Adults and Children, 4th ed. St. Louis, MO: Mosby.

11. Meiner, S.E., & Lueckenotte, A.G. (2006). *Gerontological Nursing*, 3rd ed. St. Louis, MO: Mosby/Elsevier.

12. Memory Loss & the Brain. (2008). Glossary—hypoxia/anoxia. Retrieved August 4, 2008, from http://www.memorylossonline.com/glossary/hypoxiaanoxia.html.

13. National Center for Health Statistics. (2007). Health, United States, 2007, with chartbook on trends in the health of Americans. Retrieved July 31, 2008, from http://www.cdc.gov/nchs/data/hus/hus07.pdf#032.

14. National Institute on Deafness and Other Communication Disorders (NIDCD). (2008). Quick statistics. Retrieved August 4, 2008, from http://www.nidcd.nih.gov/health/statistics/quick.htm.

15. New York-Presbyterian Hospital. (2008). Outpatient surgery. Retrieved August 4, 2008, from http://www.nyp.org/health/surgery_outpt.html.

16. Patkin, M. (2007). Postoperative confusion: a guide to management. Retrieved August 4, 2008, from http://www.mpatkin.org/surgery_clinical/post_op_confusion.htm.

17. Petersen C. (2007). Perioperative nursing data set, the perioperative nursing vocabulary. (Revised 2nd ed.). Denver: AORN, Inc.

18. Russo, C.A., & Elixhauser, A. (2006). Hospitalizations in the elderly population, 2003. Statistical brief #6. May 2006. Agency for Healthcare Research and Quality, Rockville, MD. Retrieved August 4, 2008, from http://www.hcupus.ahrq.gov/reports/statbriefs/sb6.pdf.

19. U.S. Census Bureau. Persons 65 years old and over—characteristics by sex: 1990–2006. Retrieved July 31, 2008, from www.census.gov/compendia/statab/tables/08s0034.pdf.

20. Van Wagner, K. (2008). Crystallized intelligence definition. Retrieved August 4, 2008, from http://psychology.about.com/od/cindex/g/def_crystalinte.htm.

21. Wikipedia. (2008a). Robert J. Havighurst. Retrieved August 4, 2008, from http://en.wikipedia.org/wiki/Robert_J._Havighurst.

22. Wikipedia. (2008b). Maslow's hierarchy of needs. Retrieved August 4, 2008, from http://en.wikipedia.org/wiki/Maslow's_hierarchy_of_needs.

23. Winters, A. (2008). Erickson's Theory of Human Development. Retrieved July 11, 2008, from http://ezinearticles.com/?Ericksons-Theory-of-Human-Development&id=20117.

Index

Page numbers followed by f indicate figures. Page numbers followed by t indicate tables. Page numbers followed by n indicate footnotes.